Disposition of Toxic Drugs and Chemicals in Man

Fourth Edition

Disposition of Toxic Drugs and Chemicals in Man

Fourth Edition

RANDALL C. BASELT, Ph.D.
Director, Chemical Toxicology Institute
Foster City, California

ROBERT H. CRAVEY, B.S.
Chief Toxicologist (Retired)
County of Orange
Santa Ana, California

CHEMICAL TOXICOLOGY INSTITUTE
FOSTER CITY, CALIFORNIA

Library of Congress Catalog Card No. 94-69572

ISBN 0-9626523-1-8

Preface to the Fourth Edition

We are pleased to present our latest effort to summarize current information on the fate of toxic drugs and chemicals in the human body. Much new data has been compiled in the last five or six years, and many new agents continue to make their appearance, despite the proliferation of legal restrictions aimed at protecting man and his environment.

Once again we must pay our respects to our many colleagues who have supported our work through their comments, constructive criticism, contributions to the scientific literature and their use of this book as a reference tool.

Randall C. Baselt
Robert H. Cravey

"My part of the work has been mainly selective and detective, in the endeavor to compile as accurate and as practical a book as possible."

William Boericke
Materia Medica, 1901

Preface to the Third Edition

With this latest edition of *Disposition of Toxic Drugs and Chemicals in Man*, we welcome Robert Cravey as co-author. Bob brings with him many years of experience in forensic toxicology and took on the task of preparing monographs for the numerous agents recently added to the work, as well as reviewing the extensive changes made to the older sections of the text.

We trust that our work will continue to be useful to our colleagues and, as always, we welcome your suggestions for further improvement of this presentation and any unpublished data that may help to fill gaps in our knowledge of the fate of toxic substances in humans.

Preface to the Second Edition

I have greatly appreciated the warm reception given the first edition of this work and the many helpful suggestions for improvements offered by my colleagues.

The organizational changes in this new edition are a reflection of those valuable comments, and I trust that this compilation will continue to be of use to analytical toxicologists.

The amount of new information on the fate of drugs and chemicals in man appearing in the four years since publication of the first edition is gratifying but somewhat overwhelming. The longer I delayed the revision, the more formidable seemed the task. The present volume contains information on 305 substances, a 60% greater number than before. Data on volume of distribution (Vd), fraction bound to plasma protein (Fb), plasma half-life (T½) and pKa value have been included wherever possible to aid in the evaluation of substance concentrations in biological specimens.

The reader should be aware, however, that these values are generally based on healthy adults in normal circumstances. They should not be viewed as constants for a given substance, but as measurements often dependent on dose, disease state, and interindividual variation.

Preface to the First Edition

The purpose of this two-volume work is to present in a single, convenient source the current essential information on the disposition of the chemicals and drugs most frequently encountered in episodes of human poisoning. The data included relate to the body fluid concentrations of substances in normal or therapeutic situations, concentrations in fluids and tissues in instances of toxicity and the known metabolic fate of these substances in man. Brief mention is made of specific analytical procedures which are applicable to the determination of each substance and its active metabolites in biological specimens. It is expected that such information will be of particular interest and use to toxicologists, pharmacologists and clinical chemists who have need either to conduct an analytical search for these materials in specimens of human origin or to interpret analytical data resulting from such a search.

Volume 1 is devoted to licit and illicit drugs affecting the central nervous system, while Volume 2 will comprise peripherally-acting drugs and common toxic chemicals. As an aid to the student and to the author, the substances have been grouped primarily by pharmacologic class and secondarily by chemical structure. Occasionally a material appears not in the category for which it was therapeutically intended but in one which is more consistent with its major toxic effect. The failure to discuss a particular agent is generally the result of insufficient information regarding its human disposition to warrant its inclusion. The author would greatly appreciate any communication regarding errors of omission or commission.

I gratefully acknowledge the assistance and patient understanding in the preparation of this work of my dear friend and colleague, Robert H. Cravey.

Contents

Acetaldehyde

T½: ?
Vd: ?
Fb: ?

CH_3CHO

Occurrence and Usage. Acetaldehyde is a volatile liquid used in the manufacture of a number of synthetic chemical products, including certain plastics, dyes, and resins. It is also present in fairly high concentrations in cigarette smoke. The current threshold limit value is 100 ppm (180 mg/m^3) in the industrial atmosphere.

Blood Concentrations. Acetaldehyde has not been determined in the blood of persons exposed to the vapor. The substance is a metabolite of ethanol and paraldehyde, however, and has been measured following the administration of these drugs. Endogenous blood acetaldehyde levels probably do not exceed 0.2 mg/L. An acute oral dose of ethanol to volunteers produces blood acetaldehyde concentrations of 0.9–1.3 mg/L, whereas in chronic alcoholics, these levels may range from 1.7–2.5 mg/L (Korsten et al., 1975). Following co-administration of ethanol and an inhibitor of acetaldehyde metabolism, such as disulfiram or calcium carbamide, acetaldehyde blood concentrations may increase 5–10 fold over normal levels (Truitt and Walsh, 1971; Stowell et al., 1980).

Metabolism and Excretion. The major portion of a dose of acetaldehyde is metabolized to acetic acid and then to carbon dioxide. Urinary excretion of acetaldehyde during periods of elevated blood levels has been suggested, but not documented (Truitt and Walsh, 1971). A certain portion is also excreted unchanged in the expired breath. A single acute dose of ethanol (78 mL/70 kg) produces maximal breath acetaldehyde concentrations of 0.007–0.010 mg/L (Freund and O'Hollaren, 1965).

Toxicity. Low to moderate air concentrations of acetaldehyde (50–200 ppm) cause eye irritation and upper respiratory discomfort. Higher concentrations may cause dyspnea and central nervous system depression. The characteristic disulfiram-alcohol reaction is believed due to the toxic accumulation of acetaldehyde in imbibers of alcohol (Truitt and Walsh, 1971); in non-alcoholics, this flushing reaction begins at blood acetaldehyde levels of 1.8–2.6 mg/L (Johnsen et al., 1992).

An alcoholic patient who attempted suicide by ingesting large amounts of cyanamide and ethanol lost consciousness, but recovered with supportive therapy; his blood acetaldehyde concentration 11 hours after ingestion was 18 mg/L (Kobayashi et al., 1983).

Analysis. Procedures have been described for the analysis of blood or urine acetaldehyde by ultraviolet spectrophotometry (Burbridge et al., 1950), headspace (Eriksson et al., 1977) and direct-injection gas chromatography (Brien and Loomis, 1978), and liquid chromatography following derivatization (Helander et al., 1993). It should be noted that acetaldehyde is formed nonenzymatically during processing or storage of whole blood specimens containing ethanol (Eriksson, 1980); enzymatic destruction may also occur, apparently due to aldehyde dehydrogenase in erythrocytes (Tomita et al., 1987).

References

J.F. Brien and C.W. Loomis. Gas-liquid chromatographic determination of ethanol and acetaldehyde in blood. Clin. Chim. Acta 87: 175–180, 1978.

T.N. Burbridge, C.H. Hine and A.F. Schick. A simple spectrophotometric method for the determination of acetaldehyde in blood. J. Lab. Clin. Med. 35: 983–987, 1950.

C.J.P. Eriksson, H.W. Sippel and O.A. Forsander. The determination of acetaldehyde in biological samples by head-space gas chromatography. Anal. Biochem. 80: 116–124, 1977.

C.J.P. Eriksson. Elevated blood acetaldehyde levels in alcoholics and their relatives: a reevaluation. Science 207: 1383–1384, 1980.

G. Freund and P. O'Hollaren. Acetaldehyde concentrations in alveolar air following a standard dose of ethanol in man. J. Lipid Res. 6: 471–477, 1965.

A. Helander, C. Lowenmoand M. Johannson. Distribution of acetaldehyde in human blood: effects of ethanol and treatment with disulfiram. Alcohol Alcoholism 28: 461–468, 1993.

J. Johnsen, A. Stowell and J. Morland. Clinical responses in relation to blood acetaldehyde levels. Pharm. Tox. 70: 41–45, 1992.

M. Kobayashi, A. Watanabe, N. Hobara et al. Survival after a blood acetaldehyde concentration of 1750 μg/dL. Lancet 3: 1138, 1983.

M.A. Korsten, S. Matsuzaki, L. Feinman and C.S. Lieber. High blood acetaldehyde levels after ethanol administration. New Eng. J. Med. 292: 386–389, 1975.

M. Tomita, I. Ijiri, K. Shimosato and S. Kawai. Simple and sensitive method for the determination of acetaldehyde in blood by gas chromatography. J. Chrom. 414: 454–459, 1987.

E.B. Truitt, Jr. and M.J. Walsh. In *The Biology of Alcoholism*, Vol. 1 (B. Kissin and H. Begleiter, eds.), Plenum Press, New York, 971, pp. 161–195.

Acetaminophen

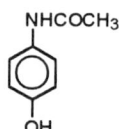

T½: 1–3 hr
Vd: 0.8–1.0 L/kg
Fb: 0.25
pKa: 9.5

Occurrence and Usage. Acetaminophen (paracetamol, N-acetyl-p-aminophenol, Tylenol) is available in pure form as numerous tradename preparations for oral use, in amounts of up to 500 mg. It is also found combined in over 200 preparations with other drugs, such as codeine and propoxyphene. Acetaminophen has become a popular alternative to aspirin as a result of its lower potential for undesirable side effects. The compound has analgesic and antipyretic effects but lacks anti-inflammatory properties. It is generally a safe drug in therapeutic amounts but has been found to produce acute hepatic necrosis after overdosage. Ingestion of less than 20 g of the drug may be lethal to an adult.

Blood Concentrations. Plasma concentrations averaged 4.2 mg/L (range, 2.4–6.4) 6 hours after a single 324 mg dose of acetaminophen (Thomas et al., 1972). Following oral administration of 1000 mg, serum concentrations averaged 9 mg/L at 1, 2 and 3 hours (Weikel, 1958). Thirty minutes after the ingestion of 1300 mg, serum concentrations ranged from 4.8–13 mg/L in 4 volunteers (Fletterick et al., 1979). One hour after administration of 1800 mg of the drug to 8 subjects, plasma concentrations averaged 26 mg/L and ranged from 5.6–52 mg/L (Prescott et al., 1968). Both the half-life and volume of distribution of acetaminophen in children are comparable to those in adults (Peterson and Rumack, 1978). The drug may exhibit nonlinear kinetics when doses exceed 18 mg/kg (1260 mg/70 kg) (Sahajwalla and Ayres, 1991).

Metabolism and Excretion. In therapeutic usage the drug is excreted largely in the urine as various conjugates: 45–55% as a glucuronide conjugate, 20–30% as a sulfate, and 15–55% as cysteine and mercapturic acid conjugates. Approximately 2% of a dose is excreted unchanged in the urine. Glutathione is required for the formation of the cysteine and mercapturic acid conjugates; following overdosage, saturation of conjugation pathways occurs and glutathione stores become depleted, resulting in the formation of a highly reactive acetaminophen metabolite, possibly an epoxide. This toxic intermediate combines irreversibly with hepatocyte constituents causing cell damage (Davis et al., 1976; Andrews et al., 1976). The amount of unchanged acetaminophen excreted in urine after overdosage may increase to as much as 10–14% of a dose (Slattery and Levy, 1979).

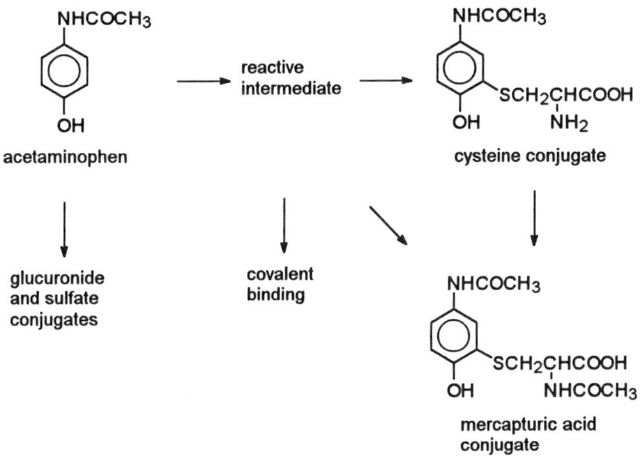

NHCOCH$_3$

OH

acetaminophen

→ reactive intermediate →

NHCOCH$_3$

OH — SCH$_2$CHCOOH — NH$_2$

cysteine conjugate

glucuronide and sulfate conjugates

covalent binding

NHCOCH$_3$

OH — SCH$_2$CHCOOH — NHCOCH$_3$

mercapturic acid conjugate

Toxicity. Hepatotoxicity following therapeutic doses of acetaminophen has occurred in infants who accumulated toxic amounts of the drug (Greene et al., 1983), in alcoholic patients with impaired liver function (Kaysen et al., 1985), and in persons taking phenobarbital, which causes enzyme induction (Pirotte, 1984). Plasma concentrations of acetaminophen in overdosed patients may range from 30 to over 300 mg/L; the plasma half-life of the drug is considered to be the best indicator of serious toxicity, i.e., liver damage. Patients developing hepatotoxicity usually ingest at least 10–15 g of drug, exhibit a drug half-life greater than the normal 2 hours, and have a plasma drug concentration greater than 300 mg/L at 4 hours post-ingestion. Treatment with an antidote such as N-acetylcysteine may be warranted if the half-life exceeds 4 hours (Prescott et al., 1971; Peterson and Rumack, 1977). This must be accomplished within the first 10 hours to be effective. Intravenous administration of N-acetylcysteine may have advantages over oral administration in patients with nausea and vomiting (Prescott, 1981). The use of a nomograph relating plasma drug concentration, time since ingestion, and hepatotoxicity is helpful in evaluating the need for antidotal treatment (Rumack and Peterson, 1978).

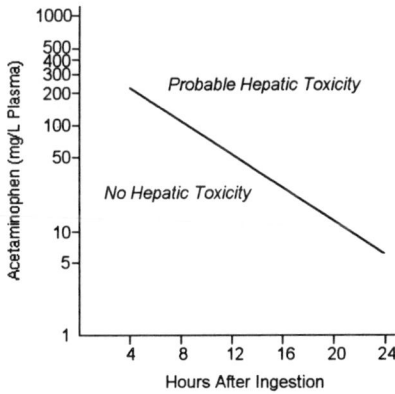

A 3.5 year old child who died of hepatic and renal failure following inadvertent cumulative overdosage with acetaminophen had a serum level of 53 mg/L approximately 14 hours after the last dose (Nogen and Brenner, 1978). The distribution of acetaminophen in 6 adults who succumbed to overdosage of the drug is shown in the following table (Robinson et al., 1977; Ashton, 1979; Holzbecher et al., 1981):

Acetaminophen Concentrations in Fatalities (mg/L or mg/kg)

	Blood	Liver	Bile	Kidney	Urine	Gastric
Average	248	264	560	190	406	1744 mg
(Range)	(160–387)	(90–385)	(180–900)	(190)	(140–830)	(14–5000)

Analysis. Numerous methods have been published for the analysis of acetaminophen in biological fluids, many of which have been recently reviewed by Wiener (1978). Colorimetric techniques have been frequently employed in clinical laboratories (Routh et al., 1968; Glynn and Kendal, 1975; Walberg, 1977; Miceli et al., 1979; Liu and Oka, 1980), but these may be subject to interference by acetaminophen metabolites, salicylate, phenacetin or uremic or icteric serum (Stewart et al., 1979). Gas chromatography, with (Prescott, 1971; Thoma et al., 1978; Wahl and Rejent, 1978) or without (Grove, 1971; Jeevanandam et al., 1980) derivatization, is a more specific technique. High-pressure liquid chromatography is both sensitive and specific for clinical purposes (Horvitz and Jatlow, 1977; Gotelli et al., 1977; Black and Sprague, 1978; Fletterick et al., 1979; Manno et al., 1981; West, 1981; Kordoba and Petruzzi, 1984) and has the advantage of being applicable to the measurement of the conjugated metabolites of acetaminophen in plasma, urine (Howie et al., 1977; Knox and Jurand, 1978; Adriaenssens and Prescott, 1978; Jung and Zafar, 1985) and tissue homogenates (Colin et al., 1987).

References

P.I. Adriaenssens and L.F. Prescott. High performance liquid chromatographic estimation of paracetamol metabolites in plasma. Brit. J. Clin. Pharm. 6: 87–88, 1978.

R.S. Andrews, C.C. Bond, J. Burnett et al. Isolation and identification of paracetamol metabolites. J. Int. Med. Res. (Suppl. 4) 4: 34–39, 1976.

P.G. Ashton. Personal communication, 1979.

M. Black and K. Sprague. Rapid micromethod for acetaminophen determination in serum. Clin. Chem. 24: 1288–1289, 1978.

P. Colin, G. Sirois and S. Chakrabarti. Rapid high-performance liquid chromatographic assay of acetaminophen in serum and tissue homogenates. J. Chrom. 413: 151–160, 1987.

M. Davis, D. Labadarios and R.S. Williams. Metabolism of paracetamol after therapeutic and hepatotoxic doses in man. J. Int. Med. Res. (Suppl. 4) 4: 40–45, 1976.

C.G. Fletterick, T.H. Grove and D.C. Hohnadel. Liquid-chromatographic determination of acetaminophen in serum. Clin. Chem. 25: 409–412, 1979.

J.P. Glynn and S.E. Kendal. Paracetamol measurement. Lancet l: 1147–1148, 1975.

G.R. Gotelli, P.M. Kolia and L.J. Marton. Determination of acetaminophen and phenacetin in plasma by high-pressure liquid chromatography. Clin. Chem. 23: 957–959, 1977.

J.W. Green, L. Craft and F. Ghishan. Acetaminophen poisoning in infancy. Am. J. Dis. Child. 137: 386–387, 1983.

J. Grove. Gas-liquid chromatography of N-acetyl-p-aminophenol (paracetamol) in plasma and urine. J. Chrom. 59: 289–295, 1971.

M. Holzbecher, R.A. Perry and H.S. Ellenberger. Acetaminophen fatality — a case report. J. Can. Soc. For. Sci. 14: 32–33, 1981.

R.A. Horvitz and P.I. Jatlow. Determination of acetaminophen concentrations in serum by high-pressure liquid chromatography. Clin. Chem. 23: 1596–1598, 1977.

D. Howie, P.I. Adriaenssens and L.F. Prescott. Paracetamol metabolism following overdosage: application of high performance liquid chromatography. J. Pharm. Pharmac. 29: 235–237, 1977.

M. Jeevanandam, B. Novic, R. Savich and E. Wagman. Serum acetaminophen assay using activated charcoal adsorption and gas chromatography without derivatization. J. Anal. Tox. 4: 124–126, 1980.

D. Jung and N.V. Zafar. Micro high-performance liquid chromatographic assay of acetaminophen and its major metabolites in plasma and urine. J. Chrom. 339: 198–202, 1985.

G.A. Kayson, S.M. Pond, M.H. Roper et al. Combined hepatic and renal injury in alcoholics during therapeutic use of acetaminophen. Arch. Int. Med. 145: 2019–2023, 1985.

J.H. Knox and J. Jurand. Determination of paracetamol and its metabolites in urine by high-performance liquid chromatography using ion-pair systems. J. Chrom. 149: 297–312, 1978.

C.A. Kordoba and R.F. Petruzzi. High-performance liquid chromatographic method for the determination of trace amounts of acetaminophen in plasma. J. Pharm. Sci. 73: 117–119, 1984.

T.Z. Liu and K.H. Oka. Spectrophotometric screening method for acetaminophen in serum and plasma. Clin. Chem. 26: 69–71, 1980.

B.R. Manno, J.E. Manno, C.A. Dempsey and M.A. Wood. A high-pressure liquid chromatographic method for the determination of N-acetyl-p-aminophenol (acetaminophen) in serum or plasma using a direct injection technique. J. Anal. Tox. 5: 24–28, 1981.

J. Miceli, M. Aravind and A. Done. A rapid simple acetaminophen spectrophotometric determination. Pediatrics 63: 609–610, 1979.

A.G. Nogen and J.E. Bremmer. Fatal acetaminophen overdosage in a young child. Pediatrics 92: 832–833, 1978.

R.G. Peterson and B.H. Rumack. Treating acute acetaminophen poisoning with acetylcysteine. J. Am. Med. Asso. 237: 2406–2407, 1977.

R.G. Peterson and B.H. Rumack. Pharmacokinetics of acetaminophen in children. Pediatrics 62: Part 2 (Suppl.) 877–879, 1978.

J.H. Pirotte. Apparent potentiation by phenobarbital of hepatotoxicity from small doses of acetaminophen. Ann. Int. Med. 101: 403, 1984.

L.F. Prescott, M. Sansur, W. Levin and A.H. Conney. The comparative metabolism of phenacetin and N-acetyl-p-aminophenol in man, with particular reference to effects on the kidney. Clin. Pharm. Ther. 9: 605–614, 1968.

L.F. Prescott. The gas-liquid chromatographic estimation of phenacetin and paracetamol in plasma and urine. J. Pharm. Pharmac. 23: 11–115, 1971.

L.F. Prescott, N. Wright, P. Roscoe and S.S. Brown. Plasma-paracetamol half-life and hepatic necrosis in patients with paracetamol overdosage. Lancet 1: 519–522, 1971.

L.F. Prescott. Treatment of severe acetaminophen poisoning with intravenous acetylcysteine. Arch. Int. Med. 141: 386–389, 1981.

A.E. Robinson, H. Sattar, R.D. McDowall et al. Forensic toxicology of some deaths associated with the combined use of propoxyphene and acetaminophen (paracetamol). J. For. Sci. 22: 708–717, 1977.

J.I. Routh, N.A. Shane, E.G. Arredondo and W.D. Paul. Determination of N-acetyl-p-aminophenol in plasma. Clin. Chem. 14: 882–889, 1968.

B.H. Rumack and R.G. Peterson. Acetaminophen overdosage: incidence, diagnosis, and management in 416 patients. Pediatrics 62: Part 2 (Suppl.) 898–903, 1978.

C.G. Sahajwalla and J.W. Ayres. Multiple-dose acetaminophen pharmacokinetics. J. Pharm. Sci. 80: 855–860, 1991.

J.T. Slattery and G. Levy. Acetaminophen kinetics in acutely poisoned patients. Clin. Pharm. Ther. 25: 185–195, 1979.

M.J. Stewart, P.I. Adriaenssens, D.R. Jarvie and L.F. Prescott. Inappropriate methods for the emergency determination of plasma paracetamol. Ann. Clin. Biochem. 16: 89–95, 1979.

J.J. Thoma, M. McCoy, T. Ewald and N. Myers. Acetaminophen — an improved gas chromatographic assay. J. Anal. Tox. 2: 226–228, 1978.

B.H. Thomas, B.B. Coldwell, W. Zeitz and G. Solomonraj. Effect of aspirin, caffeine, and codeine on the metabolism of phenacetin and acetaminophen. Clin. Pharm. Ther. 13: 906–910, 1972.

K.C. Wahl and T.A. Rejent. Quantitative gas chromatographic determination of acetaminophen using trimethylanilinium hydroxide as a derivatizing agent. J. For. Sci. 23: 14–20, 1978.

C.B. Walberg. Determination of acetaminophen in serum. J. Anal. Tox. 1: 79–80, 1977.

J.H. Weikel, Jr. A comparison of human serum levels of acetylsalicylic acid, salicylamide, and N-acetyl-p-aminophenol following oral administration. J. Am. Pharm. Asso. 47: 477–479, 1958.

J.C. West. Rapid HPLC analysis of paracetamol (acetaminophen) in blood and postmortem viscera. J. Anal. Tox. 5: 118–121, 1981.

K. Wiener. A review of methods for plasma paracetamol estimation. Ann. Clin. Biochem. 15: 187–196, 1978.

Acetohexamide

T½: 0.3–1.3 hr
Vd: 0.2 L/kg
Fb: 0.75
pKa: 6.6

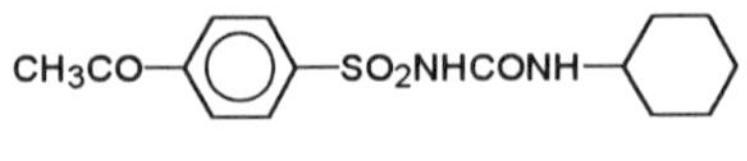
CH3CO
SO2NHCONH

Occurrence and Usage. Acetohexamide (Dymelor) is a sulfonylurea derivative that was first synthesized in 1962 as an oral hypoglycemic agent. It is administered once or twice per day, in total daily doses of 250–1500 mg.

Blood Concentrations. It was found that chronic 500 mg daily doses of acetohexamide produced an average serum concentration of 42 mg/L in 18 subjects of normal weight when measured 3–5 hours after the dose; a daily dose of 1000 mg given in 2 equal parts produced an average serum level of 67 mg/L. The average serum concentration in 24 patients exhibiting a good response to daily doses of 500–2000 mg of the drug was 37 mg/L, with a range of 21–56 mg/L (Sheldon et al., 1965). Hydroxyhexamide concentrations in subjects receiving a single 750 mg oral dose of acetohexamide reached an average peak of about 30 mg/L at 4 hours post-administration (Kleber et al., 1977).

Metabolism and Excretion. Acetohexamide is metabolized in man by reduction of the acetyl group with the production of an alcoholic compound known as hydroxyhexamide. This metabolite is pharmacologically active and has a half-life of 6 hours, compared to 1.3 hours for its parent (Smith et al., 1965). An average of 49% of a dose is excreted in the 24 hour urine as unconjugated hydroxyhexamide (Welles et al., 1961), while other inactive hydroxylated metabolites and unchanged drug account for an additional 25% (Galloway et al., 1967).

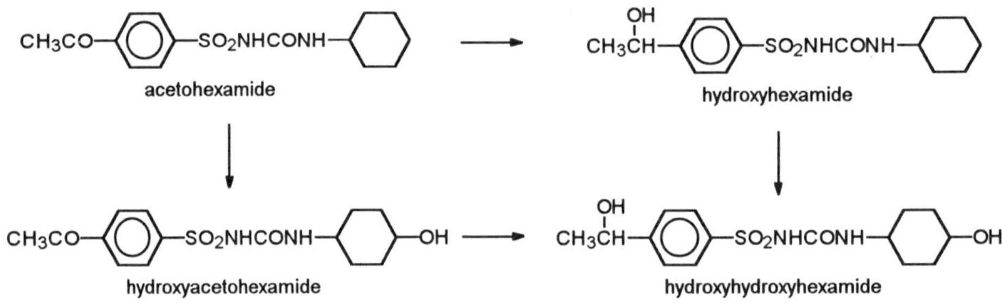
CH3CO
SO2NHCONH
acetohexamide
OH
CH3CH
SO2NHCONH
hydroxyhexamide
CH3CO
SO2NHCONH
OH
hydroxyacetohexamide
OH
CH3CH
SO2NHCONH
OH
hydroxyhydroxyhexamide

Toxicity. Severe hypoglycemia has been produced in certain individuals by administration of therapeutic amounts of acetohexamide. This is especially likely to occur in patients with reduced renal function, and may result from renal retention of active drug metabolites (Lampe, 1967). Peritoneal dialysis with 4.5% dextrose solution has been found to control the hypoglycemic state but was not effective in removing the drug or its major metabolite (Skoutakis et al., 1977).

Analysis. Acetohexamide has been assayed in biological fluids by relatively non-specific colorimetric procedures designed for the sulfonylurea derivatives (Carmichael, 1959; Wiseman et al., 1964). Ultraviolet spectrophotometry (Smith et al., 1965), fluorimetry (Girgis-Takla and Chroneos, 1979) and gas chromatography (Kleber et al., 1977; Hartvig et al., 1980) have also been applied to the determination of this drug.

References

R.H. Carmichael. A method for the routine determination of chlorpropamide in plasma. Clin. Chem. 5: 597–602, 1959.

J.A. Galloway, R.E. McMahon, H.W. Culp et al. Metabolism, blood levels and rate of excretion of acetohexamide in human subjects. Diabetes 16: 118–127, 1967.

P. Girgis–Takla and L. Chroneos. Fluorimetric determination of acetohexamide in plasma and tablet formulations using 1-methylnicotinamide. Analyst 104: 117–123, 1979.

P. Hartvig, C. Fagerlund and O. Gyllenhaal. Electron-capture gas chromatography of plasma sulphonylureas after extractive methylation. J. Chrom. 181: 17–24, 1980.

J.W. Kleber, J.A. Galloway and B.E. Rodda. GLC determination of acetohexamide and hydroxyhexamide in biological fluids. J. Pharm. Sci. 66: 635–638, 1977.

W.T. Lampe. Hypoglycemia due to acetohexamide. Arch. Int. Med. 120: 239–241, 1967.

J. Sheldon, J. Anderson and L. Stoner. Serum concentration and urinary excretion of oral sulfonylurea compounds. Diabetes 14: 362–367, 1965.

V.A. Skoutakis, W.D. Black, S.R. Acchiardo and G.C. Wood. Peritoneal dialysis in the treatment of acetohexamide-induced hypoglycemia. Am. J. Hosp. Pharm. 34: 68–70, 1977.

D.L. Smith, T.J. Vecchio and A.A. Forist. Metabolism of antidiabetic sulfonylureas in man. Metabolism 14: 229–240, 1965.

J.S. Welles, M.A. Root and R.C. Anderson. Metabolic reduction of 1-(p-acetylbenzenesulfonyl)-3-cyclohexylurea (acetohexamide) in different species. Proc. Soc. Exp. Biol. Med. 107: 583–585, 1961.

E.H. Wiseman, J. Chiaini and R. Pinson, Jr. Determination of sulfamylurea hypoglycemic agents and their metabolites in biological fluids. J. Pharm. Sci. 53: 766–769, 1964.

Acetone

T½: 3–5 hr
Vd: 0.8 L/kg
Fb: 0

CH_3COCH_3

Occurrence and Usage. Acetone is frequently employed as a solvent for paints, plastics and adhesives and as a chemical intermediate. The current threshold limit value for industry is 750 ppm (1780 mg/m³) of the vapor in the air. Acetone is produced endogenously in man and is also found as a metabolite of isopropanol.

Blood Concentrations. In healthy adults, endogenous acetone blood levels (up to 10 mg/L) are unmeasurable by routine gas chromatographic techniques. Acetone concentrations are markedly elevated during diabetic or fasting ketoacidosis and may range from 100–700 mg/L (Ramu et al., 1978). Blood acetone levels in 8 volunteers peaked at 20 and 100 mg/L at the end of a 2 hour exposure to 100 and 500 ppm, respectively, of acetone vapor. The levels declined with an apparent half-life of 3 hours (DiVincenzo et al., 1973). A volunteer who ingested 10 g of acetone on an empty stomach developed a maximal blood concentration of 327 mg/L after 10 minutes; on a full stomach, a maximal concentration of about 200 mg/L was measured at 1 hour. The concentrations declined according to first-order kinetics, with an elimination half-life of 5 hours (Widmark, 1981).

Some accumulation occurs when acetone is breathed on a daily basis; in a subject exposed to air containing 2100 ppm for 8 hours daily, accumulation occurred for 3 days until steady-state was attained. The peak blood level (at the end of the 8 hour day) was 182 mg/L and the trough level measured 16 hours later was 91 mg/L. Intoxication was not observed in subjects with blood concentrations as high as 330 mg/L (Haggard et al., 1944).

Metabolism and Excretion. Acetone is metabolized by oxidation to acetate and formate at a relatively slow rate, 1–3 mg/kg/hr in most subjects tested. At higher blood concentrations, the majority of the chemical is removed by excretion, primarily in the breath and to a lesser extent (3% of a dose) in the urine. Reduction to isopropanol is considered to be a minor metabolic pathway in humans (Lewis et al., 1984). The average blood/breath acetone concentration ratio is 330 (range, 322–339), whereas the average ratio between urine and blood is 1.34 (Haggard et al., 1944). Urinary acetone shows a linear correlation to the environmental air concentration, such that a person exposed to 50 ppm acetone vapor for 8 hours would be expected to produce an end-of-shift urine specimen containing 20 mg/L acetone (Kawai et al., 1990).

Toxicity. Acetone is considered to be relatively nontoxic, causing eye irritation at air concentrations of 1000–6000 ppm and central nervous system depression at concentrations exceeding 10,000 ppm. Several workers who developed symptoms of acute intoxication (dizziness and muscular weakness) on exposure to air concentrations of at least 12,000 ppm exhibited urine acetone concentrations of 46–72 mg/L (Ross, 1973). Hyperglycemia has been noted as a frequent finding during acetone intoxication resulting from either ingestion or inhalation of the chemical (Gitelson et al., 1966). An individual who ingested acetone and became lethargic was noted to have a blood acetone level of 2500 mg/L, which declined with a half-life of 31 hours (Ramu et al., 1978).

Analysis. Widmark (1919) described a sensitive titrimetric method for measurement of acetone in biological fluids. Most of the gas chromatographic techniques cited in the section on ethanol are applicable to acetone determination.

References

G.D. DiVincenzo, F.J. Yanno and B.D. Astill. Exposure of man and dog to low concentrations of acetone vapor. Am. Ind. Hyg. Asso. J. 34: 329–336, 1973.

S. Gitelson, A. Werczberger and J.B. Herman. Coma and hyperglycemia following drinking of acetone. Diabetes 15: 810–811, 1966.

H.W. Haggard, L.A. Greenberg and J.M. Turner. The physiological principles governing the action of acetone together with determination of toxicity. J. Ind. Hyg. Tox. 5: 133–151, 1944.

T. Kawai, T. Yasugi, Y. Uchida et al. Urinary excretion of unmetabolized acetone as an indication of occupational exposure to acetone. Int. Arch. Occ. Env. Health 62: 165–169, 1990.

G.D. Lewis, A.K. Laufman, B.H. McAnalley and J.C. Garriott. Metabolism of acetone to isopropyl alcohol in rats and humans. J. For. Sci. 29: 541–549, 1984.

A. Ramu, J. Rosenbaum and T.F. Blaschke. Disposition of acetone following acute acetone intoxication. West. J. Med. 129: 429–432, 1978.

D.S. Ross. Acute acetone intoxication involving eight male workers. Ann. Occ. Hyg. 16: 73–75, 1973.

E.M.P. Widmark. Studies in the acetone concentration in blood, urine, and alveolar air. Biochem. J. 13: 430–445, 1919.

E.M.P. Widmark. *Principles and Applications of Medicolegal Alcohol Determination*, Biomedical Publications, Davis, California, 1981, pp. 61–62.

Acetonitrile

T½: 32 hr
Vd: 0.7 L/kg   CH3CN
Fb: 0

Occurrence and Usage. Acetonitrile, or methyl cyanide, is a clear liquid used as a laboratory and industrial solvent, a synthetic intermediate and an ingredient of glue removers for artificial fingernails. The current threshold limit value is 40 ppm (67 mg/m^3) in the industrial atmosphere, which is approximately the odor threshold of the vapor.

Blood Concentrations. Acetonitrile has not been measured in blood or plasma in nontoxic situations. However, the metabolites of acetonitrile, cyanide and thiocyanate, may be determined in blood as an index of exposure. In normal persons, blood cyanide is usually less then 0.04 mg/L and plasma thiocyanate levels less then 12 mg/L. Cyanide was not detected in the blood of volunteers exposed to a concentration of 160 ppm acetonitrile vapor for 4 hours (Pozzani, 1959).

Metabolism and Excretion. Acetonitrile is known to undergo biotransformation to cyanide, which is further metabolized to thiocyanate. It has been estimated that at least 12% of an inhaled dose of the chemical is metabolized in this manner, and undoubtedly a substantial portion is exhaled unchanged in the breath. In normal subjects, thiocyanate urine levels may range from 1–17 mg/L. Urine thiocyanate concentrations were not significantly elevated in volunteers exposed to a concentration of 160 ppm acetonitrile vapor for 4 hours (Pozzani, 1959).

Toxicity. Acetonitrile vapor concentrations of up to 500 ppm cause irritation of mucous membranes, whereas higher concentrations may produce weakness, nausea, convulsions and death. Blood cyanide concentrations of 3–11 mg/L and serum thiocyanate levels of 160–230 mg/L were observed in 2 workers suffering severe toxicity due to exposure to high concentrations of acetonitrile. Serum thiocyanate concentrations of less than 120 mg/L were associated with less severe symptoms such as weakness, nausea and abdominal pain in other subjects (Amdur, 1959). A 30 year old man who ingested 5 mL acetonitrile intentionally was treated and survived; he attained a peak serum acetonitrile level of 80 mg/L about 5 hours post-ingestion and a peak blood cyanide level of 17 mg/L at 24 hours (Michaelis et al., 1991).

Five individuals who died following either accidental ingestion (doses of 0.5–2.4 g/kg) or prolonged vapor inhalation had postmortem blood acetonitrile concentrations that averaged 710 mg/L (range, 560–800) and blood cyanide concentrations that averaged 4.5 mg/L (range, 2.4–8.0) (Amdur, 1959; Caravati and Litovitz, 1988; Jones et al., 1992; Swanson, 1992).

Analysis. Acetonitrile may be determined in biological specimens by gas chromatography with flame-ionization detection (Michaelis et al., 1991; Jones et al., 1992) or by gas chromatography-mass spectrometry (Jones et al., 1992). Some gas chromatographic methods may not be capable of distinguishing acetonitrile from ethanol. Procedures are presented for the analysis of blood cyanide and plasma and urine thiocyanate in the section on cyanide.

References

M.L. Amdur. Accidental group exposure to acetonitrile. J. Occ. Med. 1: 627–633, 1959.

E.M. Caravati and T.L. Litovitz. Pediatric cyanide intoxication and death from an acetonitrile-containing cosmetic. J. Am. Med. Asso. 260: 3470–3473, 1988.

A.W. Jones, A. Lofgren, A. Eklund and R. Grundin. Two fatalities from ingestion of acetonitrile: limited specificity of analysis by headspace gas chromatography. J. Anal. Tox. 16: 104–106, 1992.

H.C. Michaelis, C. Clemens, H. Kijewski et al. Acetonitrile serum concentrations and cyanide blood levels in a case of suicidal oral acetonitrile ingestion. Clin. Tox. 29: 447–458, 1991.

U.C. Pozzani, C.P. Carpenter, P.E. Palm et al. Mammalian toxicity of acetonitrile. J. Occ. Med. 1: 634–642, 1959.

J.R. Swanson. An acetonitrile related death. Presented at the 44th annual meeting of the American Academy of Forensic Sciences, New Orleans, February 21, 1992.

Acetylmethadol

T½: 32–116 hr
Vd: ?
Fb: ?
pKa: 8.8

$$CH_3CH_2CH-\underset{\underset{CH_3COO}{|}}{C}-CH_2\underset{\underset{CH_3}{|}}{C}HN(CH_3)_2$$

Occurrence and Usage. The synthesis of acetylmethadol (methadyl acetate) from methadone was reported in 1948 following a search for active narcotic analgesics based on the methadone structure. Although there are 4 optical isomers of this compound, most of the recent interest has centered on α–l-acetylmethadol, which is less active than its α–d enantiomorph but produces a delayed response in animals and humans. This compound has been extensively investigated as a long-acting alternative to methadone in the treatment of narcotic addicts. The compound is administered orally in doses of approximately 40–80 mg once every 2–3 days. Its demethylation to noracetylmethadol and dinoracetylmethadol is a bioactivation process that is believed to partly account for the long duration of action of the drug. Acetylmethadol may also be metabolized to methadol and normethadol, both of which are less active than their parent.

Blood Concentrations. Following a single oral administration of 60 mg of acetylmethadol, plasma concentrations (average of 5 subjects) of intact drug peaked at 0.13 mg/L at 6 hours, while noracetylmethadol (half-life of 13 hours) and dinoracetylmethadol (half-life of over 100 hours) peak concentrations were 0.04 and 0.02 mg/L, respectively. Half-lives for acetylmethadol ranged from 32–116 hours and averaged 53 hours (Henderson et al., 1977a). With chronic administration of the same dose, the steady-state plasma concentrations of parent, nor-, and dinoracetylmethadol were on the order of 0.06, 0.14 and 0.22 mg/L, respectively. These data show accumulation of the 2 metabolites, but not of the parent (Henderson et al., 1977b). The pharmacologic effects of the drug appear to correlate best with the noracetylmethadol plasma concentration (Kaiko and Inturissi, 1975).

Metabolism and Excretion. An average of 28% of administered acetylmethadol was excreted in the 48 hour urine of 4 subjects as unchanged drug (1.8%), noracetylmethadol (8.2%), dinoracetylmethadol (13%), and methadol (4.8%) (Kaiko et al., 1975). Other metabolites may include glucuronide or acetyl conjugates of these materials, and fecal excretion may also account for a portion of the dosage.

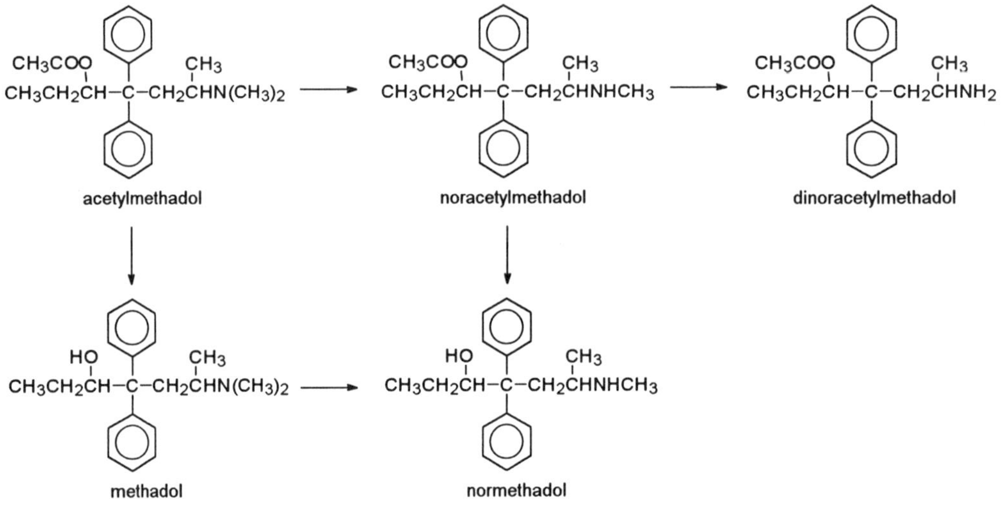

acetylmethadol   noracetylmethadol   dinoracetylmethadol

methadol   normethadol

Toxicity. A female heroin addict who ingested 75 mg of acetylmethadol collapsed in respiratory distress and was admitted to hospital in coma. Her blood acetylmethadol concentration remained at 0.02 mg/L for the first 3 days and at 0.01 mg/L for the subsequent 3 days, while concentrations of the 2 nor-metabolites were approximately twice those values. Urine concentrations of the 3 compounds generally remained at less than 0.5 mg/L.

A 24 year old male addict who one week previously had been placed on a thrice weekly oral acetylmethadol dose of 55–65 mg developed coma at home and died after 24 hours in the hospital. The following concentrations were obtained from the postmortem tissues (Chinn et al., 1979):

Concentrations in an Acetylmethadol Fatality (mg/L or mg/kg)

Drug	Blood	Brain	Lung	Liver	Kidney
Acetylmethadol	0.03	0.24	2.49	0.48	0.37
Noracetylmethadol	0.06	0.42	6.00	1.43	0.64
Dinoracetylmethadol	0.06	0.34	8.52	2.00	0.83

Analysis. Thin-layer chromatographic systems for the separation of a number of acetylmethadol metabolites and congeners have been described (Kuttab et al., 1976; Flor and Inturissi, 1977). The quantitative analysis of acetylmethadol and its metabolites is often performed using gas-liquid chromatography, and usually involves conversion of the metabolites to halogenated derivatives (Henderson et al., 1977b; Tse and Welling, 1980) or intramolecular amide formation (Kaiko and Inturissi, 1975). Gas chromatography employing a capillary column and nitrogen-specific detection provides a sensitive method for the detection and quantitation of acetylmethadol and its metabolites in serum (Verebey et al., 1985). Detection by mass spectrometry has increased the specificity of the gas chromatographic assay (Jindal et al., 1978; Jennison et al., 1979), while a comprehensive liquid chromatographic procedure for the parent drug and its 4 major active metabolites has been reported (Kiang et al., 1981).

References

D.M. Chinn, B.S. Finkle, D.J. Crouch and T.A. Jennison. The biodisposition of l-alpha-acetylmethadol and its principal metabolites: some fatal and nonfatal cases. J. Anal. Tox. 3: 143–149, 1979.

S.C. Flor and C.E. Inturrisi. Separation of radiolabeled acetylmethadol and metabolites by thin-layer chromatography. J. Anal. Tox. 1: 75–76, 1977.

G.L. Henderson, B.K. Wilson and D.H.M. Lau. Plasma l-α-acetylmethadol (LAAM) after acute and chronic administration. Clin. Pharm. Ther. 21: 16–25, 1977a.

G.L. Henderson, J.A. Weinberg, W.A. Hargreaves et al. Accumulation of l-α-acetylmethadol (LAAM) and active metabolites in plasma following chronic administration. J. Anal. Tox. 1: 1–5, 1977b.

T.A. Jennison and B.S. Finkle. The quantitative analysis of l-α-acetylmethadol and its principal metabolites in biological specimens by gas chromatography-chemical ionization-multiple ion monitoring mass spectrometry. J. Chrom. Sci. 17: 64–74, 1979.

S.P. Jindal, P. Vestergaard and T. Lutz. Mass fragmentographic determination of methadyl acetate in urine using stable isotope labeled analog as internal standard. J. Pharm. Sci. 67: 1483–1485, 1978.

R.F. Kaiko, N. Chatterjie and C.E. Inturrisi. Simultaneous determination of acetylmethadol and its active biotransformation products in human biofluids. J. Chrom. 109: 247–258, 1975.

R.F. Kaiko and C.E. Inturrisi. Disposition of acetylmethadol in relation to pharmacologic action. Clin. Pharm. Ther. 18: 96–103, 1975.

C. Kiang, S. Campos-Flor and C.E. Inturrisi. Determination of acetylmethadol and metabolites by use of high-performance liquid chromatography. J. Chrom. 222: 81–93, 1981.

S.H. Kuttab, H. North-Root and G.L. Henderson. Extraction method and thin-layer chromatographic system for the determination of α-l-acetylmethadol and metabolites in biological fluids. J. Chrom. 117: 193–198, 1976.

F.L.S. Tse and P.G. Welling. Pharmacokinetics of acetylmethadols I: gas-liquid chromatographic determination of l-α-acetylmethadol and its major metabolites in plasma. Biopharm. Drug Disp. 1: 203–209, 1980.

K. Verebey, A. DePace and S.J. Mule. Quantitation of l-α-acetylmethadol and its metabolites in human serum by capillary gas-liquid chromatography and nitrogen detection. J. Chrom. 343: 339–348, 1985.

Acetylsalicylic Acid

T½: 13–20 min
    3–20 hr for salicylic acid (dose-dependent)
Vd: 0.15–0.20 L/kg
    0.13 L/kg for salicylic acid
Fb: 0.04–0.12
    0.40–0.80 for salicylic acid
pKa: 3.5

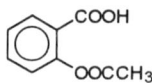

Occurrence and Usage. Acetylsalicylic acid (aspirin, ASA) remains one of the most commonly used therapeutic chemicals, both in pure form and in combination with many other drug substances. Oral doses of 325–975 mg, either as the free acid or a calcium or magnesium salt, are commonly administered to adults for analgesic and antipyretic effects, and amounts of 3000–5000 mg daily are often used for the antiinflammatory treatment of rheumatoid arthritis. More recently, aspirin has been frequently employed for its anticoagulant properties in low, chronic doses for selected patients.

Blood Concentrations. Most procedures used for the measurement of salicylate in biological specimens do not differentiate between acetylsalicylic acid and its major active metabolite, salicylic acid. The few studies that have distinguished between these 2 compounds have found that plasma acetylsalicylic acid concentrations after ingestion of 600–900 mg of the drug do not exceed 10 mg/L and decline rapidly, with a half-life of approximately 15 minutes (Thomas et al., 1973; Rance et al., 1975). It is therefore customary to report plasma concentrations in terms of total salicylate, representing both parent drug and salicylic acid.

Single oral doses of 1000 mg of aspirin were found to produce an average peak serum salicylic acid level of 77 mg/L (range, 31–114 mg/L) 2 hours after ingestion, declining to 51 and 26 mg/L by 6 and 10 hours, respectively (Hollister and Kanter, 1965). Arthritic patients maintained on a divided daily dosage of 50 mg/kg (3000 mg for a 70 kg male) exhibited plateau serum salicylate concentrations ranging from 44–330 mg/L (Gupta et al., 1975). The non-linear kinetics exhibited by salicylate cause the elimination half-life to increase from about 3 hours to 20 hours as the dose is increased from 300 mg to 20 g (Levy, 1979); at the same time, the volume of distribution increases, probably due to the decreased plasma protein binding with increasing plasma salicylate concentration (Levy and Yaffe, 1974).

Metabolism and Excretion. Virtually the total dose of aspirin is hydrolyzed by both liver and blood esterases to salicylic acid, an active analgesic that accounts for most or all of the pharmacological activity of the parent drug. Nearly all of a single dose is eliminated in the urine as salicylic acid (5%) and as salicylic acid conjugates: salicyluric acid (80%), salicyl phenolic glucuronide (10%) and salicyl acyl glucuronide (5%). Salicylic acid is also ring-hydroxylated in trace amounts to form di- and tri-hydroxy derivatives (Davison, 1971).

Toxicity. The ingestion of only 1 or 2 aspirin tablets has been known to produce sudden death in hypersensitive asthmatics (Dysart, 1933; Francis et al., 1935). Unintentional salicylate intoxication may play a role in the development of Reye's syndrome in children (Starko and Mullick, 1983). Serum salicylate concentrations exceeding 500 mg/L are indicative of salicylate toxicity. Done (1960) has presented a nomogram that relates serum salicylate and elapsed time since ingestion to the theoretical serum concentration at time zero, providing a guide to the severity of the intoxication.

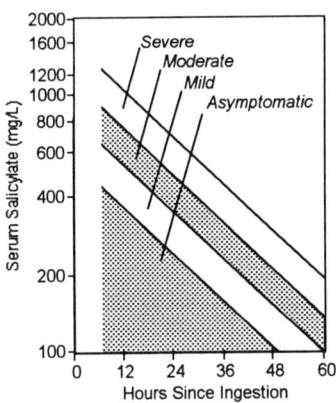

In aspirin overdosage, salicylic acid conjugation pathways become saturated and larger relative amounts of free salicylic acid are excreted in the urine (Levy et al., 1972). In the treatment of overdosage, the alkalinization of urine by intravenous administration of bicarbonate can greatly increase the renal clearance of salicylic acid and may shorten the duration of intoxication (Done, 1968). This also serves to enhance the ionization of salicylate in plasma, encouraging movement of drug out of the central nervous system (Done, 1978). In an overdosed patient, the fraction of salicylate bound to plasma protein was observed to increase from 0.4–0.8 as the plasma salicylate concentration declined from 925–83 mg/L (Alvan et al., 1981). The elimination half-life of salicylate was 17 hours in a woman who survived the ingestion of 81 g of aspirin (James and Martinak, 1975), and 27 hours in a woman who died following ingestion of an unknown amount (Ferguson and Boutros, 1970); in each case the maximal plasma salicylate concentration was approximately 1400 mg/L.

An acute dose of 16.25 g (50 tablets of 325 mg each) has been fatal in an adult. The following distribution data were derived from a report of 62 cases of fatal salicylate poisoning (Rehling, 1967):

Salicylate Concentrations in Fatalities (mg/L or mg/kg)

	Blood	Brain	Liver	Kidney	Urine
Average	661	218	420	390	557
Range	(61–7320)	(22–700)	(2.5–1000)	(1.7–1200)	(19–1350)

Analysis. The customary procedure for determination of salicylate in blood or plasma is the direct colorimetric technique of Trinder (1954), which is subject to interference from salicylate metabolites and other plasma consitutents. A more elaborate colorimetric technique involving solvent extraction and differential hydrolysis makes possible the measurement of both aspirin and salicylic acid (Muni et al., 1978). Numerous other methods are in use, such as ultraviolet spectrophotometry (Ungar et al., 1952); fluorimetry, both with solvent extraction (Chirigos and Udenfriend, 1959) and without (Baselt and Stewart, 1976); and gas chromatography with silyl derivative formation (Thomas et al., 1973; Walter et al., 1974; Rance et al., 1975). These latter GC procedures are capable of distinguishing aspirin from salicylic acid. High-pressure liquid chromatography is probably more suitable for this purpose, and is also capable of determining the conjugated metabolites of salicylic acid (Blair et al., 1978; Amick and Mason, 1979; Cham et al., 1980a, 1980b; Buskin, 1982; Chubb et al., 1986; Kwong, 1987). Goehl et al. (1981) have warned against the loss of salicylic acid by sublimation during the evaporation of organic solvents in methods employing solvent extraction.

References

G. Alvan, U. Bergman and L.L. Gustafsson. High unbound fraction of salicylate in plasma during intoxication. Brit. J. Clin. Pharm. 11: 625–626, 1981.

E.N. Amick and W.D. Mason. Determination of aspirin, salicylic acid, salicyluric acid, and gentisic acid in human plasma and urine by high pressure liquid chromatography. Anal. Letters 12: 629–640, 1979.

R.C. Baselt and C.B. Stewart. Rapid fluorometric analysis of unbound salicylate in whole blood. Res. Comm. Chem. Path. Pharm. 15: 351–360, 1976.

D. Blair, B.H. Rumack and R.G. Peterson. Analysis for salicylic acid in serum by high-performance liquid chromatography. Clin. Chem. 24: 1543–1544, 1978.

J.N. Buskin, R.A. Upton and R.L. Williams. Improved liquid-chromatography of aspirin, salicylate, and salicyluric acid in plasma, with a modification for determining aspirin metabolites in urine. Clin. Chem. 28: 1200–1203, 1982.

B.E. Cham, F. Bochner, D.M. Imhoff et al. Simultaneous liquid-chromatographic quantitation of salicylic acid, salicyluric acid, and gentisic acid in urine. Clin. Chem. 26: 111–114, 1980a.

B.E. Cham, L. Ross-Lee, F. Bochner and D.M. Imhoff. Measurement and pharmacokinetics of acetylsalicylic acid by a novel high performance liquid chromatographic assay. Ther. Drug Mon. 2: 365–372, 1980b.

M.A. Chirigos and S. Udenfriend. A simple fluorometric procedure for determining salicylic acid in biologic tissues. J. Lab. Clin. Med. 54: 769–772, 1959.

S.A.P. Chubb, R.S. Campbell and C.P. Price. Rapid method of measuring salicylate in serum by high-performance liquid chromatography. J. Chrom. 380: 163–169, 1986.

C. Davison. Salicylate metabolism in man. Ann. N.Y. Acad. Sci. 179: 249–268, 1971.

A.K. Done. Salicylate intoxication. Pediatrics 26: 800–807, 1960.

A.K. Done. Treatment of salicylate poisoning: review of personal and published experiences. Clin. Tox. 4: 451–467, 1968.

A.K. Done. Aspirin overdosage: incidence, diagnosis, and management. Pediatrics 62: Part 2 (Suppl.) 890–897, 1978.

B.R. Dysart. Death following ingestion of five grains of acetylsalicylic acid. J. Am. Med. Asso. 101: 446, 1933.

R.K. Ferguson and A.R. Boutros. Death following self-poisoning with aspirin. J. Am. Med. Asso. 213: 1186–1188, 1970.

N. Francis, O.T. Ghent and S.S. Bullen. Death from ten grains of aspirin. J. Allergy 6: 504–506, 1935.

T.J. Goehl, C.T. DeWoody and G.M. Sundaresan. Sublimation losses of salicylic acid from plasma during analysis. Clin. Chem. 27: 776, 198l.

N. Gupta, E. Sarkissian and H.E. Paulus. Correlation of plateau serum salicylate level with rate of salicylate metabolism. Clin. Pharm. Ther. 18: 350–355, 1975.

G.E. Hollister and S.L. Kanter. Studies of delayed-action medication. IV. Salicylates. Clin. Pharm. Ther. 6: 5–13, 1965.

S.H. James and J.F. Martinak. Recovery following massive self-poisoning with aspirin. N.Y. State J. Med. 75: 1512–1514, 1975.

T.C. Kwong. Analysis of acetylsalicylic acid and its metabolites by liquid chromatography. J. Liq. Chrom. 10: 305–321, 1987.

G. Levy. Pharmacokinetics of salicylate in man. Drug Met. Rev. 9: 3–19, 1979.

G. Levy, T. Tsuchiya and L.P. Amsel. Limited capacity for salicyl phenolic glucuronide formation and its effect on the kinetics of salicylate elimination in man. Clin. Pharm. Ther. 13: 258–268, 1972.

G. Levy and S.J. Yaffe. Relationship between dose and apparent volume of distribution of salicylate in children. Pediatrics 54: 713–717, 1974.

I.A. Muni, J.L. Leeling, R.J. Helms et al. Improved colorimetric determination of aspirin and salicylic acid concentrations in human plasma. J. Pharm. Sci. 67: 289–291, 1978.

M.J. Rance, B.J. Jordan and J.D. Nichols. A simultaneous determination of acetylsalicylic acid, salicylic acid and salicylamide in plasma by gas liquid chromatography. J. Pharm. Pharmac. 27: 425–429, 1975.

C.J. Rehling. Poison residues in human tissues. In *Progress in Chemical Toxicology*, Vol. 3 (A. Stolman, ed.), Academic Press, New York, 1967, pp. 363–386.

K.M. Starko and F.G. Mullick. Hepatic and cerebral pathology findings in children with fatal salicylate intoxication: further evidence for a causal relation between salicylate and Reye's syndrome. Lancet 1: 326–329, 1983.

B.H. Thomas, G. Solomonraj and B.B. Coldwell. The estimation of acetylsalicylic acid and salicylate in biological fluids by gas–liquid chromatography. J. Pharm. Pharmac. 25: 201–204, 1973.

P. Trinder. Rapid determination of salicylate in biological fluids. Biochem. J. 57: 301–303, 1954.

G. Ungar, E. Damgaard and W.K. Wong. Determination of salicylate acid and related substances in serum by ultraviolet spectrophotometry. Proc. Soc. Exp. Biol. Med. 80: 45–47, 1952.

L.J. Walter, D.F. Biggs and R.T. Coutts. Simultaneous GLC estimation of salicylic acid and aspirin in plasma. J. Pharm. Sci. 63: 1754–1758, 1974.

Acrylonitrile

T½: ? $CH_2=CHCN$
Vd: ?
Fb: ?

Occurrence and Usage. Acrylonitrile (vinyl cyanide) is used extensively in the manufacture of plastics, synthetic fibers and adhesives. It is also employed as a chemical intermediate and as a fumigant, and is a component of cigarette smoke. The current threshold limit value for the vapor is 2 ppm (4.3 mg/m^3). Acrylonitrile has been classified as a suspected human carcinogen by the American Conference of Governmental Industrial Hygienists.

Blood Concentrations. The compound is readily absorbed following inhalation of the vapor or during dermal contact with the liquid. Acrylonitrile has not been detected in the blood of workers occupationally exposed to the vapor. The metabolites of acrylonitrile, cyanide and thiocyanate, may be measured in blood as an index of exposure, however (Brieger et al., 1952). In normal unexposed subjects, blood cyanide is usually less than 0.04 mg/L and plasma thiocyanate levels less than 12 mg/L. Plasma thiocyanate achieves a maximum at the end of an exposure to acrylonitrile; Lawton et al. (1943) stated that levels exceeding 20 mg/L in non-smokers and 30 mg/L in smokers were indicative of overexposure to the chemical.

Metabolism and Excretion. Acrylonitrile is known to produce cyanide *in vivo*, with further metabolism to thiocyanate. The extent of this biotransformation is unknown, and it is likely that a portion of an absorbed dose of the chemical is exhaled unchanged in the breath. A positive correlation has been found between occupational air concentrations of acrylonitrile and urine acrylonitrile levels in workers; an 8 hour exposure to 0.13 ppm in air resulted in an average urine concentration of 39 µg/L (Houthuijs et al., 1982).

Attempts to relate urine thiocyanate concentrations to the level of exposure to acrylonitrile vapor were unsuccessful due to the wide normal range of thiocyanate in urine (Brieger et al., 1952). However, Lawton et al. (1943) found that urinary thiocyanate levels reached a maximum 24–48 hours after an exposure, and that levels exceeding 2 mg/24 hours in non-smokers and 16 mg/24 hours in smokers were indicative of overexposure to the chemical.

Toxicity. Mild cases of intoxication due to acrylonitrile usually involve eye irritation, headache, nausea and weakness. Severe toxicity results in asphyxia and death due to cyanide poisoning. Exposure to concentrations exceeding 150 ppm for 4 hours has caused serious toxicity in monkeys (Dudley et al., 1942). One child died following inhalation of acrylonitrile used as a room fumigant (Grunske, 1949) and another after dermal absorption of the compound used as a pediculicide (Lorz, 1950). The autopsy findings in both cases were suggestive of cyanide poisoning.

Analysis. Procedures for the analysis of blood cyanide and plasma and urine thiocyanate are cited in the section on cyanide. Acrylonitrile has been measured in biological specimens using gas chromatography with nitrogen-phosphorus detection (Houthuijs et al., 1982; Freshour and Melcher, 1983).

References

H. Brieger, F. Rieders and W.A. Hodes. Acrylonitrile: spectrophotometric determination, acute toxicity, and mechanism of action. Arch. Ind. Hyg. Occ. Med. 6: 128–140, 1952.

H.C. Dudley, T.R. Sweeney and J.W. Miller. Toxicology of acrylonitrile (vinyl cyanide). J. Ind. Hyg. Tox. 24: 255–258, 1942.

N.L. Freshour and R.G. Melcher. Analytical method for the determination of acrylonitrile in rat plasma at the nanograms per milliliter level. J. Anal. Tox. 7: 103–105, 1983.

F. Grunske. Ventox und Ventox-Vergiftung. Deut. Med. Wochenschr. 74: 1081–1083, 1949.

D. Houthuijs, B. Remijn, H. Willems et al. Biological monitoring of acrylonitrile exposure. Am. J. Ind. Med. 3: 313–320, 1982.

A.H. Lawton, T.R. Sweeney and H.C. Dudley. Toxicology of acrylonitrile (vinyl cyanide). J. Ind. Hyg. Tox. 25: 13–19, 1943.

H. Lorz. Ueber perkutane Vergiftung mit Akrylnitril. Deut. Med. Wochenschr. 75: 1087–1088, 1950.

Albuterol

T½: 2–7 hr
Vd: 2.2 L/kg
Fb: ?
pKa: 9.3 (acid), 10.3 (base)

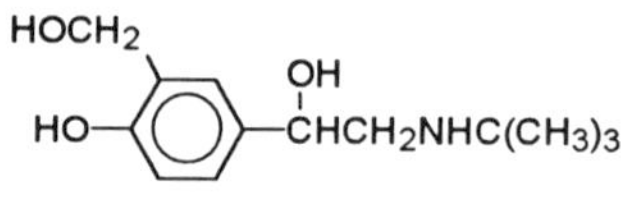

Occurrence and Usage. Albuterol (salbutamol, Proventil, Ventolin) is a sympathomimetic beta$_2$-agonist that is widely used for the treatment of bronchial asthma. It is available as an inhalation aerosol with each actuation delivering 90 µg, as a syrup containing 2 mg/5 mL, and as tablets containing 2–4 mg of the sulfate salt.

Blood Concentrations. Inhalation of 3 mg of aerosolized albuterol in asthmatic patients produced an average peak plasma level of 2.1 µg/L (range, 1.4–3.2) at 0.5 hours (PDR, 1993). A single 4 mg oral dose given to adults resulted in an average peak plasma concentration of 7.2 µg/L (Maconochie and Fowler, 1983).

Twelve healthy adult volunteers weighing 66–87 kg received a 4 mg albuterol tablet every 6 hours for 5 days; steady-state plasma albuterol concentrations on the third day showed a mean maximum concentration of 15 µg/L and a mean minimum concentration of 9.9 µg/L (Powell et al., 1986).

Metabolism and Excretion. Little is known of the metabolism of albuterol. Its metabolites include the 4-O-sulfate ester (Kucharczyk and Segelman, 1985). Following intravenous administration, approximately 64% of the dose is eliminated unchanged in the urine. Up to 90% of a dose is excreted over 72 hours (Morgan et al., 1986).

Toxicity. Manifestations of overdose may include anginal pain, hypertension, hypokalemia, cardio-vascular palpitations, tremor, nausea and dizziness. A 22 month old infant recovered uneventfully with supportive care following ingestion of up to 30 mg of albuterol (King et al., 1992). A suicide attempt in an adult who ingested 240 mg did not result in a fatal outcome (Prior et al., 1981).

A 2 month old child, found dead after a prescription error that resulted in his receiving 6 times the recommended oral dose, had a postmortem blood albuterol concentration of 31 µg/L (Keen, 1993).

Analysis. A specific radioimmunoassay for the determination of albuterol has been described (Loo et al., 1987). Albuterol may be determined in plasma and other biological samples employing liquid chromatography with electrochemical (Emm et al., 1988; Sagar et al., 1993) or fluorescence detection (Miller and Greenblatt, 1986; Ong et al., 1989; Bland et al., 1990; McCarthy et al., 1993). Gas chromatography-mass spectrometry offers specificity in the analysis of the compound (Lindberg and Jonsson, 1982; Weisberger et al., 1983).

References

R.E. Bland, R.J.N. Tanner, W.H. Chern et al. Determination of albuterol concentrations in human plasma using solid-phase extraction and high-performance liquid chromatography with fluorescence detection. J. Pharm. Biomed. Anal. 8: 591–596, 1990.

T. Emm, L.J. Lesko, J. Leslie and M.B. Perkal. Determination of albuterol in human serum by reversed-phase high-performance liquid chromatography with electrochemical detection. J. Chrom. 427: 188–194, 1988.

P. Keen. Personal communication, 1993.

W.D. King, M. Holloway and P.A. Palmisano. Albuterol overdose: a case report and differential diagnosis. Pediat. Emer. Care 8: 268–271, 1992.

N. Kucharczyk and F.H. Segelman. Drug level monitoring of antiasthmatic drugs. J. Chrom. 340: 243–271, 1985.

C. Lindberg and S. Jonsson. Simultaneous determination of terbutaline and salbutamol in plasma by selected ion monitoring. Biomed. Mass Spec. 6: 493–494, 1982.

J.C.K. Loo, N. Beaulieu, N. Jordan et al. A specific radio-immunoassay (RIA) for salbutamol (albuterol) in human plasma. Res. Comm. Chem. Path. Pharm. 55: 283–286, 1987.

J.G. Maconochie and P. Fowler. Plasma concentrations of salbutamol after an oral slow-release preparation. Curr. Med. Res. Opin. 8: 634–639, 1983.

P.T. McCarthy, S. Atwal, A.P. Sykes and J.G. Ayres. Measurement of terbutaline and salbutamol in plasma by high performance liquid chromatography with fluorescence detection. Biomed. Chrom. 7: 25–28, 1993.

L.G. Miller and D.J. Greenblatt. Determination of albuterol in human plasma by high-performance liquid chromatography with fluorescence detection. J. Chrom. 381: 205–208, 1986.

D.J. Morgan, J.D. Paull, B.H. Richmond et al. Pharmacokinetics of intravenous and oral salbutamol and its sulphate conjugate. Brit. J. Clin. Pharm. 22: 587–593, 1986.

H. Ong, A. Adam, S. Perreault et al. Analysis of albuterol in human plasma based on immunoaffinity chromatographic cleanup combined with high-performance liquid chromatography with fluorimetric detection. J. Chrom. 497: 213–222, 1989.

Physicians' Desk Reference, Medical Economics Company, Montvale, New Jersey, 1993, pp. 582–585.

M.L. Powell, M. Chung, M. Weisberger et al. Multiple-dose albuterol kinetics. J. Clin. Pharm. 26: 643–646, 1986.

J.G. Prior, G.M. Cochrane, S.M. Raper et al. Self-poisoning with oral salbutamol. Brit. Med. J. 282: 1932, 1981.

K.A. Sagar, M.T. Kelly and M.R. Smyth. Simultaneous determination of salbutamol and terbutaline at overdose levels in human plasma by high performance liquid chromatography with electrochemical detection. Biomed. Chrom. 7: 29–33, 1993.

M. Weisberger, J.E. Patrick and M.L. Powell. Quantitative analysis of albuterol in human plasma by combined gas chromatography chemical ionization mass spectrometry. Biomed. Mass Spec. 10: 556–558, 1983.

Aldrin

T½: 50–167 days
Vd: ?
Fb: ?

Occurrence and Usage. Aldrin (octalene) is a chlorinated naphthalene derivative that has been used as an insecticide since 1950. It is closely related to 2 other members of the cyclodiene class, dieldrin and endrin. Aldrin has been banned from use in some countries due to its persistence in the environment and its potential for chronic toxicity. The current threshold limit value for industrial exposure is 0.25 mg/m^3.

Blood Concentrations. Blood concentrations of dieldrin, an aldrin metabolite, averaged 0.0014 mg/L in 10 persons with no occupational exposure to insecticides. About 80% of whole blood dieldrin was restricted to the plasma. Serum concentrations in persons with low to high occupational exposure to aldrin and dieldrin averaged 0.0007–0.0023 mg/L for aldrin and 0.0094–0.0270 mg/L for dieldrin (Dale et al., 1966). Plasma concentrations in apparently asymptomatic industrial aldrin formulators who had direct contact with the chemical averaged 0.030 mg/L for aldrin and 0.183 mg/L for dieldrin (Mick et al., 1972). The average half-life of dieldrin in blood is 97 days, with a range of 50–167 days (Brown et al., 1964).

Metabolism and Excretion. Aldrin is metabolized in man by epoxide formation, converting it to dieldrin. Aldrin and dieldrin are approximately equitoxic, but it is as dieldrin that the compound accumulates in the body fat of man and other animals. Concentrations of dieldrin in fat from 131 autopsies in England averaged 0.21 mg/kg (range, 0–1.29), with no significant correlation to sex, age, place of abode or cause of death (Hunter et al., 1963). In industrially exposed workers, dieldrin concentrations in fat averaged 6.12 mg/kg (range, 0.60–32). Aldrin is slowly eliminated from the body, primarily as unknown hydrophilic metabolites, in feces and to a slight extent in urine. Unchanged aldrin is not found in the urine of workers exposed to the chemical, although dieldrin concentrations may range up to 0.07 mg/L (Hayes and Curley, 1968).

aldrin   dieldrin   hydrophilic metabolites

Toxicity. Aldrin produces central nervous system excitation after both acute and chronic overexposure; poisoning is manifested by nausea, dizziness, headache, involuntary movements, convulsions and loss of consciousness. Blood dieldrin concentrations of 4 aldrin workers who displayed moderate to severe symptoms of chronic intoxication ranged from 0.04–0.53 mg/L; fat concentrations in 2 of these subjects 2–3 weeks after the last exposure were 60 and 149 mg/kg (Kazantzis et al., 1964). Brown et al. (1964) established a threshold blood dieldrin concentration of 0.16–0.25 mg/L for the expression of signs of intoxication due to aldrin or dieldrin. Avar and Czegledi-Janko (1970), in a similar study, described several workers who exhibited symptoms of poisoning at blood dieldrin levels of 0.10 mg/L and higher, and others who were asymptomatic at levels of 0.25 mg/L.

   An individual who ingested aldrin was found to have characteristic signs of poisoning and aldrin and dieldrin plasma concentrations of 0.036 and 0.279 mg/L, respectively, 18 hours after ingestion; after 20 days, when recovering, these concentrations had fallen to 0.002 and 0.090 mg/L, respectively (Dale et al., 1966). A young man who inhaled aldrin powder over a 2 day period while repackaging the substance had a convulsive seizure on the evening of the second day; 2 weeks later a fat biopsy showed a dieldrin concentration of 40 mg/kg (Bell, 1960). The acute lethal dose of aldrin in man is believed to range from 3–7 g of the compound (Spiotta, 1951).

Analysis. Aldrin and dieldrin may be determined in biological specimens by electron-capture gas chromatography, using a scheme that includes many other organochlorine insecticides (Dale et al., 1966; Barquet et al., 1981).

References

P. Avar and G. Czegledi-Janko. Occupational exposure to aldrin: clinical and laboratory findings. Brit. J. Ind. Med. 27: 279–282, 1970.

A. Barquet, C. Morgade and C.D. Pfaffenberger. Determination of organochlorine pesticides and metabolites in drinking water, human blood serum, and adipose tissue. J. Tox. Env. Health 7: 469–479, 1981.

A. Bell. Aldrin poisoning: a case report. Med. J. Aust. 2: 698–700, 1960.

V.K.H. Brown, C.G. Hunter and A. Richardson. A blood test diagnostic of exposure to aldrin and dieldrin. Brit. J. Ind. Med. 21: 283–286, 1964.

W.E. Dale, A. Curley and C. Cueto, Jr. Hexane extractable chlorinated insecticides in human blood. Life Sci. 5: 47–54, 1966.

W.J. Hayes and A. Curley. Storage and excretion of dieldrin and related compounds. Arch. Env. Health 16: 155–162, 1968.

C.G. Hunter, J. Robinson and A. Richardson. Chlorinated insecticide content of human body fat in southern England. Brit. Med. J. 1: 221–224, 1963.

G. Kazantzis, A.I.G. McLaughlin and P.F. Prior. Poisoning in industrial workers by the insecticide aldrin. Brit. J. Ind. Med. 21: 46–51, 1964.

D.L. Mick, K.R. Long and D.P. Bonderman. Aldrin and dieldrin in the blood of pesticide formulators. Am. Ind. Hyg. Asso. J. 33: 94–99, 1972.

E.J. Spiotta. Aldrin poisoning in man. Arch. Ind. Hyg. Occ. Med. 4: 560–566, 1951.

Alfentanil

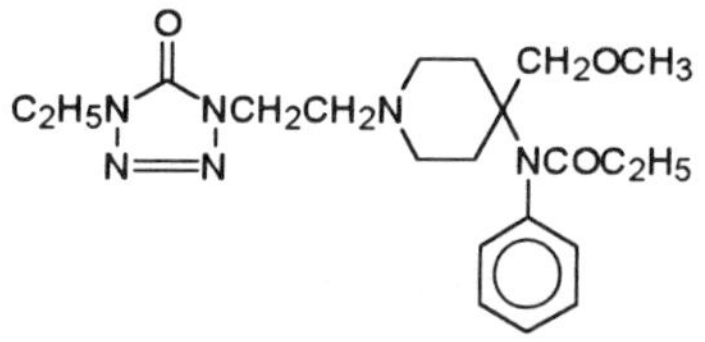

T½: 1–2 hr
Vd: 0.3–1.0 L/kg
Fb: 0.92
pKa: 6.5

Occurrence and Usage. Alfentanil (Alfenta, Rapifen), chemically related to fentanyl, is an intravenous narcotic analgesic characterized by very rapid onset and short duration of action. It has been used as an adjunct to surgical anesthesia, often in combination with nitrous oxide; initial doses may range from 8–50 µg/kg or higher. The drug is available as the hydrochloride salt in a 500 µg/mL solution (expressed as the free base) intended for intravenous injection.

Blood Concentrations. Five surgical patients, aged 33–55 and weighing 46–72 kg, were given a bolus dose of 120 µg/kg alfentanil by intravenous injection; the average plasma concentration was 565 µg/L at 2 minutes, 229 µg/L at 15 minutes, and 81 µg/L at 60 minutes (Camu et al., 1982).

Ten patients were given a mean total dose of 1379 µg/kg (96.5 mg/70 kg) as a continuous infusion during cardiac surgery; plasma alfentanil concentrations averaged 1000–1200 µg/L, postoperative unconsciousness averaged 2.6 hours, and the plasma alfentanil concentration at the time of awakening averaged 460 µg/L (Hynynen et al., 1986).

Young children have been found to exhibit shorter half-lives (average, 0.7 hr) and smaller volumes of distribution (average, 0.16 L/kg) than adults (1.6 hours and 0.46 L/kg, respectively) (Meistelman et al., 1987). Older adults do not differ significantly from younger adults in terms of pharmacokinetic parameters, but they often demonstrate increased sensitivity to the narcotic effects of alfentanil (Scott and Stanski, 1987).

Metabolism and Excretion. Alfentanil undergoes extensive metabolism via N- and O-dealkylation, ring hydroxylation, amide hydrolysis and conjugation. The metabolites of alfentanil appear to have no pharmacologic activity (Niemegeers and Janssen, 1981). Less than 1% of a dose is excreted unchanged in the 24 hour urine, while 31% is present as noralfentanil, 16% as free and conjugated O-demethylnoralfentanil, 6.4% as free and conjugated N-(4-hydroxyphenyl)propanamide, and 6.0% as free and conjugated N-(4-hydroxyphenyl)acetamide (Meuldermans et al., 1988).

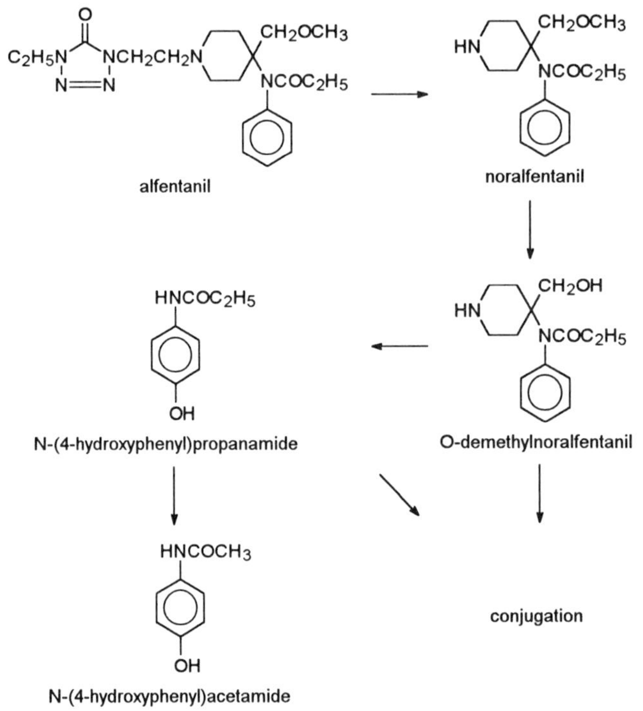

Toxicity. Alfentanil is capable of producing severe respiratory depression, hypotension and coma. Respiratory depression occurs at serum concentrations greater than 100–200 µg/L (Stanski and Hug, 1982), although occasionally patients exhibit prolonged or delayed effects at lower levels. Two surgical patients who developed respiratory arrest within 45–60 min post-infusion had plasma alfentanil levels of 87 and 95 ng/mL (Sebel et al., 1984; Mahla et al., 1988).

Analysis. Gas chromatography with nitrogen-phosphorus detection (Gillespie et al., 1981; Hynynen et al., 1986; Bjorkman et al., 1989) has been used in the determination of alfentanil in biological specimens. Gas chromatography-mass spectrometry offers both a sensitive and specific method of analysis for alfentanil and its metabolites in plasma (Lin et al., 1981; van Rooy et al., 1981). The drug may also be measured by a specific radioimmunoassay (Michiels et al., 1983).

References

S. Bjorkman, N. Aziz, D. Stein and D.R. Stanski. Determination of alfentanil in serum by radioimmunoassay or capillary column gas-liquid chromatography. Acta Pharm. Nord. 1: 211–220, 1989.

F. Camu, E. Gepts, M. Rucquoi and J. Heykants. Pharmacokinetics of alfentanil in man. Anesth. Anal. 61: 657–661, 1982.

T.J. Gillespie, A.J. Gandolfi, R.M. Maiorino and R.W. Vaughn. Gas chromatographic determination of fentanyl and its analogues in human plasma. J. Anal. Tox. 5: 133–137, 1981.

M. Hynynen, O. Takkunen, M. Salmenpera et al. Continuous infusion of fentanyl or alfentanil for coronary artery surgery. Brit. J. Anaesth. 58: 1252–1259, 1986.

S.N. Lin, T.P. Wang, R.M. Caprioli and B.P.N. Mo. Determination of plasma fentanyl by GC-mass spectrometry and pharmacokinetic analysis. J. Pharm. Sci. 70: 1276–1278, 1981.

M.E. Mahla, S.E. White and M.D. Moneta. Delayed respiratory depression after alfentanil. Anesthesiology 69: 593–595, 1988.

C. Meistelman, C. Saint-Maurice, M. Lepaul et al. A comparison of alfentanil pharmacokinetics in children and adults. Anesthesiology 66: 13–16, 1987.

W. Meuldermans, A. Van Peer, J. Hendrickx et al. Alfentanil pharmacokinetics and metabolism in humans. Anesthesiology 69: 527–534, 1988.

M. Michiels, R. Hendricks and J. Heykants. Radioimmunoassay of the new opiate analgesics alfentanil and sufentanil. Preliminary pharmacokinetic profile in man. J. Pharm. Pharmac. 35: 86–93, 1983.

C.J.E. Niemegeers and P.A.J. Janssen. Alfentanil (R39209), a particularly short-acting intravenous narcotic analgesic in rats. Drug Dev. Res. 1: 83–88, 1981.

J.S. Scott and D.R. Stanski. Decreased fentanyl and alfentanil dose requirements with age. J. Pharm. Exp. Ther. 240: 159–166, 1987.

P.S. Sebel, J.M. Labor, P.J. Flynn and B.A. Simpson. Respiratory depression after alfentanil infusion. Brit. Med. J. 289: 1581–1582, 1984.

D.R. Stanski and C.C. Hug. Alfentanil: a kinetically predictable narcotic analgesic. Anesthesiology 57: 435–438, 1982.

H.H. van Rooy, N.P.E. Vermeulen and J.G. Bovill. The assay of fentanyl and its metabolites in plasma of patients using gas chromatography-mass spectrometry. J. Chrom. 223: 85–93, 1981.

Alphaprodine

T½: 1.6–2.6 hr
Vd: 1.9 L/kg
Fb: ?
pKa: 8.7

Occurrence and Usage. Alphaprodine (Nisentil) is a synthetic narcotic analgesic, similar in chemical structure and potency to meperidine. It has a relatively short duration of action, 1–2 hours, and is used primarily in obstetrics and for minor surgical procedures. Doses of 40–60 mg are commonly given by subcutaneous or intravenous injection; the drug is supplied as a powder or solution.

Blood Concentrations. A single intravenous 35 mg dose of alphaprodine given to 6 adults produced an initial average peak plasma concentration of 0.87 mg/L, declining with a half-life of 2.2 hours (range, 1.6–2.6) to 0.07 mg/L by 5 hours after injection (Fung et al., 1980). A 120 mg intravenous dose in 5 surgical patients produced a mean peak plasma concentration of 1.0 mg/L, declining to 0.25 mg/L at 4.2 hours (Burns, 1963).

Metabolism and Excretion. Little data is available on the disposition of alphaprodine in man. In dogs, the drug is rapidly N-demethylated to noralphaprodine, which appears in plasma soon after drug administration and remains at a constant level for at least 4 hours. The pharmacological activity of noralphaprodine has not been reported. Approximately 42% of a dose is excreted by dogs in the 24 hour urine; unchanged drug accounts for 5%, noralphaprodine for 5–6%, and unidentified conjugated metabolites for the remainder (Abdel-Monem et al., 1972).

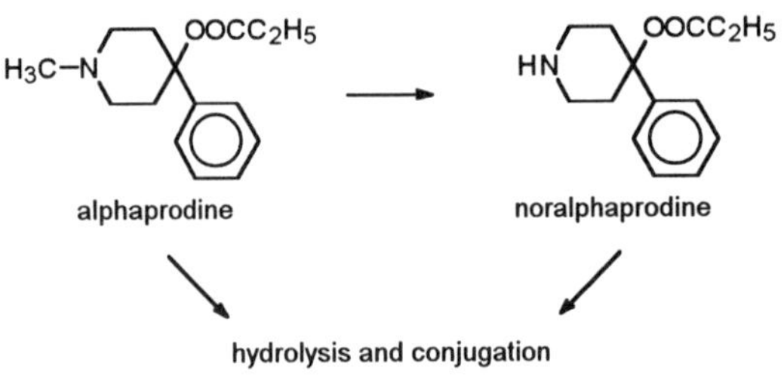

alphaprodine   noralphaprodine

hydrolysis and conjugation

Toxicity. Alphaprodine toxicity is manifested by stupor, hypotension, coma, convulsions and cardiorespiratory arrest. A 215 pound male adult, the victim of superficial knife wounds, was admitted to a hospital and administered 40 mg alphaprodine intravenously. He died 1 hour later; alphaprodine concentrations of 0.62 and 0.30 mg/L were found in postmortem blood and urine, respectively, and 0.17 g/dL ethanol in blood (Griesemer, 1973). A dental hygienist was found dead after self-administering alphaprodine by injection; the following concentrations were measured in postmortem specimens (Turner, 1986):

Alphaprodine Concentrations in a Fatal Case (mg/L or mg/kg)

Blood	Brain	Liver	Urine	Gastric
3.3	10	12	2	0.15 mg

Analysis. Most procedures designed for the analysis of meperidine in biological specimens are applicable as well to alphaprodine. Methods specific for alphaprodine have utilized gas chromatography with detection by flame-ionization (Fung et al., 1980) or mass spectrometry (Kuhnert et al., 1988).

References

M.M. Abdel-Monem, P.A. Harris and P.S. Portoghese. Pharmacokinetics, metabolism, and urinary excretion of (^{3}H)alphaprodine in dogs. J. Med. Chem. 15: 706–708, 1972.

J.J. Burns. Role of biotransformation. In *Uptake and Distribution of Anesthetic Agents* (E.M. Papper and R.J. Kitz, eds.), McGraw-Hill, New York, 1963, pp. 177–188.

D.L. Fung, J.H. Asling, J.H. Eisele and R. Martucci. A comparison of alphaprodine and meperidine pharmacokinetics. J. Clin. Pharm. 20: 37–41, 1980.

E. Griesemer. Personal communication, 1973.

B.R. Kuhnert, W.T. Brashear and C.D. Syracuse. Measurement of alphaprodine by selected-ion monitoring. J. Chrom. 426: 392–398, 1988.

J. Turner. Personal communication, 1986.

Alprazolam

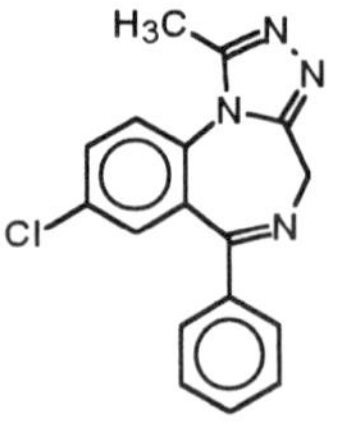

T½: 6–27 hr (average, 11)
Vd: 0.9–1.3 L/kg
Fb: 0.65–0.75
pKa: ?

Occurrence and Usage. Alprazolam (Xanax), a triazolobenzodiazepine derivative, is a short-acting antidepressant and anxiolytic agent. The drug has also been found effective in the treatment of agoraphobia, panic attacks and panic disorders. Doses of 0.75–4 mg daily are effective for generalized anxiety, while doses of 6–9 mg daily have been used for phobic and panic disorders. The drug is supplied as the free base in tablets of 0.25–1.0 mg.

Blood Concentrations. Following a single 1 mg oral dose in 6 male patients, peak plasma concentrations averaged 19 µg/L at 1.3 hours after dosing (Ciraulo et al., 1986). Steady-state serum concentrations of 25–55 µg/L were reported in 6 patients taking daily oral doses of 1.5–6 mg (McCormick et al., 1984). Plasma concentrations appear to be proportional to the dose given; patients given 3 mg/day reached an average steady-state plasma concentration of 29 µg/L, those on 6 mg/day averaged 61 µg/L and those on 9 mg/day, 102 µg/L (Ciraulo et al., 1986). α–Hydroxyalprazolam and 4-hydroxyalprazolam have approximately 66% and 19% of the parent drug's potency, respectively, but are present in plasma (in unconjugated form) at less than 10% of the alprazolam level, even with chronic dosing (Smith and Kroboth, 1987).

Metabolism and Excretion. Alprazolam is extensively metabolized by oxidation and conjugation. The principal metabolites are α–hydroxyalprazolam of a dose (17%), 4-hydroxyalprazolam (0.3%) and α,4-dihydroxyalprazolam (0.2%). Cleavage of the 5,6-azomethine bond forms the 3-hydroxy-5-methyltriazolyl (17%) analogue of chlorobenzophenone (HMTBP) (Eberts et al., 1980). Approximately 94% of a radiolabeled dose is excreted within 72 hours, with 80% in the urine and 7% in the feces; about 20% of a dose is eliminated in the urine as unchanged alprazolam (Dawson et al., 1984). The major urinary species include the parent drug and conjugates of α–hydroxyalprazolam and HMTBP (Joern and Joern, 1987).

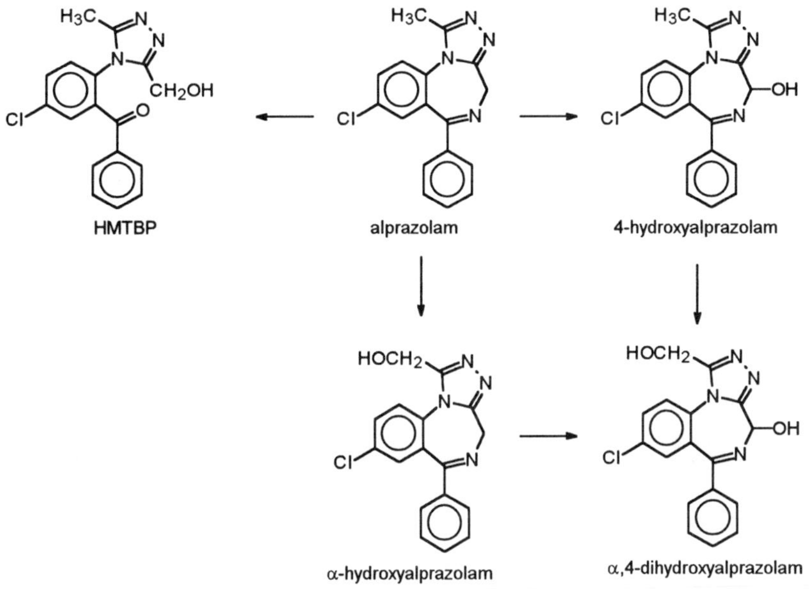

HMTBP   alprazolam   4-hydroxyalprazolam

α-hydroxyalprazolam   α,4-dihydroxyalprazolam

Toxicity. Adverse reactions to alprazolam include drowsiness, confusion, hypotension, tachycardia, palpitations, nausea and muscle tremors (Dawson et al., 1984). Anger, hostility, manic symptoms, insomnia, nightmares, and self-mutilatory impulses have also been reported (Medical Letter, 1986). Withdrawal symptoms including delerium and seizures may occur following abrupt discontinuance of chronic therapy (Brier et al., 1984; Levy, 1984; Vital-Herne et al., 1985).

A study of 102 instances of individuals driving under the influence of alprazolam showed blood alprazolam concentrations in the suspects ranging from 8–642 µg/L, with 30% of the values exceeding 100 µg/L (Drugs & Driving Committee, 1993).

In 5 apparent cases of suicide by alprazolam ingestion, postmortem blood concentrations of 122–390 µg/L (average, 236) were observed (Stafford, 1984; Edinboro and Backer, 1985; Howell, 1985; Munoz, 1988; Reynolds, 1988).

Analysis. Alprazolam has been determined in biological specimens by gas chromatography with electron-capture (Greenblatt et al., 1981, 1990) or nitrogen-phosphorus detection (Watts and Simonick 1986; Joern and Joern, 1987). Liquid chromatography has been used for the analysis of the drug and its metabolites in serum and plasma (Gill et al., 1986; Miller and DeVane, 1988; Atta-Politou et al., 1991; Schmith et al., 1991). A gas chromatographic-mass spectrometric procedure has also been described (Javaid and Liskevych, 1986). Immunoassays that detect alprazolam and/or its metabolites are commercially available (Fraser, 1987; Fraser and Bryan, 1991). 4-Hydroxyalprazolam has been shown to be unstable in aqueous solution when stored at room temperature or at an acid pH (Schmith et al., 1991).

References

J. Atta-Politou, M. Parissi-Poulou, A. Dona and A. Koutselinis. A simple and rapid reversed phase high performance liquid chromatographic method for quantification of alprazolam and α–hydroxyalprazolam in plasma. J. Liq. Chrom. 14: 3531–3546, 1991.

A. Breier, D.S. Charney and J.C. Nelson. Seizures induced by abrupt discontinuation of alprazolam. Am. J. Psych. 141: 1606–1607, 1984.

D.A. Ciraulo, J.G. Barnhill, H.G. Boxenbaum et al. Pharmacokinetics and clinical effects of alprazolam following single and multiple oral doses in patients with panic disorder. J. Clin. Pharm. 26: 292–298, 1986.

G.W. Dawson, S.G. Jue and R.N. Brogden. Alprazolam. A review of its pharmacodynamic properties and efficacy in the treatment of anxiety and depression. Drugs 27: 132–147, 1984.

Drugs & Driving Committee, American Academy of Forensic Sciences Toxicology Section, 1993.

F.S. Eberts, Y. Philopoulos, L.M. Reineki and R.W. Vliek. Disposition of ^{14}C-alprazolam, a new anxiolytic-antidepressant in man. Pharmacologist 22: 279, 1980.

L.E. Edinboro and R.C. Backer. Preliminary report on the application of a high performance liquid chromatographic method for alprazolam in postmortem blood specimens. J. Anal. Tox. 9: 207–208, 1985.

A.D. Fraser. Urinary screening for alprazolam, triazolam and their metabolites with the EMIT d.a.u. benzodiazepine metabolite assay. J. Anal Tox. 11: 263–266, 1987.

A.D. Fraser and W. Bryan. Evaluation of the Abbott ADx and TDx serum benzodiazepine immunoassay for analysis of alprazolam. J. Anal. Tox. 15: 63–65, 1991.

R. Gill, B. Law and J.P. Gibbs. High-performance liquid chromatography systems for the separation of benzodiazepines and their metabolites. J. Chrom. 356: 37–46, 1986.

D.J. Greenblatt, M. Divoll, L.J. Moschitto and R.I. Shader. Electron-capture gas chromatographic analysis of the triazolobenzodiazepines alprazolam and triazolam. J. Chrom. 225: 202–207, 1981.

D.J. Greenblatt, J.I. Javaid, A. Locniskar et al. Gas chromatographic analysis of alprazolam in plasma: replicability, stability and specificity. J. Chrom. 534: 202–207, 1990.

S. Howell. Personal communication, 1985.

J.I. Javaid and U. Liskevych. Quantitative analysis of alprazolam in human plasma by combined capillary gas chromatography/negative ion chemical ionization mass spectrometry. Biomed. Env. Mass Spec. 13: 129–132, 1986.

W.A. Joern and A.B. Joern. Detection of alprazolam (Xanax) and its metabolites in urine using dual capillary column, dual nitrogen detector gas chromatography. J. Anal. Tox. 11: 247–251, 1987.

A.B. Levy. Delerium and seizures due to abrupt alprazolam withdrawal: case report. J. Clin. Psych. 45: 38–39, 1984.

Medical Letter on Drugs and Therapeutics 28: 81–86, 1986.

S.R. McCormick, J. Nielsen and P. Jatlow. Quantification of alprazolam in serum or plasma by liquid chromatography. Clin. Chem. 30: 1652–1655, 1984.

R.L. Miller and C.L. DeVane. Alprazolam, α–hydroxy- and 4-hydroxyalprazolam analysis in plasma by high-performance liquid chromatography. J. Chrom. 430: 180–186, 1988.

M. Munoz. Personal communication, 1988.

P. Reynolds. Personal communication, 1988.

V.D. Schmith, S.R. Cox, M.A. Zemaitis and P.D. Kroboth. New high-performance liquid chromatographic method for the determination of alprazolam and its metabolites in serum: instability of 4-hydroxyalprazolam. J. Chrom. 568: 253–260, 1991.

R.B. Smith and P.D. Kroboth. Influence of dosing regimen on alprazolam and metabolite serum concentrations and tolerance to sedative and psychomotor effects. Psychopharmacology 93: 105–112, 1987.

D.T. Stafford. Xanax (alprazolam)—an overdose death. Presented at the annual meeting of the American Academy of Forensic Sciences, Anaheim, California, February 23, 1984.

J. Vital-Herne, R. Brenner and M. Lesser. Another case of alprazolam withdrawal syndrome. Am. J. Psych. 142: 1515, 1985.

V.W. Watts and T.F. Simonick. Screening of basic drugs in biological samples using dual column capillary chromatography and nitrogen-phosphorus detectors. J. Anal. Tox. 10: 198–204, 1986.

Alprenolol

T½: 2.3 hr
Vd: 3 L/kg
Fb: 0.85
pKa: 9.6

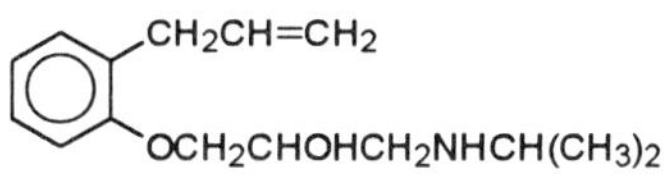

Occurrence and Usage. Alprenolol (Aptin) is a beta-blocking agent that has been used in the treatment of hypertension in European countries since about 1969. Like its relatives, oxprenolol and propranolol, it is normally administered orally every 6 hours, in single doses of 50–100 mg as the hydrochloride salt. Sustained release oral preparations are available as well, and the drug may also be given by intravenous injection at a recommended dose of 5–10 mg.

Blood Concentrations. After a 100 mg oral dose given to 5 adults, plasma alprenolol concentrations reached peak levels of 0.01–0.06 mg/L at 30 minutes in 4 of the subjects; the fifth subject demonstrated a peak level that exceeded 0.10 mg/L at 2 hours. Maximal plasma concentrations 30 minutes after an intravenous injection of 0.1 mg/kg (7 mg/70 kg) ranged from 0.02–0.05 mg/L, and declined with an average half-life of 2.3 hours (Bodin et al., 1974; Ervik, 1969). Ablad et al. (1972) showed that increasing the oral dose of alprenolol from 50–200 mg produced a disproportionately larger increase in the serum level of the drug, possibly due to saturation of the metabolizing enzymes. 4-Hydroxyalprenolol, an active metabolite, reaches higher plasma levels than its parent in the first 2 hours after oral administration, but is eliminated more quickly (T½=0.8 hour); this metabolite is not observed in serum after intravenous administration (Collste et al., 1979).

Steady-state plasma concentrations of alprenolol in 16 patients receiving 600 mg daily averaged 0.04 mg/L, ranging from 0.01–0.14 mg/L (Collste et al., 1976).

Metabolism and Excretion. About 91% of an oral dose of alprenolol is eliminated in the 24 hour urine, with less than 1% being excreted in unchanged form (Bodin et al., 1974). The known urinary metabolites include 4-hydroxyalprenolol, in both conjugated (39%) and free (5%) form, conjugated alprenolol (34%), and conjugated noralprenolol (1%). Unknown metabolites account for the remainder of a dose (Bodin, 1974).

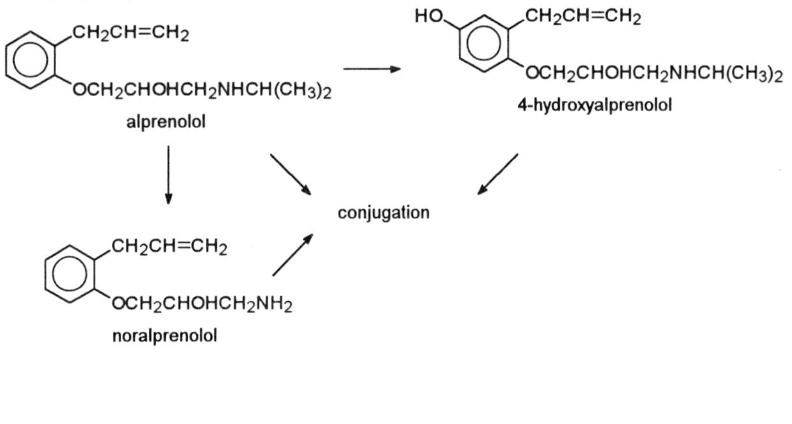

Toxicity. Four adults, who died in as little as 5 hours after the intentional ingestion of 4–22 g of alprenolol, had the following drug concentrations in their postmortem tissues (Alha, 1976; Dickson et al., 1978):

Alprenolol Concentrations in Fatal Cases (mg/L or mg/kg)

	Blood	Brain	Liver	Kidney	Urine
Average	43	25	203	174	19
(Range)	(40–48)	(16–33)	(72–324)	(119–228)	(19)

Analysis. Therapeutic plasma concentrations of alprenolol have been measured by gas chromatography after trifluoroacetylation (Ervik, 1969; Delbeke et al., 1988) or transboronation (Poole et al., 1980; Yamaguchi et al., 1982). Dickson et al. (1978) described flame-ionization gas chromatographic analysis of toxic levels of the drug in forensic specimens. Liquid chromatography is suitable for the determination of therapeutic serum concentrations (Duchateau et al., 1986).

References

B. Ablad, M. Ervik, J. Hallgren et al. Pharmacological effects and serum levels of orally administered alprenolol in man. Eur. J. Clin. Pharm. 5: 44–52, 1972.

A. Alha. Personal communication, 1976.

N. Bodin. Identification of the major urinary metabolite of alprenolol in man, dog and rat. Life Sci. 14: 685–692, 1974.

N. Bodin, K.O. Borg, R. Johansson et al. Absorption, distribution and excretion of alprenolol in man, dog and rat. Acta Pharm. Tox. 35: 261–269, 1974.

P. Collste, K. Haglund, M. Frisk-Holmberg et al. Pharmacokinetics and pharmacodynamics of alprenolol in the treatment of hypertension. Eur. J. Clin. Pharm. 10: 89–95, 1976.

P. Collste, K. Borg, H. Astrom and C. von Bahr. Contribution of 4-hydroxy-alprenolol to adrenergic beta receptor blockade of alprenolol. Clin. Pharm. Ther. 25: 416–422, 1979.

F.T. Delbeke, M. Debackere, N. Desmet and F. Maertens. Qualitative gas chromatographic and gas chromatographic-mass spectrometric screening for β–blockers in urine after solid-phase extraction using Extrelut-1 columns. J. Chrom. 426: 194–201, 1988.

S.J. Dickson, J.M. Muirhead and P.E. Nelson. The gas chromatographic determination of alprenolol in human postmortem liver and blood samples. J. Anal. Tox. 2: 242–244, 1978.

G.S.M.J.E. Duchateau, W.M. Albers and H.H. van Rooij. Rapid and simple determination of alprenolol in serum. J. Chrom. 383: 212–217, 1986.

M. Ervik. Gas chromatographic determination of the secondary amine alprenolol, as its trifluoroacetyl derivative, at nanogram levels in biological fluids. Acta Pharm. Suecica 6: 393–400, 1969.

C.F. Poole, L. Johansson and J. Vessman. Formation of electron-capturing derivatives of alprenolol by transboronation. J. Chrom. 194: 365–377, 1980.

T. Yamaguchi, Y. Morimoto, Y. Sekine and M. Hashimoto. Determination of β–adrenergic blocking drugs as cyclic boronates by gas chromatography with nitrogen-selective detection. J. Chrom. 239: 609–615, 1982.

Aluminum

T½: ?
Vd: ?   Al
Fb: 0.6–0.7

Occurrence and Usage. Aluminum is the most abundant metal in the earth's crust and is found in all human tissues, but its biological role, if any, is unknown. Due to the presence of aluminum in most foods and its widespread use in food packaging, as a food additive and in cooking utensils, the intake of the metal by persons in industrialized countries may range from as little as 4 to as much as 80 mg per day. The oral ingestion of aluminum hydroxide as an antacid (or as a phosphate-binding agent in renal failure) can easily increase the daily intake to several grams. The current threshold limit value for industrial exposure is 5 mg/m³ for welding fumes and 10 mg/m³ for metal dust.

Blood Concentrations. Serum or plasma aluminum concentrations in 12 different studies of normal adults have been reported to range from 2–1800 µg/L, even using highly specific techniques such as atomic absorption spectrometry and neutron activation analysis. This large disparity is believed due primarily to technical difficulties in specimen collection and analysis. The most recent studies support the view that the normal serum level is in the range of 1–4 µg/L (Alderman and Gitelman, 1980; Versieck and Cornelis, 1980; Wang et al., 1991). The blood/plasma ratio for aluminum is approximately 0.95 (van der Voet and Wolf, 1985). Industrial exposure to aluminum powder did not significantly alter serum aluminum levels in workers in one study (Valentin et al., 1976), but was found to raise the blood levels of another group to an average of 12 µg/L (Ljunggren et al., 1991). Ingestion of aluminum-containing antacids has increased serum levels to an average of 17 µg/L (Kaehny et al., 1977).

Metabolism and Excretion. Only about 2–6% of the aluminum in antacid preparations is absorbed from the gastrointestinal tract. Urine aluminum concentrations averaged 17 µg/L (range, 4–31) in normal subjects, 39 µg/L (range, 11–220) in aluminum-exposed workers, and 83 µg/L in an individual ingesting 1 g of aluminum (as aluminum hydroxide) daily (Valentin et al., 1976; Gorsky et al., 1979). Apparently, only a very small amount of the aluminum that is absorbed is excreted via the urine. Urinary elimination half-lives vary from days to years depending on the interval between cessation of exposure and the half-life determination, possibly due to a multiphasic, multi-compartmental elimination process (Sjogren et al., 1988; Elinder et al., 1991).

The following tissue aluminum concentrations were found in 4 normal adults at autopsy (McLaughlin et al., 1968):

Aluminum Concentrations in Normal Adults (mg/kg)

	Brain	Lung	Liver
Average	0.25	21	0.70
(Range)	(0.23–0.29)	(16–24)	(0.61–0.76)

Toxicity. The administration of aluminum to experimental animals is known to produce an encephalopathy similar to that seen in Alzheimer's disease in man, a progressive dementia that occurs after age 40. Patients with renal failure who receive dialysis therapy (and who often receive large amounts of aluminum antacids to lower serum phosphate) occasionally develop a psychosis known as dialysis dementia. It has been demonstrated that the serum of dialysis patients contains elevated aluminum concentrations (27–347 µg/L), as does the brain of those dying of dialysis dementia (8.9 vs. 1.3 mg/kg in controls), but a cause and effect relationship has not been established (Alfrey et al., 1976; Alderman and Gitelman, 1980; Gorsky and Dietz, 1981). Aluminum toxicity in dialysis patients is mainly associated with serum aluminum levels exceeding 100 µg/L; to prevent excessive exposure, dialysate aluminum concentrations should be kept below 5 µg/L (de Wolff and van der Voet, 1986). Three infants with renal failure receiving chronic oral aluminum hydroxide (but not dialysis) developed osteomalacia and serum aluminum concentrations of 345–595 µg/L (Andreoli et al., 1984).

A number of cases, some fatal, of pulmonary fibrosis due to chronic industrial inhalation of aluminum powder have been described (Mitchell et al., 1961). A man who had worked in an aluminum powder factory for 13 years developed encephalopathy with epileptiform attacks. He was admitted to hospital, but gradually deteriorated and died of bronchopneumonia. An autopsy showed cerebral edema, pulmonary fibrosis, and the following tissue aluminum concentrations (McLaughlin et al., 1962):

Aluminum Concentrations in a Fatal Case (mg/kg)

Brain	Lung	Liver	Bone
5	430	90	30

Analysis. The preferred technique for determination of aluminum in biological specimens is graphite-furnace atomic absorption spectrometry. Several investigators have published such methods, stressing the need to avoid contamination during analysis (Alderman and Gitelman, 1980; Smeyers-Verbeke et al., 1980; Oster, 1981; D'Haese et al., 1985; Anderson and Reimert, 1986; Wang et al., 1991). Glass containers and serum-separator tubes may cause aluminum contamination of the specimen and should be avoided (Leung and Henderson, 1983; Jaudon et al., 1985; Wilhelm and Ohnesorge, 1990).

References

F.R. Alderman and H.J. Gitelman. Improved electrothermal determination of aluminum in serum by atomic absorption spectroscopy. Clin. Chem. 26: 258–260, 1980.

A.C. Alfrey, G.R. LeGendre and W.D. Kaehny. The dialysis encephalopathy syndrome. New Eng. J. Med. 294: 184–188, 1976.

S.P. Andreoli, J.M. Bergstein and D.J. Sherrard. Aluminum intoxication from aluminum-containing phosphate binders in children with azotemia not undergoing dialysis. New Eng. J. Med. 310: 1079–1085, 1984.

J.R. Anderson and S. Reimert. Determination of aluminum in human tissues and body fluids by Zeeman-corrected atomic absorption spectrometry. Analyst 111: 657–660, 1986.

F.A. de Wolff and G.B. van der Voet. Biological monitoring of aluminium in renal patients. Clin. Chim. Acta 160: 183–188, 1986.

P.C. D'Haese, F.L. Van der Vyver, F.A. de Wolff and M.E. De Broe. Measurement of aluminum in serum, blood, urine, and tissues of chronic hemodialyzed patients by use of electrothermal atomic absorption spectrometry. Clin. Chem. 31: 24–29, 1985.

C.G. Elinder, L. Ahrengart, V. Lidums et al. Evidence of aluminium accumulation in aluminium welders. Brit J. Ind. Med. 48: 735–738, 1991.

J.E. Gorsky, A.A. Dietz, H. Spencer and D. Osis. Metabolic balance of aluminum studied in six men. Clin. Chem. 25: 1739–1743, 1979.

J.E. Gorsky and A.A. Dietz. Aluminum concentrations in serum of hemodialysis patients. Clin. Chem. 27: 932–935, 1981.

M.C. Jaudon, B.L. Coz and J.P. Clavel. More on Al contamination of samples for Al analysis. Clin. Chem. 31: 660, 1985.

W.D. Kaehny, A.P. Hegg and A.C. Alfrey. Gastrointestinal absorption of aluminum from aluminum-containing antacids. New Eng. J. Med. 296: 1389–1390, 1977.

F.Y. Leung and A.R. Henderson. Quality-control sera for routine determination of aluminum by electrothermal atomic absorption analysis. Clin. Chem. 29: 1966–1968, 1983.

K.G. Ljunggren, V. Lidums and B. Sjogren. Blood and urine concentrations of aluminium among workers exposed to aluminium flake powders. Brit. J. Ind. Med. 48: 106–109, 1991.

A.I.G. McLaughlin, G. Kazantzis, E. King et al. Pulmonary fibrosis and encephalopathy associated with the inhalation of aluminium dust. Brit. J. Ind. Med. 19: 253–263, 1962.

J. Mitchell, G.B. Manning, M. Molyneux and R.E. Lane. Pulmonary fibrosis in workers exposed to finely powdered aluminium. Brit. J. Ind. Med. 18: 10–20, 1961.

O. Oster. The aluminium content of human serum determined by atomic absorption spectroscopy with a graphite furnace. Clin. Chim. Acta 114: 53–60, 1981.

B. Sjogren, C.G. Elinder, V. Lidums and G. Chang. Uptake and urinary excretion of aluminum among welders. Int. Arch. Occ. Env. Health 60: 77–79, 1988.

J. Smeyers-Verbeke, D. Verbeelen and D.L. Massart. The determination of aluminum in biological fluids by means of graphite furnace atomic absorption spectrometry. Clin. Chim. Acta 108: 67–73, 1980.

H. Valentin, P. Preusser and K.H. Schaller. Die Analyse von Aluminium im Serum und Urin zur Ueberwachung exponierter Personen. Int. Arch. Occ. Env. Health 38: 1–17, 1976.

G.B. van der Voet and F.A. de Wolff. Distribution of aluminium between plasma and erythrocytes. Hum. Tox. 4: 643–648, 1985.

J. Versieck and R. Cornelis. Measuring aluminum levels. New Eng. J. Med. 302: 468, 1980.

S.T. Wang, S. Pizzolato and H.P. Demshar. Aluminum levels in normal human serum and urine as determined by Zeeman atomic absorption spectrometry. J. Anal. Tox. 15: 66–70, 1991.

M. Wilhelm and F.K. Ohnesorge. Influence of storage conditions on aluminum concentrations in serum, dialysis fluid, urine, and tap water. J. Anal. Tox. 14: 206–210, 1990.

Amantadine

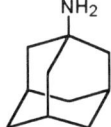

T½: 7–37 hr
Vd: 4.4 L/kg
Fb: 0.67
pKa: 10.1

Occurrence and Usage. Amantadine (Symmetrel) is a synthetic antiviral and anti-Parkinsonism agent first described in 1964. It is a water-soluble tricyclic amine of unusual structure, unrelated to any of the other antimicrobial agents. The adult daily dosage for prophylaxis and treatment of influenza A virus respiratory tract disease is 200 mg as a single or divided dose. For the treatment of Parkinsonism, the usual dose is 100 mg twice a day when used alone. After one to several weeks, it may be necessary to increase the dose up to 400 mg daily in divided doses. Amantadine hydrochloride is available in 100 mg capsules and in a 50 mg/5 mL syrup.

Blood Concentrations. After a single 200 mg oral dose of amantadine, maximal plasma concentrations of 0.3–0.6 mg/L occur in 1–4 hours (Sande and Mandell, 1985). Steady-state plasma concentrations averaged 0.08 mg/L (range, 0.06–0.10) in subjects given 50 mg of the drug daily, 0.29 mg/L (range, 0.26–0.31) in those given 200 mg, and 0.77 mg/L (range, 0.59–0.97) in those given 300 mg (Aoki et al., 1979). The elimination half-life has been reported to average 12 hours (range, 10–15) in healthy young adults (Horadam et al., 1981) and 29 hours (range, 19–45) in healthy elderly males (Aoki and Sitar, 1985). The blood/plasma ratio for amantadine averages 1.43 (Daugirdas et al., 1984).

Metabolism and Excretion. Amantadine is rapidly and almost completely absorbed from the gastrointestinal tract. Approximately 86% of an orally administered dose is excreted in the 96 hour urine in unchanged form (Bleidner et al., 1965). As many as 8 urinary metabolites have been identified, including N-acetylamantadine (5–15% of a dose), N-methylamantadine and N,N-dimethylamantadine (Koppel and Tenczer, 1985).

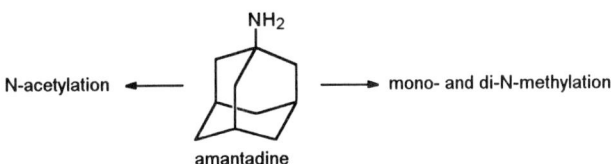

Toxicity. The most frequently occurring serious adverse reactions to amantadine are depression, congestive heart failure, urinary retention, orthostatic hypotensive episodes and psychosis. Plasma concentrations of 1–5 mg/L are associated with central nervous system toxicity, including confusion, hallucinations, seizures and coma (Sande and Mandell, 1985). Minor neurological symptoms may be seen in as many as 5% of the patients with normal renal function who receive 200 mg or more daily (LaMontagne and Galasso, 1979). Aggressive behavior was noted in 4 patients receiving 300 mg daily who developed steady-state plasma levels of 0.68–1.01 mg/L (Rizzo et al., 1973). Patients with renal failure tend to accumulate amantadine; 4 such individuals, 2 of whom died, developed confusion, unusual neurological abnormalities, hallucinations and plasma amantadine levels of 1.5–3.0 mg/L (Ing et al., 1979). A 61 year old man who attempted suicide by ingesting 2.8 g of the drug developed an admission blood amantadine concentration (40 hour post-ingestion) of 2.4 mg/L; he remained agitated, incoherent and disoriented for 3 days before recovering (Fahn et al., 1971).

A 37 year old woman who ingested 12 g had an admission serum amantadine concentration of 23 mg/L; she developed seizures, hyperthermia, and muscle rigidity and died of respiratory failure after several days (Brown et al., 1987). The following tissue concentrations were determined in 3 cases of apparent suicide in adults (Reynolds and Van Meter, 1984; Cook et al., 1986; Priddis, 1986).

Amantadine Concentrations in Fatal Cases (mg/L or mg/kg)

	Blood	Liver	Urine	Gastric
Average	33	198	1330	7.9 mg
(Range)	(21–48)	(135–260)	(1330)	(4.8–11)

Analysis. Amantadine has been analyzed in biological samples by gas chromatography (Biandrate et al., 1972; Reynolds and Van Meter, 1984; Stumph et al., 1985). The pentafluoropropionic anhydride derivative of amantadine has been analyzed by gas chromatography-mass spectrometry (Priddis, 1986).

References

F.Y. Aoki, D.S. Sitar and R.I. Ogilvie. Amantadine kinetics in healthy young subjects after long-term dosing. Clin. Pharm. Ther. 26: 729–736, 1979.

F.Y. Aoki and D.S. Sitar. Amantadine kinetics in healthy elderly men: implications for influenza prevention. Clin. Pharm. Ther. 37: 137–144, 1985.

P. Biandrate, G. Tognoni, G. Belvedere et al. A gas chromatographic method for the determination of amantadine in human plasma. J. Chrom. 74: 31–34, 1972.

W.E. Bleidner, J.B. Harmon, W.E. Herves et al. Absorption, distribution and excretion of amantadine hydrochloride. J. Pharm. Exp. Ther. 150: 484–490, 1965.

C.R. Brown, S. Hernandez and M.T. Kelly. Hyperthermia and death from amantadine overdose. Vet. Hum. Tox. 29: 463, 1987.

P.E. Cook, W.D. Stanley and T. McGurk. Fatal overdose with amantadine. Can. J. Psych. 318: 757–758, 1986.

S. Fahn, G. Craddock and G. Kamin. Acute toxic psychosis from suicidal overdosage of amantadine. Arch. Neurol. 25: 45–48, 1971.

V.W. Horadam, J.G. Sharp, J.D. Smilack et al. Pharmacokinetics of amantadine hydrochloride in subjects with normal and impaired renal function. Ann. Int. Med. 94: 454–458, 1981.

T.S. Ing, J.T. Daugirdas, L.S. Soung et al. Toxic effects of amantadine in patients with renal failure. Can. Med. Asso. J. 120: 695–698, 1979.

C. Koppel and J. Tenczer. A revision of the metabolic disposition of amantadine. Biomed. Mass Spec. 12: 499–501, 1985.

J.R. LaMontagne and G.J. Galasso. Report of a workshop on clinical studies of the efficacy of amantadine and rimantadine against influenza virus. J. Infect. Dis. 138: 928–931, 1979.

C. Priddis. Personal communication, 1986.

P.C. Reynolds and S. Van Meter. A death involving amantadine. J. Anal. Tox. 8: 100, 1984.

M. Rizzo, P. Biandrate, G. Tognoni and P.L. Morselli. Amantadine in depression: relationship between behavioral effects and plasma levels. Eur. J. Clin. Pharm. 5: 226–228, 1973.

M.A. Sande and G.L. Mandell. Antimicrobial agents. In *The Pharmacological Basis of Therapeutics*, 7th ed. (A.G. Gilman, L.S. Goodman, T.W. Rall and F. Murad, eds.), Macmillan, New York, 1985, p. 1232.

M.J. Stumph, M.W. Noall and V. Knight. Urine amantadine by gas chromatography. In *Methodology for Analytical Toxicology*, Vol. III (I. Sunshine, ed.), CRC Press, Boca Raton, Florida, 1985, pp. 13–16.

Amikacin

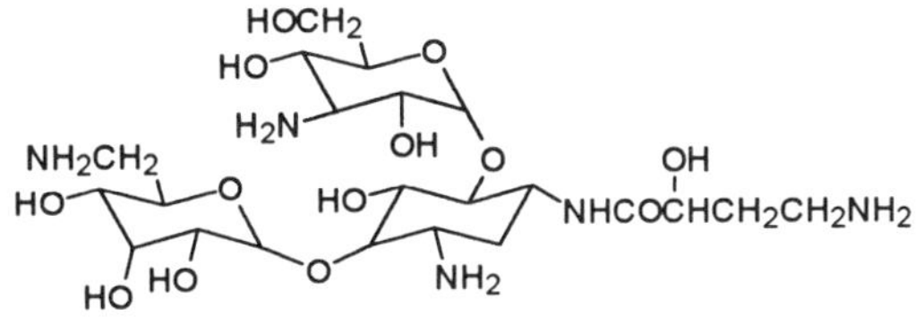

T½: 1.9–2.8 hr
Vd: 0.28 L/kg
Fb: 0
pKa: ?

Occurrence and Usage. Amikacin (BB-K8, Amikin) is a semisynthetic aminoglycoside antibiotic, available since 1973, that exhibits broad-spectrum antimicrobial activity. It is especially useful against bacterial strains with resistance to gentamicin, kanamycin, and tobramycin. The drug is usually administered as the sulfate salt in doses of 5–15 mg/kg at 12 hour intervals, by 30 minute intravenous infusion or intramuscular injection.

Blood Concentrations. A 1 hour intravenous infusion of 3.3 mg/kg amikacin produced peak serum concentrations at the end of infusion averaging 15 mg/L (range, 13–17). The intramuscular injection of 7.5 mg/kg resulted in an average peak serum level of 20 mg/L (range, 17–23) between 0.75 and 2 hours after administration (Clarke et al., 1974). The half-life of amikacin averages 2 hours in healthy subjects, but may range up to 150 hours in patients with impaired renal function. To avoid drug accumulation in such patients, the dosage must be lowered (or the dosing interval extended) in proportion to the reduction from normal of the creatinine clearance (Regeur et al., 1977). Optimal peak serum concentrations of amikacin have been suggested to lie between 15 and 25 mg/L; pre-dose specimens should have trough levels of less than 10 mg/L to avoid drug toxicity (Black et al., 1976).

Metabolism and Excretion. Approximately 98% of an administered dose of amikacin is excreted unchanged in the 24 hour urine. The drug's renal clearance, 84 mL/min, suggests that about 30% undergoes tubular reabsorption after being filtered at the glomerulus (Clarke et al., 1974). With chronic dosing, about 10% of the total administered dose remains in the body, sequestered largely in skeletal muscle (40%), kidney (26%) and bone (13%). It has been shown that this accumulation of amikacin occurs independently of renal function, and that the true elimination half-life of the drug is on the order of 7–10 days. The following table shows the tissue drug concentrations in a chronically-treated individual who died 5 days after the last amikacin dose (French et al., 1981):

Amikacin Tissue Concentrations in a Treated Patient (mg/L or mg/kg)

Serum	Heart	Lung	Liver	Kidney	Muscle	Bone	Fat
2.2	20	48	30	794	11	22	2.8

Toxicity. As with gentamicin, ototoxicity and renal damage are common in patients treated chronically with amikacin, especially if the drug is used in combination with certain diuretic agents. Ototoxicity appeared in 57% of patients with peak serum concentrations exceeding 32 mg/L and in 55% with trough levels exceeding 10 mg/L (Black et al., 1976). Nephrotoxicity occurred in 8% of a group of patients studied by Smith et al. (1977).

Analysis. Microbiological assays for amikacin and other aminoglycoside antibiotics have largely been supplanted by more sensitive and specific tests involving enzyme immunoassay, radioimmunoassay, and enzymatic radiochemical assay (Maitra et al., 1979; Bleske et al., 1987). Fluorometry (Csiba, 1979), gas chromatography (Mayhew and Gorbach, 1978), and liquid chromatography (Anhalt and Brown, 1978; Barends et al., 1983; Kabra et al., 1984; Wichert et al., 1991) have also been investigated. Serum specimens for amikacin analysis from patients receiving concurrent therapy with carbenicillin or ticarcillin should be stored refrigerated or frozen, if not analyzed immediately, due to *in vitro* inactivation of the drug by these beta-lactam antibiotics (Pickering and Gearhart, 1979).

References

J.P. Anhalt and S.D. Brown. High-performance liquid-chromatographic assay of aminoglycoside antibiotics in serum. Clin. Chem. 24: 1940–1947, 1978.

D.M. Barends, J.S. Blauw, M.H. Smits and A. Hulsoff. Determination of amikacin in serum by high-performance liquid chromatography with ultraviolet detection. J. Chrom. 276: 385–394, 1983.

R.E. Black, W.K. Lau, R.J. Weinstein et al. Ototoxicity of amikacin. Antimicrob. Agents Chemother. 9: 956–961, 1976.

B.E. Bleske, T.A. Larson and J.C. Rotschafer. Observed differences in amikacin pharmacokinetic parameters and dosage recommendations determined by enzyme immunoassay and fluorescence polarization immunoassay. Ther. Drug Mon. 9: 48–52, 1987.

J.T. Clarke, R.D. Libke, C. Regamey and W.M.M. Kirby. Comparative pharmacokinetics of amikacin and kanamycin. Clin. Pharm. Ther. 15: 610–616, 1974.

A. Csiba. Spectrofluorimetric method for aminoglycoside antibiotics. J. Pharm. Pharmac. 31: 115–116, 1979.

M.A. French, F.B. Cerra, M.E. Plaut and J.J. Schentag. Amikacin and gentamicin accumulation pharmacokinetics and nephrotoxicity in critically ill patients. Antimicrob. Agents Chemother. 19: 147–152, 1981.

P.M. Kabra, P.K. Bhatnager and M.A. Nelson. Liquid chromatographic determination of amikacin in serum with spectrophotometric detection. J. Chrom. 307: 224–229, 1984.

S.K. Maitra, T.T. Yoshikawa, L.B. Guze and M.C. Schotz. Determination of aminoglycoside antibiotics in biological fluids: a review. Clin. Chem. 25: 1361–1367, 1979.

J.W. Mayhew and S.L. Gorbach. Gas-liquid chromatographic method for the assay of aminoglycoside antibiotics in serum. J. Chrom. 151: 133–146, 1978.

L.K. Pickering and P. Gearhart. Effect of time and concentration upon interaction between gentamicin, tobramycin, netilmicin, or amikacin and carbenicillin or ticarcillin. Antimicrob. Agents Chemother. 15: 592–596, 1979.

L. Regeur, H. Colding, H. Jensen and J.P. Kampmann. Pharmacokinetics of amikacin during hemodialysis and peritoneal dialysis. Antimicrob. Agents Chemother. 11: 214–218, 1977.

C.R. Smith, K.L. Baughman, C.Q. Edwards et al. Controlled comparison of amikacin and gentamicin. New Eng. J. Med. 296: 349–353, 1977.

B. Wichert, H. Schreier and H. Derendorf. Sensitive liquid chromatography assay for the determination of amikacin in human plasma. J. Pharm. Biomed. Anal. 9: 251–254, 1991.

Amiodarone

T½: 3–80 hr (single dose)
     35–68 days (chronic therapy)
Vd: 18–148 L/kg
Fb: 0.94
pKa: 6.6

Occurrence and Usage. Amiodarone (Cordarone) is a potent antianginal drug used to suppress and prevent recurrence of life-threatening ventricular arrhythmias. Because of its delayed onset of action, complex dosing schedule and potentially serious side effects, amiodarone is used only when other agents are ineffective or cannot be tolerated. Amiodarone is available in tablets of 100 and 200 mg as the hydrochloride salt. The usual oral adult loading dose is 800–1600 mg per day for 1–

3 weeks until an initial therapeutic response or side effects occur. Oral maintenance doses are approximately 400 mg per day.

Blood Concentrations. Following a single oral dose of 1400–1800 mg in 6 patients ranging in age from 35–73 and weighing 68–136 kg (average, 87), the peak serum concentration ranged from 3.0–14 mg/L (average, 6.9) in 3–6 hours (average, 4.9). In 12 patients given 800–1800 mg oral amiodarone daily for 2–8 weeks, there was a complete suppression of ventricular tachyarrhythmias. The serum concentrations after the initial suppression of the arrhythmias were between 0.9 and 12 mg/L (average, 3.8) (Kannan et al., 1982).

Amiodarone and noramiodarone concentrations in the serum of an adult patient on long-term oral therapy of 1400 mg/daily were: on day 1, 0.66 and 0.25 mg/L, respectively; on day 10, 2.8 and 1.9 mg/L, respectively; and on day 25, the concentrations of both were 2.7 mg/L (Kannan et al., 1982). The desired plasma amiodarone concentration has been reported to be from 1.0–3.5 mg/L, but antiarrhythmic effect is difficult to predict by means of plasma concentrations (Nygaard et al., 1986). The whole blood/plasma concentration ratio for the drug averages 0.73, but there can be a significant variation in this figure on an individual basis or within the same person over time (Maling et al., 1989).

Metabolism and Excretion. Little is known about the fate of amiodarone in man. A metabolite, noramiodarone, appears in the plasma within hours after both oral and intravenous administration, but its concentration remains lower than that of the parent drug for the first few days of therapy (Heger et al., 1983; Berdeaux et al., 1984; Plomp et al., 1984; Escoubet et al., 1985). The elimination half-life of noramiodarone is longer than that of the parent drug, but it is not known if the metabolite is pharmacologically active (Mason, 1987). Neither amiodarone nor its desethyl metabolite are present in significant amounts in the 24 hour urine; less than 0.7% of a dose is present as iodine-containing metabolites (Latini et al., 1984). Seven patients on long-term therapy who died of other causes were found to have postmortem plasma concentrations in a normal range (0.6–2.3 mg/L for amiodarone and 0.4–2.5 mg/L for noramirodarone), but varied over a wide range with regard to liver concentrations (7–890 mg/kg and 64–6500 mg/kg for the drug and its metabolite, respectively) (Plomp et al., 1984).

amiodarone   noramiodarone

Toxicity. The use of amiodarone is associated with a wide variety of adverse reactions, including delerium, hepatitis, exacerbation of arrhythmia, exacerbation of congestive heart failure, and pulmonary toxicity (Nademanee and Singh, 1982; Dean et al., 1987; Mason, 1987; Trohman et al., 1988). A slate-gray or bluish skin discoloration often occurs. The most consistent complication of oral amiodarone therapy is the development of yellowish-brown granular corneal deposits (Nygaard et al., 1986). Adverse effects may occur even at therapeutic plasma amiodarone concentrations, but are more common at concentrations over 2.5 mg/L. A female adult who ingested 8 g of the drug in a suicide attempt never developed any adverse effects, despite being followed for 3 months; her highest blood concentrations of amiodarone and noramiodarone (measured 12 hour post-ingestion) were 1.1 and 0.5 mg/L, respectively (Bonati et al., 1983).

Analysis. Reported methods for the analysis of amiodarone and its major metabolite in plasma, serum or urine have been limited to liquid chromatography (Mostow et al., 1983; Plomp et al., 1983; Gupta and Connolly, 1984; Menius et al., 1987; Ou et al., 1990). Amiodarone and noramiodarone concentrations were observed to decline in stored serum by 8% and 4%, respectively, after 24 hours and by 32% and 16%, respectively, after 2 weeks; refrigeration or freezing did not improve stability of the drugs (Vuagnat et al., 1993).

References

A. Berdeaux, A. Roche, T. Labaille et al. Tissue extraction of amiodarone and N-desethylamiodarone in man after a single oral dose. Brit. J. Clin. Pharm. 18: 759–763, 1984.

M. Bonati, V. D'Aranno, F. Gallefi et al. Acute overdosage of amiodarone in a suicide attempt. Clin. Tox. 20: 181–186, 1983.

J.F. Brien, S. Jimmo and P.W. Armstrong. Rapid high performance liquid chromatographic analysis of amiodarone and N-desethylamiodarone in serum. Can. J. Physiol. Pharm. 61: 245–248, 1983.

P.J. Dean, K.D. Groshart, J.G. Porterfield et al. Amiodarone-associated pulmonary toxicity. Am. J. Clin. Path. 87: 7–13, 1987.

B. Escoubet, P. Coumel, J.M. Poirier et al. Suppression of arrhythmias within hours after a single oral dose of amiodarone and relation to plasma and myocardial concentrations. Am. J. Cardiol. 55: 696–702, 1985.

R.J. Flanagan, G.C.A. Storey and D.W. Holt. Rapid high performance liquid chromatographic method for the measurement of amiodarone in blood plasma or serum at the concentrations attained during therapy. J. Chrom. 187: 391–398, 1980.

R.N. Gupta and S. Connolly. Liquid chromatographic determination of amiodarone and its N-desethyl metabolite in plasma. Clin. Chem. 30: 1423–1424, 1984.

J.J. Heger, E.N. Prystowsky and D.P. Zipes. Relationships between amiodarone dosage, drug concentrations and adverse side effects. Am. Heart J. 106: 931–935, 1983.

R. Kannan, K. Nademanee, J.A. Hendrickson et al. Amiodarone kinetics after oral doses. Clin. Pharm. Ther. 31: 438–451, 1982.

R. Latini, G. Tognoni and R.E. Kates. Clinical pharmacokinetics of amiodarone. Clin. Pharmacokin. 9: 136–156, 1984.

T.J.B. Maling, R.W.L. Siebers, C.D. Burgess et al. Individual variability of amiodarone distribution in plasma and erythrocytes: implications for therapeutic monitoring. Ther. Drug Mon. 11; 121–126, 1989.

J.W. Mason. Amiodarone. New Eng. J. Med. 316: 455–466, 1987.

J.A. Menius, D.J. Schumacher, E.A. Hull-Ryde et al. Quantitation of amiodarone and desethylamiodarone from blood serum and myocardium using reverse phase HPLC. J. Liq. Chrom. 10: 2625–2637, 1987.

N.D. Mostow, D.L. Noon, C.M. Myers et al. Determination of amiodarone and its N-deethylated metabolite in serum by high-performance liquid chromatography. J. Chrom. 277: 229–237, 1983.

K. Nademanee and B.N. Singh. Advances in artiarrhythmic therapy. J. Am. Med. Asso. 247: 217–222, 1982.

T.W. Nygaard, T.D. Sellers, T.S. Cook and J.P. DiMarco. Adverse reactions to antiarrhythmic drugs during therapy for ventricular arrhythmias. J. Am. Med. Asso. 256: 55–57, 1986.

C.N. Ou, C.L. Rognerud, L.T. Dyong and V.L. Frawley. Liquid-chromatographic determination of amiodarone and N-desethylamiodarone in serum. Clin. Chem. 36: 532–534, 1990.

T.A. Plomp, M. Engles, E.O. Robles de Medina and R.A.A. Maes. Simultaneous determination of amiodarone and its major metabolite desethylamiodarone in plasma, urine and tissues by high-performance liquid chromatography. J. Chrom. 273: 379–392, 1983.

T.A. Plomp, J.M. van Rossum, E.O. Robles de Medina et al. Pharmacokinetics and body distribution of amiodarone in man. Arz. Forsch. 34: 513–520, 1984.

T.A. Plomp, E.O. Robles de Medina and R.A.A. Maes. Tissue concentrations of amiodarone and desethylamiodarone in post-mortem cases and surgical patients. In *Topics in Forensic and Analytical Toxicology* (R.A.A. Maes, ed.), Elsevier, New York, 1984, pp. 105–111.

G.C.A. Storey and D.W. Holt. High-performance liquid chromatographic measurement of amiodarone and desethylamiodarone in plasma or serum at the concentrations attained following a single 400-mg dose. J. Chrom. 245: 377–380, 1982.

R.G. Trohman, D. Castellanos, A. Castellanos and K.M. Kessler. Amiodarone-induced delerium. Ann. Int. Med. 108: 68–69, 1988.

A. Vuagnat, L. Goedel-Meinem, E. Gries et al. Stability of amiodarone in serum samples under various storage conditions. Arz. Forsch. 43: 327–330, 1993.

Amitriptyline

T½: 8–51 hr
Vd: 6–10 L/kg
Fb: 0.94
pKa: 9.4

Occurrence and Usage. Amitriptyline (Elavil, Endep) is a tricyclic antidepressant drug that was first synthesized in 1960 and released for clinical use in 1961. The compound is administered either orally or by intramuscular injection in maintenance doses of up to 150 mg daily for outpatients or up to 300 mg daily for hospitalized patients. It is available as the hydrochloride salt in tablets of 10–150 mg and as a 10 mg/mL injectable solution; the drug is also marketed in combination with chlordiazepoxide (Limbitrol) and perphenazine (Etrafon, Triavil).

Blood Concentrations. Following a single oral 50 mg dose of amitriptyline, peak serum concentrations of 0.016–0.035 mg/L were achieved at 2–4 hours; nortriptyline concentrations were less than 0.014 mg/L (Garland, 1977). Patients receiving a chronic daily dosage of 150 mg developed steady-state plasma concentrations of 0.095 mg/L amitriptyline (range, 0.038–0.162) and 0.106 mg/L nortriptyline (range, 0.022–0.242) (Cooper et al., 1976). Twenty-seven patients on doses of 1.2–4.2 mg/kg/day developed steady-state plasma concentrations that averaged 0.113 mg/L for amitriptyline, 0.102 mg/L for nortriptyline, 0.015 mg/L for unconjugated trans-10-hydroxyamitriptyline, and 0.124 mg/L for unconjugated trans-10-hydroxynortriptyline (Bock et al., 1982).

The serum half-life of amitriptyline has been found to range from 9–25 hours in patients, with a mean of 15 hours (Jorgensen and Staehr, 1976), while values of 8–51 hours have been determined in normal subjects (Garland, 1977; Rogers et al., 1978). Optimal patient response appears to be achieved when plasma concentrations of amitriptyline plus nortriptyline lie between 0.080 and 0.200 mg/L (Montgomery et al., 1979). The maximal plasma nortriptyline concentration occurs within 8–24 hours after oral amitriptyline and within 24–48 hours after intramuscular administration (Mellstrom et al., 1982).

The whole blood/plasma concentration ratio averages 1.0–1.1 for amitriptyline and 1.5–1.7 for nortriptyline (Maguire et al., 1980).

Metabolism and Excretion. Amitriptyline is extensively metabolized to a series of more polar compounds; these include nortriptyline, a major plasma constituent which may be largely responsible for the antidepressant effects of its parent (Bickel and Brodie, 1964), and dinortriptyline (desmethylnortriptyline), which may be active and is found to a certain extent in plasma. Two hydroxylated metabolites, 10-hydroxyamitriptyline and 10-hydroxynortriptyline, have also been found in plasma but probably do not contribute significantly to the overall effects of the drug (Kraak and Bijster, 1977; Garland et al., 1979). All of these metabolites as well as amitriptyline-N-oxide and 10-hydroxydinortriptyline have been detected in urine (Eschenhof and Rieder, 1969). Although as much as 35% of a dose of amitriptyline is eliminated as metabolites in the 24 hour urine and up to 80% is excreted within 11 days, only 0.2% is present as unchanged drug (Diamond, 1965; Braithwaite and Whatley, 1970). Under conditions of acid urine, nearly 2% of a dose is eliminated unchanged in the 72 hour urine (Karkkainen and Neuvonen, 1986). The following percentages of a single 25 mg oral dose were excreted by 2 subjects in the 72 hour urine: 38% as 10-hydroxynortriptyline (free plus conjugated), 8% as 10-hydroxydinortriptyline (free plus conjugated), 7% as dinortriptyline, 4% as 10-hydroxynortriptyline (free plus conjugated), and 3% as nortriptyline (Biggs et al., 1979).

The following drug concentrations were measured in the tissues of 14 patients who died of unrelated causes while on amitriptyline therapy (Bailey and Shaw, 1980):

Drug Concentrations in 14 Amitriptyline Patients (mg/L or mg/kg)

	Blood	Liver	Myocardium
Amitriptyline			
Average	0.18	4.7	0.7
(Range)	(0.01–0.50)	(0.4–17)	(0.3–1.6)
Nortriptyline			
Average	0.30	8.9	2.2
(Range)	(0.02–1.20)	(0.3–28)	(0.1–8.6)

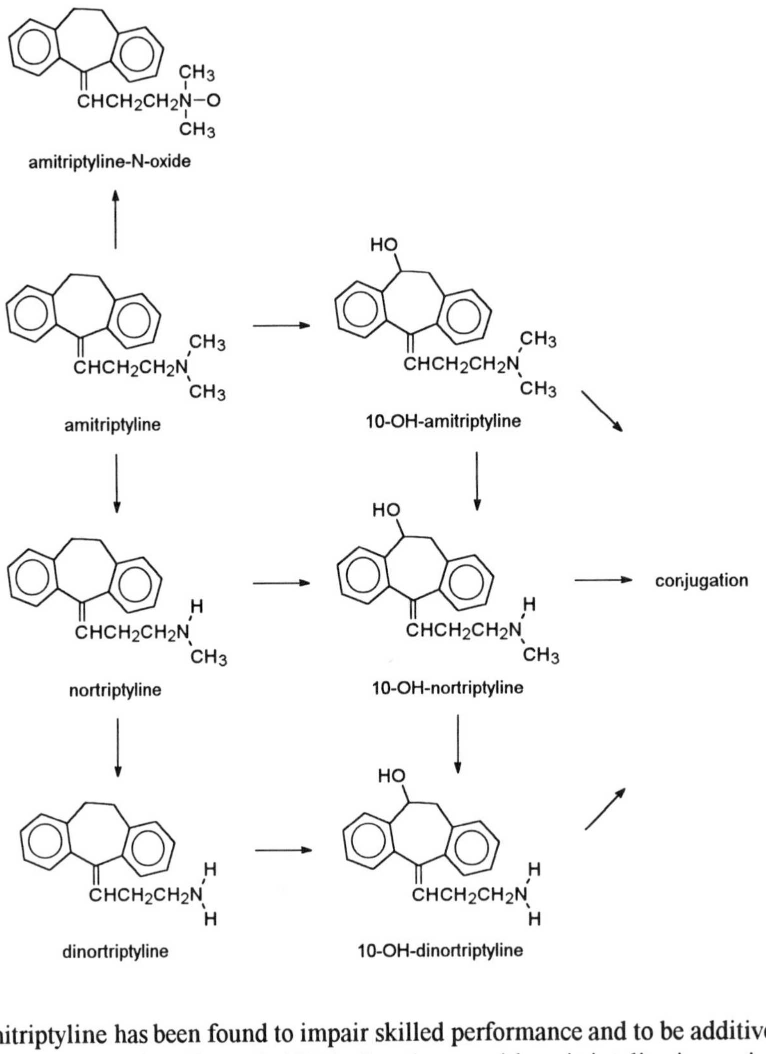

Toxicity. Amitriptyline has been found to impair skilled performance and to be additive with ethanol in its adverse effects (Linnoila et al., 1984). Overdosage with amitriptyline is a serious situation since the manifestations of poisoning are severe and difficult to control. Plasma concentrations slightly exceeding 2 mg/L have been observed in patients who ingested up to 2000 mg of amitriptyline and who survived the accompanying coma, seizures and cardiac abnormalities (Biggs et al., 1977). The kinetics of elimination of amitriptyline are apparently unchanged after overdosage, although nortriptyline does accumulate in plasma and body tissues (Hurst and Jarboe, 1981). Physostigmine, a cholinergic drug, has been used successfully in the diagnosis and antidotal therapy of poisoning with amitriptyline and other tricyclic antidepressants (Burks et al., 1974).

Many fatalities have occurred, after ingestion of as little as 600 mg of the drug by an adult (Bickel, 1975). In several fatalities involving the ingestion of 3–5 g of drug, concentrations of unchanged amitriptyline averaged 9 mg/L (range, 3–15) in the blood and 250 mg/kg (range, 92–420) in liver (Baselt and Cravey, 1977). Bonnichsen et al. (1970), reporting on a large series of amitriptyline-related deaths, concluded that liver concentrations (of amitriptyline plus nortriptyline) greater than 50 mg/kg were indicative of acute intoxication, while concentrations less than that were consistent with therapeutic doses. In 32 fatal overdoses, myocardium concentrations of amitriptyline and nortriptyline averaged 11.3 and 6.4 mg/kg, respectively; these levels were approximately 5 times the respective average blood concentrations (Bailey and Shaw, 1980).

Amitriptyline is subject to postmortem redistribution, due to continued diffusion from the gastrointestinal tract or release from drug-rich tissues such as the lung and liver; heart blood/peripheral blood concentration ratios in 30 cases averaged 3.1 (range, 0.6–15) for amitriptyline and 2.3 (range, 0.5–8.4) for nortriptyline (Apple and Bandt, 1988; Anderson and Prouty, 1989; Hilberg et al., 1993).

The following body distribution of amitriptyline and its major active metabolites was derived by gas chromatographic analysis of specimens from 4 fatal cases (Baselt, 1977):

Drug Concentrations in Amitriptyline Fatalities (mg/L or mg/kg)

	Blood	Brain	Liver	Kidney	Urine	Gastric
Amitriptyline						
Average	3.7	11	130	22	3.4	60 mg
Range	(2.7–4.7)	(2.6–18)	(13–317)	(12–31)	(0.4–7.9)	(23–92)
Nortriptyline						
Average	1.1	3.9	25	13	0.3	0.1 mg
Range	(0.5–1.7)	(0–7.7)	(7.5–64)	(1–25)	(0–0.6)	(0–0.4)

Analysis. Several authors have stressed the need to avoid serum separator tubes and certain types of evacuated tubes when collecting clinical specimens for monitoring therapeutic tricyclic levels (Cochran et al., 1978; Veith et al., 1978; Orsulak and Gerson, 1980; Nyberg and Martensson, 1986; Levy et al., 1987).

Analytical procedures for amitriptyline and nortriptyline by gas chromatography have involved flame-ionization detection (Norheim, 1974; Nyberg and Martensson, 1977) or nitrogen-phosphorus detection of the underivatized drugs (Bailey and Jatlow, 1976; Cooper et al., 1976; Witts and Turner, 1977) or of the N-acetyl derivative of nortriptyline (Jorgensen, 1975; Dhar and Kutt, 1979); and mass spectrometric detection of underivatized amitriptyline and the N-trifluoroacetyl derivative of nortriptyline (Garland, 1977; Wilson et al., 1977; Chinn et al., 1980).

High-pressure liquid chromatography has become very popular for the clinical determination of the tricyclics, and numerous methods have been published (Wallace et al., 1981; Edelbroek et al., 1982; Suckow and Cooper, 1982; Rop et al., 1986; Lin and Frade, 1987; El-Yazigi and Raines, 1993).

References

W.H. Anderson and R.W. Prouty. Postmortem redistribution of drugs. In *Advances in Analytical Toxicology* (R.C. Baselt, ed.), Vol. 2, YearBook Medical, Chicago, 1989, pp. 70–102.

F.S. Apple and C.M. Bandt. Liver and blood postmortem tricyclic antidepressant concentrations. Am. J. Clin. Path. 89: 794–796, 1988.

D.N. Bailey and P.I. Jatlow. Gas-chromatographic analysis for therapeutic concentrations of amitriptyline and nortriptyline in plasma, with use of a nitrogen detector. Clin. Chem. 22: 777–781, 1976.

D.N. Bailey and R.F. Shaw. Interpretation of blood and tissue concentrations in fatal self-ingested overdose involving amitriptyline: an update (1978–1979). J. Anal. Tox. 4: 232–236, 1980.

R.C. Baselt. Unpublished results, 1977.

R.C. Baselt and R.H. Cravey. A compendium of therapeutic and toxic concentrations of toxicologically significant drugs in human biofluids. J. Anal. Tox. 1: 81–103, 1977.

M.H. Bickel and B.B. Brodie. Structure and antidepressant activity of imipramine analogues. Int. J. Neurobiol. 3: 611–621, 1964.

M.H. Bickel. Poisoning by tricyclic antidepressant drugs. Int. J. Clin. Pharm. 11: 145–176, 1975.

J.T. Biggs, D.G. Spiker, J.M. Petit and V.E. Ziegler. Tricyclic antidepressant overdose. J. Am. Med. Asso. 237: 135–138, 1977.

S.R. Biggs, L.F. Chasseaud, D.R. Hawkins and I. Midgley. Determination of amitriptyline and its major basic metabolites in human urine by high-performance liquid chromatography. Drug Met. Disp. 7: 233–236, 1979.

J.L. Bock, E. Giller, S. Gray and P. Jatlow. Steady-state plasma concentrations of cis- and trans-10-OH amitriptyline metabolites. Clin. Pharm. Ther. 31: 609–616, 1982.

R. Bonnichsen, A.C. Maehly and G. Skold. A report on autopsy cases involving amitriptyline and nortriptyline. Z. Rechtsmed. 67: 190–200, 1970.

R.A. Braithwaite and J.A. Whatley. Specific gas chromatographic determination of amitriptyline in human urine following therapeutic doses. J. Chrom. 49: 303–307, 1970.

J.S. Burks, J.E. Walker, B.H. Rumack and J.E. Ott. Tricyclic antidepressant poisoning. J. Am. Med. Asso. 230: 1405–1407, 1974.

D.M. Chinn, T.A. Jennison, D.J. Crouch et al. Quantitative analysis for tricyclic antidepressant drugs in plasma or serum by gas chromatography-chemical-ionization mass spectrometry. Clin. Chem. 26: 1201–1204, 1980.

E. Cochran, J. Carl, I. Hanin et al. Effect of Vacutainer stoppers on plasma tricyclic levels: a reevaluation. Comm. Psychopharm. 2: 495–503, 1978.

T.B. Cooper, D. Allen and G.M. Simpson. A sensitive method for the determination of amitriptyline and nortriptyline in human plasma. Comm. Psychopharm. 2: 105–116, 1976.

A.K. Dhar and H. Kutt. An improved gas-liquid chromatographic procedure for the determination of amitriptyline and nortriptyline levels in plasma using nitrogen-sensitive detectors. Ther. Drug Mon. 1: 209–216, 1979.

S. Diamond. Human metabolization of amitriptyline tagged with carbon 14. Curr. Ther. Res. 7: 170–175, 1965.

P.M. Edelbroek, E.J.M. de Haas and F.A. de Wolff. Liquid-chromatographic determination of amitriptyline and its metabolites in serum, with adsorption onto glass minimized. Clin. Chem. 28: 2143–2148, 1982.

A. El-Yazigi and D.A. Raines. Concurrent liquid chromatographic measurement of fluoxetine, amitriptyline, imipramine, and their active metabolites in plasma. Ther. Drug Mon. 15: 305–309, 1993.

V.E. Eschenhof and J. Rieder. Untersuchungen ueber das Schicksal des Antidepressivums Amitriptylin im Organismus der Ratte und des Menschen. Arz. Forsch. 19: 957–966, 1969.

W.A. Garland. Quantitative determination of amitriptyline and its principal metabolite, nortriptyline, by GLC-chemical ionization mass spectrometry. J. Pharm. Sci. 66: 77–81, 1977.

W.A. Garland, R.R. Muccino, B.H. Min et al. A method for the determination of amitriptyline and its metabolites nortriptyline, 10-hydroxyamitriptyline, and 10-hydroxynortripyline in human plasma using stable isotope dilution and gas chromatography-chemical ionization mass spectrometry (GC-CIMS). Clin. Pharm. Ther. 25: 844–856, 1979.

T. Hilberg, A. Bugge, K.M. Beylich et al. An animal model of postmortem amitriptyline redistribution. J. For. Sci. 38: 81–90, 1993.

H.E. Hurst and C.H. Jarboe. Clinical findings, elimination pharmacokinetics, and tissue drug concentrations following a fatal amitriptyline intoxication. Clin. Tox. 18: 119–125, 1981.

A. Jorgensen. A gas chromatographic method for the determination of amitriptyline and nortriptyline in human serum. Acta Pharm. Tox. 36: 79–90, 1975.

A. Jorgensen and P. Staehr. On the biological half-life of amitriptyline. J. Pharm. Pharmac. 28: 62–64, 1976.

J.C. Kraak and P. Bijster. Determination of amitriptyline and some of its metabolites in blood by high-pressure liquid chromatography. J. Chrom. 143: 499–512, 1977.

S. Karkkainen and P.J. Neuvonen. Pharmacokinetics of amitriptyline influenced by oral charcoal and urine pH. Int. J. Clin. Pharm. Ther. Tox. 24: 326–332, 1986.

A.B. Levy, M. Walters and S.L. Stern. Reduced serum tricyclic levels due to gel separators. J. Clin. Psychopharm. 7: 423–424, 1987.

M. Linnoila, J. Johnson, K. Dubyoski et al. Effects of antidepressants on skilled performance. Brit. J. Clin. Pharm. 18: 109S–120S, 1984.

W.N. Lin and P.D. Frade. Simultaneous quantitation of eight tricyclic antidepressants in serum by high-performance liquid chromatography. Ther. Drug Mon. 9: 448–455, 1987.

K.P. Maguire, G.D. Burrows, T.R. Norman and B.A. Scoggins. Blood/plasma distribution ratios of psychotropic drugs. Clin. Chem. 26: 1624–1625, 1980.

B. Mellstrom, G. Alvan, L. Bertilsson et al. Nortriptyline formation after single oral and intramuscular doses of amitriptyline. Clin. Pharm. Ther. 32: 664–667, 1982.

S.A. Montgomery, R. McAuley, S.J. Rani et al. Amitriptyline plasma concentration and clinical response. Brit. Med. J. 1: 230–231, 1979.

G. Norheim. The simultaneous determination of amitriptyline and nortriptyline in postmortem blood and urine using gas-liquid chromatography. J. Chrom. 88: 403–406, 1974.

G. Nyberg and E. Martensson. Quantitative analysis of tricyclic antidepressants in serum from psychiatric patients. J. Chrom. 143: 491–497, 1977.

G. Nyberg and E. Martensson. Preparation of serum and plasma samples for determination of tricyclic antidepressants. Ther. Drug Mon. 8: 478–482, 1986.

P.J. Orsulak and B. Gerson. Therapeutic monitoring of tricyclic antidepressants: quality-control considerations. Ther. Drug Mon. 2: 233–242, 1980.

H.J. Rogers, P.J. Morrison and I.D. Bradbrook. The half-life of amitriptyline. Brit. J. Clin. Pharm. 6: 181–183, 1978.

P.P. Rop, T. Conquy, F. Gouezo et al. Determination of metapramine, imipramine, trimipramine and their major metabolites in plasma by reversed-phase column liquid chromaotgraphy. J. Chrom. 375: 339–347, 1986.

R.F. Suckow and T.B. Cooper. Simultaneous determination of amitriptyline, nortriptyline and their respective isomeric 10-hydroxy metabolites in plasma by liquid chromatography. J. Chrom. 230: 391–400, 1982.

R.C. Veith, V.A. Raisys and C. Perera. The clinical impact of blood collection methods on tricyclic antidepressants as measured by GC/MS-SIM. Comm. Psychopharm. 2: 491–494, 1978.

J.E. Wallace, E.L. Shimek, Jr. and S.C. Harris. Determination of tricyclic antidepressants by high-performance liquid chromatography. J. Anal. Tox. 5: 20–23, 1981.

J.M. Wilson, L.J. Williamson and V.A. Raisys. Simultaneous measurement of secondary and teritiary tricyclic antidepressants by GC/MS chemical ionization mass fragmentography. Clin. Chem. 23: 1012–1017, 1977.

D.J. Witts and P. Turner. A single comprehensive gas chromatographic assay for tricyclic and tetracyclic antidepressant drugs and their metabolites in plasma. Brit. J. Clin. Pharm. 4: 249–252, 1977.

Amobarbital

T½: 15–40 hr (dose-dependent)
Vd: 0.9–1.4 L/kg
Fb: 0.59
pKa: 7.9

Occurrence and Usage. Amobarbital (amylobarbitone, Amytal) is a barbiturate derivative of intermediate duration of action first prepared in 1924. The compound is available as either the sodium salt or the free acid in oral dosage forms of 15–200 mg for use as a sedative or hypnotic, and in ampules of 65–500 mg for intravenous or intramuscular injection for the control of seizures. It is also found in combination with other drugs such as secobarbital, amphetamine and ephedrine.

Blood Concentrations. Following a single oral administration of 120 mg of amobarbital, serum concentrations peaked at about 1.8 mg/L at 2 hours, and declined slowly thereafter with a half-life of approximately 24 hours (Inaba et al., 1976). An increase of about 40% was seen in the 10 hour post-drug plasma level after 7 days of amobarbital administration at the rate of 200 mg per day to 15 volunteers (Tansella et al., 1975). The serum concentrations of the major metabolite, 3'-hydroxyamobarbital, attained a maximum level 26 hours after a dose of 200 mg and generally did not exceed 0.5 mg/L (Grove and Toseland, 1970), although in uremic patients there was accumulation of this compound with chronic usage of the drug to levels as high as 8 mg/L (Balasubramaniam et al., 1972). After an oral dosage of 600 mg of amobarbital distributed over 3 hours, a maximal average blood level of 8.7 mg/L (range, 6.4–12.3) was observed at 0.5 hour, with a decline to 4.1 mg/L (range, 2.6–5.4) by 18 hours (Parker et al., 1970).

Metabolism and Excretion. Amobarbital undergoes extensive metabolism to more polar compounds by a saturable process that is best described by zero-order kinetics throughout the range of doses normally used (Garrett et al., 1974). The drug induces its own metabolism to only a slight degree in normal doses (Baldeo et al., 1979). The major metabolites are 3'-hydroxyamobarbital, which has one-third the hypnotic potency of its parent, and N-glucosylamobarbital. Up to 92% of a single dose is eliminated in the urine and 5% in the feces over a period of 6 days; from 1–3% of a dose is excreted unchanged in the urine, while 30–50% is present as free 3'-hydroxyamobarbital, 29% as N-glucosylamobarbital and 5% as 3'-carboxyamobarbital (Grove and Toseland, 1970; Tang et al., 1975; Tang et al., 1978; Kalow et al., 1978; Baldeo et al., 1979). Other authors have reported finding 3'-hydroxyamobarbital present in the urine partly as a conjugate (Balasubramaniam et al., 1970), but this has been disputed (Grove and Toseland, 1971). After a single 600 mg oral dose, only 0.4% was excreted unchanged within 21 hours in 3 subjects, while peak urine concentrations of the drug ranged from 2.5–3.7 mg/L at various times during the period (Parker et al., 1970).

Toxicity. Addiction with the development of tolerance to this drug and to other barbiturates is a complication of chronic usage. Blood concentrations of 8–21 mg/L were developed by chronic drug users who were titrated to the point of mild toxicity with oral amobarbital doses of 700–1400 mg at a rate of 200 mg per hour (Comstock, 1974). Four patients who were admitted for amobarbital overdosage developed maximum plasma levels of 43–66 mg/L during coma; their plasma concentrations upon awakening ranged from 14–32 mg/L, and 2 of the subjects demonstrated a marked reduction in the plasma half-life of the drug during the course of the intoxication (Prescott et al., 1973).

The minimum lethal dose in man is estimated as 1500 mg, although an individual has recovered with treatment after the ingestion of 20 g (Terplan and Unger, 1966). In a series of 55 fatal cases reported by Gupta and Kofoed (1966), blood concentrations of 13–96 mg/L were observed. Blood concentrations averaging 47 mg/L (range, 29–68) and liver concentrations averaging 219 mg/kg (range, 106–580) were determined for 6 deaths due to amobarbital ingestion (Baselt and Cravey, 1977). Concentrations of 3'-hydroxyamobarbital were quite low (1–5 mg/L or mg/kg) in body fluids and tissues in 3 cases of fatal amobarbital overdosage (Robinson and McDowall, 1979). The following 2 cases are illustrative of the distribution of amobarbital in body tissues after overdosage (Rehling, 1967; Clarke, 1969):

Amobarbital Distribution in Fatal Cases (mg/L or mg/kg)

	Blood	Brain	Liver	Kidney	Urine
Case I	81	172	414	210	98
Case 2*	163	119	362		7

*Involved ingestion of 11 g of drug within 4 days

Analysis. The classical procedure for the quantitative analysis of barbiturates in biological media is ultraviolet spectrophotometry (Goldbaum, 1948). This method alone is insufficient for qualitative purposes and must be accompanied by a separation technique for complete identification. Numerous gas chromatographic techniques have evolved for the assay of the common barbiturate derivatives. Some of these have involved flame-ionization detection of the underivatized drugs (Street, 1971; Berry, 1973) or of the methyl (Stewart et al., 1969; Brochmann-Hanssen and Oke, 1969; Kananen et al., 1972) or ethyl derivatives (MacGee, 1971); electron-capture detection of the 2-chloroethyl (Dilli and Pillai, 1977) or pentafluorobenzyl derivatives (Walle, 1975); and nitrogen-selective detection of the drugs in their native state (Toseland et al., 1975). High-pressure liquid chromatography has been applied successfully to the separation of 12 of the common barbiturates (Atwell et al., 1975) and to sedative-hypnotic drugs in general (Kabra et al., 1978). Various immunoassay procedures are commercially available for the detection of barbiturates in body fluids, but these methods cross-react with most barbiturate derivatives and the results must be confirmed by qualitative testing.

References

S.H. Atwell, V.A. Green and W.G. Haney. Development and evaluation of a method for simultaneous determination of phenobarbital and diphenylhydantoin in plasma by high-pressure liquid chromatography. J. Pharm. Sci. 64: 806–809, 1975.

K. Balasubramaniam, S.B. Lucas, G.E. Mawer and P.J. Simons. The kinetics of amylobarbitone metabolism in healthy men and women. Brit. J. Pharm. 39: 564–572, 1970.

K. Balasubramaniam, G.E. Mawer, J.E.F. Phol and P.J.G. Simons. Impairment of cognitive function associated with hydroxyamylobarbitone accumulation in patients with renal insufficiency. Brit. J. Pharm. 45: 360–367, 1972.

W.C. Baldeo, J.N.T. Gilbert and J.W. Powell. A multi-dose study on the human metabolism of amylobarbitone. Xenobiotica 9: 205–208, 1979.

R.C. Baselt and R.H. Cravey. A compendium of therapeutic and toxic concentrations of toxicologically significant drugs in human biofluids. J. Anal. Tox. 1: 81–103, 1977.

D.J. Berry. Gas chromatographic analysis of the commonly prescribed barbiturates at therapeutic and overdose levels in plasma and urine. J. Chrom. 86: 89–105, 1973.

E. Brochmann-Hanssen and T. Oke. Gas chromatography of barbiturates, phenolic alkaloids, and xanthine bases: flash-heater methylation by means of trimethylanilinium hydroxide. J. Pharm. Sci. 58: 370–371, 1969.

E.G.C. Clarke (ed.). In *Isolation and Identification of Drugs*, Pharmaceutical Press, London, 1969, pp. 195–196.

E. Comstock. Personal communication, 1974.

S. Dilli and D.N. Pillai. Relative electron capture response of the 2-chloroethyl derivatives of some barbituric acids and anticonvulsant drugs. J. Chrom. 137: 111–117, 1977.

E.R. Garrett, J. Bres, K. Schnelle and L.L. Rolf, Jr. Pharmacokinetics of saturably metabolized amobarbital. J. Pharm. Biopharm. 2: 43–103, 1974.

L.R. Goldbaum. An ultraviolet spectrophotometric procedure for the determination of barbiturates. J. Pharm. Exp. Ther. 94: 68–75, 1948.

J. Grove and P.A. Toseland. The gas-liquid chromatography of hydroxyamylobarbitone in plasma and urine. Clin. Chim. Acta 29: 253–260, 1970.

J. Grove and P.A. Toseland. The excretion of hydroxyamylobarbitone in man after oral administration of amylobarbitone and hydroxyamylobarbitone. J. Pharm. Pharmac. 23: 936–940, 1971.

R.C. Gupta and J. Kofoed. Toxicological statistics for barbiturates, other sedatives, and tranquillizers in Ontario. Can. Med. Asso. J. 94: 863–865, 1966.

T. Inaba, B.K. Tang, L. Endrenyi and W. Kalow. Amobarbital — a probe of hepatic drug oxidation in man. Clin. Pharm. Ther. 20: 439–444, 1976.

P.M. Kabra, H.Y. Koo and L.J. Marton. Simultaneous liquid-chromatographic determination of 12 common sedatives and hypnotics in serum. Clin. Chem. 24: 657–662, 1978.

W. Kalow, B.K. Tang, D. Kadar and T. Inaba. Distinctive patterns of amobarbital metabolites. Clin. Pharm. Ther. 24: 576–582, 1978.

G. Kananen, R. Osiewicz and I. Sunshine. Barbiturate analysis — a current assessment. J. Chrom. Sci. 10: 283–287, 1972.

J. Macgee. Rapid identification and quantitative determination of barbiturates and glutethimide in blood by gas-liquid chromatography. Clin. Chem. 17: 587–591, 1971.

K.D. Parker, H.W. Elliott, J.A. Wright et al. Blood and urine concentrations of subjects receiving barbiturates, meprobamate, glutethimide, or diphenylhydantoin. Clin. Tox. 3: 131–145, 1970.

L.F. Prescott, P. Roscoe and J.A.H. Forrest. Plasma concentrations and drug toxicity in man. In *Biological Effects of Drugs in Relation to Their Plasma Concentrations* (D.S. Davies and B.N.C. Prichard, eds.), University Park Press, Baltimore, 1973, pp. 51–81.

C.J. Rehling. Poison residues in human tissues. In *Progress in Chemical Toxicology*, Vol. 3 (A. Stolman, ed.), Academic Press, New York, 1967, pp. 363–386.

A.E. Robinson and R.D. McDowall. The distribution of amylobarbitone, butobarbitone, pentobarbitone and quinalbarbitone and the hydroxylated metabolites in man. J. Pharm. Pharmac. 31: 357–365, 1979.

J.T. Stewart, G.B. Duke and J.E. Willcox. Rapid micromethod for the gas chromatographic determination of methylated barbiturates in biological samples. Anal. Letters 2: 449–456, 1969.

H.V. Street. Determination of barbiturates in blood by GLC. Clin. Chim. Acta 34: 357–364, 1971.

B.K. Tang, T. Inaba and W. Kalow. N-hydroxyamobarbital: the second major metabolite of amobarbital in man. Drug Met. Disp. 3: 479–486, 1975.

B.K. Tang, W. Kalow and A.A. Grey. Amobarbital metabolism in man: N-glucoside formation. Res. Comm. Chem. Path. Pharm. 21: 45–53, 1978.

M. Tansella, O. Siciliani and L. Burti. N-desmethyldiazepam and amylobarbitone sodium as hypnotics in anxious patients. Plasma levels, clinical efficacy and residual effects. Psychopharmacologia 41: 81–85, 1975.

M. Terplan and A.M. Unger. Survival following massive barbiturate ingestion. J. Am. Med. Asso. 198: 322–323, 1966.

P.A. Toseland, M. Albani and F.D. Gauchel. Organic nitrogen-selective detector used in gas-chromatographic determination of some anticonvulsant and barbiturate drugs in plasma and tissues. Clin. Chem. 21: 98–103, 1975.

T. Walle. Electron-capture gas chromatography of barbituric acids and diphenylhydantoin after pentafluorobenzylation. J. Chrom. 114: 345–350, 1975.

Amoxapine

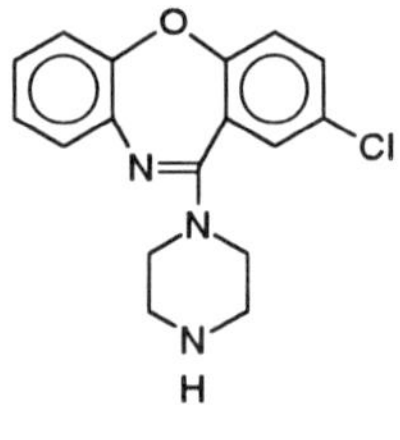

T½: 8 hr (33 hr for 8-hydroxyamoxapine)
Vd: ?
Fb: 0.90
pKa: ?

Occurrence and Usage. Amoxapine (Asendin) is a newer antidepressant of the dibenzoxazepine class, closely related to loxapine (N-methylamoxapine). Its therapeutic and toxic effects are quite similar to those of the tricyclic antidepressants. Amoxapine is available as the free base in tablets of 25–150 mg for oral administration; recommended daily maintenance doses range from 150–600 mg.

Blood Concentrations. A single 50 mg oral dose given to 26 subjects produced an average peak serum amoxapine concentration of 0.030 mg/L at 1.5 hours, declining to 0.003 mg/L by 24 hours; the active metabolite, 8-hydroxyamoxapine, also attained a peak concentration of 0.030 mg/L at 1.5 hours but was still at a level of approximately 0.014 mg/L by 24 hours; and another metabolite, 7-hydroxyamoxapine, reached a peak level of about 0.008 mg/L at 1.5 hours and was undetectable by 10 hours after ingestion (Cooper and Kelly, 1979). Serum concentrations in 12 patients stabilized on 300 mg daily oral doses ranged from 0.017–0.093 mg/L for amoxapine and 0.158–0.512 mg/L for 8-hydroxyamoxapine. The investigator concluded that optimal patient response occurred at combined serum concentrations of amoxapine and 8-hydroxyamoxapine of 0.200–0.400 mg/L (Boutelle, 1980).

Metabolism and Excretion. Little information is available on the human disposition of amoxapine. It is known to be metabolized by 7- and 8-hydroxylation, both metabolites appearing in urine as glucuronide conjugates (Cooper and Kelly, 1979).

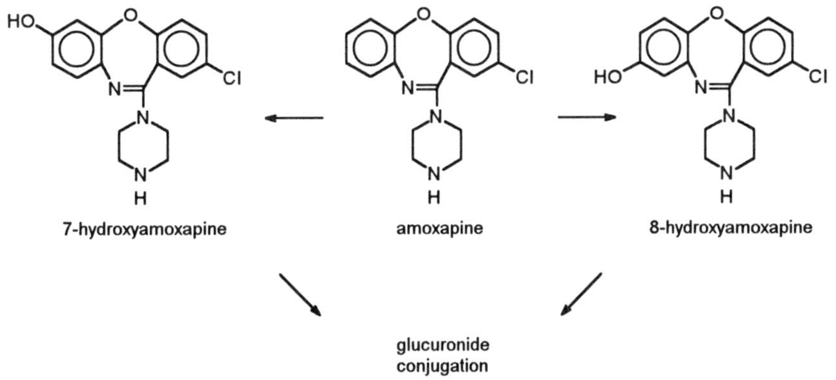

7-hydroxyamoxapine   amoxapine   8-hydroxyamoxapine

glucuronide
conjugation

Toxicity. Individuals have reportedly taken up to 2.7 g of amoxapine acutely without serious adverse effect. However, published reports of 10 adults who ingested from 0.8–6 g of the drug and developed peak serum amoxapine concentrations of 0.31–2.90 mg/L (average, 1.58) have described seizures, coma, severe metabolic acidosis and tachycardia, with recovery occurring in 2–14 days (Bock et al., 1982; Goldberg and Spector, 1982; Kulig et al., 1982; Lopez and Russell, 1983; Rodgers and Hurst, 1983; Tasset and Pesce, 1984).

The following postmortem concentrations were measured in 16 adults who died following acute overdosage with amoxapine (Sedgwick et al., 1982; Taylor et al., 1982; Peclet, 1983; Wu Chen et al., 1983; Rejent, 1984; Stajic, 1985; Winek, 1985; Rohrig and Backer, 1986):

Amoxapine Concentrations in Fatal Cases (mg/L or mg/kg)

	Blood	Liver	Urine	Gastric
Average	6.9	97	15	920 mg
(Range)	(0.9–20)	(17–348)	(11–22)	(2.7–3600)

Amoxapine may be subject to postmortem redistribution; heart blood/peripheral blood concentration ratios in 7 cases averaged 1.8 and ranged from 1.1–2.5 (Anderson and Prouty, 1989).

Analysis. Cooper and Kelly (1979) described an electron-capture gas chromatographic method for amoxapine and its hydroxylated metabolites in serum and urine that required trifluoroacetylation of the secondary amine functions and trimethylsilylation of the phenolic groups. Several liquid chromatographic techniques have also been published (Tasset and Hassan, 1982; Wong and Waugh, 1983; Suckow and Cooper, 1985).

References

W.H. Anderson and R.W. Prouty. Postmortem redistribution of drugs. In *Advances in Analytical Toxicology* (R.C. Baselt, ed.), Vol. 2, YearBook Medical, Chicago, 1989, pp. 70–102.

J.L. Bock, K.C. Cummings and P.I. Jatlow. Amoxapine overdose: a case report. Am. J. Psych. 139: 1619–1620, 1982.

W.E. Boutelle. Clinical response and blood levels in the treatment of depression with a new antidepressant drug, amoxapine. Neuropharmacology 19: 1229–1231, 1980.

T.B. Cooper and R.G. Kelly. GLC analysis of loxapine, amoxapine, and their metabolites in serum and urine. J. Pharm. Sci. 68: 216–219, 1979.

M.J. Goldberg and R. Spector. Amoxapine overdose: report of two patients with severe neurologic damage. Ann. Int. Med. 96: 463–464, 1982.

K. Kulig, B.H. Rumack, J.B. Sullivan, Jr. et al. Amoxapine overdose. J. Am. Med. Asso. 248: 1092–1094, 1982.

L.M. Lopez and W.L. Russell. Amoxapine overdose: case report and pharmacokinetic profile. Clin. Tox. 20: 101–105, 1983.

C. Peclet. Personal communication, 1983.

G.C. Rodgers and H.E. Hurst. Amoxapine overdose. Vet. Hum. Tox. 25: 280, 1983.

T.P. Rohrig and R.C. Backer. Amoxapine overdose: report of two cases. J. Anal. Tox. 10: 211–212, 1986.

P. Sedgwick, V.R. Spiehler and D.R. Lowe. Toxicological findings in amoxapine overdose. J. Anal. Tox. 6: 82–84, 1982.

M. Stajic. Personal communication, 1985.

R.F. Suckow and T.B. Cooper. Determination of amoxapine and metabolites in plasma by liquid chromatography with electrochemical detection. J. Chrom. 338: 225–229, 1985.

J.J. Tasset and F.M. Hassan. Liquid-chromatographic determination of amoxapine and 8-hydroxyamoxapine in human serum. Clin. Chem. 28: 2154–2157, 1982.

J.J. Tassett and A.J. Pesce. Amoxapine in human overdose. J. Anal. Tox. 8: 124–128, 1984.

R.L. Taylor, C.R. Crooks and Y.H. Caplan. The determination of amoxapine in human fatal overdoses. J. Anal. Tox. 6: 309–311, 1982.

S.H.Y. Wong and S.W. Waugh. Determination of the antidepressants maprotiline and amoxapine, and their metabolites, in plasma by liquid chromatography. Clin. Chem. 29: 314–318, 1983.

W.B. Wu Chen, M.I. Schaffer, R.L. Lin et al. Analysis of blood and tissue for amoxapine and trimipramine. J. For. Sci. 28: 116–121, 1983.

Amphetamine

T½: 7–34 hr (urine pH-dependent)
Vd: 3.2–5.6 L/kg
Fb: 0.16
pKa: 9.9

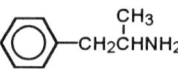

Occurrence and Usage. Amphetamine (Benzedrine, Dexedrine) is a sympathomimetic phenethylamine derivative with prominent central stimulant activity. The compound was first synthesized in 1887 and has been used since 1935 in the treatment of obesity, narcolepsy and hypotension. It is available as the d- or dl-isomeric form, the d-isomer having 3–4 times the central activity of the l-form. The drug is commonly administered as the sulfate salt in single oral doses of 5–15 mg and occasionally in sustained-release form. Amphetamine is frequently abused for its stimulant effects and may be self-administered either orally or by intravenous injection in amounts of up to 2000 mg daily by tolerant addicts.

Blood Concentrations. Following a single oral dosage of 10 mg of d-amphetamine sulfate in a 66 kg adult, blood concentrations reached a peak of about 0.035 mg/L at 2 hours and declined with a half-life of 11–13 hours (Rowland, 1969). The plasma half-life for the l-isomer has been found to be up to 39% longer, indicating that it is metabolized at a slower rate. Additionally, the half-lives of both isomers are reduced to about 7 hours by enhancing elimination via acidification of the urine (Matin et al., 1977; Wan et al., 1978). Nine hyperactive children, age 5–12 years, who received a single oral dose of 0.5 mg/kg (14 mg/28 kg) d-amphetamine exhibited peak plasma levels averaging 0.070 mg/L at 4 hours, with a decline to 0.064 mg/L by 8 hours (Brown et al., 1980). After oral administration of 30 mg of amphetamine base to 8 adults, an average peak plasma level of 0.111 mg/L was observed at 2.5 hours and this diminished to 0.084 mg/L by 4.5 hours (Ebert et al., 1976).

Metabolism and Excretion. Amphetamine is largely inactivated during metabolism, being deaminated to phenylacetone which is subsequently oxidized to benzoic acid and excreted as conjugates. However, a small amount is converted by oxidation to norephedrine, and this compound and its parent are p-hydroxylated. These latter 3 metabolites are pharmacologically active and may contribute to the effects of the drug, especially during chronic usage. Probably the entire dose of amphetamine is eliminated in the urine over a period of several days; normally about 30% is excreted unchanged in the 24 hour urine, but this may increase to as much as 74% in acid urine and may decrease to 1% in alkaline urine. Under normal conditions 0.9% is excreted as phenylacetone, 16–28% as hippuric acid, 4% as benzoylglucuronide, 2% as norephedrine, 0.3% as conjugated p-hydroxynorephedrine, and 2–4% as conjugated p-hydroxyamphetamine (Beckett and Rowland, 1965; Dring et al., 1970; Sever et al., 1973).

Toxicity. Changes in the amplitude and frequency of the electroencephalographic alpha-rhythm pattern appear at plasma amphetamine levels of 0.005 mg/L, while peripheral effects such as increased heart rate and blood pressure require a threshold level of 0.020 mg/L (Morselli et al., 1976). Tolerance builds rapidly during high-dose intravenous use, but chronic usage is associated with a high incidence of weight loss, hallucinations, and paranoid psychosis (Kramer et al., 1967). Plasma concentrations as high as 0.590 mg/L were seen in a chronic user one hour after the intravenous administration of 160 mg of dl-amphetamine (Anggard et al., 1970). A steady-state blood level of 2.0–3.0 mg/L was maintained by a tolerant addict who orally consumed an average of 1000 mg of the drug daily (Baselt and Cravey, 1977).

There are reports of at least 11 fatalities having resulted from the acute oral or intravenous administration of amphetamine for which analytical data is available. Death does not usually ensue immediately but after a period of several hours, during which the subject experiences agitation, hyperthermia, convulsions, unconsciousness, and respiratory and/or cardiac failure; postmortem findings often include organ congestion and hemorrhage. In most instances, the amphetamine dosage has not been determined, but in one case the oral ingestion of 3750 mg was well-documented and in another the intravenous injection of 750–1500 mg was suspected; the following distribution was noted in the 11 known fatal cases (Adjutantis et al., 1975; Bailey, 1976; Baselt and Cravey, 1977; DiMaio and Garriott, 1977; Finkle, 1973; Orrenius and Maehly, 1970; Richards and Stephens, 1973; van Hoof et al., 1974):

Amphetamine Concentrations in Fatalities (mg/L or mg/kg)

	Blood	Brain	Liver	Kidney	Urine
Average	8.6	2.9	30	17	237
(Range)	(0.5–4l)	(2.8–3.0)	(4.3–74)	(3.2–52)	(25–700)
No. of Values	II	2	II	6	8

Analysis. Gas chromatography is the procedure of choice in most situations and this has been accomplished with flame-ionization detection of the native drug (Campbell, 1969) or its N-acetyl derivative (Toseland and Scott, 1969; Lebish et al., 1970) and by mass spectrometric detection of various halogenated derivatives (Hornbeck and Czarny, 1989; Hughes et al., 1991; Melgar and Kelly, 1993). Derivatization with certain chiral reagents allows gas chromatographic differentiation of the optical isomers of the drug (Wells, 1970; Matin et al., 1977). Liquid chromatography has been applied to measurement of therapeutic amounts of amphetamine in plasma and urine (Farrell and Jeffries, 1983). Various immunoassay techniques are now commercially available; these methods may exhibit cross-reactivity with other sympathomimetic amines and with prescription drugs such as labetolol, ranitidine and selegiline.

References

G. Adjuntantis, A. Coutselinis and G. Dimopoulous. Fatal intoxication with amphetamines. Med. Sci. Law 15: 62–63, 1975.

E. Anggard, L.M. Gunne and F. Niklasson. Gas chromatographic determination of amphetamine in blood, tissue and urine. Scand. J. Clin. Lab. Invest. 26: 137–143, 1970.

M. Bailey. Personal communication, 1976.

R.C. Baselt and R.H. Cravey. A compendium of therapeutic and toxic concentrations of toxicologically significant drugs in human biofluids. J. Anal. Tox. 1: 81–103, 1977.

A.H. Beckett and M. Rowland. Urinary excretion kinetics of amphetamine in man. J. Pharm. Pharmac. 17: 628–639, 1965.

G.L. Brown, M.H. Ebert, E.J. Mikkelson and R.D. Hunt. Behavior and motor activity response in hyperactive children and plasma amphetamine levels following a sustained release preparation. J. Am. Acad. Child Psych. 19: 225–239, 1980.

D.B. Campbell. A method for the measurement of therapeutic levels of (+)-amphetamine in human plasma. J. Pharm. Pharmac. 21: 129–131, 1969.

V.J.M. DiMaio and J.C. Garriott. Death due to ingestion of dextroamphetamine. For. Sci. Gaz. 8: 1–2, 1977.

L.G. Dring, R.L. Smith and R.T. Williams. The metabolic fate of amphetamine in man and other species. Biochem. J. 116: 425–435, 1970.

M.H. Ebert, D.P. Van Kammen and D.L. Murphy. Plasma levels of amphetamine and behavioral response. In *Pharmacokinetics of Psychoactive Drugs* (L.A. Gottschalk and S. Merlis, eds.), Spectrum Publications, New York, 1976, pp. 157–169.

B.M. Farrell and T.M. Jeffries. An investigation of high-performance liquid chromatographic methods for the analysis of amphetamines. J. Chrom. 272: 111–128, 1983.

B. Finkle. Personal communication, 1973.

C.L. Hornbeck and R.J. Czarny. Quantitation of methamphetamine and amphetamine in urine by capillary GC/MS. J. Anal. Tox. 13: 144–149, 1989.

R.O. Hughes, W.E. Bronner and M.L. Smith. Detection of amphetamine and methamphetamine in urine by gas chromatography/mass spectrometry following derivatization with (-)-menthyl chloroformate. J. Anal. Tox. 15: 256–259, 1991.

J.C. Kramer. Amphetamine abuse. J. Am. Med. Asso. 201: 89–93, 1967.

P. Lebish, B.S. Finkle and J.W. Brackett, Jr. Determination of amphetamine, methamphetamine, and related amines in blood and urine by gas chromatography by hydrogen-flame ionization detector. Clin. Chem. 16: 195–200, 1970.

S.B. Matin, S.H. Wan and J.B. Knight. Quantitative determination of enantiomeric compounds. Biomed. Mass Spec. 4: 118–121, 1977.

R. Melgar and R.C. Kelly. A novel GC/MS derivatization method for amphetamines. J. Anal. Tox. 17: 399–402, 1993.

P.L. Morselli, G.F. Placid, C. Maggini et al. An integrated approach for the evaluation of psychotropic drugs in man. Psychopharmacologia 46: 211–217, 1976.

S. Orrenius and A.C. Maehly. Lethal amphetamine intoxication. Z. Rechtsmed. 67: 184–189, 1970.

H.G.H. Richards and A. Stephens. Sudden death associated with the taking of amphetamines by an asthmatic. Med. Sci. Law 13: 35–38, 1973.

M. Rowland. Amphetamine blood and urine levels in man. J. Pharm. Sci. 58: 508–509, 1969.

P.S. Sever, J. Caldwell, L.G. Dring and R.T. Williams. The metabolism of amphetamine in dependent subjects. Eur. J. Clin. Pharm. 6: 177–180, 1973.

P.A. Toseland and P.H. Scott. Determination of amphetamine as its N-acetyl derivative by gas-liquid chromatography. Clin. Chim. Acta 25: 75–78, 1969.

F. van Hoof and J. Timperman. Report of a human fatality due to amphetamine. Arch. Tox. 32: 307–312, 1974.

S.H. Wan, S.B. Matin and D.L. Azarnoff. Kinetics, salivary excretion of amphetamine isomers, and effect of urinary pH. Clin. Pharm. Ther. 23: 585–590, 1978.

V.W. Watts and T.F. Simonick. Screening of basic drugs in biological samples using dual column capillary chromatography and nitrogen-phosphorus detectors. J. Anal. Tox. 10: 198–204, 1986.

C.E. Wells. GLC determination of the optical isomers of amphetamine. J. Asso. Off. Anal. Chem. 53: 113–115, 1970.

Amygdalin

T½: 44–157 min
Vd: 0.3 L/kg
Fb: 0

Occurrence and Usage. Amygdalin ("laetrile," "vitamin B-17," Amygdalina, Kemdalin) is a cyanogenic glycoside that occurs in the kernels of almonds, apricots, cherries, peaches, and other fruits. Laetrile, a term often mistakenly used synonymously with amygdalin, is actually mandelonitrile glucuronide. Attempts to duplicate the patented syntheses of laetrile from amygdalin have been unsuccessful, and it is generally recognized that all the commercial forms of laetrile marketed for use in the treatment of cancer are actually amygdalin. The substance is available in tablets of 250 and 500 mg for oral administration and 3 g/10 mL solutions for intravenous or intramuscular injection. The dosage forms often contain only 55–85% of the stated amount, and some imported injectable solutions have been found to contain microbial and particulate contaminants (Davignon, 1977; Fenselau et al., 1977; Cairns et al., 1978). The usual daily adult dose is 500–2500 mg orally or 3000–6000 mg by injection. A typical therapeutic course includes 3 weeks of daily injections followed by daily oral doses for an indefinite period.

Crude forms of amygdalin are also available for oral usage and usually consist of ground apricot kernels (Apriken, Apricaps). Cassava root, used as a major dietary staple in certain tropical countries, contains prunasin, an amygdalin derivative.

Blood Concentrations. In 6 patients taking 1500 mg of amygdalin daily by oral ingestion (500 mg before each meal) for 7 days, plasma amygdalin concentrations reached peak levels of less than 1 mg/L within 30–60 minutes. Blood cyanide levels after the second day's morning dose reached peak levels of 0.4–2.1 mg/L (average, 1.0) at 1.5–2.0 hours, remaining fairly stable over the course of therapy; plasma thiocyanate concentrations continued to increase until the last day, reaching an average level of 25 mg/L and remaining at that value for at least a week after cessation of therapy (Moertel et al., 1981).

Following the intramuscular injection of 6000 mg in an adult male, a peak plasma amygdalin concentration of 180 mg/L was observed at 1.25 hours, declining to about 50 mg/L by 8 hours (Ames et al., 1978). Plasma amygdalin concentrations as high as 1160 mg/L were produced in 3 subjects who received a daily 4500 mg/m² intravenous dose; elimination half-lives ranged from 44–157 minutes. Cyanide was not detected in the blood of these patients during a 21 day course of intravenous therapy, nor were any toxic reactions observed, although plasma thiocyanate concentrations were slightly elevated (Moertel et al., 1981). Normal blood cyanide and plasma thiocyanate levels are presented in the section on cyanide.

Metabolism and Excretion. Amygdalin may be hydrolyzed enzymatically or by acid or alkali first to mandelonitrile-beta-glucoside (prunasin) and glucose, then to mandelonitrile and glucose, and finally to benzaldehyde and hydrogen cyanide. This reaction is catalyzed by a group of enzymes known as emulsin, present in the kernels of fruits that contain amygdalin, when the kernels are ground and moistened (or masticated). The reaction also proceeds, somewhat more slowly, in the acid environment of the stomach when pure amygdalin is ingested orally. It may also occur in the intestine due to the presence of bacterial hydrolytic enzymes. When injected parenterally, only small amounts are hydrolyzed. Amygdalin contains 6% cyanide by weight (Haisman and Knight, 1967; Schmidt et al., 1978; Moertel et al., 1981).

Nearly an entire intramuscularly or intravenously injected dose of amygdalin may be recovered unchanged in the 24 hour urine. With oral administration, only 8–32% is eliminated unchanged in the urine. Urine cyanide and thiocyanate concentrations are not significantly elevated after either intravenous or oral administration of amygdalin (Moertel et al., 1981).

Toxicity. A 3 year old child who was receiving both oral and intravenous therapy with amygdalin was also given 3 enemas with 3.5 g of the intravenous form of the drug; vomiting and diarrhea developed after the second enema and after the third he became lethargic, unresponsive and cyanotic. Five hours after admission to a hospital, a blood cyanide concentration of 2.1 mg/L was measured. The child recovered with supportive therapy over a 12 hour period (Ortega and Creek, 1978). The daily ingestion of 1500 mg of amygdalin by an adult has produced toxicity and a blood cyanide level of 10 mg/L (Smith et al., 1977). The acute ingestion of 500–2500 mg by an infant produced a blood cyanide level of 0.29 mg/L at admission, with death after 72 hours (Humbert et al., 1977); and the acute ingestion of 3500 mg by a 17 year old girl caused her death within 24 hours (Sadoff et al., 1978).

Acute intoxication occurred in 9 children, 2 of whom died, following the ingestion of apricot seeds capable of releasing 217 mg of cyanide per 100 g of moist seed; the authors cite 9 other poisonings involving fruit seeds (Sayre and Kaymakcalan, 1964). A similar episode occurred in 1977 involving 8 children, one of whom died (Lasch and El Shawa, 1981).

Cancer patients often ingest almonds or apricot kernels as a supplement or replacement to the usual oral or intravenous amygdalin therapy. Moertel et al. (1981) showed that patients receiving normal oral doses of amygdalin remained asymptomatic, with blood cyanide concentrations below 1 mg/L, but that on addition of almonds (which contain β-glucosidase) to this regimen the blood cyanide level increased to as much as 2.0 mg/L, with resulting symptoms of nausea, vomiting, headache, dizziness, and profound weakness. Peak blood cyanide concentrations of 2.0 and 3.2 mg/L were observed in 2 such intoxicated women, one of whom exhibited a cyanide blood half-life of 44 hours; both patients recovered after intravenous sodium nitrite and sodium thiosulfate therapy (Rubino and Davidoff, 1979; Shragg et al., 1982). Another woman died under similar circumstances, with a postmortem blood cyanide concentration of 3.8 mg/L (Herbert, 1979).

Analysis. Amygdalin may be determined in plasma or urine by ultraviolet spectrophotometry after enzyme hydrolysis to benzaldehyde (Ames et al., 1978; Flora et al., 1978). Gas chromatography has been used, with either flame-ionization or electron-capture detection, to assay amygdalin as a silyl derivative (Ames et al., 1978) or amygdalin-derived benzaldehyde as a halogenated derivative (Kawai et al., 1981). Liquid chromatography has also been employed (Balkon, 1982). Methods for the analysis of cyanide and thiocyanate are discussed in the section on cyanide.

References

M.M. Ames, J.S. Kovach and K.P. Flora. Initial pharmacologic studies of amygdalin. Res. Comm. Chem. Path. Pharm. 22: 175–185, 1978.

J. Balkon. Methodology for the detection and measurement of amygdalin in tissues and fluids. J. Anal. Tox. 6: 244–246, 1982.

T. Cairns, J.E. Froberg, S. Gonzales et al. Analytical chemistry of amygdalin. Anal. Chem. 50: 317–322, 1978.

J.P. Daviginon. Contaminated laetrile: a heath hazard. New Eng. J. Med. 297: 1355–1356, 1977.

C. Fenselau, S. Pallante, R.P. Batzinger et al. Mandelonitrile β-glucuronide: synthesis and characterization. Science 198: 625–627, 1977.

K.P. Flora. J.C. Cradock and M.M. Ames. A simple method for the estimation of amygdalin in urine. Res. Comm. Chem. Path. Pharm. 20: 367–378, 1978.

D.R. Haisman and D.J. Knight. The enzymic hydrolysis of amygdalin. Biochem. J. 103: 528–534, 1967.

V. Herbert. Laetrile: the cult of cyanide-promoting poison for profit. Am. J. Clin. Nutri. 32: 1121–1158, 1979.

J.R. Humbert, J.H. Tress and K.T. Braico. Fatal cyanide poisoning: accidental ingestion of amygdalin. J. Am. Med. Asso. 238: 482, 1977.

S. Kawai, K. Kobayashi and Y. Takayama. Gas chromatographic enzymic determination of amygdalin. J. Chrom. 210: 342–345, 1981.

E.E. Lasch and R. El Shawa. Multiple cases of cyanide poisoning by apricot kernels in children from Gaza. Pediatrics 68: 5–7, 1981.

C.G. Moertel, M.M. Ames, J.S. Kovach et al. A pharmacologic and toxicological study of amygdalin. J. Am. Med. Asso. 245: 591–594, 1981.

J.A. Ortega and J.E. Creek. Acute cyanide poisoning following administration of laetrile enemas. J. Pediat. 93: 1059, 1978.

M.J. Rubino and F. Davidoff. Cyanide poisoning from apricot seeds. J. Am. Med. Asso. 241: 359, 1979.

L. Sadoff, K. Fuchs and J. Hollander. Rapid death associated with laetrile ingestion. J. Am. Med. Asso. 239: 1532, 1978.

J.W. Sayre and S. Kaymakcalan. Cyanide poisoning from apricot seeds among children in central Turkey. New Eng. J. Med. 270: 1113–1115, 1964.

E.S. Schmidt, G.W. Newton, S.M. Sanders et al. Laetrile toxicity studies in dogs. J. Am. Med. Asso. 239: 943–947, 1978.

T.A. Shragg, T.E. Albertson and C.J. Fisher, Jr. A case of severe cyanide poisoning after bitter almond ingestion treated with sodium nitrite and sodium thiosulfate. West. J. Med. 136: 65–69, 1982.

F.P. Smith, T.P. Butler, S. Cohan and P.S. Schein. Laetrile toxicity: a report of two cases. J. Am. Med. Asso. 238: 1361, 1977.

Anileridine

T½: 1–3 hr
Vd: ?
Fb: ?
pKa: 3.7, 7.5

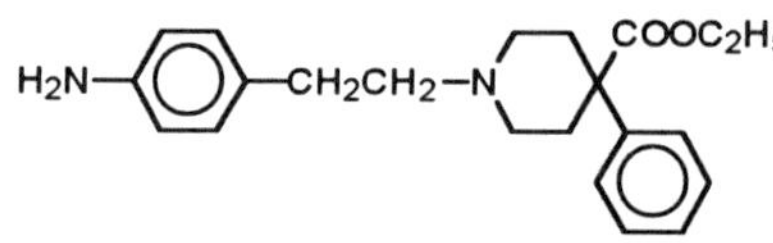

H_2N—⬡—CH_2CH_2—N⟨$COOC_2H_5$⟩

Occurrence and Usage. Anileridine (Leritine) is a synthetic narcotic analgesic similar in structure to but several times more potent than meperidine. It is supplied as the dihydrochloride in 25 mg tablets for oral administration (25–50 mg every 4–6 hours) and as the phosphate in a 25 mg/mL injectable solution (5–10 mg intravenously or 25–50 mg subcutaneously).

Blood Concentrations. Therapeutic blood or plasma concentrations of anileridine have not been established in man. By analogy with meperidine, they probably do not exceed 0.5 mg/L.

Metabolism and Excretion. Anileridine is metabolized in man by deesterification and N-acetylation. About 5% of a single dose is eliminated unchanged in the 24 hour urine, 7–14% as anileridine acid, 1–2% as acetylanileridine acid, and 0.5–2% as acetylanileridine. Another 15–35% of a dose has been tentatively identified as p-acetylaminophenylacetic acid, which could represent a product of N-dealkylation of anileridine (Porter, 1957). The other product of this reaction, noranileridine (or normeperidine), has been identified in human urine (Lin and Way, 1965).

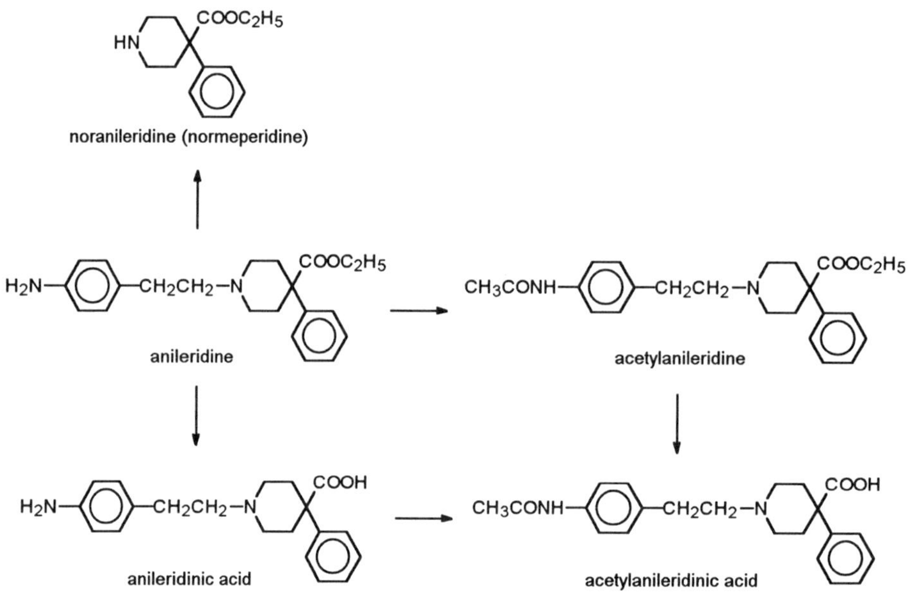

noranileridine (normeperidine)

anileridine   acetylanileridine

anileridinic acid   acetylanileridinic acid

Toxicity. Two fatal cases believed due primarily to intentional ingestion of an overdose of anileridine have been reported, with the following tissue distribution of drug (Peat, 1979; Peclet, 1981):

Anileridine Concentrations in Fatalities (mg/L or mg/kg)

	Blood	Liver	Bile	Kidney	Urine	Gastric
Case 1*	0.9		2.4		11	3 mg
Case 2**	2.0	12		3.0		2400 mg

 * Blood diazepam, 1.1 mg/L; nordiazepam, 0.7 mg/L
 ** Blood secobarbital, 8 mg/L

Analysis. Anileridine may be analyzed in biological specimens using procedures designed for meperidine or codeine.

References

S.C. Lin and E.L. Way. N-dealkylation of anileridine to normeperidine. J. Pharm. Exp. Ther. 150: 309–315, 1965.

M.A. Peat. Personal communication, 1979.

C. Peclet. Personal communication, 1981.

C.C. Porter. The absorption and metabolism of anileridine, ethyl-1-(4-aminophenethyl)-4-phenylisonipecotate. J. Pharm. Exp. Ther. 120: 447–454, 1957.

Aniline

T½: 2–7 hr
Vd: ?
Fb: ?
pKa: 4.6

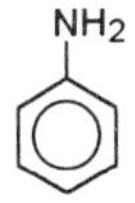

Occurrence and Usage. Aniline is a colorless aromatic liquid that tends to darken on exposure to light. The compound is widely used as a chemical intermediate and solvent and in the manufacture of synthetic dyes. The threshold limit value in the industrial atmosphere is currently 2 ppm (7.6 mg/m^3). Exposure to aniline is commonly by inhalation of the vapor or by cutaneous absorption of the liquid; probably the latter mode is of the greatest toxicological importance in industry (Piotrowski, 1977).

Blood Concentrations. Aniline has not been measured in blood except in experimental studies with animals. In man, blood methemoglobin levels are often measured as an index of exposure to aniline.

Metabolism and Excretion. Aniline has not been found in the exhaled air of subjects exposed to it. Less than 1% of an absorbed dose of aniline is excreted unchanged in the urine. From 15–60% is oxidized to p-aminophenol, which is excreted in the urine as glucuronide and sulfate conjugates, primarily in the first 24 hours after exposure. The production of this metabolite is more efficient at higher doses of aniline (Piotrowski, 1977). A minor metabolite, phenylhydroxylamine, is apparently responsible for many of the toxic effects associated with aniline (Jenkins et al., 1972). Linch (1974) considers that a urinary p-aminophenol concentration of 10 mg/L is a warning of potentially toxic exposure to aniline and that a concentration of 20 mg/L indicates the need for medical intervention. Piotrowski (1977) has shown that the rate of urinary excretion of p-aminophenol in a timed urine specimen taken at the end of an exposure period may be used to estimate the amount of aniline absorbed by a subject, over a range of 10–100 mg. At the former threshold limit value of 5 ppm, an 8 hour exposure would result in the absorption of approximately 150 mg of aniline and would lead to a p-aminophenol urinary excretion rate over the last 2 hours of exposure of 13 mg/hour. The urinary p-aminophenol concentration also appears to be directly related to blood methemoglobin levels in workers exposed to aniline (Pacseri, 1961).

Toxicity. Acute or chronic exposure to aniline may produce symptoms of headache, dizziness and nausea. Single oral 15 mg doses of the chemical given to volunteers caused no effects, whereas a dose of 25 mg produced an increase in blood methemoglobin of 2% and a dose of 65 mg increased methemoglobin by 16%. A methemoglobin level of 15% is consistent with clinical cyanosis, and levels exceeding 60% may be life-threatening. A woman who ingested 80 mL of aniline achieved a blood aniline (plus diazotizable metabolites) concentration of 25 mg/L and a methemoglobin level of 50%, but survived the intoxication after hemodialysis and methylene blue administration (Lubash et al., 1964). Exchange transfusion was used successfully to treat a 4.5 year old child who ingested approximately 5 mL of aniline and developed a blood methemoglobin level of 77% at 13 hours post-ingestion (Mier, 1988).

Analysis. A procedure has been described for the determination of blood methemoglobin content by visible spectrophotometry (Evelyn and Malloy, 1938). This procedure, modified by Leahy and Smith (1960), is also useful for assessment of exposure to other amino and nitro compounds that cause methemoglobinemia, such as nitrobenzene. p-Aminophenol may be determined in urine, following acid hydrolysis of conjugates, by a colorimetric procedure (Greenberg and Lester, 1948; Chang et al., 1993). It should be noted that urinary p-aminophenol concentrations may reach values as high as 200 mg/L following the ingestion of either acetaminophen or phenacetin, and therefore the use of these drugs must be ruled out when performing aniline exposure tests (Piotrowski, 1977; Chang et al., 1993).

References

M.J.W. Chang, G.I. Kao and C.T. Tsai. Biological monitoring of exposure to low dose aniline, p-aminophenol, and acetaminophen. Bull. Env. Cont. Tox. 51: 494–500, 1993.

K.A. Evelyn and H.T. Malloy. Microdetermination of oxyhemoglobin, methemoglobin, and sulfhemoglobin in a single sample of blood. J. Biol. Chem. 126: 655–662, 1938.

L.A. Greenberg and D. Lester. The metabolic fate of acetanilid and other aniline derivatives. J. Pharm. Exp. Ther. 88: 87–98, 1948.

F.P. Jenkins, J.A. Robinson, J.B.M. Gellatly and G.W.A. Salmond. The no-effect dose of aniline in human subjects and a comparison of aniline toxicity in man and the rat. Food Cosmet. Tox. 10: 671–679, 1972.

T. Leahy and R. Smith. Notes on methemoglobin determination. Clin. Chem. 6: 148–152, 1960.

A.L. Linch. Biological monitoring for industrial exposure to cyanogenic aromatic nitro and amino compounds. Am. Ind. Hyg. Asso. J. 35: 426–432, 1974.

G.D. Lubash, R.E. Phillips, J.D. Shields and R.W. Bonsnes. Acute aniline poisoning treated by hemodialysis. Arch. Int. Med. 114: 530–532, 1964.

R.J. Mier. Treatment of aniline poisoning with exchange transfusion. Clin. Tox. 26: 357–364, 1988.

J. Pacseri. p-Aminophenol excretion as an index of aniline exposure. Pure Appl. Chem. 3: 313–314, 1961.

J.K. Piotrowski. *Exposure Tests for Organic Compounds in Industrial Toxicology*, U.S. Government Printing Office, Washington, D.C., 1977, pp 70–75.

Antimony

T½: 38 days
Vd: ?   Sb
Fb: ?

Occurrence and Usage. Various salts of both trivalent and pentavalent antimony have been used for centuries as drugs, and they continue to be available as parasiticides for parenteral administration. Inorganic salts of antimony are used as pigments, abrasives and for flame-proofing fabrics, whereas metallic antimony is found in a number of alloys. Industrial exposure is usually via inhalation. The current threshold limit value for compounds of antimony is 0.5 mg/m^3 in air, calculated as the metal.

Blood Concentrations. Since trivalent antimony is largely bound to erythrocytes when present in blood, and pentavalent antimony is primarily found in plasma, whole blood is the preferred specimen for assay. Whole blood antimony concentrations in healthy subjects not exposed to the metal rarely exceed 0.01 mg/L. During intravenous therapy with sodium antimonyl tartrate (20 mg antimony administered once every 48 hours for 42 days), blood antimony concentrations averaged 0.52 mg/L at 1 hour after injection and 0.07 mg/L at 48 hours after injection. These levels did not fluctuate significantly throughout the course of therapy (Ozawa, 1956).

Metabolism and Excretion. Soluble forms of trivalent or pentavalent antimony, when administered by inhalation or parenteral injection, appear to be rapidly absorbed and eliminated, largely in urine and to a slight extent in feces. On the other hand, inhalation of insoluble forms or oral ingestion of soluble forms usually results in slow absorption and therefore prolonged elimination from the body. In general, the excretion of pentavalent antimony is more rapid than that of the trivalent form. The liver contains the highest concentration of antimony of any organ in the body during therapeutic administration of antimonials and has the ability to reduce the pentavalent form to the trivalent form. Lung, liver and kidney concentrations in normal individuals average 0.33, 0.02 and 0.01 mg/kg, respectively (Yukawa et al., 1980).

Urine antimony concentrations in persons not exposed to the metal occupationally are usually less than 0.001 mg/L. Occupationally exposed but asymptomatic individuals may develop urine concentrations of up to 0.3 mg/L. During therapy with antimonials, however, urine concentrations may reach 2 mg/L within the first 24 hours after an injection and antimony may still be detectable 100 days after the discontinuation of therapy (Ozawa, 1956; Stemmer, 1976; Taylor, 1966). A smelter worker with antimony pneumoconiosis showed a urine antimony level of 0.05 mg/L 7 months after retirement, and a level of 0.03 mg/L over 3 years later (McCallum, 1963).

Toxicity. The effects of acute or chronic antimony poisoning are similar to those produced by arsenic and include abdominal pain, dyspnea, nausea, vomiting, dermatitis and visual disturbances. There is some indication that the body burden of antimony increases with prolonged exposure, although this apparently does not occur to the same extent as with many other toxic metals. Occupational poisoning is most frequently related to the inhalation of antimony compounds, such as the oxide or trichloride, either as fumes or as dusts. In these cases, the air concentrations of antimony have ranged from 5–73 mg/m^3 and urine concentrations have reached 5 mg/L (Renes, 1953; Taylor, 1966). Exposure to antimony hydride (stibine) is especially hazardous due to the gaseous nature of this compound and its very rapid pulmonary absorption.

A woman who died 48 hours after accidental ingestion of a bottle of antimony trichloride solution had the following tissue levels at autopsy (Ryall, 1978):

Antimony Concentrations in a Fatal Case (mg/L or mg/kg)

Blood	Brain	Lung	Liver	Bile	Kidney	Fat
4.6	6	6	45	404	32	5

Analysis. Urine antimony levels may be useful in the diagnosis of acute or chronic poisoning, and may be determined by colorimetric (Kneip et al., 1976; Taylor, 1977) or atomic absorption procedures (Kneip et al., 1977; Collett et al., 1978). The latter technique is also useful for blood level measurements, which are especially recommended during suspected acute intoxication. Procedures for wet or dry ashing of biological specimens are cited in the section on arsenic.

References

D.L. Collett, D.E. Fleming and G.A. Taylor. Determination of antimony by stibine generation and atomic-absorption spectrophotometry using a flame-heated silica furnace. Analyst 103: 1074–1075, 1978.

T.J. Kneip, R.S. Ajemian, J.N. Driscoll et al. Analytical method for antimony in air and urine. Health Lab. Sci. 13: 90–94, 1976.

T.J. Kneip, R.S. Ajemian, J.N. Driscoll et al. Arsenic, selenium and antimony in urine and air: analytical method by hydride generation and atomic absorption spectroscopy. Health Lab. Sci. 14: 53–58, 1977.

R.I. McCallum. The work of an occupational hygiene service in environmental control. Ann. Occ. Hyg. 6: 55–64, 1963.

K. Ozawa. Studies on the therapy of schistosomiasis japonica. Tohoku J. Exp. Med. 65: 1–9, 1956.

L.E. Renes. Antimony poisoning in industry. Arch. Ind. Hyg. Occ. Med. 7: 99–108, 1953.

J.E. Ryall. Personal communication, 1978.

K.L. Stemmer. Pharmacology and toxicology of heavy metals: antimony. Pharm. Ther. 1: 157–160, 1976.

D.G. Taylor. *NIOSH Manual of Analytical Methods*, 2nd ed., National Institute for Occupational Safety and Health, Cincinnati, 1977, pp. 107–1 to 107–6.

P.J. Taylor. Acute intoxication from antimony trichloride. Brit. J. Ind. Med. 23: 318–321, 1966.

M. Yukawa, K. Amano, M. Suzuki-Yasumoto and M. Terai. Distribution of trace elements in the human body determined by neutron activation analysis. Arch. Env. Health 35: 36–44, 1980.

Antipyrine

T½: 7–15 hr
Vd: 0.56 L/kg
Fb: 0.03
pKa: 1.4

Occurrence and Usage. Antipyrine (phenazone) is a weakly basic non-narcotic analgesic, in use since 1884, that also exhibits anti-inflammatory and antipyretic effects. Daily oral doses of 1200–2400 mg are given, in the form of tablets or capsules. Due to the greater popularity of the salicylates, antipyrine is rarely used today except as a clinical tool in the determination of total body water or hepatic microsomal enzyme status.

Blood Concentrations. Whole blood and plasma have been found to be approximately equivalent in regard to antipyrine concentration, since the drug exhibits negligible plasma protein binding and distributes in total body water. Four hours after a single oral dose of 10 mg/kg (700 mg/70 kg), plasma concentrations in 3 subjects averaged 13 mg/L (range, 10–16), declining thereafter with an average half-life of 9.8 hours. The behavior of the drug was best described by a one-compartment open model (van Boxtel et al., 1976). Three hours after an 18 mg/kg (1260 mg/70 kg) oral dose, plasma concentrations in 12 individuals ranged from 12–25 mg/L (Vesell et al., 1975). Peak plasma levels may not appear until 6 hours after drug ingestion in some subjects (Huffman et al., 1974).

Metabolism and Excretion. Antipyrine is extensively metabolized in man, primarily by 4-hydroxylation and glucuronide conjugation. N-demethylation and oxidation of the 3-methyl group also occur. The compound is eliminated in the 24 hour urine as conjugated 4-hydroxyantipyrine (30–40%), 3-hydroxymethylantipyrine (10%), conjugated norantipyrine (6%), and unchanged drug (5%). The half-life of appearance of 4-hydroxyantipyrine (an inactive compound that does not accumulate in plasma) in the urine is equivalent to the plasma half-life of the parent drug (Brodie and Axelrod, 1950; Baty and Price Evans, 1973; Huffman et al., 1974; Stafford et al., 1974). p-Hydroxyantipyrine has also been found in urine, representing 2–4% of a dose (Inaba et al., 1981).

Toxicity. Hypersensitive individuals may develop serious skin eruptions or generalized anaphylactic reactions after therapeutic ingestion of antipyrine. An 87 year old woman was given 500 mg of the drug intravenously for total body water determination and suffered a cardiac arrest; the postmortem blood antipyrine concentration of 22 mg/L was within the expected range (Travers, 1991). Overdosage causes nausea, fainting, cyanosis due to methemoglobinemia, coma and convulsions. Antipyrine is not believed to produce agranulocytosis as does its 4-dimethylamino derivative, aminopyrine.

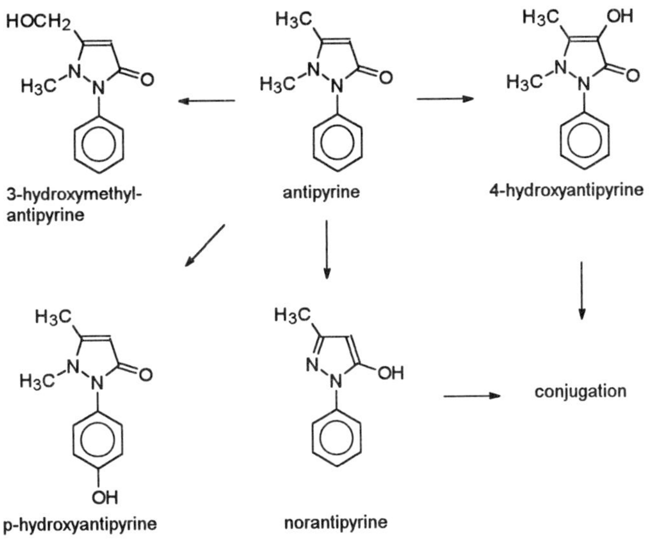

3-hydroxymethyl-antipyrine

antipyrine

4-hydroxyantipyrine

p-hydroxyantipyrine

norantipyrine

conjugation

A 60 year old man who apparently committed suicide with an overdose of antipyrine was found to have a postmortem blood concentration of 110 mg/L (Peclet, 1981).

Analysis. Antipyrine has been frequently measured in biological fluids by a somewhat tedious spectrophotometric method requiring derivatization (Brodie et al., 1949). More specific techniques include gas chromatography (Prescott et al., 1973; Abernethy et al., 1981) and high-pressure liquid chromatography (Eichelbaum and Spannbrucker, 1977; Shargel et al., 1979).

References

D.R. Abernethy, D.J. Greenblatt and A.M. Zumbo. Antipyrine determination in human plasma by gas-liquid chromatography using nitrogen-phosphorus detection. J. Chrom. 223: 432–437, 1981.

J.D. Baty and D.A. Price Evans. Norphenazone, a new metabolite of phenazone in human urine. J. Pharm. Pharmac. 25: 83–84, 1973.

B.B. Brodie, J. Axelrod, R. Soberman and B.B. Levy. The estimation of antipyrine in biological materials. J. Biol. Chem. 179: 25–29, 1949.

B.B. Brodie and J. Axelrod. The fate of antipyrine in man. J. Pharm. Exp. Ther. 98: 97–104, 1950.

M. Eichelbaum and N. Spannbrucker. Rapid and sensitive method for the determination of antipyrine in biological fluids by high-pressure liquid chromatography. J. Chrom. 140: 288–292, 1977.

D.H. Huffman, D.W. Shoeman and D.L. Azarnoff. Correlation of the plasma elimination of antipyrine and the appearance of 4-hydroxyantipyrine in the urine of man. Biochem. Pharm. 23: 197–201, 1974.

T. Inaba, H. Uchino and W. Kalow. Identification of p(4')-hydroxyantipyrine as a metabolite of antipyrine in man. Res. Comm. Chem. Path. Pharm. 33: 3–8, 1981.

C. Peclet. Personal communication, 1981.

L.F. Prescott, K.K. Adjepon-Yamoah and E. Roberts. Rapid gas-liquid chromatographic estimation of antipyrine in plasma. J. Pharm. Pharmac. 25: 205–207, 1973.

L. Shargel, W. Cheung and A.B.C. Yu. High-pressure liquid chromatographic analysis of antipyrine in small plasma samples. J. Pharm. Sci. 68: 1052–1054, 1979.

M. Stafford, G. Kellerman, R.N. Stillwell and M.G. Horning. Metabolism of antipyrine by the epoxide-diol pathway in the rat, guinea pig and human. Res. Comm. Chem. Path. Pharm. 8: 593–606, 1974.

A.F. Travers. A fatality after antipyrine administration. Clin. Pharm. Ther. 49: 695–696, 1991.

C.J. van Boxtel, J.T. Wilson, S. Lindgren and F. Sjoqvist. Comparison of the half-life of antipyrine in plasma, whole blood and saliva of man. Eur. J. Clin. Pharm. 9: 327–332, 1976.

E.S. Vesell, G.T. Passananti, P.A. Glenwright and B.H. Dvorchik. Studies on the disposition of antipyrine, aminopyrine, and phenacetin using plasma, saliva and urine. Clin. Pharm. Ther. 18: 259–272, 1975.

Aprobarbital

T½: 14–34 hr
Vd: ?
Fb: 0.55–0.70
pKa: 8.1

Occurrence and Usage. Aprobarbital (5-allyl-5-isopropylbarbituric acid) is a barbiturate deriva-tive of intermediate duration of action that was synthesized in 1923. The compound is used only occasionally in the United States in the form of an elixir. It is administered orally at a dose of 40 mg 3 times daily for sedation or in a single dose of 40–160 mg to induce sleep. The drug is also found in one preparation in combination with butabarbital and phenobarbital.

Blood Concentrations. A single oral dose of 750 mg of aprobarbital produced in 3 subjects an average peak plasma concentration of 15 mg/L (range, 12–18) 12 hours after ingestion, with a slow decline to 10 mg/L (range, 4–14) after 36 hours (Lous, 1954a).

Metabolism and Excretion. The extent and nature of the biotransformation of aprobarbital in man are unknown. From 7.5–17.5% of a single dose is excreted unchanged in the urine over a 4 day period (Lous, 1954a; Svendsen and Brochmann-Hanssen, 1962).

Toxicity. A series of 50 cases of overdosage with aprobarbital has been described in which only 4 patients died (Lous, 1954b). Serum concentrations of 40–150 mg/L were observed 24 hours after drug intake in these patients, and those who survived awoke when their serum concentrations fell to 16–54 mg/L. The deaths occurred after the ingestion of 2.5–7.7 g of the drug and the victims developed antemortem serum concentrations of 120–150 mg/L. An average blood concentration of 50 mg/L and liver concentration of 83 mg/kg were found for 9 cases of fatal overdosage with aprobarbital (Bonnichsen et al., 1961).

Analysis. Methods for the determination of barbiturates are cited in the section on amobarbital.

References

R. Bonnichsen, A.C. Maehly and A. Frank. Barbiturate analysis: method and statistical survey. J. For. Sci. 6: 411–443, 1961.
P. Lous. Plasma levels and urinary excretion of three barbituric acids after oral administration to man. Acta Pharm. 10: 147–165, 1954a.
P. Lous. Barbituric acid concentrations in serum from patients with severe acute poisoning. Acta Pharm. Tox. 10: 261–280, 1954b.
A.B. Svendsen and E. Brochmann-Hanssen. Gas chromatography of barbiturates II. Application to the study of their metabolism and excretion in humans. J. Pharm. Sci. 51: 494–495, 1962.

Arsenic

T½: 7 hr
Vd: 0.2 L/kg
Fb: ?

As

Occurrence and Usage. Arsenic is the twentieth most abundant element in the earth's crust and is present in all living organisms. In certain areas of the United States and Canada, fresh water sup-plies contain up to 1.4 mg/L, substantially in excess of the acceptable limit of 0.01 mg/L. Seafood can contain from 2 mg/kg for freshwater fish up to 22 mg/kg for lobsters, most of which is organically bound. The average adult dietary intake of arsenic is 0.025–0.033 mg/kg/day. The largest source of human exposure to arsenic today is arsenical pesticides, which account for over 80% of the industrial consumption of arsenic. These compounds are derived from arsenic trioxide and include arsenic acid, dimethylarsinic acid (cacodylic acid) and salts of arsenite, arsenate and methanearsonate. Other important uses are in pharmaceuticals, in the ceramic and glass industry and in metallurgy. Arsine gas is occasionally encountered accidentally in industrial processes. Arsenic compounds are absorbed into the body following inhalation, ingestion or dermal contact (especially organo-arsenic compounds). The threshold limit value for inorganic arsenic compounds is currently set at 0.2 mg/m^3 (expressed as arsenic).

Blood Concentrations. Arsenic is a trace element that is present in all human tissues, probably bound to proteins. In blood, it is evenly distributed between plasma and erythrocytes; blood concentrations in normal subjects vary due to dietary and environmental influence and have been found to range from 0.002–0.062 mg/L in some populations (Heydorn, 1970). Mean blood levels ranged from 0.003–0.005 mg/L in 4 U.S. communities with normal (0.006–0.098 mg/L) arsenic concentrations in their drinking water, and averaged 0.013 mg/L in a community where the water contained 0.393 mg/L of arsenic (Valentine et al., 1979). Asymptomatic workers using dimethylarsinic acid as an herbicide developed maximal blood concentrations of 0.27 mg/L (Wagner and Weswig, 1974).

Metabolism and Excretion. An administered dose of arsenic is distributed throughout the body, with the largest amount found in the muscles; excretion by the kidney is nearly complete within 6 days and accounts for over 90% of a dose, only a trace amount appearing in the feces (Hunter et al., 1942). The majority of a dose of dietary trivalent arsenic is rapidly excreted in urine as dimethylarsinic acid (50%), methylarsonic acid (14%), pentavalent arsenic (8%) and trivalent arsenic (8%); organo-arsenic compounds, as found in crab meat, are excreted unchanged in urine (Crecelius, 1977). A single dose of pentavalent arsenic was excreted in the 7 day urine of volunteers as dimethylarsinic acid (57–69%), methylarsonic acid (9–18%), pentavalent arsenic (9–10%) and trivalent arsenic (12–15%) (Johnson and Farmer, 1991).

Urine arsenic concentrations of unexposed persons may range from 0.01–0.30 mg/L. Subjects who ate a seafood meal developed maximal urine arsenic concentrations of 0.2–1.7 mg/L within 4 hours, with over 90% present as dimethylarsinic acid. Workers occupationally exposed to arsenic trioxide dust had urine concentrations ranging from 0.02–2.00 mg/L (Schrenk and Schreibeis, 1958; Pinto et al., 1976; Arbouine and Wilson, 1992). Concentrations in urine of asymptomatic forest workers applying organic arsenic herbicides averaged 0.36–0.62 mg/L, with a range of 0.07–2.50 mg/L; the concentrations tended to increase toward the end of the week, but returned to normal by the next Monday (Tarrant and Allard, 1972).

Concentrations in other tissues of 50 trauma victims ranged as follows (Gerin and de Zorzi, 1961):

Arsenic Concentrations in Normal Tissues (mg/kg)*

	Brain	Lung	Liver	Kidney	Hair	Nails
Average	0.009	0.007	0.033	0.011	0.307	0.252
(Range)	(0–0.025)	(0–0.085)	(0–0.092)	(0–0.068)	(0–1.92)	(0–1.70)

*By a colorimetric technique; detectability limit, 0.005 mg/kg

Toxicity. With chronic low-level worker exposure to arsenic, epidemiological evidence suggests that a significant increase in the incidence of respiratory and skin cancers will occur (Pinto and Nelson, 1976). Chronic arsenic poisoning often results in cardiovascular abnormalities and neurological effects and has been attributed to the drinking of contaminated well water or excessive occupational exposure; this is best diagnosed by a measurement of hair or urine arsenic concentrations. Concentrations in hair of normal persons are less than 1 mg/kg (average, 0.5), whereas concentrations in subjects with chronic poisoning are often in the 1–5 mg/kg region and may range as high as 47 mg/kg (Hindmarsh et al., 1977).

The inhalation of arsine gas may produce rapid death, with massive hemolysis leading to renal failure. The maximum allowable atmospheric concentration of arsine is 0.05 ppm, and a concentration of 25–50 ppm is believed to be lethal within 30 minutes. Arsenic concentrations in blood and urine of a subject who survived an arsine exposure were initially as high as 1.6 and 1.9 mg/L, respectively (Pinto, 1976), although in other nonfatal cases, when specimens were not collected immediately, urine concentrations have ranged from only 0.04 up to 0.97 mg/L (Parish et al., 1979; Rathus et al., 1979; Hesdorffer et al., 1986). Concentrations of arsenic in the tissues of 3 men who died within 1 hour to 6 days of exposure to arsine fumes were as follows (Teitelbaum and Kier, 1969; Pothel and Brosseau, 1976):

Arsenic Concentrations in Fatal Arsine Poisoning (mg/L or mg/kg)

	Blood	Brain	Liver	Spleen	Kidney	Urine
Average	0.4	0.6	2.7	2.1	1.4	0.2
(Range)	(0.1–0.6)	(0.5–0.8)	(1.4–4.0)	(0.7–3.4)	(0.3–2.8)	(0.1–0.4)

The acute ingestion of only 200 mg of arsenic trioxide may be fatal to an adult, death occurring within a few hours or after many days. A 2 year old child who swallowed an unknown amount of sodium arsenite solution was hospitalized and received BAL therapy for 28 days; urine arsenic concentrations on days 6, 10 and 21 were 17.8, 2.3 and 0.1 mg/L, respectively (Petery et al., 1970). A hair concentration of approximately 200 mg/kg was determined in a man who died 6 days after the ingestion of 8 g of arsenic trioxide (Wyttenbach et al., 1967). The following tissue concentrations were compiled from a series of 49 fatalities due to accidental or intentional arsenic overdosage (Rehling, 1967):

Arsenic Concentrations in Fatal Cases (mg/L or mg/kg)

	Blood	Brain	Liver	Spleen	Kidney
Average	3.3	1.7	29	8.8	15
(Range)	(0.6–9.3)	(0.2–4.0)	(2.0–120)	(0.5–62)	(0.2–70)

Analysis. Since most methods for arsenic determination require prior destruction of organic matter, procedures for wet or dry ashing of biologic specimens are required. Wet ashing does not require special equipment (other than a fume hood) but is suitable only for inorganic arsenic (Taylor, 1977); dry ashing requires a muffle furnace and is the preferred procedure for total arsenic (inorganic plus organic) determination (Stahr, 1977; George, 1973).

A colorimetric technique employing silver diethyldithiocarbamate as a complexing reagent for the arsine that is generated is preferred by many analysts for its simplicity and reliability (George et al., 1973; Crawford and Tavares, 1974). This method has been adapted to the differential analysis of various species of arsenic (Lakso et al., 1979).

There are numerous techniques based on atomic absorption detection of arsenic; the most convenient for toxicological purposes require a graphite furnace and involve direct injection of an ashed sample (Freeman et al., 1976) or of a solution of borohydride-generated and diethyldithiocarbamate-complexed arsine (Shaikh and Tallman, 1977). Other procedures use chelation and solvent extraction of the chelate (Mushak et al., 1977; Thiex, 1980) or direct introduction of arsine into the furnace (Peter et al., 1979; Cox, 1980).

An electron-capture gas chromatographic method for the differential determination of inorganic and organic arsenic in urine has also been described (Daughtrey et al., 1975), but more commonly techniques for differentiation of the various arsenic species involve liquid chromatography separation prior to atomic absorption analysis (Arbouine and Wilson, 1992; Nixon and Moyer, 1992).

References

M.W. Arbouine and H.K. Wilson. The effect of seafood consumption on the assessment of occupational exposure to arsenic by urinary arsenic speciation measurements. J. Trace Elem. 6: 153–160, 1992.

D.H. Cox. Arsine evolution-electrothermal atomic absorption method for the determination of nanogram levels of total arsenic in urine and water. J. Anal. Tox. 4: 207–211, 1980.

G.M. Crawford and O. Tavares. Simple hydrogen sulfide trap for the Gutzeit arsenic determination. Anal. Chem. 46: 1149, 1974.

E.A. Crecelius. Changes in the chemical speciation of arsenic following ingestion by man. Env. Health Persp. 19: 147–150, 1977.

E.H. Daughtrey, Jr., A.W. Fitchett and P. Mushak. Quantitative measurements of inorganic and methyl arsenicals by gas-liquid chromatography. Anal. Chim. Acta 79: 199–206, 1975.

H. Freeman, J.F. Uthe and B. Flemming. A rapid and precise method for the determination of inorganic and organic arsenic with and without wet ashing using a graphite furnace. At. Abs. Newsl. 15: 49–50, 1976.

G.M. George, L.J. Frahm and J.P. McDonnell. Dry ashing method for the determination of total arsenic in animal tissues: collaborative study. J. Asso. Off. Anal. Chem. 56: 793–797, 1973.

C. Gerin and C. de Zorzi. The arsenic content in the organs of the human body. Zacchia 36: 1–19, 1961.

C.S. Hesdorffer, F.J. Milne, J. Terblanche and A.M. Meyers. Arsine gas poisoning: the importance of exchange transfusions in severe cases. Brit. J. Ind. Med. 43: 353–355, 1986.

K. Heydorn. Environmental variation of arsenic levels in human blood determined by neutron activation analysis. Clin. Chim. Acta 28: 349–357, 1970.

J.T. Hindmarsh, O.R. McLetchie, L.P.M. Heffernan et al. Electromyographic abnormalities in chronic environmental arsenicalism. J. Anal. Tox. 1: 270–276, 1977.

F.T. Hunter, A.F. Kip and J.W. Irvine, Jr. Radioactive tracer studies on arsenic injected as potassium arsenite. J. Pharm. Exp. Ther. 76: 207–220, 1942.

L.R. Johnson and J.G. Farmer. Use of human metabolic studies and urinary arsenic speciation in assessing arsenic exposure. Bull. Env. Cont. Tox. 46: 53–61, 1991.

J.U. Lakso, L.J. Rose, S.A. Peoples and D.Y. Shirachi. A colorimetric method for the determination of arsenite, arsenate, monomethylarsonic acid, and dimethylarsinic acid in biological and environmental samples. J. Agr. Food Chem. 27: 1229–1233, 1979.

P. Mushak, K. Dessauer and E.L. Walls. Flameless atomic absorption (FAA) and gas-liquid chromatographic studies in arsenic bioanalysis. Env. Health Persp. 19: 5–10, 1977.

D.E. Nixon and T.P. Moyer. Arsenic analysis II. Rapid separation and quantification of inorganic arsenic plus metabolites and arsenobetaine from urine. Clin. Chem. 38: 2479–2483, 1992.

G.G. Parish, R. Glass and R. Kimbrough. Acute arsine poisoning in two workers cleaning a clogged drain. Arch. Env. Health 34: 224–227, 1979.

F. Peter, G. Growcock and G. Strunc. Determination of arsenic in urine by atomic absorption spectrometry with electrothermal atomization. Anal. Chim. Acta 104: 177–180, 1979.

J.S. Petery, O.M. Rennert, H. Choi and S. Wolfson. Arsenic poisoning in childhood. Clin. Tox. 3: 519–526, 1970.

S.S. Pinto. Arsine poisoning: evaluation of the acute phase. J. Occ. Med. 18: 633–635, 1976.

S.S. Pinto and K.W. Nelson. Arsenic toxicology and industrial exposure. Ann. Rev. Pharm. 16: 95–100, 1976.

S.S. Pinto, M.O. Varner, K.W. Nelson et al. Arsenic trioxide absorption and excretion in industry. J. Occ. Med. 18: 677–680, 1976.

C. Pothel and A. Brosseau. Acute arsine poisoning: report of two cases in the Montreal region. J. Can. Soc. For. Sci. 9: 87–93, 1976.

E. Rathus, R.G. Stinton and J.L. Putman. Arsine poisoning, country style. Med. J. Aust. 1: 163–166, 1979.

C.J. Rehling. Poison residues in human tissues. In *Progress in Chemical Toxicology*, Vol. 3 (A. Stolman, ed.), Academic Press, New York, 1967, pp. 363–386.

H.H. Schrenk and L. Schreibeis, Jr. Urinary arsenic levels as an index of industrial exposure. Am. Ind. Hyg. Asso. J. 19: 225–228, 1958.

A.U. Shaikh and D.E. Tallman. Determination of sub-microgram per liter quantities of arsenic in water by arsine generation followed by graphite furnace atomic absorption spectrometry. Anal. Chem. 49: 1093–1096, 1977.

H.M. Stahr (ed.). Arsenic. In *Analytical Toxicology Methods Manual*, Iowa State University Press, Ames, Iowa, 1977, pp. 80–83.

R.F. Tarrant and J. Allard. Arsenic levels in urine of forest workers applying silvicides. Arch. Env. Health 24: 277–280, 1972.

D.G. Taylor (ed.). *NIOSH Manual of Analytical Methods*, 2nd ed., Vol. 1, National Institute for Occupational Safety and Health, Cincinnati, 1977, pp. 140–141.

D.T. Teitelbaum and L.C. Kier. Arsine poisoning. Arch. Env. Health 19: 133–143, 1969.

N. Thiex. Solvent extraction and flameless atomic absorption determination of arsenic in biological materials. J. Asso. Off. Anal. Chem. 63: 496–499, 1980.

J.L. Valentine, H.K. Kang and G. Spivey. Arsenic levels in human blood, urine, and hair in response to exposure via drinking water. Env. Res. 20: 24–32, 1979.

S.L. Wagner and P. Weswig. Arsenic in blood and urine of forest workers. Arch. Env. Health 28: 77–79, 1974.

A. Wyttenbach, P. Barthe and E.P. Martin. The content of arsenic in the hair in a case of acute lethal arsenic poisoning. J. For. Sci. Soc. 7: 194–197, 1967.

Atenolol

T½: 4–12 hr
Vd: 1.3 L/kg
Fb: 0.05
pKa: 9.6

CH_2CONH_2

$OCH_2CHOHCH_2NHCH(CH_3)_2$

Occurrence and Usage. Atenolol (ICI-66082, Tenormin) is a cardioselective beta-blocking agent that has been used in the treatment of hypertension in the United States since about 1982. Single oral doses of 25–100 mg of the free base are administered, with chronic daily intake ranging from 100–400 mg. The drug is also available as a 5 mg/10 mL solution for intravenous infusion in acute care situations.

Blood Concentrations. Plasma atenolol reached average peak concentrations of 0.14, 0.28, and 0.65 mg/L within 2–3 hours of a single oral dose of 25, 50, or 100 mg, respectively, in 12 subjects. A 50 mg dose given as a 12 minute intravenous infusion produced an average peak plasma level of 2–3 mg/L measured after the end of the infusion. The concentrations declined with an average half-life of 6 hours, and the kinetics of the drug were best explained using a 3-compartment model with predominantly renal elimination from the central compartment (Mason et al., 1979). During chronic oral administration of 100 mg daily, peak plasma concentrations averaged 0.54 mg/L in patients with normal renal function and 1.49 mg/L in those with severe renal impairment; the average elimination half-lives in these 2 patient groups were 9.2 and 36.8 hours, respectively (Kirch et al., 1981). Chronic daily doses of 300 or 600 mg of atenolol resulted in average peak blood concentrations of 1.48 and 2.75 mg/L, respectively, in 35 patients; the degree of beta-blockade correlated with the blood levels of the drug (Amery et al., 1977).

Metabolism and Excretion. Only 46–62% of an oral dose of atenolol is absorbed, even when administered as a solution. Over a 24 hour period, an average of 36% of a dose is eliminated (unabsorbed) in feces and 39% in urine. Approximately 88% of the urinary excretion products were

$HOCHCONH_2$

$OCH_2CHOHCH_2NHCH(CH_3)_2$
hydroxyatenolol

CH_2CONH_2

$OCH_2CHOHCH_2NHCH(CH_3)_2$
atenolol

⟶ glucuronide conjugation

accounted for by unchanged atenolol, with another 2% as atenolol glucuronide. Hydroxyatenolol, only one-tenth as active as its parent, was identified as a minor (2–3%) urinary metabolite. From 70–77% of a single intravenous dose appears in the 24 hour urine, mostly as parent drug (Reeves et al., 1978).

Toxicity. Side-effects of atenolol include dizziness, nausea, bradycardia and hypotension. In overdosage it causes bronchoconstriction, hypotension, and cardiac failure. Individuals have survived the acute ingestion of as much as 5 g of the drug. A 52 year old woman who self-administered an unknown dose developed a blood atenolol concentration of 2.6 mg/L; her bradycardia and hypotension were successfully treated with supportive measures (Gerkin and Curry, 1987).

Analysis. Atenolol has been measured in biological fluids by electron-capture gas chromatography after derivatization (Scales and Copsey, 1975; Ervik et al., 1980), or liquid chromatography (Yee et al., 1979; Bhamra et al., 1983; Miller and Greenblatt, 1986; Alebic-Kolbah et al., 1989; Morris et al., 1991).

References

T. Alebic-Kolbah, F. Plavsic and A. Wolf-Coporda. Determination of serum atenolol using HPLC with forensic detection following solation with activated charcoal. J. Pharm. Biomed. Anal. 7: 1777–1781, 1989.

A. Amery, J. De Plaen, P. Lijnen et al. Relationship between blood level of atenolol and pharmacologic effect. Clin. Pharm. Ther. 21: 691–699, 1977.

R.K. Bhamra, K.J. Thorley, J.A. Vale and D.W. Holt. High-performance liquid chromatographic measurement of atenolol: methodology and clinical applications. Ther. Drug Mon. 5: 313–318, 1983.

M. Ervik, K. Klyberg-Hanssen and P. Lagerstrom. Electron-capture-gas chromatographic determination of atenolol in plasma and urine, using a simplified procedure with improved selectivity. J. Chrom. 182: 341–347, 1980.

R. Gerkin and S. Curry. Significant bradycardia following acute self-poisoning with atenolol. Vet. Hum. Tox. 29: 479, 1987.

W. Kirch, H. Koehler, E. Mutschler and M. Schaefer. Pharmacokinetics of atenolol in relation to renal function. Eur. J. Clin. Pharm. 19: 65–71, 1981.

W.D. Mason, N. Winer, G. Kochak et al. Kinetics and absolute bioavailability of atenolol. Clin. Pharm. Ther. 25: 408–415, 1979.

L.G. Miller and D.J. Greenblatt. Determination of atenolol in plasma by high-performance liquid chromatography with application to single-dose pharmacokinetics. J. Chrom. 381: 201–204, 1986.

R.G. Morris, N.C. Saccoia, B.C. Sallustio and R. Zacest. Improved high-performance liquid chromatography assay for atenolol in plasma and urine using fluorescence detection. Ther. Drug Mon. 13: 345–349, 1991.

P.R. Reeves, J. McAinsh, D.A.D. McIntosh and M.J. Winrow. Metabolism of atenolol in man. Xenobiotica 8: 313–320, 1978.

B. Scales and P.B. Copsey. The gas chromatographic determination of atenolol in biological samples. J. Pharm. Pharmac. 27: 430–433, 1975.

Y. Yee, P. Rubin and T.F. Blaschke. Atenolol determination by high-performance liquid chromatography and fluorescence detection. J. Chrom. 171: 357–362, 1979.

Atracurium

T½: 17–26 min
Vd: 0.14–0.29 L/kg
Fb: ?
pKa: ?

Occurrence and Usage. Atracurium (Tracrium) is a non-depolarizing skeletal muscle relaxant used to facilitate endotracheal intubation and to provide skeletal muscle relaxation during surgery or mechanical ventilation. Atracurium is available as a 10 mg/mL solution of the besylate salt for intravenous administration. A 0.4–0.5 mg/kg intravenous bolus injection is the recommended initial dose for most patients.

Blood Concentrations. In 8 normal patients following injection of 0.5 mg/kg of atracurium, an average plasma concentration of 9.7 mg/L was measured 2 minutes following injection, dropping to 0.2 mg/L in 60 minutes (deBros et al., 1986). Following intravenous infusion of 15.8 µg/kg/min of atracurium for 6–11 minutes to anesthetized patients of all ages, the mean steady-state plasma concentration in infants was 0.36 mg/L; in children, 0.44 mg/L; and in adults, 0.43 mg/L (Fisher et al., 1990). In a study of 20 adults undergoing major surgery, atracurium was infused to maintain 90% paralysis; steady-state plasma concentrations ranged from 0.73–1.47 mg/L (average, 1.13) (Beemer et al., 1990).

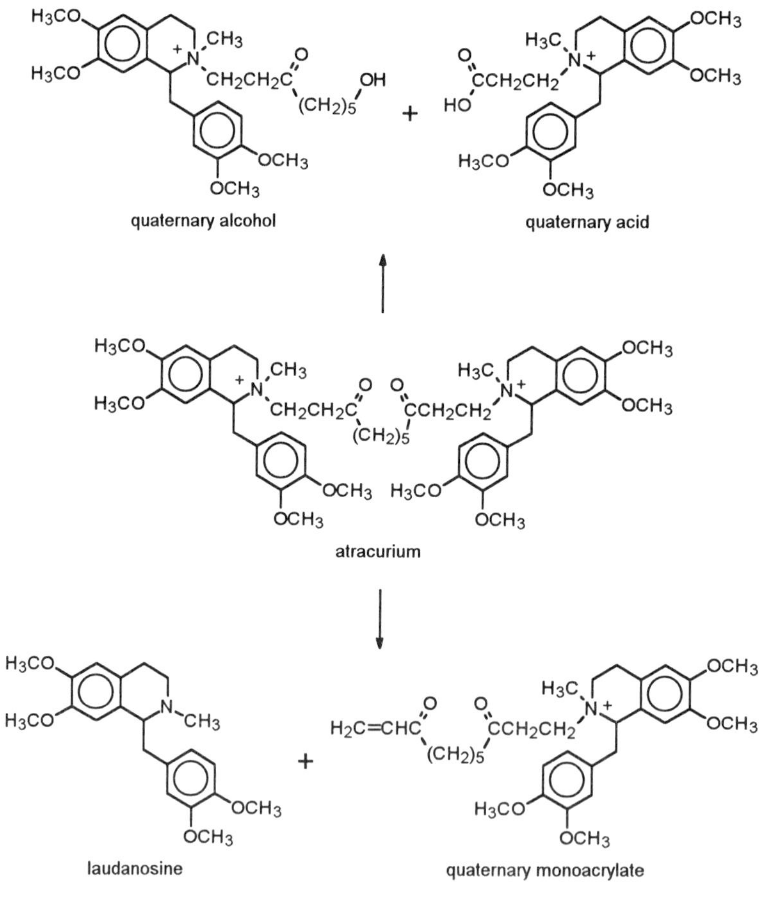

quaternary alcohol   quaternary acid

atracurium

laudanosine   quaternary monoacrylate

Metabolism and Excretion. Atracurium is biotransformed via enzymatic and nonenzymatic hydrolysis, by which the quaternary alcohol and acid are formed, in combination with a spontaneous temperature and pH-dependent degradation pathway, yielding laudanosine and an acrylate moiety (Stenlake et al., 1983; Vandenbrom et al., 1990).

Biliary and urinary excretion account for 90% of a radioactive dose in 7 hours, with parent drug representing only a minor fraction. Vandenbrom et al. (1990) found that 11% of a single dose is excreted unchanged in the urine within 19 hours.

Toxicity. Adverse effects from atracurium include itching, wheezing, hives, bronchospasm, laryngospasm, prolonged neuromuscular block, hypotension, anaphylactic reaction, respiratory failure, and death.

Analysis. Since atracurium contains 2 quaternary amine functions, it will neither extract into nonpolar organic liquids nor chromatograph on most gas chromatographic columns. Liquid chromatography, however, lends itself to the analysis of the compound in biological fluids (Neill and Jones, 1983; Uges et al., 1984; Stiller et al., 1985; Schopfer and Benakis, 1990; Vandenbrom et al., 1990; Varin et al., 1990).

References

G.H. Beemer, A.R. Bjorksten, and D.P. Crankshaw. Pharmacokinetics of atracurium during continuous infusion. Brit. J. Anaesth. 65: 668–674, 1990.

F.M. deBros, A. Lai, R. Scott et al. Pharmacokinetics and pharmacodynamics of atracurium during isoflurane anesthesia in normal and anephric patients. Anesth. Anal. 65: 743–746, 1986.

D.M. Fisher, P.C. Canfell, M.J. Spellman, and R.D. Miller. Pharmacokinetics and pharmacodynamics of atracurium in infants and children. Anesthesiology 73: 33–37, 1990.

E.A.M. Neill and C.R. Jones. Determination of atracurium in plasma by HPLC. J. Chrom. 274: 409–412, 1983.

C. Schopfer and A. Benakis. Simplified method for the determination of atracurium and laudanoside in pig plasma by high performance liquid chromatography and fluorimetric detection. J. Chrom. 526: 223–227, 1990.

J.B. Stenlake, R.D. Waigh, J. Urwin et al. Atracurium: conception and inception. Brit. J. Anaesthesia 55: 3S–10S, 1983.

R.L. Stiller, B.W. Brandom and D.R. Cook. Determination of atracurium in plasma by high-performance liquid chromatography. Anesth. Anal. 54: 58, 1985.

D.R.A. Uges, H. Bloemhof and S. Agoston. The determination of atracurium and its metabolite laudanosine in serum by HPLC. Pharm. Weekblad 6: 265, 1984.

R.H.G. Vandenbrom, J.M.K.H. Wieda and S. Agoston. Pharmacokinetics and neuromuscular blocking effects of atracurium besylate and two of its metabolites in patients with normal and impaired renal function. Clin. Pharmacokin. 19: 230–240, 1990.

F. Varin, J. Ducharme, J.G. Besner and Y. Theoret. Determination of atracurium and laudanosine in human plasma by high-performance liquid chromatography. J. Chrom. 529: 319–328, 1990.

Atropine

T½: 2–3 hr
Vd: 2.3–3.6 L/kg
Fb: 0.18
pKa: 9.8

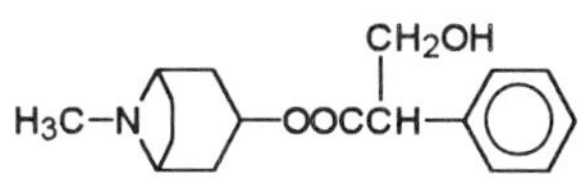

Occurrence and Usage. Atropine (dl-hyoscyamine) is an alkaloid derived from certain plants, especially *Atropa belladonna* (deadly nightshade) and *Datura stramonium* (Jimson weed), which also contain scopolamine. It is a potent anticholinergic agent, with nearly all the pharmacological activity being attributed to the l-isomer (hyoscyamine), and has been used for centuries as a drug and poison.

Atropine is available as the sulfate salt in the form of tablets, capsules, injectable solutions and ophthalmic solutions. It is also found combined with diphenoxylate, a narcotic analgesic, to help prevent abuse of that drug. Atropine is used as a preanesthetic medication to reduce salivary and bronchial secretions, for relaxation of the gastrointestinal tract in certain spastic conditions, as an antidote to poisoning by cholinesterase inhibitors, and to produce mydriasis in ophthalmic procedures. Oral doses of 0.5–1.0 mg and intramuscular or intravenous doses of 0.4–0.6 mg are frequently used for routine purposes, but treatment of anticholinesterase poisoning may require hourly doses of 1–6 mg.

Blood Concentrations. Three volunteers given 0.32 mg intravenous doses of atropine exhibited initial plasma concentrations (by radioimmunoassay) as high as 0.070 mg/L, very rapidly declining to about 0.002 mg/L within 5 minutes; thereafter, the levels declined with a half-life of 2–3 hours (Hayden et al., 1979). Atropine blood concentrations (by bioassay) in 14 pregnant women given 0.0125 mg/kg (0.875 mg/70 kg) of the drug by intravenous injection averaged 0.035 mg/L after 2–3 minutes, 0.009 mg/L after 5–9 minutes, and 0.005 mg/L after 20–33 minutes (Onnen et al., 1979). Serum concentrations (by radioimmunoassay) in 6 subjects receiving 1 mg intravenously averaged over 0.200 mg/L within the first few minutes and fell to 0.005 mg/L by 20 minutes; 4 subjects who were given a 1 mg intramuscular dose achieved an average peak serum concentration of 0.003 mg/L by 30 minutes, with a decline to 0.002 mg/L by 2 hours (Berghem et al., 1980). The elimination half-life of atropine is increased in young children (average, 4.8 hours) and in the elderly (average, 10 hours) (Virtanen et al., 1982).

Metabolism and Excretion. Up to 93% of a single dose of labeled atropine is eliminated in the 24 hour urine (Kalser and McLain, 1970). Approximately 50% of a dose is excreted as unchanged drug after intravenous injection, 30% after intramuscular administration, and only about 13% after oral administration. About 24% of a dose is present in urine as noratropine, 15% as atropine-N-oxide, 3% as tropic acid and 2% as tropine (Tonnesen, 1950; Gosselin et al., 1960; Kalser, 1971; Van der Meer et al., 1986).

Toxicity. As little as 1–2 mg of atropine produces toxic symptoms in hypersensitive individuals; systemic toxicity has developed even after the therapeutic use of a 1% atropine ophthalmic solution (German and Siddiqui, 1970). In most persons, atropine doses exceeding 10 mg cause moderate to severe symptoms of toxicity, and doses greater than 50 mg can be fatal. Physostigmine is a specific antidote for both the central and peripheral effects of the drug. A 20 year old male who ingested 500 mg of atropine in a suicide attempt exhibited tachycardia, hypertension, fever, delerious behavior, and pulmonary edema; he recovered with supportive treatment after 2–3 days (Comroe, 1933). Similar effects may be observed in persons who ingest or smoke Jimson weed, a plant that is found throughout much of the United States (Rodgers and Van Kanel, 1993). A pharmacy student who may have ingested up to 1 g of atropine while under the influence of alcohol developed a serum atropine level of 0.13 mg/L; he survived with physostigmine administration and supportive care (Michelson et al., 1991).

An 18 year old male who died after ingesting an unknown number of 30 mg atropine tablets for recreational purposes was found to have postmortem blood and urine atropine concentrations of 0.2 and 1.5 mg/L, respectively (Corbett, 1978).

Analysis. Atropine has been analyzed in biological specimens by extraction and bioassay (Tonnesen, 1948; Onnen et al., 1979), by radioimmunoassay (Wurzburger et al., 1977) and by radioreceptor assay (Ensing et al., 1987). Gas chromatography employing flame-ionization (Corbett, 1978), electron-capture (Green, 1982) or mass spectrometric detection (Eckert and Hinderling, 1981; Palmer et al., 1981; Saady and Poklis, 1989) has also been performed. Liquid chromatographic methods have employed fluorescence (Li and Khalil, 1990) or ultraviolet detection (Okuda et al., 1991).

References

L. Berghem, U. Bergman, B. Schildt and B. Sorbo. Plasma atropine concentrations determined by radioimmunoassay after single-dose i.v. and i.m. administration. Brit. J. Anaesth. 52: 597–601, 1980.

B.I. Comroe. Atropine poisoning: recovery after 7% grains of atropine sulphate by mouth. J. Am. Med. Asso. 101: 446–447, 1933.

B.W. Corbett. Personal communication, 1978.

M. Eckert and P.H. Hinderling. Atropine: a sensitive gas chromatography-mass spectrometry assay and prepharmacokinetic studies. Agents Actions 11: 520–545, 1981.

K. Ensing, R.A. deZeeuw, V. Hornchen et al. Detection of atropine in plasma by a direct radioreceptor assay. Pharm. Weekblad 9: 321–323, 1987.

E. German and N. Siddiqui. Atropine toxicity from eyedrops. New Eng. J. Med. 282: 689, 1970.

R.E. Gosselin, J.D. Gabourel and J.H. Wills. The fate of atropine in man. Clin. Pharm. Ther. 1: 597–603, 1960.

M.D. Green. Determination of atropine through an electron capture gas chromatographic procedure. Proc. West. Pharm. Soc. 25: 15–17, 1982.

P.W. Hayden, S.M. Larson and S. Lakshminarayanan. Atropine clearance from human plasma. J. Nucl. Med. 20: 366–367, 1979.

S.C. Kalser. The fate of atropine in man. Ann. N.Y. Acad. Sci. 179: 667–683, 1971.

S.C. Kalser and P.L. McLain. Atropine metabolism in man. Clin. Pharm. Ther. 11: 214–227, 1970.

S. Li and S.K.W. Khalil. An HPLC method for detection of atropine in human plasma. J. Liq. Chrom. 13: 1339–1350, 1990.

E.A. Michaelson, S.M. Schneider and T.G. Martin. Adult inadvertent massive oral atropine overdose. Vet. Hum Tox. 33: 360, 1991.

T. Okuda, M. Nishida, I. Sameshima et al. Detection of atropine in biological specimens by high-performance liquid chromatography. J. Chrom. 567: 141–149, 1991.

I. Onnen, G. Barrier, S. Sureau and G. Olive. Placental transfer of atropine at the end of pregnancy. Eur. J. Clin. Pharm. 15: 443–446, 1979.

L. Palmer, J. Edgar, G. Lundgren et al. Atropine in mouse brain and plasma quantified by mass fragmentography. Acta Pharm. Tox. 49: 72–76, 1981.

G.C. Rodgers and R.L. Von Kanel. Conservative treatment of Jimsonweed ingestion. Vet. Hum. Tox. 35: 32–33, 1993.

J.J. Saady and A. Poklis. Determination of atropine in blood by gas chromatography/mass spectrometry. J. Anal. Tox. 13: 296–299, 1989.

M. Tonnesen. Chemical and biological methods for determination of small concentrations of atropine and allied alkaloids in forensic analyses. Acta Pharm. 4: 186–198, 1948.

M. Tonnesen. The excretion of atropine and allied alkaloids in urine. Acta Pharm. 6: 147–164, 1950.

M.J. Van der Meer, H.K.L. Hundt and F.O. Muller. The metabolism of atropine in man. J. Pharm. Pharmac. 38: 781–784, 1986.

R.J. Wurzburger, R.L. Miller, H.G. Boxenbaum and S. Spector. Radioimmunoassay of atropine in plasma. J. Pharm. Exp. Ther. 203: 435–441, 1977.

R. Virtanen, J. Kanto, E. Iisalo et al. Pharmacokinetic studies on atropine with special reference to age. Acta Anaesth. Scand. 26: 297–300, 1982.

Azide

T½: ?
Vd: ?   N₃⁻
Fb: ?
pKa: 4.7

Occurrence and Usage. Hydrazoic acid (hydrogen azide, triazoic acid) and its sodium and lead salts are used industrially in the manufacture of explosives and as preservatives for diagnostic reagents. Sodium azide was at one time was investigated as a potential antihypertensive agent in oral doses of 0.01–0.03 mg/kg. Hydrazoic acid is a flammable and volatile liquid (b.p., 37° C.) with a characteristic pungent odor. The current threshold limit value for sodium azide in air is 0.3 mg/m³.

Blood Concentrations. Azide concentrations in blood or serum of persons receiving the drug therapeutically, or in workers occupationally exposed to the chemical, have not been reported. Single oral sodium azide doses of 0.7–1.3 mg causes a rapid fall in blood pressure that lasts 10–15 minutes (Graham, 1949). Hypertensive patients receiving daily oral sodium azide doses of 0.7–3.9 mg for up to 2.5 years exhibited no adverse effects other than headache (Black et al., 1954).

Metabolism and Excretion. Little is known of the fate of azide in the human body.

Toxicity. Azide is considered to have a degree of toxicity similar to that of cyanide and, like that ion, is believed to cause many of its toxic effects through the inhibition of cytochrome oxidase. Acutely, inhalation of the vapor or ingestion of the salt can initially produce respiratory stimulation and tachycardia, followed by metabolic acidosis, hypotension, respiratory depression, bradycardia, convulsions and death. Five laboratory workers who accidentally ingested 20–80 mg of sodium azide developed symptoms lasting 2 hours and ranging from faintness to severe chest pains (Edmonds and Bourne, 1982). A patient accidentally administered 50–60 mg of sodium azide orally collapsed, briefly lost consciousness and complained of a severe headache lasting overnight (Richardson et al., 1975). Chemists preparing acidified sodium azide solutions have inhaled sufficient hydrazoic acid to cause dizziness, weakness, faintness, cough and shortness of breath (Reinhardt and Brittelli, 1981; Senecal et al., 1991).

An adult male died about 30 hours afrer oral ingestion of 10–20 g of sodium acide, despite resuscitative efforts (Albertson et al., 1986). An individual accidentally administered 700–800 mg of sodium azide orally at first exhibited nausea, vomiting, diarrhea and confusion, but her condition gradually worsened to include cardiac arrhythmia, seizures, hypotension and respiratory distress; she died 3.5 days after the incident with a urine azide level of 0.14 mg/L (Howard et al. 1990). A male student found dead after apparent intentional oral ingestion of sodium azide had a postmortem blood azide level of 40 mg/L (Peclet, 1991).

Analysis. Azide may be analyzed in biological specimens using the microdiffusion process often employed for the isolation of cyanide, followed by detection either by ultraviolet spectrometry at 214 nm or colorimetry using ferric chloride (Reinhardt and Britelli, 1981). Liquid chromtography has also been described (Swarin and Waldo, 1982).

References

T.E. Albertson, S. Reed and A. Siefkin. A case of fatal sodium azide ingestion. Clin. Tox. 24: 339–351, 1986.

M.M. Black, B.W. Sweifach and F.D. Speer. Comparison of hypotensive action of sodium azide in hypertensive patients. Proc. Soc. Exp. Biol. Med. 85: 11–16, 1954.

O.P. Edmonds and M.S. Bourne. Sodium azide poisoning in five laboratory technicians. Brit. J. Ind. Med. 39: 308–309, 1982.

J.D.P. Graham. Actions of sodium azide. Brit. J. Pharm. 4: 1–6, 1949.

J.D. Howard, K.J. Skogerboe, G.A. Case et al. Death following accidental sodium azide ingestion. J. For. Sci. 35: 193–196, 1990.

C. Peclet. Personal communication, 1991.

C.F. Reinhardt and M.R. Brittelli. Heterocyclic and miscellaneous nitrogen compounds. In *Patty's Industrial Hygiene and Toxicology*, Vol. IIA (G.D. Clayton and F.E. Clayton, eds.), Wiley & Sons, New York, 1981, pp. 2778–2784.

S.C.N. Richardson, C. Giles and C.H.J. Swan. Two cases of sodium azide poisoning by accidental ingestion of Isoton. J. Clin. Path. 28: 350–351, 1975.

P.E. Senecal, J.E. Dyer, J.D. Osterloh and K.R. Olson. Toxic volatile hydrazoic acid (HN_3) from contact of sodium azide (NaN_3) with acids. Vet. Hum. Tox. 33: 364, 1991.

S.J. Swarin and R.A. Waldo. Liquid chromatographic determination of azide as the 3-5-dinitrobenzoyl derivative. J. Liq. Chrom. 5: 597–604, 1982.

Baclofen

T½: 2.5–4.0 hr
Vd: ?
Fb: 0.30
pKa: 3.9, 9.6

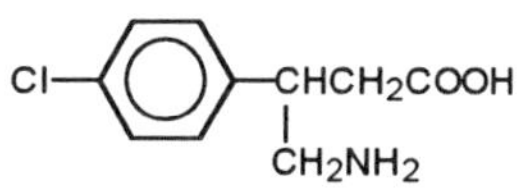

Occurrence and Usage. Baclofen (Atrofen, Lioresal) is an analog of the putative inhibitory neurotransmitter gamma-aminobutyric acid (GABA). It is used for the alleviation of signs and symptoms of spasticity resulting from multiple sclerosis. The dosage titration schedule is 5 mg 3 times a day for 3 days, increasing by 5 mg every 3 days until the desired effect is achieved. The total daily dose should not exceed 80 mg. Baclofen is available in tablets containing 10–20 mg of the free acid for oral administration.

Blood Concentrations. After a single oral dose of 40 mg to 1 subject, a peak plasma concentration of 0.6 mg/L of baclofen was attained in 2 hours (Faigle and Keberle, 1972). Following single doses of 15–90 mg, trough plasma baclofen concentrations ranging from 0.1–0.4 mg/L have been reported (Nugent et al., 1986).

Metabolism and Excretion. Approximately 15% of a dose is deaminated to β–(p-chlorophenyl)-α–hydroxybutyric acid in the liver. Elimination of baclofen is primarily renal with 85% of the dose excreted unchanged in the urine. Trace amounts of the drug may be excreted in the feces. About 40% of the dose is usually excreted within 6 hours and excretion is generally complete within 72 hours (Nugent et al., 1986).

Toxicity. Acute intoxication with baclofen causes drowsiness, dizziness, confusion, palpitation, diplopia, seizures, respiratory depression and coma. Nonfatal overdoses have involved blood levels of 1.1–3.5 mg/L.

In a fatal case attributed to baclofen overdose in an adult male, serum and urine concentrations measured in hospital admission specimens were 17 and 760 mg/L, respectively (Fraser et al., 1991).

Analysis. Baclofen has been detected in plasma and urine following fluorescent derivatization by thin-layer chromatography (Krauss et al., 1988). Liquid chromatography appears to be the method of choice in the determination of baclofen in biological specimens (Wuis et al., 1987; Sallerin-Caute et al., 1988; Spahn et al., 1988; Wall and Baker, 1989; Fraser et al., 1991). Gas chromatography-mass spectrometry has also been described (Fraser et al., 1991).

References

J.W. Faigle and H. Keberle. The chemistry and kinetics of Llioresal. Postgrad. Med. J. 48 (Suppl): 9–13, 1972.

A.D. Fraser, W. MacNeil and A.F. Isner. Toxicological analysis of a fatal baclofen (Lioresal) ingestion. J. For. Sci. 36: 1596–1602, 1991.

D. Krauss, H. Spahn and E. Mutschler. Quantification of baclofen and its fluoro analogue in plasma and urine after fluorescent derivatisation with benoxaprofen chloride and thin-layer chromatographic separation. Arz. Forsch. 38: 1533–1536, 1988.

S. Nugent, M.D. Katz and T.E. Little. Baclofen overdose with cardiac conduction abnormalities: case report and review of the literature. Clin. Tox. 24: 321–328, 1986.

B. Sallerin-Caute, B. Monsarrat, Y. Lazorthes et al. A sensitive method for the determination of baclofen in human CSF by high performance liquid chromatography. J. Liq. Chrom. 11: 1753–1761, 1988.

H. Spahn, D. Krauss and E. Mutschler. Enantiospecific high-performance liquid chromatographic (HPLC) determination of baclofen and its fluoro analogue in biological material. Pharm. Res. 5: 107–112, 1988.

G.M. Wall and J.K. Baker. Determination of baclofen and α-baclofen in rat liver homogenate and human urine using solid-phase extraction, o-phthalaldehyde-tert-butyl thiol derivatization and high-performance liquid chromatography with amperometric detection. J. Chrom. 491: 151–162, 1989.

E.W. Wuis, L.E.C. Van Beijsterveldt, R.J.M. Dirks et al. Rapid simultaneous determination of baclofen and its α-hydroxymetabolite in urine by high-performance liquid chromatography with ultraviolet detection. J. Chrom. 420: 212–216, 1987.

Barbital

T½: 2 days
Vd: 0.4–0.6 L/kg
Fb: 0.25
pKa: 7.8

Occurrence and Usage. The 5,5-diethyl derivative of barbituric acid is known as barbital, a compound that was prepared in 1903 and was once used frequently as a sedative and hypnotic. It is no longer therapeutically available in the United States, but is a common constituent of buffer solutions in laboratories and is occasionally abused.

Blood Concentrations. Following a single oral dose of 1500 mg administered to 4 subjects, an average peak plasma level of 26 mg/L (range, 21–31) was found at 12 hours and this declined to 21 mg/L (range, 19–23) by 36 hours (Lous, 1954a). Plasma barbital concentrations were found to decline with a half-life of approximately 2 days in 1 volunteer (Varin et al., 1980).

Metabolism and Excretion. Barbital is believed to undergo negligible, if any, metabolism in man. After a single dose 33% is excreted unchanged in the urine within 2 days, and up to 95% by 13 days. Traces of the drug are still found in the urine 16 days after a single 300 mg dose (Lous, 1954a; Svendsen and Brochmann-Hanssen, 1962).

Toxicity. The minimum lethal dose of barbital in man is estimated as 2 g, although a subject has survived the ingestion of 22 g with treatment; a plasma concentration of 500 mg/L and urine concentration of 240 mg/L were observed in this case, which was treated by charcoal hemoperfusion (Yatzidis et al., 1965). Serum concentrations of 43–1202 mg/L were observed in 8 persons suffering from barbital intoxication; the comatose individuals were able to be aroused after their serum levels had fallen below 160 mg/L. In one patient the serum half-life of the drug was estimated to be 46.5 hours (Bailey and Jatlow, 1975). Other cases of clinical intoxication reviewed by the previous authors indicated that subjects with grade IV coma exhibited serum barbital concentrations of 412–685 mg/L (average, 387).

The blood concentrations in fatal cases have ranged from 100–579 mg/L (Lous, 1954b; Solomons, 1975; Oram, 1984). In 3 fatalities, the blood concentrations averaged 133 mg/L (range, 90–225) and the liver, 509 mg/kg (range, 108–932). The following tissue distribution was found in 2 of those cases (Cravey, 1975):

Barbital Tissue Distribution in Fatal Cases (mg/L or mg/kg)

Blood	Brain	Lung	Liver	Kidney
90	63	127	108	142
225	380	932	320	

Analysis. Barbital may be assayed in biological specimens using many of the techniques described under amobarbital.

References

D.N. Bailey and P.I. Jatlow. Barbital overdose and abuse. Am. J. Clin. Path. 64: 291–296, 1975.

R.H. Cravey. Personal communication, 1975.

P. Lous. Plasma levels and urinary excretion of three barbituric acids after oral administration to man. Acta Pharm. Tox. 10: 147–165, 1954a.

P. Lous. Barbituric acid concentration in serum from patients with severe acute poisoning. Acta Pharm. Tox. 10: 261–280, 1954b.

J. Oram. Personal communication, 1984.

E.T. Solomons. Personal communication, 1975.

A.B. Svendsen and E. Brochmann-Hanssen. Gas chromatography of barbiturates II. Application to the study of their metabolism and excretion in humans. J. Pharm. Sci. 51: 494–495, 1962.

F. Varin, C. Marchand, P. Larochelle and K.K. Midha. GLC-mass spectrometric procedure with selected-ion monitoring for determination of plasma concentrations of unlabeled and labeled barbital following simultaneous oral and intravenous administration. J. Pharm. Sci. 69: 640–643, 1980.

H. Yatzidis, S. Voudiclari, D. Oreopoulos et al. Treatment of severe barbiturate poisoning. Lancet 2: 216–217, 1965.

Barium

T½: 3.6 days
Vd: ?
Fb: ?

Ba

Occurrence and Usage. Inorganic compounds of barium are utilized in industry as pigments and dyes and for numerous miscellaneous applications. The sulfide has been used in depilatories, and the water-insoluble sulfate is currently employed in clinical medicine as an X-ray contrast agent in the diagnosis of gastrointestinal tract disorders. Industrial exposure to the compounds is usually via inhalation and rarely by oral ingestion. The current threshold limit value for soluble barium salts in the industrial atmosphere is 0.5 mg/m^3 (expressed as barium).

Blood Concentrations. Barium is present in trace amounts in all human tissues and some studies indicate that it is an element essential to proper growth. Gooddy et al. (1975) showed that normal human blood concentrations by arc spectrography range from 0.08–0.40 mg/L, although by plasma emission spectrometry the values in 13 healthy subjects were less than 0.001 mg/L (Mauras and Allain, 1979).

Metabolism and Excretion. The tissue distribution of absorbed barium is best described by a 3 compartment model, with half-lives of 3.6, 34 and 1033 days (Rundo, 1967). About 90% of the total body burden is contained in bone. The predominant route of excretion is via the feces, with renal elimination accounting for a relatively minor portion (less than 3%) of a dose. Unexposed persons excrete from 0.006–0.022 mg/day in the urine according to Sutton and Shepherd (1973), while Mauras and Allain (1979) found normal urine to contain an average of 0.004 mg/L. The following tissue concentrations were determined in normal humans (Schroeder et al., 1972):

Barium Concentrations in Normal Tissues (mg/kg)

Brain	Lung	Heart	Liver	Kidney	Bone
0.004	0.160	0.009	0.003	0.016	2.0

Toxicity. Inhalation of insoluble barium compounds may result in a benign pneumoconiosis, known as baritosis. This occurs chiefly in workers involved in the processing of barium ores. The inhalation or ingestion of soluble salts in toxic amounts produces gastroenteritis, ventricular fibrillation and muscular paralysis. The lethal dose for such compounds is estimated at from 1–15 g, and death may be expected to occur rapidly or after several days. Serious hypokalemia occurs in barium poisoning; its reversal by intravenous administration of potassium appears to accelerate recovery (Diengott et al., 1964; Gould et al., 1973).

In 1 case of accidental barium poisoning (apparently nonfatal), a blood concentration of 0.26 mg/L and a urine concentration of 0.28 mg/L were observed (Mauras and Allain, 1979). In 2 cases of intentional but nonfatal poisoning with barium chloride or barium carbonate, serum barium concentrations of 3.4 and 7.8 mg/L were measured (Phelan et al., 1984; Boehnert et al., 1985).

Two individuals who died 14 and 31 hours after the suicidal ingestion of barium sulfide had barium levels of 132 and 141 mg/kg in liver and 160 and 162 mg/kg in kidney (Jobba and Rengei, 1971). Several patients who died within a few hours of accidental administration of a soluble barium salt during a diagnostic procedure had liver and kidney barium concentrations in the neighborhood of 1200–2120 mg/kg (Baisane et al., 1979). An adult who died within hours of ingesting 11.5 g of barium as the sulfide exhibited the following tissue concentrations (Suero et al., 1987):

Barium Concentrations in a Fatal Case (mg/L or mg/kg)

Blood	Brain	Liver	Bile	Spleen	Kidney	Vitreous
1.9	0.4	1.6	6.1	5.9	7.5	0.5

Analysis. Barium may be determined in biological specimens by colorimetry (Chou and Chin, 1943), arc spectrography (Baisane et al., 1979), and atomic absorption spectrometry (Berman, 1980). Methods for wet and dry ashing of specimens were cited in the section on arsenic.

References

S.O. Baisane, V.S. Chincholkar and B.N. Mattoo. Spectrographic determination of barium in biological material. For. Sci. Int. 12: 127–129, 1979.

E. Berman. *Toxic Metals and Their Analysis*, Heyden, London, 1980, pp. 44–47.

M. Boehnert, N. Shore, R. Timperi and F.H. Lovejoy. Measurement of serum levels in acute barium chloride overdose. Vet. Hum. Tox. 28: 291, 1985.

C. Chou and Y.C. Chin. The absorption, fate and concentration in serum of barium in acute experimental poisoning. Chin. Med. J. 61: 313–322, 1943.

D. Diengott, O. Rozsa, N. Levy and S. Muammar. Hypokalaemia in barium poisoning. Lancet 2: 343–344, 1964.

W. Gooddy, E.I. Hamilton and T.R. Williams. Spark-source mass spectrometry in the investigation of neurological disease. Brain 98: 65–70, 1975.

D.B. Gould, M.R. Sorrell, and A.D. Lupariello. Barium sulfide poisoning. Arch. Int. Med. 132: 891–894,
1973.

G. Jobba and B. Rengei. Ueber die Neopol-Vergiftung. Arch. Tox. 27: 106–110, 1971.

Y. Mauras and P. Allain. Dosage du baryum dans l'eau et les liquides biologiques par spectrometrie d'emission
avec source plasma haute frequence. Anal. Clin. Acta 110: 271–177, 1979.

D.M. Phelan, S.R. Hagley and M.D. Guerin. Is hypokalemia the cause of paralysis in barium poisoning? Brit.
Med. J. 289: 882, 1984.

J. Rundo. The retention of barium-133 in man. Int. J. Radiat. Biol. 13: 301–302, 1967.

H.A. Schroeder, I.H. Tipton and A.P. Nason. Trace metals in man: strontium and barium. J. Chron. Dis. 25:
491–517, 1972.

M.E. Suero, M.I. Schaffer and L.W. Blum. Distribution of barium in postmortem tissues after a suicidal
ingestion of "Magic Shaving Powder" depilatory. Presented at the annual meeting of the American Academy of Forensic Sciences, San Diego, California, February 19, 1987.

A. Sutton and H. Shepherd. Urinary barium excretion in man and its reduction by alginate. Health Physics 25:
182–184, 1973.

Benzene

T½: 8 hr
Vd: ?
Fb: ?

Occurrence and Usage. Benzene is a common laboratory and industrial chemical that produces a
unique spectrum of acute and chronic toxic effects in man. It is found in gasoline, paint removers
and many commercial solvents. The recommended threshold limit value for benzene in the workplace is currently 10 ppm (32 mg/m³), and the chemical is listed as a potential carcinogen in man.
The odor threshold for the compound has been reported as 1–5 ppm in air.

Blood Concentrations. Blood benzene concentrations from environmental exposure in European
citizens average 0.2 µg/L in nonsmokers and 0.4–0.6 µg/L in smokers (Hajimiragha et al., 1989;
Brugnone et al., 1992). A 2 hour exposure to 25 ppm benzene produced an average maximal blood
benzene concentration of approximately 200 µg/L in 3 subjects, measured at the end of exposure
(Sato and Fujiwara, 1972). Blood benzene concentrations of 8–204 µg/L were observed in specimens collected near the end of the work day in 9 workers exposed to low levels of benzene (Braier
et al., 1981).

Metabolism and Excretion. Following human exposure to benzene, only about 12% of a dose is
exhaled unchanged by the lungs and about 0.1% is excreted unchanged in the urine. The remainder
is eventually metabolized in the liver to highly toxic oxidation products. The kinetics of benzene
elimination in man can be described by a 2 compartment open model, with half-lives of 1–3 hours
and 9–24 hours (Piotrowski, 1977). Since benzene is 20–50 times more soluble in fat than in other
tissues, adipose tissue may act as a third, deep compartment (Sato and Fujiwara, 1972). Within 48
hours, from 51–87% is excreted in the urine as phenol (Hunter and Blair, 1972), 6% as catechol,
and 2% as hydroquinone (Teisinger et al., 1952); these phenolic metabolites are eliminated largely
in conjugated form. Other minor metabolites include 1,2,4-trihydroxybenzene, muconic acid,
phenylmercapturic acid and carbon dioxide (Parke and Williams, 1953).

Industrial exposure to benzene is sometimes monitored by determination of urinary phenol levels; normally, these levels are less then 10 mg/L in the nonexposed individual, they do not exceed
30 mg/L in persons chronically exposed to 0.5–4.0 ppm of benzene (Roush and Ott, 1977), and they
average 200 mg/L during exposure to 25 ppm (Walkley et al., 1961). Certain drugs such as Pepto-

Bismol and Chloraseptic are known to elevate urine phenol concentrations to as much as 270 mg/L, obscuring interpretation of urine monitoring results (Fishbeck et al., 1975). Another, older index of exposure is the urinary inorganic/organic sulfate ratio, normally at least 80%, but which drops to less than this figure during the excretion of sulfate-conjugated metabolites of benzene. Organic sulfates are also excreted in urine following the ingestion of phenolic drugs or certain foods (Hamilton and Hardy, 1974). Other means for monitoring exposure to benzene have included the measurement in urine of intact benzene (Ghittori et al., 1993), 1,2,4-trihydroxybenzene (Inoue et al., 1989), muconic acid (Bechtold et al., 1991) and phenylmercapturic acid (Jongeneelen et al., 1987).

Benzene in the breath of unexposed urban nonsmokers averaged 2.5 ppb and, in unexposed smokers, 6.8 ppb (Wester et al., 1986). Breath concentrations have been found to average 2 ppm at the end of a 4.5 hour sedentary exposure to 25 ppm of benzene, and averaged 0.2 ppm 16 hours later (Sherwood and Carter, 1970).

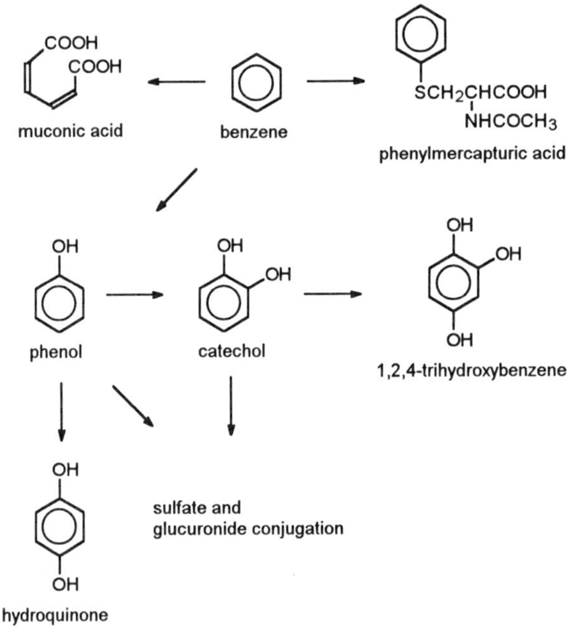

Toxicity. Chronic benzene poisoning is manifested by hematopoietic system injury and has been produced by occupational exposure to concentrations as low as 30 ppm. It is estimated that several hundred cases of fatal aplastic anemia due to chronic exposure to benzene at levels of 6–470 ppm occurred prior to 1963 (ACGIH, 1971). The acute toxic effects of benzene, however, are due either to central nervous system depression or to myocardial sensitization to epinephrine (Nahum and Hoff, 1934). Atmospheric concentrations of 7500 ppm may cause death within 30 minutes, and concentrations of 20,000 ppm may prove fatal within 5 minutes. The following tissue concentrations of benzene were observed in 8 acute fatalities due to inhalation or oral ingestion (Bonnichsen et al., 1966; Collom and Winek, 1970; Tauber, 1970; Winek and Collom, 1971; Alha, 1975; Avis and Hutton, 1993):

Benzene Concentrations in Fatal Cases (mg/L or mg/kg)

	Blood	Brain	Liver	Kidney	Urine	Gastric
Average	38	72	34	16	10	9 g
(Range)	(0.9–120)	(14–253)	(15–105)	(5.5–21)	(0.6–20)	(9)

Analysis. Benzene is frequently determined in blood and tissues by gas chromatography with headspace sampling (Collom and Winek, 1970; Angerer et al., 1973; Withey and Martin, 1974; Sato et al., 1975; Gruenke et al., 1986; Pekari et al., 1989) or after solvent extraction (Snyder et al., 1977; Jirka and Bourne, 1982). Losses of up to 48% of blood benzene have been noted after 1–2 days storage of specimens in rubber-stoppered (Collom and Winek, 1970) or plastic containers (Baselt, 1974). Urinary phenols have been conveniently determined colorimetrically (Walkley et al., 1961) or by gas chromatography (Van Haaften and Sie, 1965; Sherwood and Carter, 1970; Buchet et al., 1972; Baldwin et al., 1981; Van Roosmalen et al., 1981), and the urinary sulfate ratio is frequently measured by turbidimetry before and after acid hydrolysis (Sperber, 1948). A gas chromatographic method for the determination of benzene and 9 of its potential metabolites in rabbit urine has been briefly described (Nomiyama and Nomiyama, 1969).

References

ACGIH. *Documentation of the Threshold Limit Values*, American Conference of Governmental Industrial Hygienists, Cincinnati, Ohio, 1971, p. 22.

P. Alha. Personal communications, 1975.

J. Angerer, D. Szadkowski, A. Manz et al. Chronische Loesungsmittelbelastung am Arbeitsplatz. Int. Arch. Arbeitsmed. 31: 1–8, 1973.

S.P. Avis and C.J. Hutton. Acute benzene poisoning: a report of 3 fatalities. J. For. Sci. 38: 599–602, 1993.

M.K. Baldwin, M.A. Selby and H. Bloomberg. Measurement of phenol in urine by the method of Van Haaften and Sie: a critical appraisal. Analyst 106: 763–767, 1981.

R.C. Baselt. Blood benzene stability in plastic containers. Clin. Chem. 20: 1477–1478, 1974.

W.E. Bechtold, G. Lucier, L.S. Birnbaum et al. Muconic acid determinations in urine as a biological exposure index for workers occupationally exposed to benzene. Am. Ind. Hyg. Asso. J. 52: 473–478, 1991.

R. Bonnichsen, A.C. Maehly and M. Moeller. Poisoning by volatile compounds. I. Aromatic hydrocarbons. J. For. Sci. 11: 186–204, 1966.

L. Braier, A. Levy, K. Dror and A. Pardo. Benzene in blood and phenol in urine in monitoring benzene exposure in industry. Am. J. Ind. Med. 2: 119–123, 1981.

F. Brugnone, L. Perbellini, G. Maranelli et al. Reference values for blood benzene in the occupationally unexposed general population. Int. Arch. Occ. Env. Health 64: 179–184, 1992.

J.P. Buchet, R. Lauwerys and M. Cambier. An improved gas chromatographic method for the determination of phenol in urine. Eur. J. Tox. 5: 27–30, 1972.

W.D. Collom and C.L. Winek. Detection of glue constituents in fatalities due to "glue sniffing." Clin. Tox. 3: 125–130, 1970.

W.A. Fishbeck, R.R. Langner and R.J. Kociba. Elevated urinary phenol levels not related to benzene exposure. Am. Ind. Hyg. Asso. J. 36: 820–824, 1975.

S. Ghittori, M.L. Fiorentino, L. Maestri et al. Urinary excretion of unmetabolized benzene as an indicator of benzene exposure. J. Tox. Env. Health 38: 233–243, 1993.

L.D. Gruenke, J.C. Craig, R.C. Wester and H.I. Maibach. Quantitative analysis of benzene by selected ion monitoring/gas chromatography/mas spectrometry. J. Anal. Tox. 10: 225–232, 1986.

H. Hajimiragha, U. Ewers, A. Brockhaus and A. Boettger. Levels of benzene and other volatile aromatic compounds in the blood of non-smokers and smokers. Int. Arch. Occ. Env. Health 61: 513–518, 1989.

A. Hamilton and H.L. Hardy. *Industrial Toxicology*, 3rd ed., Publishing Sciences Group, Acton, MA, 1974, p. 274.

C.G. Hunter and D. Blair. Benzene: pharmacokinetic studies in man. Ann. Occ. Hyg. 15: 193–199, 1972.

O. Inoue, K. Seiji, H. Nakatsuka et al. Excretion of 1,2,4-benzenetriol in the urine of workers exposed to benzene. Brit. J. Ind. Med. 46: 559–565, 1989.

A.M. Jirka and S. Bourne. Gas-chromatographic analysis for benzene in blood. Clin. Chem. 28: 1492–1494, 1982.

F.J. Jongeneelen, H.A.A.M. Dirven, C.M. Leijdekkers et al. 5-Phenyl-N-acetylcysteine in urine of rats and workers after exposure to benzene. J. Anal. Tox. 11: 100–104, 1987.

L. H. Nahum and H.E. Hoff. The mechanism of sudden death in experimental acute benzol poisoning. J. Pharm. Exp. Ther. 50: 336–345, 1934.

K. Nomiyama and H. Nomiyama. Gas-liquid chromatographic determination of benzene metabolites. J. Chrom. 44: 386–388, 1969.

D.V. Parke and R.T. Williams. Studies in detoxication. 49. The metabolism of benzene containing ($^{14}C_1$) benzene. Biochem. J. 54: 231–238, 1953.

K. Pekari, M.L. Riekkola and A. Aitio. Simultaneous determination of benzene and toluene in the blood using head-space gas chromatography. J. Chrom. 491: 309–320, 1989.

J.K. Piotrowski. *Exposure Tests for Organic Compounds in Industrial Toxicology*, U.S. Government Printing Office, Washington, D.C., 1977, pp. 41–47.

G.J. Roush and M.G. Ott. A study of benzene exposure versus urinary phenol levels. Am. Ind. Hyg. Asso. J. 38: 67–75, 1977.

A. Sato and Y. Fujiwara. Elimination of inhaled benzene and toluene in man. Jap. J. Ind. Health 14: 224–225, 1972.

A. Sato, T. Nakajima and Y. Fujiwara. Determination of benzene and toluene in blood by means of a syringe-equilibration method using a small amount of blood. Brit. J. Ind. Med. 32: 210–214, 1975.

R.J. Sherwood and F.W.G. Carter. The measurement of occupational exposure to benzene vapour. Ann. Occ. Hyg. 13: 125–146, 1970.

C.A. Snyder, M.N. Erlichman, B.D. Goldstein and S. Laskin. An extractive method for determination of benzene in tissue by gas chromatography. Am. Ind. Hyg. Asso. J. 38: 272–276, 1977.

I. Sperber. A direct turbidimetric method for determining ethereal sulfates in urine. J. Biol. Chem. 172: 441–444, 1948.

J.B. Tauber. Instant benzol death. J. Occ. Med. 12: 520–523, 1970.

J. Teisinger, V. Fiserova-Bergerova and J. Kudrna. The metabolism of benzene in man. Prac. Lek. 4: 175–188, 1952.

A.B. Van Haaften and S.T. Sie. The measurement of phenol in urine by gas chromatography as a check on benzene exposure. Am. Ind. Hyg. Asso. J. 26: 52–58, 1965.

P.B. Van Roosmalen, J. Purdham and I. Drummond. An improved method for the determination of phenol in the urine of workers exposed to benzene or phenol. Int. Arch. Occ. Env. Health 48: 159–163, 1981.

J.E. Walkley, L.D. Pagnotto and H.B. Elkins. The measurement of phenol in urine as an index of benzene exposure. Am. Ind. Hyg. Asso. J. 22: 362–367, 1961.

R.C. Wester, H.I. Maibach, L.D. Gruenke and J.C. Craig. Benzene levels in ambient air and breath of smokers and nonsmokers in urban and pristine environments. J. Tox. Env. Health 18: 567–573, 1986.

C.L. Winek and W.D. Collom. Benzene and toluene fatalities. J. Occ. Med. 13: 259–261, 1971.

R.T. Withey and L. Martin. A sensitive micro method for the analysis of benzene in blood. Bull. Env. Cont. Tox. 12: 659–664, 1974.

Benzidine

T½: 5 hr
Vd: ?
Fb: ?
pKa: ?

H_2N—⟨○⟩—⟨○⟩—NH_2

Occurrence and Usage. Benzidine (4,4-diaminobiphenyl) is widely employed in the manufacture of dyes. Prior to the recognition of its carcinogenic properties, it was a common laboratory reagent. As a carcinogen, benzidine does not have a threshold limit value assigned for its presence in the industrial atmosphere. Dermal absorption is often the major route of entry into the body, although inhalation and ingestion may also occur.

Blood Concentrations. The determination of benzidine or its metabolites in blood is not routinely performed. The intravenous administration of 0.2 mg/kg of labeled benzidine to dogs produced initial blood concentrations as high as 0.2 mg/L, declining to about 0.01 mg/L by 24 hours. An early elimination half-life of 4 hours and a terminal half-life of 88 hours were apparent (Kellner et al., 1973).

Metabolism and Excretion. Of an absorbed dose of benzidine, it has been estimated that urinary excretion accounts for 4–10% as the parent compound; another 7–16% is excreted as mono- and diacetylbenzidine and much of the remainder as the sulfate conjugate of 3-hydroxybenzidine (Sciarini and Meigs, 1961; Piotrowski, 1977).

The measurement of unchanged benzidine in urine has been used as an index of exposure to the compound. The maximum rate of excretion occurs 2–3 hours after an exposure, and urinary levels decline with a half-life of 5–6 hours. Urine benzidine concentrations average 0.009 mg/L in workers exposed to air levels of 0.007–0.011 mg/m³; they have ranged from 0.100–0.200 mg/L in workers exposed to air containing 0.150–0.400 mg/m³ of the chemical (Piotrowski, 1977). Slow acetylators develop urinary benzidine levels nearly twice those of rapid acetylators following an 8 hour occupational exposure (Dewan et al., 1986).

benzidine — monoacetylbenzidine

3-hydroyxbenzidine — diacetylbenzidine

Toxicity. Chronic exposure to benzidine is known to produce urinary bladder cancer in man. It is believed that exposure must last for at least 6 months, and that tumors may appear after a latency period of from 2–42 years (Haley, 1975). Workers exhibiting a high incidence of bladder tumors had urine benzidine concentrations of less than 0.160 mg/L (Zavon et al., 1973).

Analysis. A colorimetric method was described for the analysis of unchanged benzidine in urine that has a detection limit of 0.020 mg/L (Glassman and Meigs, 1951). More sensitive or more specific chromatographic methods have been published, involving paper chromatography (Laham et al., 1970) and liquid chromatography (Rice and Kissinger, 1979), that are applicable as well to the determination of benzidine metabolites. A radioimmunoassay has been described for diacetylbenzidine in urine (Johnson et al., 1981). Meal et al. (1981) have shown, using gas chromatography/mass spectrometry, that free benzidine may be detected in the urine of workers exposed to benzidine-derived dyes if the urine is first treated by acid hydrolysis.

References

A. Dewan, J.P. Jani, K.S. Shah and S.K. Kashyap. Urinary excretion of benzidine in relation to the acetylator status of occupationally exposed subjects. Hum. Tox. 5: 95–97, 1986.

J.M. Glassman and J.W. Meigs. Benzidine (4,4'-diaminobiphenyl) and substituted benzidines. Arch. Ind. Hyg. Occ. Med. 4: 519–532, 1951.

T.J. Haley. Benzidine revisited: a review of the literature and problems associated with the use of benzidine and its congeners. Clin. Tox. 8: 13–42, 1975.

H.J. Johnson, Jr., S.F. Cernosek, Jr., R.M. Gutierrez-Cernosek and L.L. Brown. Validation of a radioimmunoassay procedure for N,N'-diacetylbenzidine, a metabolite of the chemical carcinogen benzidine, in urine. J. Anal. Tox. 5: 157–161, 1981.

H.M. Kellner, O.E. Christ and K. Lotzsch. Animal studies on the kinetics of benzidine and 3,3'-dichlorobenzidine. Arch. Tox. 31: 61–79, 1973.

S. Laham, J. Farant and M. Potvin. Biochemical determination of urinary bladder carcinogens in human urine. Occ. Health Rev. 21: 14–23, 1970.

P.F. Meal, J. Cocker, H.K. Wilson and J.M. Gilmour. Search for benzidine and its metabolites in urine of workers weighing benzidine-derived dyes. Brit. J. Ind. Med. 38: 191–193, 1981.

J.K. Piotrowski. *Exposure Tests for Organic Compounds in Industrial Toxicology*, U.S. Government Printing Office, Washington, D.C., 1977, pp. 81–85.

J.R. Rice and P.T. Kissinger. Determination of benzidine and its acetylated metabolites in urine by liquid chromatography. J. Anal. Tox. 3: 64–66, 1979.

L.J. Sciarini and J. W. Meigs. The biotransformation of benzidine. Arch. Env. Health. 2: 423–428, 1961.

M.R. Zavon, U. Hoegg and E. Bingham. Benzidine exposure as a cause of bladder tumors. Arch. Env. Health 27: 1–7, 1973.

Benzphetamine

T½: ?
Vd: ?
Fb: ?
pKa: 6.6

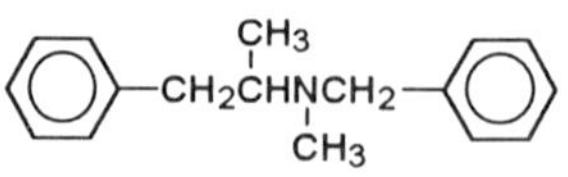

Occurrence and Usage. Benzphetamine (Didrex) is a sympathomimetic amine used medically in the treatment of obesity. It differs from amphetamine in that it has both a benzyl and a methyl group on the nitrogen, reducing the stimulant and cardiovascular effects of the drug while retaining anorectic efficacy. The drug is available as the hydrochloride salt for oral use in 25 and 50 mg tablets, which may be taken 1–3 times daily.

Blood Concentrations. Blood benzphetamine concentrations have not been determined following therapeutic administration in man.

Metabolism and Excretion. Benzphetamine is extensively metabolized in animals and man to methamphetamine and amphetamine with little, if any, excreted as unchanged drug (Vree and van Rossum, 1970; Budd and Jain, 1978). Following a single 20 mg dose in a healthy adult male, peak urine concentrations of 1.06 mg/L methamphetamine and 0.69 mg/L amphetamine were observed at 3.7 hours (Budd and Jain, 1978).

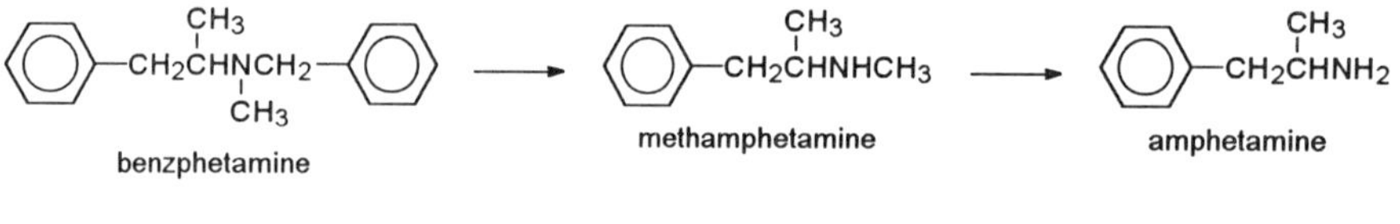

Toxicity. Benzphetamine in overdosage causes confusion, anxiety, cardiac arrhythmias, hallucinations, circulatory collapse, convulsions and coma. The following concentrations were observed in a 16 year old male who died after intentionally ingesting a large amount of the drug (Brooks et al., 1982):

Benzphetamine Concentrations in a Fatality (mg/L or mg/kg)

Blood	Brain	Liver	Bile	Kidney	Urine*	Adipose	Gastric
14	31	106	83	38	8	17	53 mg

* Amphetamine and methamphetamine were also present in the urine.

Analysis. Benzphetamine and its metabolites have been determined in biological samples by gas chromatography with either flame-ionization (Jain et al, 1977; Brooks et al., 1982; Niwaguchi et al., 1982) or mass spectrometric detection (Niwaguchi et al. 1982). The analytical techniques cited for amphetamine are applicable for the most part to the simultaneous assay of benzphetamine and its metabolites.

References

J.P. Brooks, M. Phillips, D.T. Stafford and J.S. Bell. A case of benzphetamine poisoning. Am. J. For. Med. Path. 3: 245–247, 1982.

R.D. Budd and N.C. Jain. Metabolism and excretion of benzphetamine: sources of error in reporting results. J. Anal. Tox. 2: 241, 1978.

N.C. Jain, T.C. Sneath, R.D. Budd and B.A. Olson. Mass screening and confirmation of seven sympathomimetic amine drugs by EMIT-gas chromatography. J. Anal. Tox. 1: 233–235, 1977.

T. Niwaguchi, T. Inoue and S. Suzuki. The metabolism of 1-phenyl-2-(N-methyl-N-benzylamino)propane (benzphetamine) in vivo in the rat. Xenobiotica 12: 617–625, 1982.

T.B. Vree and J.M. Rossum. Kinetics of metabolism and excretion of amphetamines in man. In *Amphetamines and Related Compounds* (E. Costa and S. Garattini, eds.), Raven Press, New York, 1970, pp. 165–190.

Benztropine

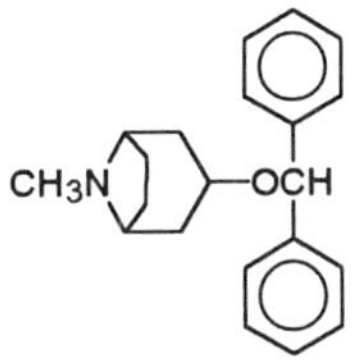

T½: ?
Vd: ?
Fb: ?
pKa: 10.0

Occurrence and Usage. Benztropine (Cogentin) is a synthetic compound resulting from the combination of the active portions of atropine and diphendydramine. It is used in the treatment of all forms of Parkinsonism and in the control of extrapyramidal disorders (except tardive dyskinesia) due to neuroleptic drugs. It is available as the mesylate in tablets of 1 and 2 mg, which are used orally in doses of up to 6 mg/day. It is also available in ampules containing 1 mg/mL for intravenous or intramuscular administration.

Blood Concentrations. A 2 mg dose in a patient produced a plasma benztropine level of 6.7 µg/L at 12 hours post-dose (Selinger et al., 1989). Four patients on benztropine therapy with 4 mg per day were found to have plasma concentrations ranging from 80–126 µg/L (average, 99) (Jindal et al., 1981).

Metabolism and Excretion. The metabolism of benztropine in man has not been reported. Urine benztropine concentrations in 4 patients on daily therapy with 4 mg of the drug ranged from 5–123 µg/L (Jindal et al., 1981).

Toxicity. Overdose results in symptoms typical of those seen in atropine poisoning or antihistamine overdosage, including central nervous system depression, delirium, coma, shock, convulsions, respiratory arrest and death. Psychosis characterized by mental confusion and bizarre behavior has been reported (Ananth and Jain, 1973; Woody et al., 1974) and it has been suggested that the drug may be abused for its hallucinogenic and euphoriant effects (Craig and Rosen, 1981). A man who ingested an unknown dose exhibited a serum benztropine concentration of 100 µg/L on the second hospital day; his anticholinergic symptoms persisted for 8 days but he survived with physostigmine administration and supportive treatment (Arnold et al., 1987).

The following tissue levels were observed in 4 adults who died after acute ingestion of unknown amounts of benztropine (del Vilar, 1976; Sims, 1989; Rosano et al., 1993):

Benztropine Concentrations in Fatal Cases (mg/L or mg/kg)

	Blood	Liver	Urine	Gastric
Average	0.4	3.1	4.0	2 mg
(Range)	(0.2–0.7)	(1.6–5.3)	(0.8–7.1)	(0–4)

Analysis. Gas chromatography-mass spectrometry has been used for the determination of benztropine in plasma and urine (Jindal et al., 1981). Liquid chromatography with ultraviolet detection has also been described (Selinger et al., 1989).

References

J.V. Ananth and R.C. Jain. Benztropine psychosis. Can. Psych. Asso. J. 18: 409–414, 1973.

P. Arnold, D. Beaird and S. Curry. Serial plasma benztropine concentrations after overdose. Vet. Hum. Tox. 29: 482, 1987.

D.H. Craig and P. Rosen. Abuse of antiparkinsonian drugs. Ann. Emer. Med. 10: 98–100, 1981.

G. del Villar. Personal communication, 1976.

S.P. Jindal, T. Lutz, C. Hallstrom and P. Vestergaard. A stable isotope dilution assay for the antiparkinsonian drug benztropine in biological fluids. Clin. Chim. Acta 112: 267–273, 1981.

T.G. Rosano, J.M. Meola, S.P. Jindal et al. Benztropine identification and quantitation in a suicidal overdose case. Presented at the annual meeting of the Society of Forensic Toxicologists, October 15, 1993, Phoenix, Arizona.

K. Selinger, G. Lebel, H.M. Hill and C. Discenza. High-performance liquid chromatographic method for the analysis of benztropine in human plasma. J. Chrom. 491: 248–252, 1989.

D.N. Sims. Personal communication, 1989.

G.E. Woody and C.P. O'Brien. Anticholinergic toxic psychosis in drug abusers treated with benztropine. Comp. Psych. 15: 439–442, 1974.

Benzyl Alcohol

T½: ?
Vd: ?
Fb: ?

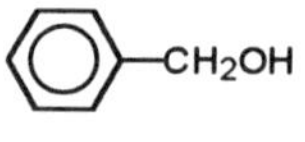

Occurrence and Usage. Benzyl alcohol at concentrations of 0.9–2.0% is commonly used as an antibacterial agent in a variety of pharmaceutical formulations intended for intravenous administration. The compound is also used in organic synthesis and as a solvent for various substances, including cellulose acetate and shellac. It is also found in jasmine, hyacinth and at least several dozen other essential oils. As a local anesthetic/disinfectant, it has been used topically in concentrations of up to 10%.

Blood Concentrations. Blood concentrations of benzyl alcohol following exposure in non-symptomatic individuals have not been reported.

Metabolism and Excretion. Benzyl alcohol is rapidly oxidized to benzoic acid, which is conjugated with glycine to form hippuric acid and excreted in the urine; a small portion of a dose may be excreted as the glucuronide (Snapper et al., 1924; Bray et al., 1951). Neonates excrete approximately 82% of a single intravenous dose as hippuric acid in the 24 hour urine (LeBel et al., 1988).

Toxicity. Single 32 mL intravenous doses of a methylprednisolone sodium succinate formulation containing 0.9% benzyl alcohol as a preservative given to 28 healthy, young males produced no serious side effects (Novak et al., 1972). Symptoms of neurologic deterioration, severe metabolic acidosis, hematologic abnormalities, respiratory distress, hepatic and renal failure, hypotension, and cardiovascular collapse have resulted from benzyl alcohol intoxication in neonates (Brown et al., 1982; Gershanik et al., 1982). In one study, 10 premature infants received multiple intravenous injections of solutions containing 0.9% benzyl alcohol; analysis of blood samples from 6 of the infants with respiratory distress showed benzyl alcohol concentrations ranging from 66–148 mg/L. Urine samples from 5 of these infants contained hippuric acid in concentrations approximately twice those of unexposed controls (Gershanik et al., 1982).

Analysis. Benzyl alcohol in blood and urine has been determined by gas chromatography, although no details of the procedure were reported (Gershanik et al., 1982). Methods for the analysis of benzoic acid in urine are cited in the section on toluene. A liquid chromatographic method for both benzyl alcohol and benzoic acid has been described (Tan et al., 1991).

References

H.G. Bray, W.V. Thorpe and K. White. Kinetic studies of the metabolism of foreign organic compounds. Biochem. J. 48: 88–96, 1951.

W.J. Brown, N.R.M. Buist, H.T.C. Gipson et al. Fatal benzyl alcohol poisoning in a neonatal intensive care unit. Lancet 1: 1250, 1982.

J. Gershanik, B. Boecler, H. Ensley et al. The gasping syndrome and benzyl alcohol poisoning. New Eng. J. Med. 307: 1384–1388, 1982.

M. LeBel, L. Ferron, M. Masson et al. Benzyl alcohol metabolism and elimination in humans. Dev. Pharm. Ther. 11: 347–356, 1988.

E. Novak, S.S. Stubbs, E.C. Sanborn and R.M. Eustice. The tolerance and safety of intravenously administered benzyl alcohol in methylprednisolone sodium succinate formulations in normal human subjects. Tox. Appl. Pharm. 23: 54–61, 1972.

J. Snapper, A. Grunbaum and S. Sturkop. Uber die Spaltung und die Oxydation von Benzylalkohol und Benzylestern im Menschlichen Organismus. Biochem. Z. 155: 163–173, 1924.

H.S.I. Tan, M.A. Manning, M.K. Hahn et al. Determination of benzyl alcohol and its metabolite in plasma by reversed-phase high-performance liquid chromatography. J. Chrom. 568: 145–155, 1991.

Beryllium

T½: ?
Vd: ?
Fb: 0.7

Be

Occurrence and Usage. Beryllium and its compounds are important ingredients in the manufacture of alloys, many electrical components and ceramic heat-shields for space vehicles. Exposure is generally via inhalation of beryllium dusts or fumes created during manufacturing processes, and occasionally by dermal contact. The current threshold limit value is 0.002 mg/m^3 of beryllium in the industrial atmosphere, and the metal is listed as a suspected carcinogen.

Blood Concentrations. The normal blood beryllium concentration averaged 0.001 mg/L in 10 unexposed persons (Stiefel et al., 1980).

Metabolism and Excretion. Up to 90% of an absorbed dose of beryllium is excreted in the urine over a period of several days. Urine concentrations in unexposed nonsmokers average 0.0009 mg/L and in smokers, about 0.002 mg/L. Beryllium concentrations in urine (in mg/L) closely approximate the beryllium concentrations in room air (in mg/m^3) in exposed workers (Stiefel et al., 1980).

When inhaled, the metal or its insoluble salts are deposited in the lung and appear to be slowly absorbed and excreted. It can be found in urine of workers up to 10 years after cessation of exposure.

Small doses favor deposition in bone, whereas larger doses deposit initially in the liver and are slowly mobilized to bone. The biological half-life of beryllium is inversely related to the dose (Reeves, 1979).

Toxicity. Dermal exposure to beryllium may produce contact dermatitis. Inhalation can cause bronchitis and severe pneumonitis. Chronic beryllium disease is often manifested by dyspnea, cough, fatigue, loss of weight, hepatomegaly and pulmonary granulomatosis. The development of the disease does not appear to be dose-related, and may involve a hypersensitivity reaction (Reeves, 1977).

The beryllium content of lung tissue in 66 individuals with beryllium diesase averaged 1.19 mg/kg of dried tissue (range, 0.004–45.7), whereas in 6 control subjects this averaged 0.005 mg/kg (range, 0.003–0.010). The finding of beryllium in dried lung tissue at concentrations greater than 0.02 mg/kg is indicative of significant exposure. The test is diagnostically useful, although low or negative results do not preclude the possibility of beryllium disease (Sprince et al., 1976).

The urine of 25 subjects with beryllium disease was found to contain beryllium at concentrations of 0–1.7 mg/L, compared to levels of 0–0.6 mg/L for 6 asymptomatic workers. The excretion of beryllium in the urine is quite variable from day to day (Dutra et al., 1949) and does not necessarily correlate with the severity of lung disease or extent of exposure (Klemperer et al., 1951).

Analysis. Beryllium may be determined in urine by fluorimetry after reaction with morin (Walkley, 1959). More specific procedures involve flame (Borkowski, 1968) or flameless (Lockwood and Limtiaco, 1975; Stiefel et al., 1976; Hurlbut, 1978) atomic absorption spectrometry. Procedures for wet or dry-ashing of biological specimens were cited in the section on arsenic.

References

D.L. Bokowski. Rapid determination of beryllium by a direct-reading atomic absorption spectrophotometer. Am. Ind. Hyg. Asso. J. 29: 474–481, 1968.

F.R. Dutra, J. Cholak and D.M. Hubbard. The value of beryllium determination in the diagnosis of berylliosis. Am. J. Clin. Path. 19: 229–234, 1949.

J.A. Hurlbut. Determination of beryllium in biological tissues and fluids by flameless atomic absorption spectroscopy. At. Abs. Newsl. 17: 121–124, 1978.

F.W. Klemperer, A.P. Martin and J. Van Riper. Beryllium excretion in humans. Am. Ind. Hyg. Asso. J. 4: 251–256, 1951.

T.H. Lockwood and L.P. Limtiaco. Determination of beryllium, cadmium, and tellurium in animal tissues using electronically excited oxygen and atomic absorption spectrophotometry. Am. Ind. Hyg. Asso. J. 36: 57–62, 1975.

A.L. Reeves. Beryllium in the environment. Clin. Tox. 10: 37–48, 1977.

A.L. Reeves. Beryllium. In *Handbook on the Toxicology of Metals*, (L. Friberg et al., eds.), Elsevier, New York, 1979, pp. 329–343.

N.L. Sprince, H. Kazemi and H.L. Hardy. Current (1975) problem of differentiating between beryllium disease and sarcoidosis. Ann. N.Y. Acad. Sci. 278: 654–664, 1976.

T. Stiefel, K. Schulze, G. Toelg and H. Zorn. Ein Verbundverfahren zur Bestimmung von Beryllium in Biologischen Matrices durch flammenlose Atomabsorptionsspektrometrie. Anal. Chim. Acta 87: 67–78, 1976.

T. Stiefel, K. Schulze, H. Zorn and G. Toelg. Toxicokinetic and toxicodynamic studies of beryllium. Arch. Tox. 45: 81–92, 1980.

J. Walkley. A study of the morin method for the determination of beryllium in air samples. Am. Ind. Hyg. Asso. J. 20: 241–245, 1959.

Bismuth

T½: 5 days
Vd: ?
Fb: ?

Bi

Occurrence and Usage. Bismuth is used industrially in the production of low-melting alloys, pigments, and chemical additives. Various compounds of low solubility, including the aluminate, carbonate, gallate, nitrate, and salicylate sub-salts, have been used therapeutically as astringents, antacids, skin powders, radio-opaque agents, and in the treatment of ulcers, diarrhea, syphilis, and warts. Bismuth subsalicylate (Pepto-Bismol, Pabizol), commonly prescribed for indigestion and diarrhea as a 1.75% solution, yields 200 mg of bismuth per single 30 mL dose or 1600 mg if the recommended maximum of 8 doses is ingested.

Blood Concentrations. Background bismuth blood concentrations in 33 peptic ulcer patients ranged from 0.001–0.012 mg/L, averaging 0.004 mg/L. After 6 weeks of daily therapy with 1120 mg of bismuth complexed with protein, these same patients reached steady-state blood bismuth levels averaging 0.012 mg/L, ranging from 0.004–0.030 mg/L (Serfontein et al., 1979). Levels averaging 0.017–0.038 mg/L were developed by groups of subjects receiving 12–20 g daily oral doses of the phosphate, polysilicate, or subnitrate salts of bismuth for 5–10 days (Conso et al., 1975).

Metabolism and Excretion. The poorly soluble bismuthyl compounds used as oral medicines are excreted largely unabsorbed in the feces. Bismuth compounds given by parenteral injection (usually the subsalicylate, thioglycollate, or triglycollamate) are eliminated primarily in urine over a period of several weeks. Normal human brain, lung and liver contain less than 0.040 mg/kg bismuth, while kidney concentrations average 0.400 mg/kg (Fowler and Vouk, 1979). Normal urine concentrations average 0.018 mg/L (range, 0.010–0.023), while during a course of therapy with a bismuth ulcer drug urine levels ranged from 0.020–0.940 mg/L (Serfontein et al., 1979).

The following tissue distribution was noted in 22 patients who received intramuscular injections of bismuth subsalicylate (60–2100 mg of bismuth) for syphilis within 1–251 days of death (Sollman et al., 1938):

Average Bismuth Concentrations in Treated Patients (mg/L or mg/kg)

Blood	Brain	Lung	Liver	Bile	Kidney	Urine
0.5	0.6	0.9	6.8	3.9	33	1.2

Toxicity. The toxic effects of bismuth are similar to those of lead and mercury. Salivation, mucosal swelling, discoloration of the tongue, gums, or skin, and abdominal pain and nausea are common early symptoms. Renal damage is the major result of bismuth overdosage, although encephalopathy and peripheral neuropathy have also been frequently noted.

Nausea, vomiting and nephrotoxicity occurred in 2 children who received therapeutic intramuscular doses of bismuth thioglycollate for weeks; normal renal function returned within several weeks (Grybowski and Gotoff, 1961; Chamberlain and Franks, 1963). A similar incident involving the oral ingestion of 21 tablets of bismuth triglycollamate (1.5 g bismuth) occurred in a 19 year old, who recovered within 2 weeks (Czerwinski and Ginn, 1964). Bismuth subgallate (a fecal deodorizer and stool-firming agent) has produced muscle tremors, ataxia, loss of memory, confusion, irritability and blurring of vision in colostomy patients taking the drug chronically by mouth (Burns et al., 1974; Coffey and Graham, 1974; Robertson, 1974). Chronic usage of bismuth subsalicylate by a 60 year old man resulted in encephalopathy and a blood bismuth level of 0.072 mg/L (Hasking and Duggan, 1982).

Bismuth concentrations in toxic situations arising from chronic oral administration of bismuth subnitrate have ranged from 0.05–1.60 mg/L in blood and from 0.15–1.25 mg/L in urine. All persons who survived the initial 7–14 days after appearance of toxic symptoms, regardless of the form of bismuth involved, have recovered without permanent injury (Serfontein and Mekel, 1979).

Analysis. A colorimetric technique for bismuth in blood has been described that has a detectability limit of 0.05 mg/L (Palliere and Gernez, 1980). Atomic absorption spectrometry using flame (Willis, 1962; Hall and Farber, 1972), graphite furnace (Allain, 1975; Slikkerveer et al., 1993) or hydride generation (Chou et al., 1984; Froomes et al., 1988) is the preferred technique for determination of trace levels of bismuth in biological specimens. Methods for wet and dry-ashing of specimens are cited in the section on arsenic.

References

P. Allain. Le dosage du bismuth dans les milieux biologiques par absorption atomique sans flamme. Clin. Chim. Acta 64: 281–286, 1975.

R. Burns, D.W. Thomas and V.J. Barron. Reversible encephalopathy possibly associated with bismuth subgallate ingestion. Brit. Med. J. 1: 220–223, 1974.

J.L. Chamberlain and R.C. Franks. Nephropathy resulting from bismuth. South. Med. J. 56: 509–510, 1963.

P.P. Chou, P.K. Jaynes and J.L. Bailey. Determination of bismuth in urine by atomic absorption with hydride generation. J. Anal. Tox. 8: 158–160, 1984.

G.L. Coffey and J.W. Graham. Mental illness or metal illness? Bismuth subgallate. Med. J. Aust. 2: 885, 1974.

F. Conso, R. Boudon, M. Gaultier and F. Prouillet. Resorption digestive chez l'homme de differents sels insolubles de bismuth. Nouv. Presse Med. 4: 1293–1295, 1975.

A.W. Czerwinski and H.E. Ginn. Bismuth nephrotoxicity. Am. J. Med. 37: 969–975, 1964.

B.A. Fowler and V. Vouk. Bismuth. In *Handbook on the Toxicology of Metals* (L. Friberg et al., eds.), Elsevier, New York, 1979, pp. 345–353.

P.R.A. Froomes, A.T. Wan, P.M. Harrison and A.J. McLean. Improved assay for bismuth in biological samples by atomic absorption spectrophotometry with hydride generation. Clin. Chem. 34: 382–384, 1988.

J.D. Gryboski and S.P. Gotoff. Bismuth nephrotoxicity. New Eng. J. Med. 265: 1289–1291, 1961.

R. J. Hall and T. Farber. Determination of bismuth in body tissues and fluids after administration of controlled doses. J. Asso. Off. Anal. Chem. 55: 639–642, 1972.

G. Hasking and J. Duggan. Encephalopathy from bismuth subsalicylate. Med. J. Aust. 2: 167, 1982.

M. Palliere and G. Gernez. Dosage des traces de bismuth dans le sang. Ann. Pharm. Fran. 38: 123–126, 1980.

J.F. Robertson. Mental illness or metal illness? Bismuth subgallate. Med. J. Aust. 61: 887–888, 1974.

W.J. Serfontein, R. Mekel, S. Bank et al. Bismuth toxicity in man — I. Res. Comm. Chem. Path. Pharm. 26: 383–389, 1979.

W.J. Serfontein and R. Mekel. Bismuth toxicity in man — II. Res. Comm. Chem. Path. Pharm. 26: 391–411, 1979.

A. Slikkerveer, R.B. Helmich and F.A. deWolff. Analysis for bismuth in tissue by electrothermal atomic absorption spectrometry. Clin. Chem. 39: 800–803, 1993.

Sollmann, H.N. Cole, K. Henderson et al. Clinical excretion of bismuth. Am. J. Syphilis 22: 555–583, 1938.

J.B. Willis. Determination of lead and other heavy metals in urine by atomic absorption spectroscopy. Anal. Chem. 34: 614–617, 1962.

Borate

T½: 12–27 hr
Vd: 0.17–0.50 L/kg
Fb: ?
pKa: 9.2

$BO_3^{-3}, B_4O_7^{-2}$

Occurrence and Usage. The borate ion is a weak germicide in aqueous solution and has been commonly employed in the household, in medical therapy and in industry for over a century. Boric acid is frequently used as an antiseptic for external use and may be found in eyewashes, mouthwashes, skin powders, ointments and irrigating solutions to the extent of 0.5–5%. Sodium borate (borax) is contained in cleaning agents, wood preservatives and fungicides. Borates were once used as food preservatives but have been replaced by less toxic agents for this purpose. Current threshold limit values for the borates range from 1–5 mg/m³ in the industrial atmosphere.

Blood Concentrations. Borate is found in trace amounts in normal tissue. Blood borate concentrations in 34 children with no known exposure to boric acid averaged 1.43 mg/L (range, 0–7.15) (Fisher and Freimuth, 1958). Imbus et al. (1963) found that blood boron concentrations, expressed as borate, in normal men averaged 0.6 mg/L with a range of 0.2–2.0. Boric acid is well-absorbed through broken skin surfaces or from mucous membranes, but not from intact skin (Goldbloom and Goldbloom, 1953). The daily use of a boric acid mouthwash raised the blood borate concentrations in 4 adults from an average of 0.4 mg/L to 0.8–1.1 mg/L after a week. Similar concentrations were attained within 1–2 hours of the ingestion of wine or raisins, foods high in boron content (Edwall et al., 1979).

Metabolism and Excretion. Borates are excreted unchanged largely by the kidney; from 85–100% of a dose may be eliminated in the urine over a period of 5–7 days, with small amounts found in sweat and feces (Pfeiffer et al., 1945; Locksley and Sweet, 1954; Jansen et al., 1984).

Toxicity. Occupational exposure to borax dusts has caused dermatitis, cough, irritation of mucous membranes and shortness of breath in workers (ACGIH, 1977). The remarkable number of human systemic poisonings associated with the borates is undoubtedly due in part to the popular belief that the compounds are relatively innocuous (Valdes-Dapena and Arey, 1962). It is true that relatively large amounts are necessary to produce toxicity in adults. An intravenous dose of 14–20 g of sodium borate was administered for the purposes of neutron capture therapy to 10 patients, who experienced immediate nausea, vomiting, defecation, and occasionally seizures and respiratory depression (Locksley and Farr, 1955). The duration of exposure to borates is apparently of more significance in the manifestation of toxicity than the serum borate concentration, since acute ingestion of up to 20 g of boric acid by infants has produced serum borate levels of 80–580 mg/L and caused only emesis and diarrhea (Linden et al., 1986), while ingestion of 4–30 g over a 4–10 week period has caused seizures in infants who developed serum borate levels of 15–49 mg/L (O'Sullivan and Taylor, 1983).

The application of boric acid powder for diaper rash has produced neurological disorders, severe erythema of the skin, gastrointestinal symptoms and deaths in infants (Goldbloom and Goldbloom, 1953); one such child developed a serum borate concentration of at least 303 mg/L, which fell to 32 mg/L after 54 hours of peritoneal dialysis with marked improvement in the patient (Baliah et al., 1969). The same manifestations were observed in 11 infants who ingested boric acid inadvertently mixed into their formula; from 2–4.5 g of the compound was ingested by 6 of the survivors, who developed serum borate levels of 20–150 mg/L, while the 5 infants who ingested larger amounts (4.5–14 g) exhibited levels of 200–1600 mg/L and died within 3 days (Wong et al., 1964). A 28 year old female recovered following the intentional ingestion of 297 g of a 99% boric acid insecticide; her serum borate concentration 2 hours after ingestion was 49 mg/L. A 35 year old female survived the ingestion of 80 g of boric acid in a suicide attempt; serum borate concentrations were 2320 mg/L after 1 hour and 1360 mg/L after 13 hours (Linden et al., 1986).

Brain and liver concentrations in children who have died of boric acid poisoning have ranged from 126–540 mg/kg (Young et al., 1949; Baker and Wilson, 1963; Rubenstein and Musher, 1970). A serum borate level of 440 mg/L was measured in a man who died after ingesting a large quantity of boric acid (Litovitz et al., 1991). Postmortem concentrations of borate in 2 fatal cases, one of which involved the inadvertent administration of about 15 g of boric acid to an adult by instillation into connective tissue, are illustrative of the generalized tissue distribution of this agent (Rehling, 1967; Hauck and Henn, 1969):

Borate Concentrations in Fatal Cases (mg/L or mg/kg)

Blood	Brain	Liver	Kidney
381	588	515	562
620	515	735	453

Analysis. Borate concentrations in biological fluids and tissues have been frequently determined using a colorimetric procedure that employs carminic acid (Hatcher and Wilcox, 1950; Smith et al., 1955; Rieders and Frere, 1963). The method is not sufficiently sensitive to detect endogenous levels of borate ion. A more sensitive colorimetric technique employs low temperature ashing of specimens and formation of a complex with curcumin (Mair and Day, 1972).

References

ACGIH. *Documentation of the Threshold Limit Values*, American Conference of Governmental Industrial Hygienists, Cincinnati, Ohio, 1977, pp. 356–357.

D.H. Baker and R.E. Wilson. The lethality of boric acid in the treatment of burns. J. Am. Med. Asso. 186: 1169–1170, 1963.

T. Baliah, H. MacLeish and K.N. Drummond. Acute boric acid poisoning. Can. Med. Asso. J. 101: 166–168, 1969.

L. Edwall, B. Karlen and A. Rosen. Absorption of boron after mouthwash treatment with Bocosept. Eur. J. Clin. Pharm. 15: 417–420, 1979.

R.S. Fisher and H.C. Freimuth. Blood boron levels in human infants. J. Invest. Derm. 30: 85–86, 1958.

R.B. Goldbloom and A. Goldbloom. Boric acid poisoning. J. Pediat. 43: 631–643, 1953.

J.T. Hatcher and L.V. Wilcox. Colorimetric determination of boron using carmine. Anal. Chem. 22: 567–569, 1950.

G. Hauck and R. Henn. Histopathologische und chemische-toxikologische Befunde bei einer akuten toedlichen Borsaeurevergiftung. Arch. Tox. 25: 83–88, 1969.

H.R. Imbus, J. Cholak, L.H. Miller and T. Sterling. Boron, cadmium, chromium and nickel in blood and urine. Arch. Env. Health. 6: 286–295, 1963.

J.A. Jansen, J. Andersen and J.S. Schou. Boric acid single dose pharmacokinetics after intravenous administration to man. Arch. Tox. 55: 64–67, 1984.

C.H. Linden, A.H. Hall, K.W. Kulig and B.H. Rumack. Acute ingestions of boric acid. Clin. Tox. 24: 269–279, 1986.

T.L. Litovitz, K.M. Baily and B.F. Schmitz. Annual report of the AAPCC National Data Collection System. Am. J. Emer. Med. 9: 461–509, 1991.

H.B. Locksley and W.H. Sweet. Tissue distribution of boron compounds in relation to neutron-capture therapy of cancer. Proc. Soc. Exp. Biol. Med. 86: 56–63, 1954.

H.B. Locksley and L.E. Farr. The tolerance of large doses of sodium borate intravenously by patients receiving neutron capture therapy. J. Pharm. Exp. Ther. 114: 484–489, 1955.

J.W. Mair, Jr. and H.G. Day. Curcumin method for spectrophotometric determination of boron extracted from radio frequency ashed animal tissues using 2-ethyl-1,3-hexanediol. Anal. Chem. 44: 2015–2017, 1972.

K. O'Sullivan and M. Taylor. Chronic boric acid poisoning in infants. Arch. Dis. Child. 58: 737–749, 1988.

C.C. Pfeiffer, L.F. Hallman and I. Gersh. Boric acid ointment. J. Am. Med. Asso. 128: 266–274, 1945.

C.J. Rehling. Poison residues in human tissues. In *Progress in Chemical Toxicology*, Vol. 3 (A. Stolman, ed.), Academic Press, New York, 1967, pp. 363–386.

F. Rieders and F.J. Frere. Detection and estimation of toxicologically significant amounts of borate, chlorate and oxalate in biological material. J. For. Sci. 8: 46–53, 1963.

A.D. Rubenstein and D.M. Musher. Epidemic boric acid poisonings simulating staphylococcal toxic epidermal necrolysis of the newborn infant: Ritter's disease. J. Pediat. 77: 884–887, 1970.

W.C. Smith, Jr., A.J. Goudie and J.N. Sivertson. Colorimetric determination of trace quantities of boric acid in biological materials. Anal. Chem. 27: 295–297, 1955.

M.A. Valdes-Dapena and J.B. Arey. Boric acid poisoning. J. Pediat. 61: 531–546, 1962.

L.C. Wong, M.D. Heimbach, D.R. Truscott and B.D. Duncan. Boric acid poisoning: report of 11 cases. Can. Med. Asso. J. 90: 1018–1023, 1964.

E.G. Young, R.P. Smith and O.C. MacIntosh. Boric acid as a poison. Can. Med. Asso. J. 61: 447–450, 1949.

Bromazepam

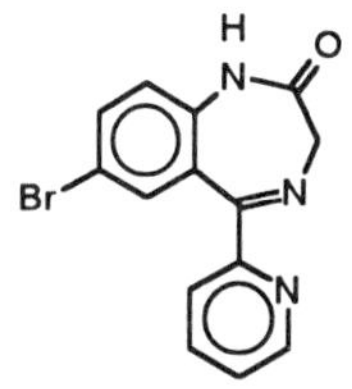

T½: 8–19 hr
Vd: 0.9 L/kg
Fb: 0.70
pKa: 2.9, 11.0

Occurrence and Usage. Bromazepam (Lectopam, Lexotan, Ro5-3350) is a benzodiazepine derivative that was synthesized in 1963. It is available in many European countries for use as an antianxiety agent in single oral doses of 3–12 mg as the free base.

Blood Concentrations. Following a single 12 mg oral dose administered to 10 subjects, an average peak plasma bromazepam concentration of 0.131 mg/L (range, 0.107–0.173) was achieved between 1 and 4 hours, declining with an average half-life of 11.9 hours (range, 7.9–19.3). During chronic oral administration of 9 mg daily, steady-state plasma levels averaged 0.120 mg/L (range, 0.081–0.154) by a specific gas chromatographic method (Kaplan et al., 1976).

Metabolism and Excretion. Bromazepam is metabolized primarily by 3-hydroxylation and cleavage of the 7-membered ring, followed by glucuronide conjugation of the hydroxylated metabolites.

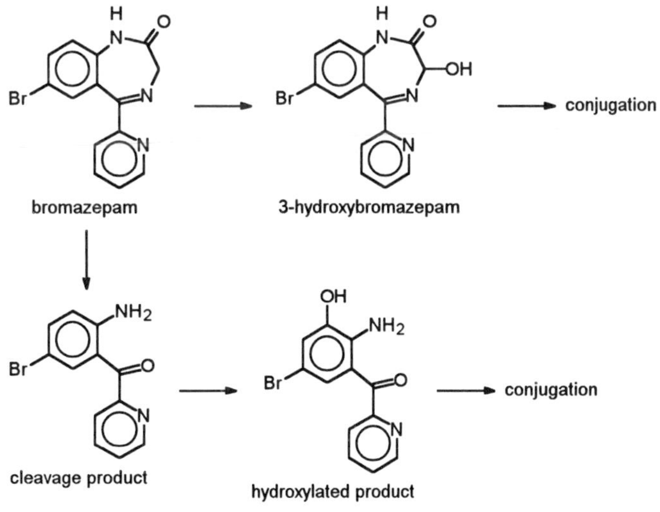

bromazepam   3-hydroxybromazepam   conjugation

cleavage product   hydroxylated product   conjugation

Intact bromazepam is the major blood constituent. About 2% of a dose is excreted in the 72 hour urine as unchanged bromazepam, 0.4% as the ring cleavage product, 27% as conjugated 3-hydroxybromazepam and 40% as the hydroxylated and conjugated cleavage product (Schwartz et al., 1973; de Silva et al., 1974; Kaplan et al., 1976).

Toxicity. A woman who was found dead after apparently ingesting an overdose had a postmortem blood bromazepam concentration of 5 mg/L (Brehmer, 1992).

Analysis. Bromazepam may be analyzed in biological specimens by electron-capture gas chromatography of either the intact drug (deSilva et al., 1974; Friedman et al., 1986), its hydrolysis product (Cano et al., 1975), or the N-methyl derivative (Klotz, 1981). Liquid chromatography has also been used (Hirayama et al., 1983; Heizman et al., 1984).

References

C. Brehmer, Personal communication, 1992.
J.P. Cano, A.M. Baille, A. Viala and J. Covo. Determination of bromazepam in plasma with an internal standard by gas-liquid chromatography. Arz. Forsch. 25: 1012–1026, 1975.
J.A. deSilva, I. Bekersky, M.A. Brooks et al. Determination of bromazepam in blood by electron-capture glc and its major urinary metabolites by differential pulse polarography. J. Pharm. Sci. 63: 1440–1445, 1974.
H. Friedman, D.J. Greenblatt and E.S. Burstein. Underivatized measurement of bromazepam by gas chromatography-electron capture detection with application to single-dose pharmacokinetics. J. Chrom. 387: 473–477, 1986.
P. Heizman, R. Geschke and K. Zinapold. Determination of bromazepam in plasma and of its main metabolites in urine by reversed-phase high-performance liquid chromatography. J. Chrom. 310: 129–137, 1984.
H. Hirayama, Y. Kasuya and T. Suga. High-performance liquid chromatographic determination of bromazepam in human plasma. J. Chrom. 277: 414–418, 1983.
S.A. Kaplan, M.L. Jack, R.E. Weinfeld et al. Biopharmaceutical and clinical pharmacokinetic profile of bromazepam. J. Pharm. Biopharm. 4: 1–16, 1976.
U. Klotz. Determination of bromazepam by gas-liquid chromatography and its application for pharmacokinetic studies in man. J. Chrom. 222: 501–506, 1981.
M.A. Schwartz, E. Postma, S.J. Kolis and A.S. Leon. Metabolites of bromazepam, a benzodiazepine, in the human, dog, rat, and mouse. J. Pharm. Sci. 62: 1776–1779, 1973.

Bromide

T½: 9–15 days
Vd: 0.35–0.48 L/kg   Br⁻
Fb: 0

Occurrence and Usage. The ammonium, calcium, potassium and sodium salts of bromide have been used therapeutically since 1835 and were first recognized as antiepileptic drugs in 1857. Around the turn of the century bromides were used indiscriminately as sedatives for various neuroses, being available without prescription. Non-prescription preparations such as Bromo-Seltzer and Nervine have not contained bromide since 1971 in the U.S., although a number of preparations such as triple bromide, a combination of the calcium, potassium, and sodium salts, are still obtainable in other countries. Bromides continue to be used outside the U.S. in the treatment of grand mal and focal epilepsy, in daily oral doses of 3–6 g.

Certain organic bromides, such as carbromal (a sedative), halothane (an anesthetic), and methyl bromide (a fumigant), are covered in separate sections. These materials are known to release bromide ion *in vivo* in various amounts.

Blood Concentrations. Normal background blood bromide concentrations in humans average 3–4 mg/L (Soremark, 1960a; Cross and Smith, 1978). Plasma bromide concentrations after an oral dose of 0.1 g/kg (7 g/70 kg) reached an average peak of 230 mg/L after 36 hours; this dose had no pharmacological effect on the 20 individuals involved (Haerer et al., 1964). Plasma levels of 750–1500 mg/L have been found to be effective in the treatment of epilepsy, although many patients may show signs of toxicity at these concentrations (Woodbury, 1972).

Metabolism and Excretion. Bromide is neither bound to plasma protein nor sequestered in cells; it occupies essentially the same volume of distribution as chloride, and competes with that ion for excretion by the kidney. An average of 4.3% of a dose is excreted in the daily urine, so that the elimination half-life is approximately 12 days (Soremark, 1960a, 1960b). Loss of bromide also occurs in feces, sweat and hair.

Toxicity. Acute intoxication with bromide is rare, apparently due to the nausea, vomiting and diarrhea produced by overdosage. Chronic intoxication generally takes 2–4 weeks to develop, usually involves women aged 40–60 years, and is often mistaken for numerous other diseases affecting the central nervous system. Common symptoms include fatigue, irritability, loss of appetite, stomach pain, skin pigmentation and rash, rapid respiration, stupor, and delerium with both auditory and visual hallucinations. Treatment involves proper hydration and the administration of chloride and/or diuretics to promote bromide excretion; these procedures are capable of reducing the plasma half-life from the usual 12 days to 65 hours or less (Moses and Klawans, 1979). In severe cases, hemodialysis has reduced the half-life to 1–2 hours (Wieth and Funder, 1963). Rarely, bromide intoxication has occurred in patients chronically receiving the hydrobromide salts of drugs such as pyridostigmine or dextromethorphan (Rothenberg et al., 1990).

In a series of 400 instances of chronic bromide intoxication, blood bromide concentrations ranged from 500–4280 mg/L, with 44% of the patients in the 500–1000 mg/L range. No deaths were reported even though several patients exceeded the 33% level of replacement of plasma chloride by bromide (2637 mg/L for a serum chloride of 100 mmol/L) considered to be life-threatening (Hanes and Yates, 1938).

Analysis. Inorganic bromide in biological fluids has been customarily measured by a gold chloride colorimetric procedure (Sunshine, 1975) that has a detectability limit of about 50 mg/L. A more specific colorimetric test has been proposed (Street, 1960), as well as several gas chromatographic (Archer, 1972; Wells and Cimbura, 1973; Corina et al., 1979) and liquid chromatographic procedures (Miller and Cappon, 1984; Goewie and Hogendoorn, 1985). Bromide-specific electrodes have been developed that are capable of measuring even the endogenous plasma bromide levels (Degenhart et al., 1972; Poser et al., 1974). Many clinical laboratory methods for serum chloride are subject to interference by bromide; spuriously high chloride values in a patient should raise the suspicion of bromism (Wenk et al., 1976).

References

A.W. Archer. A gas-chromatographic method for the determination of increased bromide concentrations in blood. Analyst 97: 428–432, 1972.

D.L. Corina, K.E. Ballard, D. Grice et al. Bromide measurement in serum and urine by an improved gas chromatographic method. J. Chrom. 162: 382–387, 1979.

J.D. Cross and H. Smith. Bromine in human tissue. For. Sci. 11: 147–153, 1978.

H.J. Degenhart, G. Abeln, B. Bevaart and J. Baks. Estimation of Br⁻ in plasma with a Br⁻ selective electrode. Clin. Chim. Acta 38: 217–220, 1972.

C.E. Goewie and E.A. Hogendoorn. Liquid chromatographic determination of bromide in human milk and plasma. J. Chrom. 344: 157–165, 1985.

A.F. Haerer, W.W. Tourtellotte, K.A. Richard et al. A study of the blood-cerebrospinal fluid-brain barrier in multiple sclerosis. Neurology 14: 345–354, 1964.

F.M. Hanes and A. Yates. An analysis of four hundred instances of chronic bromide intoxication. South. Med. J. 31: 667–671, 1938.

M.E. Miller and C.J. Cappon. Anion-exchange chromatographic determination of bromide in serum. Clin. Chem. 30: 781–783, 1984.

H. Moses and H.L. Klawans. Bromide intoxication. Hdbk. Clin. Neurol. 36: 291–318, 1979.

S. Poser, W. Poser and B. Muller-Oerlinghausen. Use of bromide electrodes for rapid screening of elevated bromide concentrations in biological fluids. Z. Klin. Chem. Klin. Biochem. 12: 350–351, 1974.

D.M. Rothenberg, A.S. Berns, R.Barkin and R.H. Glantz. Bromide intoxication secondary to physostigmine bromide therapy. J.Am. Med. Asso. 263: 1121–1122, 1990.

R. Soremark. The biological half-life of bromide ions in human blood. Acta Physiol. Scand. 50: 119–123, 1960a.

R. Soremark. Excretion of bromide ions by human urine. Acta Physiol. Scand. 50: 306–310, 1960b.

H.V. Street. Determination of bromide in blood. Clin. Chim. Acta 5: 938–941, 1960.

I. Sunshine (ed.). Bromide. Type A procedure. In *Methodology for Analytical Toxicology*, CRC Press, Cleveland, 1975, pp. 54–55.

J. Wells and G. Cimbura. The determination of elevated bromide levels in blood by gas chromatography. J. For. Sci. 18: 437–440, 1973.

R.E. Wenk, J.A. Lustgarten, J. Pappas et al. Serum chloride analysis, bromide detection, and the diagnosis of bromism. Am. J. Clin. Path. 64: 49–57, 1976.

J.O. Wieth and J. Funder. Treatment of bromide poisoning. Lancet 2: 327–329, 1963.

D.M. Woodbury. Bromides. In *Antiepileptic Drugs* (D.M. Woodbury, J.K. Penry and R.P. Schmidt, eds.), Raven Press, New York, 1972, pp. 519–527.

Brompheniramine

T½: 15–22 hr
Vd: ?
Fb: ?
pKa: ?

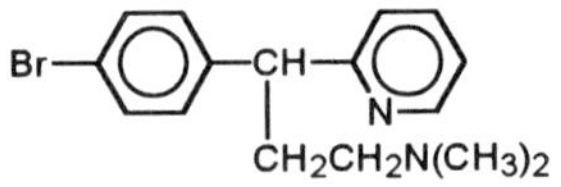

Occurrence and Usage. Brompheniramine (Dimetane, Puretane) has been used frequently as an antihistamine since its synthesis in 1951. It is available as the maleate salt of either the racemic mixture the racemic mixture or the d-isomer, dexbrompheniramine, which has approximately twice the potency of the dl-form. Brompheniramine is available in ampules for intravenous or intramuscular injection in doses of 5–20 mg, and in tablet and elixir preparations which are administered orally in doses of 4–12 mg. Dexbrompheniramine is marketed in tablets of 2–6 mg, alone or in combination with pseudoephedrine.

Blood Concentrations. Blood concentrations in 2 subjects after oral administration of 8 mg averaged 0.015 mg/L at 3 hours, 0.012 mg/L at 7 hours and 0.005 mg/L at 24 hours (Bruce et al., 1968a). Twelve adult males given 2 mg of dexbrompheniramine orally every 4 hours (12 mg/day) for 7 days developed average steady-state plasma concentrations of 0.018 (trough) to 0.022 mg/L (peak), with the peak levels occurring 5–7 hours after the last dose (Lin et al., 1985).

Metabolism and Excretion. Brompheniramine is biotransformed principally by mono- and di-N-demethylation. Deamination also occurs with formation of a carboxylic acid. About 53% of a labeled dose is excreted in urine over a 5 day period, with less than 3% appearing in the feces. The urinary products consist of unchanged drug (10.5%), norbrompheniramine (11.5%), dinorbrompheniramine (9.9%), beta-(p-bromophenyl)-2-pyridinepropionic acid (4.2%) and its glycine conjugate (1.6%). Other unidentified polar metabolites were also present (Bruce et al., 1968b).

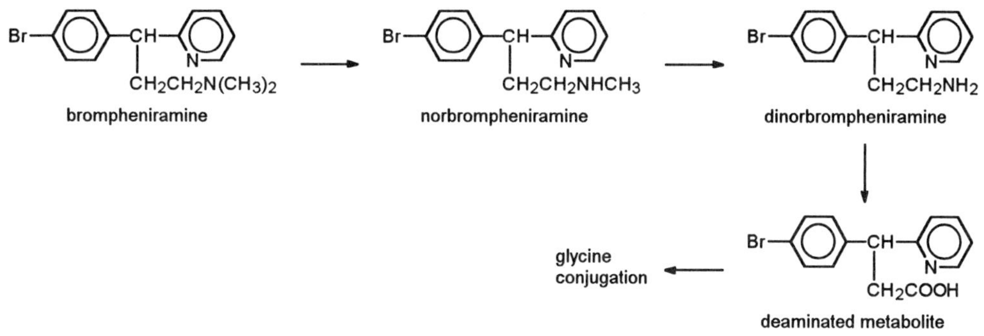

Toxicity. Concentrations of 0.2 mg/L in blood and 4.5 mg/kg in liver were found in a case of fatal overdosage with dexbrompheniramine and 3 other drugs (Baselt et al., 1977).

Analysis. A gas chromatographic method that has the necessary sensitivity to detect therapeutic concentrations in blood has been described, and involves electron-capture detection of a permanganate oxidation product (Bruce et al., 1968a; Lin et al., 1985). The drug may also be determined at higher concentrations by flame-ionization detection without derivatization.

References

R.C. Baselt, E. Shaskan and E.M. Gross. Tranylcypromine concentrations and monoamine oxidase activity in tissues from a fatal poisoning. J. Anal. Tox. 1: 168–170, 1977.

R.B. Bruce, J.E. Pitts and F.M. Pinchbeck. Determination of brompheniramine in blood and urine by gas-liquid chromatography. Anal. Chem. 40: 1246–1250, 1968a.

R.B. Bruce, L.B. Turnbull, J.H. Newman and J.E. Pitts. Metabolism of brompheniramine. J. Med. Chem. 11: 1031–1034, 1968b.

C.C. Lin, H.K. Kim, J. Lim et al. Steady-state bioavailability of dexbrompheniramine and pseudoephedrine from a repeat-action combination tablet. J. Pharm. Sci. 74: 25–28, 1985.

Buformin

T½: 1.8–3.8 hr
Vd: 1.5 L/kg
Fb: 0
pKa: 11.3

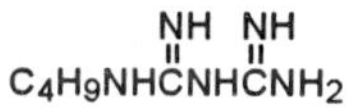

$$C_4H_9NHC(NH)NHC(NH)NH_2$$

Occurrence and Usage. Buformin (1-butylbiguanide, Silubin, Sindiatil) is a biguanide derivative that has been in clinical use in Europe since the 1960s as an oral hypoglycemic agent in the treatment of maturity-onset diabetes. It is closely related to metformin and phenformin. Daily oral doses of 100–600 mg of the hydrochloride salt, as a normal or sustained-release preparation, are common.

Blood Concentrations. Maximum plasma concentrations averaged 0.38 mg/L in 6 adults at 2 hours after the oral administration of 100 mg of buformin as a sustained-release preparation. The elimination half-life was 7.2 hours (Gutsche et al., 1976), as compared to an average of 2.2 hours for the normal preparation (Beckmann and Huebner, 1965). Therapeutic plasma levels in maintenance patients are believed to lie within 0.2–0.6 mg/L (De Groot et al., 1980).

Metabolism and Excretion. Buformin is apparently not metabolized in man (Beckman, 1966). Up to 98% of a dose is excreted unchanged in the 12 hour urine (Beckman, 1968); with the sustained-release form, 36% is eliminated in urine and 28% in feces within 24 hours (Gutsche et al., 1976).

Toxicity. Severe lactic acidosis has been produced in hundreds of patients who have either become chronically intoxicated or who suffered an acute reaction due to hypersensitivity or an overdose. The survival rate in these individuals has been on the order of only 50% (Luft et al., 1978). Six patients who survived serious lactic acidosis following chronic buformin therapy had maximum plasma concentrations averaging 1.7 mg/L (range, 1.1–2.4), while 4 patients who died showed an average of 2.5 mg/L and a range of 1.0–3.4 mg/L (Berger et al., 1976; Butt and Reitinger, 1977; Althoff et al., 1978).

One subject ingested 2100 mg of the drug in an unsuccessful suicide attempt and developed a plasma level of 5.4 mg/L (Berger et al., 1976). The following tissue distribution was noted in a woman who died of lactic acidosis that developed during treatment (De Groot et al., 1980):

Buformin Concentrations in a Fatal Case (mg/L or mg/kg)

Plasma	Lung	Liver	Bile	Kidney
3.2	2.8	5.2	6.3	98

Analysis. A spectrophotometric procedure for the analysis of buformin in biological fluids has been described, but does not have sufficient sensitivity for the measurement of therapeutic plasma concentrations (Beckmann and Huebner, 1965). Two gas chromatographic methods have appeared, based on acylation of the drug and conversion to a triazine derivative, with electron-capture (Matin et al., 1975) or nitrogen-specific detection (De Groot et al., 1980).

References

P.H. Althoff, W. Fassbinder, M. Neubauer et al. Haemodialyse bei der behandlung der biguanid-induzierten Lactacidose. Deut. Med. Wochenshr. 103: 61–68, 1978.

R. Beckmann. Zum biologischen Abbau von 1-Butyl-biguanid-[14C]-hydrochlorid (Silubin-[14C]). Arch. Int. Pharm. 160: 161–172, 1966.

R. Beckmann. The fate of biguanides in man. Ann. N.Y. Acad. Sci. 148: 820–832, 1968.

R. Beckmann and G. Huebner. Zur Pharmakokinetik von 1-Butyl-biguanid-hydrochlorid und einer Retard-Form dieser Substanz. Arz. Forsch. 15: 765–770, 1965.

W. Berger, S. Mehner-Aner, K. Muelly et al. 10 Faelle von Lactatazidose unter Biguanidtherapie (Buformin und Phenformin). Schweiz. Med. Wochenshr. 106: 1830–1834, 1976.

H. Butt and J. Reitinger. Lactatacidose und Biguanidtherapie. Med. Klin. 72: 708–711, 1977.

G. De Groot, R.A.A. Maes, B. Sangster et al. Gas chromatographic determination of buformin in body fluids and tissues, using a nitrogen phosphorus detector: application to a postmortem case. J. Anal. Tox. 4: 281–285, 1980.

H. Gutsche, L. Blumenbach, W. Losert and H. Wiemann. Plasmakonzentration und Elimination von 14C-1-Butyl-biguanid-HCl bei Diabetikern nach Einnahme der Substanz in einer neuen Zubereitung. Arz. Forsch. 26: 1227–1229, 1976.

D. Luft, R.M. Schmuelling and M. Eggstein. Lactic acidosis in biguanide-treated diabetics. Diabetologia 14: 75–87, 1978.

S.B. Matin, J.H. Karam and P.H. Forsham. Simple electron capture gas chromatographic method for the determination of oral hypoglycemic biguanides in biological fluids. Anal. Chem. 47: 545–548, 1975.

Bupivacaine

T½: 1.3–2.8 hr
Vd: 0.4–1.0 L/kg
Fb: 0.92
pKa: 8.1

Occurrence and Usage. Bupivacaine (Marcaine) is a long-acting amide local anesthetic that was first synthesized in 1957 and that is structurally related to mepivacaine and lidocaine. It is supplied as the hydrochloride in solutions of 0.25–0.75%, with or without epinephrine, for caudal, epidural or peripheral nerve block. Single doses of 12–225 mg are commonly administered, with daily doses of up to 400 mg.

Blood Concentrations. Plasma bupivacaine concentrations at delivery averaged 0.22 mg/L in 11 mothers who received 25 mg of the drug for pudendal block (Belfrage et al., 1973). The administration of 150 mg of bupivacaine to 12 patients for peridural anesthesia produced a mean peak plasma level of 1.14 mg/L after 20 minutes, with an observed plasma half-life of 2.8 hours; cerebrospinal fluid concentrations in 5 of these patients reached an average maximum of 31 mg/L at 30 minutes and declined with a half-life of 2.6 hours (Wilkinson and Lund, 1970). After bilateral intercostal nerve block with 400 mg of the drug in 10 patients, arterial plasma concentrations reached an average peak of 3.29 mg/L (range, 1.72–4.00) and venous plasma concentrations achieved an average peak of 2.52 mg/L (range, 1.40–3.45) within 10–20 minutes (Moore et al., 1976).

Metabolism and Excretion. The pathways of metabolism of bupivacaine in man have not been fully investigated, but are probably similar to those of mepivacaine. Less than 1% of a dose is excreted unchanged in the 24 hour urine; substantially larger amounts are present as norbupivacaine (2,6-pipecoloxylidide, normepivacaine), which is not believed to be pharmacologically active. 4'-Hydroxybupivacaine has been reported to be a minor urinary metabolite, accounting for 0.1% of a dose (Kuhnert et al., 1981; Lindberg et al., 1986).

4'-OH-bupivacaine   bupivacaine   norbupivacaine

Toxicity. Bupivacaine administered intravenously is several times more toxic than etidocaine or lidocaine (Scott, 1975). Plasma concentrations as low as 1.5–2.3 mg/L are capable of causing dizziness, ringing in the ears, and hypotension (Hollmen et al., 1969; Matouskova and Hanson, 1979). Blood concentrations of 9 and 12 mg/L were noted 5 minutes after intercostal nerve block with 3 mg/kg (210 mg/70 kg) of the drug without epinephrine in 2 patients who developed muscular rigidity (Yoshikawa et al., 1968). Convulsions occurred in one patient at an arterial bupivacaine concentration of 5.4 mg/L, following accidental intravascular injection of the drug (Moore et al., 1979). Hypotension, bradycardia, cyanosis, loss of consciousness, convulsions and delayed respiratory arrest have occurred in several patients with blood or plasma bupivacaine levels of 0.3–1.8 mg/L (Holmboe and Kongsrud, 1982; Rosenberg et al., 1983; Hasselstrom and Mogensen, 1984). At least 10 cases of fatal cardiac arrest have occurred following bupivacaine administration for obstetric epidural anesthesia; since 1983, the 0.75% concentration of the drug has not been recommended for this purpose (Anonymous, 1983; Marx, 1986).

Analysis. Bupivacaine may be conveniently analyzed in body fluids by gas chromatography with flame–ionization (Thomas et al., 1969; Tucker, 1970; Zylber-Katz et al., 1978; Verheesen et al.,

1980) or nitrogen-selective detection (Lesko et al., 1980; Park et al., 1980; LeNormand et al., 1986). Liquid chromatography has also been employed (Lindberg and Pihlajamaki, 1984; Wiegand et al., 1984; Michaelis et al., 1990).

References

Anonymous. Adverse reactions with bupivacaine. FDA Drug Bulletin 13(3): 23, 1983.

P. Belfrage, A. Berlin, M. Lindstedt and N. Raabe. Plasma levels of bupivacaine following pudendal block in labour. Brit. J. Anaesth. 45: 1067–1069, 1973.

L.J. Hasselstrom and T. Mogensen. Toxic reaction of bupivacaine at low plasma concentration. Anesthesiology 61: 99–100, 1984.

H. Hollmen, M. Korhonen and A. Ojala. Bupivacaine in paracervical block — plasma levels and changes in maternal and foetal acid-base balance. Brit. J. Anaesth. 41: 603–608, 1969.

J. Holmboe and F. Kongsrud. Delayed respiratory arrest after bupivacaine. Anaesthesia 37: 60–62, 1982.

P.M. Kuhnert, B.R. Kuhnert, J.M. Stitts and T.L. Gross. The use of a selected ion monitoring technique to study the disposition of bupivacaine in mother, fetus, and neonate following epidural anesthesia for Cesarean section. Anesthesiology 55: 611–617, 1981.

L.J. Lesko, J. Ericson, G. Ostheimer and A. Marion. Simultaneous determination of bupivacaine and 2,6-pipecoloxylidide in serum by gas-liquid chromatography. J. Chrom. 182: 226–231, 1980.

Y. LeNormand, C. DeVillepoix, A. Athovel et al. Determination of bupivacaine in human plasma by capillary gas chromatography with nitrogen-selective detector. J. Chrom. 383: 232–235, 1986.

R.L.P. Lindberg and K.K. Pihlajamaki. High-performance liquid chromatographic determination of bupivacaine in human serum. J. Chrom. 309: 369–374, 1984.

R.L.P. Lindberg, J.H. Kanto and K.K. Pihlajamaki. Simultaneous determination of bupivacaine and its two metabolites, desbutyl- and 4'-hydroxybupivacaine, in human serum and urine. J. Chrom. 383: 357–364, 1986.

G.F. Marx. Bupivacaine cardiotoxicity — concentration or dose? Anesthesiology 65: 116, 1986.

A. Matouskova and B. Hanson. Continuous mini-infusion of bupivacaine into the epidural space during labor. Acta Obs. Gyn. Scand. Suppl. 83: 31–41, 1979.

H.C. Michaelis, W. Geng, G.F. Kahl and H. Foth. Sensitive determination of bupivacaine in human plasma by high-performance liquid chromatography. J. Chrom. 527: 201–207, 1990.

D.C. Moore, L.E. Mather, L.D. Bridenbaugh et al. Arterial and venous plasma levels of bupivacaine following peripheral nerve blocks. Anesth. Anal. 55: 763–768, 1976.

D.C. Moore, R.I. Balfour and D. Fitzgibbons. Convulsive arterial plasma levels of bupivacaine and the response to diazepam therapy. Anesthesiology 50: 454–456, 1979.

G.B. Park, P.E. Erdtmansky, R.R. Brown et al. Analysis of mepivacaine, bupivacaine, etidocaine, lidocaine, and tetracaine. J. Pharm. Sci. 69: 603–605, 1980.

P.H. Rosenberg, E.A. Kalso, M.K. Tuominen and H.B. Linden. Acute bupivacaine toxicity as a result of venous leakage under the tourniquet cuff during a Bier block. Anesthesiology 58: 95–98, 1983.

D.B. Scott. Evaluation of the toxicity of local anaesthetic agents in man. Brit. J. Anaesth. 47: 56–61, 1975.

J. Thomas, C.R. Climie and L.E. Mather. The maternal plasma levels and placental transfer of bupivacaine following epidural analgesia. Brit. J. Anaesth. 41: 1035–1040, 1969.

G.T. Tucker. Determination of bupivacaine (Marcaine) and other anilide-type local anesthetics in human blood and plasma by gas chromatography. Anesthesiology 32: 255–260, 1970.

P.E. Verheesen, P.J. Brombacher, H.M.H.G. Cremers and R. de Boer. Determination of low levels of bupivacaine (Marcaine) in plasma during epidural analgesia. J. Clin. Chem. Clin. Biochem. 18: 351–353, 1980.

V.W. Wiegand, R.C. Chou, E. Lanz and E. Jahnchen. Determination of bupivacaine in human plasma by high-performance liquid chromatography. J. Chrom. 311: 218–222, 1984.

G.R. Wilkinson and P.C. Lund. Bupivacaine levels in plasma and cerebrospinal fluid following peridural administration. Anesthesiology 33: 482–486, 1970.

K. Yoshikawa, T. Mima and J. Egawa. Blood level of Marcaine (LAC-43) in axillary plexus blocks, intercostal nerve blocks and epidural anaesthesia. Acta Anaesth. Scand. 12: 1–4, 1968.

E. Zylber-Katz, L. Granit and M. Levy. Gas-liquid chromatographic determination of bupivacaine and lidocaine in plasma. Clin. Chem. 24: 1573–1575, 1978.

Buprenorphine

T½: 2–4 hr
Vd: 2.5 L/kg
Fb: 0.96
pKa: 8.5, 10.0

Occurrence and Usage. Buprenorphine (Buprenex) is a synthetic thebaine derivative that has both analgesic and opioid antagonist properties. As an analgesic, it is about 25 to 40 times more potent than morphine. When used as an antagonist, it is equivalent in potency to naltrexone. The usual dose is 0.3–0.6 mg given parenterally, or 0.2–0.4 mg by the sublingual route, every 6 to 8 hours. It is supplied as the hydrochloride in 0.3 mg/mL ampules for parenteral administration.

Blood Concentrations. Five adult patients were given 0.4 mg sublingual doses of buprenorphine 3 hours after a single 0.3 mg intravenous dose; plasma buprenorphine concentrations 2 hours after the sublingual dose ranged from 0.45–0.84 μg/L (average, 0.61). Six and a half hours after the sublingual dose, the plasma concentrations ranged from 0.36–0.58 μg/L (average, 0.47) and, after 10 hours, the concentrations ranged from 0.25–0.36 μg/L (average, 0.31) (Bullingham et al., 1982).

Nine patients with a mean age of 66 years and mean weight of 63 kg were given an intravenous dose of 0.3 mg of buprenorphine and an average plasma concentration of 0.5 μg/L was present 2 hours post-dose; another group of 10 patients, mean age 60 years and mean weight of 72 kg, was given a 0.6 mg dose and at 2 hours the average plasma concentration was almost twice that of the 0.3 mg dose group (Watson et al., 1982).

Metabolism and Excretion. Buprenorphine is metabolized in man primarily by N-dealkylation and conjugation to form norbuprenorphine, which is pharmacologically active, and conjugates of buprenorphine and norbuprenorphine (Cone et al., 1984). Within 144 hours of a single intramuscular dose of radiolabeled drug, 95% is eliminated, with 68% of the radioactivity in the feces and 27% in the urine (Brewster et al., 1981). Concentrations of free buprenorphine and norbuprenorphine in urine may be less than 1 μg/L after therapeutic administration, but can range up to 20 μg/L in abuse situations (Debrabandere et al., 1991).

Toxicity. Symptoms of overdosage include confusion, dizziness, pinpoint pupils, hallucinations, hypotension, respiratory difficulty, seizures and coma. One case has been reported in which the patient took as much as 16 mg of buprenorphine in a suicide attempt and became drowsy, but had an uneventful recovery; blood concentrations were not given (Banks, 1979).

Analysis. Buprenorphine may be measured in biological specimens using a commercially available immunoassay. The drug and its metabolites have been determined by gas chromatography with detection by electron-capture (Cone et al., 1985; Martinez et al., 1990) or mass spectrometry (Blom and Bondesson, 1985; Ohtani et al., 1989). Liquid chromatography has also been used (Garrett and Chandran, 1985; Tebbett, 1985; Debrabandere et al., 1991; Ho et al., 1991).

References

C.D. Banks. Overdosage of buprenorphine: case report. New Zeal. Med. J. 89: 256–257, 1979.

Y. Blom and U. Bondesson. Analysis of buprenorphine and its N-dealkylated metabolite in plasma and urine by selected-ion monitoring. J. Chrom. 338: 89–98, 1985.

D. Brewster, M.J. Humphrey and M.A. McLeavy. Biliary excretion, metabolism and enterohepatic circulation of buprenorphine. Xenobiotica 11: 189–196, 1981.

R.E.S. Bullingham, H.J. McQuay, E.J.B. Porter et al. Sublingual buprenorphine used post-operatively: ten hour plasma drug concentration analysis. Brit. J. Clin. Pharm. 13: 665–673, 1982.

E.J. Cone, C.W. Gorodetzky, D. Yousefnejad et al. The metabolism and excretion of buprenorphine in humans. Drug Met. Disp. 12: 577–581, 1984.

E.J. Cone, C.W. Gorodetzky, D. Yousefnejad and W.D. Darwin. [63]Ni-electron-capture gas chromatographic assay for buprenorphine and metabolites in human urine and feces. J. Chrom. 337: 291–300, 1985.

L. Debrabandere, M. Van Boven and P. Daenens. High-performance liquid chromatography with electrochemical detection of buprenorphine and its major metabolite in urine. J. Chrom. 564: 557–566, 1991.

E.R. Garrett and V.R. Chandran. Pharmacokinetics of morphine and its surrogates VI: bioanalysis, solvolysis kinetics, solubility, pKa values, and protein binding of buprenorphine. J. Pharm. Sci. 74: 515–524, 1985.

S.T. Ho, J.J. Wang, W. Ho and O.Y. Hu. Determination of buprenorphine by high-performance liquid chromatography with fluorescence detection. J. Chrom. 570: 349–350, 1991.

D. Martinez, M.C. Jurado and M. Repetto. Analysis of buprenorphine in plasma and urine by gas chromatography. J. Chrom. 528: 459–463, 1990.

M. Ohtani, F. Shibuya, H. Kotaki et al. Quantitative determination of buprenorphine and its active metabolite, norbuprenorphine, in human plasma by gas chromatography-chemical ionization mass spectrometry. J. Chrom. 487: 469–475, 1989.

I.R. Tebbett. Analysis of buprenorphine by high-performance liquid chromatography. J. Chrom. 347: 411–413, 1985.

P.J.Q. Watson, H.J. McQuay, R.E.S. Bullingham et al. Single-dose comparison of buprenorphine 0.3 and 0.6 mg i.v. given after operation: clinical effects and plasma concentrations. Brit. J. Anaesth. 54: 37–43, 1982.

Bupropion

T½: 4–24 hr
Vd: 40 L/kg
Fb: 0.85
pKa: 8.0

Occurrence and Usage. Bupropion (Wellbutrin), patented in 1974, has been available in the United States since 1990. It is an antidepressant that possesses neither sympathomimetic nor anticholinergic properties, and does not induce monoamine oxidase inhibition, cardiovascular problems or sedation. It is administered in tablets of 75 and 100 mg as the hydrochloride salt; daily oral doses may range from 200–450 mg.

Blood Concentrations. Twenty-four healthy male subjects, 19 to 43 years of age, weighing 56–95 kg (average, 69), were given a 0.46–0.78 mg/kg (32–55 mg/70 kg) oral dose of bupropion following a 12 hour fast; peak plasma concentrations ranged from 64–125 µg/L and occurred within 3 hours (Findlay et al., 1981). Following a single 100 mg oral dose of bupropion, a healthy adult male volunteer exhibited a peak plasma concentration of about 140 µg/L at 3 hours, declining to 50 µg/mL after 6 hours; measurement was by radioimmunoassay (Lai and Schroeder, 1983). Six healthy adult males were given a single oral dose of 200 mg of bupropion following an overnight fast; peak plasma concentrations ranged from 126–388 µg/L and occurred within 100 minutes. Three metabolites appeared later in plasma and were present in all subjects; peak plasma concentrations of hydroxybupropion ranged from 94–486 µg/L and that of the threoamino metabolite, from 27–213 µg/L. The erythroamino metabolite was not quantitated in all subjects (Laizure et al., 1985).

Sixty-one patients, aged 18–82 years, were treated with bupropion in daily doses beginning with 300 mg and gradually increasing to 750 mg by day 14. The minimum effective plasma concentration appeared to be about 25 µg/L and response appeared to diminish above 100 µg/L; maximum improvement in these patients occurred at plasma concentrations between 50 and 100 µg/L (Preskorn, 1983).

Metabolism and Excretion. Bupropion is rapidly and extensively absorbed, widely distributed in the tissues despite more than 80% plasma protein binding, and readily metabolized by hydroxylation and reduction. The metabolites generally show less activity than the parent drug, are not concentrated in the tissues, and are mainly excreted in urine (Schroeder, 1983). However, the 3 major metabolites have somewhat longer elimination half-lives than their parent and generally exceed the plasma bupropion concentration in patients on chronic therapy (Goodnick, 1991). Less than 0.5% of an oral dose is excreted unchanged in urine (Lai and Schroeder, 1983). Urinary elimination of the hydroxy, threoamino and erythroamino metabolites accounts for approximately 4%, 7% and 2% of a dose, respectively, over 48 hours (Devane et al., 1990).

erythro- and threo-amino metabolites — bupropion — hydroxybupropion

Toxicity. Serious side effects were not reported during clinical trials of bupropion. Vivid imagery and dreams, subjective perceptual changes, and dry mouth have been noted in some patients (Becker and Dufresne, 1982; Zung, 1983; Posner et al., 1985). Overdosage often results in seizures, tachycardia, lethargy, confusion, tremors and vomiting (Spiller et al., 1992).

Five fatalities have been reported involving adults who ingested from 4–15 g of the drug; post-mortem bupropion levels averaged 7.3 mg/L (range, 4.0–13) in blood and 11 mg/kg (range, 8.7–14) in liver (Goldberger, 1992; Meeker, 1992; Rohrig and Ray, 1992; Friel et al., 1993).

Analysis. Bupropion may be assayed in biological fluids by radioimmunoassay (Bunz et al., 1981; Mehta and Musso, 1986). Both the parent drug and its major metabolites may be determined by liquid chromatography (Schroeder et al., 1978; Cooper et al., 1984). Gas chromatography has been employed with either nitrogen-phosphorus (Rohrig and Ray, 1992) or mass spectrometric detection (Fogel et al., 1984; Friel et al., 1993). The concern regarding postmortem redistribution stated for amitriptyline also applies to bupropion (Rohrig and Ray, 1992).

References

R.E. Becker and R.L. Dufresne. Perceptual changes with bupropion, a novel antidepressant. Am. J. Psych. 139: 1200–1201, 1982.

R.F. Bunz, D.H. Schroeder, R.M. Welch et al. Radioimmunoassay and pharmacokinetic profile of bupropion in the dog. J. Pharm. Exp. Ther. 217: 602–610, 1981.

T.B. Cooper, R.F. Suckow and A. Glassman. Determination of bupropion and its major basic metabolites in plasma by liquid chromatography with dual-wavelength ultraviolet detection. J. Pharm. Sci. 73: 1104–1107, 1984.

C.L. DeVane, S.C. Laizure, J.T. Stewart et al. Disposition of bupropion in healthy volunteers and subjects with alcoholic liver disease. J. Clin. Psychopharm. 10: 328–332, 1990.

J.W.A. Findlay, J.V.W. Fleet, P.G. Smith et al. Pharmacokinetics of bupropion, a novel antidepressant agent, following oral administration to healthy subjects. Eur. J. Clin. Pharm. 21: 127–135, 1981.

P. Fogel, O.A. Mamer, G. Chouinard and P.G. Farrell. Determination of plasma bupropion and its relationship to therapeutic effect. Biomed. Mass Spec. 11: 629–632, 1984.

P.N. Friel, B.K. Logan and C.L. Fligner. Three fatal drug overdoses involving bupropion. J. Anal. Tox. 17: 436–438, 1993.

B.A. Goldberger. Personal communication, 1992.

P.J. Goodnick. Pharmacokinetics of second generation antidepressants: bupropion. Psychopharm. Bull. 27: 513–519, 1991.

A.A. Lai and D.H. Schroeder. Clinical pharmacokinetics of bupropion: a review. J. Clin. Psych. 44: 82–84, 1983.

S.C. Laizure, S.L. DeVane, J.T. Stewart et al. Pharmacokinetics of bupropion and its major basic metabolites in normal subjects after a single dose. Clin. Pharm. Ther. 38: 586–589, 1985.

J.E. Meeker. Personal communication, 1992.

N.B. Mehta and D.L. Musso. Design and synthesis of a hapten for the radioimmunoassay of bupropion. J. Pharm. Sci. 75: 410–412, 1986.

J. Posner, A. Bye, K. Dean et al. The disposition of bupropion and its metabolites in heathy male volunteers after single and multiple doses. Eur. J. Clin. Pharm. 29: 97–103, 1985.

S.H. Preskorn. Antidepressant response and plasma concentrations of bupropion. J. Clin. Psych. 44: 137–139, 1983.

T.P. Rohrig and N.G. Ray. Tissue distribution of bupropion in a fatal overdose. J. Anal. Tox. 16: 343–345, 1992.

D.H. Schroeder, M.L. Hinton, P.G. Smith et al. A method for analysis for bupropion and its disposition in animals and man. Fed. Proc. 37: 691, 1978.

D.H. Schroeder. Metabolism and kinetics of bupropion. J. Clin. Psych. 44: 79–81, 1983.

H.A. Spiller, E.A. Ramoska, E.P. Krenzelok et al. Bupropion in overdose: a three year multi-center retrospective evaluation. Vet. Hum. Tox. 34: 335, 1992.

W.W.K. Zung. Review of placebo controlled trials with bupropion. J. Clin. Psych. 44: 104–114, 1983.

Buspirone

T½: 1.3–6.6 hr
Vd: ?
Fb: 0.95
pKa: ?

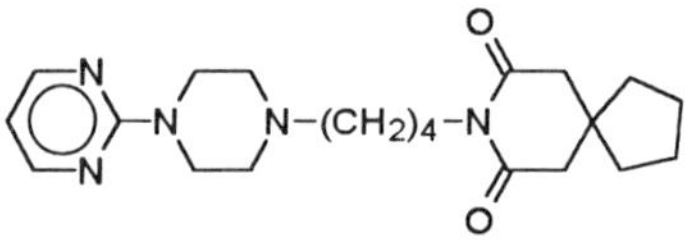

Occurrence and Usage. Buspirone (BuSpar) is an anxiolytic agent that has been available in the United States since 1986. It is the first such drug in a chemical group known as the azaspirodecanediones, which are chemically unrelated to other existing anxiolytic or antipsychotic agents. Buspirone is indicated for the management of anxiety disorders. The initial dose is 5 mg three times daily and the maximum daily dose should not exceed 60 mg. The drug is available as the hydrochloride salt in 5 and 10 mg tablets for oral administration.

Blood Concentrations. Following a single oral dose of 20 mg of buspirone in 12 healthy subjects, the average maximum plasma concentration was 1.15 µg/L (range, 0.49–3.07) at 0.5–1.0 hours. A second peak was observed in 7 of the volunteers averaging 0.47 µg/L (range, 0.21–1.03) between 2 and 4 hours after administration (Dalhoff et al., 1987). Plasma concentrations of a metabolite, 1-PP, are approximately twice those of buspirone after a single oral dose (Sciacca et al., 1988).

Metabolism and Excretion. Buspirone is metabolized primarily by oxidation, producing several hydroxylated derivatives and a pharmacologically active metabolite, 1-pyrimidinylpiperazine (1-PP). The 2 major metabolites are a 5-hydroxy derivative and a glucuronide. From 29–63% of a dose is excreted in the 24 hour urine, primarily as metabolites. Fecal excretion accounts for about 18–38% of the dose (Mayol et al., 1985; Dalhoff et al., 1987).

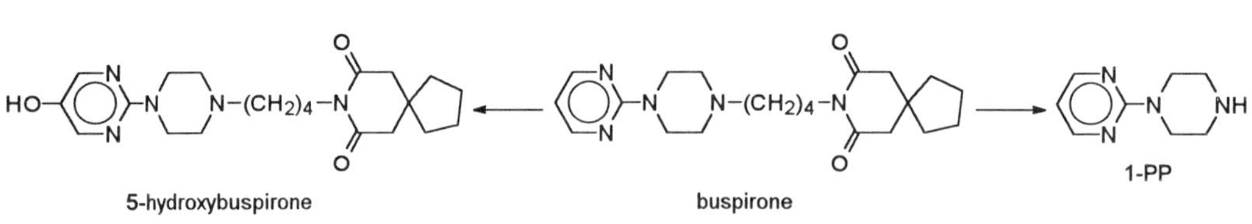

5-hydroxybuspirone   buspirone   1-PP

Toxicity. In overdose, buspirone causes nausea, vomiting, dizziness, drowsiness, miosis and gastric distress. No fatal cases have yet been reported.

Analysis. A radioimmunoassay has been described that is sufficiently sensitive to measure buspirone in plasma following a single therapeutic dose (Mayol et al., 1981). Buspirone can be determined in biological specimens using liquid chromatography (Diaz-Marot et al., 1989; Franklin, 1990; Kristjansson, 1991; Turcant et al., 1991; Betto et al., 1992) or gas chromatography-mass spectrometry (Gammans et al., 1985; Kerns et al., 1986; Sciacca et al., 1988).

References

P. Betto, A. Meneguz, G. Ricciarello and S. Pichini. Simultaneous high-performance liquid chromatographic analysis of buspirone and its metabolite 1-(2-pyrimidinyl)piperazine in plasma using electrochemical detection. J. Chrom. 575: 117–122, 1992.

K. Dalhoff, H.E. Poulsen, P. Garred et al. Buspirone pharmacokinetics in patients with cirrhosis. Brit. J. Clin. Pharm. 24: 547–550, 1987.

A. Diaz-Marot, E. Puigdellivol, C. Salvatella et al. Determination of buspirone and 1-(2-pyrimidinyl)piperazine in plasma samples by high-performance liquid chromatography. J. Chrom. 490: 470–473, 1989.

M. Franklin. Determination of plasma buspirone by high-performance liquid chromatography with coulometric detection. J. Chrom. 526: 590–596, 1990.

R.E. Gammans, E.H. Kerns and W.W. Bullen. Capillary gas chromatographic-mass spectrometric determination of buspirone in plasma. J. Chrom. 345: 285–297, 1985.

E.H. Kerns, W.W. Bullen and R.E. Gammans. Quantitative analysis of 1-(2-pyrimidinyl)piperazine in plasma by capillary gas chromatography-mass spectrometry. J. Chrom. 377: 195–203, 1986.

F. Kristjansson. Sensitive determination of buspirone in serum by solid-phase extraction and two-dimensional high-performance liquid chromatography. J. Chrom. 566: 250–256, 1991.

R.F. Mayol, C.J. Marvel and J.A. La Budde. Development and validation of a radioimmunoassay for buspirone. Fed. Proc. 40: 684, 1981.

R.F. Mayol, D.S. Adamson, R.E. Gammans and J.A. La Budde. Pharmacokinetics and disposition of C-14 buspirone HCl after intravenous and oral dosing in man. Clin. Pharm. Ther. 37: 210, 1985.

M.A. Sciacca, G.F. Duncan, J.P. Shea et al. Simultaneous quantitation of buspirone and 1-(2-pyrimidinyl)piperazine in human plasma and urine by capillary gas chromatography-mass spectrometry. J. Chrom. 428: 265–274, 1988.

A. Turcant, A. Premel-Cabic, A. Cailleux and P. Allain. Toxicological screening of drugs by microbore high-performance liquid chromatography with photodiode-array detection and ultraviolet spectral library searches. Clin. Chem. 37: 1210–1215, 1991.

Butabarbital

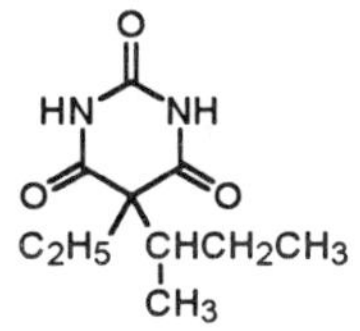

T½: 34–42 hr
Vd: ?
Fb: 0.26
pKa: 7.9

Occurrence and Usage. Butabarbital (secbutobarbitone, 5-ethyl-5-secbutylbarbituric acid, Butisol) is a short to intermediate-acting barbiturate derivative that was prepared in 1932 and is now frequently used as a sedative and hypnotic. In the United States it is available in amounts of 15–100 mg either alone or in combination with other drugs, in at least 10 different preparations containing analgesic, antihypertensive, antispasmodic or diuretic agents. The compound is easily confused with butethal (butobarbitone, 5-ethyl-5-n-butylbarbituric acid), a closely related drug that is in common use in Europe.

Blood Concentrations. In 5 subjects administered the unusually large dose of 600 mg of butabarbital over a 3 hour period, blood concentrations reached an average maximum of 12.3 mg/L (range, 7.6–16.9) at 0.5 hours after the last dose and diminished to 9.9 mg/L (range, 8.8–10.3) by 18 hours (Parker et al., 1970).

Metabolism and Excretion. Butabarbital is metabolized by oxidation of the secondary butyl side chain with formation of a carboxylic acid, a ketone and an alcohol. The stereochemistry of the metabolically produced alcohol, which may exist as diastereoisomers, has not been determined. A single dose is excreted slowly in the urine over a period of 9 days as unchanged drug (5–9%), 2'-hydroxybutabarbital (2–3%), 2'-oxobutabarbital (0.5%) and the carboxylic acid (24–34%) (Gilbert et al., 1975). Urine concentrations of unchanged drug ranged from 4–17 mg/L during the first 21 hours after a 600 mg oral dose (Parker et al., 1970).

butabarbital → 2'-carboxybutabarbital

2'-hydroxybutabarbital → 2'-oxobutabarbital

Toxicity. A 19 year old who ingested an overdose of butabarbital in an unsuccessful suicide attempt was admitted to the hospital in a comatose state. A maximum blood concentration of 39 mg/L was reached 26 hours after admission, and declined thereafter with a half-life of 17 hours. He was arousable when the level fell to about 32 mg/L and became talkative at 19 mg/L (Houts et al., 1981).

Four fatalities due to the ingestion of the drug were reported, with blood concentrations averaging 58 mg/L (range, 30–88) and liver concentrations averaging 112 mg/kg (range, 51–250) (Baselt and Cravey, 1977).

Analysis. Butabarbital is amenable to analysis by the techniques discussed for amobarbital. In addition, Jain et al. (1976) have described several gas chromatographic procedures for the differentiation of butabarbital and butalbital, which are often difficult to separate with common chromatographic systems.

References

R.C. Baselt and R.H. Cravey. A compendium of therapeutic and toxic concentrations of toxicologically significant drugs in human biofluids. J. Anal. Tox. 1: 81–103, 1977.

J.N.T. Gilbert, J.W. Powell and J. Templeton. A study of the human metabolism of secbutobarbitone. J. Pharm. Pharmac. 27: 923–927, 1975.

M. Houts, R.C. Baselt and R.H. Cravey. *Courtroom Toxicology*, Vol. 3, Matthew Bender, New York, 1981.

N.C. Jain, T.Sneath, R. Budd et al. Gas chromatographic separation of allylbarbital and butabarbital. J. Chrom. 116: 194–196, 1976.

K.D. Parker, H.W. Elliott, J.A. Wright et al. Blood and urine concentrations of subjects receiving barbiturates, meprobamate, glutethimide, or diphenylhydantoin. Clin. Tox. 3: 131–145, 1970.

Butalbital

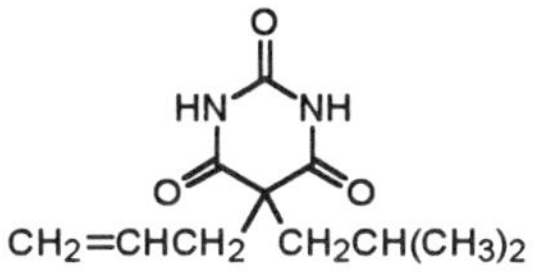

T½: 35–88 hr
Vd: ?
Fb: ?
pKa: 7.6

$$CH_2=CHCH_2 \quad CH_2CH(CH_3)_2$$

Occurrence and Usage. Butalbital (allylbarbital, allylbarbitone, itobarbital, 5-allyl-5-isobutylbarbituric acid, Sandoptal) is an occasionally-encountered short-acting barbiturate closely related to talbutal and less closely to aprobarbital and secobarbital. At one time it was available as a sole agent for sedative-hypnotic use, but at this time it is found only in combination with other drugs such as acetaminophen, aspirin, caffeine, codeine and phenacetin. These "analgesic-sedative" mixtures may contain from 30–50 mg of butalbital and are intended for oral administration.

Blood Concentrations. A single oral 100 mg dose in 5 adults resulted in an average peak blood butalbital concentration of 2.1 mg/L (range, 1.7–2.6) at 2 hours, with a decline to 1.5 mg/L (range, 1.3–1.7) by 24 hours. The elimination half-life averaged 61 hours and the blood/plasma concentration ratio averaged 1.0 (Drost and Walter, 1988).

Metabolism and Excretion. The disposition of butalbital has not been studied in man. In dogs, 92% of a labeled dose is excreted in the 48 hour urine; 50% was present as 5-isobutyl-5-(2,3-dihydroxypropyl) barbituric acid, 10% as 5-allyl-5-(3-hydroxy-2-methyl-1-propyl) barbituric acid, 3% as unchanged drug, and the remainder as unidentified metabolites (Dain et al., 1980).

Toxicity. Intoxication with butalbital can result in lethargy, confusion, disorientation and ataxia. Butalbital blood concentrations in 64 persons arrested for driving under the influence of drugs averaged 8.5 mg/L, with a range of 0.1–28 mg/L (Flores, 1988).

The following concentrations were observed in 2 cases of suicide involving adults (Baselt and Cravey, 1977; Gottschalk and Cravey, 1980):

Butalbital Concentrations in Fatal Cases (mg/L or mg/kg)

Blood	Liver	Urine	Gastric
26*	50	51	28 mg
13	305		

* Also: salicylate, 45 mg/L; caffeine, 25 mg/L

Analysis. Methods for the analysis of this and other barbiturates are discussed under amobarbital. Special gas chromatographic conditions for the separation of butalbital and butabarbital have been described by Jain et al. (1976).

References

R.C. Baselt and R.H. Cravey. A compendium of therapeutic and toxic concentrations of toxicologically significant drugs in human biofluids. J. Anal. Tox. 1: 81–103, 1977.

J.G. Dain, S.I. Bhuta, R.A. Coombs et al. Metabolism of butalbital, 5-allyl-5-isobutylbarbituric acid, in the dog. Drug Met. Disp. 8: 247–252, 1980.

M.L. Drost and L. Walter. Blood and plasma concentrations of butalbital following single oral doses in man. J. Anal. Tox. 12: 322–324, 1988.

J. Flores. Personal communication, 1988.

L.A. Gottschalk and R.H. Cravey. *Toxicological and Pathological Studies on Psychoactive Drug-Involved Deaths*, Biomedical Publications, Davis, California, 1980, pp. 123–124.

N.C. Jain, T. Sneath, R. Budd et al. Gas chromatographic separation of allylbarbital and butabarbital. J. Chrom. 116: 194–196, 1976.

Butaperazine

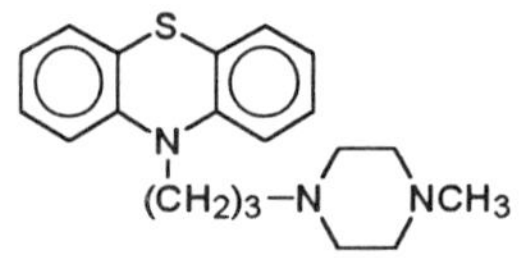

T½: 5–33 hr
Vd: ?
Fb: ?
pKa: ?

Occurrence and Usage. Butaperazine (Repoise) is a commonly used antipsychotic phenothiazine derivative of the piperazine group that was synthesized in 1961. It is administered in daily oral doses of 15–100 mg as the dimaleate salt.

Blood Concentrations. After a single 40 mg oral dose of butaperazine, an average peak plasma concentration of 0.279 mg/L (range, 0.070–0.690) was achieved at approximately 3 hours, with a terminal half-life of 12.4 hours (Garver et al., 1976). In 8 patients receiving 20–100 mg of the drug on a chronic daily basis, plasma concentrations 24 hours after the last dose ranged from 0–0.428 mg/L with an average of 0.110 mg/L (Cooper et al., 1975). During chronic administration of 20 mg daily, the average steady-state serum butaperazine concentration 12 hours after the last dose was 0.229 mg/L; at a chronic dosage of 40 mg daily, the average serum concentration was approximately twice this level (Davis et al., 1974). At a chronic daily dosage of 80 mg, the steady-state plasma levels in 13 patients not responding to the drug ranged from 0.02–0.15 mg/L, and in 11 responders, from 0.10–3.00 mg/L (Smith et al., 1979).

Metabolism and Excretion. Very little is known regarding the human metabolism or excretion of this drug. A sulfoxide has been identified (Simpson et al., 1973) and other unidentified metabolites have been detected in patient plasma (Manier et al., 1974). In dogs, 2–9% of a dose is excreted in urine and 36–71% in feces over a 48 hour period; the major metabolites are products of ring hydroxylation and N-demethylation (Bruce et al., 1974).

Toxicity. Instances of butaperazine poisoning in man have not been reported.

Analysis. A fluorometric procedure has been described for the analysis of butaperazine in biological fluids; the specificity has been investigated by both countercurrent distribution and thin-layer chromatography, with no apparent interference by metabolites (Davis et al., 1974; Garver et al., 1976). At least 3 other variations of the fluorometric technique have appeared and have been applied to clinical determinations of the unchanged drug in plasma (Simpson et al., 1973; Manier et al., 1974; Dekirmenjian et al., 1980). A gas chromatographic method using nitrogen-selective detection has also been developed (Javaid et al., 1979).

References

R.B. Bruce, L.B. Turnbull, J.H. Newman et al. Butaperazine dimaleate metabolism. Xenobiotica 4: 197–207, 1974.

T.B. Cooper, G.M. Simpson, E.J. Haher and P.E. Bergner. Butaperazine pharmacokinetics. Arch. Gen. Psych. 32: 903–905, 1975.

J.M. Davis, D.S. Janowski, H.J. Sekerke et al. The pharmacokinetics of butaperazine in serum. In *The Phenothiazines and Structurally Related Drugs* (I.S. Forrest, C.J. Carr and E. Usdin, eds.), Raven Press, New York, 1974, pp. 433–443.

H. Dekirmenjian, J.I. Javaid, U. Liskevych and J.M. Davis. Determination of butaperazine in plasma and red blood cells by fluorometry. Anal. Biochem. 105: 6–13, 1980.

D.L. Garver, J.M. Davis, H. Dekirmenjian et al. Pharmacokinetics of red blood cell phenothiazine and clinical effects. Arch. Gen. Psych. 33: 862–866, 1976.

J.I. Javaid, H. Dekirmenjian, U. Liskevych and J.M. Davis. Determination of butaperazine in biological fluids by gas chromatography using nitrogen specific detection system. J. Chrom. Sci. 17: 666–670, 1979.

D.H. Manier, J. Sekerke, J.V. Dingell and M.K. El-Yousef. A fluorometric method for the measurement of butaperazine in human plasma. Clin. Chim. Acta 57: 225–230, 1974.

G.M. Simpson, R. Lament, T.B. Cooper et al. The relationship between blood levels of different forms of butaperazine and clinical response. J. Clin. Pharm. 13: 288–297, 1973.

R.C. Smith, J. Crayton, H. Dekirmenjian et al. Blood levels of neuroleptic drugs in nonresponding chronic schizophrenic patients. Arch. Gen. Psych. 36: 579–584, 1979.

Butethal

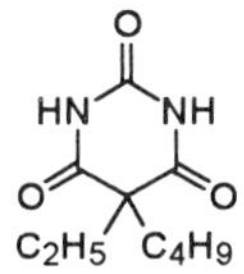

T½: 34–42 hr
Vd: 0.78 L/kg
Fb: 0.26
pKa: 7.9

Occurrence and Usage. Butethal (butobarbitone, butobarbital, 5-ethyl-5-n-butylbarbituric acid, Neonal) is a sedative-hypnotic of intermediate to long duration that was first introduced in 1931. It is not clinically available in the United States but is used frequently in many European countries in oral doses of 50–200 mg for the induction of sleep.

Blood Concentrations. After a single oral dose of 200 mg given to 5 volunteers, peak plasma butethal concentrations of 2.9–4.1 mg/L were attained between 0.6 and 2.0 hours and declined slowly thereafter with an average half-life of 38 hours. During chronic dosing with 50–200 mg of the drug once daily, accumulation in the plasma was noted after the first few days, but this was offset by a 20–25% reduction in the plasma half-life; this latter effect was believed to be the result of induction of drug-metabolizing enzymes (Breimer, 1976).

Metabolism and Excretion. Butethal is metabolized extensively by oxidation of the n-butyl sidechain to alcoholic, keto, and carboxylic acid biotransformation products. Up to 54% of a dose is excreted in the urine over a period of 9 days as unchanged drug (7%), 3'-hydroxybutethal (27%), 3'-oxobutethal (14%) and 3'-carboxybutethal (6%) (Gilbert et al., 1974; Grove et al., 1974).

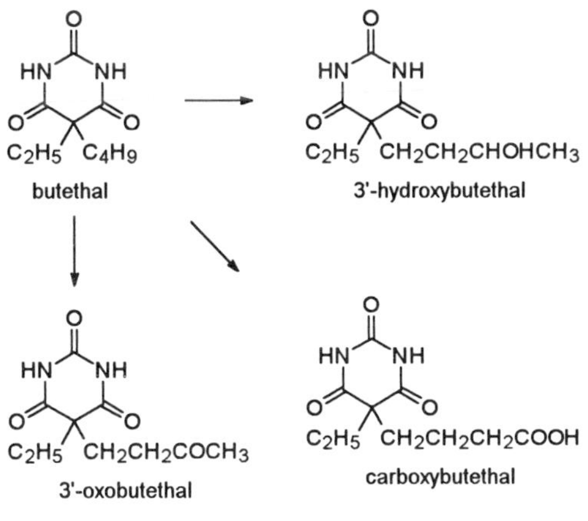

Toxicity. Plasma concentrations as high as 118 mg/L were measured in a barbiturate addict who was admitted in a comatose condition after butethal overdosage; the patient regained consciousness after 16 hours when the plasma level fell to 61 mg/L. The plasma half-life of the drug in this subject was only 12 hours, indicating substantial induction of metabolic enzymes (Prescott et al., 1973).

A blood concentration of 166 mg/L and liver concentration of 155 mg/kg were observed in a fatal case due to ingestion of at least 30 g of the drug (Leung and Ho, 1975). The following concentration ranges for butethal (B) and 3'-hydroxybutethal (HB) were determined in the tissues of 3 victims of fatal overdosage (Robinson and McDowall, 1979):

Drug Concentrations in Butethal Fatalities (mg/L or mg/kg)

Drug	Blood	Lung	Liver	Bile	Kidney	Urine
B	18–49	19–52	47–83	27–131	23–72	4–38
HB	0–3	8–19	2–17	4–312	8–12	5–259

Analysis. Analytical procedures for the quantitation of barbiturates in tissues have been reviewed under amobarbital. Additionally, butethal and its metabolite(s) have been analyzed by gas chromatography (Robinson and McDowall, 1979) and gas chromatography-mass spectrometry (Gilbert and Powell, 1974).

References

D.D. Breimer. Pharmacokinetics of butobarbital after single and multiple oral doses in man. Eur. J. Clin. Pharm. 10: 263–271, 1976.

J.N.T. Gilbert and J.W. Powell. Mass spectrometric determination of butobarbitone and its metabolites in man. Biomed. Mass Spec. 1: 142–144, 1974.

J.N.T. Gilbert, T. Natunen, J.W. Powell and L. Saunders. A kinetic study of human urinary excretion results for butobarbitone and its metabolites. J. Pharm. Pharmac. 26: 16P–23P, 1974.

J. Grove, P.A. Toseland, G.H. Draffan et al. Butobarbitone metabolism in man: identification of 3'-ketobutobarbitone. J. Pharm. Pharmac. 26: 175–178, 1974.

L.C. Leung and K.H. Ho. Personal communication, 1975.

L.F. Prescott, P. Roscoe and J.A.H. Forrest. Plasma concentrations and drug toxicity in man. In *Biological Effects of Drugs in Relation to Their Plasma Concentrations* (D.S. Davies and B.N.C. Prichard, eds.), University Park Press, Baltimore, 1973, pp. 51–81.

A.E. Robinson and R.D. McDowall. The distribution of amylobarbitone, butobarbitone, pentobarbitone and quinalbarbitone and the hydroxylated metabolites in man. J. Pharm. Pharmac. 31: 357–365, 1979.

Butorphanol

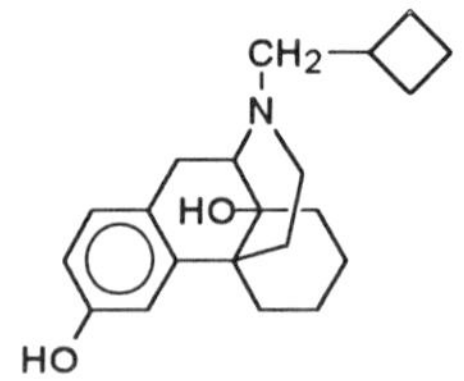

T½: 2.7 hr
Vd: 5 L/kg
Fb: 0.83
pKa: 8.6

Occurrence and Usage. Butorphanol (Stadol) is a synthetic narcotic analgesic, structurally related to levorphanol, that has narcotic antagonist properties. It has analgesic potency 5–8 times greater than that of morphine and 30–40 times that of meperidine. The drug is available as the tartrate salt, in 1–2 mg/mL solutions for intramuscular or intravenous administration and as a 10 mg/mL nasal spray solution. Doses of 0.5–4 mg may be given every 3–4 hours.

Blood Concentrations. Plasma butorphanol concentrations in 6 subjects averaged as high as 1.3 μg/L within 15 minutes of a 1 mg intravenous injection and declined to 0.6 μg/L by 1 hour (Gaver et al., 1980). One hour after a 2 mg intravenous dose, serum concentrations in 3 volunteers averaged 1.5 μg/L, with a range of 1.1–1.7 μg/L (Pittman et al., 1980). A 2 mg intramuscular dose produced peak plasma levels of 2 μg/L after 45 minutes, declining to about 1.3 μg/L by 4 hours (Gaver et al., 1980).

Metabolism and Excretion. Butorphanol is metabolized by hydroxylation of the cyclobutyl ring or by N-dealkylation. A total of 72% of a dose is eliminated in the 96 hour urine, with 14% in the feces. Elimination products consist of free butorphanol (4–5% of a single dose), free hydroxybutorphanol (36%), and free (4%) and conjugated (4%) norbutorphanol. Hydroxybutorphanol, an inactive metabolite, is also found in plasma in concentrations similar to those of the parent drug (Gaver et al., 1980).

butorphanol → hydroxybutorphanol

norbutorphanol → conjugation

Toxicity. Adverse reactions to butorphanol have included sedation, dizziness, nausea, vomiting and insomnia. Overdosage may cause respiratory depression and coma. Instances of toxicity involving butorphanol have not been reported.

Analysis. Butorphanol has been analyzed in biological fluids by radioimmunoassay (Pittman et al., 1980), electron-capture gas chromatography with heptafluorobutyric anhydride derivatization (Gaver et al., 1980; Pfeffer et al., 1980), and gas chromatography-mass spectrometry with trimethylsilyl derivatization (Pittman et al., 1980).

References

R.C. Gaver, M. Vasiljev, H. Wong et al. Disposition of parenteral butorphanol in man. Drug Met. Disp. 8: 230–235, 1980.

M. Pfeffer, R.D. Smyth, K.A. Pittman and P.A. Nardella. Pharmacokinetics of subcutaneous and intramuscular butorphanol in dogs. J. Pharm. Sci. 69: 801–803, 1980.

K.A. Pittman, R.D. Smyth and R.F. Mayol. Serum levels of butorphanol by radioimmunoassay. J. Pharm. Sci. 69: 160–163, 1980.

Butyl Nitrite

T½: ? $C_4H_9NO_2$
Vd: ?
Fb: ?

Occurrence and Usage. Butyl nitrite (n-butyl nitrite or isobutyl nitrite, Locker Room, Rush) is a volatile liquid sold ostensibly as a room odorizer but widely abused by inhalation for its euphoric effects. It is closely related to amyl nitrite, a drug administered by inhalation to produce coronary vasodilation in heart patients and methemoglobinemia in victims of cyanide poisoning.

Butyl nitrite is available without a prescription, in bottles or ampules, in amounts of 2–15 mL. Most brands contain isobutyl nitrite, although n-butyl nitrite is also found. The iso derivative is slightly more potent than the straight-chain compound, and has a boiling point of 67° C. versus 78° C. The LD50 of n-butyl nitrite, orally in rats, has been established as 83 mg/kg (Wood and Cox, 1981). Commercial forms have been found to contain minor amounts of the corresponding butanol isomer (possibly as a degradation product) and 8–10% isoamyl nitrite.

Blood Concentrations. Six volunteers who inhaled isobutyl nitrite for 6–12 minutes developed blood concentrations of the chemical that ranged from 0.5–4.0 mg/L during the exposure; the blood methemoglobin level in these subjects was raised from a baseline of 0.05–0.07 g/dL to 0.2–1.2 g/dL. The subjects experienced dizziness, facial flushing and nasal congestion, which disappeared 5 minutes after inhalation stopped (Horne et al., 1979).

Metabolism and Excretion. The fate of butyl nitrite in man has not been investigated. By analogy to amyl nitrite, it probably rapidly decomposes *in vivo* to butanol and nitrite ion, with a small amount excreted unchanged in the breath. This decomposition can occur in the acid medium of the stomach when the chemical is ingested.

Toxicity. Butyl nitrite or its congeners can cause light-headedness, nausea, ataxia, headache, sedation, syncope, hypotension, cutaneous flushing, pulmonary irritation, methemoglobinemia, and death when inhaled to excess (Sigell et al., 1978). One individual developed severe tracheobronchitis after inhaling isobutyl nitrite over a 1 week period (Covalla et al., 1981), and others have lost consciousness after ingesting a 12 mL bottle of the chemical, developing methemoglobin levels of 54–62% (Smith et al., 1980; Steiner and Manoguerra, 1980). Methemoglobin is normally cleared from the blood with a half-life of 1 hour, but in methemoglobin-reductase deficient persons the half-life is on the order of 2 hours (Horne et al., 1979). The intravenous administration of 100 mg of methylene blue can very rapidly reverse methemoglobinemia (Smith et al., 1980).

Two deaths have occurred following the oral ingestion of isobutyl nitrite; the first individual lived for 2 hours in the hospital and had a postmortem blood methemoglobin level of 95% (O'Toole et al., 1987). The second person also lived for 2 hours, but received methylene blue; his postmortem methemoglobin level was 38%, and nitrite ion was found in the following amounts (Dixon et al., 1981; Shesser et al., 1981):

Nitrite Levels in an Isobutyl Nitrite Fatality (mg/L or mg/kg)

Blood	Brain	Lung	Liver	Kidney	Gastric
22	3	14	9	11	900

Analysis. Intact isobutyl nitrite has been measured in biological specimens by gas chromatography, although details of the method have not been published (Horne et al., 1979). The analysis of nitrite ion is discussed in the section on nitrite, and methods for methemoglobin determination are cited in the section on aniline.

References

J.R. Covalla, C.V. Strimlan and J.G. Lech. Severe tracheobronchitis from inhalation of an isobutyl nitrite preparation. Drug Int. Clin. Pharm. 15: 51–52, 1981.

D.S. Dixon, R.F. Reisch and P.H. Santinga. Fatal methemoblobinemia resulting from ingestion of isobutyl nitrite, a "room odorizer" widely used for recreational purposes. J. For. Sci. 26: 587–593, 1981.

M.K. Horne, M.R. Waterman, L.M. Simon et al. Methemoglobinemia from sniffing butyl nitrite. Ann. Int. Med. 91: 417–418, 1979.

J.B. O'Toole, G.B. Robbins and D.S. Dixon. Ingestion of isobutyl nitrite, a recreational chemical of abuse, causing fatal methemoglobinemia. J. For. Sci. 32: 1811–1812, 1987.

R. Shesser, J. Mitchell and S. Edelstein. Methemoglobinemia from isobutyl nitrite preparations. Ann. Emer. Med. 10: 262–264, 1981.

L.T. Sigell, F.T. Kapp, G.A. Fusaro et al. Popping and snorting volatile nitrites: a current fad for getting high. Am. J. Psych. 135: 1216–1218, 1978.

M. Smith, T. Stair and M.A. Rolnick. Butyl nitrite and a suicide attempt. Ann. Int. Med. 92: 719–720, 1980.

R.W. Steiner and A.S. Manoguerra. Butyl nitrite and methemoglobinemia. Ann. Int. Med. 92: 570, 1980.

R.W. Wood and C. Cox. Acute oral toxicity of butyl nitrite. J. Appl. Tox. 1: 30–31, 1981.

Cadmium

T½: 16 yr (total body)
Vd: ?   Cd
Fb: ?

Occurrence and Usage. Exposure to cadmium is a common occurrence in industry, where it is incorporated into a variety of alloys and metal platings; the inhalation of cadmium dust or fumes constitutes a hazard during heating, grinding, welding and soldering operations involving cadmium-containing metal products. The general populace is exposed to cadmium via food, water, air and cigarette smoking (average, 1.9 µg per pack absorbed), and daily intake of 2–200 µg of the metal is normal. Body accumulation of cadmium, which begins from birth, has been suggested to play a role in hypertension. The threshold limit value for cadmium in air, as a dust or fume, is 0.05 mg/m³.

Blood Concentrations. Mean serum cadmium concentrations in healthy unexposed persons have ranged from 0.0005–0.0020 mg/L in separate studies; whole blood contains nearly twice as much cadmium as serum. Although no relationship was observed between age, sex or smoking history and serum cadmium levels (PetitClerc et al., 1977; Bernard et al., 1977), other investigators have found such associations. For instance, Pleban and Pearson (1979) found that 20 nonsmokers, aged 21–29, had an average blood cadmium concentration of 0.0004 mg/L versus 0.0011 mg/L for a similar group of smokers. Blood cadmium concentrations averaged 0.009 mg/L in asymptomatic workers exposed to cadmium fumes, versus 0.004 mg/L in unexposed subjects (Baker et al., 1979). Blood cadmium concentrations in 102 brazers working with cadmium-containing hard solder ranged from <0.001–0.113 mg/L and correlated only with the length of the brazed splice rather than with factors such as age, sex, smoking or exposure time (Lundberg et al., 1984).

Metabolism and Excretion. After administration of cadmium by inhalation or injection, the metal is known to accumulate in lungs, liver and kidney, with slow excretion in the urine (Potts et al., 1950). In liver and kidney it is bound to a small protein called metallothionein. Due to this accumulation, kidney cadmium concentrations have been shown to correlate positively with age (Schroeder,

1967). Average concentrations for autopsy specimens in England are 2.0 mg/kg (range, 1.2–3.7) for liver and 11.7 mg/kg (range, 2.1–22.0) for kidney (Curry and Knott, 1970), whereas liver concentrations of 23–145 mg/kg and kidney concentrations of 13–80 mg/kg were observed in 4 workers who died 3–9 years after having been occupationally exposed to cadmium for periods of 18–26 years (Friberg, 1957). Normal urine cadmium levels are on the order of 0.0001–0.0002 mg/L (Perry et al., 1975).

The following average concentrations were found in the tissues of normal residents of the United States (Kowal et al., 1979):

Cadmium Concentrations in Normal Subjects (mg/L or mg/kg)

	Blood	Liver	Renal Cortex	Fat	Urine	Hair
Nonsmokers	0.0009	1.0	13	0.03	0.0006	1.0
Smokers	0.0015	1.3	24	0.04	0.0007	0.5

Toxicity. Industrial contamination of water supplies by cadmium, with accumulation of the metal by shellfish, caused an epidemic of cadmium poisoning in Japan known as "itai-itai" disease. Renal damage leading to disturbances in calcium and phosphorus metabolism were believed responsible for the resulting skeletal deformities and severe leg and back pain (Friberg et al., 1971). It has been estimated by several groups of investigators that a cadmium concentration in the range of 100–400 mg/kg in the renal cortex represents a critical level for manifestation of cadmium toxicity during chronic exposure (Ellis et al., 1981).

Early signs of renal damage were observed in 19 cadmium workers whose cadmium levels averaged 0.033 mg/L in blood and 48 μg/g creatinine in urine (Lauwerys et al., 1974). Five men exposed chronically to cadmium fumes at an average air concentration of 0.1 mg/m^3 exhibited symptoms of fatigue, coughing, chest pain and a burning sensation of the throat; urine cadmium levels ranged from 0.01–0.05 mg/L in these workers (Hardy and Skinner, 1947). In 5 nonfatal cases of acute exposure to cadmium fumes, blood and urine concentrations ranged from 1.2–3.0 mg/L and 0.10–0.36 mg/L, respectively (Cotter and Cotter, 1951).

As little as 4 mg of cadmium may be fatal to an adult when inhaled; by ingestion, the lethal dose is estimated to be several hundred milligrams of a soluble salt. Lung cadmium concentrations of 1.5–4.1 mg/kg (normal, 0.5–1.3) were found in several victims of acute fatal exposure to cadmium fume; liver and kidney concentrations were well within the normal ranges, however (Beton et al., 1966; Blejer et al., 1966; Patwardhan and Finckh, 1976). In 3 fatal cases related to chronic cadmium poisoning, concentrations of the metal averaged 128 mg/kg (range, 5–200) in liver and 180 mg/kg (range, 70–300) in kidney (Curry and Knott, 1970). A man who ingested 5 g of cadmium iodide and survived for 7 days developed an initial urine concentration of 5.6 mg/L, declining to 0.1 mg/L on the seventh day (0.5 g EDTA administered daily to hasten excretion); concentrations found in autopsy specimens are as follows (Wisniewska-Knypl et al., 1971):

Cadmium Concentrations in a Fatal Case (mg/L or mg/kg)

Blood*	Brain	Liver	Renal Cortex	Renal Medulla
1.1	0.5	80	80	8.9

* Sampled 3 days after ingestion

Analysis. Prior to the acceptance of atomic absorption spectrophotometry for trace metal analysis, the dithizone colorimetric method was most frequently used for the determination of cadmium in biologic specimens (Stolman, 1961). Atomic absorption procedures include flame (Berman, 1967; Delves, 1977) and graphite furnace techniques (Perry et al., 1975; Lagesson and Andrasko, 1979;

Pleban and Pearson, 1979; Subramanian and Meranger, 1981); most methods require initial sample digestion. Special precautions must be taken in performing these analyses due to the very low concentrations of cadmium in normal biological specimens and the presence of the metal in common laboratory reagents and glassware.

References

E.L. Baker, W.A. Peterson, J.L. Holtz et al. Subacute cadmium intoxication in jewelry workers: an evaluation of diagnostic procedures. Arch. Env. Health 39: 173–177, 1979.

E. Berman. Determination of cadmium, thallium and mercury in biological materials by atomic absorption. At. Abs. Newsl. 6: 57–60, 1967.

A. Bernard, H.A. Roels, J.P. Buchet et al. α_1-Antitrypsin levels in workers exposed to cadmium. In *Clinical Chemistry and Chemical Toxicology of Metals* (S.S. Brown, ed.), Elsevier, New York, 1977, pp. 161–164.

D.C. Beton, G.S. Andrews, H.J. Davies et al. Acute cadmium fume poisoning. Brit. J. Ind. Med. 23: 292–301, 1966.

H.P. Blejer, P.E. Caplan and A.E. Alcocer. Acute cadmium fume poisoning in welders—a fatal and a nonfatal case in California. Calif. Med. 105: 290–296, 1966.

L.H. Cotter and B.H. Cotter. Cadmium poisoning. Arch. Ind. Hyg. Occ. Med. 3: 495–504, 1951.

A.S. Curry and A.R. Knott. "Normal" levels of cadmium in human liver and kidney in England. Clin. Chim. Acta 30: 115–118, 1970.

H.T. Delves. A simple matrix modification procedure to allow the direct determination of cadmium in blood by flame micro-sampling atomic-absorption spectrophotometry. Analyst 102: 403–405, 1977.

K.J. Ellis, W.D. Morgan, I. Zanzi et al. Critical concentrations of cadmium in human renal cortex: dose-effect studies in cadmium smelter workers. J. Tox. Env. Health 7: 691–703, 1981.

L. Friberg. Deposition and distribution of cadmium in man in chronic poisoning. Arch. Ind. Health 16: 27–29, 1957.

L. Friberg, M. Piscator and G. Nordberg. *Cadmium in the Environment*, CRC Press, Cleveland, 1971.

H.L. Hardy and J.B. Skinner. The possibility of chronic cadmium poisoning. J. Ind. Hyg. Tox. 29: 321–324, 1947.

N.E. Kowal, D.E. Johnson, D.F. Kraemer and H.R. Pahren. Normal levels of cadmium in diet, urine, blood, and tissues of inhabitants of the United States. J. Tox. Env. Health 5: 995–1014, 1979.

V. Lagesson and L. Andrasko. Direct determination of lead and cadmium in blood and urine by flameless atomic absorption spectrophotometry. Clin. Chem. 25: 1948–1953, 1979.

R.R. Lauwerys, J.P. Buchet, H.A. Roels et al. Epidemiological survey of workers exposed to cadmium. Arch. Env. Health 28: 145–148, 1974.

I. Lundberg, B. Sjogren, V. Hallne et al. Environmental factors and uptake of cadmium among brazers using cadmium-containing hard solders. Am. Ind. Hyg. Asso. J. 45: 353–359, 1984.

J.R. Patwardhan and E.S. Finckh. Fatal cadmium-fume pneumonitis. Med. J. Aust. 1: 962–966, 1976.

E.F. Perry, S.R. Koirtyohann and H.M. Perry, Jr. Determination of cadmium in blood and urine by graphite furnace atomic absorption spectrophotometry. Clin. Chem. 21: 626–629, 1975.

C. PetitClerc, L. Munan, A. Kelly and M. Cote. Serum cadmium concentrations in patients from a cardiac clinic and in healthy controls. In *Clinical Chemistry and Chemical Toxicology of Metals* (S.S. Brown, ed.), Elsevier, New York, 1977, pp. 157–160.

P.A. Pleban and K.H. Pearson. Determination of cadmium in whole blood and urine by Zeeman atomic absorption spectroscopy. Clin. Chim. Acta 99: 267–277, 1979.

A.M. Potts, F.P. Simon, J.M. Tobias et al. Distribution and fate of cadmium in the animal body. Arch. Ind. Hyg. Occ. Med. 2: 175–188, 1950.

H.A. Schroeder. Cadmium, chromium and cardiovascular disease. Circulation 35: 570–582, 1967.

A. Stolman. Chemical tests for metallic poisons. In *Toxicology, Mechanisms and Analytical Methods*, Vol. 2 (C.P. Stewart and A. Stolman, eds.), Academic Press, New York, 1961, pp. 639–679.

K.S. Subramanian and J.C. Meranger. A rapid electrothermal atomic absorption spectrophotometric method for cadmium and lead in human whole blood. Clin. Chem. 27: 1866–1871, 1981.

J.M. Wisniewska-Knypl, J. Jablonska and Z. Myslak. Binding of cadmium on metallothionein in man: an analysis of a fatal poisoning by cadmium iodide. Arch. Tox. 28: 46–55, 1971.

Caffeine

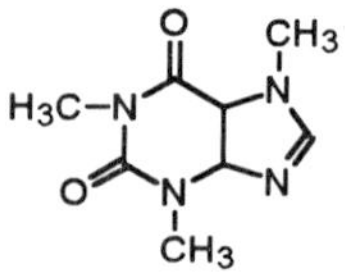

T½: 2.3–12 hr
Vd: 0.4–0.6 L/kg
Fb: 0.35
pKa: 0.8

Occurrence and Usage. Caffeine (1,3,7-trimethylxanthine) is a mild central nervous system stimulant that also produces diuresis, myocardial and respiratory stimulation, and coronary vessel dilation. Its central stimulant actions are more prominent than those of its dimethylxanthine congeners, theophylline and theobromine. Caffeine is a weakly basic alkaloid that occurs naturally in coffee and cocoa beans, kola nuts and tea leaves in amounts of up to 2% by weight. An average cup of coffee or tea in the United States contains 40–100 mg of the drug whereas a 12 oz. cola drink may contain from 35–55 mg. It is believed that chronic usage of caffeine results in tolerance and habituation to this agent. Caffeine is frequently administered orally in analgesic mixtures, migraine remedies and antisoporific preparations in amounts of 32–200 mg; it is occasionally used to reverse central depression in adults by intramuscular injection of 0.5–1.0 g or apnea in premature infants by intravenous injection of 15–20 mg/kg.

Blood Concentrations. After oral ingestion of 120 mg of caffeine by 13 subjects, peak plasma concentrations averaged 3.0 mg/L (range, 2.0–4.0) at 1 hour and fell to 2.5 mg/L by 2 hours (Routh et al., 1969). Following a single oral 300 mg dose, peak plasma levels averaged 7.9 mg/L (range, 6.0–9.0) of caffeine at 1 hour and 0.17 mg/L of theophylline, a metabolite, at 7.5 hours in 4 volunteers (Sved et al., 1976). A single oral administration of 500 mg produced a peak plasma concentration of 14 mg/L at 0.5 hours, declining to 8 mg/L after 3 hours; the plasma half-life of the drug was found to average 3.1 hours (range, 2.3–4.5) (Sant'Ambrogio et al., 1964). Another study has reported an average plasma half-life in 12 subjects of 5.8 hours (range, 3.2–12) (Levy and Zylber-Katz, 1983). Plasma caffeine levels found to be effective in preventing neonatal apnea ranged from 12–36 mg/L (Gorodischer and Karplus, 1982).

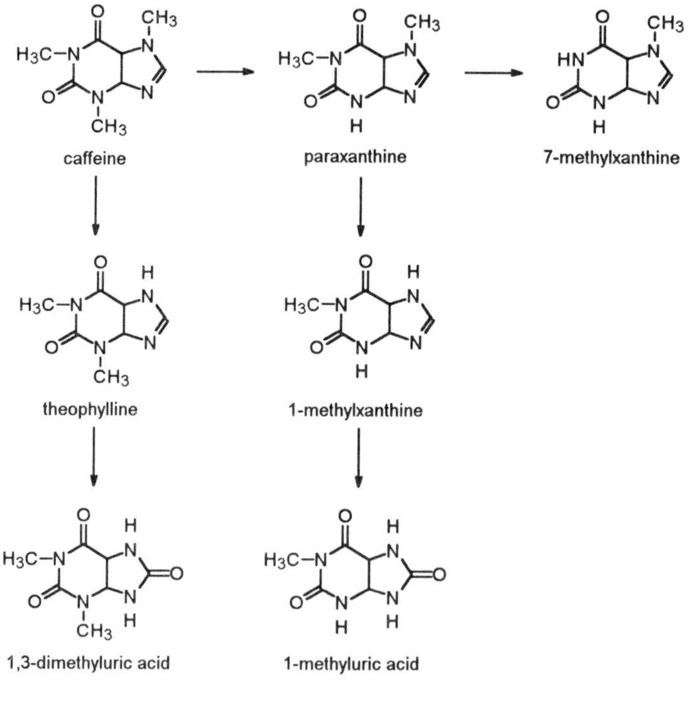

caffeine   paraxanthine   7-methylxanthine

theophylline   1-methylxanthine

1,3-dimethyluric acid   1-methyluric acid

Metabolism and Excretion. Metabolism of caffeine is extensive and involves N-demethylation and oxidation of the 8-carbon to uric acid derivatives. The following amounts of metabolites (expressed as a percentage of the dose) are excreted in the 48 hour urine: 1% caffeine, 4% paraxanthine, 6% 7-methylxanthine, 16% 1-methylxanthine, 9% 1,3-dimethyluric acid and 26% 1-methyluric acid. Uric acid itself has not been found after caffeine administration (Cornish and Christman, 1957). Newborns excrete up to 85% of a dose as unchanged caffeine in the urine, and exhibit a plasma half-life of about 4 days; they gradually develop the ability to metabolize the drug, reaching an adult-like excretion pattern by the age of 8 months (Aldridge et al., 1979). Urinary caffeine concentrations averaged 5.8 mg/L (range, 0–15) in a group of 85 coffee drinkers; the authors concluded that levels greater than 15 mg/L in athletes may represent abuse of caffeine for stimulant purposes (Delbeke and Debackere, 1984).

Toxicity. Caffeine taken in excess can cause flushing or chills, irritability, loss of appetite, weakness, tremor, tachycardia, vomiting, fever, convulsions, cardiac arrhythmias, coma, and death. A newborn who received 375 mg of caffeine for treatment of apnea developed tremor, rapid breathing, and a serum caffeine level of 55 mg/L by 26 hours after birth; this level declined with a half-life of about 60 hours and the child recovered with supportive treatment (Kulkarni and Dorand, 1979). A 1 year old child who ingested from 1–1.5 g of caffeine exhibited emesis, agitation, tachycardia, diuresis, and hyperglycemia; a serum caffeine concentration of 46 mg/L was measured 9 hours after ingestion, and the patient was discharged after several days (Sullivan, 1977). Two adults admitted to a hospital after intentional overdosage with caffeine had maximal serum levels of 49 and 59 mg/L; their symptoms of central nervous system stimulation were successfully treated with sedatives (Baselt, 1980). Two other adults developed tachycardia and one became comatose after intentional ingestion of large amounts (24 g in one case) of caffeine; serum caffeine levels of 200 and 400 mg/L were observed in these patients, both of whom survived (Benowitz et al., 1982; Tisdell et al., 1986).

Fatal caffeine poisoning is a relatively rare event, but several instances have been recorded, usually after accidental or intentional ingestion of very large amounts. The death of an adult occurred following the intravenous injection of 3.2 g of drug (Jokela and Vartiainen, 1959). The following data are derived from 14 cases of fatal overdosage that resulted from the oral administration of 5.3–50 g of caffeine (Borkowski, 1972; Alstott et al., 1973; Grusz-Harday, 1973; Di Maio and Garriott, 1974; Turner and Cravey, 1977; McGee, 1980; Bryant, 1981; Garriott et al., 1985; Winek et al., 1985; Hanzlick et al., 1986).

Caffeine Concentrations in Fatalities (mg/L or mg/kg)

	Blood	Brain	Liver	Kidney	Urine
Mean	183	114	241	184	165
(Range)	(79–344)	(75–188)	(58–670)	(104–352)	(21–542)

Analysis. Caffeine has been analyzed in biological fluids and tissues by ultraviolet spectrophotometry after solvent extraction with measurement at 273 nm (Axelrod and Reichenthal, 1953; Routh et al., 1969). It may also be included in chromatographic assays designed for theophylline; both gas chromatography (Bailey et al., 1976) and liquid chromatography (Blanchard et al., 1980; Haughey et al., 1982; Hartley et al., 1984; Setchell et al., 1987; Tanaka, 1992) have been used successfully in the separation of the major xanthine derivatives. Caffeine may also be analyzed using a commercial enzyme immunoassay (Aranda et al., 1987).

References

A. Aldridge, J.V. Aranda and A.H. Neims. Caffeine metabolism in the newborn. Clin. Pharm. Ther. 25: 447–453, 1979.

A.L. Alstott, A.J. Miller and R.B. Forney. Report of a human fatality due to caffeine. J. For. Sci. 18: 135–137, 1973.

J.V. Aranda, K. Beharry, J. Rex et al. Caffeine enzyme immunoassay in neonatal and pediatric drug monitoring. Ther. Drug Mon. 9: 97–103, 1987.

J. Axelrod and J. Reichenthal. The fate of caffeine in man and a method for its estimation in biological material. J. Pharm. Exp. Ther. 107: 519–523, 1953.

D.G. Bailey, H.L. Davis and G.E. Johnson. Improved theophylline serum analysis by an appropriate internal standard for gas chromatography. J. Chrom. 121: 263–268, 1976.

R.C. Baselt. Unpublished results, 1980.

N.L. Benowitz, J. Osterloh, N. Goldschlager et al. Massive catecholamine release from caffeine poisoning. J. Am. Med. Asso. 248: 1097–1098, 1982.

J. Blanchard, J.D. Mohammadi and K.A. Conrad. Improved liquid-chromatographic determination of caffeine in plasma. Clin. Chem. 26: 1351–1354, 1980.

T. Borkowski. Personal communication, 1972.

J. Bryant. Suicide by ingestion of caffeine. Arch. Path. Lab. Med. 105: 685–686, 1981.

H.H. Cornish and A.A. Christman. A study of the metabolism of theobromine, theophylline and caffeine in man. J. Biol. Chem. 228: 315–323, 1957.

F.T. Delbeke and M. Debackere. Caffeine: use and abuse in sports. Int. J. Sports Med. 5: 179–182, 1984.

V.J.M. Di Maio and J.C. Garriott. Lethal caffeine poisoning in a child. For. Sci. 3: 275–278, 1974.

J.C. Garriott, L.M. Simmons, A. Poklis and M.A. MacKell. Five cases of fatal overdose from caffeine-containing "look-alike" drugs. J. Anal. Tox. 9: 141–143, 1985.

R. Gorodischer and M. Karplus. Pharmacokinetic aspects of caffeine in premature infants with apnoea. Eur. J. Clin. Pharm. 22: 47–52, 1982.

E. Grusz-Harday. Personal communication, 1973.

R. Hanzlick, G.T. Gowitt and W. Wall. Deaths due to caffeine in "look-alike" drugs. J. Anal. Tox. 10: 126, 1986.

R. Hartley, J.R. Cookman and I.J. Smith. Simultaneous determination of caffeine and its N-demethylated metabolites in umbilical cord plasma using high-performance liquid chromatography. J. Chrom. 306: 191–203, 1984.

D.B. Haughey, R. Greenberg, S.F. Schaal and J.J. Lima. Liquid chromatographic determination of caffeine in biologic fluids. J. Chrom. 229: 387–395, 1982.

S. Jokela and A. Vartiainen. Caffeine poisoning. Acta Pharm. Tox. 15: 331–334, 1959.

P.B. Kulkarni and R.D. Dorand. Caffeine toxicity in a neonate. Pediatrics 64: 254–255, 1979.

M. Levy and E. Zylber-Katz. Caffeine metabolism and coffee-attributed sleep disturbances. Clin. Pharm. Ther. 33: 770–775, 1983.

M.B. McGee. Caffeine poisoning in a 10 year old female. J. For. Sci. 25: 29–32, 1980.

R.I. Routh, N.A. Shane, E.G. Arredondo and W.D. Paul. Determination of caffeine in serum and urine. Clin. Chem. 15: 661–668, 1969.

G. Sant'Ambrogio, P. Mognoni and L. Ventrella. Plasma levels of caffeine after oral, intramuscular and intravenous administration. Arch. Int. Pharm. 150: 259–263, 1964.

K.D.R. Setchell, M.B. Welsh, M.J. Klooster and W.F. Balistreri. Rapid high-performance liquid chromatography assay for salivary and serum caffeine following an oral load. An indicator of liver function. J. Chrom. 385: 267–274, 1987.

J.L. Sullivan. Caffeine poisoning in an infant. J. Pediat. 90: 1022–1023, 1977.

S. Sved, R.D. Hossie and I.J. McGilveray. The human metabolism of caffeine to theophylline. Res. Comm. Chem. Path. Pharm. 13: 185–192, 1976.

E. Tanaka. Simultaneous determination of caffeine and its primary demethylated metabolites in human plasma by high-performance liquid chromatography. J. Chrom. 575: 311–314, 1992.

R. Tisdell, M. Iacobucci and W.R. Snodgrass. Caffeine poisoning in an adult. Vet. Hum. Tox. 28: 492, 1986.

J.E. Turner and R.H. Cravey. A fatal ingestion of caffeine. Clin. Tox. 10: 341–344, 1977.

C.L. Winek, W. Wahba, K. Williams et al. Caffeine fatality: a case report. For. Sci. Int. 29: 207–211, 1985.

W.M. Williams, D.C. May, C.H. Jarboe et al. Toxicology screening by gas chromatography-mass spectrometry: three years experience. J. Kent. Med. Asso. 81: 822–825, 1983.

Camphor

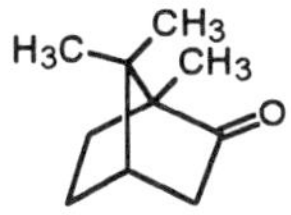

T½: ?
Vd: ?
Fb: 0.61

Occurrence and Usage. Camphor (2-camphenone) is a cyclic ketone obtained by distillation of bark from the tree *Cinnamomum camphora*. Now produced synthetically, it was used for centuries as a medicine by the Chinese, and up until about 1930 was administered parenterally as a cardiovascular stimulant by western physicians. It is now present in a number of over-the-counter medications, for external application as a rubefacient. These liniments contain from 0.3–20% camphor, and include such products as Vicks Vaporub (4.8%), Campho-Phenique (11%), and camphorated oil (20%). The current threshold limit value for industrial exposure is 2 ppm (12 mg/m^3) in the environmental air.

Blood Concentrations. Concentrations of camphor found in blood or plasma after therapeutic usage of the substance have not been reported.

Metabolism and Excretion. Camphor is well-absorbed after inhalation, ingestion, or application to the skin. Its solubility in oil suggests that it would tend to localize in adipose tissue. The compound is believed to be oxidized to an alcohol, campherol, which is then conjugated with glucuronic acid and excreted in the urine (Weiss and Catalano, 1973).

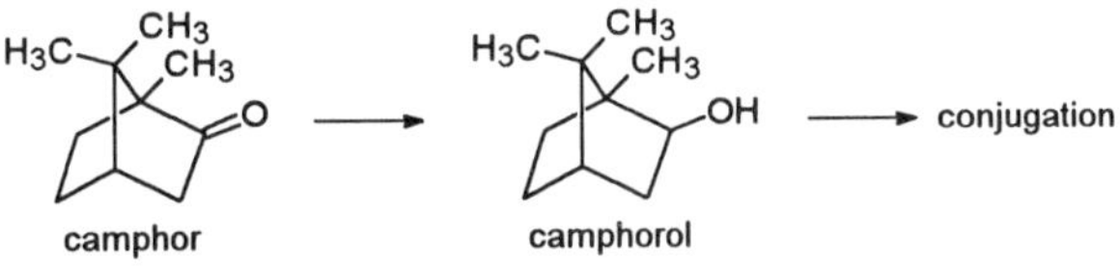

camphor   →   camphorol   →   conjugation

Toxicity. Camphor is a mild local anesthetic when applied to the skin. When ingested in large amounts, it causes nausea, vomiting, central nervous system stimulation, hallucinations, convulsions, coma, and death (Siegel and Watson, 1986). Ingestion of as little as 0.7 g has proven fatal in children, but an adult has survived a dose of 15 g. Twenty children age 4–10 years survived the ingestion of 1–1.5 tablespoons of camphorated oil (mistaken for castor oil), after developing symptoms ranging from nausea to muscular rigidity, coma, and convulsions (Benz, 1919). A 3 year old girl ingested 0.7 g of camphor and became moderately intoxicated; serum taken 7 hours after the ingestion contained 19.5 mg/L camphor (Phelan, 1976). Two adults ingested 6–10 g and developed extreme agitation and hallucinations; serum concentrations of 0.3 and 0.4 mg/L were observed (Koppel et al., 1982). An adult who ingested about 18 g of camphor and developed severe intoxication was treated successfully with resin hemoperfusion and anticonvulsants; his plasma camphor concentration 12 hours after ingestion and just before hemoperfusion was started was 1.7 mg/L (Kopelman et al., 1979).

A 19 month old child died 5 days after the ingestion of 1 teaspoon of camphorated oil; autopsy findings included congestion of the major organs, pulmonary atelectasis and edema, and severe anoxic changes of the brain (Smith and Margolis, 1954).

Analysis. Camphor has been measured in biological fluids by flame-ionization gas chromatography (Kelly et al., 1979) and liquid chromatography (Gallicano et al., 1985).

References

R.W. Benz. Camphorated oil poisoning with no mortality. J. Am. Med. Asso. 72: 1217–1218, 1919.

K.D. Gallicano, H.Y. Park and L.M. Young. A sensitive liquid chromatography procedure for the analysis of camphor in equine urine and plasma. J. Anal. Tox. 9: 24–30, 1985.

R.C. Kelly, R.C. Kopelman and I. Sunshine. A simple gas chromatographic procedure for the determination of camphor in plasma. J. Anal. Tox. 3: 76–77, 1979.

R. Kopelman, S. Miller, R. Kelly and I. Sunshine. Camphor intoxication treated by resin hemoperfusion. J. Am. Med. Asso. 241: 727–728, 1979.

C. Koppel, J. Tenczer, T. Schirop and K. Ibe. Abuse of camphor as a stimulant. Arch. Tox. 51: 101–106, 1982.

W.J. Phelan. Camphor poisoning: over-the-counter dangers. Pediatrics 57: 428–431, 1976.

E. Siegel and S. Watson. Camphor toxicity. Pediat. Clin. N. Am. 33: 375–379, 1986.

A.G. Smith and G. Margolis. Camphor poisoning. Am. J. Path. 30: 857–869, 1954.

J. Weiss and P. Catalano. Camphorated oil intoxication during pregnancy. Pediatrics 52: 713–714, 1973.

Captopril

T½: 1–2 hr
Vd: 0.7 L/kg
Fb: 0.30
pKa: 3.7, 9.8

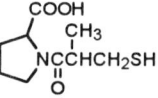

Occurrence and Usage. Captopril (Capoten, Capozide) is a dipeptide analog that was first synthesized in 1976. It was the first of a new class of drugs for the treatment of hypertension, a specific competitive inhibitor of angiotensin I-converting enzyme (ACE). Captopril is also effective in the management of congestive heart failure. The initial dose is 25 mg twice a day, which may be increased as necessary to a maximum daily dose of 450 mg. The drug is available as the free acid in tablets of 12.5–100 mg for oral administration.

Blood Concentrations. Following a single oral dose of 100 mg to 10 adults, peak blood concentrations of 0.51–1.31 mg/L (average, 0.80) of captopril and 0.11–0.49 mg/L (average, 0.23) of captopril disulfide were observed at 0.5–1.5 hours (Kripalani et al., 1980). After the oral administration of 25 mg 3 times daily (75 mg/day) to 12 subjects, a mean maximum steady-state captopril concentration of 0.14 mg/L was found 0.9 hour after a dose (Cody et al., 1982). Ten healthy volunteers were given 100 mg doses for 6 consecutive days of treatment; following the initial dose, the average peak blood concentration was 0.88 mg/L and, after the repeated doses, was 0.82 mg/L, indicating no accumulation of parent drug in man (Duchin et al., 1988).

Metabolism and Excretion. Captopril contains a sulfhydryl group and binds readily to albumin and other plasma proteins. It also forms mixed disulfides with thiol-containing compounds (i.e., cysteine, glutathione), as well as the disulfide dimer of the parent compound; these conjugates are reversible. The following metabolites have been identified: captopril disulfide, captopril S-methyl, captopril S-methyl sulfoxide, captopril glutathione, captopril cysteine, and captopril-N-acetylcysteine (Duchin et al., 1988). Over a 24 hour period, more than 95% of a dose is eliminated in the urine, with about 38% present as unchanged captopril and 1.5% as captopril disulfide (Kripalani et al., 1980; Williams, 1988).

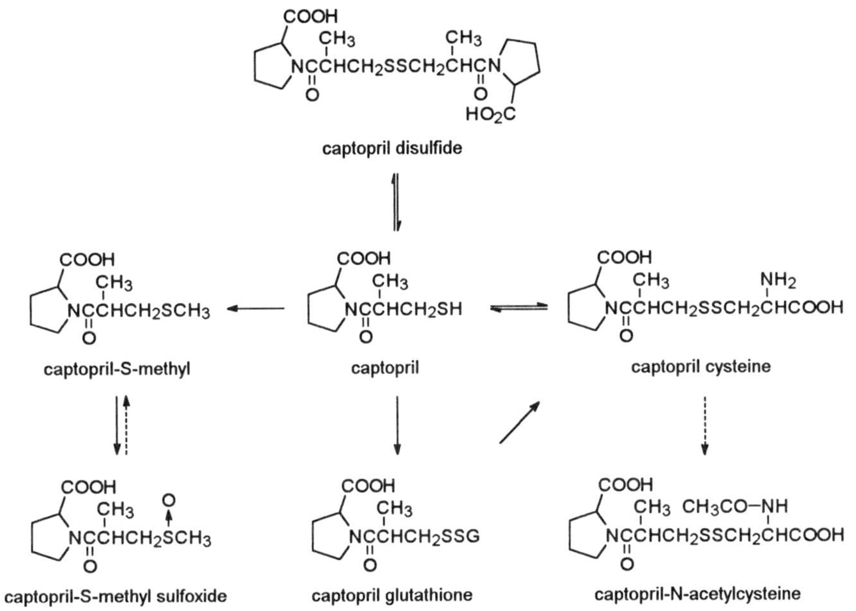

captopril disulfide

captopril-S-methyl   captopril   captopril cysteine

captopril-S-methyl sulfoxide   captopril glutathione   captopril-N-acetylcysteine

Toxicity. Adverse reactions to captopril include skin rash, proteinuria, hematologic disorders, hypotension and angioedema (potentially fatal if it involves the upper airways). A serum captopril concentration of 20 mg/L was measured in a 43 year old man about 7 hours after oral ingestion of 5–7.5 g of drug in an unsuccessful suicide attempt (Lechleitner et al., 1990). A 33 year old woman who ingested 500–730 mg of captopril in a suicide attempt exhibited a plasma captopril concentration of 6.0 mg/L after 6 hours; on the third hospital day, the concentration had dropped to 0.07 mg/L (Augenstein et al., 1988).

In a fatal case involving a 75 year old man with previous suicide attempts found dead in bed, the postmortem blood concentration was 60 mg/L (Park et al., 1990).

Analysis. Captopril has been determined in biological specimens employing gas chromatography with flame-ionization (Matsuki et al., 1980), electron-capture (Bathala et al., 1984) and mass spectrometric detection (Funke et al., 1980; Drummer et al., 1984; Ito et al., 1987). Liquid chromatography has been used for the determination of both captopril and its metabolites (Jarrott et al., 1981; Hayashi et al., 1985; Pereira and Tam, 1988; Colin and Scherer, 1989; Klein et al., 1990; Shen et al., 1992).

References

W.L. Augenstein, K.W. Kulig and B.H. Rumack. Captopril overdose resulting in hypotension. J. Am. Med. Asso. 259: 3302–3305, 1988.

M.S. Bathala, S.H. Weinstein, F.S. Meeker et al. Quantitative determination of captopril in blood and captopril and its disulfide metabolites in plasma by gas chromatogaphy. J. Pharm. Sci. 73: 340–344, 1984.

R.J. Cody, G.L. Schaer, A.B. Covitt et al. Captopril kinetics in chronic congestive heart failure. Clin. Pharm. Ther. 32: 721–726, 1982.

P. Colin and E. Sherer. Simple high performance liquid chromatography determination of captopril in human plasma and cerebrospinal fluid. J. Liq. Chrom. 12: 629–643, 1989.

O.H. Drummer, B. Jarrott and W.J. Louis. Combined gas chromatographic-mass spectrometric procedure for the measurement of captopril and sulfur-conjugated metabolites of captopril in plasma and urine. J. Chrom. 305: 83–89, 1984.

K.L. Duchin, D.N. McKinstry, A.I. Cohen and B.H. Migdalof. Pharmacokinetics of captopril in healthy subjects and in patients with cardiovascular diseases. Clin. Pharmacokin. 14: 241–259, 1988.

P.T. Funke, E. Ivashkiv, M.F. Malley and A.I. Cohen. Gas chromatography-selected ion monitoring mass spectrometric determination of captopril in human blood. Anal. Chem. 52: 1086–1089, 1980.

K. Hayashi, M. Miyamoto and Y. Sekine. Determination of captopril and its mixed disulphides in plasma and urine by high-performance liquid chromatography. J. Chrom. 388: 161–169, 1985.

T. Ito, Y. Matsuki and H. Kurihara. Sensitive method for determination of captopril in biological fluids by gas chromatography-mass spectrometry. J. Chrom. 417: 79–88, 1987.

B. Jarrott, A. Anderson, R. Hooper and W.J. Louis. High-performance liquid chromatographic analysis of captopril in plasma. J. Pharm. Sci. 70: 665–667, 1981.

J. Klein, P. Colin. E. Sherer et al. Simple measurement of captopril in plasma by high-performance liquid chromatography with ultraviolet detection. Ther. Drug Mon. 12: 105–110, 1990.

K.J. Kripalani, D.N. McKinstry, S.M. Singhvi et al. Disposition of captopril in normal subjects. Clin. Pharm. Ther. 27: 636–641, 1980.

P. Lechleitner, A. Dzien, D. Haring and H. Glossmann. Uneventful self-poisoning with a very high dose of captopril. Toxicology 64: 325–329, 1990.

Y. Matsuki, K. Fukuhara, T. Ito et al. Determination of captopril in biological fluids by gas-liquid chromatography. J. Chrom. 188: 177–183, 1980.

H. Park, G.V. Purnell and H.G. Mirchandani. Suicide by captopril overdose. Clin. Tox. 28: 379–382, 1990.

C.M. Pereira and Y.K. Tam. Simplified determination of captopril in plasma by high-performance liquid chromatography. J. Chrom. 425: 208–213, 1988.

G. Shen, W.R. Tian and S.X. Wang. Simple high-performance liquid chromatographic method for the determination of captopril in biological fluids. J. Chrom. 582: 258–262, 1992.

J.A. Williams. Converting-enzyme inhibitors in the treatment of hypertension. New Eng. J. Med. 319: 1517–1525, 1988.

Carbamazepine

T½: 18–65 hr (single dose)
Vd: 0.8–1.8 L/kg
Fb: 0.75
pKa: 7.0

$CONH_2$

Occurrence and Usage. Carbamazepine (Tegretol) is structurally related to the tricyclic antidepressants yet shares few of the pharmacologic properties of that group of drugs. The compound was synthesized in the 1950's, released in the United States for the treatment of trigeminal neuralgia in 1968, and approved for use as an anticonvulsant in 1974. It is supplied in the form of a 100 mg/5 mL suspension or 100 and 200 mg tablets as the free base. The daily oral dose may range from 200–1600 mg in adults.

Blood Concentrations. A single 6 mg/kg (420 mg/70 kg) oral dose given to 5 subjects produced an average peak serum concentration of 6.5 mg/L after 3.2 hours, declining with an average half-life of 31 hours (Levy et al., 1975). The optimal plasma concentration of carbamazepine is thought to lie between 4 and 8 mg/L. A metabolite, carbamazepine-10,11-epoxide, has anticonvulsant activity similar to that of the parent drug, and a plasma half-life that averages 6.1 hours (Tomson et al., 1983).

In 25 epileptic patients receiving a chronic oral dosage ranging from 5.3–20 mg/kg (average, 12.5), plasma concentrations of carbamazepine averaged 5.4 mg/L (range, 1.4–12) and of the epoxide metabolite, 1.1 mg/L (range, 0.2–2.0) (Eichelbaum et al., 1976). In 19 patients receiving an average dose of 17.5 mg/kg, serum carbamazepine concentrations averaged 7.6 mg/L with a range of 1.7–15 (Johannessen and Strandjord, 1973). The blood/plasma concentration ratio for carbamazepine during therapy averages 0.59 (Pynnonen and Yrjana, 1977) and the brain/plasma concentration ratio averages 1.1 (Morselli et al., 1977). The elimination half-life carbamazepine tends to decline with chronic administration, exhibiting values of 5–26 hours for adults and 10–14 hours in children (Morselli, 1989).

Metabolism and Excretion. Carbamazepine has a plasma half-life of 18–65 hours after a single dose and 8–20 hours in epileptic patients on maintenance therapy. Significant self-induction of metabolism occurs with chronic administration (McNamara et al., 1979). It is extensively metabolized, and only 1% of an administered dose is eliminated unchanged in urine. The major pathway of biotransformation is via 10,11-epoxide formation with subsequent hydrolysis to 10,11-dihydroxycarbamazepine and conjugation. A minor pathway results in iminostilbene formation. The identified urinary metabolites (free plus conjugated) consist of 10,11-dihydroxycarbamazepine (10–20%), carbamazepine-10,11-epoxide (2%) and iminostilbene (0.5%) An additional 28% of the dose is eliminated in the feces (Morselli and Frigerio, 1975). Other metabolites identified in urine but not quantitated include carbamazepine-N-glucuronide and a number of mono-, di- and trihydroxycarbamazepine isomers (Lynn et al., 1978; Lertratanangkoon and Horning, 1982).

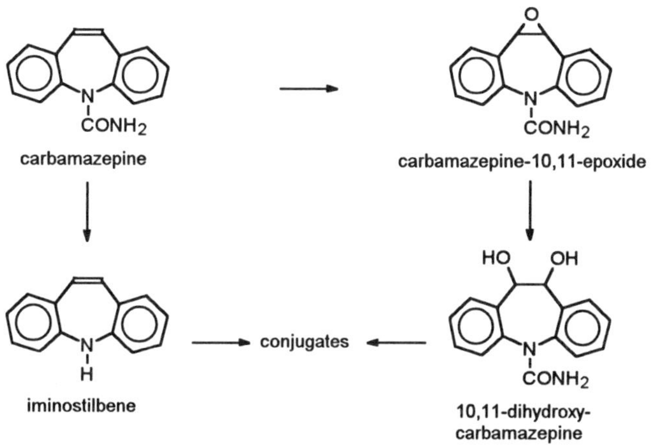

Toxicity. Carbamazepine can cause alopecia, photosensitivity, hepatitis, skin rash, and blood dyscrasias in therapeutic amounts; a number of fatal reactions have occurred during therapy (Zucker et al., 1977; Moore et al., 1985). One case of overdosage involved the intentional ingestion of 5.8 g of the drug; a plasma sample taken while the patient was in a comatose state, 36 hours after ingestion, was found to contain 10 mg/L carbamazepine (Saloman and Pippenger, 1975). In a case involving the ingestion of 20 g of carbamazepine, a maximal blood concentration of nearly 25 mg/L was observed at least 60 hours post-ingestion; the patient did not awaken until the sixth day, at which time the carbamazepine blood concentration had fallen to 9 mg/L (Gruska et al., 1971). Another 24 nonfatal cases have been reported in which peak plasma carbamazepine levels ranged from 12–77 mg/L and carbamazepine-10,11-epoxide levels from 4–34 mg/L; symptoms of intoxication included cyclic coma, seizures, nystagmus, hyper- and hyporeflexia, and tachycardia. Charcoal hemoperfusion or charcoal given frequently by nasogastric tube has been used successfully to accelerate recovery (de Zeeuw et al., 1979; Drenck and Risbo, 1980; Chan et al., 1981; Gary et al., 1981; Lehrman and Bauman, 1981; Rockoff and Baselt, 1981; Sullivan et al., 1981; Hundt et al., 1983; Leslie et al., 1983; Deng et al., 1986; Vree et al., 1986; Spiller and Durbin, 1991).

   A 19 year old male ingested 50 g of carbamazepine and exhibited seizures, hypotension and a plasma drug level of 120 mg/L; cardiorespiratory arrest occurred about 14 hours after admission, at which time the plasma level was 90 mg/L (Vuignier et al., 1986). A 34 year old man ingested an overdose and exhibited seizures, delerium and an admission carbamazepine serum level of 54 mg/L; within 6 hours he developed respiratory difficulty with cyanosis and was declared dead after 4 days in a comatose condition (Fisher and Cysyk, 1988). A 20 year old male epileptic was found dead in bed; postmortem blood contained 53 mg/L carbamazepine and 0.19 g/dL ethanol (Rousseau, 1981).

Analysis. Carbamazepine has been analyzed by gas chromatography, although the drug and its active metabolite are unstable under most chromatographic conditions. The parent compound has been measured as the dimethylformamide dimethylacetal derivative (Perchalski and Wilder, 1974; Millner and Taber, 1979), the pentafluorobenzamide derivative (Schwertner et al., 1978), the N-cyano derivative (Gerardin et al., 1975), the trimethylsilyl derivative (Least et al., 1975; Lensmeyer, 1977) and as the underivatized drug with variable decomposition to iminostilbene (Sheehan and Beam, 1975; Cocks et al., 1981). As the 10,11-epoxide metabolite is easily degraded, the preferred procedure for the simultaneous assay of the parent drug and metabolite is liquid chromatography (Mihaly et al., 1977; Astier et al., 1979; MacKichan, 1980; Sawchuk and Cartier, 1982; Hartley et al., 1986; Bonato et al., 1992).

References

A. Astier, M. Maury and J Barbizet. Simultaneous, rapid high-performance liquid chromatographic microanalysis of plasma carbamazepine and its 10,11-epoxide metabolite. J. Chrom. 164: 235–240, 1979.

P.S. Bonato, V.L. Lanchote, D. deCarvalho and P. Ache. Measurement of carbamazepine and its main biotransformation products in plasma by HPLC. J. Anal. Tox. 16: 88–92, 1992.

K. Chan, J.J. Aguanno, R. Jansen and D.N. Dietzler. Charcoal hemoperfusion for treatment of carbamazepine poisoning. Clin. Chem. 27: 1300–1302, 1981.

D.A. Cocks, T.F. Dyer and K. Edgar. Simple and rapid gas-liquid chromatographic method for estimating carbamazepine in serum. J. Chrom. 222: 496–500, 1981.

J.F. Deng, J.R. Shipe, A.D. Rogol et al. Carbamazepine toxicity: comparison of measurement of drug levels by HPLC and EMIT and model of carbamazepine kinetics. Clin. Tox. 24: 281–294, 1986.

R.A. de Zeeuw, H.G.M. Westenberg, E. van der Kleijn and J.S.F. Gimbrere. An unusual case of carbamazepine poisoning with a near-fatal relapse after two days. Clin. Tox. 14: 263–269, 1979.

N.E. Drenck and A. Risbo. Carbamazepine poisoning, a surprisingly severe case. Anaesth. Int. Care 8: 203–205, 1980.

M. Eichelbaum, L. Bertilsson, L. Lund et al. Plasma levels of carbamazepine and carbamazepine-10,11-epoxide during treatment of epilepsy. Eur. J. Clin. Pharm. 9: 417–421, 1976.

R.S. Fisher and B. Cysyk. A fatal overdose of carbamazepine: case report and review of literature. Clin. Tox. 26: 477–486, 1988.

N.E. Gary, W.M. Byra and R.P. Eisinger. Carbamazepine poisoning: treatment by hemoperfusion. Nephron 27: 202–203, 1981.

A. Gerardin, F. Abadie and J. Laffont. GLC determination of carbamazepine suitable for pharmacokinetic studies. J. Pharm. Sci. 64: 1940–1942, 1975.

H. Gruska, K.H. Beyer, S. Kubicki and H. Schneider. Klinik, Toxikologie und Therapie einer schweren Carbamazepin-Vergiftung. Arch. Tox. 27: 193–203, 1971.

R. Hartley, M. Lucock, J.R. Cookman et al. High-performance liquid chromatographic determination of carbamazepine and carbamazepine 10,11-epoxide in plasma and saliva following solid-phase sample extraction. J. Chrom. 380: 347–356, 1986.

H.K.L. Hundt, A.K. Aucamp and F.O. Muller. Pharmacokinetic aspects of carbamazepine and its two major metabolites in plasma during overdosage. Hum. Tox. 2: 607–614, 1983.

S.I. Johannessen and R.E. Strandjord. Concentration of carbamazepine (Tegretol) in serum and in cerebrospinal fluid in patients with epilepsy. Epilepsia 14: 373–379, 1973.

C.J. Least, G.F. Johnson and H.M. Solomon. Therapeutic monitoring of anticonvulsant drugs: gas-chromatographic simultaneous determination of primidone, phenylethylmalonamide, carbamazepine, and diphenylhydantoin. Clin. Chem. 21: 1658–1662, 1975.

S.N. Lehrman and M.L. Bauman. Carbamazepine overdose. Am. J. Dis. Child. 135: 768–769, 1981.

G.L. Lensmeyer. Isothermal gas chromatographic method for the rapid determination of carbamazepine ("Tegretol") as its TMS derivative. Clin. Tox. 11: 443–454, 1977.

K. Lertratanangkoon and M.G. Horning. Metabolism of carbamazepine. Drug Met. Disp. 10: 1–10, 1982.

P.J. Leslie, R. Heyworth and L.F. Prescott. Cardiac complications of carbamazepine intoxication: treatment by haemoperfusion. Brit. Med. J. 286: 1018, 1983.

R.H. Levy, W.H. Pitlick, A.S. Troupin et al. Pharmacokinetics of carbamazepine in normal man. Clin. Pharm. Ther. 17: 657–668, 1975.

R.K. Lynn, R.G. Smith, R.M. Thompson et al. Characterization of glucuronide metabolites of carbamazepine in human urine by gas chromatography and mass spectrometry. Drug Met. Disp. 6: 494–501, 1978.

J.J. MacKichan. Simultaneous liquid chromatographic analysis for carbamazepine and carbamazepine 10,11-epoxide in plasma and saliva by use of double internal standardization. J. Chrom. 181: 373–383, 1980.

P.J. McNamara, W.A. Colburn and M. Gilbaldi. Time course of carbamazepine self-induction. J. Pharm. Biopharm. 7: 63–68, 1979.

G.W. Mihaly, J.A. Phillips, W.J. Louis and F.J. Vajda. Measurement of carbamazepine and its epoxide metabolite by high-performance liquid chromatography, and a comparison of assay techniques for the analysis of carbamazepine. Clin. Chem. 23: 2283–2287, 1977.

S.N. Millner and C.A. Taber. Rapid gas chromatographic determination of carbamazepine for routine therapeutic monitoring. J. Chrom. 163: 96–102, 1979.

N.C. Moore, B. Lerer, E. Meyendorff and S. Gershon. Three cases of carbamazepine toxicity. Am. J. Psych. 142: 974–975, 1985.

P.L. Morselli. Carbamazepine. In *Antiepileptic Drugs*, 3rd ed. (R. Levy, R. Mattson, B. Meldrum et al., eds), Raven Press, New York, 1989, pp. 473–490.

P.L. Morselli and A. Frigerio. Metabolism and pharmacokinetics of carbamazepine. Drug Met. Rev. 4: 97–113, 1975.

P.L. Morselli, A. Baruzzi, M. Gerna et al. Carbamazepine and carbamazepine-10,11-epoxide concentrations in human brain. Brit. J. Clin. Pharm. 4: 535–540, 1977.

R.J. Perchalski and B.J. Wilder. Rapid gas-liquid chromatographic determination of carbamazepine in plasma. Clin. Chem. 20: 492–493, 1974.

S. Pynnonen and T. Yrjana. The significance of the simultaneous determination of carbamazepine and its 10,11-epoxide from plasma and human erythrocytes. Int. J. Clin. Pharm. 15: 222–226, 1977.

S. Rockoff and R. Baselt. Severe carbamazepine poisoning. Clin. Tox. 18: 935–939, 1981.

M. Rousseau. Personal communication, 1981.

M. Saloman and C.E. Pippenger. Acute carbamazepine encephalopathy. J. Am. Med. Asso. 231: 915, 1975.

R.J. Sawchuk and L.L. Cartier. Simultaneous liquid-chromatographic determination of carbamazepine and its epoxide metabolite in plasma. Clin. Chem. 28: 2127–2130, 1982.

H.A. Schwertner, H.E. Hamilton and J.E. Wallace. Analysis for carbamazepine in serum by electron-capture gas chromatography. Clin. Chem. 24: 895–899, 1978.

M. Sheehan and R.E. Beam. GLC determination of underivatized carbamazepine in whole blood. J. Pharm. Sci. 64: 2004–2006, 1975.

H.A. Spiller and D.R. Durbin. Massive carbamazepine overdose with cranial nerve abnormalities. Vet. Hum. Tox. 33: 357, 1991.

J.B. Sullivan, Jr., B.H. Rumack and R.G. Peterson. Acute carbamazepine toxicity resulting from overdose. Neurology 31: 621–624, 1981.

T. Tomson, G. Tybring and L. Bertilsson. Single-dose kinetics and metabolism of carbamazepine-10,11-epoxide. Clin. Pharm. Ther. 33: 58–65, 1983.

B.I. Vuignier, O.F. Woo and C.E. Becker. Fatal carbamazepine overdose with seizures: role of charcoal hemoperfusion. Vet. Hum. Tox. 28: 504, 1986.

T.B. Vree, T.J. Janssen, Y.A. Hekster et al. Clinical pharmacokinetics of carbamazepine and its epoxy and hydroxy metabolites in humans after an overdose. Ther. Drug Mon. 8: 297–304, 1986.

P. Zucker, F. Daum and M.I. Cohen. Fatal carbamazepine hepatitis. J. Pediat. 91: 667–668, 1977.

Carbaryl

T½: ?
Vd: ?
Fb: ?

Occurrence and Usage. Carbaryl (Sevin) is a carbamate derivative of 1-naphthol that is used as a short-acting insecticide. Human exposure is usually via inhalation, although the compound is also absorbed through the skin. The current threshold limit value is 5 mg/m³.

Blood Concentrations. Intact carbaryl is not routinely measured in human blood. Blood or plasma cholinesterase levels are frequently used to monitor exposure to carbaryl and other cholinesterase inhibitors. Professional applicators wearing no protective equipment exhibited no net decrease in serum or erythrocyte cholinesterase after a 25 minute spray application (Leavitt et al., 1982).

Metabolism and Excretion. Carbaryl is known to be metabolized by ring hydroxylation, hydrolysis and conjugation. The hydrolysis pathway results in the urinary excretion of free and conjugated 1-naphthol, which accounts for over 20% of an ingested dose and which may be measured as an index of exposure to the chemical. Another 4% of a dose is excreted as conjugated p-hydroxycarbaryl (Knaak et al., 1967).

Urine concentrations of 1-naphthol in unexposed subjects average less than 0.01 mg/L and do not exceed 0.23 mg/L (Kutz et al., 1978). Exposed but asymptomatic workers exhibited 1-naphthol urine concentrations of less than 0.1 to more than 42 mg/L; air concentrations of carbaryl during these exposures ranged from 0.2–31 mg/m³ (Best and Murray, 1962). In another study of formulating plant workers, asymptomatic individuals excreted 1-naphthol in urine at concentrations of 0.2–65 mg/L, averaging 8.9 mg/L (Comer et al., 1975).

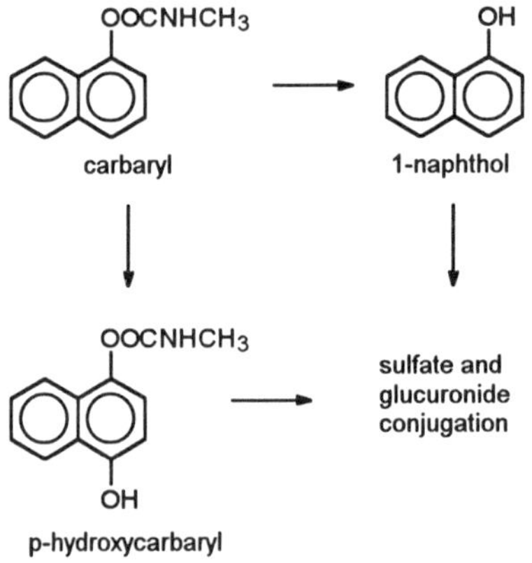

Toxicity. The inactivation of cholinesterase by carbaryl produces symptoms of intoxication that include blurred vision, salivation, sweating, nausea, vomiting and convulsions. The effects of the carbamate insecticides in general do not persist as long as those of the organophosphates. Volunteers who ingested doses of carbaryl of up to 0.13 mg/kg daily for 6 weeks were asymptomatic (Wills et al., 1968). Workers exposed to air concentrations of the chemical of up to 31 mg/m³ were also asymptomatic but did exhibit occasional depression of blood cholinesterase activity (Best and Murray, 1962).

A 1.5 year old child who ingested an unknown amount of carbaryl became moderately intoxicated and was treated with atropine; the urine, collected 18 hours after the incident, contained 31 mg/L 1-naphthol (Best and Murray, 1962). Ingestion of 250 mg has caused severe poisoning in an adult who recovered after administration of 3 mg atropine (Hayes, 1963). A man who ingested 27 g of carbaryl was comatose for 24 hours but survived with treatment; he experienced severe peripheral neuropathy that persisted for 9 months (Dickoff et al., 1987).

Three adults who died within hours after intentionally ingesting an unknown amount of carbaryl had the following tissue concentrations of the chemical (Farago, 1967; Duck and Woolias, 1985; Simmons, 1989):

Carbaryl Concentrations in Fatalities (mg/L or mg/kg)

	Blood	Brain	Liver	Kidney	Urine
Average	16	4.6	21	13	31
(Range)	(6–27)	(4.6)	(12–29)	(1.9–25)	(31)

Analysis. Cholinesterase activity in blood or brain, which has been found to correlate well with carbaryl concentration in these tissues (Mount et al, 1981), may be determined by colorimetry (Fleisher and Pope, 1954) or by an electrometric method (Michel, 1949). Carbaryl itself has been analyzed in biological specimens by a nonspecific colorimetric technique involving diazotization (Farago, 1967) and by electron-capture gas chromatography after derivatization with heptafluorobutyric anhydride (Mount and Oehme, 1980). The measurement of 1-naphthol in urine is generally accomplished by colorimetry (Best and Murray, 1962) or by gas chromatography (Shafik et al., 1971). Liquid chromatography has also been employed (DeBerardinis and Wargin, 1982; Duck and Woolias, 1985).

References

E.M. Best and B.L. Murray. Observations on workers exposed to Sevin insecticide: a preliminary report. J. Occ. Med. 10: 507–517, 1962.

S.W. Comer, D.C. Staiff, J.F. Armstrong and H.R. Wolfe. Exposure of workers to carbaryl. Bull. Env. Cont. Tox. 13: 385–391, 1975.

M. DeBernardinis and W.A. Wargin. High-performance liquid chromatographic determination of carbaryl and 1-naphthol in biological fluids. J. Chrom. 246: 89–94, 1982.

D.J. Dickoff, O. Gerber and Z. Turovsky. Delayed neurotoxicity after ingestion of carbamate pesticide. Neurology 37: 1229–1231, 1987.

B.J. Duck and M. Woolias. Reversed-phase high performance liquid chromatographic determination of carbaryl in postmortem specimens. J. Anal. Tox. 9: 177–179, 1985.

A. Farago. Suicidale, toedliche Sevin-(1-Naphthyl-N-methyl-karbamat-) Vergiftung. Arch. Tox. 24: 309–315, 1969.

J.H. Fleisher and E.J. Pope. Colorimetric method for determination of red blood cell cholinesterase activity in whole blood. Arch. Ind. Hyg. Occ. Med. 9: 323–334, 1954.

W.J. Hayes, Jr. *Clinical Handbook on Economic Poisons*, U.S. Government Printing Office, Washington, DC, 1963, p. 45.

J.B. Knaak, L.J. Sullivan and J.H. Wills. Metabolism of carbaryl in man. Tox. Appl. Pharm. 10: 390, 1967.

F.W. Kutz, R.S. Murphy and S.C. Strassman. Survey of pesticide residues and their metabolites in urine from the general population. In *Pentachlorophenol* (K.R. Rao, ed.), Plenum Press, New York, 1978, pp. 363–369.

J.R.C. Leavitt, R.E. Gold, T. Holcslaw and D. Tupy. Exposure of professional pesticide applicators to carbaryl. Arch. Env. Cont. Tox. 11: 57–62, 1982.

H.O. Michel. An electrometric method for the determination of red blood cell and plasma cholinesterase activity. J. Lab. Clin. Med. 34: 1564–1568, 1949.

M.E. Mount and F.W. Oehme. Microprocedure for determination of carbaryl in blood and tissues. J. Anal. Tox. 4: 286–292, 1980.

M.E. Mount, A.D. Dayton and F.W. Oehme. Carbaryl residues in tissues and cholinesterase activities in brain and blood of rats receiving carbaryl. Tox. Appl. Pharm. 58: 282–296, 1981.

M.T. Shafik, H.C. Sullivan and H.F. Enos. A method for the determination of 1-naphthol in urine. Bull. Env. Cont. Tox. 6: 34–39, 1971.

V.C.G. Simmons. Personal communication, 1989.

J.H. Wills, E. Jameson and F. Coulston. Effect of oral doses of carbaryl in man. Clin. Tox. 1: 265–271, 1968.

Carbon Disulfide

T½: less than 1 hr
Vd: ?   CS$_2$
Fb: ?

Occurrence and Usage. Carbon disulfide is widely used as an industrial solvent and as an insecticide. It is also a chemical byproduct in the production of viscose rayon, and is a human metabolite of disulfiram and other dithiocarbamates. Exposure is usually via inhalation of the vapor or by dermal contact. The current threshold limit value for carbon disulfide is 10 ppm (31 mg/m^3).

Blood Concentrations. Carbon disulfide blood concentrations reached maximum levels after 2 hours of exposure to about 30 ppm of the vapor in air and ranged from 0.15–0.28 mg/L (Teisinger and Soucek, 1949). Blood concentrations of 0.10–0.70 mg/L were observed during exposure to air concentrations on the order of 80 ppm. The half-life for disappearance of the substance from blood is estimated at less than 1 hour (Piotrowski, 1977).

Metabolism and Excretion. From 50–90% of an absorbed dose of carbon disulfide is metabolized in the body. From 8–20% of the dose may be eliminated unchanged in the exhaled breath and only about 0.5% in the urine. About two-thirds of that which is excreted unchanged in urine is in bound form, and requires acidification and aeration of urine for its release (McKee et al., 1948; Teisinger and Soucek, 1949; Piotrowski, 1977). The metabolized carbon disulfide appears primarily in the urine as inorganic sulfates, thiourea, 2-mercapto-2-thiazolin-5-one and 2-thiothiazolidine-4-carboxylic acid (TTCA); the latter 2 compounds are conjugates with glycine and cysteine, respectively (Pergal et al., 1972a; Pergal et al., 1972b; van Doorn et al., 1981). Urinary TTCA accounts for 1–2% of an absorbed dose of carbon disulfide (Rosier et al., 1987), but its concentrations do not appear to correlate well with the extent of environmental exposure to the chemical (Kitamura et al., 1993).

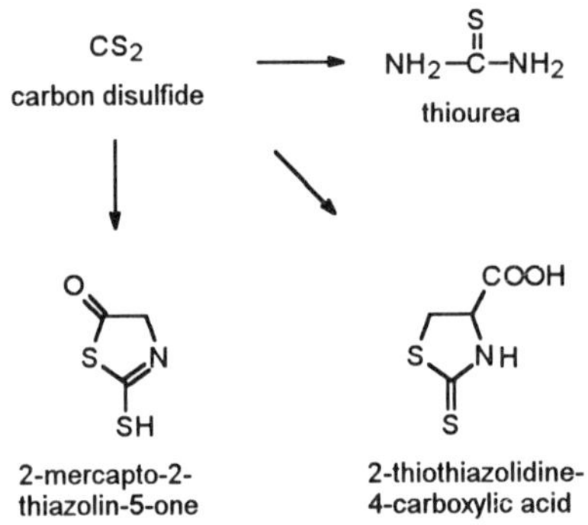

Toxicity. Mild exposure to carbon disulfide causes dizziness and headache, while moderate exposure may produce nervousness, fatigue and weight loss. Chronic intoxication has been reported to result in permanent damage to the central and peripheral nervous systems, atherosclerotic tendencies, electrocardiographic abnormalities, and liver and kidney damage (Gordy and Trumper, 1938). Symptoms of moderate to severe intoxication have appeared in individuals chronically exposed to vapor concentrations averaging slightly in excess of 20 ppm (Kleinfeld and Tabershaw, 1955). Exposure to carbon disulfide concentrations of 300 ppm or more can cause serious pathologic changes after only a few days.

Acute ingestion of only 15 mL may be fatal to an adult. The victims of fatal poisoning have exhibited breathing difficulty, collapse, hypothermia, cyanosis, convulsions, coma, and respiratory paralysis (Davidson and Feinleib, 1972).

Analysis. Intact carbon disulfide may be measured in biological fluids by colorimetry (McKee, 1941) or gas chromatography (Herber and Poppe, 1976). For the routine assessment of industrial exposure, the iodine-azide test for urinary metabolites of carbon disulfide is customarily performed (Djuric et al., 1965; Djuric, 1967). Other methods applicable to carbon disulfide determination are cited in the section on disulfiram.

References

M. Davidson and M. Feinleib. Carbon disulfide poisoning: a review. Am. Heart J. 83: 100–114, 1972.

D. Djuric. Determination of carbon disulfide and its metabolites in biological material. In *Toxicology of Carbon Disulphide* (H. Brieger and J. Teisinger, eds.), Excerpta Medica, Amsterdam, 1967, pp. 52–61.

D. Djuric, N. Surducki and I. Berkes. Iodine-azide test on urine of persons exposed to carbon disulphide. Brit. J. Ind. Med. 22: 321–323, 1965.

S.T. Gordy and M. Trumper. Carbon disulfide poisoning. J. Am. Med. Asso. 110: 1543–1549, 1938.

R.F.M. Herber and H. Poppe. A new method for the estimation of exposure to carbon disulphide. J. Chrom. 118: 23–34, 1976.

S. Kitamura, F. Ferrari, G. Vides and D.C.M. Filho. Biological monitoring of workers occupationally exposed to carbon disulphide in a rayon plant in Brazil. Int. Arch. Occ. Env. Health 65: S177–S180, 1993.

M. Kleinfeld and I.R. Tabershaw. Carbon disulfide poisoning. J. Am. Med. Asso. 159: 677–679, 1955.

R.W. McKee. A quantitative microchemical colorimetric determination of carbon disulfide in air, water and biological fluids. J. Ind. Hyg. Tox. 23: 151–158, 1941.

R.W. McKee, C. Kiper, J.H. Fountain et al. A solvent vapor, carbon disulfide. J. Am. Med. Asso. 122: 217–222, 1948.

M. Pergal, N. Vukojevic, N. Cirin-Popov et al. Carbon disulfide metabolites excreted in the urine of exposed workers. Arch. Env. Health 25: 38–41, 1972a.

M. Pergal, N. Vukojevic, N. Sad and D. Djuric. II. Isolation and identification of thiocarbamide. Arch. Env. Health 25: 42–44, 1972b.

J.K. Piotrowski. *Exposure Tests for Organic Compounds in Industrial Toxicology*, U.S. Government Printing Office, Washington, D.C., 1977, pp. 102–106.

J. Rosier, H. Veulemans, R. Masschelein et al. Experimental human exposure to carbon disulfide. Int. Arch. Occ. Env. Health 59: 243–250, 1987.

T. Teisinger and B. Soucek. Absorption and elimination of carbon disulfide in man. J. Ind. Hyg. Tox. 2: 67–73, 1949.

R. van Doorn, L.P.C. Delbressine, C.M. Leijdekkers et al. Identification and determination of 2-thiothiazolidine-4-carboxylic acid in urine of workers exposed to carbon disulfide. Arch. Tox. 47: 51–58, 1981.

Carbon Monoxide

T½: 4–5 hr
Vd: ?   CO
Fb: ?

Occurrence and Usage. Carbon monoxide is an odorless, colorless gas that has approximately the same density as air. The compound is produced from the incomplete combustion of organic fuels, and it represents the most abundant air pollutant in the lower atmosphere. Common sources of the gas are cigarette smoke, which contains about 4% carbon monoxide, automobile exhaust, which contains from 0.5–10%, and various industrial processes. The metabolism of dichloromethane provides an unexpected source of CO. Atmospheric CO concentrations range from 2–50 ppm along expressways and in smoke-filled rooms, and may exceed 100 ppm during temperature inversions and in heavy urban traffic. The current occupational threshold limit value is 25 ppm (29 mg/m³).

Blood Concentrations. Carbon monoxide is produced endogenously by the catabolism of heme at an average rate of 0.4 mL/hour in resting male subjects; this amount is sufficient to establish a background carboxyhemoglobin (COHb) saturation of 0.4–0.7% (Stewart, 1975). COHb averages 1–2% in urban nonsmokers and 5–6% in smokers (Stewart et al., 1974). Sitting in a smoky room for 1.5 hours caused a 38% increase in the COHb saturation of nonsmokers (Seppanen, 1977). Exposure to a constant air concentration of carbon monoxide results in a constant COHb level after an equilibration period of some hours, the time required being inversely proportional to the CO concentration. Atmospheric concentrations of 50, 100 and 200 ppm produce approximate equilibrium COHb saturations of 8, 16 and 30%, respectively (Peterson and Stewart, 1970).

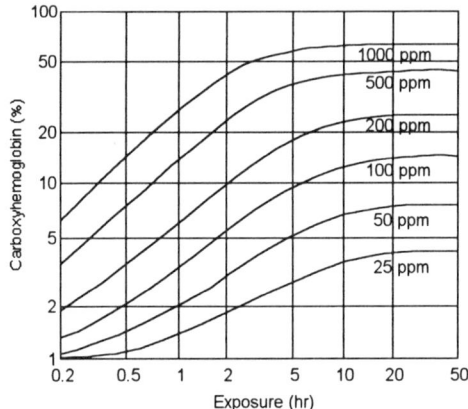

Metabolism and Excretion. Carbon monoxide is eliminated substantially unchanged by pulmonary excretion, with less than 1% oxidized by metabolic processes to carbon dioxide. The half-life of carboxyhemoglobin in resting adults at sea level is 4–5 hours, but may be reduced to approximately 80 minutes by the administration of pure oxygen, and may be further reduced to 24 minutes by using oxygen at 3 atmospheres pressure (Stewart, 1975).

Toxicity. The reversible binding of carbon monoxide with the hemoglobin molecule results in a mild to severe hypoxia, which can produce symptoms of headache, nausea, weakness, confusion, stupor and coma.

It has been shown in a number of studies that COHb concentrations of 10% or less adversely affect a person's ability to perform complex tasks as well as strenuous manual labor (Coburn et al., 1977). Blood COHb concentrations of 5–10% may aggravate pre-existing heart disease, while concentrations of 15–25% often cause dizziness and nausea (Grace and Platt, 1981; Allred et al., 1991). Levels of carboxyhemoglobin that exceed 50% saturation are considered as life-threatening. If the concentrations are attained rapidly by exposure to very high levels of carbon monoxide, the resulting physiological effects are not as intense as if the concentrations are attained gradually. It is believed that prolonged hypoxia as well as the delayed entry of CO into cells account for this lack of correlation (Sokal, 1975; Somogyi et al., 1981).

Persons who die in fires usually succumb as a result of the carbon monoxide and, possibly, hydrogen cyanide produced during the combustion process. In 85 victims of fire, postmortem COHb concentrations ranged from 25–85% with an average value of 59% (Dominguez, 1962). In victims of flash fires, however, carboxyhemoglobin levels may not be significantly elevated (Hirsh et al., 1977). Analysis of a series of 41 fatalities due to the accidental or intentional inhalation of automobile exhaust gases has revealed COHb concentrations ranging from 48–93%, with an average of 72% (Baselt, 1978).

Analysis. Whole blood specimens for carbon monoxide analysis should be preserved with sodium fluoride and stored in the dark at 4° C. (or frozen), since bacterial action can result in both the production of CO and the denaturation of hemoglobin. The aging of blood results in the spontaneous production of methemoglobin with marked increases in the apparent concentration of COHb by some analytical procedures. Treatment of old or postmortem blood specimens with sodium hydrosulfite (10 mg/5 mL) to convert methemoglobin to hemoglobin is recommended prior to CO measurement regardless of the procedure used (Dominguez et al., 1964; Blackmore, 1974).

Prior to 1960, quantitative estimations of carboxyhemoglobin involved primarily spectrophotometric, colorimetric and gasometric techniques (Maehly, 1962). Automated visible spectrophotometry is now a widely used procedure (Freireich and Landau, 1971; Dubowski and Luke, 1973), and gas chromatography has largely replaced other less accurate and less specific methods. However, several manual spectrophotometric techniques are available that are especially useful for routine monitoring of low-level employee exposure, requiring only a finger-prick blood specimen (Commins and Lawther, 1965; Buchwald, 1969; Rodkey et al., 1979), while others have been adapted to the requirements of forensic analysis (Hayashi and Nanikawa, 1978; Pannell et al., 1981; Siek and Rieders, 1984; Lopez-Rivadulla et al., 1989).

Gas chromatographic techniques usually involve release of the carbon monoxide with ferricyanide reagent, followed by separation on a molecular sieve column and thermal conductivity detection (Dominguez et al., 1959; Hessel and Modglin, 1967; Vreman et al., 1984; Goldbaum et al., 1986). Calculation of COHb saturation may be based on the total CO-binding capacity of the specimen, although other authors suggest that determination of total hemoglobin by a cyanmethemoglobin or total iron method provides a more accurate means of assessing COHb in postmortem or aged samples (Ainsworth et al., 1967; Blackmore, 1970; Kupferschmidt and Perrigo, 1977; Sato et al., 1990). Gas chromatographic procedures for the determination of very low levels of COHb in fresh blood specimens have utilized vacuum or vortex gas extraction (McCredie and Jose, 1967; Dahms and Horvath, 1974), or catalytic reduction of CO to methane and subsequent flame-ionization detection (Collison et al., 1968; Baretta et al., 1978; Griffin, 1979; Cardeal et al., 1993).

References

C.A. Ainsworth, E.L. Schoegel, T.J. Domanski and L.R. Goldbaum. A gas chromatographic procedure for the determination of carboxyhemoglobin in postmortem samples. J. For. Sci. 12: 529–537, 1967.

E.N. Allred, E.R. Bleecker, B.R. Chaitman et al. Effects of carbon monoxide on myocardial ischemia. Env. Health Persp. 91: 89–132, 1991.

E.D. Baretta, R.D. Stewart, S.A. Graff and K.K. Donahoo. Methods developed for the mass sampling analysis of CO and carboxyhemoglobin in man. Am. Ind. Hyg. Asso. J. 39: 202–209, 1978.

R.C. Baselt. Unpublished results, 1978.

D.J. Blackmore. The determination of carbon monoxide in blood and tissue. Analyst 95: 439–458, 1970.

D.J. Blackmore. Interpretation of carbon monoxide levels found at post-mortem. In *Forensic Toxicology* (B. Ballantyne, ed.), John Wright & Sons, Bristol, 1974, pp. 114–120.

H. Buchwald. A rapid and sensitive method for estimating carbon monoxide in blood and its application in problem areas. Am. Ind. Hyg. Asso. J. 30: 564–569, 1969.

Z.L. Cardeal, D. Pradeau, M. Hamon et al. New calibration method for gas chromatographic assay of carbon monoxide in blood. J. Anal. Tox. 17: 193–195, 1993.

R.F. Coburn, E.R. Allen, S.M. Ayres et al. *Carbon Monoxide*, National Academy of Sciences, Washington, D.C., 1977.

H.A. Collison, F.L. Rodkey and J.D. O'Neal. Determination of carbon monoxide in blood by gas chromatography. Clin. Chem. 14: 162–171, 1968.

B.T. Commins and P.J. Lawther. A sensitive method for the determination of carboxyhaemoglobin in a finger prick sample of blood. Brit. J. Ind. Med. 22: 139–143, 1965.

T.E. Dahms and S.M. Horvath. Rapid, accurate technique for determination of carbon monoxide in blood. Clin. Chem. 20: 533–537, 1974.

A.M. Dominguez, H.E. Christensen, L.R. Goldbaum and V.A. Stembridge. A sensitive procedure for determining carbon monoxide in blood or tissue utilizing gas-solid chromatography. Tox. Appl. Pharm. 1: 135–143, 1959.

A.M. Dominguez. Problems of carbon monoxide in fires. J. For. Sci. 7: 379–392, 1962.

A.M. Dominguez, J.R. Halstead and T.J. Domanski. The effect of postmortem changes on carboxyhemoglobin results. J. For. Sci. 9: 330–341, 1964.

K.M. Dubowski and J.L. Luke. Measurement of carboxyhemoglobin and carbon monoxide in blood. Ann. Clin. Lab. Sci. 3: 53–65, 1973.

A.W. Freireich and D. Landau. Carbon monoxide determination in postmortem clotted blood. J. For. Sci. 16: 112–119, 1971.

L.R. Goldbaum, D.H. Chace and N.T. Lappas. Determination of carbon monoxide in blood by gas chromatography using a thermal conductivity detector. J. For. Sci. 31: 133–142, 1986.

T.W. Grace and F.W. Platt. Subacute carbon monoxide poisoning. J. Am. Med. Asso. 246: 1698–1700, 1981.

B.R. Griffin. A sensitive method for the routine determination of carbon monoxide in blood using flame ionization gas chromatography. J. Anal. Tox. 3: 102–104, 1979.

T. Hayashi and R. Nanikawa. Further study on spectrophotometric determination of CO-Hb in post-mortem blood. For. Sci. 11: 127–134, 1978.

D.W. Hessel and F.R. Modglin. The determination of carbon monoxide in blood by gas-solid chromatography. J. For. Sci. 12: 123–131, 1967.

C.S. Hirsch, R.O. Bost, S.R. Gerber et al. Carboxyhemoglobin concentrations in flash fire victims. Am. J. Clin. Path. 68: 317–320, 1977.

G.J. Kupferschmidt and B. Perrigo. Carbon monoxide and hemoglobin determination in autopsy blood samples. Can. Soc. For. Sci. J. 10: 13–25, 1977.

M. Lopez-Rivadulla, A.M. Bermejo, P. Fernandez et al. Direct carboxyhemoglobin determination by derivative spectroscopy. For. Sci. Int. 40: 261–266, 1989.

A.C. Maehly. Quantitative determination of carbon monoxide. In *Methods of Forensic Science*, Vol. 1 (F. Lundquist, ed.), Interscience Publishers., New York, 1962, pp. 539–592.

R.M. McCredie and A.D. Jose. Analysis of blood carbon monoxide and oxygen by gas chromatography. J. Appl. Physiol. 22: 863–866, 1967.

L.K. Pannell, B.M. Thomson and L.F. Wilkinson. A modified method for the analysis of carbon monoxide in postmortem blood. J. Anal. Tox. 5: 1–5, 1981.

J.E. Peterson and R.D. Stewart. Absorption and elimination of carbon monoxide by inactive young men. Arch. Env. Health 21: 165–171, 1970.

F.L. Rodkey, T.A. Hill, L.L. Pitts and R.F. Robertson. Spectrophotometric measurement of carboxyhemoglobin and methemoglobin in blood. Clin. Chem. 25: 1388–1393, 1979.

K. Sato, K. Tamaki, H. Hattori et al. Determination of total hemoglobin in forensic blood samples with special reference to carboxyhemoglobin analysis. For. Sci. Int. 48: 89–96, 1990.

A. Seppanen. Smoking in closed space and its effect on carboxyhaemoglobin saturation of smoking and non-smoking subjects. Ann. Clin. Res. 9: 281–283, 1977.

T.J. Siek and F. Rieders. Determination of carboxyhemoglobin in the presence of other blood hemoglobin pigments by visible spectrophotometry. J. For. Sci. 29: 39–54, 1984.

J.A. Sokal. Lack of the correlation between biochemical effects on rats and blood carboxyhemoglobin concentrations in various conditions of single acute exposure to carbon monoxide. Arch. Tox. 34: 331–336, 1975.

E. Somogyi, I. Balogh, G. Rubanyi et al. New findings concerning the pathogenesis of acute carbon monoxide (CO) poisoning. Am. J. For. Med. Path. 2: 31–39, 1981.

R.D. Stewart, E.D. Baretta, L.R. Platte et al. Carboxyhemoglobin levels in American blood donors. J. Am. Med. Asso. 229: 1187–1195, 1974.

R.D. Stewart. The effect of carbon monoxide on humans. Ann. Rev. Pharm. 15: 409–422, 1975.

H.J. Vreman, L.K. Kroong and D.K. Stevenson. Carbon monoxide in blood: an improved microliter blood-sample collection system, with rapid analysis by gas chromatography. Clin. Chem. 30: 1382–1386, 1984.

Carbon Tetrachloride

T½: ?
Vd: ? CCl_4
Fb: ?

Occurrence and Usage. Carbon tetrachloride has for years been widely used as a dry-cleaning chemical, degreasing agent and fire extinguisher, although recent United States Food and Drug Administration regulations against its commercial sale have restricted it to laboratory and industrial usage. The fact that it was once used as an antihelmintic drug for humans in oral doses of 2–4 mL is now alarming in view of its acute toxicity (minimal lethal dose, 3–5 mL) and the severe hepatorenal effects seen in subacute and chronic exposures. It is now employed as a grain fumigant, solvent and a chemical intermediate in the manufacture of fluorocarbons. The current threshold limit value for industrial environments is 5 ppm (30 mg/m³). The odor threshold of the compound is about 50 ppm.

Blood Concentrations. Using an analytical method that had a 5 mg/L limit of sensitivity, Stewart et al. (1961) were unable to detect carbon tetrachloride in the blood of men exposed to 11 ppm of the vapor for 3 hours or to 49 ppm for 1.2 hours. Monkeys exposed to 46 ppm of the vapor developed maximal blood concentrations of 1.7 mg/L after 4.5 hours (McCollister et al., 1951).

Metabolism and Excretion. The metabolism of carbon tetrachloride has not been studied in man. In monkeys, at least 51% of the absorbed dose was eliminated in the expired air as carbon tetrachloride (40%) and carbon dioxide (11%) in the 29 days after exposure; significant amounts were excreted in urine and feces as metabolic products, including urea and carbonates (McCollister et al., 1951). It is believed that the metabolic conversion of the molecule to a highly reactive free radical accounts for its ability to cause tissue necrosis.

Carbon tetrachloride concentrations in the breath of men exposed to 10 ppm of the vapor for 3 hours averaged 2–3 ppm at the end of the exposure, 0.7 ppm after 1 hour and less than 0.3 ppm after 5 hours. Following a 70 minute exposure to 49 ppm, these concentrations were 10–20 ppm, less than 2 ppm and less than 0.3 ppm, respectively (Stewart et al., 1961).

Toxicity. Carbon tetrachloride has produced numerous cases of acute and chronic poisoning, by virtue of its central nervous system depressant and nephro- and hepatotoxic effects (Hardin, 1954). Prolonged exposure to vapor concentrations of 25 ppm or more may cause severe kidney and liver damage. Acute renal damage leading to death has resulted from exposure to concentrations of 1000–2000 ppm for 30–60 minutes. Excessive alcohol usage may potentiate the toxic effects of carbon tetrachloride. The chemical is suspected of having carcinogenic potential in man.

An adult who ingested 30 mL of the chemical and recovered had a serum carbon tetrachloride level of 20 mg/L on admission to the hospital; the first 24 hour urine specimen was found to contain 8 mg/L of the compound (Clarke, 1969). Nineteen patients admitted to hospital with symptoms of acute carbon tetrachloride poisoning had blood concentrations ranging from 0.1–32 mg/L; all patients recovered except one (Ruprah et al., 1985). A 29 year old woman who ingested up to 300 mL of carbon tetrachloride was successfully treated by gastric lavage, mannitol diuresis, and hemodialysis; she eliminated the chemical with a half-life of about 2 days, as measured by analysis of the expired air (Stewart et al., 1963).

An adult who committed suicide by inhaling carbon tetrachloride vapors had a postmortem blood concentration of 260 mg/L (Cravey, 1978). A 32 year old worker who died of liver and kidney failure 18 hours after a 1 day exposure to the vapor had a postmortem blood level of 288 mg/L (Maravelias et al., 1985). The following concentrations were determined in the tissues of an adult who died 7 days after a single inhalation exposure to carbon tetrachloride (Korenke and Pribilla, 1969):

Carbon Tetrachloride Concentrations in a Fatal Case (mg/L or mg/kg)

Muscle	Lung	Liver	Kidney	Gastric
46	39	142	32	2.3 mg

Analysis. Carbon tetrachloride may be determined colorimetrically after steam distillation from biological specimens using a modification of the Fujiwara method (Freimuth, 1961). Gas chromatographic techniques have relied on headspace sampling with flame-ionization detection or solvent extraction with electron-capture detection (Dubowski, 1975; Reddrop et al., 1980; Vierke et al., 1982).

References

E.G.C. Clarke (ed.). *Isolation and Identification of Drugs*, Pharmaceutical Press, London, 1969, p. 240.

R.H. Cravey. Personal communication, 1978.

K.M. Dubowski. Organic volatile substances. In *Methodology for Analytical Toxicology* (I. Sunshine, ed.), CRC Press, Cleveland, 1975, pp. 407–411.

H.C. Freimuth. Identification and estimation of volatile poisons. In *Toxicology, Mechanisms and Analytical Methods*, Vol. 2 (C.P. Stewart and A. Stolman, eds.), Academic Press, New York, 1961, pp. 75–77.

B.L. Hardin, Jr. Carbon tetrachloride poisoning—a review. Ind. Med. Surg. 23: 93–105, 1954.

H.D. Korenke and O. Pribilla. Suicid durch einmalige Inhalation von Tetrachlorkohlenstoff (CCl₄) mit Leukoencephalopathie. Arch. Tox. 25: 109–126, 1969.

C. Maravelias, S. Athanaselis and A. Koutselinis. A fatal case involving the inhalation of chlorinated hydrocarbon solvent. In *Proceedings of the International Association of Forensic Toxicologists*, Brighton, England, 1985, pp. 373–376.

D.D. McCollister, W.H. Beamer, G.J. Atchison and H.C. Spencer. The absorption, distribution and elimination of radioactive carbon tetrachloride by monkeys upon exposure to low vapor concentrations. J. Pharm. Exp. Ther. 102: 112–124, 1951.

C.J. Reddrop, W. Riess and T.F. Slater. Two rapid methods for the simultaneous gas-liquid chromatographic determination of carbon tetrachloride and chloroform in biological material and expired air. J. Chrom. 193: 71–82, 1980.

M. Ruprah, T.G.K. Mant and R.J. Flannagan. Acute carbon tetrachloride poisoning in 19 patients: implications for diagnosis and treatment. Lancet 1: 1027–1029, 1985.

R.D. Stewart, H.H. Gay, D.S. Erley et al. Human exposure to carbon tetrachloride vapor. J. Occ. Med. 3: 586–590, 1961.

R.D. Stewart, E.A. Boettner, R.R. Southworth and J.C. Cerny. Acute carbon tetrachloride intoxication. J. Am. Med. Asso. 183: 994–997, 1963.

W. Vierke, J. Gellert and R. Teschke. Head-space gas chromatographic analysis for rapid quantitative determination of carbon tetrachloride in blood and liver of rats. Arch. Tox. 51: 91–99, 1982.

Carbromal

T½: 7–15 hr
Vd: ?
Fb: ?

$(C_2H_5)_2CBrCONHCONH_2$

Occurrence and Usage. Carbromal (bromodiethylacetylurea, Adalin, ingredient of Carbrital) is a monoureide derivative used as a mild short-acting sedative. Other less commonly used bromoureides include acetylcarbromal and bromisoval (bromvaletone, Bromural). Although carbromal is considered to be largely obsolete, its continued availability and relatively high toxicity occasionally result in episodes of acute or chronic intoxication. It is administered orally in doses of 130–520 mg alone or in combination with 49–195 mg of pentobarbital; the latter preparation (Carbrital) is marketed in the United States as both a capsule and an elixir.

Blood Concentrations. A 1000 mg single oral dose of carbromal produced a maximal serum concentration of the intact drug of 6.0 mg/L at 0.5 hours, declining rapidly to 4.3 mg/L at 2 hours and 1.0 mg/L by 9 hours; concentrations of bromoethylbutyramide, an active metabolite, reached a peak of 3.1 mg/L at 2 hours and declined more slowly than the parent drug; serum concentrations of total bromide reached 13 mg/L by 9 hours and were still increasing (Vohland et al., 1976). Inorganic bromide blood concentrations in subjects administered 650–2275 mg of carbromal for up to 10 days reached as high as 100 mg/L (Shaw and Shaw, 1959).

Metabolism and Excretion. Carbromal is metabolized by hydrolysis to bromoethylbutyramide, which is further metabolized by oxidation of an ethyl group to 2-bromo-2-ethyl-3-hydroxybutyramide. Debromination of the parent also occurs with formation of 2-ethylbutyrylurea and the release of bromide ion. The overall sedative effect of the drug during chronic usage is due to the combined actions of carbromal, bromoethylbutyramide and bromide ion. The metabolites are excreted in the urine in undetermined quantity (Butler, 1964; Curry, 1960; Sticht and Kaferstein, 1976).

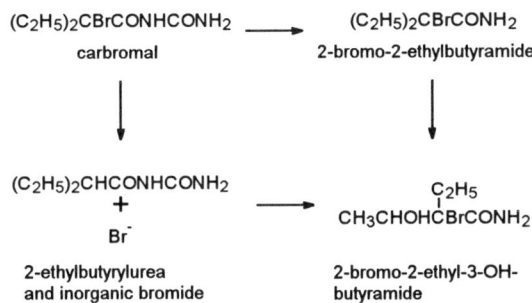

Toxicity. Acute intoxication with carbromal causes central nervous system depression. Chronic use can result in hallucinations, delerium, speech defects, emotional disturbances and motor incoordination.

Inorganic bromide blood concentrations in patients intoxicated with carbromal tend to be lower than those seen in poisonings with inorganic bromide salts, primarily due to the smaller amount of bromide administered. Serum bromide levels in five chronic carbromal abusers, who had symptoms ranging from anxiety to ataxia, were between 400 and 1250 mg/L (Kessell, 1969). Other patients have been studied, however, who presented with acute delerium and who had serum bromide levels, obtained through chronic abuse, of 1500–3500 mg/L (Trethowan and Pawloff, 1962).

Although most fluid and tissue concentrations in cases involving carbromal have been reported in terms of total bromide, in acute poisonings the predominant drug species are carbromal and bromoethylbutyramide. Uges and Bouma (1979) described the case of a 16 year old girl who ingested an overdose and was comatose at a serum carbromal concentration of 49 mg/L; this level subsequently rose to 105 mg/L 6 hours later, and the girl awoke 2 days later when the serum level had declined to 37 mg/L. Carbromal concentrations in the serum of patients with moderate to severe acute intoxication have ranged from 24–110 mg/L, while serum levels of bromoethylbutyramide were approximately twice as high (Vohland et al., 1978; Maes et al., 1985).

A number of deaths have been documented following the ingestion of as little as 10 g of carbromal. Two cases were described in which serum carbromal concentrations as high as 400 and 920 mg/L were determined during the course of intoxication; both patients died after several days in coma, when the serum concentrations had fallen to 158 and 71 mg/L, respectively (Gruska et al., 1970; Gruska et al., 1971). Turner (1959) has found liver bromide concentrations of 80–502 mg/kg (average, 306) in 5 fatal cases due to combined ingestion of carbromal and bromisoval. The same author determined that liver pentobarbital concentrations in instances of death due to pentobarbital alone were considerably higher than those in cases due to the combined ingestion of pentobarbital and carbromal, indicating that carbromal contributes significantly to the toxicity of this popular combination. In 4 cases of death due to overdosage with carbromal, blood bromide concentrations averaged 1611 mg/L (range, 1285–2450) and cerebrospinal fluid, 887 mg/L (range, 570–1050); a urine bromide concentration of 1100 mg/L was observed in one of these cases (Steel and Johnstone, 1959; Clarke, 1969; Baselt, 1976).

Analysis. The inorganic bromide released during carbromal therapy may be determined in biological specimens by colorimetric procedures (Street, 1960; Sunshine, 1975) or by gas chromatography (Wells and Cimbura, 1973). Organic bromide (representing carbromal, bromoethylbutyramide and bromoethylhydroxybutyramide) may be separately determined by a titration procedure following the precipitation of inorganic bromide (Rauws, 1969). A spectrophotometric procedure provides for the measurement of carbromal (together with certain metabolites) in urine (Schuetz et al., 1974). Gas chromatography has been applied to the analysis of carbromal and its active organic metabolites using both flame-ionization and electron-capture detection of the underivatized compounds (Vohland et al., 1976). More recently, liquid chromatographic methods that have been reported allow the differential measurement of carbromal and its major metabolites (Hobel and Bender, 1977; Eichelbaum et al., 1978; Uges and Bouma, 1979).

References

R. Baselt. Unpublished results, 1976.

T.C. Butler. The metabolic fate of carbromal (2-bromo-2-ethylbutyrylurea). J. Pharm. Exp. Ther. 143: 23–29, 1964.

E.G.C. Clarke (ed.). *Isolation and Identification of Drugs*, Pharmaceutical Press, London, 1969, pp. 241–242.

A.S. Curry. A metabolite of carbromal. Nature 188: 58, 1960.

M. Eichelbaum, B. Sonntag and G. von Unruh. Determination of monoureides in biological fluids by high-pressure-liquid-chromatography. Arch. Tox. 41: 187–193, 1978.

H. Gruska, V. Becker, K.H. Beyer et al. Klinik, Toxicologie und Therapie einer schweren Carbromalvergiftung mit letalem Ausgang. Arch. Tox. 26: 149–160, 1970.

H. Gruska, K.H. Beyer, G. Grosse and E. Wolbergs. Klinik und Toxikologie einer mit extrakorporaler Haemodialyse behandelten Carbromal-Vergiftung mit letalem Ausgang. Arch. Tox. 28: 149–158, 1971.

M. Hobel and G. Bender. Separation and quantitative determination of acecarbromal, carbromal, and bromisoval as well as their main metabolites by means of high-pressure liquid chromatographic analysis. Arch. Tox. 37: 307–312, 1977.

A. Kessell. Serum bromide levels in a mental health unit. Med. J. Aust. 1: 1073–1075, 1969.

V. Maes, L. Huyghens, J. Dekeyser and C. Sevens. Acute and chronic intoxication with carbromal preparations. Clin. Tox. 23: 341–346, 1985.

A.G. Rauws. The determination of bromisoval and carbromal in biological material. J. Pharm. Pharmac. 21: 283–286, 1969.

C. Schuetz, Y.D. Ha, D. Post and H. Schuetz. Untersuchungen zum UV-photometrischen Nachweis der kurzzeitig zurueckliegenden Einnahme therapeutischer und suicidaler Dosen von Carbromal (Adalin) im Harn. Arch. Tox. 31: 271–278, 1974.

F.H. Shaw and E. Shaw. A new outlook on carbromal. Aust. J. Pharm. 40: 214–218, 1959.

M. Steel and J.M. Johnstone. Addiction to carbromal. Brit. Med. J. 2: 118, 1959.

G. Sticht and H. Kaferstein. Strukturnachweis von bromhaltigen Carbromalmetaboliten. Arch. Tox. 35: 263–273, 1976.

H.V. Street. Determination of bromide in blood. Clin. Chim. Acta 5: 938–941, 1960.

I. Sunshine (ed.). Bromide. Type A procedure. In *Methodology for Analytical Toxicology*, CRC Press, Cleveland, 1975, pp. 54–55.

W.H. Trethowan and T. Pawloff. A clinical and experimental study of bromide intoxication, with special reference to bromureides. Med. J. Aust. 1: 229–232, 1962.

L.K. Turner. Poisoning by carbromal and bromvaletone. Med. J. Aust. 46: 729–731, 1959.

D.R.A. Uges and P. Bouma. Determination of monoureides in biological fluids by high-pressure-liquid-chromatography. Arch. Tox. 42: 85–86, 1979.

H.W. Vohland, S. Hadisoemarto and B. Wanke. Zur Toxikologie von Carbromal. Arch. Tox. 36: 31–42, 1976.

H.W. Vohland, T. Schirop, D. Barckow et al. Zur Toxikologie von Carbromal. Arch. Tox. 40: 211–229, 1978.

J. Wells and G. Cimbura. The determination of elevated bromide levels in blood by gas chromatography. J. For. Sci. 18: 437–440, 1973.

Carisoprodol

T½: 8 hr
Vd: ?
Fb: ?

$$\underset{\underset{C_3H_7}{|}}{\overset{\overset{CH_3}{|}}{NH_2COOCH_2CCH_2OCONHCH(CH_3)_2}}$$

Occurrence and Usage. Carisoprodol (N-isopropylmeprobamate, Soma) is a carbamate derivative first synthesized in 1959. It is used primarily as a muscle relaxant, and is administered orally in doses of 200–350 mg. In certain preparations it is found in combination with such drugs as phenacetin, caffeine and codeine.

Blood Concentrations. Plasma concentrations of carisoprodol reached an average peak in 18 subjects after ingestion of 350 mg of 2.1 mg/L at 1 hour, declining to 1.1 mg/L by 3 hours and 0.24 mg/L by 6 hours (Kucharczyk et al., 1986).

Metabolism and Excretion. Carisoprodol is known to be metabolized to meprobamate and hydroxymeprobamate (Adams et al., 1975). Based on animal studies, hydroxycarisoprodol may also be a major biotransformation product (Douglas et al., 1962). Less than 1% of a single 350 mg oral dose is excreted unchanged in the 24 hour urine, with meprobamate accounting for 4.7% of the dose (Baselt, 1975). Meprobamate and the hydroxylated metabolites may be partially excreted as conjugates (Ludwig et al., 1961).

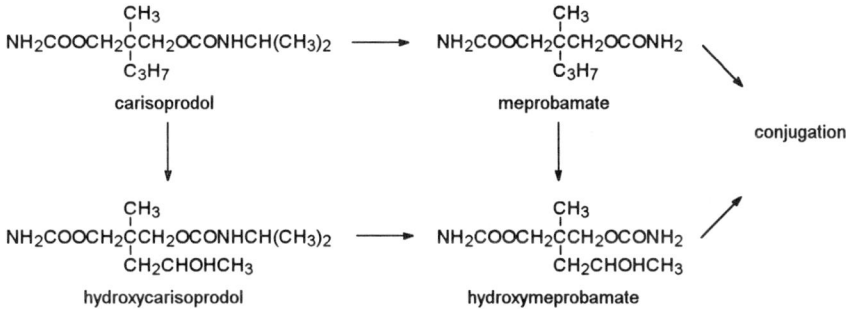

Toxicity. Overdosage with carisoprodol has resulted in several isolated instances of drug intoxication. One stuporous patient was found to have a blood concentration of 31 mg/L using a specific gas chromatographic method (Maes et al., 1970). By means of a similar procedure, serum concentrations of 36 and 15 mg/L, respectively, were found for carisoprodol and its active metabolite, meprobamate, 4.5 hours after the ingestion of 3500 mg of the drug by a 5 year old child; at the same time urine concentrations of 24 and 166 mg/L were observed for the 2 drugs. The patient remained comatose until his death approximately 40 hours after ingestion (Adams et al., 1975). Two adults who ingested 8.4 and 9.5 g of carisoprodol and survived were observed to develop maximal serum carbamate concentrations of 37–38 mg/L, as measured by a nonspecific method (Goldberg, 1969).

A woman who intentionally ingested an overdose had postmortem blood levels of 39 and 40 mg/L for carisoprodol and meprobamate, respectively (Backer et al., 1990). A fatality due solely to the ingestion of carisoprodol was investigated by Maes et al. (1969), who found the following tissue distribution by gas chromatography:

Carisoprodol Concentrations in a Fatal Case (mg/L or mg/kg)

Blood	Liver	Bile	Kidney	Urine
110	127	64	110	165

Analysis. Carisoprodol may be assayed by the colorimetric technique of Hoffman and Ludwig (1959), although this procedure does not differentiate between the drug and its major metabolites. Specific gas chromatographic methods that distinguish the parent drug, meprobamate and hydroxymeprobamate have been reported (Adams et al., 1975; Douglas et al., 1969; Maes et al., 1970; Kucharczyk et al., 1986; Kintz et al., 1988).

References

H.R. Adams, I. Kerzee and C.D. Morehead. Carisoprodol-related death in a child. J. For. Sci. 20: 200–202, 1975.

R.C. Backer, R. Zumwalt, P. McFeeley et al. Carisoprodol concentrations from different anatomical sites: three overdose cases. J. Anal. Tox. 14: 332–334, 1990.

R.C. Baselt. Unpublished results, 1975.

J.F. Douglas, B.J. Ludwig and A. Schlosser. The metabolic fate of carisoprodol in the dog. J. Pharm. Exp. Ther. 138: 21–27, 1962.

J.F. Douglas, N.B. Smith and J.A. Stockage. Gas chromatographic determination of mebutamate, carisoprodol, and tybamate in plasma and urine. J. Pharm. Sci. 58: 145–146, 1969.

D. Goldberg. Carisoprodol toxicity. Mil. Med. 134: 597–601, 1969.

A.J. Hoffman and B.J. Ludwig. An improved colorimetric method for the determination of meprobamate in biological fluids. J. Am. Pharm. Asso. 48: 740–742, 1959.

P. Kintz, P. Mangin, A.A.J. Lugnier and A.J. Chaumont. A rapid and sensitive gas chromatographic analysis of meprobamate or carisoprodal in urine and plasma. J. Anal. Tox. 12: 73–74, 1988.

N. Kucharczyk, F.H. Segelman, E. Kelton et al. Gas chromatographic determination of carisoprodol in human plasma. J. Chrom. 377: 384–390, 1986.

B.J. Ludwig, J.F. Douglas, L.S. Powell et al. Structures of the major metabolites of meprobamate. J. Med. Pharm. Chem. 3: 53–61, 1961.

R. Maes, N. Hodnett, H. Landesman et al. The gas chromatographic determination of selected sedatives (ethchlorvynol, paraldehyde, meprobamate, and carisoprodol) in biological material. J. For. Sci. 14: 235–254, 1969.

R. Maes, R. Bouche and L. Laruelle. Determination quantitative de meprobamate et de carisoprodol par chromatographie en phase gazeuse, dans differents cas d'intoxications. Eur. J. Tox. 3: 140–143, 1970.

Chloral Hydrate

T½: 6–10 hr (trichloroethanol)
Vd: 0.6 L/kg
Fb: 0.35 (trichloroethanol) $CCl_3CH(OH)_2$
pKa: 10.0

Occurrence and Usage. Chloral hydrate (Noctec) was first prepared in 1832 and utilized clinically in 1869. Although it was once a very popular hypnotic agent, it is now used relatively infrequently. The drug may be administered rectally in doses of 325–975 mg or orally in amounts of 250–1000 mg. Oral doses of 30–75 mg/kg are occasionally employed in pediatric dentistry as a sedative.

Blood Concentrations. Concentrations of trichloroethanol in blood after a single 1000 mg oral dose of chloral hydrate given to 5 adult subjects averaged 8.0 mg/L (range, 2.0–12) at 1 hour, 7.6 mg/L (range, 6.5–8.0) at 2 hours and 4.5 mg/L (range, 3.0–6.3) at 6 hours (Kaplan et al., 1967). An oral sedative dose of 50 mg/kg given to young children produced an average peak plasma chloral hydrate concentration of 3.9 mg/L at 0.7 hour and an average peak trichloroethanol level of 27 mg/L at 2.2 hours (Mayers et al., 1991). The blood half-life of trichloroethanol averages 7 hours in adults (Breimer et al., 1974), but is increased to 10 hours in young children and 28 hours in neonates (Mayers et al., 1991).

Metabolism and Excretion. Chloral hydrate *in vivo* is rapidly converted (half-life of 4 minutes) by reduction to trichloroethanol, its major active metabolite. This reaction is catalyzed by liver alcohol dehydrogenase and also by erythrocytes. Virtually no parent drug is observed in blood or plasma following normal dosages. Trichloroethanol is further metabolized by oxidation to trichloroacetic acid, an inactive compound with a half-life of 4–5 days, and by conjugation with glucuronic acid. Both trichloroacetic acid and trichloroethanol glucuronide (urochloralic acid) are present in blood or plasma during chloral hydrate administration at levels that equal or exceed those of trichloroethanol. Plasma trichloroacetic acid concentrations rose to 82 mg/L over an 8 day period of daily administration of 15 mg/kg of chloral hydrate (Sellers et al., 1978). Only about 0.7% of a dose is excreted in the 24 hour urine as free trichloroethanol and about 28% as trichloroethanol glucuronide. Most of the remainder of a dose is excreted in urine as trichloroacetic acid over a period of many days (Marshall and Owens, 1954; Sellers et al., 1972; Breimer et al., 1974; Berry, 1975).

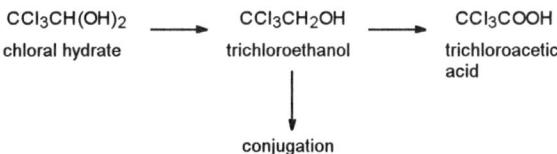

Toxicity. Chloral hydrate may cause respiratory depression, coma, convulsions, cardiac arrhythmias and death. A case of chloral hydrate dependence was described in which daily ingestion of 7.5–10 g of the drug was continued for a year by a woman with a history of sleeping during the day and stumbling over furniture (Stone and Okun, 1978). A 2 year old child suffered cardiorespiratory arrest after a 250 mg oral dose, but eventually recovered (Granoff et al., 1971). A comatose woman who had ingested 38 g of the drug had a peak plasma trichloroethanol concentration of 330 mg/L after 2 hours; hemodialysis succeeded in reducing the plasma half-life from 35 hours to 6 hours (Stalker et al., 1978).

As little as 3 g of chloral hydrate has been fatal to an adult, although tolerant individuals have been known to consume up to 25 g daily without mishap. Blood trichloroethanol concentrations ranging from 20–240 mg/L (average, 119) were reported in 14 cases of death due to chloral hydrate overdosage (Rehling, 1967). In 4 cases known to involve the acute ingestion of 15–30 g of the drug, postmortem blood trichloroethanol concentrations averaged 265 mg/L (range, 100–640) (Baselt and Cravey, 1977). The following tissue distribution of trichloroethanol (TCE) was observed in the case of a 25 year old woman who died within 3 hours of the ingestion of a large amount of chloral hydrate (Poklis, 1973):

TCE Concentrations in a Chloral Hydrate Death (mg/L or mg/kg)

Blood	Brain	Liver	Urine	Gastric
55	91	200	30	5 g

Analysis. Various modifications have been made to the Fujiwara reaction to allow its use in the differential measurement of chloral hydrate and its metabolites by visible spectrophotometry (Butler, 1948; Friedman and Cooper, 1958; Cabana and Gessner, 1967; McBay et al., 1980). A number of sensitive and specific gas chromatographic procedures have also been published for the analysis of this drug and its metabolites in biological specimens and nearly all have employed electron-capture detection; the techniques involve solvent extraction (Garrett and Lambert, 1966; Wells and Cimbura, 1972; Flanagan et al., 1978; van der Hoeven et al., 1979; Gorecki et al., 1990), headspace analysis (Breimer et al., 1974), or direct injection of the specimen after dilution with an internal standard (Jain et al., 1967; Berry, 1975). Gas chromatography-mass spectrometey has also been employed (Heller et al., 1992). Several other pertinent methods are cited in the section on trichloro-ethylene.

References

R.C. Baselt and R.H. Cravey. A compendium of therapeutic and toxic concentrations of toxicologically significant drugs in human biofluids. J. Anal. Tox. 1: 81–103, 1977.

D.J. Berry. Determination of trichloroethanol at therapeutic and overdose levels in blood and urine by electron capture gas chromatography. J. Chrom. 107: 107–114, 1975.

D.D. Breimer, H.C.J. Ketelaars and J.M. Van Rossum. Gas chromatographic determination of chloral hydrate, trichloroethanol and trichloroacetic acid in blood and in urine employing head-space analysis. J. Chrom. 88: 55–63, 1974.

T.C. Butler. The metabolic fate of chlorol hydrate. J. Pharm. Exp. Ther. 92: 49–58, 1948.

B.E. Cabana and P.K. Gessner. Determination of chloral hydrate, trichloroacetic acid, trichloroethanol, and urochloralic acid in the presence of each other and in tissue homogenates. Anal. Chem. 39: 1449–1452, 1967.

R.J. Flanagan, T.D. Lee and D.M. Rutherford. Analysis of chlormethiazole, ethchlorvynol and trichloroethanol in biological fluids by gas-liquid chromatography as an aid to the diagnosis of acute poisoning. J. Chrom. 153: 473–479, 1978.

P.J. Friedman and J.R. Cooper. Determination of chloral hydrate, trichloroacetic acid, and trichloroethanol. Anal. Chem. 30: 1674–1676, 1958.

E.R. Garrett and H.J. Lambert. Gas chromatographic analysis of trichloroethanol, chloral hydrate, trichloroacetic acid, and trichloroethanol glucuronide. J. Pharm. Sci. 55: 812–817, 1966.

D.K.J. Gorecki, K.W. Hindmarsh, C.A. Hall et al. Determination of chloral hydrate metabolism in adult and neonate biological fluids after single-dose administration. J. Chrom. 528: 333–341, 1990.

D.M. Granoff, D.B. McDaniel and S.P. Borkouf. Cardiorespiratory arrest following aspiration of chloral hydrate. Am. J. Dis. Child. 122: 170–171, 1971.

P.F. Heller, B.A. Goldberger and Y.H. Caplan. Chloral hydrate overdose: trichloroethanol detection by gas chromatography/mass spectrometry. For. Sci. Int. 52: 231–234, 1992.

N.C. Jain, H.L. Kaplan, R.B. Forney and F.W. Hughes. A rapid gas chromatographic method for the determination of chloral hydrate and trichloroethanol in blood and other biological materials. J. For. Sci. 12: 497–508, 1967.

H.L. Kaplan, R.B. Forney, F.W. Hughes and N.C. Jain. Chloral hydrate and alcohol metabolism in human subjects. J. For. Sci. 12: 295–304, 1967.

E.K. Marshall and A.H. Owens, Jr. Absorption, excretion and metabolic fate of chloral hydrate and trichloroethanol. Bull. Johns Hopkins Hosp. 95: 1–81, 1954.

D.J. Mayers, K.W. Hindmarsh, K. Sankaran et al. Chloral hydrate disposition following single-dose administration to critically ill neonates and children. Dev. Pharm. Ther. 16: 71–77, 1991.

A.J. McBay, V.R. Boling, Jr. and P.C. Reynolds. Spectrophotometric determination of trichloroethanol in chloral hydrate poisoning. J. Anal. Tox. 4: 99–101, 1980.

A. Poklis. Personal communication, 1973.

C.J. Rehling. Poison residues in human tissues. In *Progress in Chemical Toxicology*, Vol. 3 (A. Stolman, ed.), Academic Press, New York, 1967, pp. 363–386.

E.M. Sellers, M. Lang, J. Koch-Weser et al. Interaction of chloral hydrate and ethanol in man. Clin. Pharm. Ther. 13: 37–49, 1972.

E.M. Sellers, M. Lang-Sellers and J. Koch-Weser. Comparative metabolism of chloral hydrate and triclofos. J. Clin. Pharm. 18: 457–461, 1978.

N.E. Stalker, J.G. Gambertoglio, C.J. Fukumitsu et al. Acute massive chloral hydrate intoxication treated with hemodialysis: a clinical pharmacokinetic analysis. J. Clin. Pharm. 18: 136–142, 1978.
C.B. Stone and R. Okun. Chloral hydrate dependence: report of a case. Clin. Tox. 12: 377–380, 1978.
R. van der Hoeven, R.H. Drost, R.A.A. Maes et al. Improved method for the electron-capture gas chromatographic determination of trichloroacetic acid in human serum. J. Chrom. 164: 106–108, 1979.
J. Wells and G. Cimbura. Determination of chloral hydrate and trichloroethanol in biological tissue. J. For. Sci. 17: 674–677, 1972.

Chloramphenicol

T½: 1.6–3.3 hr
Vd: 0.57 L/kg
Fb: 0.44
pKa: 5.5

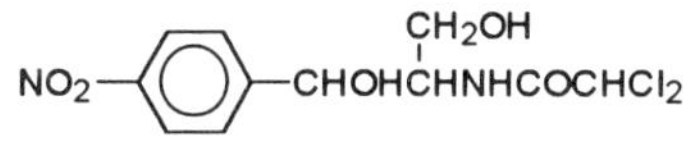
CH2OH
NO2
CHOHCHNHCOCHCl2

Occurrence and Usage. Chloramphenicol (Chloromycetin) is a broad-spectrum antibiotic that was first isolated in 1947. It is especially useful in the treatment of meningitis, typhoid fever, cystic fibrosis, and various anerobic infections. The drug is available for oral use in 250 mg capsules, or in a liquid suspension (150 mg/5 mL) as the palmitate ester. The latter is hydrolyzed in the stomach to chloramphenicol prior to absorption. An intravenous preparation contains 100 mg/mL of the sodium succinate ester when reconstituted; this form also readily hydrolyzes *in vivo* to yield active chloramphenicol. Both oral and intravenous doses range from 25–100 mg/kg/day.

Blood Concentrations. A 1 g oral dose given every 6 hours to adults produced an average initial peak serum chloramphenicol concentration of 11 mg/L after 1 hour; this peak level rose to 18 mg/L by the fifth dose due to drug accumulation. Therapeutic concentrations of 10–20 mg/L are generally maintained by either oral or intravenous administration of 50 mg/kg/day, in equally divided doses every 6 hours, to healthy adults. Individuals with hepatic or renal disease or infants with immature liver enzyme systems may have drug half-lives substantially longer than the normal value of 1.6–3.3 hours and may require a lower dose to prevent drug accumulation (PDR, 1981).

Metabolism and Excretion. Chloramphenicol is extensively metabolized by glucuronide conjugation and, to a lesser extent, by hydrolysis of the amide linkage. A total of 93% of a dose is excreted in the 24 hour urine, largely as inactive metabolites (Glazko et al., 1949b). Urine collected for 8 hours after a single 500 mg oral dose contained 6.0% of the dose as free chloramphenicol, 48% as chloramphenicol glucuronide, and 4.3% as p-nitrophenyl-2-amino-1,3-propanediol (Nakagawa et al., 1975). Another metabolite, p-nitrophenyl-2-hydroxyacetamido-1,3-propanediol, was found in the urine of newborns in an unstated amount; the compound had only 4% of the antimicrobial activity of chloramphenicol and a very low order of toxicity (Dill et al., 1960).

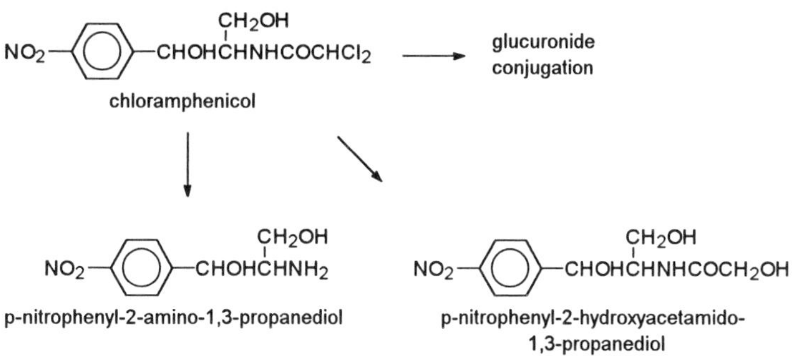
CH2OH
NO2
CHOHCHNHCOCHCl2
glucuronide
conjugation
chloramphenicol
CH2OH
NO2
CHOHCHNH2
p-nitrophenyl-2-amino-1,3-propanediol
CH2OH
NO2
CHOHCHNHCOCH2OH
p-nitrophenyl-2-hydroxyacetamido-
1,3-propanediol

Toxicity. Symptoms of chloramphenicol toxicity include headache, confusion, delerium, nausea, vomiting, and skin rash. Serious bone marrow depression leading to aplastic anemia, thrombocytopenia, or granulocytopenia occurs in rare instances. The "gray baby syndrome" usually occurs in newborns who develop excessive serum concentrations of the drug, producing pallid cyanosis, vasomotor collapse, respiratory difficulty, and death.

Infants with this syndrome have shown serum chloramphenicol concentrations of 28–108 mg/L; charcoal hemoperfusion has been used successfully to clear excess drug from the system (Craft et al., 1974; Mauer et al., 1980; Mulhall et al., 1983). Adults who develop hematologic toxicity after chloramphenicol administration tend to have impaired plasma clearance of the drug and higher serum drug concentrations than individuals who do not experience such reactions (McCurdy, 1963; Suhrland and Weisberger, 1969). Chloramphenicol half-lives as long as 19–36 hours have been measured in patients with hepatic or renal disease (Koup et al., 1979).

A 26 year old woman accidentally received a total of 21 g of chloramphenicol intravenously within 12 hours and went into shock; her plasma drug concentration 5.5 hours after the last dose was 201 mg/L, and she eventually recovered. A 70 year old woman received a similar amount of drug and died after 11 hours (Thompson et al., 1975). A 5 week old child accidentally received 1100 mg, developed a serum chloramphenicol level of 180 mg/L, and died 48 hours later (Stevens et al., 1981.)

Analysis. Chloramphenicol in biological fluids has been frequently measured by microbiological assay (de Louvois et al., 1980) or colorimetry (Glazko et al., 1949a). Gas chromatography after trimethylsilyl derivatization may be accomplished with either flame-ionization (Least et al., 1977) or electron-capture detection (Pickering et al., 1979). Numerous procedures for liquid chromatographic analysis of the drug have also appeared (Crechiolo and Hill, 1979; Petersdorf et al., 1979; Triebig et al., 1979; Aravind et al., 1980; Burke et al., 1980; Gal et al., 1980; Oseekey et al., 1980; Ferrell et al., 1981; Velagapudi et al., 1982).

References

M.K. Aravind, J.N. Miceli, R.E. Kauffman et al. Simultaneous measurement of chloramphenicol and chloramphenicol succinate by high-performance liquid chromatography. J. Chrom. 221: 176–181, 1980.

J.T. Burke, W.A. Wargin and M.R. Blum. High-pressure liquid chromatographic assay for chloramphenicol, chloramphenicol-3- monosuccinate, and chloramphenicol-1-monosuccinate. J. Pharm. Sci. 69: 909–912, 1980.

A.W. Craft, J.T. Brocklebank, E.N. Hey and R.H. Jackson. The "grey toddler" — chloramphenicol toxicity. Arch. Dis. Child. 49: 235–237, 1974.

J. Crechiolo and R.E. Hill. Determination of serum chloramphenicol by high-performance liquid chromatography. J. Chrom. 162: 480–484, 1979.

J. de Louvois, A. Mulhall and R. Hurley. Comparison of methods available for assay of chloramphenicol in clinical specimens. J. Clin. Path. 33: 575–580, 1980.

W.A. Dill, E.M. Thompson, R.A. Fisken and A.J. Glazko. A new metabolite of chloramphenicol. Nature: 185: 535–537, 1960.

W.J. Ferrell, M.P. Szuba, P.R. Miluk and K.D. McClatchey. Determination of serum chloramphenicol by high performance liquid chromatography. J. Liq. Chrom. 4: 171–176, 1981.

J. Gal, P.D. Marcell and C.M. Tarascio. High-performance liquid chromatographic micro-assay for chloramphenicol in human blood plasma and cerebrospinal fluid. J. Chrom. 181: 123–126, 1980.

A.J. Glazko, L.M. Wolf and W.A. Dill. Biochemical studies on chloramphenicol (Chloromycetin). I. Colorimetric methods for the determination of chloramphenicol and related nitro compounds. Arch. Biochem. 23: 411–418, 1949a.

A.J. Glazko, L.M. Wolf, W.A. Dill and A.C. Bratton, Jr. Biochemical studies on chloramphenicol (chloromycetin). II. Tissue distribution and excretion studies. J. Pharm. Exp. Ther. 96: 445–459, 1949b.

J.R. Koup, A.H. Lau, B. Brodsky and R.L. Slaughter. Chloramphenicol pharmacokinetics in hospitalized patients. Antimicrob. Agents Chemother. 15: 651–657, 1979.

C.J. Least, Jr., N.J. Wiegand, G.F. Johnson and H.M. Solomon. Quantitative gas-chromatographic flame-ionization method for chloramphenicol in human serum. Clin. Chem. 23: 220–222, 1977.

S.M. Mauer, B.M. Chavers and C.M. Kjellstrand. Treatment of an infant with severe chloramphenicol intoxication using charcoal-column hemoperfusion. J. Pediat. 96: 136–139, 1980.

P.R. McCurdy. Plasma concentration of chloramphenicol and bone marrow suppression. Blood 21: 363–372, 1963.

A. Mulhall, J. de Louvois and R. Horley. Chloramphenicol toxicity in neonates; its incidence and prevention. Brit. Med. J. 287: 1424–1427, 1983.

T. Nakagawa, M. Masada and T. Uno. Gas chromatographic determination and gas chromatographic-mass spectrometric analysis of chloramphenicol, thiamphenicol and their metabolites. J. Chrom. 111: 355–364, 1975.

K.B. Oseekey, K.L. Rowse and H.B. Kostenbauder. High-performance liquid chromatographic determination of chloramphenicol and its monosuccinate ester in plasma. J. Chrom. 182: 459–464, 1980.

S.H. Petersdorf, V.A. Raisys and K.E. Opheim. Micro-scale method for liquid-chromatographic determination of chloramphenicol in serum. Clin. Chem. 25: 1300–1302, 1979.

Physicians' Desk Reference, Medical Economics, Oradell, New Jersey, 1981, pp. 1335–1336.

L.K. Pickering, J.L. Hoecker, W.G. Kramer et al. Assays for chloramphenicol compared: radioenzymatic, gas chromatographic with electron capture, and gas chromatographic-mass spectrometric. Clin. Chem. 25: 300–305, 1979.

D.C. Stevens, M.B. Kleiman, P.S. Lietman and R.L. Schreiner. Exchange transfusion in acute chloramphenicol toxicity. J. Pediat. 99: 651–653, 1981.

L.G. Suhrland and A.S. Weisberger. Delayed clearance of chloramphenicol from serum in patients with hematologic toxicity. Blood 34: 466–471, 1969.

W.L. Thompson, S.E. Anderson, Jr., J.J. Lipsky and P.S. Lietman. Overdoses of chloramphenicol. J. Am. Med. Asso. 234: 149–150, 1975.

G. Triebig, K. Gobler and M. Klinger. Micromethod for the quantitation of chloramphenicol in body fluids by high-pressure liquid chromatography. Fresenius Z. Anal. Chem. 299: 271–272, 1979.

R. Velagapudi, R.V. Smith, T.M. Ludden and R. Sagraves. Simultaneous determination of chloramphenicol and chloramphenicol succinate in plasma using high-performance liquid chromatography. J. Chrom. 228: 23–428, 1982.

Chlordane

T½: 88 days
Vd: ?
Fb: ?

Occurrence and Usage. Chlordane (Ortho-Klor, Octachlor) is an organochlorine insecticide that has been commercially available since 1949. The technical product is a mixture of 2 chlordane isomers (60–75%) and related products (chlordene, heptachlor and nonachlor) and has been widely employed in agriculture and in households. It is frequently used in the form of a dust containing 5% or a solution containing 50% active ingredients. The compound is readily absorbed following inhalation, ingestion or dermal contact. Chlordane, closely related structurally to heptachlor, has come under severe restrictions in some countries due to its persistence in the environment. The current threshold limit value is 0.5 mg/m³.

Blood Concentrations. Concentrations of cis and trans-chlordane in the blood of nonexposed Japanese subjects have been found to range from 0.01–0.26 µg/L for each of the isomers; similar levels were reported for cis and trans-nonachlor and levels of 0.10–0.75 µg/L for oxychlordane (Wariishi et al., 1986). The blood levels of total chlordane metabolites (trans-nonachlor, oxychlordane and heptachlor epoxide) in pest control operators spraying a 40% emulsifiable chlordane concentrate ranged from 0.3 µg/L for those with only 1 spraying day to 5.6 µg/L for those with 27 days (Saito et al., 1986).

Metabolism and Excretion. Over a period of 2.5 days, rats excreted 1% of an injected dose of chlordane in the urine and 29% in the feces, primarily as water-soluble metabolites (Poonawalla and Korte, 1964). Oxychlordane, a major metabolite, is the predominant species in tissues during chronic feeding studies, accounting for 90% of the chlordane residue in fat and 40–60% in liver and kidney (Barnett and Dorough, 1974).

The disposition of the compound has not been studied in man, but oxychlordane is found in the adipose tissue of the general population at concentrations of 0.03–0.40 mg/kg (Biros and Enos, 1973). Both oxychlordane and nonachlor, an ingredient of technical chlordane, have been found in the breast milk of women in several industrialized nations at concentrations of about 1 µg/L (Miyazaki et al., 1980).

Toxicity. Chlordane is a persistent, fat-soluble central nervous system stimulant. Acute intoxication produces symptoms of confusion, delirium, nausea, convulsions and death. Chronic exposure is known to cause liver and kidney damage.

Thirteen persons exhibited signs of mild acute poisoning for a period of 36–48 hours after exposure to domestic water contaminated with chlordane in concentrations of up to 0.1%. Serum oxychlordane concentrations were unmeasureable initially in all but one of these individuals, but 4 months later the levels ranged from 0.2–1.3 µg/L (Harrington et al., 1978). Several cases of chronic poisoning have been reported in which the victims had monocytic leukemia (Collins and Crawford, 1976) or megaloblastic anemia (Furie and Trubowitz, 1976). Acute nonfatal incidents have generally involved ingestion of less than 2 g of chlordane and resulted in collapse and convulsions (Lensky and Evans, 1952; Dadey and Kammer, 1953; Barnes, 1967), although an adult survived the ingestion of 215 g after achieving a blood chlordane level of 5 mg/L (Olanoff et al., 1983).

A 20 month old child ingested chlordane and developed seizures within an hour; after 3 hours, chlordane concentrations of 2.7 mg/L in serum and 3.1 mg/kg in fat were measured, and after 3 months these values had decreased to 0.02 mg/L and increased to 26 mg/kg, respectively. Less than 50 µg of chlordane was excreted in the first 24 hour urine specimen (Curley and Garrettson, 1969). A 4 year old child who experienced convulsions after chlordane ingestion exhibited an initial serum concentration of 3.4 mg/L, with a serum half-life of 88 days (Aldrich and Holmes, 1969). In both of these cases the victims recovered within 24–48 hours of ingestion, and urine concentration of unchanged chlordane were very low (0.3 mg/L or less).

Two deaths in adults have been due to chlordane poisoning; one occurred about an hour after massive dermal exposure and the other 9.5 days after ingestion of 6 g of the compound (Derbes et al., 1955). A 59 year old man died 1.3 hours after ingesting an unknown amount of chlordane; his postmortem blood and urine contained 4.4 and 0.2 mg/L, respectively, of the compound (Bost, 1978). The following concentrations were found in the tissues of a 66 year old male who ingested approximately 400 mL of a 70% commercial chlordane solution and died after 40 hours (Morano, 1978) and in a 59 year old male who died shortly after ingesting an unknown amount of chlordane (Kutz et al., 1983):

Chlordane Concentrations in Fatalities (mg/L or mg/kg)

Blood	Liver	Kidney	Urine	Fat	Reference
1.7	43	14	0.6	378	Morano, 1978
4.9	60	14	0.2	22	Kutz et al., 1983

Analysis. Concentrations of chlordane in biological material may be determined by an electron-capture gas chromatographic procedure designed for chlorinated hydrocarbon insecticides (Dale et al., 1966; Dale et al., 1967) or by one developed specifically for chlordane (Saito et al., 1985).

References

A.D. Aldrich and J.H. Holmes. Acute chlordane intoxication in a child. Arch. Env. Health 19: 129–132, 1969.

R. Barnes. Poisoning by the insecticide chlordane. Med. J. Aust. 1: 972–973, 1967.

J.R. Barnett and H.W. Dorough. Metabolism of chlordane in rats. J. Agr. Food Chem. 22: 612–619, 1974.

F.J. Biros and H.F. Enos. Oxychlordane residues in human adipose tissue. Bull. Env. Cont. Tox. 5: 257–260, 1973.

R.O. Bost. Personal communication, 1978.

I.S. Collins and W.A. Crawford. Chlordane. Med. J. Aust. 1: 762, 1976.

A. Curley and L.K. Garrettson. Acute chlordane poisoning. Arch. Env. Health 18: 211–215, 1969.

J.L. Dadey and A.G. Kammer. Chlordane intoxication. J. Am. Med. Asso. 153: 723–725, 1953.

W.E. Dale, A. Curley and C. Cueto, Jr. Hexane extractable chlorinated insecticides in human blood. Life Sci. 5: 47–54, 1966.

W.E. Dale, A. Curley and W.J. Hayes, Jr. Determination of chlorinated insecticides in human blood. Ind. Med. Surg. 36: 275–280, 1967.

V.J. Derbes, J.H. Dent, W.W. Forrest and M.F. Johnson. Fatal chlordane poisoning. J. Am. Med. Asso. 158: 1367–1369, 1955.

B. Furie and S. Trubowitz. Insecticides and blood dyscrasias. J. Am. Med. Asso. 235: 1720–1722, 1976.

J.M. Harrington, E.L. Baker, Jr., D.S. Folland et al. Chlordane contamination of a municipal water system. Env. Res. 15: 155–159, 1978.

F.W. Kutz, S.C. Strassman, J.F. Sperling et al. A fatal chlordane poisoning. Clin. Tox. 20: 167–174, 1983.

P. Lensky and H.L. Evans. Human poisoning by chlordane. J. Am. Med. Asso. 149: 1394–1395, 1952.

T. Miyazaki, K. Akiyama, S. Kaneko et al. Chlordane residues in human milk. Bull. Env. Cont. Tox. 25: 518–523, 1980.

R. Morano. Personal communication, 1978.

L.S. Olanoff, W.J. Bristow, J. Colcolough and J.R. Reigart. Acute chlordane intoxication. Clin. Tox. 20: 291–306, 1983.

N.H. Poonawalla and F. Korte. Metabolism of insecticides, VIII (I): excretion, distribution and metabolism of α–chlordan-^{14}C by rats. Life Sci. 3: 1497–1500, 1964.

I. Saito, N. Kawamura, K. Uno and Y. Takeuchi. Determination of chlordane in human blood by gas chromatography. Analyst 110: 263–267, 1985.

I. Saito, N. Kawamura, K. Uno et al. Relationship between chlordane and its metabolites in blood of pest control operators and spraying conditions. Int. Arch. Occ. Env. Health 58: 91–97, 1986.

M. Wariishi, Y. Suzuki and K. Nishiyama. Chlordane residues in normal human blood. Bull. Env. Cont. Tox. 36: 635–643, 1986.

Chlordecone

T½: 63–148 days
Vd: ?
Fb: ?

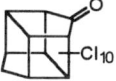

Occurrence and Usage. Chlordecone (Kepone) is a chlorinated hydrocarbon pesticide, first developed in 1952, that is closely related to mirex. Most of the chlordecone produced in the United States has been exported for the control of agricultural pests, but inadequate precautions during manufacturing led in 1975 to a number of human poisonings and extensive environmental contamination in the manufacturing area. The compound is well-absorbed following oral, respiratory or dermal administration. A threshold limit value for occupational exposure has not been set for chlordecone.

Blood Concentrations. Of 216 blood samples obtained from healthy members of the general population living within a 1 mile radius of a chlordecone manufacturing facility, 40 were found to contain detectable amounts of chlordecone ranging from 0.005-0.033 mg/L (Anonymous, 1976). Serum concentrations of chlordecone in 11 occupationally exposed subjects ranged from 0.120-

2.109 mg/L and averaged 0.734 mg/L. The average serum half-life was found to be 96 days (range, 63-148) and the average blood/serum concentration ratio, 0.57 (Adir et al., 1978).

Metabolism and Excretion. Quantitative estimates of chlordecone excretion have not been made in man, but a reduction product, chlordecone alcohol, and its glucuronide conjugate have been identified in human bile (Fariss et al., 1980). The comound is primarily eliminated in bile, but is largely reabsorbed, so that the overall elimination rate is only 0.075% of the total body burden per day. Negligible amounts are excreted in urine and sweat (Cohn et al., 1976). A single oral dose administered to rats was slowly excreted over a period of 84 days in feces (66%) and urine (1.6%), apparently as unchanged chlordecone (Egle et al., 1978).

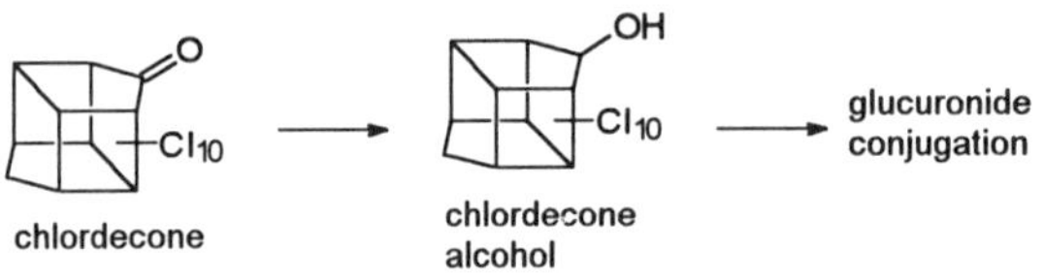

Toxicity. Chronic toxicity due to chlordecone exposure is expressed as neurological, hepatic and hormonal abnormalities. The compound is carcinogenic in animals and is considered a potential human carcinogen. Oral administration of cholestyramine, an ion-exchange resin, for a period of several months has been found to reduce the blood half-life of chlordecone by 50% in poisoned workers (Cohn et al., 1978).

Chlordecone was found present in blood and biopsy tissues of 32 chemical workers exhibiting symptoms of toxicity in the following concentrations (Cohn et al., 1976):

Chlordecone Concentrations in Nonfatal Poisoning (mg/L or mg/kg)

	Blood	Liver	Fat
Average	5.8	76	22
(Range)	(0.6–32)	(13–173)	(2.2–62)

Analysis. Chlordecone has been assayed in body fluids and tissues by electron-capture gas chromatography (Blanke et al., 1977; Caplan et al., 1979) and by gas chromatography-mass spectrometry (Harless et al., 1978).

References

J. Adir, Y.H. Caplan and B.C. Thompson. Kepone serum half-life in humans. Life Sci. 22: 699–702, 1978.

Anonymous. Preliminary report of Kepone levels found in human blood from the general population of Hopewell, Virginia. Health Effects Research Laboratory, U.S. Environmental Protection Agency, Research Triangle Park, North Carolina, March 3, 1976.

R.V. Blanke, M.W. Fariss, F.D. Griffith, Jr. and P. Guzelian. Analysis of chlordecone (Kepone) in biological specimens. J. Anal. Tox. 1: 57–62, 1977.

Y.H. Caplan, B.C. Thompson and J.H. Hebb, Jr. A method for the determination of chlordecone (Kepone) in human serum and blood. J. Anal. Tox. 3: 202–205, 1979.

W.J. Cohn, R.V. Blanke, F.D. Griffith, Jr. and P.S. Guzelian. Distribution and excretion of Kepone (KP) in humans. Gastroenterology 71: 901, 1976.

W.J. Cohn, J.J. Boylan, R.V. Blanke et al. Treatment of chlordecone (Kepone) toxicity with cholestyramine. New Eng. J. Med. 298: 243–248, 1978.

J.L. Egle, S.B. Fernandez, P.S. Guzelian and J.F. Borzelleca. Distribution and excretion of chlordecone (Kepone) in the rat. Drug. Met. Disp. 6: 91–95, 1978.

M.W. Fariss, R.V. Blanke, J.J. Saady and P.S. Guzelian. Demonstration of major metabolic pathways for chlordecone (Kepone) in humans. Drug Met. Disp. 8: 434–438, 1980.

R.L. Harless, D.E. Harris, G.W. Sovocool et al. Mass spectrometric analyses and characterization of Kepone in environmental and human samples. Biomed. Mass Spec. 5: 232–237, 1978.

Chlordiazepoxide

T½: 6–27 hr
Vd: 0.3–0.5 L/kg
Fb: 0.94
pKa: 4.8

Occurrence and Usage. Chlordiazepoxide (Librium) is the prototype of the benzodiazepine class of sedative-hypnotic drugs, which are very extensively used as antianxiety agents, hypnotics, muscle relaxants and anticonvulsants. It was first synthesized in 1955 during a search for a patentable tranquilizing drug and was approved for human use in 1960. The compound is administered as the hydrochloride or the free base in doses of 5–100 mg either orally or by intramuscular injection. Daily doses are not to exceed 300 mg.

Blood Concentrations. A single oral 30 mg chlordiazepoxide dosage produces peak plasma concentrations of about 1.6 mg/L at 4 hours, with a slow decline to 1.1 mg/L by 24 hours; the plasma half-life of the drug in this study ranged from 16–27 hours (Koechlin and D'Arconte, 1963), but in another study of 6 healthy subjects, the value ranged from 7–14 hours (Boxenbaum et al., 1977a). Intramuscular chlordiazepoxide is more slowly absorbed, reaching peak levels of only 0.5–1.2 mg/L within 2–12 hours after a 50 mg dose (Greenblatt et al., 1976). During chronic therapy with 30 mg daily by mouth, plasma concentrations averaged 0.75, 0.54, and 0.36 mg/L for chlordiazepoxide, norchlordiazepoxide and demoxepam, respectively (Boxenbaum et al., 1977b). During chronic oral therapy with an average of 55 mg daily, these levels averaged 2.3, 1.4, and 0.67 mg/L, respectively (Lin and Friedel, 1979). Plasma nordiazepam concentrations during similar chronic therapy with chlordiazepoxide were found to achieve a steady-state of about 0.29–0.31 mg/L (Dixon et al., 1976).

Metabolism and Excretion. Chlordiazepoxide undergoes extensive metabolism in man, resulting in the production of at least 4 active metabolites. The compound is first N-demethylated to norchlordiazepoxide, which is then deaminated to form demoxepam. These 2 compounds are major metabolites with pharmacologic activity similar to that of their parent, and are present in plasma in concentrations comparable to chlordiazepoxide. Nordiazepam is a third active metabolite formed from the reduction of demoxepam; it accumulates in the plasma of patients on chronic therapy. Oxazepam is produced by the hydroxylation of nordiazepam and, while active, has not been detected in plasma. Several phenolic derivatives of demoxepam are produced in small quantities (Schwartz, 1973; Hackman et al., 1974; Dixon et al., 1976). Less than 1% of a dose is excreted unchanged in the urine; about 6% is excreted as demoxepam and the remainder as glucuronide conjugates of oxazepam and the other hydroxylated metabolites (Koechlin et al., 1965; Schwartz, 1973).

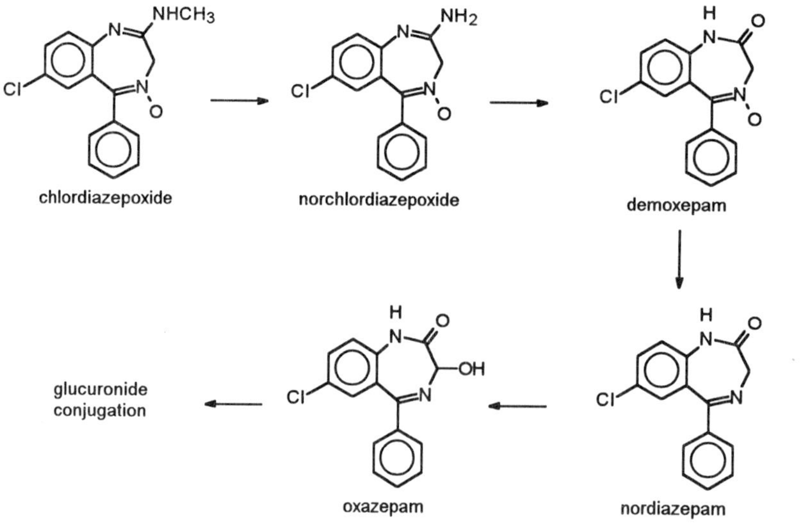

chlordiazepoxide   norchlordiazepoxide   demoxepam

glucuronide
conjugation   oxazepam   nordiazepam

Toxicity. Chlordiazepoxide toxicity is often manifested by ataxia, sedation, hyperreflexia, tachycardia, hypertension and seizures. The drug has been implicated in numerous cases of acute intoxication, but it has only been reported as the sole agent in a few fatalities. Serum concentrations of 1–66 mg/L using a spectrophotometric method were observed in 60 hospitalized patients, none of whom exhibited deep coma (Cate and Jatlow, 1973). In one comatose adult subject who ingested 1000 mg of the drug, the highest plasma concentrations observed were 20 mg/L for chlordiazepoxide at 6 hours, 12 mg/L for norchlordiazepoxide at 21 hours, and 9 mg/L for demoxepam at 51 hours (deSilva and d'Arconte, 1969).

The following distributions were observed for the drug in 2 fatal cases, the first of which was attributed solely to chlordiazepoxide (Mohseni, 1975) and the second, to a combination of amitriptyline and chlordiazepoxide (Finkle, 1975):

Chlordiazepoxide Concentrations in Fatalities (mg/L or mg/kg)

	Blood	Liver	Bile	Kidney	Urine	Gastric
Case 1*	26	10	39	11	8	21 mg
Case 2**	20	50			8	164 mg

*   By ultraviolet spectrophotometry
** By gas chromatography after acid hydrolysis

Analysis. Chlordiazepoxide is unstable in stored or decomposed biological specimens; it tends to form desoxychlordiazepoxide, which further degrades to nordiazepam (Entwhistle et al., 1986). Many techniques have been applied to the difficult problem of the quantitation of chlordiazepoxide and its metabolites in biological specimens, but few may be described as outstanding in terms of sensitivity, specificity and convenience. Ultraviolet spectrophotometry has been utilized in toxicological applications (Jatlow, 1972), but it suffers from a lack of specificity. Specific procedures involving fluorimetry (Schwartz and Postma, 1966) and polarography (Hackman et al., 1974) have been employed in research studies. A sensitive gas chromatographic method requiring acid hydrolysis of the drug is convenient but does not differentiate between the metabolites and the parent drug (deSilva et al., 1964). Intact chlordiazepoxide is thermally unstable under the conditions used in most gas chromatographic techniques, and while the decomposition product may be quantitated by flame-ionization (Baselt et al., 1977) or electron-capture detection (deSilva et al., 1976), the metabolites, if present in the same extract, will give rise to the same product. Sun and Hoffman

(1978) have avoided this problem by derivatizing with trimethylanilinium hydroxide. A number of very suitable liquid chromatographic procedures have been described (Skellern et al., 1978; Strojny et al., 1978; Peat et al., 1979; Ascalone, 1980; Foreman et al., 1980; Vree et al., 1981; Divoll et al., 1982; Puopolo et al., 1991).

References

V. Ascalone. Determination of chlordiazepoxide and its metabolites in human plasma by reversed-phase high-performance liquid chromatography. J. Chrom. 181: 141–146, 1980.

R.C. Baselt, C.B. Stewart and S.J. Franch. Toxicological determination of benzodiazepines in biological fluids and tissues by flame-ionization gas chromatography. J. Anal. Tox. 1: 10–13, 1977.

H.G. Boxenbaum, K.A. Geitner, M.L. Jack et al. Pharmacokinetic and biopharmaceutic profile of chlordiazepoxide HCl in healthy subjects: single-dose studies by the intravenous, intramuscular, and oral routes. J. Pharm. Biopharm. 5: 3–23, 1977a.

H.G. Boxenbaum, K.A. Geitner, M.L. Jack et al. Pharmacokinetics and biopharmaceutic profile of chlordiazepoxide HCl in healthy subjects: multiple-dose oral administration. J. Pharm. Biopharm. 5: 25–39, 1977b.

J.C. Cate and P.I. Jatlow. Chlordiazepoxide overdosage: interpretation of serum drug concentrations. Clin. Tox. 6: 553–561, 1973.

J.A.F. deSilva, M.A. Schwartz, V. Stefanovic et al. Determination of diazepam (Valium) in blood by gas liquid chromatography. Anal. Chem. 36: 2099–2105, 1964.

J.A.F. deSilva and L. D'Arconte. The use of spectrophotofluorometry in the analysis of drugs in biological materials. J. For. Sci. 14: 184–202, 1969.

J.A.F. deSilva, I. Bekersky, C.V. Puglisi et al. Determination of 1,4-benzodiazepines and -diazepine-2-ones in blood by electron-capture gas-liquid chromatography. Anal. Chem. 48: 10–19, 1976.

M. Divoll, D.J. Greenblatt and R.I. Schader. Liquid chromatographic determination of chlordiazepoxide and metabolites in plasma. Pharmacology 24: 261–266, 1982.

R. Dixon, M.A. Brooks, E. Postma et al. N-desmethyldiazepam: a new metabolite of chlordiazepoxide in man. Clin. Pharm. Ther. 20: 450–457, 1976.

N. Entwhistle, P. Owen, D.A. Patterson et al. The occurrence of chlordiazepoxide degradation products in sudden deaths associated with chlordiazepoxide overdosage. J. For. Sci. Soc. 26: 45–54, 1986.

B. Finkle. Personal communication, 1975.

J.M. Foreman, W.C. Griffith, P.G. Dextraze and I. Diamond. Simultaneous assay of diazepam, chlordiazepoxide, N-desmethyldiazepam, N-desmethylchlordiazepoxide, and demoxepam in serum by high performance liquid chromatography. Clin. Biochem. 13: 122–125, 1980.

D.J. Greenblatt, R.I. Shader, J. Koch-Weser and K. Franke. Clinical pharmacokinetics of chlordiazepoxide. In *Pharmacokinetics of Psychoactive Drugs* (L.A. Gottschalk and S. Merlis, eds.), Spectrum Pub., New York, 1976, pp. 127–139.

M.R. Hackman, M.A. Brooks and J.A.F. deSilva. Determination of chlordiazepoxide hydrochloride (Librium) and its major metabolites in plasma by differential pulse polarography. Anal. Chem. 46: 1075–1081, 1974.

P.I. Jatlow. Ultraviolet spectrophotometric determination of chlordiazepoxide in plasma. Clin. Chem. 18: 516–518, 1972.

B.A. Koechlin and L. D'Arconte. The determination of chlordiazepoxide (Librium) and of metabolite of lactam character in plasma of humans, dogs and rats by a specific spectrofluorometric micro method. Anal. Biochem. 5: 195–207, 1963.

B.A. Koechlin, M.A. Schwartz, G. Krol and W. Oberhausli. The metabolic fate of ^{14}C-labeled chlordiazepoxide in man, in the dog, and in the rat. J. Pharm. Exp. Ther. 148: 399–411, 1965.

K. Lin and R.O. Friedel. Relationship of plasma levels of chlordiazepoxide and metabolites to clinical response. Am. J. Psych. 136: 18–23, 1979.

H. Mohseni. Personal communication, 1975.

M.A. Peat, B.S. Finkle and M.E. Deyman. High-pressure liquid chromatographic determination of chlordiazepoxide and its major metabolites in biological fluids. J. Pharm. Sci. 68: 1467–1468, 1979.

P.R. Puopolo, M.E. Pothier, S.A. Volpicelli and J.G. Flood. Single procedure for detection, confirmation, and quantification of benzodiazepines in serum by liquid chromatography with photodiode-array detection. Clin. Chem. 37: 701–706, 1991.

M.A. Schwartz and E. Postma. Metabolic N-demethylation of chlordiazepoxide. J. Pharm. Sci. 55: 1358–1362, 1966.

M.A. Schwartz. Pathways of metabolism of the benzodiazepines. In *The Benzodiazepines* (S. Garattini, E. Mussini and L.O. Randall, eds.), Raven Press, New York, 1973, pp. 53–74.

G.G. Skellern, J. Meier, B.I. Knight and B. Whiting. The application of HPLC to the determination of some 1,4 benzodiazepines and their metabolites in plasma. Brit. J. Clin. Pharm. 5: 483–487, 1978.

N. Strojny, C.V. Puglisi and J.A.F. deSilva. Determination of chlordiazepoxide and its metabolites in plasma by high pressure liquid chromatography. Anal. Letters 2: 135–160, 1978.

S. Sun and D.J. Hoffman. Rapid GLC determination of chlordiazepoxide and metabolite in serum using on-column methylation. J. Pharm. Sci. 67: 1647–1648, 1978.

T.B. Vree, A.M. Baars, Y.A. Hekster and E. van der Kleijn. Simultaneous determination of chlordiazepoxide and its metabolites in human plasma and urine by means of reversed-phase high-performance liquid chromatography. J. Chrom. 224: 519–525, 1981.

Chlormethiazole

T½: 3–5 hr
Vd: 15 L/kg
Fb: 0.60–0.70
pKa: 3.2

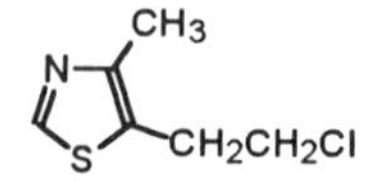

Occurrence and Usage. Chlormethiazole (clomethiazole, Heminevrin, Distraneurin) is a weakly basic thiamine derivative first investigated in 1957. It has been used as a sedative-hypnotic and anticonvulsant agent in the management of alcohol and drug withdrawal, toxemia of pregnancy, status epilepticus, and anxiety states. The drug is administered orally as the free base (192 mg capsule) or ethanedisulfonate salt (50 mg/mL syrup or 300 mg capsule) or intravenously as the ethanedisulfonate salt (8 mg/mL solution). The salt form contains 64% by weight of the free base. Daily doses range from 192–2300 mg.

Blood Concentrations. Blood concentrations of chlormethiazole in 14 volunteers reached an average peak concentration of 0.11 mg/L at 1 hour after the oral ingestion of a 192 mg capsule; the ingestion of 2 capsules (384 mg) produced an average peak level of 0.28 mg/L after 45 minutes. An oral dose of syrup containing 480 mg free base resulted in an average peak blood concentration of 0.80 mg/L after only 20 minutes. A 30 minute intravenous infusion of 192 mg (free base) of chlormethiazole as the ethanedisulfonate produced an average peak blood level of 0.75 mg/L at the end of the infusion. The elimination half-lives in these subjects ranged from 3.1–4.9 hours (average, 3.7) and the blood/plasma concentration ratio of the drug averaged 0.76. The kinetics of chlormethiazole can be described by a 2-compartment open model (Jostell et al., 1978). The half-life of the drug is significantly longer in the elderly and in patients with liver cirrhosis, averaging about 8.6 hours (Nation et al., 1976; Pentikainen et al., 1980).

Metabolism and Excretion. Chlormethiazole is extensively metabolized in man; the known metabolites, products of dechlorination and oxidation, account for only 16% of an administered dose. Less than 0.01% of a dose is excreted unchanged in the 36 hour urine; 4-methyl-5-thiazoleacetic acid accounts for 12–14%, 5-(1-hydroxyethyl)-4-methylthiazole (HEMT) for 2–3%, and 5-acetyl-4-methylthiazole (AMT) for less than 0.05% (Moore et al., 1975). Both HEMT and AMT are found in plasma at concentrations that often exceed those of the parent drug (Nation et al., 1977). The pharmacological activity of the metabolites, if any, is unknown.

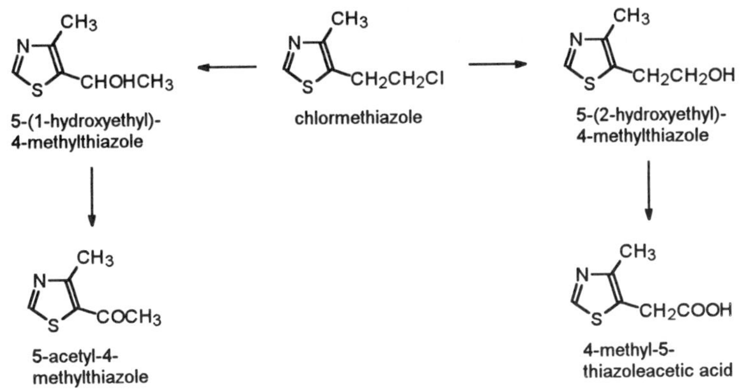

5-(1-hydroxyethyl)-
4-methylthiazole

chlormethiazole

5-(2-hydroxyethyl)-
4-methylthiazole

5-acetyl-4-
methylthiazole

4-methyl-5-
thiazoleacetic acid

Toxicity. The clinical features of acute chlormethiazole poisoning are similar to those of barbiturate intoxication, but also include increased salivation. In a controlled intravenous infusion, subjects exhibited moderately heavy sedation with amnesia at a mean plasma level of 9.2 mg/L. Other symptoms included nasal irritation and congestion, eye irritation, sneezing and flushing of the face (Seow et al., 1981). Peak plasma chlormethiazole concentrations after overdosage in 10 comatose patients ranged from 7–36 mg/L, and plasma half-lives ranged from 4–17 hours. The highest plasma concentration observed in a patient who remained conscious was 11.5 mg/L (Illingworth et al., 1979). A chronic alcoholic who was arrested after a minor traffic accident had a chlormethiazole blood concentration of 26 mg/L; no alcohol was found (Horder, 1978).

At least 6 patients have died in hospital after receiving chlormethiazole infusions to control anxiety or convulsions, but the specific role of the drug in the deaths was not elucidated (Pentikainen et al., 1976). One person is known to have died within an hour of ingesting 10 g of the drug, and the postmortem blood concentrations of 9 victims who died after the ingestion of 10–50 g ranged from 25–80 mg/L (Jakobsson, 1972). The following distribution was noted in 13 fatalities occurring after oral overdosage (Richardson, 1972; Oliver and Stewart, 1975; Horder, 1978; Robinson and McDowall, 1979):

Chlormethiazole Concentrations in Fatal Cases (mg/L or mg/kg)

	Blood	Brain	Liver	Bile	Kidney	Urine	Gastric
Average	55	134	94	91	78	43	218 mg
(Range)	(10–214)	(134)	(42–190)	(38–143)	(78)	(5–114)	(4–857)

Analysis. Determination of chlormethiazole in biological specimens may be performed by gas chromatography of the underivatized drug, with detection by flame-ionization (Frisch and Ortengren, 1966; Flanagan et al., 1978), nitrogen-phosphorus (Tsuei et al., 1980; Heipertz and Reimer, 1981), or mass spectrometry (Nation et al., 1977; Jostell et al., 1978). Liquid chromatography has also been employed (Hartley et al., 1983; Kim and Khanna, 1983; Hartley et al., 1987).

References

R.J. Flanagan, T.D. Lee and D.M. Rutherford. Analysis of chlormethiazole, ethchlorvynol and trichloroethanol in biological fluids by gas-liquid chromatography as an aid to the diagnosis of acute poisoning. J. Chrom. 153: 473–479, 1978.

E.P. Frisch and B. Ortengren. Plasma concentration of chlormethiazole following oral intake of tablets and capsules. Acta Psych. Scand. 192: 35–41, 1966.

R. Hartley, M. Becker and S.F. Leach. Determination of chlormethiazole in plasma by high-performance liquid chromatography. J. Chrom. 276: 471–477, 1983.

R. Hartley, M. Lucock and M. Becker. Improved high-performance liquid chromatographic procedure for the determination of chlormethiazole levels following solid-phase extraction from plasma. J. Chrom. 415: 357–364, 1987.

R. Heipertz and C. Reimer. A rapid gas-chromatographic method for the quantitative determination of clomethiazole in human serum. Clin. Chim. Acta 110: 131–138, 1981.

J.M. Horder. Fatal chlormethiazole poisoning in chronic alcoholics. Brit. Med. J. 1: 693–694, 1978.

R.N. Illingworth, M.J. Stewart and D.R. Jarvie. Severe poisoning with chlormethiazole. Brit. Med. J. 2: 902–903, 1979.

S.V. Jakobsson. Personal communication, 1972.

K.G. Jostell, S. Agurell, L.G. Allgen et al. Pharmacokinetics of clomethiazole in healthy adults. Acta Pharm. Tox. 43: 180–189, 1978.

C. Kim and J.M. Khanna. Determination of chlormethiazole in blood by high performance liquid chromatography. J. Liq. Chrom. 6: 907–916, 1983.

R.G. Moore, A.V. Robertson, M.P. Smyth et al. Metabolism and urinary excretion of chlormethiazole in humans. Xenobiotica 5: 687–696, 1975.

R.L. Nation, B. Learoyd, J. Barber and E.J. Triggs. The pharmacokinetics of chlormethiazole following intravenous administration in the aged. Eur. J. Clin. Pharm. 10: 407–415, 1976.

R.L. Nation, J. Vine, E.J. Triggs and B. Learoyd. Plasma level of chlormethiazole and two metabolites after oral administration to young and aged human subjects. Eur. J. Clin. Pharm. 12: 137–145, 1977.

J.S. Oliver and P.D. Stewart. Chlormethiazole poisoning (a case report). Med. Sci. Law 15: 67–68, 1975.

P.J. Pentikainen, V.V. Valtonen and T.A. Miettinen. Deaths in connection with chlormethiazole (Heminevrin) therapy. Int. J. Clin. Pharm. Biopharm. 14: 225–230, 1976.

P.J. Pentikainen, P.J. Neuvonen and K.G. Jostell. Pharmacokinetics of chlormethiazole in healthy volunteers and patients with cirrhosis of the liver. Eur. J. Clin. Pharm. 17: 275–284, 1980.

A. Richardson. Personal communication, 1972.

A.E. Robinson and R.D. McDowall. Toxicological investigations of six chlormethiazole-related deaths. For. Sci. Int. 14: 49–55, 1979.

L.T. Seow, L.E. Mather and J.G. Roberts. An integrated study of pharmacokinetics and pharmacodynamics of chlormethiazole in healthy young volunteers. Eur. J. Clin. Pharm. 19: 263–269, 1981.

S.E. Tsuei, J. Thomas and R.L. Nation. Simultaneous quantitation of chlormethiazole and two of its metabolites in blood and plasma by gas-liquid chromatography. J. Chrom. 182: 55–62, 1980.

Chlormezanone

T½: 30–53 hr
Vd: ?
Fb: 0.48

Occurrence and Usage. Chlormezanone (Trancopal) is a mild sedative and muscle relaxant first described in 1958. This neutral drug is available in tablets of 100 and 200 mg, and daily doses range from 300–800 mg.

Blood Concentrations. Plasma chlormezanone concentrations after a single 200 mg oral dose given to 5 subjects reached an average peak of 2.7 mg/L (range, 2.5–3.2) by 4 hours; the level declined to 1.6 mg/L by 24 hours (Ohya et al., 1980). A 400 mg dose given to 4 subjects produced an average peak plasma concentration of 5.3 mg/L (range, 4.8–8.8) at 2 hours, declining to 2.5 mg/L by 24 hours (McChesney et al., 1967). The elimination half-life of the drug has been found to average 38 hours in young adults and 54 hours in the elderly (Bernard et al., 1991a).

In a group of patients receiving 600 mg of chlormezanone daily for 5 days, steady-state plasma levels ranged from 10–14 mg/L (Koppell et al., 1991).

Metabolism and Excretion. Koppell et al. (1986) proposed that chlormezanone is extensively hydrolyzed in the stomach to a pharmacologically active hydrolysis product, which constitutes the principal plasma species; further metabolism yields p-chlorobenzaldehyde, p-chlorobenzoic acid, p-chlorohippuric acid and p-chlorobenzoyl-N-methylamide. More recent reports have disputed this, however, claiming that unchanged chlormezanone is the only identifiable species in plasma and urine, and that urinary excretion of parent drug represents less than 3% of a dose over 5 days (Ali and Blume, 1987; Bernard et al., 1991a).

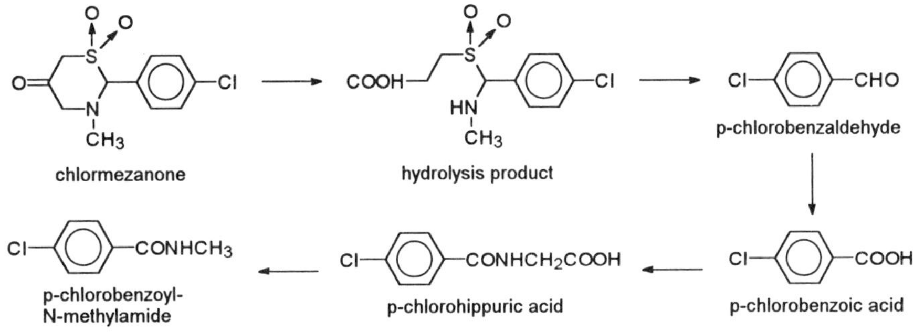

Toxicity. A daily oral 1200 mg dose of chlormezanone in adults is associated with plasma drug levels of 18–27 mg/L and usually causes muscular weakness, ataxia and tachycardia (Koppel et al., 1991). A 36 year old woman ingested 7 g of drug and developed coma but not respiratory depression; a plasma chlormezanone level of 60 mg/L was measured 10 hours after ingestion and she regained consciousness at 15 hours (Armstrong et al., 1983).

The following concentrations were found in the tissues of a woman who died after ingesting 10.8 g of chlormezanone and 200 mg of diazepam (Kristinsson, 1980):

Chlormezanone Concentrations in a Fatal Case (mg/L or mg/kg)

Blood	Brain	Liver	Urine	Blood Diazepam
53	109	88	31	1.6

Analysis. Chlormezanone is known to degrade *in vitro* to p-chlorobenzaldehyde at pH 7.35 with a half-life of 48 hours. The drug has been determined in biological specimens by colorimetry (McChesney et al., 1967), ultraviolet spectrophotometry after thin-layer chromatography purification (Kristinsson, 1980), and electron-capture gas chromatography after conversion to p-chlorobenzaldehyde (Ohya et al., 1980). Gas chromatography of the intact drug has not been successful due to thermal decomposition. The most specific procedure to date has employed liquid chromatography (Koppel et al., 1986; Ali and Blume, 1987; Bernard et al., 1991b).

References

S.L. Ali and H. Blume. Determination of chlormezanone in human plasma after administration of chlormezanone formulations. Arz. Forsch. 37: 1396–1399, 1987.

D. Armstrong, R.A. Braithwaite and J.A. Vale. Chlormezanone poisoning. Brit. Med. J. 286: 845–846, 1983.

N. Bernard, J.P. Fauvel, N. Pozet et al. Pharmacokinetics of chlormezanone in elderly patients. Eur. J. Clin. Pharm. 40: 603–607, 1991a.

N. Bernard, N. Ferry, G. Guisinaud and J. Sassard. Determination of chlormezanone in plasma and urine by high performance liquid chromatography. J. Liq. Chrom. 14: 1747–1755, 1991b.

C. Koppel, J. Tenczer and A. Wagemann. Metabolism of chlormezanone in man. Arz. Forsch. 36: 1116–1118, 1986.

C. Koppel, J. Kristinsson, A. Wagemann et al. Chlormezanone plasma and blood levels in patients after single and repeated oral doses and after suicidal drug overdose. Eur. J. Drug Met. Pharmacokin. 16: 43–47, 1991.

J. Kristinsson. Personal communication, 1980.

E.W. McChesney, W.F. Banks, Jr., G.A. Portmann and A.V.R. Crain. Metabolism of chlormezanone in man and laboratory animals. Biochem. Pharm. 16: 813–826, 1967.

K. Ohya, S. Shintani, W. Suzuki and M. Sano. Sensitive and selective method for the determination of chlormezanone in plasma by electron-capture gas chromatography. J. Chrom. 221: 67–74, 1980.

Chloroform

T½: 1.5 hr
Vd: 2.6 L/kg   CHCl₃
Fb: ?

Occurrence and Usage. Chloroform was once used extensively as an anesthetic in man, but is now considered obsolete for this application. It has also been incorporated into many pharmaceutical preparations for its solvent and local anesthetic properties, but its proven carcinogenic potential in laboratory animals has precluded its use in food or drugs in the United States. Chloroform continues to be encountered as a solvent and chemical intermediate in laboratory and industrial situations, for which the current threshold limit value is 10 ppm (49 mg/m³). The odor threshold of the compound is about 50 ppm.

Blood Concentrations. Plasma chloroform concentrations in 25 nonexposed adult women were found to range from 4–350 µg/L over a period of six months, with most subjects varying within a narrow range; 3 subjects exhibited temporary excursions of up to 1655–4000 µg/L for unknown reasons (Pfaffenberger and Peoples, 1982). A single 500 mg oral dose of chloroform administered to 2 subjects produced maximal blood concentrations of 1–5 mg/L at about 1 hour; an average elimination half-life of 1.5 hours was observed (Fry et al., 1972). An individual who inhaled chloroform vapor from an open container for 7 seconds (until he felt faint) developed a peak blood level of 4 mg/L at 20 minutes post-exposure (Allan et al., 1988). Blood specimens drawn from 58 patients undergoing chloroform anesthesia exhibited overall concentrations ranging from 20–232 mg/L with an average of 92 mg/L; samples from patients in plane 1 of stage III anesthesia averaged 71 mg/L; plane 2, 106 mg/L; plane 3, 122 mg/L; and plane 4, 165 mg/L (Morris et al., 1951). The blood/plasma concentration ratio for chloroform averages 4.0 at a blood concentration of 75 mg/L (Seto et al., 1993).

Metabolism and Excretion. Chloroform undergoes considerable biotransformation in man, with the formation of carbon dioxide and hydrochloric acid. An average of 43% (range, 18–67) of a single dose is eliminated unchanged in the expired air within 8 hours, and an average of 50% is found as exhaled CO_2 in the same time period. Less than 0.01% of the dose was found in the 8 hour urine (Fry et al., 1972). The chemical is highly lipid-soluble and tends to accumulate in adipose tissue (Vogt et al., 1980).

The following concentrations of chloroform were measured in the tissues of 9 patients who died during surgery of causes unrelated to the anesthetic agent (Gettler and Blume, 1931):

Chloroform Concentrations During Surgical Anesthesia (mg/kg)

	Brain	Lung	Liver
Average	126	100	64
(Range)	(60–182)	(22–145)	(24–88)

Toxicity. Prolonged exposure to chloroform vapor concentrations of 77–237 ppm causes weakness, mental dullness and gastrointestinal disturbances (Challen et al., 1958). Chronic exposure to concentrations of up to 205 ppm has produced a high incidence of liver abnormalities in workers (Bomski et al., 1967), and chronic addiction to the chemical has been noted to cause psychotic behavior and degenerative changes of the brain (Heilbrunn et al., 1945). Delayed hepatotoxic reactions, occasionally fatal, have been reported after use of chloroform as a surgical anesthetic (Gibberd, 1935; Lunt, 1953).

Acute ingestion of as little as 10 mL of chloroform may result in death due to central nervous system depression. Exposure to air concentrations of 100–1000 ppm for short periods may cause discomfort and dizziness, and concentrations of 7000–20,000 ppm will produce rapid loss of consciousness. Persons who survive an acute exposure to the chemical may develop hepatotoxicity within 2–5 days (Schroeder, 1965; Storms, 1973).

In 15 acute fatalities due to the intentional or forced inhalation of chloroform, the following tissue concentrations were observed (Bonnichsen and Maehly, 1966; Bidanset, 1973; Kaempe and Dalgaard, 1980; Giusti and Chiarotti, 1981; Iffland and Ramme, 1983; McGee et al., 1987; Allan et al., 1988; Rao, 1988; Ryall, 1989):

Chloroform Concentrations in Fatal Cases (mg/L or mg/kg)

	Blood	Brain	Liver	Kidney	Urine
Average	64	133	82	52	21
(Range)	(10–194)	(50–310)	(6–201)	(16–124)	(0–70)

Analysis. Chloroform may be estimated in biologic samples by means of a nonspecific colorimetric technique that is an adaptation of the Fujiwara reaction (Morris et al., 1951). Using this method, Gettler and Blume (1931) observed an 82% loss of chloroform from tissue specimens stored for a period of 42 days. Gas chromatographic procedures have entailed solvent extraction of the chloroform (Fry et al., 1972; Poobalasingam, 1976; Vogt et al., 1980) or headspace sampling (Dubowski, 1975; Reddrop et al., 1980; Allan et al., 1988; Seto et al., 1993).

References

A.R. Allan, R.C. Blackmore and P.A. Toseland. A chloroform inhalation fatality—an unusual asphyxiation. Med. Sci. Law 28: 120–122, 1988.

J. Bidanset. Presented at the annual meeting of the American Academy of Forensic Sciences, Las Vegas, February 22, 1973.

H. Bomski, A. Sobolewska and A. Strakowski. Toxische Schaedigung der Leber durch Chloroform bei Chemiebetriebswerkern. Int. Arch. Gewerbepath. Gewerbehyg. 24: 127–134, 1967.

R. Bonnichsen and A.C. Maehly. Poisoning by volatile compounds. II. Chlorinated aliphatic hydrocarbons. J. For. Sci. 11: 414–427, 1966.

P.J.R. Challen, D.E. Hickish and J. Bedford. Chronic chloroform intoxication. Brit. J. Ind. Med. 15: 243–249, 1958.

K.M. Dubowski. Organic volatile substances. In *Methodology for Analytical Toxicology* (I. Sunshine, ed.), CRC Press, Cleveland, 1975, pp. 407–411.

B.J. Fry, T. Taylor and D.E. Hathway. Pulmonary elimination of chloroform and its metabolite in man. Arch. Int. Pharm. Ther. 196: 98–111, 1972.

A.O. Gettler and H. Blume. Chloroform in the brain, lungs and liver. Arch. Path. 11: 554–560, 1931.

G.F. Gibberd. Delayed chloroform poisoning in obstetric practice. Guy's Hosp. London Reports 85: 142–160, 1935.

G.V. Giusti and M. Chiarotti. Double 'suicide' by chloroform in a pair of twins. Med. Sci. Law 21: 2–3, 1981.

R. Iffland and H. Ramme. Chloroform vergiftung eines jugendlichen Drogenkonsumenten. Arch. Tox. 53: 289–295, 1983.

G. Heilbrunn, E. Liebert and P.B. Szanto. Chronic chloroform poisoning. Arch. Neurol. Psych. 53: 68–72, 1945.

R. Iffland and H. Ramme. Chloroform Vergiftung eines jugendlichen Drogenkonsumenten. Arch. Tox. 53: 289–295, 1983.

B. Kaempe and J.B. Dalgaard. Chloroform as a tool for homicide. In *Toxicological Aspects* (A. Kovatsis, ed.), Thessaloniki, Greece, 1980, pp. 422–430.

R.L. Lunt. Delayed chloroform poisoning in obstetric practice. Brit. Med. J. 1: 489–490, 1953.

M.B. McGee. S.G. Jejurikar and L.C. VanBerkom. A double homicide as a result of chloroform poisoning. J. For. Sci. 32: 1453–1459, 1987.

L.E. Morris, E.L. Frederickson and O.S. Orth. Differences in the concentration of chloroform in the blood of man and dog during anesthesia. J. Pharm. Exp. Ther. 101: 56–62, 1951.

C.D. Pfaffenberger and A.J. Peoples. Long-term variation study of blood plasma levels of chloroform and related purgeable compounds. J. Chrom. 239: 217–226, 1982.

N. Poobalasingam. Analysis of chloroform in blood. Brit. J. Anaesth. 48: 953–956, 1976.

C. Rao. Presented at the annual meeting of the American Academy of Forensic Sciences, Philadelphia, February 18, 1988.

C.J. Reddrop, W. Riess and T.F. Slater. Two rapid methods for the simultaneous gas-liquid chromatographic determination of carbon tetrachloride and chloroform in biological material and expired air. J. Chrom. 193: 71–82, 1980.

J.E. Ryall. Personal communication, 1989.

H.G. Schroeder. Acute and delayed chloroform poisoning. Brit. J. Anaesth. 37: 972–975, 1965.

Y. Seto, N. Tsunoda, H. Ohta and T. Shinohara. Determination of chloroform levels in blood using a headspace capillary gas chromatographic method. J. Anal. Tox. 17: 415–420, 1993.

W.W. Storms. Chloroform parties. J. Am. Med. Asso. 225: 160, 1973.

C.R. Vogt, J.C. Liao and A.Y. Sun. Extraction and determination of chloroform in rat blood and tissues by gas chromatography-electron-capture detection: distribution of chloroform in the animal body. Clin. Chem. 26: 66–68, 1980.

Chloroprocaine

T½: 1.5–6.4 min
Vd: ?
Fb: ?
pKa: 9.0

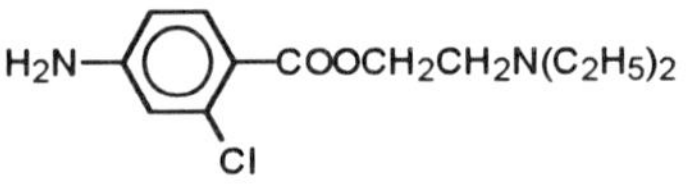

H_2N—⬡—$COOCH_2CH_2N(C_2H_5)_2$
|
Cl

Occurrence and Usage. Chloroprocaine (2-chloroprocaine, Nesacaine) is a local anesthetic of the ester type, similar in action and use to procaine but of more rapid onset of action. It is available for intravenous and intramuscular injection in solutions of 0.5–3% as the hydrochloride. Single doses are not to exceed a maximum of 800 mg without epinephrine or 1000 mg with epinephrine.

Blood Concentrations. Peak plasma concentrations of 2-chloro-4-aminobenzoic acid ranged from 3.5–4.3 mg/L in 3 subjects at the end of an intravenous infusion of 250 mg of chloroprocaine over a period of 30 minutes; chloroprocaine was not present in a detectable concentration (O'Brien et al., 1979). Doses of 220–990 mg given to obstetrical patients for epidural anesthesia produced chloroprocaine plasma concentrations that generally did not exceed 0.2 mg/L when measured within 5–10 minutes (Kuhnert et al., 1986).

Ten minutes after an inadvertent intravenous administration of 600 mg of chloroprocaine in a 23 year old 60 kg female, a chloroprocaine plasma concentration of 17 mg/L was detected; in spite of this high concentration, the patient suffered no adverse effects (Gross et al., 1981).

Metabolism and Excretion. Chloroprocaine is rapidly hydrolyzed by blood esterases into two relatively nontoxic metabolites, 2-chloro-4-aminobenzoic acid and diethylaminoethanol, which are excreted primarily in the urine (O'Brien et al., 1979).

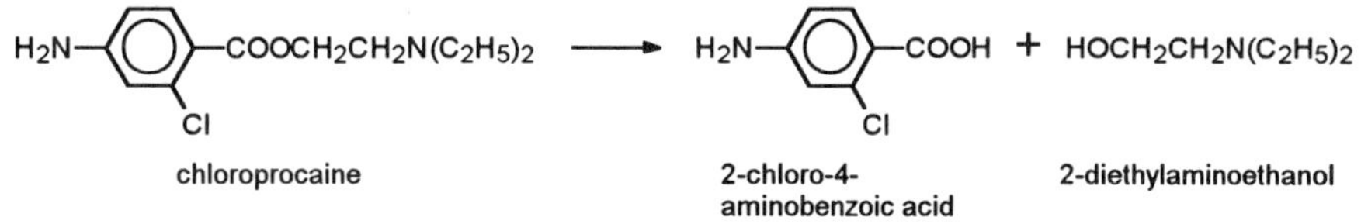

H$_2$N—⟨benzene⟩—COOCH$_2$CH$_2$N(C$_2$H$_5$)$_2$ ⟶ H$_2$N—⟨benzene⟩—COOH + HOCH$_2$CH$_2$N(C$_2$H$_5$)$_2$

chloroprocaine (Cl)	2-chloro-4-aminobenzoic acid (Cl)	2-diethylaminoethanol

Toxicity. In overdosage, chloroprocaine produces central nervous system stimulation, tremors, acidosis, bradycardia, cardiac arrhythmias, central nervous system depression, coma, convulsions, and respiratory and cardiac arrest. A number of instances of very prolonged (several weeks to several months) neural blockade following use of chloroprocaine for spinal obstetrical anesthesia have been reported; the low pH of this solution and its use in large volumes have been cited as possible causes (Ravindran et al., 1980; Reisner et al., 1980; Moore et al., 1982).

Analysis. Chloroprocaine has been determined in plasma by gas chromatography employing flame-ionization (Smith et al., 1978; O'Brien et al., 1979), nitrogen-phosphorus (Kuhnert et al., 1980) and mass spectrometric detection (Krohg and Jellum, 1981; Kuhnert et al., 1981). Precautions regarding the *in vitro* hydrolysis of ester-type local anesthetics are given in the sections on cocaine and procaine.

References

T.L. Gross, P.M. Kuhnert, B.R. Kuhnert et al. Plasma levels of 2-chloroprocaine and lack of sequelae following an apparent intravenous injection. Anesthesiology 54: 173–174, 1981.

K. Krohg and E. Jellum. Urinary metabolites of chloroprocaine studied by combined gas chromatography-mass spectrometry. Anesthesiology 54: 329–332, 1981.

B.R. Kuhnert, P.M. Kuhnert, A.L. Prochaska and T.L. Gross. Plasma levels of 2-chloroprocaine in obstetric patients and their neonates after epidural anesthesia. Anesthesiology 53: 21–25, 1980.

B.R. Kuhnert, P.M. Kuhnert and A.L.P. Reese. Measurement of 2-chloroprocaine in plasma by selected ion monitoring. J. Chrom. 224: 488–491, 1981.

D.C. Moore, J. Spierdijk, J.D. VanKleef et al. Chloroprocaine neurotoxicity: four additional cases. Anesth. Anal. 61: 155–159, 1982.

J.E. O'Brien, V. Abbey, O. Hinsvark et al. Metabolism and measurement of chloroprocaine, an ester-type local anesthetic. J. Pharm. Sci. 68: 75–79, 1979.

R.S. Ravindran, V.K. Bond, M.D. Tasch et al. Prolonged neural blockade following regional analgesia with 2-chloroprocaine. Anesth. Anal. 59: 447–451, 1980.

L.S. Reisner, B.N. Hochman and M.H. Plumer. Persistent neurologic deficit and adhesive arachnoiditis following intrathecal 2-chloroprocaine injection. Anesth. Anal. 59: 452–454, 1980.

R.H. Smith, M.A. Brewster, J.A. MacDonald and D.S. Thompson. Measurement of chloroprocaine and procaine in plasma by flame ionization gas-liquid chromatography. Clin. Chem. 24: 1599–1602, 1978.

Chloroquine

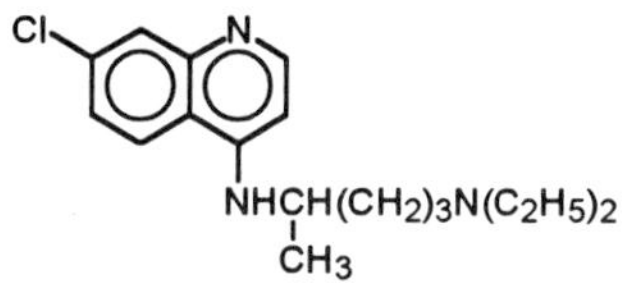

NHCH(CH$_2$)$_3$N(C$_2$H$_5$)$_2$
CH$_3$

T½: 3–14 days (dose-dependent)
Vd: 116–285 L/kg
Fb: 0.55
pKa: 8.4, 10.8

Occurrence and Usage. Chloroquine (Aralen) is an aminoquinoline derivative that was first synthesized in 1934 for use as an antimalarial agent. It may be administered by intramuscular injection of the hydrochloride in single doses of 200–250 mg; chronic oral therapy is conducted with the phosphate salt in once weekly doses of 500 mg for malaria or in daily doses of 250 mg for rheumatoid diseases.

Blood Concentrations. Steady-state plasma concentrations of 0.022, 0.049, 0.110 and 0.176 mg/L were developed by patients on daily oral chloroquine doses of 50, 100, 200 and 300 mg, respectively. Plasma concentrations in excess of 0.010 mg/L were found most effective against vivax malaria, whereas concentrations of 0.020 mg/L or higher were generally required for permanent suppression of falciparum malaria. The drug was found to have a plasma half-life of 3–14 days, a blood/plasma concentration ratio of 3.7, and to exhibit 55% binding to plasma proteins at a plasma concentration of 0.080 mg/L (Alving et al., 1948; Berliner et al., 1948; Gustafsson et al., 1983). Patients receiving a once weekly 500 mg oral dose on a chronic basis attained plasma concentrations that averaged a maximal 0.094 mg/L at 6 hours after the last dose, and a minimum of 0.012 mg/L immediately prior to the next dose (McChesney et al., 1962). Most patients receiving a daily 250 mg oral dose for at least 2 months had serum concentrations of 0.2–0.4 mg/L; the drug displayed dose-dependent kinetics when the dose was varied from 250–1000 mg (Frisk-Holmberg et al., 1979). The plasma concentrations of desethylchloroquine have been found to exceed those of its parent in patients on therapy with the drug (Bergqvist and Frisk-Holmberg, 1980).

Metabolism and Excretion. Chloroquine is metabolized by oxidation of the side chain to a series of more polar and less active compounds. No evidence has been found for the existence of phenolic metabolites. In persons on chronic therapy about 8% of a dose is eliminated in the daily feces and about 33% in the urine; the urinary products consist of unchanged drug (19%), desethylchloroquine (13%), and didesethylchloroquine (1%). An alcoholic deamination product and 4-amino-7-chloroquinoline have been found in urine but appear to be of minor quantitative importance (Berliner et al., 1948; Kuroda, 1962; McChesney et al., 1966; Brown et al., 1985).

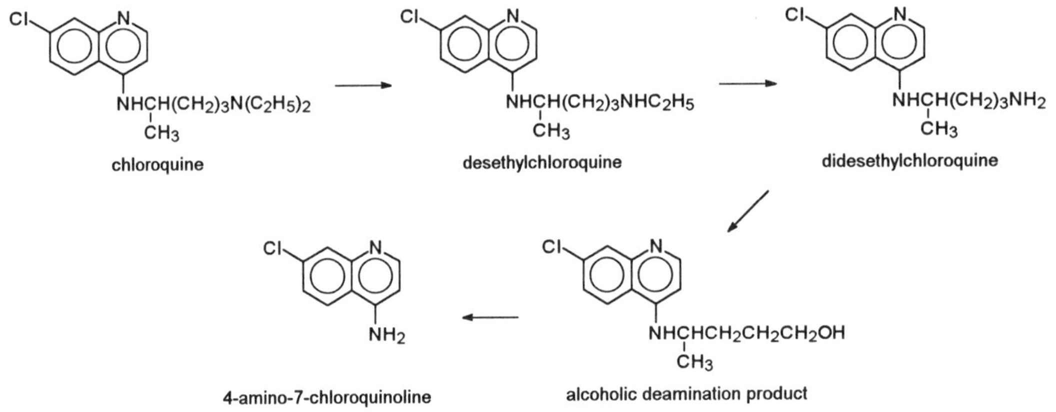

The following tissue concentrations were found in 8 adults receiving therapeutic amounts of the drug (Prouty and Kuroda, 1958):

Chloroquine Distribution During Therapy (mg/L or mg/kg)

	Brain	Liver	Kidney
Average	2.9	25	3.0
(Range)	(0.5–7.3)	(4.3–58)	(0.6–5.8)

Toxicity. In acute overdosage, chloroquine may produce respiratory depression and cardiogenic shock with hypotension. Patients on therapy with the drug generally exhibit symptoms of toxicity at plasma concentrations exceeding 0.6 mg/L; such symptoms include headache, confusion, visual disturbances, and serum creatinine increase (Frisk-Holmberg et al., 1979). Plasma chloroquine concentrations in persons who survived the ingestion of 5–20 g have been as high as 7–36 mg/L initially (Meunier et al., 1977; Czajka and Flynn, 1978; Bauer et al., 1991). Neither hemodialysis nor peritoneal dialysis has been found to be effective in treatment of overdosage (McCann et al., 1975; van Stone, 1976; Heath et al., 1983), although a combination of diazepam, epinephrine and mechanical ventilation has been successfully employed (Riou et al., 1988). The blood half-life was prolonged to 60 days in one victim of acute poisoning (Frisk-Holmberg et al., 1983).

Kiel (1964) reviewed 18 deaths due to overdosage with chloroquine and presented the following analytical data on 9 other cases of suicide following the acute ingestion of 3–44.5 g of the drug by adult males: brain, 2.8–50 mg/kg (average, 16); liver, 200–750 mg/kg (average, 410); kidney, 110–640 mg/kg (average, 303). The ingestion of 3–20 g of the drug caused the death of 5 adults, in whom the following tissue distribution was noted (Prouty and Kuroda, 1958; Bonnichsen and Maehly, 1965; Robinson et al., 1970):

Chloroquine Concentrations in Fatal Cases (mg/L or mg/kg)

	Blood	Brain	Liver	Kidney	Urine
Average	10	12	392	280	44
(Range)	(3–16)	(10–16)	(150–900)	(70–470)	(20–68)

Nine other fatal cases have been reported in which postmortem blood concentrations averaged 51 mg/L (range, 24–99), although concentrations in the other organs were generally within the ranges mentioned above (Hoole, 1966; Carson et al., 1967; Ifftsits-Simon, 1968; Pitt, 1978; Weingarten and Cherry, 1981; Wong, 1982; Rousseau, 1984). Kuhlman et al. (1991) reported that postmortem redistribution of chloroquine may artifactually increase the postmortem blood concentration; they suggested that a liver concentration exceeding 150 mg/kg is a more reliable indicator of acute fatal overdosage.

Analysis. Chloroquine may be determined in blood or plasma by fluorimetry (Alving et al., 1948; Adelusi and Salako, 1980). Ultraviolet spectrophotometry has been utilized for the measurement of toxic levels of the drug in tissue specimens (Prouty and Kuroda, 1958; Robinson et al., 1970). More specific techniques include nitrogen-selective gas chromatography (Viala et al., 1981; Churchill et al., 1983) and liquid chromatography (Bergqvist and Frisk-Holmberg, 1980; Akintonwa et al., 1983; Pussard et al., 1986; Chaulet et al., 1991; Houze et al., 1992).

References

S.A. Adelusi and L.A. Salako. Improved fluorimetric assay of chloroquine in biological samples. J. Pharm. Pharmac. 32: 711–712, 1980.

A. Akintowa, M.C. Meyer and P.T.R. Hwang. Simultaneous determination of chloroquine and desethylchloroquine in blood, plasma and urine by high-performance liquid chromatography. J. Liq. Chrom. 6: 1513–1522, 1983.

A.S. Alving, L. Eichelberger, B. Craige, Jr. et al. Studies on the chronic toxicity of chloroquine (SN-7618). J. Clin. Invest. 27: 60–65, 1948.

P. Bauer, B. Maire, M. Weber et al. Full recovery after a chloroquine suicide attempt. Clin. Tox. 29: 23–30, 1991.

Y. Bergqvist and M. Frisk-Holmberg. Sensitive method for the determination of chloroquine and its metabolite desethyl-chloroquine in human plasma and urine by high-performance liquid chromatography. J. Chrom. 221: 119–127, 1980.

R.W. Berliner, D.P. Earle, Jr., J.V. Taggart et al. Studies on the chemotherapy of the human malarias. VI. The physiological disposition, antimalarial activity, and toxicity of several derivatives of 4-aminoquinoline. J. Clin. Invest. 27: 98–107, 1948.

R. Bonnichsen and A.C. Maehly. Two fatal poisonings by chloroquine and by hydroxychloroquine. J. For. Sci. Soc. 5: 201–202, 1965.

N.D. Brown, B.T. Poon and J.D. Chulay. Chloroquine metabolism in man: urinary excretion of 7-chloro-4-hydroxyquinoline and 7-chloro-4-aminoquinoline metabolites. J. Chrom. 345: 209–214, 1985.

J.W. Carson, Jr., M.L. Barringer and R.E. Jones, Jr. Fatal chloroquine ingestion: an increasing hazard. Pediatrics 40: 449–450, 1967.

J.F. Chaulet, C. Mounier, O. Soares and J.L. Brazier. High-performance liquid chromatographic assay for chloroquine and its two major metabolites, desethylchloroquine and bidesethylchloroquine, in biological fluids. Anal. Letters 24: 665–682, 1992.

F.C. Churchill, D.L. Mount and I.K. Schwartz. Determination of chloroquine and its major metabolite in blood using perfluoroacylation followed by fused-silica capillary gas chromatography with nitrogen-sensitive detection. J. Chrom. 274: 111–120, 1983.

P.A. Czajka and P.J. Flynn. Nonfatal chloroquine poisoning. Clin. Tox. 13: 361–369, 1978.

M. Frisk-Holmberg, Y. Bergkvist, B. Domeij-Nyberg et al. Chloroquine serum concentration and side effects: evidence for dose-dependent kinetics. Clin. Pharm. Ther. 25: 345–350, 1979.

M. Frisk-Holmberg, Y. Bergkvist and U. Englund. Chloroquine intoxication. Brit. J. Clin. Pharm. 15: 502–503, 1983.

L.L. Gustafsson, O. Walker, G. Alvan et al. Disposition of chloroquine in man after single intravenous and oral doses. Brit. J. Clin. Pharm. 15: 471–479, 1983.

A. Heath, J. Ahlmen, T. Mellstrand and I. Wickstrom. Resin hemoperfusion in chloroquine poisoning. Clin. Tox. 19: 1067–1071, 1983.

A. Hoole. Personal communication, 1966.

P. Houze, A. de Reynies, F.J. Baud et al. Simultaneous determination of chloroquine and its three metabolites in human plasma, whole blood and urine by ion-pair high-performance liquid chromatography. J. Chrom. 574: 305–312, 1992.

C. Ifftsits-Simon. Fatal, suicidal chloroquine poisonings. Arch. Tox. 23: 204–208, 1968.

F.W. Kiel. Chloroquine suicide. J. Am. Med. Asso. 190: 398–400, 1964.

J.J. Kuhlman, R.W. Mayes, B. Levine et al. Chloroquine distribution in postmortem cases. J. For. Sci. 36: 1572–1579, 1991.

K. Kuroda. Detection and distribution of chloroquine metabolites in human tissues. J. Pharm. Exp. Ther. 137: 156–161, 1962.

W.P. McCann, R. Permisohn and P.A. Palmisano. Fatal chloroquine poisoning in a child: experience with peritoneal dialysis. Pediatrics 55: 536–538, 1975.

E.W. McChesney, W.F. Banks, Jr. and J.P. McAuliff. Laboratory studies of the 4-aminoquinoline antimalarials: II. Plasma levels of chloroquine and hydroxychloroquine in man after various oral dosage regimens. Antibiot. Chemo. 12: 583–594, 1962.

E.W. McChesney, W.D. Conway, W.F. Banks, Jr. et al. Studies of the metabolism of some compounds of the 4-amino-7-chloroquinoline series. J. Pharm. Exp. Ther. 151: 482–493, 1966.

J. Meunier, F.X. Girod, L. Saliou et al. Chloroquine determinations in biological fluids: results obtained in four cases of intoxication. Acta Pharm. Tox. 41 (Suppl 2): 228, 1977.

A. Pitt. Personal communication, 1978.

R.W. Prouty and K. Kuroda. Spectrophotometric determination and distribution of chloroquine in human tissues. J. Lab. Clin. Med. 52: 477–480, 1958.

E. Pussard, F. Verdier and M.C. Blayo. Simultaneous determination of chloroquine, amodiaquine and their metabolites in human plasma, red blood cells, whole blood and urine by column liquid chromatography. J. Chrom. 374: 111–118, 1986.

B. Riou, P. Barriott, A. Rimailho and F.J. Baud. Treatment of severe chloroquine poisoning. New Eng. J. Med. 318: 1–6, 1988.

A.E. Robinson, A.I. Coffer and F.E. Camps. The distribution of chloroquine in man after fatal poisoning. J. Pharm. Pharmac. 22: 700–703, 1970.

M. Rousseau. Personal communication, 1984.

J.C. van Stone. Hemodialysis and chloroquine poisoning. J. Lab. Clin. Med. 88: 87–90, 1976.

A. Viala, E. Deturmeny, M. Estadieu et al. Determination of chloroquine in blood by gas chromatography with nitrogen-selective detection using an internal standard. J. Chrom. 224: 503–506, 1981.

H.C. Weingarten and E.J. Cherry. A chloroquine fatality. Clin. Tox. 18: 959–963, 1981.

R.J. Wong. Personal communication, 1982.

Chlorothiazide

T½: 0.7–2.0 hr
Vd: ?
Fb: 0.95
pKa: 6.7, 9.5

Occurrence and Usage. Chlorothiazide (Diuril) is a thiazide derivative used as a diuretic and antihypertensive agent since 1957. It is a weakly acidic substance and a close structural analogue of the more potent hydrochlorothiazide. The drug is available in 250 or 500 mg tablets, a liquid suspension containing 250 mg/5 mL, or in vials containing 500 mg (as the sodium salt) for intravenous injection. Daily doses range from 500–2000 mg.

Blood Concentrations. Three normal subjects given a single 500 mg oral dose of radiolabeled chlorothiazide developed maximum serum concentrations averaging 2.3 mg/L after 2.3 hours; 4 subjects who received 1000 mg orally had peak concentrations that averaged 8.9 mg/L at 1.5 hours. Patients with cardiac, hepatic, or renal disease achieved somewhat lower maximum serum concentrations at later times (2.8, 3.5 or 5.0 hours, respectively). Subjects given 500 mg of the drug intravenously had initial serum concentrations of 39–201 mg/L; 1–8 hours later, these levels ranged from 4.0–5.2 mg/L (Brettell et al., 1960). Using a more specific technique, Barbhaiya et al. (1981) reported peak plasma levels of 0.4–0.9 mg/L following a single 500 mg oral dose in 3 subjects.

Metabolism and Excretion. Urine concentrations of chlorothiazide in persons receiving a 500–1000 mg oral dose generally range from 50–500 mg/L. Recovery of a labeled dose in the 24 hour urine is essentially complete after intravenous administration, but ranges from 9–58% after oral administration, indicating poor absorption from the gastrointestinal tract (Brettell et al., 1960). The bioavailability of several different commercial tablets ranged from 11–20%. Chlorothiazide is believed to be excreted in unchanged form in man (Straughn et al., 1979).

Toxicity. Adverse reactions to chlorothiazide include nausea, vomiting, dizziness, headache, hematologic disorders, hypotension, weakness, and various hypersensitivity manifestations. The drug may cause azotemia in patients with renal disease, and all persons receiving it should be monitored for possible fluid or electrolyte depletion.

Analysis. Chlorothiazide may be determined in urine by a somewhat nonspecific colorimetric method (Suria, 1978) or by liquid chromatography (Tisdall et al., 1980; Barbhaiya et al., 1981; Shah et al., 1982; Hessey et al., 1986). This determination is usually performed to monitor patient compliance or in the investigation of electrolyte imbalance of unknown etiology.

References

R.H. Barbhaiya, T.A. Phillips and P.G. Welling. High-pressure liquid chromatographic determination of chlorothiazide and hydrochlorothiazide in plasma and urine: preliminary results of clinical studies. J. Pharm. Sci. 70: 291–295, 1981.

H.R. Brettell, J.K. Aikawa and G.S. Gordon. Studies with chlorothiazide tagged with radioactive carbon (C14) in human beings. Arch. Int. Med. 106: 109–115, 1960.

G.A. Hessey, M.L. Constanzer and W.F. Bayne. Determination of chlorothiazide in urine using reversed-phase high-performance liquid chromatography with ultraviolet detection. J. Chrom. 380: 450–454, 1986.

V.P. Shah, J. Lee and V.K. Prasad. Thiazides XII: a simple hplc method for determination of thiazides in urine. Anal. Letters 15: 529–536, 1982.

A.B. Straughn, A.P. Melikian and M.C. Meyer. Bioavailability of chlorothiazide tablets in humans. J. Pharm. Sci. 68: 1099–1102, 1979.

D. Suria. Quantitative determination of thiazides in urine by a sensitive colorimetric method. Clin. Biochem. 11: 222–224, 1978.

P.A. Tisdall, T.P. Moyer and J.P. Anhalt. Liquid-chromatographic detection of thiazide diuretics in urine. Clin. Chem. 26: 702–706, 1980.

Chlorphenesin Carbamate

T½: 2.3–4.3 hr
Vd: 1.3 L/kg
Fb: ?

$$Cl-\langle O \rangle-OCH_2CHOHCH_2OCONH_2$$

Occurrence and Usage. Chlorphenesin carbamate (Maolate) is used occasionally as a sedative and muscle relaxant. Chlorphenesin, as the free alcohol, has been in use since 1949 but is no longer marketed in the United States at this time. Its carbamate derivative is still available in 400 mg tablets and may be administered in daily oral doses of up to 2400 mg.

Blood Concentrations. A mean peak serum concentration of 9.3 mg/L was determined at 1 hour after the 30th dose of a multiple-dose regimen (400 mg every 6 hours) given orally to 4 subjects (Kaiser and Shaw, 1974). A single oral 2000 mg dose administered to one subject produced a maximum serum level of 14.9 mg/L at 2 hours, declining to 7.6 mg/L by 6 hours and 3.8 mg/L by 10 hours; a biological half-life of 3.1 hours (range, 2.3–4.3) was calculated for this drug (Forist and Judy, 1971). During chronic oral administration of 2400 mg of chlorphenesin carbamate daily to 10 volunteers, an average peak serum concentration of 14.4 mg/L was observed at 2 hours after the 225th 800 mg dose; the authors found no evidence for enzyme induction after 57 days of this dosage regimen (Stoll et al., 1974).

Metabolism and Excretion. Chlorphenesin carbamate is metabolized primarily by conjugation with glucuronic acid; it is also degraded by oxidation to p-chlorophenoxylactic acid, p-chloro-phenoxyacetic acid and p-chlorophenol. Over 85% of a dose is excreted in the 24 hour urine as the O-glucuronide conjugate of the parent drug, with only minor amounts of the unchanged drug and the oxidation products present. No evidence was found for the formation of an N-glucuronide of this drug (Buhler, 1964; Buhler, 1965).

Toxicity. Chlorphenesin carbamate produces central nervous system depression in overdosage.

Analysis. Chlorphenesin carbamate has been estimated in biological fluids by a colorimetric method that uses chromotropic acid and is apparently specific for the parent drug (Morgan et al., 1957; Forist and Judy, 1971). A gas chromatographic method has been reported (Kaiser and Shaw, 1974) that is based on flame-ionization detection of the trimethylsilyl derivative of the drug.

References

D.R. Buhler. The metabolism of chlorphenesin carbamate. J. Pharm. Exp. Ther. 145: 232–241, 1964.

D.R. Buhler. Characterization of the glucuronide conjugate of chlorphenesin carbamate from the rat and from man. Biochem. Pharm. 14: 371–373, 1965.

A.A. Forist and R.W. Judy. Comparative pharmacokinetics of chlorphenesin carbamate and methocarbamol in man. J. Pharm. Sci. 60: 1686–1688, 1971.

D.G. Kaiser and S.R. Shaw. GLC determination of chlorphenesin carbamate in serum. J. Pharm. Sci. 63: 1094–1097, 1974.

A.M. Morgan, E.B. Truitt and J.M. Little. Plasma levels of mephenesin, mephenesin carbamate, guaiacol glyceryl ether, and methocarbamol (AHR-85) after oral and intravenous administration in the dog. J. Am. Pharm. Asso. 46: 374–377, 1957.

R.G. Stoll, K.A. DeSante, E. Novak et al. Chlorphenesin carbamate serum levels during subchronic administration to human (normal) volunteers. J. Clin. Pharm. 14: 520–524, 1974.

Chlorpheniramine

T½: 12–43 hr (urine pH-dependent)
Vd: 5.9 L/kg
Fb: 0.72
pKa: 9.2

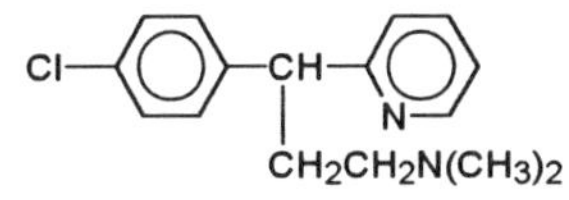

Occurrence and Usage. The p-chloro analogue of brompheniramine is known as chlorpheniramine, a potent antihistamine that has been used since 1951. The racemic mixture is available, usually as the maleate salt, in nearly 100 over-the-counter and prescription formulations. It is administered orally in doses of 0.5–4 mg (up to 8 mg in sustained-release form) and by intramuscular injection in doses of 5 mg. The more potent dextro-isomer, dexchlorpheniramine, is much less frequently encountered. Both compounds are nearly always found in combination with decongestants, antitussives, expectorants and analgesics.

Blood Concentrations. Intravenous injection of 4 mg to 7 subjects resulted in initial serum chlorpheniramine concentrations of approximately 0.010 mg/L; the serum half-life averaged 24 hours and ranged from 18–34 hours (Vallner et al., 1979). A single oral dose of 12 mg of chlorpheniramine maleate administered to 6 subjects produced a mean plasma plasma level of 0.017 mg/L at 2 hours, diminishing to 0.010 mg/L by 12 hours and 0.004 mg/L by 24 hours. The plasma half-life of the drug was found to be 12–15 hours (Peets et al., 1972). Other authors have reported a half-life of 21–43 hours (Chiou et al., 1979).

Metabolism and Excretion. Chlorpheniramine undergoes extensive metabolism in man. N-demethylation occurs with production of mono- and dinorchlorpheniramine, these compounds accumulating to a certain extent in plasma. Only about 34% of a ^{3}H-labeled dose is excreted in the 48 hour urine, with less than 1% being found in the feces. The urinary excretion products consist of unchanged drug (3%), norchlorpheniramine (2%), dinorchlorpheniramine (1%) and unidentified polar metabolites (Peets et al., 1972). Acidification of the urine may cause as much as 27% of a dose to be eliminated unchanged in the 24 hour urine, whereas alkalinization resulted in a decrease to only 0.3–0.4% of the dose (Beckett and Wilkinson, 1965). During chronic therapy with 4 mg of the drug daily, an average of 13% of the dose is excreted unchanged, 13% as norchlorpheniramine and 6% as dinorchlorpheniramine in the 24 hour urine (Kabasakalian et al., 1968).

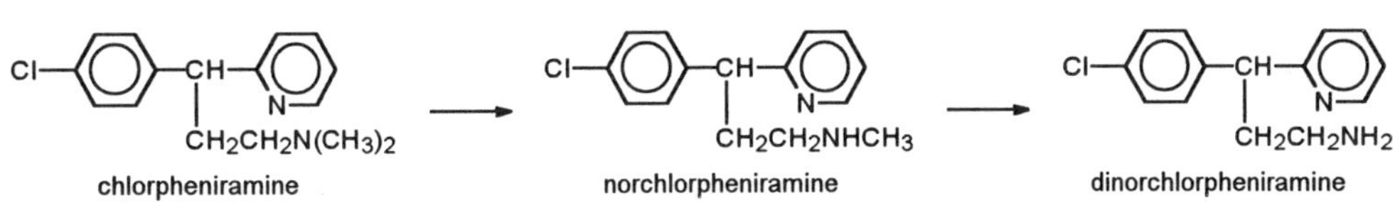

Toxicity. Chlorpheniramine produces symptoms of central nervous system depression in overdosage. One case involving the drug has been investigated in which a 63 year old woman was found dead of unknown causes; toxicological analysis of body fluids revealed only a blood chlorpheniramine level of 0.5 mg/L (Demorest, 1981). An adult male, found dead on a roadway, had a blood alcohol concentration of 0.12 g/dL and the following tissue concentrations of chlorpheniramine (Reed, 1981):

Chlorpheniramine Concentrations in a Fatal Case (mg/L or mg/kg)

Blood	Brain	Lung	Liver	Bile	Kidney	Gastric
1.1	2.5	5.2	6.6	1.5	1.4	less than 1 mg

Analysis. Gas chromatographic procedures for the determination of chlorpheniramine in biological fluids have involved detection by flame-ionization (Kabasakalian et al., 1968; Townley et al., 1970; Hanna and Tang, 1974; Ali and Beckett, 1981), electron-capture (Barnhart and Johnson, 1977), nitrogen-phosphorus (Kinsun et al., 1978; Smith et al., 1978; Masumoto et al., 1986), and mass spectrometry (Thompson and Leffert, 1980). Liquid chromatographic methods for chlorpheniramine and its demethylated metabolites have also been described (Athanikar et al., 1979; Lai et al., 1979; Midha et al., 1984).

References

H.M. Ali and A.H. Beckett. Rapid method for the determination of chlorpheniramine in urine. J. Chrom. 223: 208–212, 1981.

N.K. Athanikar, G.W. Peng, R.L. Nation et al. Chlorpheniramine. I. Rapid quantitative analysis of chlorpheniramine in plasma, saliva and urine by high-performance liquid chromatography. J. Chrom. 162: 367–376, 1979.

J.W. Barnhart and J.D. Johnson. Simplified gas chromatographic method for the determination of chlorpheniramine in serum. Anal. Chem. 49: 1085–1086, 1977.

A.H. Beckett and G.R. Wilkinson. Influence of urine pH and flow rate on the renal excretion of chlorpheniramine in man. J. Pharm. Pharmac. 17: 256–257, 1965.

W.L. Chiou, N.K. Athanikar and S. Huang. Long half-life of chlorpheniramine. New Eng. J. Med. 300: 501, 1979.

D. Demorest. Personal communication, 1981.

S. Hanna and A. Tang. GLC determination of chlorpheniramine in human plasma. J. Pharm. Sci. 63: 1954–1957, 1974.

P. Kabasakalian, M. Taggart and E. Townley. Urinary excretion of chlorpheniramine and its N-demethylated metabolites in man. J. Pharm. Sci. 57: 856–858, 1968.

H. Kinsun, A.M. Moulin and E.C. Savini. Simultaneous GLC determination of phenylpropanolamine and chlorpheniramine in urine using a nitrogen selective detector. J. Pharm. Sci. 67: 118–119, 1978.

C.M. Lai, R.G. Stoll, Z.M. Look and A. Yacobi. Urinary excretion of chlorpheniramine and pseudoephedrine in humans. J. Pharm. Sci. 68: 1243–1246, 1979.

K. Masumoto, Y. Tashiro, K. Matsumoto et al. Simultaneous determination of codeine and chlorpheniramine in human plasma by capillary column gas chromatography. J. Chrom. 381: 323–329, 1986.

K.K. Midha, G. Rauw, G. McKay et al. Subnanogram quantitation of chlorpheniramine in plasma by a new radioimmunoassay and comparison with a liquid chromatographic method. J. Pharm. Sci. 73: 1144–1147, 1984.

E.A. Peets, M. Jackson and S. Symchowicz. Metabolism of chlorpheniramine maleate in man. J. Pharm. Exp. Ther. 180: 464–474, 1972.

D. Reed. A fatal case involving chlorpheniramine. Clin. Tox. 18: 941–943, 1981.

H.T. Smith, J.T. Jacob and R.G. Achari. Trace determination of chlorpheniramine in plasma by GLC using a nitrogen-phosphorus (N-P) detector. J. Chrom. Sci. 16: 561–564, 1978.

J.A. Thompson and F.H. Leffert. Sensitive GLC-mass spectrometric determination of chlorpheniramine in serum. J. Pharm. Sci. 69: 707–710, 1980.

E. Townley, I. Perez and P. Kabasakalian. Gas-liquid chromatographic determination of chlorpheniramine in blood plasma. Anal. Chem. 42: 1759–1761, 1970.

J.J. Vallner, T.E. Needham, W. Chan and C.T. Viswanathan. Intravenous administration of chlorpheniramine to seven subjects. Curr. Ther. Res. 26: 449–453, 1979.

Chlorphentermine

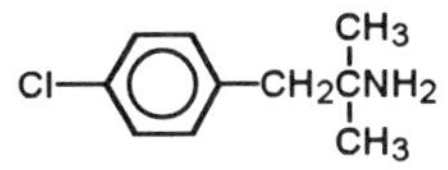

T½: 35–44 hr (urine pH-dependent)

Vd: 3.0 L/kg

Fb: ?

pKa: 9.6

$Cl-\langle\bigcirc\rangle-CH_2CNH_2$ (with two CH_3 groups on the central carbon)

Occurrence and Usage. Chlorphentermine (p-chlorophentermine, Pre-Sate) is a sympathomimetic phenethylamine derivative used as an anorexigenic agent. It is administered orally as the hydrochloride salt in single doses of 65–100 mg, and is also available as a prolonged-release preparation.

Blood Concentrations. After a single oral dosage of 100 mg, blood concentrations in 4 subjects averaged 0.32 mg/L at 4 hours and declined with an apparent half-life of 41 hours to 0.14 mg/L by 48 hours. No stimulant effect was noticed at this dosage level, although pupil dilation was evident (Jun and Triggs, 1970).

Metabolism and Excretion. Chlorphentermine is biotransformed in man to more polar compounds, primarily by N-hydroxylation and conjugation and secondarily by N-oxidation to nitroso and nitro derivatives. In normal urine over a 48 hour period, about 17% of a dose is excreted unchanged, 13% and 16% as free and conjugated N-hydroxychlorphentermine, respectively, and an additional 18% as other products of N-oxidation. When urine is maintained under acidic conditions, as much as 90% of a dose may be excreted unchanged over an extended period of time (Jun and Triggs, 1970; Beckett and Belanger, 1977).

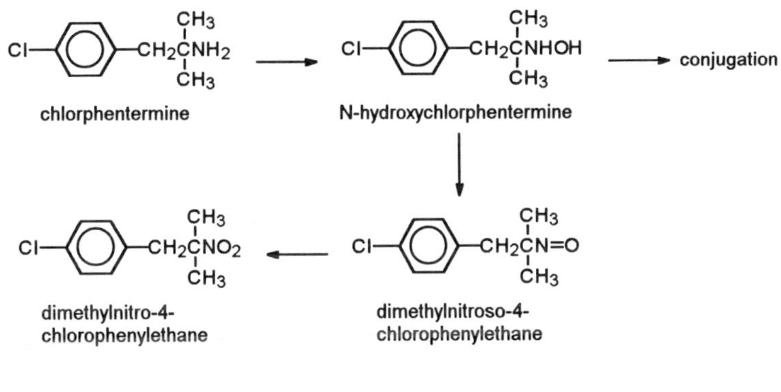

chlorphentermine → N-hydroxychlorphentermine → conjugation

dimethylnitro-4-chlorophenylethane ← dimethylnitroso-4-chlorophenylethane

Toxicity. Chlorphentermine causes symptoms of central nervous system stimulation in overdosage. No instances of toxicity have been reported.

Analysis. Chlorphentermine may be assayed using many of the gas chromatographic procedures designed for amphetamine-like drugs, including those requiring the formation of amide derivatives. It has been measured as the underivatized drug with flame-ionization detection (Jun and Triggs, 1970), whereas the N-hydroxy metabolite may be chromatographed as the trimethylsilyl derivative (Beckett and Belanger, 1974; Caldwell et al., 1975).

References

A.H. Beckett and P.M. Belanger. Metabolism of chlorphentermine and phentermine in man to yield hydroxylamino, C-nitroso- and nitro- compounds. J. Pharm. Pharmac. 26: 205–206, 1974.

A.H. Beckett and P.M. Belanger. The metabolism, distribution and elimination of chlorphentermine in man. Brit. J. Clin. Pharm. 4: 193–200, 1977.

J. Caldwell, U. Koster, R.L. Smith and R.T. Williams. Species variations in N-oxidation of chlorphentermine. Biochem. Pharm. 24: 2225–2232, 1975.

H.W. Jun and E.J. Triggs. Blood levels of chlorphentermine in man. J. Pharm. Sci. 59: 306–308, 1970.

Chlorpromazine

T½: 7–119 hr (average, 18–30)
Vd: 10–35 L/kg
Fb: 0.98
pKa: 9.3

$CH_2CH_2CH_2N(CH_3)_2$

Occurrence and Usage. Chlorpromazine (Thorazine) was first synthesized in 1952 and was found to be effective in the treatment of psychotic disorders in the same year. It is still considered one of the most useful of the numerous phenothiazine derivatives available. Chlorpromazine is available as the hydrochloride in the form of tablets or suppositories (10–300 mg), a syrup (10 mg/5 mL), a concentrate (30–100 mg/mL), and in ampules for injection (25 mg/mL). The drug is administered by oral or intramuscular administration, in single doses of 25–100 mg for acute disturbances or in chronic daily amounts of up to 2400 mg for the maintenance of mental patients.

Blood Concentrations. A single oral 25 mg dose produced an average peak plasma chlorpromazine concentration in 4 subjects of 0.001 mg/L at 2.8 hours; a radioimmunoassay was used that cross-reacted with norchlorpromazine, but this metabolite was not present in appreciable amounts (Loo et al., 1980). Following a single oral administration of 150 mg of chlorpromazine to adults, an average peak plasma concentration of 0.018 mg/L (range, 0.010–0.026) was achieved at 3 hours and declined to 0.013 mg/L by 6 hours (Hollister et al., 1970). A single intramuscular 50 mg dose given to 8 subjects produced peak plasma concentrations of 0.017–0.140 mg/L (average, 0.069) within 4 hours of the injection (Dahl and Strandjord, 1977). The pharmacokinetics of the drug were best described by a 2-compartment open model with zero-order absorption; the elimination half-life averaged 18 hours and ranged from 7–119 hours (Whitfield et al., 1978).

Five patients maintained on a 600 mg/day oral dose for several weeks had plasma chlorpromazine levels that varied, on average, from 0.020–0.080 mg/L within a single day; concentrations of the active metabolites norchlorpromazine and 7-hydroxychlorpromazine remained at an average of 17% and 34%, respectively, of the chlorpromazine concentration (Wode-Helgodt and Alfredsson, 1981). Unchanged chlorpromazine is generally the compound in highest concentration in plasma, although as many as 10 of its metabolites may be present in comparable concentrations (Chan et al., 1974). Rivera-Calimlim et al. (1973) found that psychiatric patients with plasma chlorpromazine concentrations of 0.150–0.300 mg/L or greater achieved the most significant clinical improvement; a concentration of 1.106 mg/L was measured in one patient receiving 2400 mg of the drug daily, but levels above 0.750 mg/L were found to produce tremors and convulsions in most patients. Erythrocyte chlorpromazine concentrations in patients on therapy tended to correlate with plasma drug level, but the erythrocyte/plasma concentration ratio varied from 0.61–2.00 between patients (Linnoila and Dorrity, 1978).

Metabolism and Excretion. The metabolism of chlorpromazine is exceedingly complex; 168 possible metabolites have been postulated and at least 20 of these have been isolated. The elimination of the drug from the body is very slow, and metabolites have been identified in the urine of patients as long as 18 months after discontinuation of therapy. The most common pathways of biotransformation are conversion to the sulfoxide, with probable loss of activity; demethylation to nor- and dinorchlorpromazine, which are one-fourth and one-eighth as active as the parent, respectively; phenolic hydroxylation at the 7 position to produce an active metabolite, with subsequent glucuronide conjugation; N-oxide formation; and combinations of nearly all of these mechanisms. The sulfoxidation of chlorpromazine has been found to be very efficiently catalyzed by hemoglobin in whole blood (Traficante et al., 1979). Promazine, formed by N-demethylation and dehalogenation, has been found to be a major plasma metabolite; its concentration exceeded that of its parent by 21–64% in 4 patients (Sgaragli et al., 1986).

Less than 1% of a dose of chlorpromazine is excreted unchanged in the 24 hour urine; an average of 23% of a single oral dose is excreted in the urine, primarily as metabolites, and it is believed that fecal excretion may also play an important role in the elimination of this drug. Of the total quantity of metabolites excreted in the urine, approximately 25% consists of the non-hydroxylated compounds, while the 7-hydroxylated metabolites account for 9% and their glucuronide conjugates, 66% (Hollister and Curry, 1971; Chan et al., 1974). Of the unconjugated metabolites, the one in greatest abundance in urine is dinorchlorpromazine sulfoxide; this compound is believed to account for the "pink spot" observed during thin-layer chromatographic analysis of patient urines (Wad and Closs, 1971).

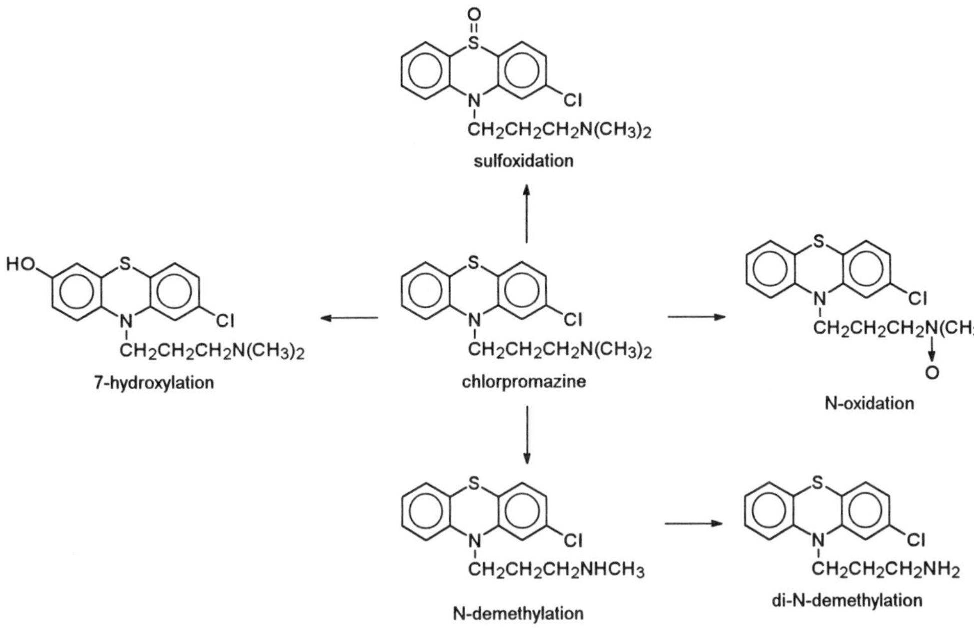

Toxicity. Chlorpromazine in overdosage causes drowsiness, fainting, hypotension, tachycardia, tremor, dizziness, electrocardiographic changes, coma, and convulsions. Serum chlorpromazine concentrations in patients who survived the acute ingestion of 1.6–1.8 g of the drug have ranged from 0.5–1.5 mg/L (Bailey and Guba, 1979).

A syndrome known as "phenothiazine sudden death" has been noted among psychiatric patients receiving large daily doses of chlorpromazine or other phenothiazines; the mechanism is believed to involve asphyxiation during a convulsive seizure, ventricular fibrillation, or cardiovascular failure during a hypotensive crisis (Hollister and Kosek, 1965; Leestma and Koenig, 1968). Death has occurred following a single acute oral ingestion of 2000 mg of the drug; blood concentrations in fatalities have ranged from 1–44 mg/L and liver concentrations have ranged from 34–190 mg/kg (Algeri et al., 1959; Cravey, 1974; Gottschalk and Cravey, 1980). Although blood concentrations of the drug during chronic high-dose therapy are often quite similar to concentrations in fatal cases (at least by spectrophotometric methods), these situations may be differentiated by determining liver concentrations, which usually do not exceed 10 mg/kg when chlorpromazine is being administered on a maintenance basis. In a series of 8 fatal cases described by Bonnichsen et al. (1970) that were analyzed by an ultraviolet spectrophotometric procedure (subject to interference by metabolites), concentrations averaged 17 mg/L (range, 3–35) in blood and 366 mg/kg (range, 54–2110) in liver. The following distribution was observed in a case of fatal intoxication after acute ingestion of an unknown amount of the drug by an adult (Baselt, 1976):

Chlorpromazine Concentrations in a Fatal Case (mg/L or mg/kg)*

Blood	Brain	Liver	Kidney	Urine	Gastric
6.6	12	84	34	1.2	21 mg

* By fluorometry after chemical oxidation; blood ethanol 0.19%

Analysis. Many analytical techniques have been applied to the analysis of chlorpromazine and its metabolites in biological specimens. Among the more practical for routine purposes are ultraviolet spectrophotometry (Wallace and Biggs, 1971) and spectrophotofluorometry after photo-oxidation (White and Frings, 1976; Kaul et al., 1976) or chemical oxidation (Ragland et al., 1965) of the drug. In general, these procedures suffer from a lack of specificity regarding the metabolites and other phenothiazines. Gas-liquid chromatography with electron-capture (Flint et al., 1971; Spirtes, 1972; Curry, 1976) or nitrogen-phosphorus detection (Linnoila and Dorrity, 1978; Bailey and Guba, 1979) offers specificity and sensitivity, although problems with artifacts and adsorption of the drug to glassware often arise. Mass fragmentography (Alfredsson et al., 1976; McKay et al., 1982) and radioimmunoassay (Kawashima et al., 1975) have also been evaluated but are not generally available. Liquid chromatographic analysis of chlorpromazine and its metabolites with either ultraviolet (Midha et al., 1981; Allender et al., 1983; Smith et al., 1987) or electrochemical detection (Murakami et al., 1982; Cooper et al., 1983) has been shown to be of value.

It has been noted by several groups of investigators that storage of plasma specimens containing chlorpromazine for a period of only one week, even at temperatures down to -20° C., often leads to extensive loss of the drug (Linnoila and Dorrity, 1978; McMullin et al., 1979). Other authors disagree, however (Gupta et al., 1981; Young and Nysewander, 1986).

References

G. Alfredsson, B. Wode-Helgodt and G. Sedvall. A mass fragmentographic method for the determination of chlorpromazine and two of its active metabolites in human plasma and csf. Psychopharmacology 48: 123–131, 1976.

E.J. Algeri, G.G. Katsas and A.J. McBay. Toxicology of some new drugs: glutethimide, meprobamate and chlorpromazine. J. For. Sci. 4: 111–135, 1959.

W.J. Allender, A.W. Archer and A.G. Dawson. Extraction and analysis of chlorpromazine and its major metabolites in post mortem material by enzymic digestion and HPLC. J. Anal. Tox. 7: 203–206, 1983.

D.N. Bailey and J.J. Guba. Gas-chromatographic analysis for chlorpromazine and some of its metabolites in human serum, with use of a nitrogen detector. Clin. Chem. 25: 1211–1215, 1979.

R.C. Baselt. Unpublished results, 1976.

R. Bonnichsen, P. Geertinger and A.C. Maehly. Toxicological data on phenothiazine drugs in autopsy cases. Z. Rechtsmed. 67: 158–169, 1970.

T.L. Chan, G. Sakalis and S. Gershon. Quantitation of chlorpromazine and its metabolites in human plasma and urine by direct spectrodensitometry of thin-layer chromatogram. In *The Phenothiazines and Structurally Related Drugs* (I.S. Forrest, C.J. Carr and E. Usdin, eds.), Raven Press, New York, 1974, pp. 323–333.

J.K. Cooper, G. McKay and K.K. Midha. Subnanogram quantitation of chlorpromazine in plasma by high-performance liquid chromatography with electrochemical detection. J. Pharm. Sci. 71: 1259–1262, 1983.

R.H. Cravey. Personal communication, 1974.

S.H. Curry. Gas-chromatographic methods for the study of chlorpromazine and some of its metabolites in human plasma. Psychopharm. Comm. 2: 1–15, 1976.

S.G. Dahl and R.E. Strandjord. Pharmacokinetics of chlorpromazine after single and chronic dosage. Clin. Pharm. Ther. 21: 437–448, 1977.

D.R. Flint, C.R. Ferullo, P. Levandoski and B. Hwang. More sensitive gas-chromatographic measurement of chlorpromazine in plasma. Clin. Chem. 17: 830, 1971.

L.A. Gottschalk and R.H. Cravey. *Toxicological and Pathological Studies on Psychoactive Drug-Involved Deaths*, Biomedical Publications, Davis, California, 1980, pp. 139–143.

R.N. Gupta, G. Bartolucci and G. Molnar. Analysis of chlorpromazine in plasma: effect of specimen storage. Clin. Chim. Acta 109: 351–354, 1981.

L.E. Hollister and J.C. Kosek. Sudden death during treatment with phenothiazine derivatives. J. Am. Med. Asso. 21: 1035–1038, 1965.

L.E. Hollister, S.H. Curry, J.E. Derr and S.L. Kanter. Studies of delayed-action medication. Clin. Pharm. Ther. 11: 49–59, 1970.

L.E. Hollister and S.H. Curry. Urinary excretion of chlorpromazine metabolites following single doses and in steady-state conditions. Res. Comm. Chem. Path. Pharm. 2: 330–338, 1971.

P.N. Kaul, L.R. Whitfield and M.L. Clark. Chlorpromazine metabolism VII: new quantitative fluorometric determination of chlorpromazine and its sulfoxide. J. Pharm. Sci. 65: 689–694, 1976.

K. Kawashima, R. Dixon and S. Spector. Development of radioimmunoassay for chlorpromazine. Eur. J. Pharm. 32: 195–202, 1975.

W.C. Landgraf. High-pressure chromatographic analysis of phenothiazine-related compounds. In *The Phenothiazines and Structurally Related Drugs* (I.S. Forrest, C.J. Carr and E. Usdin, eds.), Raven Press, New York, 1974, pp. 357–362.

J.E. Leestma and K.L. Koenig. Sudden death and phenothiazines. Arch. Gen. Psych. 18: 137–148, 1968.

M. Linnoila and F. Dorrity. Measurement of plasma and erythrocyte chlorpromazine and N-monodesmethylchlorpromazine levels by gas chromatography with a nitrogen sensitive detector. Acta Pharm. Tox. 42: 264–270, 1978.

J.C.K. Loo, K.K. Midha and I.J. McGilveray. Pharmacokinetics of chlorpromazine in normal volunteers. Comm. Psychopharm. 4: 121–129, 1980.

G. McKay, K. Hall, J.K. Cooper et al. Gas chromatographic-mass spectrometric procedure for the quantitation of chlorpromazine in plasma and its comparison with a new high performance liquid chromatographic assay with electrochemical detection. J. Chrom. 232: 275–282, 1982.

M.W. McMullin, R.D. Cohn, P. Burghart and F. Rieders. Presented at the annual meeting of the American Academy of Forensic Sciences, Atlanta, Georgia, February 15, 1979.

K.K. Midha, J.K. Cooper, A.G. Butterfield and I.J. McGilveray. An HPLC assay for nanogram determination of chlorpromazine in plasma. Pharmacologist 21: 166, 1979.

K.K. Midha, J.K. Cooper, I.J. McGilveray et al. High-performance liquid chromatography assay for nanogram determination of chlorpromazine and its comparison with a radioimmunoassay. J. Pharm. Sci. 70: 1043–1046, 1981.

K. Murakami, K. Murakami, T. Ueno et al. Simultaneous determination of chlorpromazine and levomepromazine in human plasma and urine by high-performance liquid chromatography using electrochemical detection. J. Chrom. 227: 103–112, 1982.

J.B. Ragland, V.J. Kinross-Wright and R.S. Ragland. Determination of phenothiazines in biological samples. Anal. Biochem. 12: 60–69, 1965.

L. Rivera-Calimlim, L. Castaneda and L. Lasagna. Effects of mode of management on plasma chlorpromazine in psychiatric patients. Clin. Pharm. Ther. 14: 978–986, 1973.

G. Sgaragli, R. Ninci, L. della Corte et al. A major plasma metabolite of chlorpromazine in a population of chronic schizophrenics. Drug Met. Disp. 14: 263–266, 1986.

C.S. Smith, S.L. Morgan, S.V. Greene and R.K. Abramson. Solid-phase extraction and high-performance liquid chromatographic method for chlorpromazine and thirteen metabolites. J. Chrom. 423: 207–216, 1987.

M.A. Spirtes. Artifactual contamination of control serum extracts in gas chromatographic analyses for chlorpromazine. Clin. Chem. 18: 317–318, 1972.

D. Stevenson and E. Reid. Determination of chlorpromazine and its sulfoxide and 7-hydroxy metabolites by ion-pair high pressure liquid chromatography. Anal. Letters 14: 741–761, 1981.

L.J. Traficante, G. Sakalis, J. Siekierski et al. Rapid in vitro sulfoxidation of chlorpromazine by human blood: inhibition by an endogenous plasma protein factor. Life Sci. 24: 337–346, 1979.

R.C. Young and R.W. Nysewander. Changes in plasma and erythrocyte chlorpromazine concentrations during sample storage. J. Pharm. Biomed. Anal. 4: 131–134, 1986.

N. Wad and K. Closs. NOR2 chlorpromazine sulphoxide, a "pink spot" produced in vivo and in vitro from chlorpromazine. J. Pharm. Pharmac. 23: 131–132, 1971.

J.E. Wallace and J.D. Biggs. Determination of phenothiazine compounds in biologic specimens by UV spectrophotometry. J. Pharm. Sci. 60: 1346–1350, 1971.

V.R. White and C.S. Frings. Rapid fluorimetric determination of phenothiazines employing in situ photochemical oxidation. Anal. Chem. 48: 1314–1315, 1976.

L.R. Whitfield, P.N. Kaul and M.L. Clark. Chlorpromazine metabolism. IX. Pharmacokinetics of chlorpromazine following oral administration in man. J. Pharm. Biopharm. 6: 187–196, 1978.

B. Wode-Helgodt and G. Alfredsson. Concentrations of chlorpromazine and two of its active metabolites in plasma and cerebrospinal fluid of psychotic patients treated with fixed drug doses. Psychopharmacology 73: 55–62, 1981.

Chlorpropamide

T½: 25–42 hr
Vd: 0.1–0.3 L/kg
Fb: 0.95
pKa: 4.8

$Cl-\langle\bigcirc\rangle-SO_2NHCONHC_3H_7$

Occurrence and Usage. Chlorpropamide (Diabinese) was synthesized in 1958 and has since received widespread usage as a hypoglycemic agent. It belongs to a group of weakly acidic sulfonylurea derivatives that includes acetohexamide and tolbutamide. The compound is administered orally in the form of 100 or 250 mg tablets, in daily doses of 100–500 mg.

Blood Concentrations. Plasma concentrations in 6 subjects after a single oral 250 mg dose of chlorpropamide reached an average peak of 29 mg/L at 3 hours and declined thereafter with a half-life of 33 hours. In 4 diabetic patients receiving chronic daily doses of 250–500 mg of the drug, plasma levels averaged 142 mg/L and ranged from 76–246 mg/L (Taylor, 1972). An additional 9 patients receiving daily doses of 500–1000 mg developed serum concentrations of 102–363 mg/L, averaging 228 mg/L (Knauff et al., 1959).

Metabolism and Excretion. Chlorpropamide undergoes biotransformation in man to more polar compounds whose pharmacological activity is unknown. N-dealkylation occurs with formation of p-chlorobenzenesulfonylurea; this compound is believed to degrade spontaneously to a minor extent to p-chlorobenzenesulfonamide. Oxidation of the alkyl chain also occurs with production of 2-hydroxy- and 3-hydroxychlorpropamide. During chronic administration nearly the entire daily dose is excreted in the urine as chlorpropamide (18%), p-chlorobenzenesulfonylurea (21%), p-chlorobenzenesulfonamide (2%), 2-hydroxychlorpropamide (55%) and 3-hydroxychlorpropamide (2–3%). The metabolites are found to only a minor extent in plasma (Brotherton et al., 1969; Taylor, 1972). Alkalinization of the urine in 6 subjects reduced the average plasma half-life of chlorpropamide from 50 to 13 hours, while acidification increased the half-life to 69 hours; 85% of a dose was eliminated unchanged in the 72 hour urine under alkaline conditions versus 20% for controls and less than 2% under acid conditions (Neuvonen and Karkkainen, 1983).

$Cl-\langle\bigcirc\rangle-SO_2NHCONHC_3H_7 \longrightarrow Cl-\langle\bigcirc\rangle-SO_2NHCONH_2 \longrightarrow Cl-\langle\bigcirc\rangle-SO_2NH_2$

chlorpropamide   p-chlorobenzenesulfonylurea   p-chlorobenzenesulfonamide

$Cl-\langle\bigcirc\rangle-SO_2NHCONH(CH_2)_3OH \qquad Cl-\langle\bigcirc\rangle-SO_2NHCONHCH_2CHOHCH_3$

3-hydroxychlorpropamide   2-hydroxychlorpropamide

Toxicity. Facial flushing may occur in patients receiving chlorpropamide who also ingest alcohol, due to inhibition of aldehyde dehydrogenase by the drug; this effect is more likely to occur in those with higher plasma chlorpropamide concentrations (Groop et al., 1984). Numerous instances of drug-induced hypoglycemia have been documented during chlorpropamide therapy; the condition is often related to hepatic or renal disease, advanced age, poor diet, or the co-administration of other drugs (Seltzer, 1972). Two patients admitted in coma had serum chlorpropamide concentrations of 310 and 450 mg/L (Agarwal et al., 1970).

One case of acute overdosage with this drug involved a 6 year old child who ingested an unknown amount and developed seizures. Upon admission to the hospital 36 hours after ingestion in a comatose condition, serum was drawn and was found to contain 323 mg/L of chlorpropamide. The serum concentrations declined with a half-life of 35 hours and the patient eventually recovered (Pitlick et al., 1977). In other instances of overdosage, prolonged hypoglycemic coma has been a common feature; peak plasma chlorpropamide levels of 200–750 mg/L were observed, several patients had severe neurologic sequelae, and one death occurred (Manners, 1965; Dowell and Imrie, 1972; Forrest, 1974). Peritoneal dialysis with 7% glucose solution was ineffective in removing drug from the system (Graw and Clarke, 1970). Intravenous diazoxide was effective in controlling hypoglycemia in 3 patients who developed initial plasma chlorpropamide levels of 422–523 mg/L (Meatherall et al., 1981).

A woman who died of hypoglycemic coma 8 days after accidentally ingesting chlorpropamide had a postmortem blood chlorpropamide concentration of 23 mg/L (Scala-Barnett and Donoghue, 1986).

Analysis. Chlorpropamide may be assayed in biologic fluids colorimetrically (Carmichael, 1959) or by more specific gas chromatographic techniques that require formation of a methyl derivative (Sabih and Sabih, 1970; Prescott and Redman, 1972; Aggarwal and Sunshine, 1974; Schlicht et al., 1978; Hartvig et al., 1980). High-pressure liquid chromatography has been utilized in the determination of the drug in serum (Hill and Crechiolo, 1978) and of its metabolites in urine (Taylor, 1972).

References

R.C. Agarwal, D. Kumar and L.V. Miller. Chlorpropamide-induced hypoglycemia. Diabetes 19: 376, 1970.

V. Aggarwal and I. Sunshine. Determination of sulfonylureas and metabolites by pyrolysis gas chromatography. Clin. Chem. 20: 200–204, 1974.

P.M. Brotherton, P. Grieveson and C. McMartin. A study of the metabolic fate of chlorpropamide in man. Clin. Pharm. Ther. 10: 505–514, 1969.

R.H. Carmichael. A method for the routine determination of chlorpropamide in plasma. Clin. Chem. 5: 597–602, 1959.

R.D. Dowell and A.H. Imrie. Chlorpropamide poisoning in non-diabetics. Scot. Med. J. 17: 305–309, 1972.

J.A.H. Forrest. Chlorpropamide overdosage: delayed and prolonged hypoglycemia. Clin. Tox. 7: 19–24, 1974.

R.G. Graw and R.R. Clarke. Chlorpropamide intoxication. Pediatrics 45: 106–109, 1970.

L. Groop, C.J.P. Eriksson, E. Wahlin-Boll and A. Melander. Chlorpropamide-alcohol flush: significance of body weight, sex and serum chlorpropamide level. Eur. J. Clin. Pharm. 26: 723–725, 1984.

P. Hartvig, C. Fagerlund and O. Gyllenhaal. Electron-capture gas chromatography of plasma sulphonylureas after extractive methylation. J. Chrom. 181: 17–24, 1980.

R.E. Hill and J. Crechiolo. Determination of serum tolbutamide and chlorpropamide by high-performance liquid chromatography. J. Chrom. 145: 165–168, 1978.

R.E. Knauff, S.S. Fajans, E. Ramirez and J.W. Conn. Metabolic studies of chlorpropamide in normal men and in diabetic subjects. Ann. N.Y. Acad. Sci. 74: 603–617, 1959.

J.M. Manners. Chlorpropamide overdose. Anaesthesia 20: 165–172, 1965.

R.C. Meatherall, P.T. Green, S. Kenick and N. Donen. Diazoxide in the management of chlorpropamide overdose. J. Anal. Tox. 5: 287–291, 1981.

P.J. Neuvonen and S. Karkkainen. Effects of charcoal, sodium bicarbonate, and ammonium chloride on chlorpropamide kinetics. Clin. Pharm. Ther. 33: 386–393, 1983.

W.H. Pitlick, D. Kurnit, A. Kenyon and P. Pirakitikulr. Serum chlorpropamide levels following accidental ingestion. In *Management of the Poisoned Patient* (B.H. Rumack and A.R. Temple, eds.), Science Press, Princeton, 1977, pp. 143–150.

L.F. Prescott and D.R. Redman. Gas-liquid chromatographic estimation of tolbutamide and chlorpropamide in plasma. J. Pharm. Pharmac. 24: 713–716, 1972.

K. Sabih and K. Sabih. Gas chromatographic method for determination of tolbutamide and chlorpropamide. J. Pharm. Sci. 59: 782–784, 1970.

D.M. Scala-Barnett and E.R. Donoghue. Dispensing error causing fatal chlorpropamide intoxication in a nondiabetic. J. For. Sci. 31: 293–295, 1986.

H.J. Schlicht, H.P. Gelbke and G. Schmidt. Gas chromatographic procedure for the simultaneous determination of five common antidiabetic drugs in blood. J. Chrom. 155: 178–181, 1978.

H.S. Seltzer. Drug-induced hypoglycemia. Diabetes 21: 955–966, 1972.

J.A. Taylor. Pharmacokinetics and biotransformation of chlorpropamide in man. Clin. Pharm. Ther. 13: 710–718, 1972.

Chlorprothixene

T½: 8–12 hr
Vd: 11–23 L/kg
Fb: ?
pKa: 8.8

Occurrence and Usage. Chlorprothixene (Taractan) is the thioxanthene analogue of chlorpromazine and was first synthesized in 1960. The drug is available in tablets of 10–100 mg as the free base, a 100 mg/5 mL concentrate as the lactate and hydrochloride, and in 25 mg/2 mL vials as the hydrochloride. It is an effective antipsychotic agent when administered by either intramuscular injection or orally in daily doses of 75–600 mg.

Blood Concentrations. A single 30 mg oral dose given to a single subject produced a maximum blood chlorprothixene concentration of 0.011 mg/L after 4 hours, declining to 0.004 mg/L by 10 hours. A 30 mg intravenous dose resulted in a peak blood concentration of 0.050 mg/L after 30 minutes; the levels in 3 subjects declined with an average half-life of 9.4 hours. The fluorometric method used by the author was claimed to be relatively specific for unchanged drug (Raaflaub, 1975). Other authors have reported plasma levels of 0.04–0.10 mg/L after a single 50 mg oral dose (deSilva and D'Arconte, 1969). These values are probably high, however, since the fluorometric method used is subject to interference by metabolites. Two subjects reached peak plasma levels of 0.030–0.040 mg/L at 4 hours after a single 100 mg oral dose, using a specific chromatographic technique (Brooks et al., 1985).

Metabolism and Excretion. The biotransformation of chlorprothixene is known to proceed via sulfoxidation, N-demethylation, N-oxidation and ring hydroxylation. Urinary excretion products include unchanged drug, chlorprothixene sulfoxide, norchlorprothixene, norchlorprothixene sulfoxide, chlorprothixene-N-oxide sulfoxide and their phenolic derivatives (Huus and Khan, 1967; Raaflaub, 1967; Breyer-Pfaff et al., 1985). Urinary excretion accounts for 6–29% of a dose, and up to 41% may be eliminated in the feces (Allgen et al., 1960). In 2 victims of overdosage, blood taken 24–30 hours later had the following drug concentrations: 0.13–0.24 mg/L chlorprothixene, 0.61–0.92 mg/L chlorprothixene sulfoxide and 0.06–0.22 mg/L norchlorprothixene (Brooks et al., 1985).

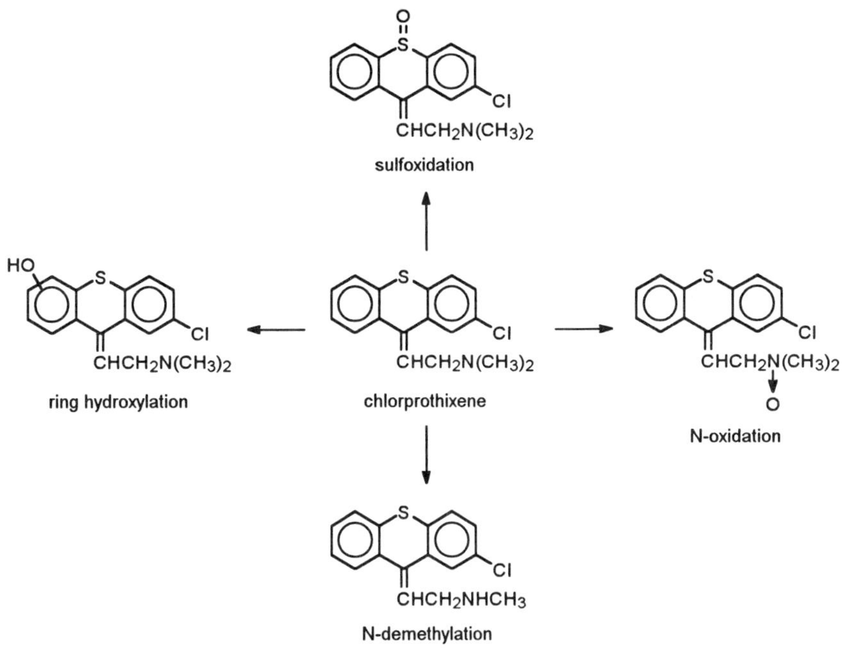

Toxicity. Ingestion of 2–3 g of chlorprothixene may be fatal, although survival after the ingestion of 12 g of the drug has been reported. In a case involving the self-administration of 7.5 g, a plasma level of 0.8 mg/L was observed 5 days later using a nonspecific fluorometric method; the patient regained consciousness when the plasma level fell to 0.08 mg/L on the 11th day (deSilva and D'Arconte, 1969).

Blood concentrations ranging from undetectable levels to 0.4 mg/L were found in 6 cases of fatal chlorprothixene overdosage, with liver concentrations of 5–42 mg/kg; of the various metabolites found in the tissues, norchlorprothixene was in highest concentration, occasionally exceeding that of its parent (Christensen, 1974). Chlorprothixene and its sulfoxide were found in postmortem blood at levels of 0.1 and 0.6 mg/L, respectively, in the case of a man who was found dead after ingesting up to 4 g of the drug (Poklis et al., 1983).

Analysis. Chlorprothixene has been analyzed in biological specimens by ultraviolet spectrophotometry (Wallace, 1967); the specificity of this technique has been improved by combining it with thin-layer chromatography, although its sensitivity barely suffices for the measurement of even toxic blood levels (Christensen, 1974). Spectrophotofluorometry has also been utilized (deSilva and D'Arconte, 1969), and one procedure in particular has the sensitivity necessary for the determination of therapeutic plasma concentrations (Mjorndal and Oreland, 1971). It is, however, subject to interference by N-demethylated metabolites. Liquid chromatography is a more sensitive and specific procedure for this purpose (Brooks et al. 1985).

References

L.G. Allgen, B. Jonsson, B. Nauckhoff et al. On the elimination of chlorprothixene in rat and man. Experientia 16: 325, 1960.

U. Breyer-Pfaff, E. Wiest, A. Prox et al. Phenolic metabolites of chlorprothixene in man and dog. Drug Met. Disp. 13: 479–489, 1985.

M.A. Brooks, G. Didonato and H.P. Blumenthal. Determination of chlorprothixene and its sulfoxide metabolite in plasma by high-performance liquid chromatography with ultraviolet and amperometric detection. J. Chrom. 337: 351–362, 1985.

H. Christensen. Chlorprothixene and its metabolites in blood, liver and urine from fatal poisoning. Acta Pharm. Tox. 34: 16–26, 1974.

J.A.F. deSilva and L. D'Arconte. The use of spectrophotofluorometry in the analysis of drugs in biological materials. J. For. Sci. 14: 184–205, 1969.

I. Huus and A.R. Khan. Studies on the metabolism of chlorprothixene (Truxal) in rats and dogs. Acta Pharm. Tox. 25: 397–404, 1967.

T. Mjorndal and L. Oreland. Determination of thioxanthenes in plasma at therapeutic concentrations. Acta Pharm. Tox. 29: 295–302, 1971.

A. Poklis, D. Maginn and M.A. MacKell. Chlorprothixene and chlorprothixene-sulfoxide in body fluids from a case of drug overdose. J. Anal. Tox. 7: 29–32, 1983.

J. Raaflaub. Zum Metabolismus des Chlorprothixen. Arz. Forsch. 17: 1393–1395, 1967.

J. Raaflaub. On the pharmacokinetics of chlorprothixene in man. Experientia 31: 557–558, 1975.

J. Wallace. Ultraviolet spectrophotometric determination of chlorprothixene in biological specimens. J. Pharm. Sci. 56: 1437–1441, 1967.

Chlorpyrifos

T½: ?
Vd: ?
Fb: ?
pKa: ?

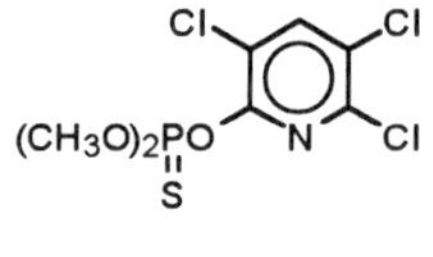

Occurrence and Usage. Chlorpyrifos (Dursban, Lorsban) is a chlorinated organophosphate used as an insecticide and ascaricide. It is generally available in powder or aerosol preparations containing 2.5% chlorpyrifos. Occupational exposure is commonly by inhalation or dermal absorption. The current threshold limit value is 0.2 mg/m^3.

Blood Concentrations. Six male subjects, 27–50 years of age, were given an oral dose of 5 mg/kg chlorpyrifos followed in 2 weeks with a 5.0 mg/kg dermal dose. Blood chlorpyrifos concentrations were less than 30 µg/L; a mean peak blood concentration of the major metabolite, 3,5,6-trichloro-2-pyridinol (3,5,6-TCP), of 0.9 mg/L occurred 6 hours after oral ingestion, while a mean peak metabolite concentration of 0.06 mg/L occurred 24 hours after dermal administration (Nolan et al., 1984).

Metabolism and Excretion. Chlorpyrifos undergoes oxidative desulfuration to form an oxon, which is 400 times more active as a cholinesterase inhibitor, and both chlorpyrifos and the oxon are rapidly hydrolyzed to 3,5,6-TCP (Sultatos and Murphy, 1983). Rats excrete 89% of an oral dose in the urine, with 3,5,6-TCP as the major metabolite (Smith et al., 1967).

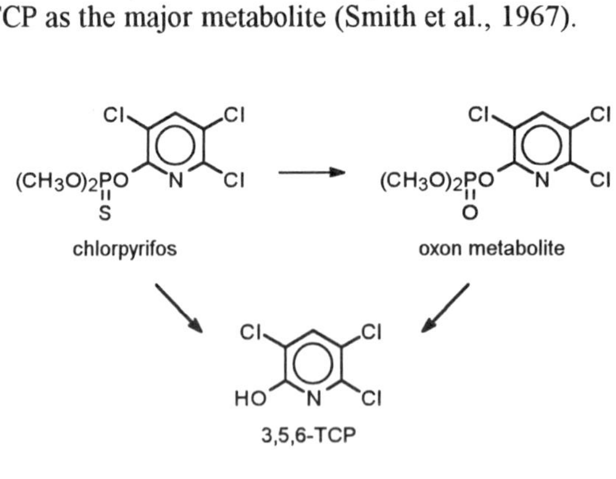

Toxicity. The principal manifestations of chlorpyrifos toxicity are due to the inhibition of cholinesterase and thus changes in plasma and erythrocyte cholinesterase activity may be used in evaluating an individual's exposure to the chemical. In cases of severe poisoning, the serum cholinesterase activity is less than 10% of normal, and victims may be unconscious, cyanotic and experience difficulty in breathing. There is a loss of the pupillary light reflex and the individual may experience flaccid paralysis (Namba et al., 1971). Two to three months are often required for recovery from overt poisoning (Whorton and Obrinsky, 1983).

A 26 year old male ingested 360 mL of Dexol (6.7% chlorpyrifos) as well as quantities of 2,4-D, MCPP and warfarin and died 30 hours later; the following chlorpyrifos concentrations were found at autopsy (Osterloh et al., 1983):

Chlorpyrifos Concentrations in a Fatal Case (mg/L or mg/kg)

Blood	Brain (Gray Matter)	Brain (White Matter)	Liver	Kidney
0	0.09	0.57	4.1	0.41

Analysis. Chlorpyrifos and its major metabolite have been determined in blood or other specimens by gas chromatography with flame-ionization (Nolan et al., 1984), electron-capture (Guinivan et al., 1981), nitrogen-phosphorus (Osterloh et al., 1983) or mass spectrometric detection (Stan and Kellner, 1982). Methods for blood chlinesterase estimation are cited in the section on carbaryl.

References

R.A. Guinivan, N.P. Thompson and P.C. Bardalaye. Simultaneous electron capture detection of chlorpyrifos and its major metabolite, 3,5,6-trichloro-2-pyridinol, after gel permeation chromatography. J. Asso. Off. Anal. Chem. 64: 1201–1204, 1981.

T. Namba, C.T. Nolte, J.J. Jackrel and D. Grob. Poisoning due to organophosphate insecticides. Am. J. Med. 50: 475–492, 1971.

R.J. Nolan, D.L. Rick, N.L. Freshour and J.H. Saunders. Chlorpyrifos: pharmacokinetics in human volunteers. Tox. Appl. Pharm. 73: 8–15, 1984.

J. Osterloh, M. Lotti and S.M. Pond. Toxicologic studies in a fatal overdose of 2,4-D, MCPP, and chlorpyrifos. J. Anal. Tox. 7: 125–129, 1983.

G.N. Smith, B.S. Watson and F.S. Fischer. Investigations on Dursban insecticide. Metabolism of (^{36}Cl) O,O-diethyl-O-3,5,6-trichloro-2-pyridyl phosphorothioate in rats. J. Agr. Food Chem. 15: 132–138, 1967.

H.J. Stan and G. Kellner. Negative chemical ionization mass spectrometry of organophosphorus pesticides. Biomed. Mass Spec. 9: 483–492, 1982.

L.G. Sultatos and S.D. Murphy. Kinetic analyses of the microsomal biotransformation of the phosphorothioate insecticides chlorpyrifos and parathion. Fund. Appl. Tox. 3: 16–21, 1983.

M.D. Whorton and D.L. Obrinsky. Persistence of symptoms after mild to moderate acute organophosphate poisoning among 19 farm field workers. J. Tox. Env. Health. 11: 347–354, 1983.

Chlorzoxazone

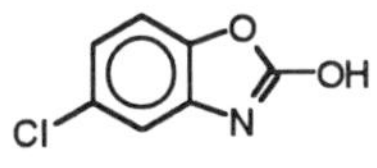

T½: 1.1 hr
Vd: ?
Fb: ?

Occurrence and Usage. Chlorzoxazone (Paraflex) has been available since 1958 for use as a skeletal muscle relaxant. It is available in tablets of 250 mg, alone or in combination with 300 mg of acetaminophen. The recommended daily dosage varies from 750–2000 mg.

Blood Concentrations. A single 600 mg oral dose of chlorzoxazone produced peak plasma concentrations of 9 and 20 mg/L in 2 subjects within 3–4 hours of ingestion; by 5.5 hours, the levels had declined to 2.8 and 5.0 mg/L, respectively (Conney and Burns, 1960). A single 750 mg oral dose given to 23 subjects resulted in an average peak plasma level of 36 mg/L at 38 minutes after administration; the levels declined with an average half-life of 1.1 hours (Desiraju et al., 1983).

Metabolism and Excretion. Chlorzoxazone is extensively metabolized by hydroxylation and conjugation. Less than 1% of a dose is excreted unchanged in the 24 hour urine, while 60–90% is excreted as conjugated 6-hydroxychlorzoxazone. Free 6-hydroxychlorzoxazone, a pharmacologically inactive metabolite, was not found in urine (Conney and Burns, 1960).

chlorzoxazone   6-OH-chlorzoxazone

Toxicity. Long-term use or abuse of chlorzoxazone has been associated with liver damage, including hepatic necrosis and hepatitis. Acute overdosage results in symptoms of central nervous system depression, nausea, vomiting, and hypotension.

Analysis. Chlorzoxazone may be determined in biological specimens by ultraviolet spectrophotometry (Conney et al., 1960) or fluorometry (Stewart and Chan, 1978). A liquid chromatographic method for the drug and its hydroxy metabolite has also been reported (Honigberg et al., 1979; Stewart and Carter, 1986).

References

A.H. Conney, N. Trousof and J.J. Burns. The metabolic fate of zoxazolamine (Flexin) in man. J. Pharm. Exp. Ther. 128: 333–339, 1960.

A.H. Conney and J.J. Burns. Physiological disposition and metabolic fate of chlorzoxazone (Paraflex) in man. J. Pharm. Exp. Ther. 128: 340–343, 1960.

R.K. Desiraju, N.L. Renzi, R.K. Nayak and K.T. Ng. Pharmacokinetics of chlorzoxazone in humans. J. Pharm. Sci. 72: 991–994, 1983.

I.L. Honigberg, J.T. Stewart and J.W. Coldren. Liquid chromatography in pharmaceutical analysis X: determination of chlorzoxazone and hydroxy metabolite in plasma. J. Pharm. Sci. 68: 253–255, 1979.

J.T. Stewart and C.W. Chan. Fluorometric determination of chlorzoxazone via chemical derivatization. Anal. Letters 11: 667–680, 1978.

J.T. Stewart and H.K. Carter. High-performance liquid chromatography with electrochemical detection of chlorzoxazone and its hydroxy metabolite in serum using solid-phase extraction. J. Chrom. 380: 177–183, 1986.

Chromium

T½: ?
Vd: ?   Cr
Fb: ?

Occurrence and Usage. Chromium is an essential nutrient for man, being required for the maintenance of normal glucose tolerance. The human diet supplies from 5–115 μg/day of the element, of which only 1–25% is absorbed from the gastrointestinal tract. Chromium has many industrial applications, including its uses in steel and nonferrous alloys, metal-plating, refractory materials, chromate pigments and chromate preservatives. Exposure to the metal and its insoluble and soluble salts is generally via inhalation of dusts or fumes; the current threshold limit values for these compounds range from 0.05–0.5 mg/m³. Chromite ore processing is listed as having carcinogenic potential, while lead and zinc chromates are suspected carcinogens.

Blood Concentrations. Serum chromium concentrations average about 0.16 μg/L (range, 0.04–0.35) in healthy subjects (Versieck et al., 1978; Kayne et al., 1978). Literature published prior to 1978 refers to normal serum chromium values ranging from 0.7–150 μg/L, due to methodological difficulties in the trace analysis of chromium.

Whole blood chromium concentrations averaged 0.90 μg/L in a group of stainless-steel welders and 0.43 μg/L in non-welders employed at the same facilities (Bonde and Christensen, 1991). The blood/plasma concentration ratio for chromium averages 0.5 (Aitio et al., 1984).

Metabolism and Excretion. Of an absorbed dose of chromium, at least 80% is excreted in the urine and a lesser amount in the feces. Hexavalent chromium, which is generally more soluble and more toxic than the trivalent form, tends to be reduced to trivalent chromium *in vivo*. Chromium does not appear to accumulate in bone or most soft tissues as a result of age, occupation or smoking history. The lung, however, usually contains the highest concentration of any organ in the body and this concentration increases with age, probably as a result of the deposition of insoluble chromium compounds present in air. Chromium concentrations in the brain, liver, and kidney of normal Japanese adults ranged on average from 0.03–0.08 mg/kg, while lung concentrations were 0.15–0.38 mg/kg; women tended to have lower levels than men (Sumino et al., 1975).

Normal urinary chromium concentrations average 0.1–0.5 μg/L and range up to 1.0 μg/L (Kiilunen et al., 1987; Stern et al., 1992). Urine chromium concentrations in stainless-steel welders averaged only 2–3 times those of non-welders in one study (Bonde and Christensen, 1991), but may range as high as 62 μg/L in tannery workers (Aitio et al., 1984). Hair chromium concentrations averaged 0.6 μg/g in normal adults, 15 μg/g in office workers at a tannery using chromate salts and 17 μg/g in the tannery workers (Saner et al., 1984). Urinary elimination of chromium following inhalation exposure to welding fumes occurs in 3 distinct phases, with half-lives of 7 hours, 15–30 days and 3–5 years (ACGIH, 1986).

Toxicity. The inhalation of insoluble chromium compounds has led to pneumoconiosis with impairment of pulmonary function; exposure to the chromite ore roasting process is suspected to have carcinogenic potential. Soluble salts of hexavalent chromium are corrosive and have produced skin ulceration, dermatitis, perforation of the nasal septum, respiratory sensitization and lung cancer. Acute poisoning with soluble salts usually results in local tissue necrosis and severe kidney damage (Baetjer et al., 1974). Antibodies to chromium have been measured in the serum of a worker who developed asthma following exposure to the metal (Novey et al., 1983). Electroplaters and paint pigment workers who expressed symptoms of cough, indigestion and dermal itching were found to have urine chromium concentrations of 91–1116 μg/L (Tandon et al., 1977). An average concentration of 37 mg/kg chromium (range, 0.5–130) was found in the lungs of 8 chromate workers with lung cancer (Tsuneta et al., 1980). The following concentrations were measured in the tissues of a worker with 30 years of exposure to hexavalent chromium, who died of lung cancer 10 years after his retirement (Hyodo et al., 1980):

Chromium Concentrations in a Chromate Worker (mg/kg)

Brain	Lung	Liver	Kidney
0.05–0.06	0.6–7.1	0.07	0.13

An adult male who ingested chromic acid solution developed gastrointestinal ulceration and renal failure and died after one month; plasma and urine collected within several days of ingestion contained 960 and 5130 μg/L of chromium, respectively (Saryan and Reedy, 1988).

Analysis. Chromium in biological specimens is frequently measured by flameless atomic absorption spectrometry (Kayne et al., 1978; Routh, 1980; Veillon et al., 1980; Ericson et al., 1986;

Kiilunen et al., 1987). Gas chromatography-mass spectrometry of a volatile chelate (Veillon et al., 1979) and neutron activation analysis (Versieck et al., 1978) have also proven sensitive and accurate.

References

A. Aitio, J. Jarvisalo, M. Kiilunen et al. Urinary excretion of chromium as an indicator of exposure to trivalent chromium sulphate in leather tanning. Int. Arch. Occ. Env. Health 54: 241–249, 1984.

American Conference of Governmental Industrial Hygienists. *Documentation of Threshold Limit Values and Biological Exposure Indices*, 5th ed., ACGIH, Cincinnati, Ohio, 1986, pp. 91–95.

A.M. Baetjer, D.J. Birmingham, P.E. Enterline et al. *Chromium*, National Academy of Sciences, Washington, D.C., 1974.

J.P. Bonde and J.M. Christensen. Chromium in biological samples from low-level exposed stainless steel and mild steel workers. Arch. Env. Health 46: 225–229, 1991.

S.P. Ericson, M.L. McHalsky, B.E. Rabinow et al. Sampling and analysis techniques for monitoring serum for trace elements. Clin. Chem. 32: 1350–1356, 1986.

K. Hyodo, S. Suzuki, N. Furuya and K. Meshizuka. An analysis of chromium, copper, and zinc in organs of a chromate worker. Int. Arch. Occ. Env. Health 46: 141–150, 1980.

F.J. Kayne, G. Komar, H. Laboda and R.E. Vanderlinde. Atomic absorption spectrophotometry of chromium in serum and urine with a modified Perkin-Elmer 603 atomic absorption spectrophotometer. Clin. Chem. 24: 2151–2154, 1978.

M. Kiilunen, J. Jarvisalo, O. Makitie and A. Aitio. Analysis, storage stability and reference values for urinary chromium and nickel. Int. Arch. Occ. Env. Health 59: 43–50, 1987.

H.S. Novey, M. Habib and I.D. Wells. Asthma and IgE antibodies induced by chromium and nickel salts. J. Allergy Clin. Imm. 72: 407–412, 1983.

M.W. Routh. Analytical parameters for determination of chromium in urine by electrothermal atomic absorption spectrometry. Anal. Chem. 52: 182–185, 1980.

G. Saner, V. Yuzbasiyan and S. Cigdem. Hair chromium concentration and chromium excretion in tannery workers. Brit. J. Ind. Med. 41: 263–266, 1984.

L.A. Saryan and M. Reedy. Chromium determinations in a case of chromic acid ingestion. J. Anal. Tox. 12: 162–164, 1988.

A.H. Stern, N.C.G. Freeman, P. Pleban et al. Residential exposure to chromium waste. Env. Res. 58: 147–162, 1992.

K. Sumino, K. Hayakawa, T. Shibata and S. Kitamura. Heavy metals in normal Japanese tissues. Arch. Env. Health 30: 487–494, 1975.

S.K. Tandon, A.K. Mathur and J.S. Gaur. Urinary excretion of chromium and nickel amoung electroplaters and pigment industry workers. Int. Arch. Occ. Env. Health 40: 71–76, 1977.

Y. Tsuneta, Y. Ohsaki, K. Kimura et al. Chromium content of lungs of chromate workers with lung cancer. Thorax 35: 294–297, 1980.

C. Veillon, W.R. Wolf and B.E. Guthrie. Determination of chromium in biological materials by stable isotope dilution. Anal. Chem. 51: 1022–1024, 1979.

C. Veillon, B.E. Guthrie and W.R. Wolf. Retention of chromium by graphite furnace tubes. Anal. Chem. 52: 457–459, 1980.

V. Versieck, J. Hoste, F. Barbier et al. Determination of chromium and cobalt in human serum by neutron activation analysis. Clin. Chem. 24: 303–308, 1978.

Cimetidine

T½: 1–4 hr
Vd: 1.4 L/kg
Fb: 0.18–0.26
pKa: 7.1

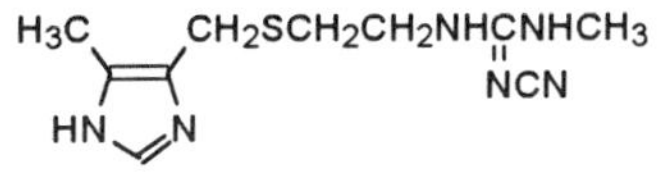
H3C
CH2SCH2CH2NHCNHCH3
NCN
HN
N

Occurrence and Usage. Cimetidine (Tagamet) is a histamine H_2-receptor antagonist that has been available since 1975 for the treatment of duodenal ulcer. The drug is available as the hydrochloride salt for oral administration (as 200 or 300 mg tablets or as a 300 mg/5 mL liquid) and for parenteral injection (as a 150 mg/mL solution). Oral, intramuscular and intravenous doses range from 1200–2400 mg/day.

Blood Concentrations. Single oral 200, 400, and 800 mg doses produced average peak plasma cimetidine concentrations of 1.1, 2.3 and 4.5 mg/L, respectively, after 3 hours in 9–10 fasting patients. A 200 mg intravenous dose resulted in an initial plasma level of about 10 mg/L, declining with an average half-life of 1.8 hours. Chronic daily therapy with 1000 mg of cimetidine in 10 patients produced an average peak plasma concentration of 2.4 mg/L (range, 1.4–4.4) after the evening 400 mg dose; the average morning pre-dose level was 0.4 mg/L (range, 0.3–0.8). The authors concluded that a morning pre-dose concentration exceeding 0.6 mg/L was indicative of renal insufficiency (Bodemar et al., 1981).

Gugler et al. (1981) found that a mean plasma cimetidine concentration of 0.78 mg/L (range, 0.54–1.04) was necessary to produce 50% inhibition of gastric acid secretion in 6 healthy subjects, and a mean of 3.9 mg/L was required for 90% inhibition. The kinetics of the drug do not differ significantly between normal subjects and ulcer patients, but the half-life is increased about 30% in older patients. The blood/plasma ratio is 0.97 (Somogyi et al., 1980).

Metabolism and Excretion. The bioavailability of cimetidine after both oral and intravenous administration is 76%. An average of 35–39% of an oral dose and 58% of an intravenous dose is eliminated unchanged in the 24 hour urine (Bodemar et al., 1981). Another 11% of a dose is excreted in urine as cimetidine sulfoxide and 4% as hydroxycimetidine. The remainder of the dose is largely accounted for as cimetidine-N'-glucuronide (Taylor et al., 1978; Mitchell et al., 1982). The following average tissue/serum concentration ratios were found in 11 patients who died of underlying diseases while at steady-state with cimetidine: kidney, 14.9; liver, 4.5; lung, 2.7; brain, 0.9; fat, 0.4 (Schentag et al., 1981).

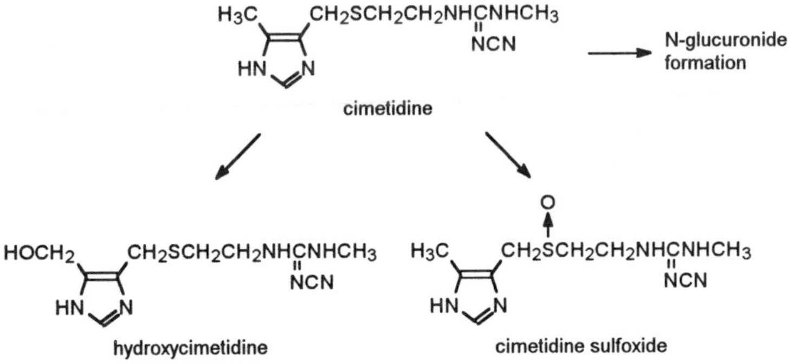
H3C
CH2SCH2CH2NHCNHCH3
NCN
HN
N
cimetidine
N-glucuronide
formation
HOCH2
CH2SCH2CH2NHCNHCH3
NCN
HN
N
hydroxycimetidine
O
H3C
CH2SCH2CH2NHCNHCH3
NCN
HN
N
cimetidine sulfoxide

Toxicity. Toxic effects of cimetidine include headache, dizziness, drowsiness, muscle pain, mental confusion, flushing of the skin and sweating. These symptoms occur in patients who take the drug in excess or in those with reduced hepatic or renal function, and are usually associated with trough cimetidine concentrations exceeding 1.25 mg/L (Schentag, 1980). The reactions have been mistaken for delerium tremens or organic psychosis in alcoholic patients receiving the drug (Arneson, 1979; Weddington et al., 1981). A manic syndrome has also been reported (Hubain et al., 1982).

An 11 year old girl became comatose after two intravenous injections of 2 mg/kg within 4 hours (Bacigalupo et al., 1978). A 35 year old man developed unconsciousness after ingesting 24 g of cimetidine, but awoke 6 hours later after treatment by gastric lavage and forced diuresis. His blood level 8 hours after ingestion was 19 mg/L; after 12 hours, 4.1 mg/L; and after 15 hours, 2.6 mg/L (van Rijthoven, 1979).

Analysis. Cimetidine is conveniently measured in biological fluids by liquid chromatography (Soldin et al., 1979; Cohen et al., 1980; Kunitani et al., 1981; Abdel-Rahim et al., 1985; Chiou et al., 1986). A comprehensive liquid chromatographic assay for cimetidine and its known metabolites has also been described (Ziemniak et al., 1981).

References

M. Abdel-Rahim, D. Ezra and J. Lazar. Liquid-chromatographic assay of cimetidine in plasma and gastric fluid. Clin. Chem. 31: 621–623, 1985.

G.A. Arneson. More on toxic psychosis with cimetidine. Am. J. Psych. 136: 1348–1349, 1979.

A. Bacigalupo, M.T. van Lint and A.M. Marmont. Cimetidine-induced coma. Lancet 2: 45–46, 1978.

G. Bodemar, B. Norlander and W. Walan. Pharmacokinetics of cimetidine after single doses and during continuous treatment. Clin. Pharmacokin. 6: 306–315, 1981.

R. Chiou, R.J. Stubbs and W.F. Bayne. Determination of cimetidine in plasma and urine by high-performance liquid chromatography. J. Chrom. 377: 441–446, 1986.

I.A. Cohen, J.K. Siepler, R. Nation et al. Relationship between cimetidine plasma levels and gastric acidity in acutely ill patients. Am. J. Hosp. Pharm. 37: 375–379, 1980.

R. Gugler, G. Fuchs, M. Dieckmann and A.A. Somogyi. Cimetidine plasma concentration-response relationships. Clin. Pharm. Ther. 29: 744–748, 1981.

P.P. Hubain, J. Sobolski and J. Mendlewicz. Cimetidine-induced mania. Neuropsychobiology 8: 223–224, 1982.

M.G. Kunitani, D.A. Johnson, R.A. Upton and S. Riegelman. Convenient and sensitive high-performance liquid chromatography assay for cimetidine in plasma or urine. J. Chrom. 224: 156–161, 1981.

S.C. Mitchell, J.R. Idle and R.L. Smith. The metabolism of [14C] cimetidine in man. Xenobiotica 12: 283–292, 1982.

J.J. Schentag. Cimetidine-associated mental confusion: further studies in 36 severely ill patients. Ther. Drug Mon. 2: 133–142, 1980.

J.J. Schentag, F.B. Cerra, G.M. Calleri et al. Age, disease, and cimetidine disposition in healthy subjects and chronically ill patients. Clin. Pharm. Ther. 29: 737–743, 1981.

S.J. Soldin, D.R. Fingold, P.C. Fenje and W.A. Mahon. High performance liquid chromatographic analysis of cimetidine in serum. Ther. Drug Mon. 1: 371–379, 1979.

A. Somogyi, H.G. Rohner and R. Gugler. Pharmacokinetics and bioavailability of cimetidine in gastric and duodenal ulcer patients. Clin. Pharmacokin. 5: 84–94, 1980.

D.C. Taylor, P.R. Cresswell and D.C. Bartlett. The metabolism and elimination of cimetidine, a histamine H2-receptor antagonist, in the rat, dog and man. Drug Met. Disp. 6: 21–30, 1978.

A.W.A.M. van Rijthoven. Cimetidine intoxication. Lancet 2: 370, 1979.

W.W. Weddington, Jr., A.E. Muelling, H.H. Moosa et al. Cimetidine toxic reactions masquerading as delirium tremens. J. Am. Med. Asso. 245: 1058–1059, 1981.

J.A. Ziemniak, D.A. Chiarmonte and J.J. Schentag. Liquid-chromatographic determination of cimetidine, its known metabolites, and creatinine in serum and urine. Clin. Chem. 27: 272–275, 1981.

Clobazam

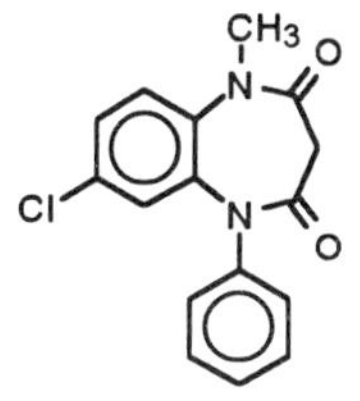

T½: 10–30 hr
Vd: 1 L/kg
Fb: 0.85

Occurrence and Usage. Clobazam (Frisium) is a 1,5-benzodiazepine derivative utilized as a sedative, anticonvulsant and antianxiety agent. Although the drug is available in a number of European countries, it is not yet marketed in the United States. Daily doses may range from 20–60 mg. The drug is formulated as 10 mg tablets or capsules of this neutral substance.

Blood Concentrations. Twelve healthy male subjects, 22–34 years of age, who took a single 20 mg dose of clobazam exhibited an average peak plasma concentration of 465 µg/L (range, 222–709) after 1.7 hours; the average plasma concentration of desmethylclobazam of 88 µg/L (range, 61–146) occurred from 24–96 hours (average, 45) post-administration (Divoll et al., 1982). Twelve healthy males aged 18–26 years given a 40 mg oral dose of clobazam developed an average peak plasma concentration at 2.5 hours of 730 µg/L, which fell to 363 µg/L at 12 hours, 180 µg/L at 48 hours and 17 µg/L at 96 hours. Desmethylclobazam was present in plasma but the concentrations were too low to measure. The average plasma half-life of clobazam in this study was 18 hours (Vallner et al., 1980).

Ten adults receiving 20 mg of the drug daily for 28 days achieved average steady-state serum levels of 333 µg/L for clobazam and 2811 µg/L for desmethylclobazam (Rupp et al., 1979).

Metabolism and Excretion. The major metabolic pathway of clobazam in humans involves N-demethylation and yields desmethylclobazam, which also has pharmacological activity (Greenblatt, 1980). Minor metabolites include 4'-hydroxyclobazam and 4'-hydroxydesmethylclobazam. Approximately 87% of a radioactive dose is excreted in the urine in 17 days, with less than 5% present as unchanged drug (Rupp et al., 1979; Volz et al., 1979).

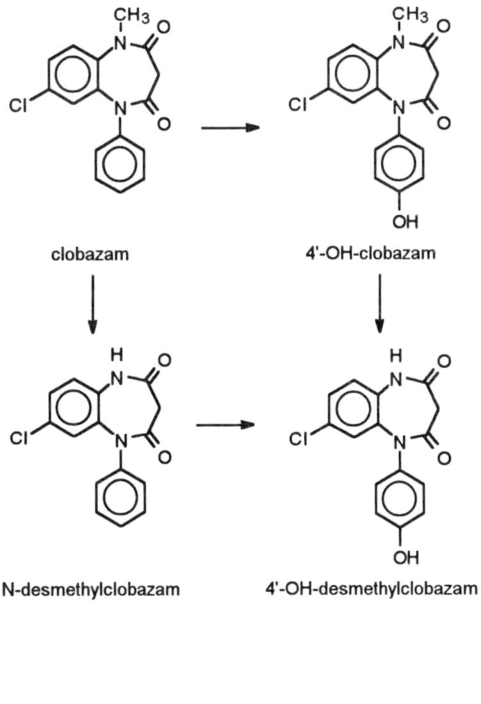

clobazam   4'-OH-clobazam

N-desmethylclobazam   4'-OH-desmethylclobazam

Toxicity. Clobazam in overdosage causes moderate sedation. A 22 year old woman who deliberately ingested 300 mg of clobazam experienced confusion, dizziness, and somnolence, but not loss of consciousness (Donlon and Singer, 1979).

Analysis. Clobazam has been measured in blood and plasma using fluorometric methods (Kotzan et al., 1979; Stewart et al., 1979). Gas chromatography with flame-ionization (Schuetz and Westenberger, 1979), electron-capture (Greenblatt, 1980), and nitrogen-phosphorus detection (Vallner et al., 1980; Pena and Lope, 1988) has been employed. Liquid chromatography has also been utilized in the determination of the drug and its metabolites (Brachet-Liermain et al., 1982; Gill et al., 1986).

References

A. Brachet-Liermain, C. Jarry, O. Faure et al. Liquid chromatography determination of clobazam and its major metabolite N-desmethylclobazam in human plasma. Ther. Drug Mon. 4: 301–305, 1982.

M. Divoll, D.J. Greenblatt, D.A. Ciraulo et al. Clobazam kinetics: intrasubject variability and effect of food on absorption. J. Clin. Pharm. 22: 69–73, 1982.

P.T. Donlon and J.M. Singer. Clobazam versus placebo for anxiety and tension in pyschoneurotic outpatients. A multicenter collaborative study. J. Clin. Pharm. 19: 297–302, 1979.

R. Gill, B. Law and J.P. Gibbs. High-pressure liquid chromatography systems for the separation of benzodiazepines and their metabolites. J. Chrom. 356: 37–46, 1986.

D.J. Greenblatt. Electron-capture GLC determination of clobazam and desmethylclobazam in plasma. J. Pharm. Sci. 69: 1451–1352, 1980.

J.A. Kotzan, T.E. Needham, I.L. Honigberg et al. Examination of blood clobazam levels and several pupillary measures in humans. J. Pharm. Sci. 68: 1002–1004, 1979.

M.I.A. Pena and E.S. Lope. Monitoring serum clobazam by isothermal gas-liquid chromatography with nitrogen detector. J. Pharm. Biomed. Anal. 6: 995–998, 1988.

W. Rupp, M. Badian, O. Christ et al. Pharmacokinetics of single and multiple doses of clobazam in humans. Brit. J. Clin. Pharm. 7: 51S–57S, 1979.

H. Schuetz and V. Westenberger. Gas chromatographic data of 31 benzodiazepines and metabolites. J. Chrom. 169: 409–411, 1979.

J.T. Stewart, I.L. Honigberg, A.Y. Tsai and P. Hajdu. Fluorometric determination of clobazam, a 1,5-benzodiazepine, in human plasma. J. Pharm. Sci. 68: 494–496, 1979.

J.J. Vallner, J.A. Kotzan, J.T. Stewart et al. Plasma levels of clobazam after 10-, 20-, and 40-mg tablet doses in healthy subjects. J. Clin. Pharm. 20: 444–451, 1980.

M. Volz, O. Christ, H.M. Kellner et al. Kinetics and metabolism of clobazam in animals and man. Brit. J. Clin. Pharm. 7: 41S–50S, 1979.

Clomipramine

T½: 12–36 hr
Vd: 17 L/kg
Fb: 0.96
pKa: 9.5

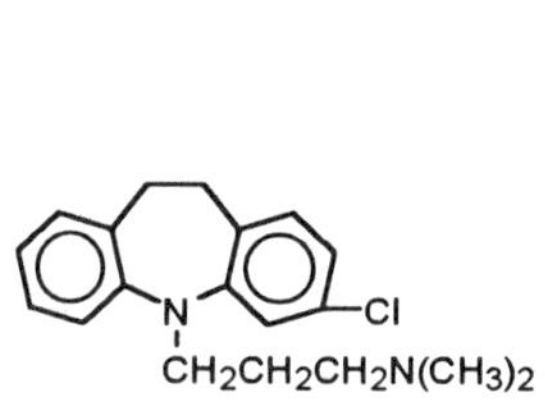

$CH_2CH_2CH_2N(CH_3)_2$

Occurrence and Usage. Clomipramine (chlorimipramine, Anafranil) is a tricyclic antidepressant that was synthesized in 1958 and has been in clinical use since 1961. It is the 3-chloro analogue of imipramine and shares many of the properties of that drug. It is available as the hydrochloride salt in tablets and capsules of 25–100 mg for oral administration and in vials for intramuscular or intravenous injection. Daily doses range from 75–300 mg.

Blood Concentrations. Average peak plasma clomipramine concentrations of 0.017 and 0.033 mg/L were attained 4 hours after the oral ingestion of 25 or 50 mg, respectively, in healthy volunteers (Read and Riad-Fahmy, 1978). After a 100 mg oral dose, peak plasma levels ranged from 0.076–0.140 mg/L, occurred within 2–5 hours, and declined with an average half-life of 23 hours (Westenberg et al., 1977).

In 8 patients who responded well to chronic oral therapy with 150 mg clomipramine daily, plasma concentrations (before the morning dose) averaged 0.126 mg/L (range, 0.082–0.236) for clomipramine and 0.189 mg/L (range, 0.083–0.316) for norclomipramine, an active metabolite. Similar averages for patients with poorer clinical response were 0.085 and 0.195 mg/L, respectively (Dencker and Nagy, 1979). Substantially higher values, averaging 0.158 mg/L (range, 0.040–0.282) for clomipramine and 0.526 mg/L (range, 0.144–1.053) for norclomipramine, were reported for 14 patients on equivalent 150 mg daily therapy by Broadhurst et al. (1977). The whole blood/plasma concentration ratio of the drug varies from 0.83–1.43 (Dubois et al., 1976).

Metabolism and Excretion. Absorption of clomipramine after oral administration is complete in man. Over a period of 14 days the drug is 92% eliminated from the body, primarily as metabolites in urine (60%) and feces (32%). Disposition of the drug after intravenous administration is very similar to that observed by the oral route (Faigle and Dieterle, 1973). Clomipramine is known to be N-demethylated to norclomipramine, which accumulates in plasma during chronic drug administration. Less than 0.2% of a dose is excreted unchanged in the 72 hour urine (Dubois et al., 1976).

Toxicity. Clomipramine in overdosage causes central nervous system depression, agitation, convulsions, hypotension, hyperpyrexia, and cardiac arrhythmias. Three fatal cases following overdosage have been reported, with postmortem blood levels of 0.54–2.1 mg/L for clomipramine and 0.58–1.4 mg/L for norclomipramine (Hucker, 1983; Meatherall et al., 1983; Fraser et al., 1986).

Analysis. Clomipramine has been measured in biological fluids by gas chromatography with nitrogen-phosphorus (Broadhurst et al., 1977) or mass spectrometric detection (Dubois et al., 1976; Alfredsson et al., 1977; Alkalay et al., 1979), and high-pressure liquid chromatography (Mellstrom and Tybring, 1977; Westenberg et al., 1977; Nielsen and Brosen, 1991).

References

D. Alkalay, J. Volk and S. Carlsen. A sensitive method for the simultaneous determination in biological fluids of imipramine and desipramine or clomipramine and N-desmethylclomipramine by gas chromatography mass spectrometry. Biomed. Mass Spec. 6: 200–204, 1979.

G. Alfredsson, F. Wiesel, B. Fyro and G. Sedvall. Mass fragmentographic analysis of clomipramine and its mono-demethylated metabolite in human plasma. Psychopharmacology 52: 25–30, 1977.

A.D. Broadhurst, H.D. James, L. Della Corte and A.F. Heeley. Clomipramine plasma level and clinical response. Postgrad. Med. J. 53: 139–145, 1977.

S.J. Dencker and A. Nagy. Single versus divided daily dosages of clomipramine. Acta Psych. Scand. 59: 326–334, 1979.

J. Dubois, W. Kung, W. Theobald and B. Wirz. Measurement of clomipramine, N-desmethylclomipramine, imipramine, and dehydroimipramine in biological fluids by selective ion monitoring, and pharmacokinetics of clomipramine. Clin. Chem. 22: 892–897, 1976.

J.W. Faigle and W. Dieterle. The metabolism and pharmacokinetics of clomipramine. J. Int. Med. Res. 1: 281–290, 1973.

A.D. Fraser, A.F. Isner and M.A. Moss. A fatality involving clomipramine. J. For. Sci. 31: 762–767, 1986.

R.S. Hucker. Personal communication, 1983.

R.C. Meatherall, D.R.P. Gray, J.L. Chalmers and J.R. Keenan. A fatal overdose with clomipramine. J. Anal. Tox. 7: 168–171, 1983.

B. Mellstrom and G. Tybring. Ion-pair liquid chromatography of steady-state plasma levels of chlorimipramine and demethylchlorimipramine. J. Chrom. 143: 597–605, 1977.

K.K. Nielsen and K. Brosen. High-performance liquid chromatography of clomipramine and metabolites in human plasma and urine. Ther. Drug. Mon. 15: 122–128, 1993.

G.F. Read and D. Riad-Fahmy. Determination of a tricyclic antidepressant, clomipramine (Anafranil), in plasma by a specific radioimmunoassay procedure. Clin. Chem. 24: 36–40, 1978.

Clonazepam

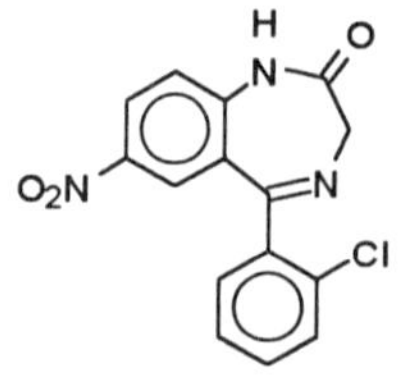

T½: 19–60 hr
Vd: 1.5–4.4 L/kg
Fb: 0.80
pKa: 1.5, 10.5

Occurrence and Usage. Clonazepam (Clonopin, Klonopin, Rivotril) is a benzodiazepine derivative that was approved for use as an anticonvulsant in the U.S. in 1975. It is the 2-chloro analogue of nitrazepam, which is a potent sedative. The drug is administered as the free base in daily oral maintenance doses of 1.5–20 mg, in the form of 0.5–2 mg tablets.

Blood Concentrations. A single oral administration of 2 mg of clonazepam resulted in an average peak plasma concentration of 0.017 mg/L (range, 0.007–0.024) between 1 and 4 hours after ingestion, with half-lives of 19–42 hours observed in the 8 volunteers (Berlin and Dahlstrom, 1975). Plasma concentrations in 25 patients on 6 mg/day chronic therapy were found to be 0.029–0.075 mg/L for clonazepam and 0.023–0.137 mg/L for its major active metabolite, 7-aminoclonazepam (Naestoft and Larsen, 1974). Substantial adverse effects (primarily drowsiness and ataxia) were noticed in most patients when plasma clonazepam concentrations exceeded 0.100 mg/L (Baruzzi et al., 1977).

Metabolism and Excretion. Clonazepam undergoes extensive biotransformation, with less than 0.5% of a dose excreted in the 24 hour urine (Kaplan et al., 1974). The major metabolite, 7-aminoclonazepam, is formed by reduction of the 7-nitro group on clonazepam. This compound achieves plasma concentrations equivalent to those of the parent drug, but it is apparently a poor anticonvulsant (Browne, 1976). It is conjugated by N-acetylation to form 7-acetamidoclonazepam, which may be found in plasma at very low concentrations (Naestoft and Larsen, 1974). Clonazepam and these two metabolites each undergo 3-hydroxylation and possible ring hydroxylation, with some conjugation. Urinary excretion accounts for 49–69% of a dose, as both free and conjugated metabolites (Eschenhof, 1973).

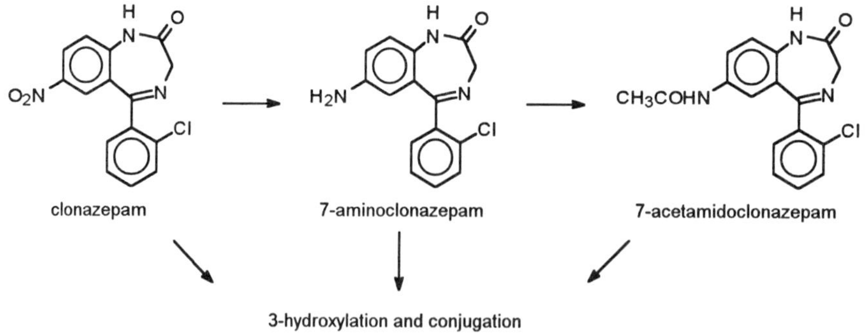

clonazepam   7-aminoclonazepam   7-acetamidoclonazepam

3-hydroxylation and conjugation

Toxicity. Overdoses of up to 60 mg of clonazepam have been taken without serious sequelae; drowsiness and ataxia were reported, but serious respiratory depression did not develop (Browne, 1976). A 4 year old boy who ingested his mother's medication cycled between a state of alert agitation and deep coma for a period of 24 hours; plasma clonazepam measured shortly after admission was 0.069 mg/L, consistent with the acute ingestion of 7–16 tablets of 2 mg each. He recovered within 36 hours of drug ingestion (Welsh et al., 1977).

Analysis. Clonazepam has been measured at therapeutic concentrations in biological fluids by radioimmunoassay, a technique that is now commercially available (Dixon and Crews, 1977). Gas chromatographic procedures have utilized nitrogen-phosphorus (Dahr and Kutt, 1981), electron-capture (Cano et al., 1977; Solow and Kenfield, 1977; Edelbroek and De Wolff, 1978; Wilson et al., 1979; Loscher and Al-Tahan, 1983; Miller et al., 1987), and mass spectrometric detection (Min et al., 1978; Wilson et al., 1979). Liquid chromatography has also been used successfully (Rovei and Sanjuan, 1980; Shaw et al., 1983; Wad, 1986; Boukhabza et al., 1990). Exposure of serum containing clonazepam to sunlight can cause up to 99% loss of the drug within 1 hour (Wad, 1986).

References

A. Baruzzi, B. Bordo, L. Bossi et al. Plasma levels of di-n-propylacetate and clonazepam in epileptic patients. Int. J. Clin. Pharm. 15: 403–408, 1977.

A. Berlin and H. Dahlstrom. Pharmacokinetics of the anticonvulsant drug clonazepam evaluated from single oral and intravenous doses and by repeated oral administration. Eur. J. Clin. Pharm. 9: 155–159, 1975.

A. Boukhabza, A.A. Lugnier, P. Kintz et al. Simple and sensitive method for monitoring clonazepam in human plasma and urine by high-performance liquid chromatography. J. Chrom. 529: 210–216, 1990.

T.R. Browne. Clonazepam. Arch. Neurol. 3: 326–332, 1976.

J.P. Cano, J. Guintrand, C. Aubert and A. Viala. Determination of flunitrazepam, desmethylflunitrazepam and clonazepam in plasma by gas liquid chromatography with an internal standard. Arz. Forsch. 27: 338–342, 1977.

A.K. Dahr and H. Kutt. Improved gas chromatographic procedure for the determination of clonazepam levels in plasma using a nitrogen-sensitive detector. J. Chrom. 222: 203–211, 1981.

R. Dixon and T. Crews. An ^{125}I-radioimmunoassay for the determination of the anticonvulsant agent clonazepam directly in plasma. Res. Comm. Chem. Path. Pharm. 18: 477–485, 1977.

P.M. Edelbroek and F.A. De Wolff. Improved micromethod for determination of underivatized clonazepam in serum by gas chromatography. Clin. Chem. 24: 1774–1777, 1978.

E. Eschenhof. Untersuchungen ueber das Schicksal des Anticonvulsivums Clonazepam im Organismus der Ratte, des Hundes und des Menschen. Arz. Forsch. 23: 390–400, 1973.

S.A. Kaplan, K. Alexander, M.L. Jack et al. Pharmacokinetic profiles of clonazepam in dog and humans and of flunitrazepam in dog. J. Pharm. Sci. 63: 527–532, 1974.

W. Loscher and F.J.O. Al-Tahan. Rapid gas chromatographic assay of underivatized clonazepam in plasma. Ther. Drug Mon. 5: 229–233, 1983.

L.G. Miller, H. Friedman and D.J. Greenblatt. Measurement of clonazepam by electron-capture gas-liquid chromatography with application to single-dose pharmacokinetics. J. Anal. Tox. 11: 55–57, 1987.

B.H. Min, W.A. Garland, K.C. Khoo and G.S. Torres. Determination of clonazepam and its amino and acetamido metabolites in human plasma by combined gas chromatography chemical ionization mass spectrometry and selected ion monitoring. Biomed. Mass Spec. 5: 692–698, 1978.

J. Naestoft and N. Larsen. Quantitative determination of clonazepam and its metabolites in human plasma by gas chromatography. J. Chrom. 93: 113–122, 1974.

R.J. Perchalski and B.J. Wilder. Determination of benzodiazepine anticonvulsants in plasma by high-performance liquid chromatography. Anal. Chem. 50: 554–557, 1978.

V. Rovei and M. Sanjuan. Simple and specific high performance liquid chromatographic method for the routine monitoring of clonazepam in plasma. Ther. Drug Mon. 2: 283–287, 1980.

W. Shaw, G. Long and J. McHan. An hplc method for analysis of clonazepam in serum. J. Anal. Tox. 7: 119–122, 1983.

E.B. Solow and C.P. Kenfield. A micromethod for the determination of clonazepam in serum by electron-capture gas-liquid chromatography. J. Anal. Tox. 1: 155–157, 1977.

N. Wad. Degradation of clonazepam in serum by light confirmed by means of a high performance liquid chromatographic method. Ther. Drug Mon. 8: 358–360, 1986.

T.R. Welch, B.H. Rumack and K. Hammond. Clonazepam overdose resulting in cyclic coma. Clin. Tox. 10: 433–436, 1977.

J.M. Wilson, P.N. Friel, A.J. Wilensky and V.A. Raisys. A methods comparison: clonazepam by gas chromatography-electron capture and gas chromatography-mass spectroscopy. Ther. Drug Mon. 1: 387–397, 1979.

Clonidine

T½: 5–13 hr
Vd: 3.2–5.6 L/kg
Fb: 0.20–0.40
pKa: 8.3

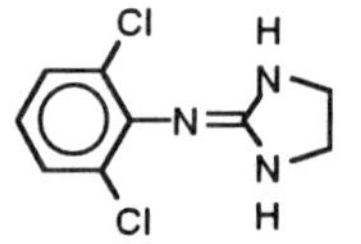

Occurrence and Usage. Clonidine (Catapres, Dixarit) is a potent antihypertensive agent, with both alpha-adrenergic blocking and agonist character, that has been in clinical use since 1966. It is available as the hydrochloride salt in 0.1–0.3 mg tablets, alone or in combination with chlorthalidone, a diuretic. Daily oral doses range from 0.2–2.4 mg. Transdermal patches are also available that contain from 2.5–7.5 mg of the drug, delivering daily doses of 0.1–0.3 mg over a 1 week period.

Blood Concentrations. A single 0.3 mg oral dose of clonidine resulted in an average peak plasma concentration of 1.0 µg/L at about 1.5 hours in 5 normal subjects. This dose produced sedation and sleep in the volunteers (Dollery et al., 1976). The same dose in hypertensive patients produced an average peak level of 1.3 µg/L, which declined with a half-life of 10 hours. Plasma drug concentrations correlated with antihypertensive effect up to a level of 1.5 µg/L; beyond this level, the effect of the drug diminished (Wing et al., 1977). A steady-state serum level of 0.30–0.35 µg/L was achieved in patients receiving 0.225 mg daily for 1 week (Keranen et al., 1978). Ten patients with essential hypertension, ranging in age from 36–64 years and weighing 51–86 kg, were treated with clonidine and the dose titrated until diastolic pressure fell below 90 or until a maximum dose of 1.2 mg/day was reached; after two weeks, plasma concentrations ranged from 0.73–3.85 µg/L (average, 2.55) (Velasquez et al., 1983).

Metabolism and Excretion. The bioavailability of oral clonidine is 75%. About 65% of a labeled dose is excreted in urine and 22% in feces within 4 days. Approximately 38% of a dose is eliminated unchanged in the 24 hour urine, together with minor amounts of several inactive oxidation products (Rehbinder and Deckers, 1969; Davies et al., 1977; Darda et al., 1978).

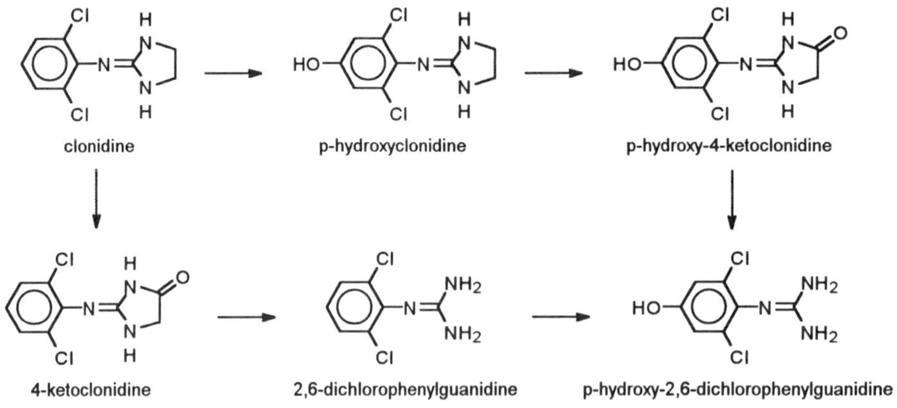

clonidine   p-hydroxyclonidine   p-hydroxy-4-ketoclonidine

4-ketoclonidine   2,6-dichlorophenylguanidine   p-hydroxy-2,6-dichlorophenylguanidine

Toxicity. Clinical symptoms seen in clonidine toxicity include hypertension or hypotension, bradycardia, convulsions, hypothermia, and coma. Although numerous cases of overdosage have been documented, recovery usually is apparent within 24–48 hours and few deaths have occurred. Dopamine or tolazoline is recommended to control hypotension, and atropine may be used to manage bradycardia (Conner and Watanabe, 1979; Anderson et al., 1981; Mathew et al., 1981; Artman and Boerth, 1983; Algren and Rodgers, 1984).

A 2 year old child who ingested 0.3 mg of the drug developed a serum clonidine concentration of 3.5 µg/L and lost consciousness; she recovered by the time the serum level had fallen (with a half-life of 5.5 hours) to 0.4 µg/L, 17 hours later (Neuvonen et al., 1979). Six other children had serum clonidine levels of 2.1–9.7 µg/L within 5 hours of drug overdose (Wasserman et al., 1992). An adult became sedated and hypotensive after ingesting 4.8 mg of clonidine; a maximal concentration of 6.0 µg/L was measured 4 hours after ingestion, declining to 4.9 µg/L by 8 hours (Moore and Phillipi, 1976). A 28 year old man survived the ingestion of 100 mg of drug, 57 mg of which was removed by gastric lavage; a plasma clonidine concentration of 230 µg/L was achieved after 1 hour (Domino et al., 1986).

A 43 year old woman who died shortly after ingesting an overdose of clonazepam had postmortem drug levels of 23 µg/L in blood, 24 µg/kg in brain and 86 µg/kg in kidney (Lukkari, 1983).

Analysis. Clonidine has been analyzed in biological specimens, after derivatization, by gas chromatography with electron-capture (Chu et al., 1979; Edlund, 1980; Nazarali et al., 1986) or mass spectrometric detection (Draffan et al., 1977; Murray et al., 1981; Haring et al., 1988).

References

J.T. Algren and G.C. Rodgers. Hypertension associated with clonidine ingestion. Vet. Hum. Tox. 26 (Suppl. 2): 32–35, 1984.

R.J. Anderson, G.R. Hart, C.P. Crumpler and M.J. Lerman. Clonidine overdose: report of six cases and review of literature. Ann. Emer. Med. 10: 107–112, 1981.

M. Artman and R.C. Boerth. Clonidine poisoning. Am. J. Dis. Child. 137: 171–174, 1983.

C.S. Conner and A.S. Watanabe. Clonidine overdose: a review. Am. J. Hosp. Pharm. 36: 906–911, 1979.

L.C. Chu, W.F. Bayne, F.T. Tao et al. Determination of submicrogram quantities of clonidine in biological fluids. J. Pharm. Sci. 68: 72–74, 1979.

S. Darda, H.J. Foerster and H. Staehle. Metabolischer Abbau von Clonidin. Arz. Forsch. 28: 255–259, 1978.

D.S. Davies, L.M.H. Wing, J.L. Reid et al. Pharmacokinetics and concentration-effect relationships of intravenous and oral clonidine. Clin. Pharm. Ther. 21: 593–601, 1977.

C.T. Dollery, D.S. Davies, G.H. Draffan et al. Clinical pharmacology and pharmacokinetics of clonidine. Clin. Pharm. Ther. 19: 11–17, 1976.

L.E. Domino, S.E. Domino and M.S. Stockstill. Relationship between plasma concentrations of clonidine and mean arterial pressure during an accidental clonidine overdose. Brit. J. Clin. Pharm. 21: 71–74, 1986.

G.H. Draffan, R.A. Clare, S. Murray et al. The determination of clonidine in human plasma. In *Advances in Mass Spectrometry in Biochemistry and Medicine*, Vol. II (A. Frigerio, ed.), Spectrum Publications, New York, 1977, pp. 389–394.

P.O. Edlund. Determination of clonidine in human plasma by glass capillary gas chromatography with electron-capture detection. J. Chrom. 187: 161–169, 1980.

N. Haring, Z. Salama, G. Reif and H. Jaeger. Gas chromatographic/mass spectrometric determination of clonidine in body fluids. Arz. Forsch. 38: 404–407, 1988.

A. Keranen, S. Nykanen and J. Taskinen. Pharmacokinetics and side-effects of clonidine. Eur. J. Pharm. 13: 97–101, 1978.

I. Lukkari. Personal communication, 1983.

P.M. Mathew, D.P. Addy and N. Wright. Clonidine overdose in children. Clin. Tox. 18: 169–173, 1981.

M.A. Moore and P. Phillipi. Clonidine overdose. Lancet 2: 694, 1976.

S. Murray, K.A. Waddell and D.S. Davies. The measurement of clonidine in human plasma and urine by combined gas chromatography mass spectrometry with ammonia chemical ionization. Biomed. Mass Spec. 8: 500–502, 1981.

A.J. Nazarali, G.B. Baker and D.P. Boisvert. Analysis of clonidine in biological tissues and body fluids by gas chromatography with electron-capture detection. J. Chrom. 380: 393–400, 1986.

P.J. Neuvonen, J. Vilska and A. Keranen. Severe poisoning in a child caused by a small dose of clonidine. Clin. Tox. 14: 369–374, 1979.

D. Rehbinder and W. Deckers. Untersuchungen zur Pharmakokinetik und zum Metabolismus des 2-(2,6-Dichlorphenylamino)-2-imidazolin-hydro chlorid (St 155). Arz. Forsch. 19: 169–175, 1969.

M.T. Velasquez, J. Rho, R.F. Maronde and J. Barr. Plasma clonidine levels in hypertension. Clin. Pharm. Ther. 34: 341–346, 1983.

G.S. Wasserman, T.T. Mydler and W.A. Watson. Pediatric clonidine levels and toxicity. Vet. Hum. Tox. 34: 335, 1992.

L.M.H. Wing, J.L. Reid, D.S. Davies et al. Pharmacokinetic and concentration-effect relationships of clonidine in essential hypertension. Eur. J. Clin. Pharm. 12: 463–469, 1977.

Clorazepate

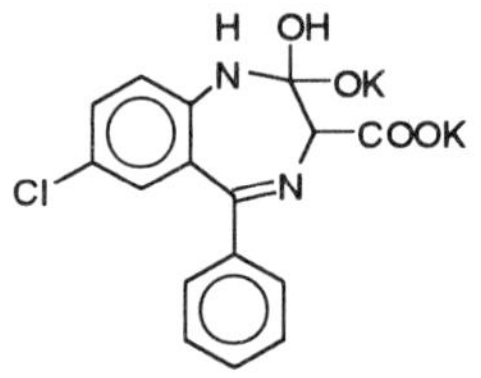

T½: 2 hr (clorazepate)
    31–97 hr (nordiazepam)
Vd: 1.1–1.7 L/kg
Fb: 0.97 (nordiazepam)
pKa: 3.5, 12.5

Occurrence and Usage. Clorazepate (Tranxene) was synthesized in 1969 and was first made available for clinical use in 1972. It is produced commercially as the dipotassium salt for oral use in tablets of 3.75–22.5 mg. Daily doses may range from 15–60 mg. The compound degrades rapidly in the acid environment of the stomach to nordiazepam, the predominant species in plasma after clorazepate administration.

Blood Concentrations. Following a single oral 15 mg dose given to volunteers, peak blood concentrations of nordiazepam averaging 0.16 mg/L were observed at 2 hours, while peak clorazepate concentrations averaging 0.02 mg/L occurred at 0.5 hours (Brooks et al., 1977). During chronic daily therapy with 22.5 mg of the drug, an average steady-state plasma nordiazepam concentration of 0.64 mg/L was attained; the half-life of nordiazepam was found to average 48 hours (Carrigan et al., 1977). Chronic daily therapy with 50 mg of clorazepate produced average steady-state plasma levels of nordiazepam averaging 1.59 mg/L (range, 1.21–2.64) in 8 psychiatric patients (Bertler et al., 1980).

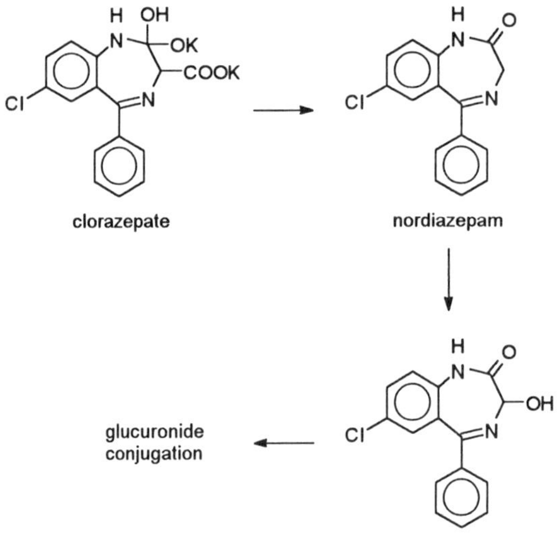

clorazepate

nordiazepam

glucuronide
conjugation

oxazepam

Metabolism and Excretion. Clorazepate is relatively stable at a pH of 7.4 or above, even in whole blood, but is decarboxylated rapidly to nordiazepam below pH 4 (Abruzzo et al., 1976). Thus, when administered orally the drug is absorbed largely as nordiazepam, its active form. Nordiazepam undergoes hydroxylation to oxazepam, which is subsequently conjugated with glucuronic acid. From 2–6% of a dose may be eliminated in the urine as unchanged clorazepate, 1% as nordiazepam and most of the remainder as oxazepam glucuronide, which is still detectable in urine 12 days after administration (Raveaux and Gros, 1969; Brooks et al., 1977).

Toxicity. Clorazepate produces symptoms of central nervous system depression in overdosage. No cases of poisoning with the drug have been reported.

Analysis. Since the primary physiologic form of clorazepate is nordiazepam, it is sufficient for most purposes to measure only the latter compound using established methods (see diazepam). However, procedures have been described for the determination of both drugs; these usually involve extraction of the nordiazepam from alkaline solution, acidification of the sample to decarboxylate clorazepate, readjustment of the pH and a second extraction of the clorazepate-derived nordiazepam (Viala et al., 1971; Hoffman and Chun, 1975; Brooks et al., 1977). The two extracts may then be analyzed by flame-ionization or electron-capture gas chromatography. The latter technique has been utilized in methods designed specifically for nordiazepam (Greenblatt, 1978; Haidukewych et al., 1980). Liquid chromatographic methods have also been described (Bertler et al., 1980; Colin et al., 1983).

References

C.W. Abruzzo, M.A. Brooks, S. Cotler and S.A. Kaplan. Differential pulse polarographic assay procedure and *in vitro* biopharmaceutical properties of dipotassium clorazepate. J. Pharm. Biopharm. 4: 29–41, 1976.

A. Bertler, S. Lindgren and H. Malmgren. Pharmacokinetics of dipotassium clorazepate in patients after repeated 50 mg oral doses. Psychopharmacology 71: 165–167, 1980.

M.A. Brooks, M.R. Hackman, R.E. Weinfeld and T. Macasieb. Determination of clorazepate and its major metabolites in blood and urine by electron capture gas-liquid chromatography. J. Chrom. 135: 123–131, 1977.

P.J. Carrigan, G.C. Chao, W.M. Barker et al. Steady-state bioavailability of two clorazepate dipotassium dosage forms. J. Clin. Pharm. 17: 18–28, 1977.

P. Colin, G. Sirois and J. Lelorier. High-performance liquid chromatography determination of dipotassium clorazepate and its major metabolite nordiazepam in plasma. J. Chrom. 273: 367–377, 1983.

D.J. Greenblatt. Determination of desmethyldiazepam in plasma by electron-capture GLC: application to pharmacokinetic studies of clorazepate. J. Pharm. Sci. 67: 427–429, 1978.

D. Haidukewych, E.A. Rodin and R. Davenport. Monitoring clorazepate dipotassium as desmethyldiazepam in plasma by electron-capture gas-liquid chromatography. Clin. Chem. 26: 142–133, 1980.

D.J. Hoffman and A.H.C. Chun. GLC determination of plasma drug levels after oral administration of clorazepate potassium salts. J. Pharm. Sci. 64: 1668–1671, 1975.

R. Raveaux and P. Gros. Etude de l'excretion du clorazepate dipotassique et de ses metabolites urinaires. Chim. Ther. 4: 481–487, 1969.

A. Viala, J.P. Cano and A. Angeletti-Philippe. Recherche toxicologique des benzodiazepines dans le sang et l'urine. Eur. J. Tox. 3: 197, 1971.

Clozapine

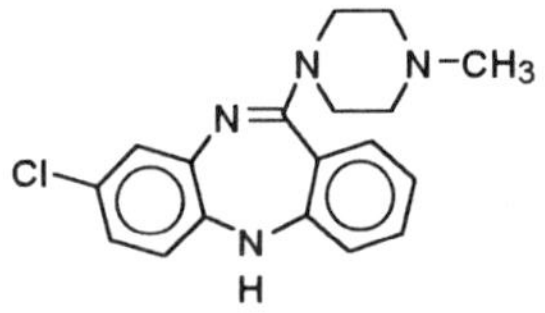

T½: 4.5–7.5 hr
Vd: 5 L/kg
Fb: 0.95
pKa: ?

Occurrence and Usage. Clozapine (Clozaril, Leponex) is an antipsychotic drug available in the U.S. since 1989 for the treatment of severely ill schizophrenic patients who do not respond to standard antipsychotic drug treatment. Due to the significant risk of agranulocytosis, the drug is available only through a distribution system that ensures weekly hematological monitoring. Clozapine is available in tablets of 25 and 100 mg as the free base for oral administration. It is recommended that therapy begin with doses of 12.5 mg once or twice a day, with a gradual increase to 300–450 mg/day by the end of 2 weeks.

Blood Concentrations. A single 100 mg dose given to 12 patients resulted in an average peak plasma clozapine level of 0.14 mg/L (range, 0.07–0.34) after 1.5 hours (Ackenheil, 1989). Plasma clozapine concentrations after the usual clinical doses range from 0.06–1.0 mg/L, with average levels of about 0.2–0.4 mg/L (Choc et al., 1987; Cheng et al., 1988; Ackenheil, 1989; Haring, 1989). In a study involving patients given an average dose of 384 mg/day, the patients who did not improve after weeks of therapy usually had a blood clozapine concentration less than 0.35 mg/L, whereas responders had a blood concentration greater than 0.35 mg/L (Perry et al., 1991). In 25 patients on chronic therapy with the drug at an average daily dose of 3.1 mg/kg (217 mg/70 kg), steady-state plasma levels averaged 0.23 mg/L for clozapine, 0.19 mg/L for norclozapine, and 0.05 mg/L for clozapine-N-oxide (Volpicelli et al., 1993).

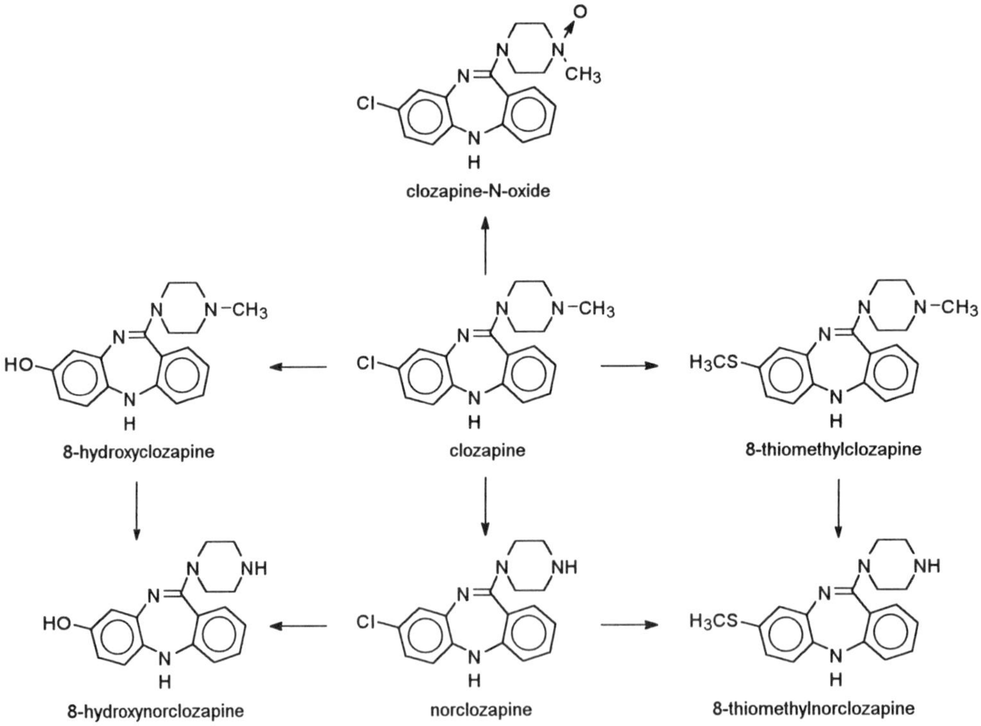

clozapine-N-oxide

8-hydroxyclozapine · clozapine · 8-thiomethylclozapine

8-hydroxynorclozapine · norclozapine · 8-thiomethylnorclozapine

Metabolism and Excretion. Clozapine is almost completely metabolized prior to excretion, undergoing N-demethylation, N-oxidation, oxidation of the chlorine-containing ring and thiomethyl conjugation (Schmutz and Eichenberger, 1982). At least 80% of the dose appears in the urine or feces as metabolites; the 2 major plasma metabolites, norclozapine and clozapine-N-oxide, are not believed to have significant pharmacological activity (Ackenheil, 1989).

Toxicity. Adverse reactions to chronic therapy with clozapine have involved hematologic disorders and tardive dyskinesia. Acute overdosage can cause hypotension, cardiac arrhythmias, respiratory depression, coma and death. Two adult patients who developed seizures after accidental overdoses with clozapine exhibited plasma levels of 1.3 and 2.2 mg/L (Simpson and Cooper, 1978). In a nonfatal suicidal attempt in which the subject ingested 2250 mg of clozapine, a blood clozapine concentration of 2.9 mg/L was determined 2.5 hours after ingestion, when the patient was somnolent yet agitated (Wolf and Otten, 1991).

In 2 deaths attributed to clozapine intoxication, a blood clozapine concentration of 4.5 mg/L was found in one, and a plasma clozapine concentration of 3.2 mg/L in the other (Vesterby et al., 1980). The following concentrations were measured postmortem in 3 adult patients following intentional overdosage; one case involved the ingestion of 2000 mg of drug (Meeker et al., 1992; Osciewicz, 1992; Sidebotham, 1992):

Clozapine Concentrations in Fatal Cases (mg/L or mg/kg)

	Blood	Brain	Liver	Urine	Gastric
Average	4.8	7.5	48	11	20 mg
(Range)	(1.6–7.1)	(7.5)	(19–82)	(11)	(1.1–54)

Analysis. Clozapine can be determined in biological specimens by gas chromatography employing nitrogen-selective detection (Heipertz et al., 1977) and by liquid chromatography (Haring et al., 1988; Humpel et al., 1989; Lovdahl et al., 1991; Weigmann and Heimke, 1992; Chung et al., 1993; Volpicelli et al., 1993). Gas chromatography-mass spectrometry offers a sensitive and specific method for the analysis of clozapine and its metabolites in biological samples (Bondesson and Lindstrom, 1988).

References

M. Ackenheil. Clozapine-pharmacokinetic investigations and biochemical effects in man. Psychopharmacology 99: S32–S37, 1989.

U. Bondesson and L.H. Lindstrom. Determination of clozapine and its N-demethylated metabolite in plasma by use of gas chromatography-mass spectrometry with single ion detection. Psychopharmacology 95: 472–475, 1988.

Y.F. Cheng, T. Lundberg, U. Bondesson et al. Clinical pharmacokinetics of clozapine in chronic schizophrenic patients. Eur. J. Clin. Pharm. 34: 445–449, 1988.

M.G. Choc, R.G. Lehr, F. Hsuan et al. Multiple-dose pharmacokinetics of clozapine in patients. Pharm. Res. 4: 402–405, 1987.

M.C. Chung, S.K. Lin, W.H. Chang and M.W. Jann. Determination of clozapine and desmethylclozapine in human plasma by high performance liquid chromatography with ultraviolet detection. J. Chrom. 613: 168–173, 1993.

C. Haring, C. Humpel, B. Auer et al. Clozapine plasma levels determined by HPLC and UV-detection. J. Chrom. 428: 160–166, 1988.

C. Haring, U. Meise, C. Humpel et al. Dose-related plasma levels of clozapine: influence of smoking behavior, sex, and age. Psychopharmacology 99: S38–S40, 1989.

R. Heipertz, H. Pilz and W. Beckers. Serum concentrations of clozapine determined by nitrogen selective gas chromatography. Arch. Tox. 37: 313–318, 1977.

C. Humpel, C. Haring and A. Saria. Rapid and sensitive determination of clozapine using high-performance liquid chromatography and amperometric detection. J. Chrom. 491: 235–239, 1989.

M.J. Lovdahl, P.J. Perry and D.D. Miller. The assay of clozapine and N-desmethylclozapine in human plasma by high-performance liquid chromatography. Ther. Drug Mon. 13: 69–72, 1991.

J.E. Meeker, P.W. Herrmann, C.W. Som and P.C. Reyno'ds. Clozapine tissue concentrations following an apparent suicidal overdose of Clozaril. J. Anal. Tox. 16: 54–56, 1992.

R. Osciewicz. Personal communication, 1992.

P.J. Perry, D. Miller, S.V.Arndt and R. Cadoret. Clozapine and norclozapine concentrations and clinical response treatment refractory schizophrenic patients. Am. J. Psych. 148: 231–235, 1991.

J. Schmutz and E. Eishenberger. Clozapine. In *Chronicles in Drug Discovery* (J.S. Bindra and D. Lednicer, eds.), Vol I, John Wiley, New York, 1982, pp. 39–59.

C. Sidebotham. Personal communication, 1991.

G.M. Simpson and T.A. Cooper. Clozapine plasma levels and convulsions. Am. J. Psych. 135: 99–100, 1978.

A. Vesterby, J.H. Pederdon, B. Kaempe and N.J. Thomsen. Sudden death during clozapine (Leponex) therapy. Ugeskr. Laeg. 142: 170–171, 1980.

A.A. Volpicelli, F. Centerrino, P.R. Pupopolo et al. Determination of clozapine, norclozapine, and clozapine-N-oxide in serum by liquid chromatography. Clin. Chem. 39: 1656–1658, 1993.

H. Weigmann and C. Heimke. Determination of clozapine and its major metabolites in human serum using automated solid-phase extraction and subsequent isocratic high performance liquid chromatography with ultraviolet detection. J. Chrom. 583: 209–216, 1992.

L.R. Wolf and E.J. Otten. A case report of clozapine overdose. Vet. Hum. Tox. 33: 370, 1991.

Cobalt

T½: ?
Vd: ?   Co
Fb: ?

Occurrence and Usage. Cobalt is an essential element for man and is supplied in the diet at an average intake of 280 µg/day. Cobalt as the metal is incorporated into certain grades of steel and into tungsten carbide tools. Compounds of cobalt are used as paint pigments and occasionally as therapeutic agents. Industrial exposure is normally via inhalation of dusts or fumes while working with cobalt-containing tools or alloys. The current threshold limit value for cobalt in air is 0.05 mg/m³, although revision of this limit to 0.02 mg/m³ is pending.

Blood Concentrations. Serum cobalt concentrations in normal subjects average 0.11 µg/L and range from 0.04–0.27 µg/L (Versieck et al., 1978). Blood cobalt concentrations reached a peak of approximately 30 µg/L in 2 normal subjects after the oral administration of 50 mg of cobaltous chloride; blood cobalt concentrations in untreated subjects in this study were 0.6–1.8 µg/L. Peak blood levels in maintenance hemodialysis patients undergoing daily oral treatment with 50 mg cobaltous chloride for 2 weeks were as high as 800 µg/L, and did not return to normal levels until 6 months following discontinuation of therapy. Toxicity in these patients was primarily limited to nausea and vomiting, although one patient later died due to suspected cobalt cardiomyopathy (Curtis et al., 1976).

Metabolism and Excretion. Of the cobalt that is ingested in the daily diet, about 86% is excreted in the urine and 14% in the feces (Schroeder et al., 1967). In normal subjects, an average of 18% of an oral dose of radioactive cobalt was eliminated in the 24 hour urine (Sorbie et al., 1971). Normal urine cobalt levels average 0.4 µg/L (Scansetti et al., 1985) and generally do not exceed 1.0 µg/L (Bouman et al., 1986). Cobalt excretion in the 24 hour urine of 2 normal subjects after an oral dose of 50 mg of cobaltous chloride reached a maximum of 500–750 µg during the first day, and fell markedly thereafter (Curtis et al., 1976). Cobalt liver and kidney concentrations in Japanese citizens were found to average 0.06 and 0.01 mg/kg, respectively (Yukawa et al., 1980).

Toxicity. Exposure to cobalt or its compounds has produced an allergic dermatitis in workers. Chronic inhalation of cobalt may result in pulmonary fibrosis, accompanied by cough and dyspnea (Bech et al., 1962). Cobalt accumulates in the serum of uremic patients and is believed to contribute to the myocardial failure often observed (Lins and Pehrsson, 1976). The metal has also been implicated in heart disease and polycythemia seen in chronic beer drinkers, at a time when cobalt was a common beer additive (Kesteloot et al., 1968).

Cobalt was qualitatively identified in a lung biopsy specimen containing metallic granules, taken from an industrial worker with a history of pulmonary fibrosis (Siegesmund et al., 1974). The following cobalt concentrations were measured in the tissues of a 41 year old metal worker with 4 years exposure to cobalt who died of cardiomyopathy; concentrations from a control case (cor pulmonale death) are included for comparison (Barborik and Dusek, 1972):

Cobalt Concentrations in Human Tissues (mg/kg)

Cause of Death	Heart	Lung	Liver	Kidney
Cardiomyopathy	0.37	0.17	0.34	0.29
Cor pulmonale	0.02	0.03	0.03	0.01

Analysis. Cobalt has been measured in biological specimens by colorimetry (Hubbard et al., 1966) and atomic absorption spectrometry (Lidums, 1979; Barfoot and Pritchard, 1980; Schumacher-Wittkopf and Angerer, 1981; Bouman et al., 1986).

References

M. Barborik and J. Dusek. Cardiomyopathy accompanying industrial cobalt exposure. Brit. Heart J. 34: 113–116, 1972.

B.A. Barfoot and J.G. Pritchard. Determination of cobalt in blood. Analyst 105: 551–557, 1980.

A.O. Bech, M.D. Kipling and J.C. Heather. Hard metal disease. Brit. J. Ind. Med. 19: 239–252, 1962.

A.A. Bouman, A.J. Platenkamp and F.D. Posma. Determination of cobalt in urine by flameless atomic absorption spectroscopy. Ann. Clin. Biochem. 23: 346–350, 1986.

J.R. Curtis, G.C. Goode, J. Herrington and L.E. Urdaneta. Possible cobalt toxicity in maintenance hemodialysis patients after treatment with cobaltous chloride: a study of blood and tissue cobalt concentrations in normal subjects and patients with terminal renal failure. Clin. Neph. 5: 61–65, 1976.

D.M. Hubbard, F.M. Creech and J. Cholak. Determination of cobalt in air and biological material. Arch. Env. Health 13: 190–194, 1966.

H. Kesteloot, J. Roelandt, J. Willems et al. An enquiry into the role of cobalt in the heart disease of chronic beer drinkers. Circulation 37: 854–864, 1968.

V.V. Lidums. Determination of cobalt in blood and urine by electrothermal atomic absorption spectrometry. At. Abs. Newsl. 18: 71–72, 1979.

L.E. Lins and K. Pehrsson. Cobalt intoxication in uraemic myocardiopathy? Lancet 1: 1191–1192, 1976.

G. Scansetti, S. Lamon, S. Talarico et al. Urinary cobalt as a measure of exposure in the hard metal industry. Int. Arch. Occ. Env. Health 57: 19–26, 1985.

H.A. Schroeder, A.P. Nason and I.H. Tipton. Essential trace elements in man: cobalt. J. Chron. Dis. 20: 869–890, 1967.

E. Schumaker-Wittkopf and J. Angerer. Praxisgerechte Methode zur Kobaltbestimmung in Harn. Int. Arch. Occ. Env. Health 49: 77–81, 1981.

K.A. Siegesmund, A. Funahashi and K. Pintar. Identification of metals in lung from a patient with interstitial pneumonia. Arch. Env. Health 28: 345–349, 1974.

J. Sorbie, D. Olatunbosun, W.E.N. Corbett and L.S. Valberg. Cobalt excretion test for the assessment of body iron stores. Can. Med. Asso. J. 104: 777–782, 1971.

J. Versieck, J. Hoste, F. Barbier et al. Determination of chromium and cobalt in human serum by neutron activation analysis. Clin. Chem. 24: 303–308, 1978.

M. Yukawa, K. Amano, M. Suzuki-Yasumoto and M. Terai. Distribution of trace elements in the human body determined by neutron activation analysis. Arch. Env. Health 35: 36–44, 1980.

Cocaine

T½: 0.7–1.5 hr
Vd: 1.6–2.7 L/kg
Fb: 0.92
pKa: 8.6

Occurrence and Usage. Cocaine is one of the most potent of the naturally-occurring central nervous system stimulants. The compound is found in the leaves of *Erythroxylon coca*, a South American shrub, in amounts of up to 2% by weight. It was first isolated in pure form in 1855, and has been widely utilized in medicine as a local anesthetic and increasingly by drug abusers for its stimulant properties. For anesthetic uses, cocaine is administered topically as the hydrochloride in 1–4% solutions for ophthalmological procedures and in 10–20% solutions for the membranes of the nose and throat. When self-administered, it is commonly taken as the hydrochloride by nasal insufflation or intravenous injection or as the free base by smoking, in doses of 10–120 mg.

Blood Concentrations. The chewing of powdered coca leaves containing 17–48 mg of cocaine produced peak plasma cocaine concentrations of 0.011–0.149 mg/L within 0.4–2 hours in 6 volunteers (Holmstedt et al., 1979). A 2 mg/kg (140 mg/70 kg) intranasal application of cocaine to 4 subjects yielded an average peak plasma concentration of 0.161 mg/L after 1 hour; an equivalent oral dose given to the same volunteers produced an average peak concentration of 0.210 mg/L at 1 hour, declining with an average half-life of 0.9 hour (Van Dyke et al., 1978). The intravenous injection of 32 mg of cocaine resulted in an average peak plasma concentration of 0.308 mg/L after 5 minutes (Javaid et al., 1978). Following the nasal topical application of 1.5 mg/kg (105 mg/70 kg) of cocaine to surgical patients, plasma concentration of the drug reached an average peak of 0.308 mg/L (range, 0.120–0.474) at 1 hour and declined to 0.206 mg/L by 3 hours (Van Dyke et al., 1976). Nasal insufflation of 106 mg of the drug by 6 subjects produced average peak plasma concentrations of 0.220 mg/L for cocaine at 0.5 hour and 0.611 mg/L for benzoylecgonine at 3.0 hours. Smoking of 50 mg of the drug in 6 subjects resulted in average peak plasma concentrations of 0.203 mg/L for cocaine at 0.08 hour and 0.151 mg/L for benzoylecgonine at 1.5 hours. The blood/plasma concentration ratio for cocaine averages 1.0 (Jeffcoat et al., 1989).

Chronic cocaine abusers given free access to cigarettes containing 75 mg each of cocaine paste developed and maintained plasma concentrations of 0.253–0.932 mg/L over a 90 minute smoking period, during which they smoked 8–10 cigarettes (Paly et al., 1982).

Metabolism and Excretion. Cocaine is rapidly inactivated in man by the hydrolysis of one or both of the ester linkages. Even in water, at pH values greater than neutrality, the drug is readily hydrolyzed to benzoylecgonine. In blood or plasma, cocaine is hydrolyzed to ecgonine methyl ester by cholinesterase; the reaction rate is highly dependent on drug concentrations and may be inhibited by freezing or by the addition of fluoride or cholinesterase inhibitors (Stewart et al., 1977). With storage at 4° C., blood containing 1 mg/L of cocaine lost 100% of the drug in 21 days, whereas with 0.5% sodium fluoride 70% of the cocaine was still intact (Baselt, 1983). A similar rate of decline was observed in stored postmortem tissues (Price, 1974). Benzoylecgonine and ecgonine methyl ester are relatively stable in fluoridated whole blood for 1 month at 4° C., but exhibit losses of 25% and 50%, respectively, when stored at 25° C. (Isenschmid et al., 1989).

Benzoylecgonine is believed to arise spontaneously *in vivo*, since neither liver nor serum esterases produce this compound from cocaine. The further production of ecgonine from benzoylecgonine, however, may be the result of enzymatic hydrolysis (Stewart et al., 1979). Each of these metabolites is highly polar and, when formed outside the central nervous system, is without pharmacological activity (Misra et al., 1975). Norcocaine, an active metabolite, has not been detected in plasma after therapeutic administration but is found in trace amounts in urine (Jatlow and Bailey, 1975; Mule et al., 1976; Jindal et al., 1978). Phenolic hydroxylation has been shown to produce a series of minor cocaine metabolites in man (Smith, 1984). Ecgonidine, methylecgonidine and methylnorecgonidine have also been reported as minor metabolites (Lowry et al., 1979; Zhang and Foltz, 1990). Cocaethylene, a substance formed when cocaine and ethanol are coadministered, is pharmacologically active and accounts for 0.7% of a cocaine dose in the 24 hour urine (Jatlow et al., 1991; de la Torre et al., 1991).

Cocaine is eliminated in the urine primarily as unchanged drug (1–9%, dependent on urine pH), benzoylecgonine (35–54%), ecgonine methyl ester (32–49%), and ecgonine (not quantitated) in a 24 hour period (Fish and Wilson, 1969; Inaba et al., 1978). After a 1.5 mg/kg intranasal application, cocaine concentrations in urine averaged 6.7 mg/L during the first hour and declined rapidly to undetectable levels by 12 hours; benzoylecgonine urine concentrations reached an average peak of 35 mg/L during the 4–8 hour period and diminished slowly to an average of 0.4 mg/L for the 48–72 hour collection period (Hamilton et al., 1977). In a similar study involving 2 subjects, ecgonine methyl ester concentrations peaked at 29–36 mg/L during the 0–8 hour period and declined rapidly to 0.1–0.2 mg/L for the 24–48 hour period (Ambre et al., 1984). Elimination half-lives based on urinary excretion data were found to average 0.8 hour for cocaine, 4.5 hours for benzoylecgonine and 3.1 hours for ecgonine methyl ester (Ambre et al., 1988).

Urinary benzoylecgonine concentrations as high as 0.06 mg/L were observed at 48 hours after dermal application of 5 mg of cocaine in a volunteer (Baselt et al., 1990) and as high as 0.07 mg/L within 13 hours in a subject who handled cocaine-contaminated paper currency (ElSohly, 1991). A 1 hour exposure to 200 mg of vaporized cocaine in an unventilated space has produced a urine benzoylecgonine concentration of 0.13 mg/L after 4–8 hours (Cone et al., 1993). Crime lab personnel who work closely with confiscated drugs may develop urinary benzoylecgonine levels as high as 1.6 mg/L (Le et al., 1992).

Drinking 1 cup of herbal tea containing 2.2 mg cocaine produced a peak urine benzoylecgonine concentration of 1.3 mg/L in a subject after 2 hours, declining to 0.1 mg/L by 29 hours (ElSohly et al., 1986). The oral ingestion of 25 mg of cocaine by a volunteer resulted in a peak urine benzoylecgonine level of 7.9 mg/L in the 6–12 hour collection period, with a decline to 0.4 mg/L by 48 hours (Baselt and Chang, 1987).

Toxicity. Overdosage with cocaine has resulted in a relatively small number of serious intoxications, considering its popularity as a recreational drug. The symptoms of acute toxicity are similar to those for amphetamine, although it is believed that a direct cardiotoxic effect may be a contributory factor in cocaine-induced deaths. Myocardial infarction, ventricular tachycardia and fibrillation, cerebrovascular accident and pulmonary dysfunction may occur with acute or chronic abuse and even with medical usage (Itkonen et al., 1984; Chiu et al., 1986; Cregler and Mark, 1986; Isner et al., 1986). Control of seizure activity with diazepam, correction of acidosis to stabilize heart rhythm and administration of a calcium-channel blocker such as nitrendipine have been recommended as treatment for acute toxic reactions (Jonsson et al., 1983; Nahas et al., 1985). One case was reported in which the unintentional rupture in the stomach of a 5 g packet of cocaine produced unconsciousness and massive convulsions; a maximal blood concentration of 5.2 mg/L was observed, but with treatment the patient survived (Suarez et al., 1977).

Cocaine concentrations observed in the tissues of victims who succumb to the drug vary greatly depending on the dosage, route of administration, period of survival and manner of storage of the specimens. Intense paranoia, bizarre and violent behavior, hyperthermia, and sudden collapse were observed in seven individuals, whose postmortem blood cocaine concentrations averaged 0.6 mg/L (range, 0.1–0.9) (Wetli and Fishbain, 1985). Blood cocaine and benzoylecgonine concentrations in 37 cocaine-related fatalities averaged 4.6 mg/L (range, 0.04–31) and 7.9 mg/L (range, 0.7–31), respectively (Spiehler and Reed, 1985). Postmortem blood concentrations averaged 3.0 mg/L in those who administered the drug intravenously, 4.4 mg/L in those practicing insufflation, and 9.2 mg/L in victims of oral overdosage (Wetli and Wright, 1979). The usually high blood cocaine concentrations of 52 and 211 mg/L were reported in 2 victims of acute massive oral overdosage (Amon et al., 1986; Winek et al., 1987). The following data summarize the analytical results of 19 fatal cases that occurred after the ingestion, inhalation or injection of from 160 mg (intravenously) to as much as 26 g (orally) of cocaine (McCurdy and Jones , 1973; Price, 1974; Griffin, 1975; Gottschalk, 1977; Lundberg et al., 1977; Prouty, 1977; Di Maio and Garriott, 1978; Bednarczyk et al., 1980; Poklis et al., 1985):

Cocaine Concentrations in Fatalities (mg/L or mg/kg)

	Blood	Brain	Liver	Kidney	Urine
Average	5.3	5.3	4.2	13	42
(Range)	(0.9–21)	(0.4–15)	(0.1–20)	(0.3–27)	(0.1–215)

Postmortem heart blood may exhibit cocaine concentrations that are 1.5–3.2 times higher than those in peripheral venous blood specimens (Hearn et al., 1991).

Analysis. Gas chromatographic techniques for the analysis of cocaine and its metabolites in urine require derivatization of the polar metabolites and have used flame-ionization, electron-capture or nitrogen-phosphorus detection (Javaid et al., 1975; Wallace et al., 1976; Jain et al., 1977; Kogan et al., 1977; von Minden and D'Amato, 1977; Ortuno et al., 1990). Gas chromatography-mass spectrometry is the method of choice for many analysts (Isenschmid et al., 1988; Hime et al., 1991; Corburt and Koves, 1994). Liquid chromatographic techniques have also been reported (Masoud and Krupski, 1980; Miller and DeVane, 1991; Rop et al., 1993). Immunoassay methods are commercially available for the qualitative detection of benzoylecgonine in urine.

References

J. Ambre, M. Fischman and T.I. Ruo. Urinary excretion of ecgonine methyl ester, a major metabolite of cocaine in humans. J. Anal. Tox. 8: 23–25, 1984.

J. Ambre, T.I. Ruo, J. Nelson and S. Belknap. Urinary excretion of cocaine, benzoylecgonine, and ecgonine methyl ester in humans. J. Anal. Tox. 12: 301–306, 1988.

C.A. Amon, L.G. Tate, R.K. Wright and W. Matusiak. Sudden death due to ingestion of cocaine. J. Anal. Tox. 10: 217–218, 1986.

R.C. Baselt. Stability of cocaine in biological fluids. J. Chrom. 268: 502–505, 1983.

R.C. Baselt and R. Chang. Urinary excretion of cocaine and benzoylecgonine following oral ingestion in a single subject. J. Anal. Tox. 11: 81–82, 1987.

R.C. Baselt, J.Y. Chang and D.M. Yoshikawa. On the dermal absorption of cocaine. J. Anal. Tox. 14: 383–384, 1990.

L.R. Bednarczyk, E.A. Gressmann and R.L. Wymer. Two cocaine-induced fatalities. J. Anal. Tox. 4: 263–265, 1980.

Y.C. Chiu, K. Brecht, D.S. DasGupta and E. Mhoon. Myocardial infarction with topical cocaine anesthesia for nasal surgery. Arch. Otolaryn. Head Neck Surg. 112: 988–990, 1986.

E.J. Cone, W.D. Darwin, R.Willis and M. Hillsgrove. Paper presented at the annual meeting of the Society of Forensic Toxicologists, Phoenix, Arizona, October 15, 1993.

M.R. Corburt and E.M. Koves. Gas chromatography-mass spectrometry for the determination of cocaine and benzoylecgonine in postmortem blood. J. For. Sci. 39: 136–149, 1994.

L.L. Cregler and H. Mark. Cardiovascular dangers of cocaine abuse. Am. J. Cardiol. 57: 1185–1186, 1986.

R. de la Torre, M. Farre, J. Ortuno et al. The relevance of urinary cocaethylene following the simultaneous administration of alcohol and cocaine. J. Anal. Tox. 15: 223, 1991.

V.J.M. Di Maio and J.C. Garriott. Four deaths due to intravenous injection of cocaine. For. Sci. Int. 12: 119–125, 1978.

M.A. ElSohly, D.F. Stanford and H.N. ElSohly. Coca tea and urinalysis for cocaine metabolites. J. Anal. Tox. 10: 256, 1986.

M.A. ElSohly. Urinalysis and casual handling of marijuana and cocaine. J. Anal. Tox. 15: 46, 1991.

F. Fish and W.D.C. Wilson. Excretion of cocaine and its metabolites in man. J. Pharm. Pharmac. 21: 135S–138S, 1969.

L.A. Gottschalk. Personal communication, 1977.

B.R. Griffin. Personal communication, 1975.

H.E. Hamilton, J.E. Wallace, E.L. Shimek, Jr. et al. Cocaine and benzoylecgonine excretion in humans. J. For. Sci. 22: 697–707, 1977.

W.L. Hearn, E.E. Keran, H. Wei and G. Hime. Site-dependent postmortem changes in blood cocaine concentrations. J. For. Sci. 36: 673–684, 1991.

G.W. Hime, W.L. Hearn, S. Rose and J. Cofino. Analysis of cocaine and cocaethylene in blood and tissues by GC-NPD and GC-ion trap mass spectrometry. J. Anal. Tox. 15: 241–245, 1991.

B. Holmstedt, J. Lindgren, L. Rivier and T. Plowman. Cocaine in blood of coca chewers. J. Ethnopharm. 1: 69–78, 1979.

T. Inaba, D.J. Stewart and W. Kalow. Metabolism of cocaine in man. Clin. Pharm. Ther. 23: 547–552, 1978.

D.S. Isenschmid, B.S. Levine and Y.H. Caplan. A method for the simultaneous determination of cocaine, benzoylecgonine, and ecgonine methyl ester in blood and urine using GC/EIMS with derivatization to produce high mass molecular ions. J. Anal. Tox. 12: 242–245, 1988.

D.S. Isenschmid, B.S. Levine and Y.H. Caplan. A comprehensive study of the stability of cocaine and its metabolites. J. Anal. Tox. 13: 250–256, 1989.

J.M. Isner, N.A.M. Esters, P.D. Thompson et al. Acute cardiac events temporally related to cocaine abuse. New Eng. J. Med. 315: 1438–1443, 1986.

J. Itkonen, S. Schnoll and J. Glassroth. Pulmonary dysfunction in 'freebase' cocaine users. Arch. Int. Med. 144: 2195–2197, 1984.

N.C. Jain, D.M. Chinn, R.D. Budd et al. Simultaneous determination of cocaine and benzoylecgonine in urine by gas chromatography with on-column alkylation. J. For. Sci. 22: 7–16, 1977.

P.I. Jatlow and D.N. Bailey. Gas-chromatographic analysis of cocaine in human plasma, with use of a nitrogen detector. Clin. Chem. 21: 1918–1921, 1975.

P. Jatlow, J.D. Elsworth, C.W. Bradberry et al. Cocaethylene: a neuropharmacologically active metabolite associated with concurrent cocaine-ethanol ingestion. Life Sci. 48: 1787–1794, 1991.

J.I. Javaid, H. Dekirmenjian, E.G. Brunngraber and J.M. Davis. Quantitative determination of cocaine and its metabolites benzoylecgonine and ecgonine by gas-liquid chromatography. J. Chrom. 110: 141–149, 1975.

J.I. Javaid, M.W. Fischman, C.R. Schuster et al. Cocaine plasma concentrations: relation to physiological and subjective effects in humans. Science 202: 227–228, 1978.

A.R. Jeffcoat, M. Perez-Reyes, J.M. Hill et al. Cocaine disposition in humans after intravenous injection, nasal insufflation (snorting), or smoking. Drug Met. Disp. 17: 153–159, 1989.

S.P. Jindal, T. Lutz and P. Vestergaard. Mass spectrometric determination of cocaine and its biologically active metabolite, norcocaine, in human urine. Biomed. Mass Spec. 5: 658–663, 1978.

S. Jonsson, M. O'Meara and J.B. Young. Acute cocaine poisoning. Am. J. Med. 75: 1061–1064, 1983.

M.J. Kogan, K.G. Verebey, A.C. DePace et al. Quantitative determination of benzoylecgonine and cocaine in human biofluids by gas-liquid chromatography. Anal. Chem. 49: 1965–1969, 1977.

S.D. Le, R.W. Taylor, D. Vidal et al. Occupational exposure to cocaine involving crime lab personnel. J. For. Sci. 37: 959–968, 1992.

W.T. Lowry, J.N. Lomonte, D. Hatchett and J.C. Garriott. Identification of two novel cocaine metabolites in bile by gas chromatography and gas chromatography/mass spectrometry. J. Anal. Tox. 3: 91–95, 1979.

G.D. Lundberg, J.C. Garriott, P.C. Reynolds et al. Cocaine-related death. J. For. Sci. 22: 402–408, 1977.

A.N. Masoud and D.M. Krupski. High-performance liquid chromatographic analysis of cocaine in human plasma. J. Anal. Tox. 4: 305–310, 1980.

H.H. McCurdy and J.K. Jones. Personal communication, 1973.

R.L. Miller and C.L. DeVane. Determination of cocaine, benzoylecgonine and ecgonine methyl ester in plasma by reversed-phase high-performance liquid chromatography. J. Chrom. 570: 412–418, 1991.

A.L. Misra, P.K. Nayak, R. Bloch and S.J. Mule. Estimation and disposition of (^{3}H) benzoylecgonine and pharmacological activity of some cocaine metabolites. J. Pharm. Pharmac. 27: 784–786, 1975.

S.J. Mule, G.A. Casella and A.L. Misra. Intracellular disposition of (^{3}H)-cocaine, (^{3}H)-norcocaine, (^{3}H)-benzoylecgonine and (^{3}H)-benzoylnorecgonine in the brain of rats. Life Sci. 19: 1585–1596, 1976.

G. Nahas, R. Trouve, J.F. Demus and M. von Sitbon. A calcium-channel blocker as antidote to the acute cardiac effects of cocaine intoxication. New Eng. J. Med. 313: 519, 1985.

J. Ortuno, R. de la Torre, J. Segura and J. Cami. Simultaneous detection in urine of cocaine and its main metabolites. J. Pharm. Biomed. Anal. 8: 911–914, 1990.

D. Paly, P. Jatlow, C. Van Dyke et al. Plasma cocaine concentrations during cocaine paste smoking. Life Sci. 30: 731–738, 1982.

A. Poklis, M.A. MacKell and M. Graham. Disposition of cocaine in fatal poisoning in man. J. Anal. Tox. 9: 227–229, 1985.

K.R. Price. Fatal cocaine poisoning. J. For. Sci. Soc. 14: 329–333, 1974.

R. Prouty. A unique cocaine fatality. Presented at the annual meeting of the American Academy of Forensic Sciences, San Diego, California, February 17, 1977.

P.P. Rop, F. Grimaldi, M. Bresson et al. Liquid chromatographic analysis of cocaine, benzoylecgonine, local anesthetic agents and some of their metabolites in biological fluids. J. Liq. Chrom. 16: 2797–2811, 1993.

R.M. Smith. Arylhydroxy metabolites of cocaine in the urine of cocaine users. J. Anal. Tox. 8: 35–37, 1984.

V.R. Spiehler and D. Reed. Brain concentrations of cocaine and benzoylecgonine in fatal cases. J. For. Sci. 30: 1003–1011, 1985.

D.J. Stewart, T. Inaba, B.K. Tang and W. Kalow. Hydrolysis of cocaine in human plasma by cholinesterase. Life Sci. 20: 1557–1564, 1977.

D.J. Stewart, I. Inaba, M. Lucassen and W. Kalow. Cocaine metabolism: cocaine and norcocaine hydrolysis by liver and serum esterases. Clin. Pharm. Ther. 25: 464–468, 1979.

C.A. Suarez, A. Arango and J. Lancelot. Cocaine-condom ingestion. J. Am. Med. Asso. 238: 1391–1392, 1977.

C. Van Dyke, P.G. Barash, P. Jatlow and R. Byck. Cocaine: plasma concentrations after intranasal application in man. Science 191: 859–861, 1976.

C. Van Dyke, P. Jatlow, J. Ungerer et al. Oral cocaine: plasma concentrations and central effects. Science 200: 211–213, 1978.

D.L. von Minden and N.A. D'Amato. Simultaneous determination of cocaine and benzoylecgonine in urine by gas-liquid chromatography. Anal. Chem. 49: 1974–1977, 1977.

J.E. Wallace, H.E. Hamilton, D.E. King et al. Gas-liquid chromatographic determination of cocaine and benzoylecgonine in urine. Anal. Chem. 48: 34–38, 1976.

C.V. Wetli and R.K. Wright. Death caused by recreational cocaine use. J. Am. Med. Asso. 241: 2519–2522, 1979.

C.V. Wetli and D.P. Fishbain. Cocaine-induced psychosis and sudden death in recreational cocaine users. J. For. Sci. 30: 873–880, 1985.

C.L. Winek, W.W. Wahba, L. Rozin and J.K. Janssen. An unusually high blood cocaine concentration in a fatal case. J. Anal. Tox. 11: 43–46, 1987.

J.Y. Zhang and R.L. Foltz. Cocaine metabolism in man. J. Anal. Tox. 14: 201–205, 1990.

Codeine

T½: 1.9–3.9 hr
Vd: 3.5 L/kg
Fb: 0.07–0.25
pKa: 8.2

Occurrence and Usage. Codeine is a narcotic analgesic occurring naturally in opium, from which it was first isolated in 1832. It is usually produced commercially by 3-O-methylation of morphine, which is present in much higher concentrations in the juice of the poppy plant, *Papaver somniferum*. Like the other narcotic analgesics, codeine is a weak base and is levorotatory in its natural form. It is considered to be 1/10 to 1/6 as potent an analgesic in man on a weight basis, but is quite effective as an antitussive. The drug is available as the phosphate or sulfate salt; single doses of 15–60 mg are given orally or by subcutaneous injection, and the total daily dose may range from 60–240 mg. Codeine is also found in numerous proprietary preparations in combination with nonnarcotic analgesics, antihistamines, and other drugs.

Blood Concentrations. Codeine is evidently well-absorbed following either oral or intramuscular administration in man (Adler et al., 1955). An average peak serum concentration of 0.03 mg/L was obtained in two subjects 2 hours after the oral administration of 15 mg of codeine base (Schmerzler et al., 1966). When plasma sampling was first performed at 1 hour after an oral dose of 60 mg of codeine sulfate, this sample contained the highest concentration of codeine, about 0.11 mg/L, and subsequent samples showed a rapid decline of concentration. Norcodeine was not present in detectable concentrations in this study (Brunson and Nash, 1975). Codeine concentrations in 20 subjects after the oral administration of 60 mg of the drug (in combination with 600 mg of acetaminophen) reached an average peak of 0.134 mg/L at 1 hour, declining with an average half-life of 2.4 hours; plasma morphine concentrations reached an average peak of 0.007 mg/L at 1.5 hours (Findlay et al., 1978). Peak plasma codeine concentrations ranged from 0.195–0.340 mg/L (average, 0.264) within the first 15–60 minutes after an intramuscular injection of 65 mg of codeine phosphate (Findlay et al., 1977). The concentration of conjugated codeine in the plasma after oral dosing has been shown to exceed that of unconjugated drug by an average factor of 5.7 (Findlay et al., 1986).

Metabolism and Excretion. Codeine is biotransformed in man via O-demethylation to morphine and via N-demethylation to norcodeine. All 3 compounds are excreted in the urine as both free drugs and as glucuronide conjugates, with over 95% of a single dose eliminated in 48 hours (Bechtel and Sinterhauf, 1978). About 7% of Caucasians are deficient in the cytochrome p-450 enzyme needed to O-demethylate codeine to morphine (Quiding et al., 1993). The following amounts were found in the 24 hour urine samples of 3 subjects receiving an oral dose of 20–22 mg of codeine base, expressed as a percentage of the dose: 5–17% free codeine, 32–46% conjugated codeine, a trace of free norcodeine, 10–21% conjugated norcodeine, a trace of free morphine, and 5–13% conjugated morphine (Adler et al., 1955). One study has reported trace amounts (0.02% of a dose) of hydrocodone in human urine after codeine ingestion (Cone et al., 1979).

Norcodeine, which appears to be equipotent with codeine in its morphine-like effects in man (Fraser et al., 1960), has been reported in serum in only trace concentrations using a very sensitive mass fragmentography technique (Brunson and Nash, 1975). Morphine may be present in serum or plasma in amounts of up to 10% of the codeine concentration within 6–8 hours after a single oral dose of codeine (Findlay et al., 1978). Inactive conjugates of codeine are found in plasma at concentrations severalfold higher than those of free codeine, soon after oral or intramuscular administration of the drug (Findlay et al., 1977).

Codeine, norcodeine and morphine concentrations in 24 hour urine samples averaged 12, 3 and 2 mg/L, respectively, for 6 persons receiving a single dose of 20–23 mg codeine base; the corresponding values for the 24 hour urine sample of a subject receiving 282 mg of codeine base (in divided doses) were 56, 38 and 19 mg/L, respectively (Adler et al., 1955). The urine concentrations of total codeine and total morphine in 4 persons who died of codeine overdosage ranged from 16–88 mg/L and 3–24 mg/L, respectively, while the urine of a codeine user who died a traumatic death contained 100 and 35 mg/L, respectively (Wright et al., 1975).

After codeine administration, the urinary codeine/morphine concentration ratio (as total drug following hydrolysis) generally exceeds 1.0 for the first 24 hours, but often falls below 1.0 by 24–30 hours; after 30 hours, only morphine may be detectable in the urine by most analytical methods (Solomon, 1974; Goenechea and Brzezinka, 1982; Dutt et al., 1983; Posey and Kimble, 1984; Cone et al., 1991). This finding has important implications for drug abuse screening programs, as quite often heroin usage is inferred from detection of morphine alone in a urine specimen.

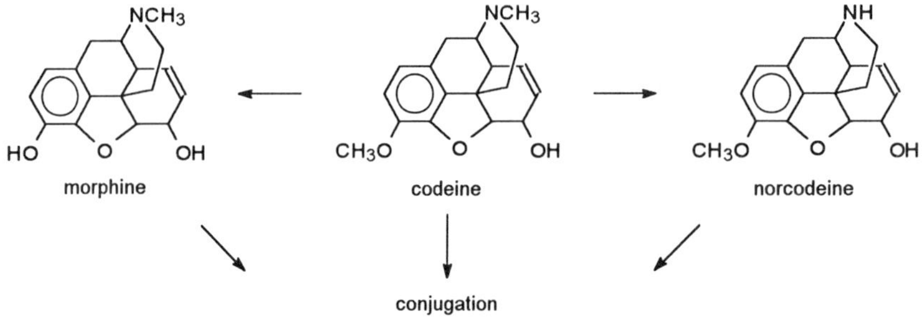

Toxicity. The acutely lethal dose of codeine for an adult has been estimated at 0.5–1.0 g. Doses of this magnitude may cause unconsciousness and convulsions, and death from respiratory failure may result in 2–4 hours. Nalorphine and naloxone are accepted antidotes to codeine poisoning. Serum concentrations exceeding 5.0 mg/L were observed in a comatose adult who had self-administered 750–900 mg of codeine intravenously; consciousness did not return until the third day when the serum level fell below 1.3 mg/L (Huffman and Ferguson, 1975). Blood codeine concentrations of 2.6 and 7.0 mg/L were detected in two individuals arrested for impaired driving ability (Cosbey, 1983; Gjerde and Morland, 1991).

One study has indicated that postmortem blood codeine concentrations in 8 persons succumbing to codeine overdosage ranged from 1.4–5.6 mg/L (Wright et al., 1975). Blood concentrations of 15 and 48 mg/L and urine concentrations of 155 and 370 mg/L were measured postmortem in 2 adults who ingested codeine in combination with alcohol (Peat and Sengupta, 1977). Pearson et al. (1979) reported a similar case with a blood level of 16 mg/L. Nakamura et al. (1976) presented a series of 39 fatal cases in which codeine was implicated and the body distribution of the drug was studied. The following table summarizes the data from 11 cases in which the blood codeine concentration exceeded or equalled 1.0 mg/L:

Drug Concentrations in Codeine Fatalities (mg/L or mg/kg)

	Blood	Bile	Liver	Kidney	Urine
Codeine					
Average	2.8	18	6.8	12	104
(Range)	(1.0–8.8)	(5.0–43)	(0.6–45)	(2.3–36)	(29–229)
Morphine					
Average	0.2	38	1.5	2.0	20
(Range)	(0–0.5)	(3.1–117)	(0–6.3)	(0.3–5.2)	(0–58)

Codeine may be subject to postmortem redistribution; heart blood/peripheral blood concentration ratios of 2.3–3.5 have been observed in fatal overdoses (Anderson and Prouty, 1989).

Analysis. Gas chromatography or gas chromatography-mass spectrometry are very well suited for the analysis of codeine and its metabolites in biological materials. The successful methods have utilized derivatization prior to chromatography; silyl (Nakamura and Way, 1975; Cone et al., 1983), heptafluorobutyryl (Ebbighausen et al., 1973), pentafluoropropionyl (Dahlstrom et al., 1977; Edlund, 1981) and acetyl derivatives (Paul et al., 1985) have been utilized. Trifluoroacetic anhydride has been used for this purpose (Wallace et al., 1974), but there is some question as to the stability of the trifluoroacetyl derivatives (Yeh, 1973). Liquid chromatographic techniques have also been described (Posey and Kimble, 1983; Stubbs et al., 1986; Persson et al., 1989; Verwey-van Vissen et al., 1991). Codeine cross-reacts in most of the commercial immunoassays for morphine; the cross-reactivity of codeine glucuronide, present in blood and urine at concentrations that often exceed those of the parent drug, has not been reported for these assays.

Acid or enzyme hydrolysis of specimens often substantially increases the amount of codeine that can be extracted with organic solvents. Goenechea et al. (1978) showed that heating of a specimen containing 5% hydrochloric acid for 30 minutes at 100° C. hydrolyzed 17% of the codeine glucuronide present, whereas 12–13% hydrochloric acid hydrolyzed 47% of the conjugated drug.

References

T.K. Adler, J.M. Fujimoto, E.L. Way and E.M. Baker. The metabolic fate of codeine in man. J. Pharm. Exp. Ther. 114: 251–262, 1955.

W.H. Anderson and R.W. Prouty. Postmortem redistribution of drugs. In *Advances in Analytical Toxicology* (R.C. Baselt, ed.), Vol 2, YearBook Medical, Chicago, 1989, pp. 70–102.

W.D. Bechtel and K. Sinterhauf. Plasma level and renal excretion of (^{3}H) codeine phosphate in man and in the dog. Arz. Forsch. 28: 308–311, 1978.

M.K. Brunson and J.F. Nash. Gas-chromatographic measurement of codeine and norcodeine in human plasma. Clin. Chem. 21: 1956–1960, 1975.

E.J. Cone, W.D. Darwin and C.W. Gorodetzky. Comparative metabolism of codeine in man, rat, dog, guinea-pig and rabbit: identification of four new metabolites. J. Pharm. Pharmac. 31: 314–317, 1979.

E.J. Cone, W.D. Darwin and W.F. Buchwald. Assay for codeine, morphine and ten potential urinary metabolites by gas chromatography-mass fragmentography. J. Chrom. 275: 307–318, 1983.

E.J. Cone, P. Welch, B.D. Paul and J.M. Mitchell. Forensic drug testing for opiates, III. J. Anal. Tox. 15: 161–166, 1991.

S.H. Cosbey. Personal communication, 1983.

B. Dahlstrom, L. Paalzow and P.O. Edlund. Simultaneous determination of codeine and morphine in biological samples by gas chromatography with electon capture detection. Acta Pharm. Tox. 41: 273–279, 1977.

M.C. Dutt, D.S.T. Lo, D.L.K. Ng and S.O. Woo. Gas chromatographic study of the urinary codeine-to-morphine ratios in controlled codeine consumption and in mass screening for opiate drugs. J. Chrom. 267: 117–124, 1983.

W.O.R. Ebbighausen, J.H. Mowat, P. Vestergaard and N.S. Kline. Stable isotope method for the assay of codeine and morphine by gas chromatography-mass spectrometry. A feasibility study. Adv. Biochem. Psychopharm. 7: 135–146, 1973.

P.O. Edlund. Determination of opiates in biological samples by glass capillary gas chromatography with electron-capture detection. J. Chrom. 206: 109–116, 1981.

J.W.A. Findlay, R.F. Butz and R.M. Welch. Codeine kinetics as determined by radioimmunoassay. Clin. Pharm. Ther. 22: 439–446, 1977.

J.W.A. Findlay, E.C. Jones, R.F. Butz and R.M. Welch. Plasma codeine and morphine concentrations after therapeutic oral doses of codeine-containing analgesics. Clin. Pharm. Ther. 24: 60–68, 1978.

J.W.A. Findlay, A.S.E. Fowle, R.F. Butz et al. Comparative disposition of codeine and pholcodine in man after single oral doses. Brit. J. Clin. Pharm. 22: 61–71, 1986.

H.F. Fraser, H. Isbell and G.D. Van Horn. Human pharmacology and addiction liability of norcodeine. J. Pharm. Exp. Ther. 129: 172–177, 1960.

H. Gjerde and J. Morland. A case of high opiate tolerance: implications for drug analyses and interpretations. Int. J. Leg. Med. 104: 239–240, 1991.

S. Goenechea, K. Kobbe and K.J. Goebel. Verhalten von Codein und Codein-6-glucuronid bei der Hydrolyse mit Salzsaeure. Arz. Forsch. 28: 1070–1071, 1978.

S. Goenechea and H. Brzezinka. Morphinnachweis im Harn nach Einnahme von Codein. Fres. Z. Anal. Chem. 313: 331–333, 1982.

D.H. Huffman and R.L. Ferguson. Acute codeine overdose: correspondence between clinical course and codeine metabolism. Johns Hopkins Med. J. 136: 183–186, 1975.

G.R. Nakamura, E.C. Griesemer and T.T. Noguchi. Antemortem conversion of codeine to morphine in man. J. For. Sci. 21: 518–524, 1976.

G.R. Nakamura and E.L. Way. Determination of morphine and codeine in post-mortem specimens. Anal. Chem. 47: 775–778, 1975.

B.D. Paul, L.D. Mell, J.M. Mitchell et al. Simultaneous identification and quantitation of codeine and morphine in urine by capillary gas chromatography and mass spectroscopy. J. Anal. Tox. 9: 222–226, 1985.

M.A. Pearson, A. Poklis and R.R. Morrison. A fatality due to the ingestion of (methyl morphine) codeine. Clin. Tox. 15: 267–271, 1979.

M.A. Peat and S. Sengupta. Toxicological investigations of cases of death involving codeine and dihydrocodeine. For. Sci. 9: 21–32, 1977.

K. Persson, B. Lindstrom, D. Spalding et al. Determination of codeine and its metabolites in human blood plasma and in microsomal incubates by high-performance liquid chromatography with ultraviolet detection. J. Chrom. 491: 473–480, 1989.

B.L. Posey and S.N. Kimble. Simultaneous determination of codeine and morphine in urine and blood by hplc. J. Anal. Tox. 7: 241–245, 1983.

B.L. Posey and S.N. Kimble. High-performance liquid chromatographic study of codeine, norcodeine, and morphine as indicators of codeine ingestion. J. Anal. Tox. 8: 68–74, 1984.

H. Quiding, G. Lundqvist, L.O. Boreus et al. Analgesic effect and plasma concentrations of codeine and morphine after two dose levels of codeine following oral surgery. Eur. J. Clin. Pharm. 44: 319–323, 1993.

E. Schmerzler, W. Yu, M.I. Hewitt and I.J. Greenblatt. Gas chromatographic determination of codeine in serum and urine. J. Pharm. Sci. 55: 155–157, 1966.

M.D. Solomon. A study of codeine metabolism. Clin. Tox. 7: 255–257, 1974.

R.J. Stubbs, R. Chiou and W.F. Bayne. Determination of codeine in plasma and urine by reversed-phase high-performance liquid chromatography. J. Chrom. 377: 447–453, 1986.

C.P.W.G.M. Verwey-van Vissen, P.M. Koupman-Kimenai and T.B. Vree. Direct determination of codeine, norcodeine, morphine and normorphine with their corresponding O-glucuronide conjugates by high-performance liquid chromatography with electrochemical detection. J. Chrom. 570: 309–320, 1991.

J.E. Wallace, H.E. Hamilton, K. Blaum and C. Petty. Determination of morphine in biologic fluids by electron capture gas-liquid chromatography. Anal. Chem. 46: 2107–2110, 1974.

J.A. Wright, R.C. Baselt and C.H. Hine. Blood codeine concentrations in fatalities associated with codeine. Clin. Tox. 8: 457–463, 1975.

S.Y. Yeh. Separation and, identification of morphine and its metabolites and congeners. J. Pharm. Sci. 62: 1827–1829, 1973.

Colchicine

T½: 9–20 hr
Vd: 10–12 L/kg
Fb: 0.31
pKa: 1.7, 12.4

Occurrence and Usage. Colchicine is a naturally-occurring alkaloid, found in the flowers of the meadow saffron (*Colchicum autumnale*) at a concentration of approximately 0.1%. It is a potent inhibitor of cellular mitosis and is used in the treatment of cancer. It is the drug of choice for acute gouty arthritis, being administered in oral doses of 0.6–1.2 mg every 2 hours (as 0.6 mg tablets) or intravenously in doses of 0.5 mg every 6 hours (as a 0.5 mg/mL solution) until relief is obtained.

Maintenance therapy usually involves daily doses of 0.5–2 mg. Some oral forms of the drug contain probenecid, a uricosuric agent.

Blood Concentrations. Plasma concentrations in 10 subjects after a 1 mg oral dose of colchicine reached an average peak of 2.2 μg/L at 2 hours; by 24 hours, the level had declined (with an elimination half-life of about 20 hours) to an average of 0.4 μg/L (Wallace and Ertal, 1973). Fifteen minutes after a 2 mg intravenous dose given to 16 patients, plasma levels averaged 11.4 μg/L (range, 4.5–33); concentrations fell quickly during the first 30 minutes, exhibiting an average distribution half-life of 19 minutes (Wallace et al., 1970).

Metabolism and Excretion. Less than 40% of a labeled dose of colchicine is excreted in the 48 hour urine. Cancer and gout patients eliminate about 4% as unchanged drug, while normal or asthmatic subjects eliminate about 28% in this manner; another 1–13% is present in the 48 hour urine as unidentified metabolites. Colchicine is believed to be metabolized by hydrolysis of the amide linkage (Walaszek et al., 1960).

Toxicity. Colchicine overdosage is often manifested by nausea, vomiting, diarrhea, confusion, fever, shock, respiratory distress, hematuria, renal failure, metabolic acidosis, and cardiovascular collapse. In later stages of acute poisoning, thrombocytopenia, granulocytopenia, consumption coagulopathy, myopathy, neuropathy and alopecia may develop. Death has occurred after administration of only 6 mg to an adult. Management of poisoned patients includes prevention of drug absorption and supportive therapy (MacLeod and Phillips, 1947; Carr, 1965; Ellwood and Robb, 1971; Heaney et al., 1976; Stapczynski et al., 1981; Kuncl et al., 1987). Plasma colchicine concentrations of 11–63 μg/L were observed within the first 4 hours after drug administration in 3 adults who survived the episode (Rochdi et al., 1992).

A 41 year old woman intentionally ingested 7.5 mg of colchicine and developed severe toxicity; her plasma colchicine levels were 21 μg/L after 6 hours and less than 5 μg/L after 24 hours. She died in cardiac asystole at about 45 hours after ingestion (Jarvie et al., 1979). A 39 year old woman ingested 20 mg of the drug and died 40 hours later; her blood colchicine concentration measured 2 hours after ingestion was 250 μg/L, but none was found in postmortem blood (Caplan et al., 1980).

Analysis. Colchicine has been quantitatively measured in biological specimens by fluorometry (Bourdon and Galliot, 1976), radioimmunoassay (Boudene et al., 1975), indirect atomic absorption spectrometry (Kovatsis et al., 1980), and liquid chromatography (Jarvie et al., 1979; Caplan et al., 1980; Lhermitte et al., 1985). The drug is unstable when exposed to light and many analytical schemes require that certain steps be performed in darkness.

References

C. Boudene, F. Duprey and C. Bohuon. Radioimmunoassay of colchicine. Biochem. J. 151: 413–415, 1975.

R. Bourdon and M. Galliot. Dosage de la colchicine dans les liquides biologiques. Ann. Biol. Clin. 34: 393–401, 1976.

Y.H. Caplan, K.G. Orloff and B.C. Thompson. A fatal overdose with colchicine. J. Anal. Tox. 4: 153–155, 1980.

A.A. Carr. Colchicine toxicity. Arch. Int. Med. 115: 29–33, 1965.

M.G. Ellwood and G.H. Robb. Self-poisoning with colchicine. Postgrad. Med. J. 47: 129–138, 1971.

D. Heaney, C.B. Derghazarian, G.F. Pineo and M.A.M. Ali. Massive colchicine overdose: a report on the toxicity. Am. J. Med. Sci. 271: 233–238, 1976.

D. Jarvie, J. Park and M.J. Stewart. Estimation of colchicine in a poisoned patient by using high performance liquid chromatography. Clin. Tox. 14: 375–381, 1979.

A. Kovatsis, M.N. Christianopoulou and V.P. Papageorgiou. Determination of colchicine in biological samples by indirect atomic absorption spectroscopy. In *Toxicological Aspects* (A. Kovatsis, ed.), Thessaloniki, Greece, 1980, pp. 220–230.

R.W. Kuncl, G. Duncan, D. Watson et al. Colchicine myopathy and neuropathy. New Eng. J. Med. 316: 1562–1568, 1987.

M. Lhermitte, J.L. Bernier, D. Mathieu et al. Colchicine quantitation by high-performance liquid chromatography in human plasma and urine. J. Chrom. 342: 416–423, 1985.

J.G. MacLeod and L. Phillips. Hypersensitivity by colchicine. Ann. Rheum. Dis. 6: 224–229, 1947.

M. Rochdi, A. Sabouraud, F.J. Baud et al. Toxicokinetics of colchicine in humans: analysis of tissue, plasma and urine data in ten cases. Hum. Exp. Tox. 11: 510–516, 1992.

J.S. Stapczynski, R.J. Rothstein, W.A. Gaye and J.T. Niemann. Colchicine overdose: report of two cases and review of the literature. Ann. Emer. Med. 10: 364–369, 1981.

E.J. Walaszek, J.J. Kocsis, G.V. Leroy and E.M.K. Geiling. Studies on the excretion of radioactive colchicine. Arch. Int. Pharm. 125: 371–382, 1960.

S.L. Wallace, B. Omokoku and N.H. Ertel. Colchicine plasma levels. Am. J. Med. 48: 443–448, 1970.

S.L. Wallace and N.H. Ertel. Plasma levels of colchicine after oral administration of a single dose. Metabolism 22: 749–753, 1973.

Copper

T½: 26 days
Vd: 2.0 L/kg   Cu
Fb: 0.95

Occurrence and Usage. Copper is an essential trace metal whose numerous metabolic functions remain to be fully delineated. The daily adult requirement is approximately 2 mg and is supplied by the diet, which averages 2–5 mg per day. Human abnormalities of copper metabolism exist that may result in gradual copper toxicity. Acute copper poisoning is usually a consequence of food contamination by copper utensils, or of the accidental or intentional ingestion of copper salts. Industrial exposure is generally by inhalation of copper fumes or dusts, which have been assigned threshold limit values of 0.2 and 1.0 mg/m^3, respectively.

Blood Concentrations. Total serum copper has been found to average 1.09 mg/L in men and 1.20 mg/L in women; erythrocyte copper averaged 0.89 mg/L of packed cells in both sexes. About 93% of the copper in serum is tightly bound to the copper enzyme, ceruloplasmin, and the remainder is loosely bound to serum protein. Serum copper values for women in the third trimester of pregnancy averaged 2.39 mg/L (Cartwright and Wintrobe, 1964).

Metabolism and Excretion. About one-third of the ingested dietary copper is absorbed. Of this amount, about 80% is excreted into the bile, about 18% passes through the intestinal wall into the bowel and 2–4% appears in the urine (Cartwright and Wintrobe, 1964). A small amount of the copper taken up by the liver is incorporated into ceruloplasmin, which is synthesized in the liver, and it soon appears in plasma in this non-diffusible form (Scheinberg and Sternlieb, 1960). Urinary excretion of copper averages only 0.052 mg daily (range, 0.026–0.064) in normal subjects (Dawson et al., 1968). Urine copper concentrations in 206 asymptomatic workers in copper smelters, where atmospheric copper levels reached as high as 30–40 mg/m^3, averaged 0.079 mg/L and ranged up to 1.145 mg/L (Wagner, 1975).

The normal tissue distribution of copper in 5 healthy subjects has been determined (Cartwright and Wintrobe, 1964):

Copper Concentrations in Normal Tissues (mg/L or mg/kg)

	Brain	Liver	Kidney	Spleen	Muscle
Average	6.3	5.1	2.0	0.8	0.9
(Range)	(5.1–8.3)	(3.0–9.5)	(1.2–3.1)	(0.2–1.1)	(0.6–1.0)

Toxicity. Chronic copper poisoning generally does not occur in normal subjects, who are able to maintain a neutral copper balance over a wide range of dietary and environmental copper intake. In persons with Wilson's disease, however, a progressive copper toxicity develops due to a hereditary metabolic abnormality; serum ceruloplasmin levels are markedly reduced and excess copper deposits in parenchymal tissues, causing damage that is eventually fatal (Scheinberg and Sternlieb, 1960). These patients may have serum copper levels that are only one-half of normal, liver concentrations 5 times normal, and urine concentrations 10 times normal (Fell et al., 1968).

The acute inhalation of copper fume during refining or welding processes may cause typical metal fume fever, with upper respiratory irritation, chills and aching muscles. A number of workers who developed copper fume fever had serum copper levels that averaged 1.26 mg/L (Cohen, 1974). The inhalation of metallic copper dust produces similar symptoms (Gleason, 1968). Chronic copper poisoning in industry is associated with anorexia, nausea, vomiting, nervous manifestations and hepatomegaly; serum copper concentrations have ranged from 0.8 to over 2.0 mg/L in such cases (Suciu et al., 1977).

Moderate gastrointestinal distress is produced by ingestion of several hundred milligrams of a copper salt, and acute symptoms of copper poisoning have been observed in persons using corroded copper utensils for preparing food (Nicholas, 1968). Increases of 15–100% in serum copper concentrations of 6 children were measured following the administration of 250 mg of copper sulfate as an emetic (Holtzman and Haslam, 1968). Serum copper levels of up to 5 mg/L were achieved during accidental intoxication by copper sulfate applied to burned skin (Holtzman et al., 1966), and serum concentrations of 13 and 27 mg/L were observed in 2 patients poisoned during hemodialysis with a unit containing a copper heating coil (Klein et al., 1972).

In a study of 48 cases of acute (usually intentional) copper sulfate poisoning, it was found that blood copper levels correlated well with the severity of intoxication, whereas serum levels did not; blood concentrations averaged 2.87 mg/L in mild poisoning cases and 7.98 mg/L in severe cases. Serum ionic copper in these patients averaged 2.57 mg/L when measured within 12 hours of ingestion and 0.23 mg/L after more than 12 hours had elapsed, with concurrent relocation of the copper into erythrocytes (Chuttani et al., 1965).

Death usually occurs within 1–7 days of the ingestion of 10–20 g of a soluble copper salt and is often preceded by vomiting, hemolysis, liver and kidney damage, and shock. The following tissue concentrations of copper were found in 9 such cases (Grusz-Harday, 1969; Richardson, 1975; Zober et al., 1978; King, 1985; Simmons, 1986; Lamont and Duflou, 1988; Gulliver, 1991):

Copper Concentrations in Fatal Cases (mg/L or mg/kg)

	Blood	Brain	Liver	Kidney
Average	36	6.8	285	39
(Range)	(2.5–66)	(2–11)	(8.3–1410)	(10–61)

Analysis. Copper may be determined in protein-free filtrates of biological specimens by a colorimetric procedure employing bathocuproine sulfonate (Zak, 1975). Atomic absorption procedures for serum or urine have been described that entail both flame (Dawson et al., 1968; Murthy et al., 1973; Sunderman, 1975; Weinstock and Uhlemann, 1981) and flameless techniques (Evenson and Warren, 1975; Halls et al., 1981; Liska et al., 1985); these procedures involve either direct sample introduction, prior sample digestion or a combination of digestion and chelation.

References

G.E. Cartwright and M.M. Wintrobe. Copper metabolism in normal subjects. Am. J. Clin. Nutr. 14: 224–232, 1964.

H.K. Chuttani, P.S. Gupta, S. Gulati and D.N. Gupta. Acute copper sulfate poisoning. Am. J. Med. 39: 849–854, 1965.

S.R. Cohen. A review of the health hazards from copper exposure. J. Occ. Med. 16: 621–624, 1974.

J.B. Dawson, D.J. Ellis and H. Newton-John. Direct estimation of copper in serum and urine by atomic absorption spectroscopy. Clin. Chim. Acta 21: 33–42, 1968.

M.A. Evenson and B.L. Warren. Determination of serum copper by atomic absorption, with use of the graphite cuvette. Clin. Chem. 21: 619–625, 1975.

G.S. Fell, H. Smith and R.A. Howie. Neutron activation analysis for copper in biological material applied to Wilson's disease. J. Clin. Path. 21: 8–11, 1968.

K.P. Gleason. Exposure to copper dust. Am. Ind. Hyg. Asso. J. 29: 461–462, 1968.

E. Grusz-Harday. Spektrophotometrische Kupferbestimmungen aus Leichenteilen bei drei Faellen von Kupfersulfatvergiftung. Arch. Tox. 24: 338–340, 1969.

J.M. Gulliver. A fatal copper sulfate poisoning. J. Anal. Tox. 15: 341–342, 1991.

D.J. Halls, G.S. Fell and P.M. Dunbar. Determination of copper in urine by graphite furnace atomic absorption spectrometry. Clin. Chim. Acta 114: 21–27, 1981.

N.A. Holtzman, D.A. Elliott and R.H. Heller. Copper intoxication. New Eng. J. Med. 275: 347–352, 1966.

N.A. Holtzman and R.H.A. Haslam. Elevation of serum copper following copper sulfate as an emetic. Pediatrics 42: 189–193, 1968.

L.A. King. Personal communication, 1985.

W.J. Klein, Jr., E.M. Metz and A.R. Price. Acute copper intoxication. Arch. Int. Med. 129: 578–582, 1972.

D.L. Lamont and J.A.L.C. Duflou. Copper sulfate. Am. J. For. Med. Path. 9: 226–227, 1988.

S.K. Liska, J. Kerkay and K.H. Pearson. Determination of copper in whole blood, plasma and serum using Zeeman effect atomic absorption spectroscopy. Clin. Chem. Acta 150: 11–19, 1985.

L. Murthy, E.E. Menden, P.M. Eller and H.G. Petering. Atomic absorption determination of zinc, copper, cadmium, and lead in tissues solubilized by aqueous tetramethylammonium hydroxide. Anal. Biochem. 53: 365–372, 1973.

P.O. Nicholas. Food-poisoning due to copper in the morning tea. Lancet 2: 40–42, 1968.

A. Richardson. Personal communication, 1975.

H. Scheinberg and I. Sternlieb. Copper metabolism. Pharm. Rev. 12: 355–381, 1960.

V.C.G. Simmons. Personal communication, 1986.

I. Suciu, V. Lazer, E. Ilea et al. Copper poisoning in the workers from a section of copper electrolysis. In *Environmental Pollution and Human Health* (S.H. Zaidu, ed.), Indian Toxicology Research Centre, Lucknow, India, 1977, p. 211.

F.W. Sunderman, Jr. Copper, type C procedure. In *Methodology for Analytical Toxicology* (I. Sunshine, ed.), CRC Press, Cleveland, 1975, pp. 109–112.

W.L. Wagner. *Environmental Conditions in U.S. Copper Smelters*, U.S. Government Printing Office, Washington, D.C., 1975.

N. Weinstock and M. Uhlemann. Automated determination of copper in undiluted serum by atomic absorption spectroscopy. Clin. Chem. 27: 1438–1440, 1981.

B. Zak. Copper, type B procedure. In *Methodology for Analytical Toxicology* (I. Sunshine, ed.), CRC Press, Cleveland, 1975, pp. 105–109.

A. Zober, M. Geldmacher-von Mallinckrodt and B. Schellmann. Akute toedliche Kupfervergiftung. Arch. Tox. 40: 263–267, 1978.

Cresol

T½: ?
Vd: ?
Fb: ?
pKa: 10.3

Occurrence and Usage. The 3 isomers of cresol are used as disinfectants (Lysol) and as chemical intermediates in the production of plasticizers and resins. Industrial exposure is usually by way of inhalation or dermal contact. The current threshold limit value for cresol in air is 5 ppm (22 mg/m³).

Blood Concentrations. Cresol concentrations in blood are not routinely measured, except in cases of severe poisoning.

Metabolism and Excretion. p-Cresol is found in the excreta of normal individuals, probably as a result of bacterial degradation of amino acids in the intestine. Following intestinal absorption, it is metabolized to glucuronide and sulfate conjugates in the liver and excreted as such in the urine. The other cresol isomers are not normal constituents of human urine (Duran et al., 1973). The p-cresol content of normal urine averages about 90 mg/L, with a range of 20–200 mg/L (Van Haaften and Sie, 1965). Whereas only about 5% of the endogenously produced p-cresol is excreted unconjugated in urine, large doses of cresol often result in excretion of substantial amounts of the unconjugated isomers.

Toxicity. Acute or chronic cresol toxicity is manifested by headache, dizziness, vomiting, rapid respiration, dyspnea, weakness, and damage to the lung, liver and kidneys. A man who survived the intentional ingestion of 50 g of technical cresol exhibited peak serum p-cresol and m-cresol concentrations of 43 and 74 mg/L, respectively, within 2 hours (Yashiki et al., 1990).

A young woman who self-administered an intrauterine injection of Lysol for the purpose of abortion died in coma within 1 day (Vance, 1945). A man who ingested at least 25 g of a cresol mixture was hospitalized and died after 4 days; a maximal serum cresol level of 90 mg/L was achieved on the first day (Arthurs et al., 1977). A 1 year old boy died within 5 hours of accidental dermal application of a cresol antiseptic fluid; the postmortem blood specimen was found to contain 120 mg/L cresols (Green, 1975). Blood and urine cresol concentrations of 190 and 304 mg/L, respectively, were found postmortem in a woman who intentionally ingested a cresol disinfectant (Bruce et al., 1976).

Analysis. Gas chromatographic methods described for determination of urinary phenol may be applicable to cresol analysis. Two of the isomers, m- and p-cresol, cannot be differentiated by these procedures (Sherwood and Carter, 1970; Duran et al., 1973). Other authors were able to adequately separate the 3 isomers by flame-ionization gas chromatography (Bruce et al., 1976; Yashiki et al., 1990). Additional procedures are cited in the section on toluene.

References

G.J. Arthurs, C.C. Wise and G.A. Coles. Poisoning by cresol. Anaesthesia 32: 642–643, 1977.

A.M. Bruce, H. Smith and A.A. Watson. Cresol poisoning. Med. Sci. Law 16: 171–176, 1976.

M. Duran, D. Ketting, P.K. De Bree et al. Gas chromatographic analysis of urinary volatile phenols in patients with gastro-intestinal disorders and normals. Clin. Chim. Acta 45: 341–347, 1973.

M.A. Green. A household remedy misused—fatal cresol poisoning following cutaneous absorption (a case report). Med. Sci. Law 15: 65–66, 1975.

R.J. Sherwood and F.W.G. Carter. The measurement of occupational exposure to benzene vapour. Ann. Occ. Hyg. 13: 125–146, 1970.

B.M. Vance. Intrauterine injection of Lysol as an abortifacient. Arch. Path. 40: 395–398, 1945.

A.B. Van Haaften and S.T. Sie. The measurement of phenol in urine by gas chromatography as a check on benzene exposure. Am. Ind. Hyg. Asso. J. 26: 52–58, 1965.

M. Yashiki, T. Kojima, T. Miyazaki et al. Gas chromatographic determination of cresols in the biological fluids of a non-fatal case of cresol intoxication. For. Sci. Int. 47: 21–29, 1990.

Cyanide

T½: 0.7–2.1 hr (whole blood)
Vd: 0.4 L/kg
Fb: ?   CN⁻
pKa: 9.1

Occurrence and Usage. Hydrocyanic acid and its sodium and potassium salts are used industrially as fumigants, insecticides, metal polishes and in electroplating solutions. The acid is a volatile liquid that boils at 26° C. The odor of its vapor can be detected at an air concentration of 1 ppm by some persons, but up to 50% of the population is unable to recognize the characteristic almond odor of cyanide. Hydrogen cyanide may be produced in relatively high concentrations in fires that involve nitrogen-containing materials. The threshold limit value for hydrogen cyanide is 10 ppm (11 mg/m³) for an 8 hour day, although as little as 110 ppm may be fatal to an adult after 1 hour. The threshold limit value for cyanide salts in air is currently 5 mg/m³. Other potential sources of cyanide (acetonitrile, acrylonitrile, amygdalin, and nitroprusside) are covered in separate sections.

Blood Concentrations. Cyanide is found in low levels in the tissues of healthy subjects as a result of normal metabolism, eating of cyanogenic foods and cigarette smoking. Plasma cyanide concentrations in healthy subjects were found to average 0.004 mg/L in nonsmokers and 0.006 mg/L in smokers (Wilson and Matthews, 1966). Whole blood cyanide, most of which is contained in erythrocytes bound to methemoglobin, in 10 nonsmokers was found to average 0.016 mg/L, whereas in 14 smokers the mean level was 0.041 mg/L; these values increased to 0.059 and 0.123 mg/L, respectively, following 1 week of storage of the blood specimens at -20° C. Blood stored at 4° C. was generally quite stable, while room temperature storage caused a significant diminution of cyanide content, to the extent of 70% loss after 15 weeks (Ballantyne, 1977a). Thiocyanate, a metabolite of cyanide, normally ranges from 1–4 mg/L in the plasma of nonsmokers and 3–12 mg/L in smokers (Pettigrew and Fell, 1972).

Metabolism and Excretion. About 80% of a cyanide dose is detoxified by conversion via the liver enzyme rhodanase to thiocyanate, which is subsequently excreted in urine. The remainder is handled by other minor routes, which include pulmonary excretion of unchanged hydrogen cyanide, trapping by hydroxocobalamin with formation of vitamin B_{12}, oxidation to formic acid and carbon dioxide, and reaction with cysteine. Normal urinary cyanide concentrations in 22 nonsmokers averaged 0.067 mg/L (range, 0–0.300) and in 80 smokers, 0.174 mg/L (range, 0.010–0.811) (Ansell and Lewis, 1970). Normal urinary thiocyanate concentrations range from 1–4 mg/L in nonsmokers and 7–17 mg/L in smokers (Maliszewski and Bass, 1955).

Toxicity. Cyanide produces hypoxia by the inhibition of cytochrome oxidase. Chronic cyanide poisoning can produce dizziness, weakness and permanent mental and motor impairment (Hardy et al., 1950). An individual who developed hemiparesis following chronic exposure to cyanide was found to have a blood cyanide concentration of 0.1 mg/L (Sandberg, 1967). Some of the effects of chronic cyanide exposure are similar to those of thiocyanate intoxication (El Ghawabi et al., 1975).

A group of workers chronically exposed to cyanide at levels of 0.2–0.8 mg/m³ who developed symptoms of mild cyanide poisoning was studied. Blood samples drawn at the end of the workshift contained cyanide at an average of 0.18 mg/L (range, 0.02–0.36) in 15 nonsmokers and 0.56 mg/L (range, 0.10–2.20) in 8 smokers; blood thiocyanate concentrations averaged 4.2 mg/L (range, 2.6–

8.3) and 4.8 mg/L (range, 1.6–9.2) in the nonsmokers and smokers, respectively. Urine thiocyanate levels in 24 hour specimens averaged 5.7 mg/L (range, 1.5–12.9) and 6.2 mg/L (range, 1.5–16.5) in these 2 groups. Each of these levels, excluding the urinary thiocyanate of smokers, was substantially elevated over those of equivalent groups of control subjects. It was concluded that the present TLV of 5 mg/m^3 for cyanide aerosols should be reviewed (Chandra et al., 1980).

Cyanide was found in the postmortem blood of 39 out of 53 fire victims, in concentrations ranging from 0.17–2.20 mg/L (Wetherell, 1966). In 89 cases of death from fire, blood cyanide concentrations averaged 1.12 mg/L, with a range of 0.01–4.36 mg/L (Caplan and Altman, 1976).

Cyanide is both a potent and very rapidly-acting poison; the minimal adult lethal dose has been estimated as 100 mg for hydrocyanic acid and 200 mg for potassium cyanide. Amyl nitrite (by inhalation), sodium nitrite, sodium thiosulfate, cobalt EDTA, and hydroxocobalamin (by intravenous injection) have been used in the therapy of acute poisoning, although vigorous nonspecific therapy is often successful (Vogel et al., 1981). Cyanide disappears from the blood of poisoning victims with a half-life of about 1 hour during the first 6 hours, but estimates of its terminal elimination half-life (which may be skewed by antidotal induction of methemoglobin) have ranged from 6–66 hours (Graham et al., 1977; Hall et al., 1987; Selden et al., 1990). A chemist who ingested 413 mg of potassium cyanide had a peak blood cyanide concentration 1 hour later of 3.8 mg/L; he was unconscious, in severe metabolic acidosis, and suffered cardiorespiratory arrest, but regained consciousness after 8 hours of supportive therapy (Edwards and Thomas, 1978). A 1.5 year old child was inadvertently given a drink containing cyanide and fell to the floor within minutes; he was admitted to a hospital in coma and severe metabolic acidosis, but recovered fully after several days with supportive therapy. A blood concentration taken within 1 hour contained 1.5 mg/L cyanide and a specimen taken about 12 hours later contained 0.07 mg/L (Baselt and Briglia, 1980). A 21 year old man ingested 600 mg of potassium cyanide, developed coma, cyanosis, pulmonary edema and lactic acidosis, and recovered with supportive therapy. Blood cyanide concentrations of 2.0, 1.6, and 1.2 mg/L were measured in specimens drawn 12, 22, and 84 hours after admission (Graham et al., 1977). A blood cyanide level of 5.1 mg/L was found in a cyanide plant worker who was successfully treated with 300 mg of cobalt EDTA (Bain and Knowles, 1967).

The tissue distribution of cyanide in fatal cases generally is in proportion to the erythrocyte content of each organ, but also demonstrates that liver concentrations following ingestion of the poison may be considerably higher than after inhalation (Ballantyne, 1974):

Cyanide Concentrations in Fatal Cases (mg/L or mg/kg)

	Blood	Brain	Liver	Spleen	Kidney	Urine
Ingestion (34 cases)						
Average	12.4	2.9	7.7	43.9	5.7	0.1
(Range)	(1.1–5.3)	(0.6–16)	(0.7–23)	(0.5–398)	(0–27)	(0.5–1.1)
Inhalation (3 cases)						
Average	7.0	1.4	0.8		1.1	2.0
(Range)	(1.0–15)	(0.1–3.4)	(0–2.0)		(1.1)	(2.0)

Another compilation of 32 fatal cases, due apparently to ingestion of cyanide, has shown a blood cyanide concentration range of 0.4–230 mg/L, with an average of 37 mg/L (Rehling, 1967).

Analysis. Cyanide is frequently determined in biologic specimens by colorimetric techniques, with isolation by aeration (Boxer and Rickards, 1951), microdiffusion (Feldstein and Klendshoj, 1954; Baar, 1966; Pettigrew and Fell, 1973; Tucker et al., 1978; Holzbecher and Ellenberger, 1985) or distillation (Tompsett, 1959; Shanahan, 1973). A sensitive electron-capture gas chromatographic procedure to detect cyanide following its conversion to cyanogen chloride has been described (Valentour et al., 1974), and an equally sensitive cyanide-specific electrode for potentiometric measurements is now commercially available (McAnalley et al., 1979; Egezeke and Oehme, 1979).

Several other recently developed techniques utilize fluorometry (Morgan and Way, 1980; Lundquist et al., 1987), nitrogen-selective gas chromatography (Darr et al., 1980; Zamecnik and Tam, 1987), liquid chromatography (Toida et al., 1984; Sano et al., 1992) and gas chromatography-mass spectrometry (Thomson and Anderson, 1980). Plasma and urine thiocyanate levels, more frequently used to monitor chronic exposure to cyanide, may be determined colorimetrically (Pettigrew and Fell, 1972; Ballantyne, 1977b, Lundquist et al., 1979).

Interestingly, toxic levels of cyanide in tissues may diminish significantly after death by mechanisms that include evaporation, thiocyanate formation and reaction with tissue components. Curry (1963) found that in a case of cyanide inhalation a blood specimen taken immediately after death contained 3.5 mg/L of cyanide, while specimens drawn subsequently at autopsy showed values of only 0.5–1.0 mg/L. With addition of cyanide to blood *in vitro*, only 67–83% is detected after 1 hour (Ballantyne et al., 1973). In rabbits sacrificed by injection of cyanide, there occurs rapid destruction of the poison after death, whether or not the tissues are removed from the animal; the concentrations declined to undetectable levels after only 2 weeks in all tissues studied except blood (Ballantyne et al., 1974). The formation of cyanide in postmortem tissues with accumulation to toxicologically significant concentrations has also been demonstrated, but can be prevented by the addition of sodium fluoride (Curry et al., 1967). This arises in part due to conversion of thiocyanate to cyanide (Egezeke and Oehme, 1980). It is apparent that temperature and cyanide concentration are important factors in the changes that occur in stored specimens; it has been suggested that blood specimens with low cyanide content be maintained at 4° C., while those with high cyanide levels be kept at -20° C. to reduce losses (Ballantyne, 1976).

References

M. Ansell and F.A.S. Lewis. A review of cyanide concentrations found in human organs. J. For. Med. 17: 148–155, 1970.

S. Baar. The micro determination of cyanide: its application to the analysis of whole blood. Analyst 91: 268–272, 1966.

J.T.B. Bain and E.L. Knowles. Successful treatment of cyanide poisoning. Brit. Med. J. 2: 763, 1967.

B. Ballantyne, J. Bright and P. Williams. An experimental assessment of decreases in measurable cyanide levels in biological fluids. J. For. Sci. Soc. 13: 111–117, 1973.

B. Ballantyne (ed). The forensic diagnosis of acute cyanide poisoning. In *Forensic Toxicology*, Wright and Sons, Bristol, 1974, pp. 99–113.

B. Ballantyne, J.E. Bright and P. Williams. The post-mortem rate of transformation of cyanide. For. Sci. 3: 71–76, 1974.

B. Ballantyne. Changes in blood cyanide as a function of storage time and temperature. J. For. Sci. Soc. 16: 305–310, 1976.

B. Ballantyne. In vitro production of cyanide in normal human blood and the influence of thiocyanate and storage temperature. Clin. Tox. 11: 173–193, 1977a.

B. Ballantyne. Factors in the analysis of whole blood thiocyanate. Clin. Tox. 11: 195–210, 1977b.

R.C. Baselt and R. Briglia. Unpublished results, 1980.

G.E. Boxer and J.C. Rickards. Chemical determination of vitamin B12. II. The quantitative isolation and colorimetric determination of millimicrogram quantities of cyanide. Arch. Biochem. 30: 372–381, 1951.

Y. Caplan and R. Altman. Microdetermination of cyanide in fire fatalities. Presented at the annual meeting of the American Academy of Forensic Sciences, Washington, D.C., February 18, 1976.

H. Chandra, B.N. Gupta, S.K. Bhargava et al. Chronic cyanide exposure—a biochemical and industrial hygiene study. J. Anal. Tox. 4: 161–165, 1980.

A.S. Curry. Cyanide poisoning. Acta Pharm. Tox. 20: 291–294, 1963.

A.S. Curry, D.E. Price and E.R. Rutter. The production of cyanide in post mortem material. Acta Pharm. Tox. 25: 339–344, 1967.

R.W. Darr, T.L. Capson and F.D. Hileman. Determination of hydrogen cyanide in blood using gas chromatography with alkali thermionic detection. Anal. Chem. 52: 1379–1381, 1980.

A.C. Edwards and I.D. Thomas. Cyanide poisoning. Lancet 1: 92–93, 1978.

J.O. Egekeze and F.W. Oehme. Direct potentiometric method for the determination of cyanide in biological materials. J. Anal. Tox. 3: 119–124, 1979.

J.O. Egekeze and F.W. Oehme. Thiocyanate to cyanide: revisited. Clin. Tox. 16: 127–128, 1980.

S.H. El Ghawabi, M.A. Gaafar, A.A. El-Saharti et al. Chronic cyanide exposure: a clinical, radioisotope, and laboratory study. Brit. J. Ind. Med. 32: 215–219, 1975.

M. Feldstein and N.C. Klendshoj. The determination of cyanide in biologic fluids by microdiffusion analysis. J. Lab. Clin. Med. 44: 166–170, 1954.

D.L. Graham, D. Laman, J. Theodore and E.D. Robin. Acute cyanide poisoning complicated by lactic acidosis and pulmonary edema. Arch. Int. Med. 137: 1051–1055, 1977.

A.H. Hall, W.H. Doutre, T. Ludden et al. Nitrite/thiosulfate treated acute cyanide poisoning: estimated kinetics after antidote. Clin. Tox. 25: 121–133, 1987.

H.L. Hardy, W.M. Jeffries, M.M. Wasserman and W.R. Waddell. Thiocyanate effect following industrial cyanide exposure. New Eng. J. Med. 242: 968–972, 1950.

M. Holzbecher and H.A. Ellenberger. An evaluation and modification of a microdiffusion method for the emergency determination of blood cyanide. J. Anal. Tox. 9: 251–253, 1985.

P. Lundquist, J. Martensson, B. Sorbo and S. Ohman. Method for determining thiocyanate in serum and urine. Clin. Chem. 25: 678–681, 1979.

P. Lundquist, H. Rosling, B. Sorbo and L. Tibbling. Cyanide concentrations in blood after cigarette smoking, as determined by a sensitive fluorometric detector. Clin. Chem. 33: 1228–1230, 1987.

T.F. Maliszewski and D.E. Bass. "True" and "apparent" thiocyanate in body fluids of smokers and nonsmokers. J. Appl. Physiol. 8: 289–291, 1955.

B.H. McAnalley, W.T. Lowry, R. Oliver and J.C. Garriott. Determination of inorganic sulfide and cyanide in blood using specific ion electrodes. J. Anal. Tox. 3: 111–114, 1979.

R.L. Morgan and J.L. Way. Fluorometric determination of cyanide in biological fluids with pyridoxal. J. Anal. Tox. 4: 78–81, 1980.

A.R. Pettigrew and G.S. Fell. Simplified colorimetric determination of thiocyanate in biological fluids, and its application to investigation of the toxic amblyopias. Clin. Chem. 18: 996–1000, 1972.

A.R. Pettigrew and G.S. Fell. Microdiffusion method for estimation of cyanide in whole blood and its application to the study of conversion of cyanide to thiocyanate. Clin. Chem. 19: 466–471, 1973.

C.J. Rehling. Poison residue in human tissues. In *Progress in Chemical Toxicology*, Vol. 3 (A. Stolman, ed.), Academic Press, New York, 1967, pp. 363–386.

C.G. Sandberg. A case of chronic poisoning with potassium cyanide? Acta Med. Scand. 181: 233–235, 1967.

A. Sano, N. Takimoto and S. Takitani. High-performance liquid chromatographic determination of cyanide in human red blood cells by pre-column fluorescence derivatization. J. Chrom. 582: 131–135, 1992.

B.S. Selden, R.F. Clark and S.C. Curry. Elimination kinetics of cyanide after acute KCN ingestion. Vet. Hum. Tox. 32: 361, 1990.

R. Shanahan. The determination of sub-microgram quantities of cyanide in biological materials. J. For. Sci. 18: 25–30, 1973.

I. Thomson and R.A. Anderson. Determination of cyanide and thiocyanate in biological fluids by gas chromatography-mass spectrometry. J. Chrom. 188: 357–362, 1980.

T. Toida, T. Togawa, S. Tanabe et al. Determination of cyanide and thiocyanate in blood plasma and red cells by high-performance liquid chromatography with fluorometric detection. J. Chrom. 308: 133–142, 1984.

S.L. Tompsett. A note on the determination and identification of cyanide in biologic materials. Clin. Chem. 5: 587–591, 1959.

R.B. Tucker, B.F. Graham and V.A. Mason. Cyanide levels in fire victims as determined by a simple microdiffusion procedure. Can. Soc. For. Sci. J. 11: 251–256, 1978.

J.C. Valentour, V. Aggarwal and I. Sunshine. Sensitive gas chromatographic determination of cyanide. Anal. Chem. 46: 924–925, 1974.

S.N. Vogel, T.R. Sultan and R.P. Ten Eyck. Cyanide poisoning. Clin. Tox. 18: 367–383, 1981.

H.R. Wetherell. The occurrence of cyanide in the blood of fire victims. J. For. Sci. 11: 167–173, 1966.

J. Wilson and D.M. Matthews. Metabolic inter-relationships between cyanide, thiocyanate and vitamin B_{12} in smokers and non-smokers. Clin. Sci. 31: 1–7, 1966.

J. Zamecnik and J. Tam. Cyanide in blood by gas chromatography with NP detector and acetonitrile as internal standard. J. Anal. Tox. 11: 47–48, 1987.

Cyclizine

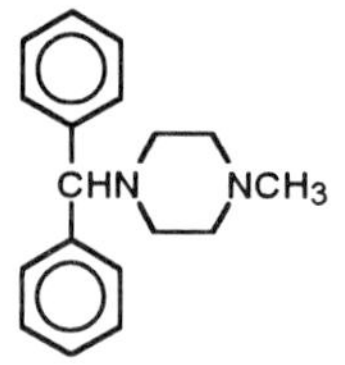

T½: 7–24 hr
Vd: ?
Fb: ?
pKa: 7.7

Occurrence and Usage. Cyclizine (Marezine) is an antihistaminic drug with antiemetic and sedative effects frequently employed in the prevention or treatment of motion sickness. The usual oral dose for motion sickness is 50 mg (as the hydrochloride salt) taken 30 minutes before travel and repeated in 4–6 hours as needed, not exceeding 200 mg daily. Cyclizine is also available as the lactate salt for intramuscular injection and is frequently used in this form for the treatment of postoperative vomiting in doses of up to 150 mg daily.

Blood Concentrations. Following the intravenous administration of 50 mg of cyclizine to a healthy adult male, a plasma concentration of more than 300 µg/L was found after 20 minutes. Two hours after administration, cyclizine was still detectable in plasma at a concentration of about 50 µg/L (Land et al., 1981). A peak blood concentration of 69 µg/L was attained 2 hours after a single 50 mg oral dose of cyclizine hydrochloride to an adult (Griffin and Baselt, 1984). On the day following termination of daily oral doses of 150 mg to 4 volunteers, a mean plasma concentration of 14 µg/L (range, 4–22) norcyclizine was reported (Kuntzman et al., 1967).

Metabolism and Excretion. Cyclizine is rapidly and extensively metabolized by N-demethylation to form norcyclizine (Kuntzman et al., 1967). Only 0.01% of a dose is excreted unchanged in the 24 hour urine (Griffin and Baselt, 1984).

cyclizine   norcyclizine

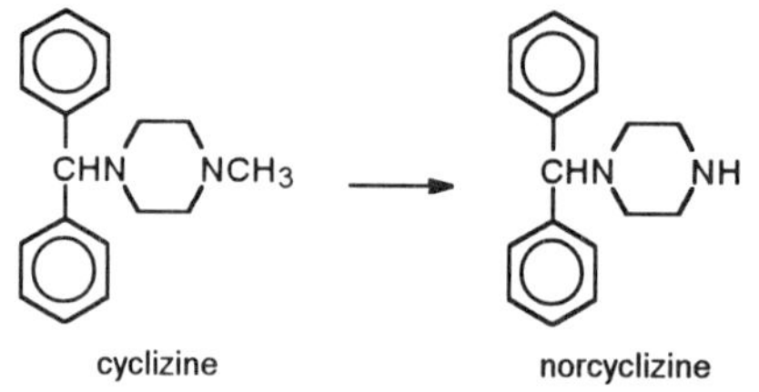

Toxicity. Cyclizine overdosage can cause central nervous system depression or stimulation, euphoria, hypertension, convulsions, coma, and death from respiratory paralysis (Gott, 1968).

A 28 year old male mental patient overdosed and suffered repeated seizures followed by respiratory arrest; cyclizine was present in postmortem specimens at concentrations of 15 mg/L in blood and 108 mg/kg in liver (Lewin et al., 1981). A young woman who intentionally ingested an overdose had a postmortem blood cyclizine concentration of 80 mg/L (Backer et al., 1989). In a suicide by injection of cyclizine and dipipanone, cyclizine was found in postmortem blood at a concentration of 1.5 mg/L (Sengupta, 1976). In the case of a 2 year old female child who ingested 800 mg and went into seizures, death occurred 4 hours after hospital admission; cyclizine was found in brain and liver at levels of 3 and 37 mg/kg, respectively (Battista et al., 1973).

Analysis. Both gas chromatography with nitrogen-phosphorus detection (Land et al., 1981; Griffin and Baselt, 1984; Patterson et al., 1984) and liquid chromatography (Patterson et al., 1984) have been applied to the analysis of cyclizine in biological specimens.

References

R.C. Backer, P. McFeeley and N. Wohlenberg. Fatality resulting from cyclizine overdosage. J. Anal. Tox. 13: 308–309, 1989.

V.H.J. Battista, R. Henn and F. Schnabel. Verlauf, morphologische und toxikologische Befunde einer todlichen Cyclizin-Vergiftung im Kindesalter. Beitr. Gerichtl. Med. 36: 429–431, 1973.

D.S. Griffin and R.C. Baselt. Blood and urine concentrations of cyclizine by nitrogen-phosphorus gas-liquid chromatography. J. Anal. Tox. 8: 97–99, 1984.

P.H. Gott. Cyclizine toxicity: intentional drug abuse of a proprietary antihistamine. New Eng. J. Med. 279: 596, 1968.

R. Kuntzman, I. Tsai and J.J. Burns. Importance of tissue and plasma binding in determining the retention of norchlorcyclizine and norcyclizine in man, dog and rat. J. Pharm. Exp. Ther. 158: 332–339, 1967.

G. Land, K. Dean and A. Bye. Determination of cyclizine and norcyclizine in plasma and urine using gas-liquid chromatography with nitrogen selective detection. J. Chrom. 222: 235–140, 1981.

J.F. Lewin. Personal communication, 1981.

S.C. Patterson, G.T. Smith and K. Fieldstead. Plasma levels of cyclizine and dipipanone as measured by HPLC and GLC after a single oral dose. Proc. Int. Asso. For. Tox., Newmarket, England, 1984.

A. Sengupta. Personal communication, 1976.

Cyclobenzaprine

T½: 1–3 days
Vd: ?
Fb: 0.97
pKa: ?

Occurrence and Usage. Cyclobenzaprine (Flexeril, Lisseril) is a tricyclic compound that differs from amitriptyline only by the addition of a double bond to the cycloheptane ring. It was synthesized in 1971 and has been available since 1977 as a centrally-acting skeletal muscle relaxant. The drug is supplied as the hydrochloride salt in 10 mg tablets for oral use; daily doses range from 30–60 mg, but are not recommended for periods longer than 2–3 weeks.

Blood Concentrations. A single 40 mg oral dose given to 4 subjects produced an average peak plasma concentration of 0.027 mg/L at 2 hours; by 8 hours, the level had only declined to 0.023 mg/L. A 3 day regimen of 30 mg of cyclobenzaprine per day with 18 subjects resulted in an average trough plasma level of 0.015 mg/L (range, 0.003–0.032); an average peak level of 0.022 mg/L (range, 0.005–0.036) was reached 4 hours after the next 10 mg dose. A similar study with a 60 mg daily dose showed trough and peak levels of 0.024 and 0.034 mg/L, respectively (Hucker et al., 1977).

Metabolism and Excretion. A total of 65% of a labeled oral dose of cyclobenzaprine is excreted in urine and feces. Only 0.2% of a dose is eliminated unchanged in the 24 hour urine, together with 0.7% as norcyclobenzaprine. However, this metabolite was not found in plasma during 3 days of drug therapy (Hucker et al., 1977).

cyclobenzaprine   norcyclobenzaprine

Toxicity. Symptoms of cyclobenzaprine toxicity include drowsiness, dry mouth, dizziness, tachycardia, blurred vision, nausea, and paresthesias. Overdosage may cause confusion, hallucinations, agitation, fever, hypotension, convulsions, coma, and cardiac arrhythmias. Physostigmine has been used sucessfully as a specific antidote (Linden et al., 1983). Cyclobenzaprine blood levels of 0.03–0.35 mg/L were measured in 11 hospitalized victims of drug overdosage (Demorest, 1987).

The following tissue distribution was noted in 2 fatal cases that involved intentional overdosage of cyclobenzaprine in combination with other sedative and narcotic analgesic drugs (Beck, 1979):

Cyclobenzaprine Concentrations in Drug Deaths (mg/L or mg/kg)

Blood	Liver	Bile	Urine	Gastric
0.46	12	12	3.2	3.1 mg
0.53	14	5.1	0.01	0.4 mg

Analysis. Cyclobenzaprine has been determined in biological specimens by gas chromatography with either flame-ionization (Hucker and Stauffer, 1976a) or nitrogen-selective detection (Hucker and Stauffer, 1976b; Constanzer et al., 1985). Liquid chromatography has also been used (Hwang et al., 1993). Cyclobenzaprine may be indistinguishable from amitriptyline with many analytical techniques (Tasset et al., 1986), although liquid chromatographic procedures utilizing dual-wavelength ultraviolet detection are capable of discriminating between these analogues (Demorest, 1987; Puopolo and Flood, 1987).

References

B.K. Beck. Personal communication, 1979.

M.L. Constanzer, W.C. Vincek and W.F. Bayne. Determination of cyclobenzaprine in plasma and urine using capillary gas chromatography with nitrogen-selective detection. J. Chrom. 339: 414–418, 1985.

D.M. Demorest. Distinguishing cyclobenzaprine from amitriptyline and imipramine. J. Anal. Tox. 11: 133–134, 1987.

H.B. Hucker and S.C. Stauffer. GLC determination of cyclobenzaprine in plasma and urine. J. Pharm. Sci. 65: 1253–1255, 1976a.

H.B. Hucker and S.C. Stauffer. Gas-liquid chromatographic determination of nanogram amounts of cyclobenzaprine in plasma using a nitrogen detector. J. Chrom. 124: 164–168, 1976b.

H.B. Hucker, S.C. Stauffer, K.S. Albert and B.W. Lei. Plasma levels of bioavailability of cyclobenzaprine in human subjects. J. Clin. Pharm. 17: 719–727, 1977.

P.T.R. Hwang, D.A. Young, A.B. Straughn and M.C. Meyer. Quantitative determination of cyclobenzaprine in human plasma by high pressure liquid chromatography. J. Liq. Chrom. 16: 1163–1171, 1993.

C.H. Linden, J.C. Mitchiner, R.D. Lindzon and B.H. Rumack. Cyclobenzaprine overdosage. Clin. Tox. 20: 281–288, 1983.

P.R. Puopolo and J.G. Flood. Detection of interference by cyclobenzaprine in liquid-chromatographic assays of tricyclic antidepressants. Clin. Chem. 33: 819–820, 1987.

J.J. Tasset, T.J. Schroeder and A.J. Pesce. Cyclobenzaprine overdosage: the importance of a clinical history in analytical toxicology. J. Anal. Tox. 10: 258, 1986.

Cyclohexane

T½: ?
Vd:?
Fb: ?

Occurrence and Usage. Cyclohexane occurs naturally in crude petroleum at a concentration of 0.5–1.0%. It is used as a solvent for lacquers and resin, as a paint remover, and as an intermediate in chemical manufacturing. The current threshold limit value for industrial exposure is 300 ppm (1030 mg/m³).

Blood Concentrations. Blood cyclohexane concentrations in specimens collected at the end of the day ranged from 29–367 µg/L in 22 shoe factory workers exposed to the chemical at air concentrations of 5–710 ppm (Perbellini and Brugnone, 1980).

Metabolism and Excretion. Up to 90% of an oral dose of cyclohexane was found to be excreted in the 48 hour urine of rabbits as cyclohexanol and cyclohexane-1,2-diol, partly as glucuronide conjugates (Elliot et al., 1959). Cyclohexanol has been identified as a human urinary metabolite (Perbellini et al., 1980), while cyclohexanone is a suspected metabolite.

Urinary cyclohexanol concentrations in specimens collected at the end of the day ranged from 0.3–7 mg/L in shoe factory workers exposed to air cyclohexane concentrations of 5–710 ppm (Perbellini and Brugnone, 1980).

cyclohexane → cyclohexanol → ? → cyclohexanone

Toxicity. Rabbits exposed to cyclohexane by inhalation developed toxicity, manifested as lethargy, narcosis, incoordination and convulsions, at concentrations of 7444 ppm and higher for 60 hours (Treon et al., 1943). Chronic administration of two cyclohexane metabolites, cyclohexanol and cyclohexanone, to rats did not cause peripheral neuropathy (Perbellini et al., 1981a), in contrast to an earlier report (Franchini et al., 1978).

Analysis. Cyclohexane in blood or breath may be measured using gas chromatography (Brugnone et al., 1978). Urinary cyclohexanol may also be analyzed by gas chromatography (Perbellini et al., 1981b; Ong et al., 1991).

References

F. Brugnone, L. Perbellini, L. Grigolini and P. Apostoli. Solvent exposure in a shoe upper factory. I. n-Hexane and acetone concentration in alveolar and environmental air and in blood. Int. Arch. Occ. Env. Health 42: 51–62, 1978.

F. Brugnone, L. Perbellini, E. Gaffuri and P. Apostoli. Biomonitoring of industrial solvent exposures in workers' alveolar air. Int. Arch. Occ. Env. Health 47: 245–261, 1980.

I. Franchini, A. Cavatorta, M. Falzoi et al. Neurotoxicite experimentale du cyclohexane et du cyclohexanone. XIX Int. Congr. Occ. Health, Dubrovnik, Yugoslavia, Sept. 25–30, 1978.

C.N. Ong, G.L. Sia, S.E. Chia et al. Determination of cyclohexanol in urine and its use in environmental monitoring of cyclohexanone exposure. J. Anal. Tox. 15: 13–16, 1991.

L. Perbellini and F. Brugnone. Lung uptake and metabolism of cyclohexane in shoe factory workers. Int. Arch. Occ. Env. Health 45: 261–269, 1980.

L. Perbellini, F. Brugnone and I. Pavan. Indentification of the metabolites of n-hexane, cyclohexane, and their isomers in men's urine. Tox. Appl. Pharm. 53: 220–229, 1980.

L. Perbellini, D. DeGrandis, F. Semenzato and L.G. Bongiovanni. Studio sperimentale sulla neurotossicita del cicloesanolo e del cicloesanone. Med. Lavoro 2: 102–107, 1981a.

L. Perbellini, F. Brugnone, R. Silvestri and E. Gaffuri. Measurement of the urinary metabolites of n-hexane, cyclohexane and their isomers by gas chromatography. Int. Arch. Occ. Env. Health 48: 99–106, 1981b.

J.F. Treon, W.E. Crutchfield and K.V. Kitzniller. The physiological response of animals to cyclohexane, methylcyclohexane, and certain derivatives of these compounds. J. Ind. Hyg. Tox. 25: 323–347, 1943.

Cyclopropane

T½: ?

Vd: ?

Fb: ?

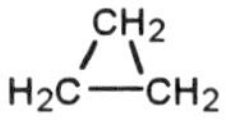

$$\begin{array}{c} CH_2 \\ / \quad \backslash \\ H_2C \text{——} CH_2 \end{array}$$

Occurrence and Usage. Cyclopropane is a colorless, flammable gas with a mild odor. It is capable of producing complete surgical anesthesia and also has moderate analgesic and muscle relaxant effects. Because cyclopropane has a low blood:gas partition coefficient, anesthetic equilibrium is attained rapidly, as is recovery after cessation of administration. It has been used extensively since 1934, but its explosive potential has tended recently to limit its application. The compound is administered with oxygen in a volumetric ratio of as high as 50:50.

Blood Concentrations. Blood concentrations of 80–180 mg/L are commonly achieved during surgical anesthesia with cyclopropane (Wollman and Smith, 1975).

Metabolism and Excretion. The compound is eliminated almost entirely by the pulmonary route, with approximately 0.5% of a dose undergoing metabolism to carbon dioxide and water. Only traces of the gas may be found in the exhaled air 3 hours after exposure. The following equilibrium distribution of cyclopropane is seen at normal body temperature (Wollman and Smith, 1975):

Partition Coefficients for Cyclopropane

Blood:Gas	Brain:Blood	Liver:Blood	Kidney:Blood	Fat:Blood
0.55	1.5–3.6	1.1	0.7	15

Toxicity. Cyclopropane is relatively safe in normal usage, although some patients have exhibited profound hypotension during recovery. This appears to be related to inadequate pulmonary ventilation with accumulation of carbon dioxide (Dripps, 1947; Buckley et al., 1953). Recreational usage of the gas has caused the death of at least 1 person (Krause and McCarthy, 1989).

Analysis. Gas chromatography is preferred for the analysis of this anesthetic gas; two of the published methods for cyclopropane in blood involve direct injection of the sample, with subsequent flame-ionization detection (Lowe, 1964; Laasberg and Etsten, 1965).

References

J.J. Buckley, F.H. Van Bergen, A.B. Dobkin et al. Postanesthetic hypotension following cyclopropane: its relationship to hypercapnia. Anesthesiology 14: 226–237, 1953.

R.D. Dripps. The immediate decrease in blood pressure seen at the conclusion of cyclopropane anesthesia: "cyclopropane shock." Anesthesiology 8: 15–35, 1947.

J.G. Krause and W.B. McCarthy. Sudden death by inhalation of cyclopropane. J. For. Sci. 34: 1011–1012, 1989.

L.H. Laasberg and B.E. Etsten. Gas chromatographic analysis of cyclopropane in whole blood. Anesthesiology 26: 216–222, 1965.

H.J. Lowe. Flame ionization detection of volatile organic anesthetics in blood, gases and tissues. Anesthesiology 25: 808–814, 1964.

H. Wollman and T.C. Smith. Uptake, distribution, elimination and administration of inhalational anesthetics. In *The Pharmacological Basis of Therapeutics*, 5th ed. (L.S. Goodman and A. Gilman, eds.), MacMillan, New York, 1975, pp. 71–80.

Cyclosporine

T½: 6–27 hr
Vd: 3.1–4.3 L/kg
Fb: 0.95
pKa: ?

$$CH_2CH=CHCH_3$$
$$CHCH_3$$
$$C_4H_9 \quad\quad C_3H_7 \quad\quad CHOH \quad C_2H_5$$
$$CH_3NCHCON(CH_3)CHCON(CH_3)CHCONHCHCON(CH_3)CH_2$$
$$CO \quad\quad\quad\quad\quad\quad\quad\quad\quad\quad\quad\quad\quad CO$$
$$CHC_4H_9 \quad\quad\quad\quad\quad\quad\quad\quad\quad\quad NHCH_3$$
$$CH_3NCOCHNHCOC(CH_3)HNHCOCHN(CH_3)COCHNHCCHC_4H_9$$
$$CH_3 \quad\quad\quad\quad\quad\quad C_4H_9 \quad\quad C_3H_7 \ O$$

Occurrence and Usage. Cyclosporine (cyclosporin A, Sandimmune) is a hydrophobic cyclic undecapeptide produced by the fungus Tolypocladium inflatum. It is a complex peptide comprised of 11 amino acid residues. The compound is an immunomodulatory substance that acts specifically at an early stage in the activation of T lymphocytes. Successful kidney, liver and heart allogenic transplants have been performed in man using cyclosporine as an immunosuppressive agent. The drug is administered either orally or intravenously; it is available as 25 or 100 mg capsules, an oral solution of 100 mg/mL, and an intravenous concentrate of 50 mg/mL. The usual oral dose is 10–15 mg/kg daily, starting a few hours before transplantation and continuing for several weeks. The dosage is then reduced gradually to a maintenance level of 5–10 mg/kg daily. The intravenous dose is usually one-third the oral dose.

Blood Concentrations. Twenty-one uremic patients (8 women and 13 men) between the ages of 18 and 66 years and weighing 50–95 kg received a single 10 mg/kg oral dose of cyclosporine following an overnight fast; the maximum concentration in blood ranged from 699–3010 µg/L and the time to reach peak concentration varied from 1–6 hours (average, 3). Twenty-four hours after the oral dose, a 2 hour intravenous infusion of cyclosporine (5 mg/kg) in saline was begun; the highest and lowest blood concentrations after cessation of the infusion were 7100 and 2800 µg/L, respectively, with a mean of 4736 µg/L. Forty-six hours after cessation of infusion, the average blood cyclosporine concentration was 67 µg/L (range, 20–122) (Lindberg et al., 1986).

The concentrations of cyclosporine and its major metabolites were measured in trough blood samples (12 hours after oral dosage) from 24 renal allograft recipients who had been administered 2–5 mg/kg of cyclosporine at 12 hour intervals as soon as they achieved good renal function. The mean whole blood cyclosporine trough concentration ranged from less than 20 to 310 µg/L (average, 125), while concentrations of the major metabolites ranged from less than 20 to 612 µg/L (Rosano et al., 1986).

The therapeutic range for cyclosporine has not been firmly established; the suggested range currently is 250–1000 µg/L when measured in whole blood using radioimmunoassay, 50–300 µg/mL in plasma using radioimmunoassay, and from 100–450 µg/mL in blood using liquid chromatography (Raisys, 1987). A minimal trough concentration of 200 µg/L in serum has been proposed as the threshold for drug toxicity, but trough concentrations lower than 100 µg/L may be associated with insufficient immunosuppression and excessive graft rejection (Calne et al., 1979; Keown et al.,

1983). About 50% of the parent compound is found in red blood cells, 40% in plasma and 10% in leukocytes (Calabresi and Parks, 1985).

Metabolism and Excretion. More than 90% of a dose of cyclosporine is metabolized by hydroxylation and N-demethylation, but there is no major metabolic pathway. Elimination is primarily biliary, with only 6% of the dose excreted in the urine and only 0.1% as unchanged drug (Maurer and Lemaire, 1986). The rate of metabolism may be affected by liver disease, age of the patient, and the presence of other drugs. None of the 12 metabolites identified so far is excreted in conjugated form, and some have been shown to possess immunosuppressive activity (Yee et al., 1986).

Toxicity. When used in high doses, cyclosporine can cause hepatotoxicity and nephrotoxicity. Occasionally, patients have developed a syndrome of thrombocytopenia and microangiopathic hemolytic anemia that may result in graft failure. Convulsions have been noted in both adult and pediatric patients receiving cyclosporine, particularly in combination with high-dose methylprednisolone (Raisys, 1987).

Analysis. A commercial radioimmunoassay kit produced by the manufacturer of cyclosporine has been widely used in analysis (Donatsch et al, 1981; Robinson et al., 1983). In an attempt to circumvent the problems associated with liquid scintillation counting, one manufacturer has synthesized ^{125}I-labeled cyclosporine and made it commercially available for use with the Sandoz kit (Mahoney and Orf, 1985; Felder et al., 1986). A fluoresence polarization assay is available that is suitable for the measurement of cyclosporine in whole blood, plasma or serum (Holt et al., 1986).

A number of liquid chromatographic methods have been published (Sawchuk and Cartier, 1981; Leyland-Jones et al., 1982; Yee et al., 1982; Carruthers et al., 1983; Robinson et al., 1983; Kates and Latini, 1984; Smith and Robinson, 1984; Lensmeyer and Fields, 1985; Annesley et al., 1986; Burckart et al., 1986; Kahn et al., 1986; Shah and Sawchuk, 1988; Sadeg et al., 1991). The potential advantage of chromatographic procedures is differential measurement of the drug and its metabolites.

Analysis of plasma requires that whole blood be incubated for 2 hours at room temperature prior to separation of plasma and erythrocytes due to a redistribution of drug into erythrocytes with decreasing temperature (Wenk et al., 1983).

References

T. Annesley, K. Matz, L. Balogh et al. Liquid-chromatographic analysis for cyclosporine with use of a microbore column and small sample volume. Clin. Chem. 32: 1407–1409, 1986.

G.J. Burckart, R. Venkataramanan, R.J. Ptachcinski et al. Cyclosporine pharmacokinetic profiles in liver, heart, and kidney transplant patients as determined by high-performance liquid chromatography. Transplant. Proc. 18: 129–136, 1986.

P. Calabresi and R.E. Parks, Jr. Antiproliferative agents and drugs used for immunosuppression. In *Goodman and Gilman's The Pharmacological Basis of Therapeutics*, 7th ed. (A.G. Gilman et al., eds), MacMillan Publishing Co., New York, 1985, pp. 1298–1299.

R.Y. Calne, K. Rolles, D.J.G. White et al. Cyclosporin A initially as the only immunosuppressant in 34 recipients of cadaveric organs: 32 kidneys, 2 pancreas, and 2 livers. Lancet 2: 1033–1036, 1979.

S.G. Carruthers, D.J. Freeman, J.C. Koegler et al. Simplified liquid-chromatographic analysis for cyclosporin A, and comparison with radioimmunoassay. Clin. Chem. 29: 180–183, 1983.

P. Donatsch, E. Abisch, M. Homberger et al. A radioimmunoassay to measure cyclosporine A in plasma and serum samples. J. Immunoassay 2: 19–32, 1981.

R.A. Felder, T.E. Mifflin and B. Bastani. An optimized method for measuring cyclosporin A with ^{125}I-labeled cyclosporin. Clin. Chem. 32: 1378–1382, 1986.

D.W. Holt, J.T. Marsden and A. Johnston. Measurement of cyclosporine: methodological problems. Transplant. Proc. 18 (Suppl. 5): 101–110, 1986.

G.C. Kahn, L.M. Shaw and M.D. Kane. Routine monitoring of cyclosporine in whole blood and in kidney tissue using high performance liquid chromatography. J. Anal. Tox. 10: 28–34, 1986.

R.E. Kates and R. Latini. Simple and rapid high-performance liquid chromatographic analysis of cyclosporine in human blood and serum. J. Chrom. 309: 441–447, 1984.

P.A. Keown, C.R. Stiller, N.R. Sinclair et al. The clinical relevance of cyclosporine blood levels as measured by radioimmunoassay. Transplant. Proc. 14: 2438–2441, 1983.

G.L. Lensmeyer and B.L. Fields. Improved liquid chromatographic determination of cyclosporine, with concomitant detection of a cell-bound metabolite. Clin. Chem. 31: 196–201, 1985.

B. Leyland-Jones, A. Clark, W. Kreis et al. High performance chromatographic determination of cyclosporine A in human plasma. Res. Comm. Chem. Path. Pharm. 37: 43–44, 1982.

A. Lindberg, B. Odlind, G. Tufveson et al. The pharmacokinetics of cyclosporine A in uremic patients. Transplant. Proc. 18: 144–152, 1986.

W.C. Mahoney and J.W. Orf. Derivatives of cyclosporin compatible with antibody-based assays: I. The generation of ^{125}I-labeled cyclosporin. Clin. Chem. 31: 459–462, 1985.

G. Maurer and M. Lemaire. Biotransformation and distribution in blood of cyclosporine and its metabolites. Transplant. Proc. 18: 25–34, 1986.

V.A. Raisys. Cyclosporine. Clin. Chem. News 13: 8–9, 1987.

W.T. Robinson, H.F. Schran and E.P. Barry. Methods to measure cyclosporine levels—high pressure liquid chromatography, radioimmunoassay, and correlation. Transplant. Proc. 14: 2403–2408, 1983.

T.G. Rosano, B.M. Freed, M.A. Pell and N. Lempert. Cyclosporine metabolites in human blood and renal tissue. Tranplant. Proc. 18 (Suppl.5): 35–40, 1986.

N. Sadeg, P.H. Chuong, J.R. Claude and M. Hamon. Micro method for liquid chromatographic determination of cyclosporin A in whole blood with use of a rapid extraction procedure. J. Anal. Tox. 15: 95–97, 1991.

R.J. Sawchuk and L.L. Cartier. Liquid chromatographic determination of cyclosporin A in blood and plasma. Clin. Chem. 27: 1368–1371, 1981.

A.K. Shah and R.J. Sawchuk. Improved liquid chromatographic determination of cyclosporine and its metabolites in blood. Clin. Chem. 34: 1467–1471, 1988.

H.T. Smith and W.T. Robinson. Semi-automated high performance liquid chromatographic method for the determination of cyclosporine in plasma and blood using column switching. J. Chrom. 305: 353–362, 1984.

M. Wenk, F. Follath and E. Abisch. Temperature dependency of apparent cyclosporin A concentrations in plasma. Clin. Chem. 29: 1865, 1983.

G.C. Yee, D.J. Gmur and M.S. Kennedy. Liquid-chromatographic determination of cyclosporine in serum with use of a rapid extraction procedure. Clin. Chem. 28: 2269–2271, 1982.

G.C. Yee, T.P. Lennon, D.G. Gmur et al. Clinical pharmacology of cyclosporine in patients undergoing bone marrow transplantation. Transplant. Proc. 18: 153–159, 1986.

Dantrolene

T½: 4–22 hr
Vd: ?
Fb: ?
pKa: 7.5

Occurrence and Usage. Dantrolene (Dantrium) was synthesized in 1967 as a peripherally-acting skeletal muscle relaxant. It is a hydantoin derivative, available as a hydrate of the sodium salt (25–100 mg capsules) for oral administration in daily doses of 25–800 mg and in 20 mg vials for intravenous injection in doses of 1–10 mg/kg. The compound has very poor water solubility and tends to hydrolyze in aqueous solution with precipitation of the free acid.

Blood Concentrations. A single oral 100 mg dose given to 8 subjects produced an average peak plasma level of 1.24 mg/L at times ranging from 1–12 hours; peak levels of 5-hydroxydantrolene averaged 0.39 mg/L at times of 4–22 hours. The average half-life of dantrolene was 6.1 hours, and that of 5-hydroxydantrolene, 15.5 hours. All subjects exhibited sedation and dizziness during the time of maximum plasma dantrolene concentrations (Meyler et al., 1979). Four patients receiving 400 mg daily on a chronic basis developed plasma concentrations of 2–3 mg/L several hours after the first morning dose (Herman et al., 1972). Plasma concentrations of two metabolites, hydroxydantrolene and acetamidodantrolene, exceeded the steady-state levels of dantrolene by several fold in 6 patients on chronic therapy with the drug (Vallner et al., 1979).

Metabolism and Excretion. Dantrolene is metabolized by reduction of the nitro group and subsequent acylation, or by hydroxylation of the hydantoin ring. Of the known metabolites, only 5-hydroxydantrolene is active, having about one-fifth the muscle-relaxant potency of its parent (Ellis and Wessels, 1978). The amino metabolite has not been detected in plasma or urine. The major metabolites in urine are 5-hydroxydantrolene and the acetamido metabolite, with small amounts of unchanged drug; only a small fraction of a single dose has been accounted for as urinary metabolites (Cox et al., 1969; Conklin and Sobers, 1973; White and Schwan, 1976).

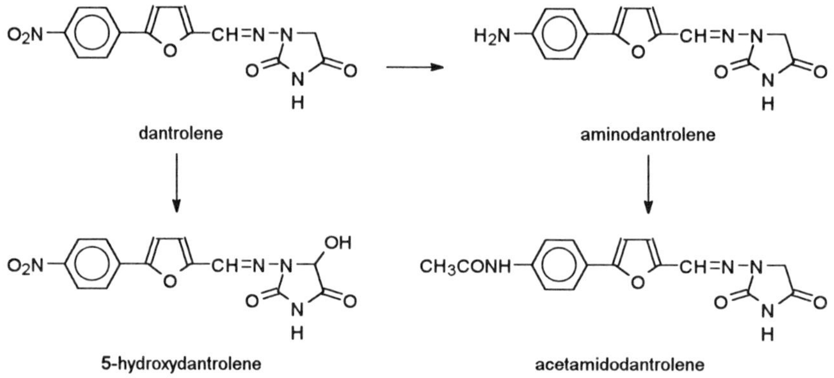

dantrolene   aminodantrolene

5-hydroxydantrolene   acetamidodantrolene

Toxicity. Toxic effects of dantrolene include loss of appetite, constipation, hepatitis, visual disturbances, headache, tachycardia, confusion, and nervousness. A 38 year old woman developed jaundice after 16 weeks of dantrolene therapy at a dose of 400 mg per day. A diagnosis of hepatitis was confirmed by liver biopsy, and the patient's liver function tests returned to normal 3 months after dantrolene discontinuation (Schneider and Mitchell, 1976). One attempt at suicide has been reported in which a large overdose of dantrolene produced temporary unconsciousness without residual neurological effect (Chyatte and Basmajian, 1973).

Analysis. A rapid fluorometric procedure for the assay of dantrolene in biological fluids has been described (Hollifield and Conklin, 1968); this technique has been modified to allow its use in the separate determination of the drug and its known metabolites (Hollifield and Conklin, 1973). A differential pulse polarographic method has also been utilized for this purpose (Cox et al., 1969). Liquid chromatography is well suited to the analysis of this drug and its metabolites (Saxena et al., 1977; Hackett and Dusci, 1979; Wuis et al., 1982; Lalande et al., 1988).

References

S.B. Chyatte and J.V. Basmajian. Dantrolene sodium: long-term effects in severe spasticity. Arch. Phys. Med. Rehab. 54: 311–315, 1973.

J.D. Conklin and R.J. Sobers. Qualitative method for dantrolene and related metabolite in urine. J. Pharm. Sci. 62: 1024–1025, 1973.

P.L. Cox, J.P. Heotis, D. Polin and G.M. Rose. Quantitative determination of dantrolene sodium and its metabolites by differential pulse polarography. J. Pharm. Sci. 58: 987–989, 1969.

K.O. Ellis and F.L. Wessels. Muscle relaxant properties of the identified metabolites of dantrolene. Arch. Pharm. 301: 237–240, 1978.

L.P. Hackett and L.J. Dusci. Determination of dantrolene sodium in human plasma using high-performance liquid chromatography. J. Chrom. 179: 222–224, 1979.

R. Herman, N. Mayer and S.A. Mecomber. Clinical pharmaco-physiology of dantrolene sodium. Am. J. Phys. Med. 51: 296–311, 1972.

R.D. Hollifield and J.D. Conklin. A spectrophotofluorometric procedure for the determination of dantrolene in blood and urine. Arch. Int. Pharm. Ther. 174: 333–341, 1968.

R.D. Hollifield and J.D. Conklin. Determination of dantrolene in biological specimens containing drug-related metabolites. J. Pharm. Sci. 62: 271–274, 1973.

M. Lalande, P. Mills and R.G. Peterson. Determination of dantrolene and its reduced and oxidized metabolites in plasma by high-performance liquid chromatography. J. Chrom. 430: 187–191, 1988.

W.J. Meyler, H.W. Mols-Thurkow and H. Wesseling. Relationship between plasma concentration and effect of dantrolene sodium in man. Eur. J. Clin. Pharm. 16: 203–209, 1979.

S.J. Saxena, I.L. Honigberg, J.T. Stewart and J.J. Vallner. Liquid chromatography in pharmaceutical analysis VII: determination of dantrolene sodium in biological fluids. J. Pharm. Sci. 66: 751–753, 1977.

R. Schneider and D. Mitchell. Dantrolene hepatitis. J. Am. Med. Asso. 235: 1590–1591, 1976.

J.J. Vallner, I.L. Honigberg, J.T. Stewart and A.B. Peyton. Dantrolene and metabolite levels in six patients on chronic therapy. Curr. Ther. Res. 25: 79–91, 1979.

R.L. White and T.J. Schwan. Synthesis of 5-hydroxy-1-((5-(p-nitrophenyl)furfurylidene)-amino)hydantoin, a metabolite of dantrolene. J. Pharm. Sci. 65: 135–136, 1976.

E.W. Wuis, A.C.L.M. Grutters, T.B. Vree and E. van der Kleyn. Simultaneous determination of dantrolene and its metabolites, 5-hydroxydantrolene and nitro-reduced acetylated dantrolene (F 490), in plasma and urine of man and dog by high-performance liquid chromatography. J. Chrom. 231: 401–409, 1982.

DDT

T½: ?
Vd: ?
Fb: ?

Occurrence and Usage. DDT (dicophane, chlorophenothane, dichlorodiphenyltrichloroethane) is a chlorinated hydrocarbon that was first synthesized in 1874 and has been employed as a contact insecticide since 1940. Technical grades of the chemical contain a mixture of p,p'-DDT (67–85%), o,p'-DDT (8–21%) and related compounds. DDT has come under severe restrictions in some countries since 1970 due to its persistence and accumulation in the food chain. The current threshold limit value for DDT in air is 1 mg/m³.

Blood Concentrations. Blood concentrations of total DDT (DDT plus DDE, a metabolite) in 44 healthy English adults with no occupational exposure to the chemical averaged 0.013 mg/L, with a range of 0.005–0.038 mg/L (Robinson and Hunter, 1966). Two subjects who ingested 10 or 20 mg of technical DDT for 183 days developed maximal serum levels of p,p'-DDT that exceeded 0.200 and 0.500 mg/L, respectively, by the end of the study (Morgan and Roan, 1971). Total DDT serum concentrations in 499 persons living downstream from a DDT factory averaged 0.159 mg/L (range, 0.001–2.821); DDE accounted for an average of 87% of the DDT-related substances in serum (Kreiss et al., 1981). A group of 18 asymptomatic DDT factory workers was found to have total DDT serum concentrations of 0.579–2.914 mg/L (average, 1.359), consisting largely of nearly equal parts of p,p'-DDT and p,p'-DDE (Poland et al., 1970).

Metabolism and Excretion. DDT is converted to a slight extent to the much less toxic DDE (dichlorodiphenyldichloroethylene) by dehydrochlorination; DDE apparently does not undergo further biotransformation, but is stored for an indefinite period of time in adipose tissues. Most of the p,p'-DDE present in human fat represents preformed dietary DDE rather than endogenously produced DDE. The major detoxification pathway of DDT is via dechlorination to DDD (dichlorodiphenyldichloroethane), an active insecticide, which readily degrades to DDA (dichlorodiphenylacetic acid), a water soluble, rapidly excreted detoxification product.

Urinary DDA represents about 47% of ingested precursor material during low exposure, but DDA excretion becomes quantitatively less important as DDT intake increases (Morgan and Roan, 1971; Roan et al., 1971). Urinary DDA concentrations correlate reasonably well with DDT storage levels in body fat; DDA was undetectable in the urine of members of the general population and ranged from 0.01–2.67 mg/L in workers with low to high exposure to DDT (Laws et al., 1967). By contrast, urine concentrations of DDT, DDE and DDD in healthy unexposed persons averaged 0.007, 0.016 and 0.003 mg/L, respectively (Cueto and Biros, 1967), and 0.011, 0.021 and 0.006 mg/L, respectively in occupationally exposed persons (Laws et al., 1967).

Fat concentrations of DDT, DDE and DDD averaged 1.3, 4.5 and 0.025 mg/kg in unexposed persons in Hawaii (Casarett et al., 1968) and 112, 73 and <0.3 mg/kg, respectively in occupationally exposed workers (Laws et al., 1967). Average fat concentrations of DDT in unexposed persons have ranged from 1.7–28 mg/kg in 12 other studies (Matsumura, 1975). An average of 72% of DDT-related material in the fat of normal persons is present as DDE (Hoffman et al., 1967). Total DDT concentrations in human milk from urban U.S. residents in 1970–1971 ranged from 0.02–0.83 mg/L, averaging 0.17 mg/L (Wilson et al., 1973).

DDT $\left[\text{Cl–C}_6\text{H}_4\text{–CH(CCl}_3\text{)–C}_6\text{H}_4\text{–Cl}\right]$ $\longrightarrow$ DDD $\left[\text{Cl–C}_6\text{H}_4\text{–CH(CHCl}_2\text{)–C}_6\text{H}_4\text{–Cl}\right]$

DDE $\left[\text{Cl–C}_6\text{H}_4\text{–C(=CCl}_2\text{)–C}_6\text{H}_4\text{–Cl}\right]$ DDA $\left[\text{Cl–C}_6\text{H}_4\text{–CH(COOH)–C}_6\text{H}_4\text{–Cl}\right]$

Toxicity. DDT is a central nervous system stimulant that in overdose can cause paresthesia of the tongue and lips, tremor, confusion and convulsions. In general, the compound is felt to be relatively safe, having an estimated lethal dose of 30 g in an adult. Men who received 35 mg daily oral doses of recrystallized DDT for a period of 21.5 months and who developed body fat concentrations of 129–659 mg/kg of DDT and 51–142 mg/kg of DDE exhibited no definite clinical or laboratory abnormalities (Hayes et al., 1971). A healthy person who self-administered an acute oral 5 g dose of technical DDT developed nausea, insomnia and excitability that diminished over a period of one week (Rappolt, 1973). Oral doses estimated at 570–1700 mg (16–120 mg/kg) produced convulsions in 6 persons accidentally poisoned with DDT (Hsieh, 1954).

Several instances of fatal DDT poisoning have been reported in humans, although the hydrocarbon vehicle involved in these cases probably contributed significantly to the deaths (Hill and Robinson, 1945; Biden-Steele and Stuckey, 1946; Hill and Damiani, 1946; Reingold and Lasky, 1947; Smith, 1948).

Analysis. Biological fluids and tissues are frequently assayed for DDT, DDE and DDD by electron-capture gas chromatography after various solvent extraction procedures (Cueto and Biros, 1967; Dale et al., 1970; Morgan and Roan, 1971). DDA has been determined in urine by colorimetry (Cueto et al., 1956) and by gas chromatography of a methyl derivative, employing either electron-capture (Laws et al., 1967; Cranmer et al., 1969; Cranmer and Copeland, 1973) or microcoulometric detection (Roan et al., 1971).

References

K. Biden-Steele and R.E. Stuckey. Poisoning by D.D.T. emulsion. Lancet 2: 235–236, 1946.

L.J. Casarett, G.C. Fryer, W.L. Yauger, Jr. and H.W. Klemmer. Organochlorine pesticide residues in human tissue—Hawaii. Arch. Env. Health 17: 306–311, 1968.

M.F. Cranmer, J.J. Carroll and M.F. Copeland. Determination of DDT and metabolites, including DDA, in human urine by gas chromatography. Bull. Env. Cont. Tox. 4: 214–223, 1969.

M.F. Cranmer and M.F. Copeland. Electron capture gas chromatographic analysis of DDA: utilization of 2-chloroethanol derivative. Bull. Env. Cont. Tox. 9: 186–192, 1973.

C. Cueto, A.G. Barnes and A.M. Mattson. Determination of DDA in urine using an ion exchange resin. J. Agr. Food Chem. 4: 943–945, 1956.

C. Cueto, Jr. and F.J. Biros. Chlorinated insecticides and related materials in human urine. Tox. Appl. Pharm. 10: 261–269, 1967.

W.E. Dale, J.W. Miles and T.B. Gaines. Quantitative method for determination of DDT and DDT metabolites in blood serum. J. Asso. Off. Anal. Chem. 53: 1287–1292, 1970.

W.J. Hayes, Jr., W.E. Dale and C.I. Pirkle. Evidence of safety of long-term, high oral doses of DDT for man. Arch. Env. Health 22: 119–135, 1971.

K.R. Hill and G. Robinson. Fatal case of D.D.T. poisoning in a child. Brit. Med. J. 2: 845–847, 1945.

W.R. Hill and C.R. Damiani. Death following exposure to DDT. New Eng. J. Med. 235: 897–899, 1946.

W.S. Hoffman, H. Adler, W.I. Fishbein and F.C. Bauer. Relation of pesticide concentrations in fat to pathological changes in tissues. Arch. Env. Health 15: 758–765, 1967.

H.C. Hsieh. D.D.T. intoxication in a family of Southern Taiwan. Arch. Ind. Hyg. Occ. Med. 10: 344–346, 1954.

K. Kreiss, M.A. Zack, R.D. Kimbrough et al. Cross-sectional study of a community with exceptional exposure to DDT. J. Am. Med. Asso. 245: 1926–1930, 1981.

E.R. Laws, Jr., A. Curley and F.J. Biros. Men with intensive occupational exposure to DDT. Arch. Env. Health 15: 766–775, 1967.

F. Matsumura. *Toxicology of Insecticides*, Plenum, New York, 1975, p. 453.

D.P. Morgan and C.C. Roan. Absorption, storage, and metabolic conversion of ingested DDT and DDT metabolites in man. Arch. Env. Health 22: 301–308, 1971.

A. Poland, D. Smith, R. Kuntzman et al. Effect of intensive occupational exposure to DDT on phenylbutazone and cortisol metabolism in human subjects. Clin. Pharm. Ther. 11: 724–731, 1970.

R.T. Rappolt, Sr. Use of oral DDT in three human barbiturate intoxications: hepatic enzyme induction by reciprocal detoxicants. Clin. Tox. 6: 147–151, 1973.

I.M. Reingold and I.I. Lasky. Acute fatal poisoning following ingestion of a solution of DDT. Ann. Int. Med. 26: 945–947, 1947.

C. Roan, D. Morgan and E.H. Paschal. Urinary excretion of DDA following ingestion of DDT and DDT metabolites in man. Arch. Env. Health 22: 309–315, 1971.

J. Robinson and C.G. Hunter. Organochlorine insecticides: concentrations in human blood and adipose tissue. Arch. Env. Health 13: 558–563, 1966.

N.J. Smith. Death following accidental ingestion of DDT. J. Am. Med. Asso. 136: 469–471, 1948.

D.J. Wilson, D.J. Locker, C.A. Ritzen et al. DDT concentrations in human milk. Am. J. Dis. Child. 125: 814–817, 1973.

Desipramine

T½: 12–54 hr
Vd: 22–59 L/kg
Fb: 0.70–0.90
pKa: 9.5

$(CH_2)_3NHCH_3$

Occurrence and Usage. Desipramine (Norpramine, Pertofrane) is the N-desmethyl metabolite of imipramine and is an active antidepressant agent in its own right. It was first synthesized in 1962 and was used clinically as early as 1963. The compound has been claimed to be faster-acting and better tolerated than its parent, although some investigators have found little difference between the two. It is available as the hydrochloride salt in tablets of 25–150 mg and is administered orally in doses of up to 300 mg daily.

Blood Concentrations. Maximal plasma desipramine concentrations of 0.008–0.015 mg/L (average, 0.012) occurred between 3 and 6 hours after a single oral 50 mg dose in 4 volunteers; peak levels of 2-hydroxydesipramine also averaged 0.012 mg/L but occurred between 2 and 4 hours.

Desipramine concentrations declined with an average half-life of 22 hours (DeVane et al., 1981). Steady-state plasma concentrations of desipramine in patients receiving 75 mg chronic daily doses have ranged from 0.010–0.280 mg/L (Hammer and Sjoqvist, 1967; Hammer et al., 1969). During chronic therapy with 1.2 mg/kg (82 mg/70 kg) daily oral doses, plasma concentrations averaged 0.043 mg/L, with a range of 0.021–0.064 mg/L (Alexanderson, 1972). A group of 54 patients receiving an average daily oral dose of 186 mg developed average steady-state plasma concentrations of 0.188 mg/L (range, 0.012–0.684) for desipramine and 0.057 mg/L (range, 0.013–0.143) for 2-hydroxydesipramine (Amsterdam et al., 1985).

The blood/plasma concentration ratio for desipramine has not been reported, but it probably falls within the range of 1.0–1.7 established for other tricyclic antidepressants (Maguire et al., 1980).

Metabolism and Excretion. The metabolism of this drug has not been quantitatively studied in man, but it is believed to be converted partially to the inactive or less active metabolites, 2-hydroxydesipramine, 10-hydroxydesipramine and iminodibenzyl, with a minor amount being N-demethylated to nordesipramine (didesmethylimipramine), which may have pharmacologic activity. The majority of a dose has not been accounted for and it is suspected that rupture of the ethylene bridge occurs with formation of unidentified metabolites. The hydroxylated metabolites are excreted for the most part as glucuronide conjugates (Crammer and Scott, 1966; Bickel et al., 1967). The 24 hour urinary excretion of unchanged desipramine does not usually exceed 1% of an administered dose, although this value may be elevated somewhat during conditions of acid urine (Sjoqvist et al., 1969).

Toxicity. Anticholinergic side-effects in patients treated with desipramine have not been found to correlate with plasma concentrations of the drug (Rudorfer and Young, 1980). The several reported cases of nonfatal desipramine overdosage involved ingestion of 1000–2500 mg of the drug, and the patients have exhibited seizures, coma, hypotension, and electrocardiographic abnormalities (Williams, 1964; Tchen et al., 1966; Colvard, 1968; Chahine and Castellanos, 1971; Lee et al., 1981, Carpenter et al., 1982). Four patients survived after ingesting as much as 2950 mg of the drug and achieving plasma concentrations of 1.2–2.0 mg/L (Biggs et al., 1977; Hughes and Rome, 1984; Sawyer et al., 1984; Spina et al., 1985).

Six deaths have occurred in adults following acute overdosage in which postmortem blood concentrations of 3–15 mg/L (average, 9.8) and liver concentrations of 50–150 mg/kg (average, 111) were observed (Robinson et al., 1979; Cravey, 1980; Chaturvedi et al., 1987; Sidebotham, 1991). The following tissue distribution was observed in an infant who died 6.5 hours following ingestion of 2500 mg of desipramine (Bickel et al., 1967):

Desipramine Concentrations in a Fatal Case (mg/L or mg/kg)

Plasma	Brain	Liver	Kidney	Urine	Gastric
10	100	125	117	0.2	118 mg

Desipramine is subject to postmortem redistribution due to continued diffusion from the gastrointestinal tract or release from drug-rich tissues such as the lung and liver; heart blood/peripheral blood concentration ratios as high as 5.7 have been observed for the drug (Apple and Bandt, 1988, Anderson and Prouty, 1989).

Analysis. Desipramine may be assayed in biological specimens using the procedures cited for imipramine. Additionally, procedures have been described specifically for desipramine using electron-capture gas chromatography after N-trifluoroacetylation (Ervik et al., 1970), nitrogen–selective gas chromatography of the free drug (Antal et al., 1980), and liquid chromatography (Kenney et al., 1989; Wanwimolruk, 1991). One investigator has drawn attention to the possibility of contamination of desipramine primary standard by imipramine and iminodibenzyl, in amounts of up to 3–4% of each (Saady et al., 1981).

References

B. Alexanderson. Pharmacokinetics of desmethylimipramine and nortriptyline in man after single and multiple oral doses—a cross-over study. Eur. J. Clin. Pharm. 5: 1–10, 1972.

J.D. Amsterdam, D.J. Brunswick, L. Potter et al. Desipramine and 2-hydroxydesipramine plasma levels in endogenous depressed patients. Arch. Gen. Psych. 42: 361–364, 1985.

W.H. Anderson and R.W. Prouty. Postmortem redistribution of drugs. In *Advances in Analytical Toxicology* (R.C. Baselt, ed.), Vol. 2, YearBook Medical, Chicago, 1989, pp. 70–102.

E. Antal, S. Mercik and P.A. Kramer. Technical considerations in the gas chromatographic analysis of desipramine. J. Chrom. 183: 149–157, 1980.

F.S. Apple and C.M. Bandt. Liver and blood postmortem tricyclic antidepressant concentrations. Am. J. Clin. Path. 89: 794–796, 1988.

M.H. Bickel, R. Brochon, B. Friolet et al. Clinical and biochemical results of a fatal case of desipramine intoxication. Psychopharmacology 10: 431–436, 1967.

J.T. Biggs, D.G. Spiker, J.M. Petit and V.E. Ziegler. Tricyclic antidepressant overdose. J. Am. Med. Asso. 237: 135–138, 1977.

P. Carpenter, F.L. Gobel and D.J. Hulsing. Desipramine cardiac toxicity. Minn. Med. 65: 231–234, 1982.

R.A. Chahine and A. Castellanos, Jr. Myocardial toxicity produced by desipramine overdosage. Chest 59: 566–568, 1971.

A.K. Chaturvedi, J.T. Hidding, N.G.S. Rao et al. Two tricyclic antidepressant poisonings. For. Sci. Int. 33: 93–101, 1987.

C. Colvard, Jr. Overdosage of desipramine hydrochloride with marked electrocardiographic abnormalities. South. Med. J. 61: 1218–1222, 1968.

J.L. Crammer and B. Scott. New metabolites of imipramine. Psychopharmacology 8: 461–468, 1966.

R.H. Cravey. Personal communication, 1980.

C.L. DeVane, M. Savett and W.J. Jusko. Desipramine and 2-hydroxy-desipramine pharmacokinetics in normal volunteers. Eur. J. Clin. Pharm. 19: 61–64, 1981.

M. Ervik, T. Walle and H. Ehrsson. Quantitative gas chromatographic determination of nanogram levels of desipramine in serum. Acta Pharm. Suecica 7: 625–634, 1970.

W. Hammer and F. Sjoqvist. Plasma levels of monomethylated tricyclic antidepressants during treatment with imipramine-like compounds. Life Sci. 6: 1895–1903, 1967.

W. Hammer and B.B. Brodie. Application of isotope derivative technique to assay of secondary amines: estimation of desipramine by acetylation with 3-acetic anhydride. J. Pharm. Exp. Ther. 157: 503–508, 1967.

W. Hammer, S. Martens and F. Sjoqvist. A comparative study of the metabolism of desmethylimipramine, nortriptyline, and oxyphenylbutazone in man. Clin. Pharm. Ther. 10: 44–49, 1969.

P.L. Hughes and J.D. Rome. Cardiopulmonary collapse associated with an overdose of desipramine. Mayo Clin. Proc. 59: 574, 1984.

J.T. Kenney, P.J. Orsulak, R.M. Kolodner and M.E. Burton. Determination of serum desipramine and 2-hydroxydesipramine for pharmacokinetic applications by HPLC with ultraviolet detection. Clin. Chem. 35: 2134–2136, 1989.

W.R. Lee, M.U. Sheikh, E.A. Covarrubias and L.M. Slotkoff. Variant ventricular tachycardia in desipramine toxicity. S. Med. J. 74: 1268–1269, 1981.

K.P. Maguire, G.D. Burrows, T.R. Norman and B.A. Scoggins. Blood/plasma distribution ratios of psychotropic drugs. Clin. Chem. 26: 1624–1625, 1980.

A.E. Robinson, R.D. McDowall, H. Satter et al. Tricyclic and tetracyclic antidepressant drugs: forensic toxicology of some autopsy cases. J. Anal. Tox. 3: 3–13, 1979.

M.V. Rudorfer and R.C. Young. Anticholinergic effects and plasma desipramine levels. Clin. Pharm. Ther. 28: 703–706, 1980.

J.J. Saady, N. Narasimhachari and R.O. Friedel. Unsuspected impurities in imipramine and desipramine standards and pharmaceutical formulations. Clin. Chem. 27: 343–344, 1981.

W.T. Sawyer, J.L. Caudill and M.J. Ellison. A case of severe acute desipramine overdose. Am. J. Psych. 141: 122–123, 1984.

C. Sidebotham. Personal communication, 1991.

F. Sjoqvist, F. Berglund, O. Borga et al. The pH-dependent excretion of monomethylated tricyclic antidepressants. Clin. Pharm. Ther. 10: 826–833, 1969.

S. Spector, N.L. Spector and M.P. Almeida, Jr. Radioimmunoassay for desmethylimipramine. Psychopharm. Comm. 1: 421–429, 1975.

E. Spina, T.K. Henthorn, L. Eleborg et al. Desmethylimipramine overdose: nonlinear kinetics in a slow hydroxylator. Ther. Drug Mon. 7: 239–241, 1985.

P. Tchen, A.D. Weatherhead and N.G. Richards. Acute intoxication with desipramine. New Eng. J. Med. 274: 1197, 1966.

S. Wanwimolruk. High performance liquid chromatographic analysis of desipramine in human plasma using a microbore column technique. J. Liq. Chrom. 14: 1805–1811, 1991.

A.J. Williams. "Desipramine" overdosage. Brit. Med. J. 1: 371–372, 1964.

Dextromethorphan

T½: 3.2–3.6 hr (rapid metabolizers)
Vd: 255–316 L/kg
Fb: ?
pKa: 8.3

Occurrence and Usage. Dextromethorphan (Romilar) is the d-isomer of 3-methoxy-N-methylmorphinan, a synthetic analogue of codeine. Although the l-isomer (levomethorphan or levorphan) is a potent narcotic analgesic, dextromethorphan is not classified as a narcotic and is used only for its antitussive effects. It is found in numerous cough syrups, tablets, and capsules as the hydrobromide salt in amounts of 2.5–20 mg per dose. The daily intake by adults may range up to 120 mg.

Blood Concentrations. Serum dextromethorphan concentrations in 12 subjects after a single 20 mg oral dose reached an average peak level of 1.8 µg/L after 2.5 hours; this declined to 1.4 µg/L by 5 hours (Barnhart and Massad, 1979). Plasma concentrations of a metabolite, conjugated dextrorphan, reached an average peak of 381 µg/L at 2 hours after a 30 mg oral dose of dextromethorphan given to 6 subjects; this declined to 263 µg/L by 4 hours. Free dextrorphan was not present in plasma at measureable levels (Ramachander et al., 1977).

With oral 30 mg doses given 4 times daily (120 mg/day) for 7 days, peak plasma dextromethorphan levels averaged 2.4 µg/L (range, 0.5–5.9) in 14 extensive metabolizers and 207 µg/L (range, 182–231) in 2 poor metabolizers (deZeeuw and Jonkman, 1988).

Metabolism and Excretion. Within a 24 hour period, 43% of an oral labeled dose of dextromethorphan is excreted in the urine and 0.1% in the feces (Calesnick and Christensen, 1967). It is known to be metabolized by both O- and N-demethylation to dextrorphan (Dromoran), an active antitussive, and to 3-methoxymorphinan and 3-hydroxymorphinan. Less than 2.5% of a dose is excreted unchanged in the 24 hour urine, while less than 1% is present as 3-methoxymorphinan; up to 15% and 30% is found as conjugated 3-hydroxymorphinan and conjugated dextrorphan, respectively (Willner, 1963; East and Dye, 1985).

A genetic polymorphism exists for the rate and extent of metabolism of dextromethorphan; rapid or extensive metabolizers exhibit plasma elimination half-lives averaging 3.4 hours, while slow or poor metabolizers, who constitute about 10% of the population, may exhibit half-lives exceeding 24 hours (Silvasti et al., 1987; Chen et al., 1990; Duche et al., 1993).

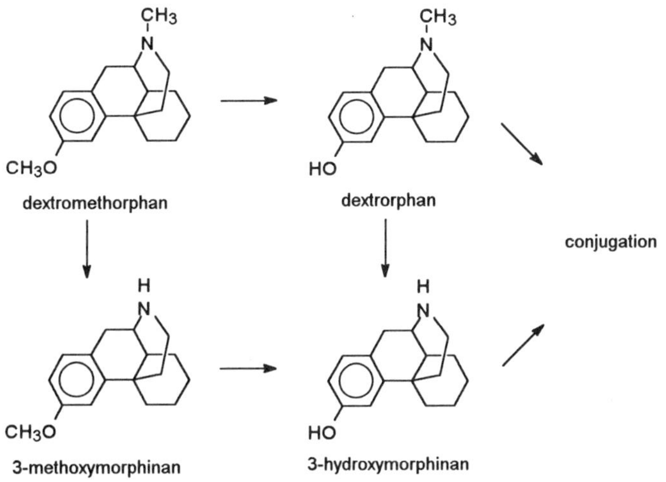

Toxicity. Dextromethorphan produces sedation in overdosage. A 1 year old child ingested 180 mg of the drug and was treated in a hospital; both dextromethorphan and dextrorphan were identified in urine in amounts representing 34% of the total dose (Versie et al., 1962). Naloxone has been used successfully to treat the respiratory depression observed with dextromethorphan overdosage (Schneider et al., 1989).

Two fatalities were reported following acute oral overdosage in adults; dextromethorphan concentrations of 3.3–9.2 mg/L in blood and 31–230 mg/kg in liver were observed (Rammer et al., 1988).

Analysis. Dextromethorphan may be measured in biological fluids by gas chromatography using flame-ionization detection for toxic levels (Noirfalise, 1974; Furlanut et al., 1977) and electron-capture detection of a pentafluorobenzyl derivative for therapeutic levels (Barnhart and Massad, 1979). The metabolite dextrorphan has been determined in plasma by fluorometry (Ramachander et al., 1977) and liquid chromatography with fluorescence detection (Gillilan et al., 1980). Liquid chromatography has also been applied to the detection of dextromethorphan and its metabolites (Park et al., 1984; East and Dye, 1985; Mascher, 1987; Johansson and Svensson, 1988; Chen et al., 1990; Marshall et al., 1992).

References

J.W. Barnhart and E.N. Massad. Determination of dextromethorphan in serum by gas chromatography. J. Chrom. 163: 390–395, 1979.

B. Calesnick and J.A. Christensen. Latency of cough response as a measure of antitussive agents. Clin. Pharm. Ther. 8: 374–380, 1967.

Z.R. Chen, A.A. Somogyi and F. Bochner. Simultaneous determination of dextromethorphan and three metabolites in plasma and urine. Ther. Drug Mon. 12: 97–104, 1990.

R.A. de Zeeuw and J.H.G. Jonkman. Genetic differences in oxidative drug metabolism. In *Proceedings of the International Association of Forensic Toxicologists*, Groningen, Netherlands, 1988, pp. 53–64.

J.C. Duche, V. Querol-Ferrer, J. Barre et al. Dextromethorphan O-demethylation and dextrorphan glucuronidation in a French population. Int. J. Clin. Pharm. Ther. Tox. 31: 392–398, 1993.

T. East and D. Dye. Determination of dextromethorphan and metabolites in human plasma and urine by high-performance liquid chromatography with fluorescence detection. J. Chrom. 338: 97–112, 1985.

M. Furlanut, L. Cima, P. Benetello and P. Giusti. Gas-liquid chromatographic determination of dextromethorphan in serum and brain. J. Chrom. 140: 270–274, 1977.

R. Gillilan, R.C. Lanman and W.D. Mason. High pressure liquid chromatographic determination of dextrorphan in human plasma. Anal. Letters 13: 381–387, 1980.

M. Johansson and C. Svensson. Determination of dextromethorphan and its metabolites in plasma by dual column liquid chromatography and fluorimetric detection. J. Pharm. Biomed. Anal. 6: 211–220, 1988.

P.S. Marshall, R.J. Straka and K. Johnson. Determination of dextromethorphan and its O-demethylated metabolite from urine. Ther. Drug Mon. 14: 402–407, 1992.

H. Masher. HPLC determination of dextrorphan and 3-hydroxymorphinan in human plasma. J. Chrom. 420: 217–222, 1987.

A. Noirfalise. Dosage du dextromethorphane dans le plasma par chromatographie en phase gazeuse. J. Chrom. 90: 392–393, 1974.

Y.H. Park, M.P. Kullberg and D.N. Hinsvark. Quantitative determination of dextromethorphan and three metabolites in urine by reverse-phase high-performance liquid chromatography. J. Pharm. Sci. 73: 24–29, 1984.

G. Ramachander, F.D. Williams and J.F. Emele. Determination of dextrorphan in plasma and evaluation of bioavailability of dextromethorphan in humans. J. Pharm. Sci. 66: 1047–1048, 1977.

L. Rammer, P. Holmgren and H. Sandler. Fatal intoxication by dextromethorphan: a report on two cases. For. Sci. Int. 37: 233–236, 1988.

S.M. Schneider, E.A. Michelson and C.D. Boucek. Dextromethorphan narcosis reversed by naloxone. Vet. Hum. Tox. 31: 376, 1989.

M. Silvasti, P. Karttunen, H. Tukiainen et al. Pharmacokinetics of dextromethorphan and dextrorphan. Int. J. Clin. Pharm. Ther. Tox. 25: 493–497, 1987.

R. Versie, A. Noirfalise, M. Neven and R. Malchair. Toxicite et metabolisme du 3 methoxy-N-methyl morphinane (Romilar) chez l'enfant. Ann. Med. Leg. 42: 561–565, 1962.

K. Willner. Ausscheidung und Abbau von (+)-3-Methoxy-N-methylmorphinan und seinen entmethylierten Derivaten beim Menschen. Arz. Forsch. 13: 26–29, 1963.

Dextromoramide

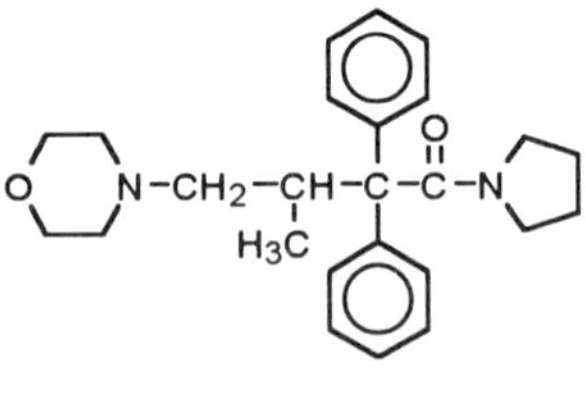

T½: 1.5–4.7 hr
Vd: 2.6 L/kg
Fb: ?
pKa: 7.0

Occurrence and Usage. Dextromoramide (Palfium) is a synthetic narcotic analgesic first prepared in 1956. The drug is approximately 5 times as potent as morphine and is used in surgery, intensive care units and at home. The compound is available in many European countries in both injectable forms and in tablets, usually as the bitartrate salt. In adults the therapeutic dose ranges from 5–20 mg, repeated as necessary.

Blood Concentrations. Following a single oral dose of 7.5 mg of dextromoramide to 9 patients, peak plasma concentrations ranged from 0.09–0.13 mg/L (average, 0.11) and occurred at 0.5–6.0 hour post-dose (Pagani et al., 1989). Plasma concentrations on the order of 0.10 mg/L were observed at 1 hour after intravenous injection of 5 mg in an adult (Kintz et al., 1988).

Metabolism and Excretion. The metabolism of dextromoramide has not been well studied. Less than 0.1% of a dose is excreted in the urine in the first 8 hours as unchanged drug (Pagani et al., 1989). It is thought that 2'-hydroxydextromoramide is a major metabolite (Caddy et al., 1979).

Toxicity. Dextromoramide in overdosage produces the usual sedative and respiratory depressant effects associated with opioid analgesics. In 4 fatal cases attributed to oral administration of dextromoramide, postmortem blood concentrations ranged from 0.14–0.50 mg/L. In 13 fatal cases following intravenous administration, blood concentrations ranged from 0.1–1.5 mg/L (Hansson, 1987; Kintz et al., 1989a, 1989b).

Analysis. Dextromoramide has been determined in biological samples by gas chromatography with nitrogen detection (Kintz, 1988), gas chromatography-mass spectrometry (Kintz et al., 1990; Pagani et al., 1989; Brewer, 1990) and liquid chromatography (Caddy et al., 1979; Hackett et al., 1987; Turcant et al., 1991; Rop et al., 1993).

References

E. Brewer. A dextromoramide-related fatality. J. For. Sci. 35: 483–489, 1990.

B. Caddy, R. Idowu, W.J. Tilstone and N.C. Thomson. Analysis and disposition of dextromoramide in body fluids. In *Proceedings of the International Association of Forensic Toxicologists* (J.S. Oliver, ed.) Croom Helm, London, 1979, pp. 126–139.

L.P. Hackett, L.J. Dusci and K.F. Iiett. Analysis of several nonopiate narcotic analgesics and cocaine in serum using high-performance liquid chromatography. J. Anal. Tox. 11: 269–271, 1987.

R.C. Hansson. Personal communication, 1986.

P. Kintz, P. Mangin, A.A. Lugnier and A.J. Chaumont. Gas chromatographic assay for dextromoramide in human plasma. J. Chrom. 432: 329–333, 1988.

P. Kintz, A. Tracqui, P. Mangin et al. Fatal intoxication by dextromoramide: a report on two cases. J. Anal. Tox. 13: 238–239, 1989a.

P. Kintz, A. Tracqui, P. Mangin et al. Toxicological findings after fatal dextromoramide injection. Clin. Tox. 27: 385–388, 1989b.

P. Kintz, P. Mangin, A.A. Lugnier and A.J. Chaumont. Determination of dextromoramide by capillary gas chromatography and electron impact mass spectrometry. J. Anal. Tox. 14: 252–253, 1990.

I. Pagani, N. Barzaghi, F. Crema et al. Pharmacokinetics of dextromoramide in surgical patients. Fund. Clin. Pharm. 3: 27–35, 1989.

P.P. Rop, F. Grimaldi, M. Bresson et al. Determination of dextromoramide in plasma and whole blood using HPLC with ultraviolet absorbance detection. J. Chrom. 573: 87–92, 1992.

A. Turcant, A. Premel-Cabic, A. Cailleux and P. Allain. Toxicological screening of drugs by microbore high-performance liquid chromatography with photodiode-array detection and ultraviolet spectral library searches. Clin. Chem. 37: 1210–1215, 1991.

Diazepam

T½: 21–37 hr
Vd: 0.7–2.6 L/kg
Fb: 0.96
pKa: 3.4

Occurrence and Usage. Diazepam (Valium, Valrelease) is the second benzodiazepine derivative to have been approved for human usage (1963) and has been one of the most frequently prescribed drugs in the United States. It is administered as an antianxiety agent, muscle relaxant or anticonvulsant, orally or by intramuscular or intravenous injection, in single doses of 2–20 mg and up to 40 mg daily. It is supplied as the free base, which is only very slightly soluble in water.

Blood Concentrations. The serum of unmedicated humans has been shown to contain diazepam and its major active metabolites at concentrations of 1–32 ng/L, possibly as a result of the natural presence of benzodiazepines in certain foods (Duthel et al., 1992). Following a single oral 10 mg dose, peak blood concentrations of diazepam averaged 0.148 mg/L at 1 hour, declining to 0.037 mg/L by 24 hours; an average peak concentration of 0.029 mg/L was achieved for the major active metabolite, nordiazepam, at 24 hours. The half-lives for diazepam and nordiazepam were estimated as 21–37 hours and 50–99 hours, respectively (Kaplan et al., 1973), although these may be prolonged to 51–122 hours and 91–182 hours, respectively, in obese subjects (Abernethy et al., 1983). In another study of the oral administration of a single 10 mg dose to 48 healthy adult males, peak plasma diazepam concentrations occurred within 0.5–2.5 hours and averaged 0.406 mg/L (range, 0.253–0.586); elimination half-lives averaged 44 hours (range, 6.5–132) (Greenblatt et al., 1989). During chronic daily oral administration of 30 mg, steady-state plasma diazepam concentrations averaged 1.03 mg/L (range, 0.70–1.50) and nordiazepam, 0.43 mg/L (range, 0.35–0.52) (van der Kleijn et al., 1971). Five schizophrenic patients receiving chronic daily 1 mg/kg (70 mg/70 kg) oral doses developed steady-state serum levels of 2–4 mg/L for diazepam, 1–2 mg/L for nordiazepam, 0.1–0.6 mg/L for temazepam and 0.05–0.40 mg/L for oxazepam (Tada et al., 1985).

Peak serum concentrations of diazepam in 6 subjects averaged 1.60 mg/L at 15 minutes after a 20 mg intravenous injection, declining to 0.44 mg/L by 2 hours; nordiazepam concentrations did not exceed 0.10 mg/L in the ensuing 72 hours. Most of the subjects fell into a comfortable, arousable sleep for the first 2 hours (Hillestad et al., 1974). Serum diazepam concentrations reached 10 mg/L in a patient receiving frequent intravenous doses of the drug to control alcohol withdrawal (Kelly et al., 1979).

The whole blood/plasma concentration ratio for diazepam averages 0.7 (Maguire et al. 1980).

Metabolism and Excretion. Diazepam undergoes N-demethylation to nordiazepam, a metabolite at least as active as its parent; both of these compounds are converted to 3-hydroxy derivatives, temazepam and oxazepam, which are also active but do not accumulate in blood or plasma to an appreciable extent. There is also evidence for phenolic hydroxylation of diazepam. Only traces of diazepam and nordiazepam are found in urine; about 33% of the dose is excreted as oxazepam glucuronide and another 20% as conjugates of nordiazepam, 4'-hydroxydiazepam and temazepam (Schwartz et al., 1965; Kaplan et al., 1973; Mahon et al., 1976).

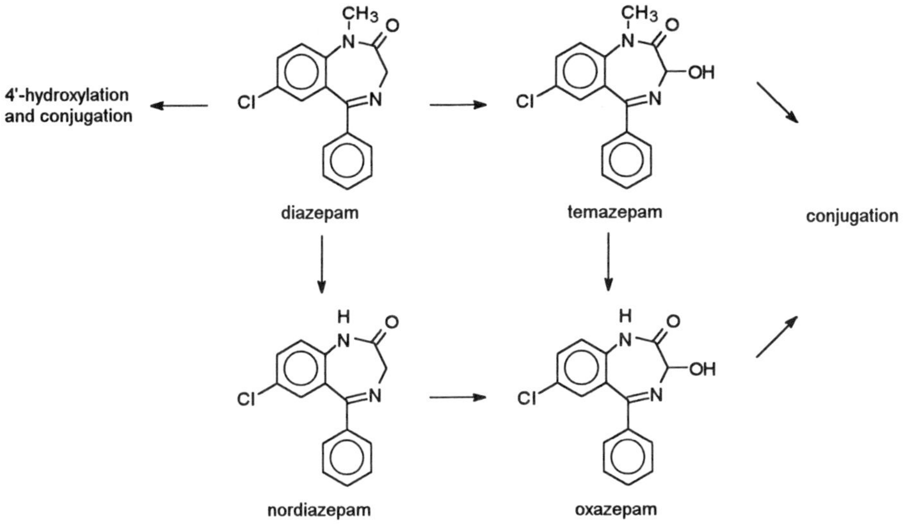

4'-hydroxylation and conjugation ← diazepam → temazepam → conjugation
diazepam → nordiazepam → oxazepam → (conjugation)

Toxicity. Overdosage with diazepam generally results in drowsiness, ataxia, and muscular weakness. Cardiac arrest was noted in a pediatric patient (Berger et al., 1975). Serum diazepam concentrations in hospitalized patients who exhibited only light coma have ranged up 20 mg/L; nordiazepam concentrations are generally lower than those of diazepam in the early stages of intoxication, but eventually achieve higher levels (Greenblatt et al., 1978; Kanto et al., 1978; Jatlow et al., 1979). Chronic usage may cause physical dependence, and grand mal seizures can occur upon withdrawal (de Bard, 1979).

Diazepam intoxication following overdosage is not an infrequent occurrence, yet there are very few well-documented fatal cases stemming from the sole use of this drug. In a nationwide survey of drug-related deaths, Dinovo et al. (1976) compiled 67 fatal cases involving diazepam and other drugs (mean blood concentration, 18 mg/L), 5 cases of diazepam-ethanol combination (mean blood concentration, 5.2 mg/L) and 3 cases involving only diazepam (mean blood concentration, 4.8 mg/L). A study of over 1200 diazepam-associated deaths revealed only 2 cases of death due to the ingestion of diazepam alone; postmortem blood concentrations of 5 and 19 mg/L were determined (Finkle et al., 1979). Cardauns and Iffland (1973) reported the following tissue distribution in a young drug addict who died after ingesting alcohol and from 0.7–3.4 g of diazepam:

Concentrations in a Diazepam-Alcohol Fatality (mg/L or mg/kg)*

	Blood	Liver	Kidney	Urine
Diazepam	30	16	0.8	3
Nordiazepam	4	4	0	7

* Blood ethanol, 0.35 g/dL

Analysis. Diazepam has been determined in body fluids by ultraviolet spectrophotometry (deSilva et al., 1966) and electron-capture gas chromatography after acid hydrolysis (deSilva et al., 1964), although these procedures are not highly specific. Gas chromatography of the intact drug and its metabolites is performed using nitrogen-phosphorus (Dhar and Kutt, 1979; Karnes et al., 1988), electron-capture (Howard et al., 1974; Arnold, 1975; Weinfeld et al., 1977; Wallace et al., 1979; Loscher, 1982) or flame-ionization detection (Baselt et al., 1977), the latter being more suitable for determination of high therapeutic or toxic levels of the drug. Gas chromatography-mass spectrometry has been used to demonstrate the presence of "endogenous" diazepam in human serum (Duthel et al., 1992). Liquid chromatography is an excellent means of simultaneously assaying diazepam and its more polar metabolites (Tjaden et al., 1980; Cotler et al., 1981; Rao et al., 1982; Tada et al., 1985; Koenigbauer et al., 1987; Lau et al., 1987; Fernandez et al., 1991). The commercially available immunoassays for benzodiazepines in urine were designed to detect oxazepam, a metabolite common to at least 6 of the benzodiazepines; several of the parent drugs, including diazepam, cross-react to a significant extent.

References

D.R. Abernethy, D.J. Greenblatt, M. Divoll and R.I. Shader. Prolonged accumulation of diazepam in obesity. J. Clin. Pharm. 23: 369–376, 1983.

E. Arnold. A simple method for determining diazepam and its major metabolites in biological fluids: application of bioavailability studies. Acta Pharm. Tox. 36: 335–352, 1975.

R.C. Baselt, C.B. Stewart and S.J. Franch. Toxicological determination of benzodiazepines in biological fluids and tissues by flame-ionization gas chromatography. J. Anal. Tox. 1: 10–13, 1977.

R. Berger, G. Green and A. Melnick. Cardiac arrest caused by oral diazepam intoxication. Clin. Pediat. 14: 842–844, 1975.

H. Cardauns and R. Iffland. Ueber eine toedliche Diazepam (Valium) Vergiftung bei einem drogenabhaengigen Jugendlichen. Arch. Tox. 31: 147–151, 1973.

S. Cotler, C.V. Puglisi and J.H. Gustafson. Determination of diazepam and its major metabolites in man and in the cat by high-performance liquid chromatography. J. Chrom. 222: 95–106, 1981.

M.L. de Bard. Diazepam withdrawal syndrome: a case with psychosis, seizure, and coma. Am. J. Psych. 136: 104–105, 1979.

J.A.F. deSilva, M.A. Schwartz, V. Stefanovic et al. Determination of diazepam (Valium) in blood by gas liquid chromatography. Anal. Chem. 36: 2099–2105, 1964.

J.A.F. deSilva, B.A. Koechlin and G. Bader. Blood level distribution patterns of diazepam and its major metabolite in man. J. Pharm. Sci. 55: 692–702, 1966.

A.K. Dhar and H. Kutt. Monitoring diazepam and desmethyldiazepam concentrations in plasma by gas-liquid chromatography, with use of a nitrogen-sensitive detector. Clin. Chem. 25: 137–140, 1979.

E.C. Dinovo, L.A. Gottschalk, F.L. McGuire et al. Analysis of results of toxicological examination performed by coroner's or medical examiner's laboratories in 2000 drug-involved deaths in nine major U.S. cities. Clin. Chem. 22: 847–850, 1976.

J.M. Duthel, H. Constant, J.J. Vallon et al. Quantitation by gas chromatography with selected-ion monitoring mass spectrometry of "natural" diazepam. J. Chrom. 579: 85–91, 1992.

P. Fernandez, L. Hermida, A.M. Bermejo et al. Simultaneous determination of diazepam and its metabolites in plasma by HPLC. J. Liq. Chrom. 14: 2587–2599, 1991.

B.S. Finkle, K.L. McCloskey and L.S. Goodman. Diazepam and drug-associated deaths. J. Am. Med. Asso. 242: 429–434, 1979.

D.J. Greenblatt, E. Woo, M.D. Allen et al. Rapid recovery from massive diazepam overdose. J. Am. Med. Asso. 240: 1872–1874, 1978.

D.J. Greenblatt, J.S. Harmatz, H. Friedman et al. A large-sample study of diazepam pharmacokinetics. Ther. Drug. Mon. 11: 652–657, 1989.

L. Hillestad, T. Hansen, H. Melsom and A. Drivenes. Diazepam metabolism in normal man. Clin. Pharm. Ther. 16: 479–484, 1974.

A.G. Howard, G. Nickless and D.M. Hailey. A rapid gas chromatographic method for the determination of diazepam and metabolites in body fluids. J. Chrom. 90: 325–329, 1974.

P. Jatlow, K. Dobular and D. Bailey. Serum diazepam concentrations in overdose. Am. J. Clin. Path. 72: 571–577, 1979.

J. Kanto, R. Sellman, M. Haataja and P. Hurme. Plasma and urine concentrations of diazepam and its metabolites in children, adults and in diazepam-intoxicated patients. Int. J. Clin. Pharm. 16: 258–264, 1978.

S.A. Kaplan, M.L. Jack, K. Alexander and R.E. Weinfeld. Pharmacokinetic profile of diazepam in man following single intravenous and oral and chronic oral administration. J. Pharm. Sci. 62: 1789–1796, 1973.

H.T. Karnes, L.A. Beightol, R.J. Serafin and D. Farthing. Improved method for the determination of diazepam and N-desmethyldiazepam in plasma. J. Chrom. 424: 398–402, 1988.

R.C. Kelly, R.M. Anthony, L. Krent et al. Toxicological determination of benzodiazepines in serum: methods and concentrations associated with high-dose intravenous therapy with diazepam. Clin. Tox. 14: 445–457, 1979.

M.J. Koenigbauer, S.P. Assenza, R.C. Willoughby et al. Trace analysis of diazepam in serum using microbore high-performance liquid chromatography and on-line preconcentration. J. Chrom. 413: 161–169, 1987.

C.E. Lau, S. Dolan and M. Tang. Microsample determination of diazepam and its three metabolites in serum by reversed-phase high-performance liquid chromatography. J. Chrom. 416: 212–218, 1987.

W. Loscher. Rapid gas chromatographic measurement of diazepam and its metabolites desmethyldiazepam, oxazepam, and 3-hydroxydiazepam (temazepam) in small samples of plasma. Ther. Drug Mon. 4: 315–318, 1982.

K.P. Maguire, G.D. Burrows, T.R. Norman and B.A. Scoggins. Blood/plasma distribution ratios of psychotropic drugs. Clin. Chem. 26: 1624–1625, 1980.

W.A. Mahon, T. Inaba, T. Umeda et al. Biliary elimination of diazepam in man. Clin. Pharm. Ther. 19: 443–450, 1976.

S.N. Rao, A.K. Dhar, H. Kutt and M. Okamoto. Determination of diazepam and its pharmacologically active metabolites in blood by Bond Elut column extraction and reversed-phase high-performance liquid chromatography. J. Chrom. 231: 341–348, 1982.

M.A. Schwartz, B.A. Koechlin, E. Postma et al. Metabolism of diazepam in rat, dog and man. J. Pharm. Exp. Ther. 149: 423–435, 1965.

K. Tada, T. Moroji, R. Sekiguchi et al. Liquid-chromatographic assay of diazepam and its major metabolites in serum, and application to pharmacokinetic study of high doses of diazepam in schizophrenics. Clin. Chem. 31: 1712–1715, 1985.

U.R. Tjaden, M.T.H.A. Meeles, C.P. Thys and M. van der Kaay. Determination of some benzodiazepines and metabolites in serum, urine and saliva by high-performance liquid chromatography. J. Chrom. 181: 227–241, 1980.

E. van der Kleijn, J.M. van Rossum, E.T.J.M. Muskens and N.V.M. Rijntjes. Pharmacokinetics of diazepam in dogs, mice and humans. Acta Pharm. Tox. 29: 109–127, 1971.

R.E. Weinfeld, H.N. Posmanter, K. Khoo and C.V. Puglisi. Rapid determination of diazepam and nordiazepam in plasma by electron capture gas-liquid chromatography. J. Chrom. 143: 581–595, 1977.

Diazinon

T½: ?
Vd: ?
Fb: ?

$(C_2H_5O)_2PO$ — S, CH$_3$, N, N, CH(CH$_3$)$_2$

Occurrence and Usage. Diazinon (dimpylate, Spectracide) is an organothiophosphate derivative widely used as an agricultural and household insecticide since its synthesis in 1953. The concentrated commercial form contains 25% diazinon and is intended to be used outdoors in a 0.05% dilution. The compound is inactivated by photochemical oxidation and therefore does not accumulate in the environment. Occupational exposure is generally by dermal contact or inhalation. The current threshold limit for diazinon is 0.1 mg/m³.

Blood Concentrations. Diazinon itself is not routinely measured in blood specimens except in cases of acute intoxication. Blood cholinesterase levels are generally used to monitor exposure to diazinon and other cholinesterase inhibitors. Oral doses of diazinon given to volunteers for 37 days at the rate of 0.02 mg/kg/day reduced plasma cholinesterase levels to 86% of pre-exposure levels; 0.05 mg/kg/day for 28 days reduced the levels to 60–65%, but neither dosage regimen affected erythrocyte cholinesterase levels (ACGIH, 1971).

Metabolism and Excretion. The metabolism of diazinon has not been specifically studied in man, but the chemical is known to be rapidly and extensively biotransformed in animals. It is activated by oxidation to diazoxon, a potent cholinesterase inhibitor, and both this compound and its parent are inactivated by hydrolysis to the corresponding phosphoric acid derivatives, diethylphosphoric acid and diethylphosphorothioic acid. Minor metabolites include hydroxy derivatives formed by oxidation of the isopropyl side chain; hydroxydiazinon is a toxic compound that is found in blood to the extent of 25–70% of the diazinon content. Diazinon itself accumulates in fat in concentrations over 100 times those in blood. Over 80% of a dose is eliminated as products of hydrolysis in the 24 hour urine of experimental animals (Nakatsugawa et al., 1969; Janes et al., 1973; Iverson et al., 1975). Urinary concentrations of diethylphosphoric acid and diethylphosphorothioic acid in members of the general population average less than 0.02 mg/L of each (Kutz et al., 1978).

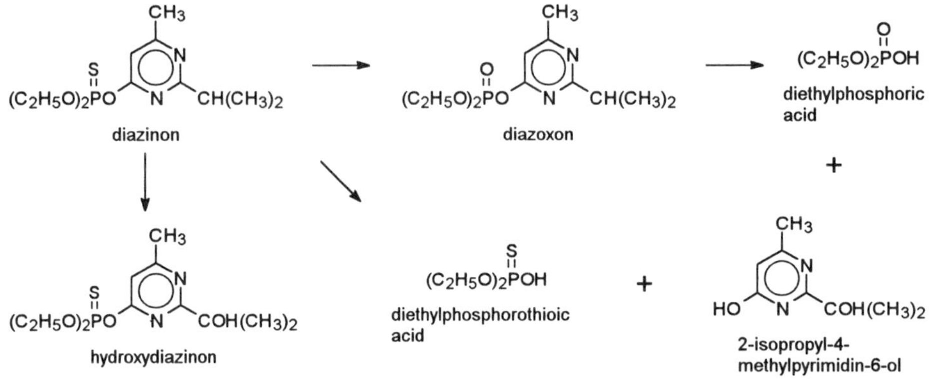

Toxicity. The estimated fatal dose of diazinon in man is 25 g by oral ingestion. Contaminated food caused the acute intoxication of 8 children, who were treated with atropine for the relief of sweating, nausea, abdominal cramps and muscle weakness; diethylphosphoric acid was found in urine specimens collected 23 and 58 days after the incident in concentrations of up to 0.22 mg/L (Reichert et al., 1977). Two subjects who survived the intentional ingestion of 60 and 100 mL of 25% diazinon solution were noted to have red blood cell cholinesterase levels within a short time of ingestion that were depressed to 19% and 39% of normal, respectively; maximal plasma diazinon concentrations noted shortly after ingestion in these 2 patients were 0.1 and 1.7 mg/L, while urine metabolite levels peaked within the first two days at 85 and 41 mg/L for diethylphosphoric acid and 101 and 35 mg/L for diethylphosphorothioic acid (Klemmer et al., 1978). Two workmen were poisoned while spraying a diazinon concentrate that had been improperly stored; analysis showed that the diazinon had been completely converted to more toxic breakdown products, including sulfotepp and thiono-TEPP (Soliman et al., 1982).

One fatal instance of diazinon poisoning was reported in which concentrations of the chemical in brain, liver and kidney ranged from 0.04–0.30 mg/kg (Heyndrickx et al., 1974). In the case of a 45 year old man who died 7 days after apparently ingesting diazinon, the chemical was only found in fat at a level of 5.1 mg/kg (Kirkbride, 1987). The following concentrations of intact diazinon were determined in the tissues of 3 adults who ingested the chemical (22 g in the second case) for suicidal purposes (Poklis et al., 1980; Wall, 1982):

Diazinon Concentrations in Fatal Cases (mg/L or mg/kg)

	Blood	Brain	Liver	Kidney	Fat	Gastric
Average	104	25	126	1.5	26	443
(Range)	(0.7–277)	(2–62)	(4–345)	(0.1–3)	(15–37)	(44–1200)

Analysis. Methods for the analysis of blood cholinesterase were cited in the section on carbaryl. Diazinon may be estimated as the intact chemical in biological material by gas chromatography with electron-capture (Reichert et al., 1977; Poklis et al., 1980) or phosphorus-specific detection

(Machin and Quick, 1969; Heyndrickx et al., 1974; Kirkbride, 1987). The phosphoric acid metabolites of diazinon have been assayed in urine by colorimetry (Mattson and Sedlak, 1960) and in blood and urine after derivatization by gas chromatography with flame photometric detection (Shafik and Enos, 1969; Shafik et al., 1973; Reid and Watts, 1981).

References

ACGIH. *Documentation of the Threshold Limit Values,* American Conference of Governmental Industrial Hygienists, Cincinnati, Ohio, 1971, pp. 70–71.

A. Heyndrickx, F. Van Hoff, L. De Wolf and C. Van Peteghem. Fatal diazinon poisoning in man. J. For. Sci. Soc. 14: 131–133, 1974.

F. Iverson, D.L. Grant and J. Lacroix. Diazinon metabolism in the dog. Bull. Env. Cont. Tox. 13: 611–618, 1975.

N.F. Janes, A.F. Machin, M.P. Quick et al. Toxic metabolites of diazinon in sheep. J. Agr. Food Chem. 21: 121–124, 1973.

K.P. Kirkbride. An estimation of diazinon in omental tissue. J. Anal. Tox. 11: 6–7, 1987.

H.W. Klemmer, E.R. Reichert and W.L. Yauger, Jr. Five cases of intentional ingestion of 25 percent diazinon with treatment and recovery. Clin. Tox. 12: 435–444, 1978.

F.W. Kutz, R.S. Murphy and S.C. Strassman. Survey of pesticide residues and their metabolites in urine from the general population. In *Pentachlorphenol* (K.R. Rao, ed.), Plenum Press, New York, 1978, pp. 363–369.

A.F. Machin and M.P. Quick. The rapid determination of diazinon and its oxygen analogue in animal tissues by gas chromatography. Analyst 94: 221–225, 1969.

A.M. Mattson and V.A. Sedlak. Ether-extractable urinary phosphates in man and rats derived from malathion and similar compounds. J. Agr. Food Chem. 8: 107–110, 1960.

T. Nakatsugawa, N.M. Tolman and P.A. Dahm. Oxidative degradation of diazinon by rat liver microsomes. Biochem. Pharm. 18: 685–688, 1969.

A. Poklis, F.W. Kutz, J.F. Sperling and D.P. Morgan. A fatal diazinon poisoning. For. Sci. Int. 15: 135–140, 1980.

E.R. Reichert, W.L. Yauger, Jr., M.N. Rashad et al. Diazinon poisoning in eight members of related households. Clin. Tox. 11: 5–11, 1977.

S.J. Reid and R.R. Watts. A method for the determination of dialkyl phosphate residues in urine. J. Anal. Tox. 5: 126–132, 1981.

M.T. Shafik and H.F. Enos. Determination of metabolic and hydrolytic products of organophosphorus pesticide chemicals in human blood and urine. J. Agr. Food Chem. 17: 1186–1189, 1969.

T. Shafik, D.E. Bradway, H.F. Enos and A.R. Yobs. Human exposure to organophosphorus pesticides. A modified procedure for the gas-liquid chromatographic analysis of alkyl phosphate metabolites in urine. J. Agr. Food Chem. 21: 625–629, 1973.

S.A. Soliman, G.W. Sovocool, A. Curley et al. Two acute human poisoning cases resulting from exposure to diazinon transformation products in Egypt. Arch. Env. Health 37: 207–212, 1982.

W.H. Wall. Personal communication, 1982.

Dibenzepine

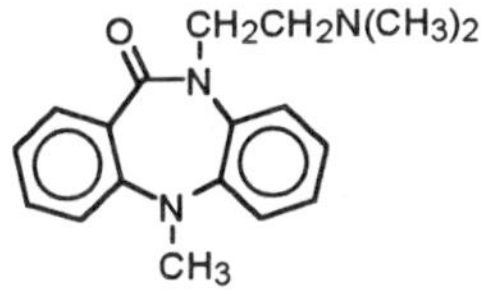

T½: ?
Vd: ?
Fb: ?
pKa: 8.5

Occurrence and Usage. Dibenzepine (dibenzepin, Noveril) is a tricyclic antidepressant drug that has been in clinical use in European countries since 1966. It is supplied as the hydrochloride salt in 40–240 mg tablets for oral administration; daily doses often range from 240–720 mg.

Blood Concentrations. In 12 adult patients receiving daily oral therapy with 8 mg/kg (560 mg/70 kg) for 22 days, steady-state plasma levels averaged 0.18 mg/L for dibenzepine and 0.28 mg/L for metabolite II (Gauch and Modestin, 1973).

Metabolism and Excretion. Dibenzepine is extensively metabolized in man. From 20–30% of a single dose is excreted as free and conjugated metabolites in the 24 hour urine. Since there are 3 nitrogen atoms in the molecule, each subject to N-dealkylation, nomenclature of the metabolites is somewhat of a problem unless lengthy chemical names are used. The only metabolites identified thus far in human urine are the five N-demethylated compounds, although metabolites with phenolic hydroxyl groups are known to be excreted in conjugated form. About 1% of a dose is eliminated in the 24 hour urine as unchanged dibenzepine; about 10% as metabolite II; about 5% as metabolite IV; about 2% as metabolite VI; about 2% as metabolite V; and about 0.3% as metabolite III (Lehner et al., 1967; De Leenheer and Heyndrickx, 1973).

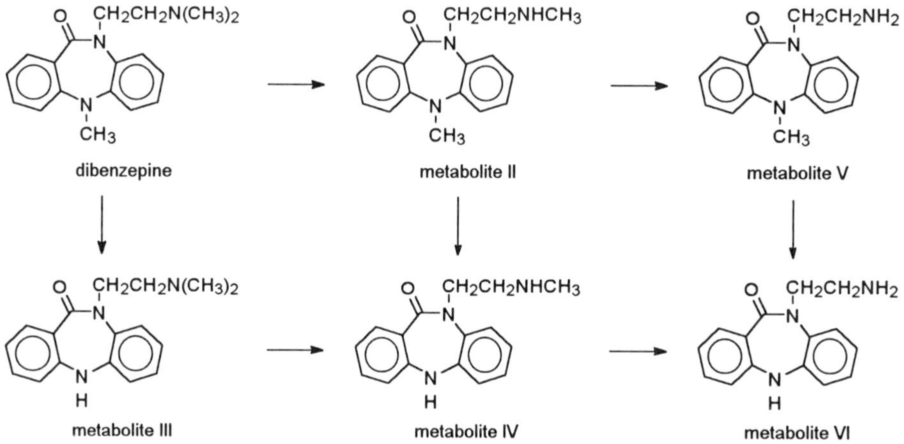

Toxicity. Overdosage with dibenzepine results in severe hypotension and circulatory collapse, coma, respiratory depression, and disturbances in cardiac rhythm (Vest et al., 1969). The following tissue distribution of dibenzepine and its metabolites was observed in the case of an individual who died after the ingestion of 3.6 g of the drug (Schlicht and Gelbke, 1978):

Concentrations in a Dibenzepine Fatality (mg/L or mg/kg)

Drug	Blood	Brain	Liver	Bile	Kidney	Urine
Dibenzepine	23	42	130	113	63	350
Metabolite II		8.3	120	80	28	180
Metabolite III		3.7	9	21	6.2	39
Metabolite IV		trace	1	36	3.2	34
Metabolite V		trace	4	trace	0.7	3
Metabolite VI		0	trace	trace	trace	2

Another 20 deaths due to acute ingestion of 2–16 g of the drug have been reported, with the following postmortem concentrations of dibenzepine (Brochon et al., 1969; Vest et al., 1969; McLinden, 1970; Bonnichsen and Shubert, 1971; Klug, 1972; Robinson et al., 1974; Christensen and Felby, 1975; Boesche and Gelbke, 1977):

Dibenzepine Concentrations in Fatalities (mg/L or mg/kg)

	Blood	Brain	Liver	Kidney	Urine
Average	32	37	185	58	80
(Range)	(1–135)	(9–76)	(10–550)	(7–170)	(4–200)
Number	20	4	19	8	10

Analysis. Determination of dibenzepine and its demethylated metabolites in biological specimens has been accomplished in overdose cases by thin-layer chromatography and ultraviolet spectrophotometry (Christensen and Felby, 1975) or by nitrogen-selective gas chromatography after trifluoroacetylation (Schlicht and Gelbke, 1978).

References

R. Bonnichsen and B. Schubert. Determination of dibenzepine in autopsy material. Z. Rechtsmed. 68: 257–260, 1971.

J. Boesche. Gas chromatographic determination of dibenzepine and its metabolites after lethal overdosage. Presented at the annual meeting of the International Association of Forensic Toxicologists, Leipzig, East Germany, August 24–26, 1977.

R. Brochon, H. Lehner, R. Gauch and O. Rudin. The detection and determination of dibenzepine and its metabolites in autopsy material. Arch. Tox. 24: 249–259, 1969.

H. Christensen and S. Felby. Dibenzepine and its metabolites in blood, muscle, liver, vitreous body and urine from fatal poisoning. Acta Pharm. Tox. 37: 393–401, 1975.

A. De Leenheer and A. Heyndrickx. Improved method for determining dibenzepine and its N-demethylated metabolites in human urine. J. Pharm. Sci. 62: 31–36, 1973.

R. Gauch and J. Modestin. Zur Pharmakokinetic von Dibenzepin. Arz. Forsch. 23: 687–690, 1973.

E. Klug. Chemische Befunde bei einigen seltenen Vergiftungen. Z. Rechtsmed. 71: 27–36, 1972.

H. Lehner, R. Gauch and W. Michaelis. Zum Stoffwechsel von 5-Methyl-10-beta-dimethylaminoaethyl-10,11-dihydro-11-oxo-5H-dibenzo- (b,e)(1,4)-diazepin-HCl. Arz. Forsch. 17: 185–189, 1967.

V.J. McLinden. Dibenzepin poisoning. J. For. Sci. Soc. 10: 135–138, 1970.

A.E. Robinson, A.I. Coffer and R.D. McDowall. Toxicology of some autopsy cases involving tricyclic antidepressant drugs. Z. Rechtsmed. 74: 261–266, 1974.

H.J. Schlicht and H.P. Gelbke. Gas chromatographic determination of dibenzepine and its basic metabolites in biological material. J. Chrom. 166: 599–603, 1978.

M. Vest, H.R. Hirt, A. Olafsson and J. Girard. Zwei toedliche Vergiftungen mit Imipramin (Tofranil) und Dibenzepin (Noveril) bei Kleinkindern. Schweiz. Med. Wochenshr. 99: 1157–1162, 1969.

p-Dichlorobenzene

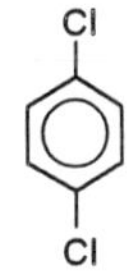

T½: ?
Vd: ?
Fb: ?

Occurrence and Usage. p-Dichlorobenzene (Paracide) has been widely used as a deodorant, disinfectant and insecticide. Occupational exposure usually occurs during manufacturing processes and results from inhalation of the vapor or particulate matter. The current threshold limit value is 75 ppm (451 mg/m^3) in the industrial atmosphere.

Blood Concentrations. Whole blood p-dichlorobenzene concentrations in 6 Tokyo residents averaged 0.010 mg/L, ranging from 0.004–0.016 mg/L (Morita and Ohi, 1975).

Metabolism and Excretion. In rats, p-dichlorobenzene is metabolized by oxidation to 2,5-dichlorophenol and 2,5-dichloroquinol; these metabolites account for 80% and 6% of the dose, respectively, as urinary sulfate and glucuronide conjugates within 6 days of a single dose (Azouz et al., 1955; Hawkins et al., 1980).

Workers employed in the manufacture of p-dichlorobenzene and exposed to air concentrations of the chemical ranging from 7–49 ppm had urinary 2,5-dichlorophenol levels of 10–233 mg/L. The urine metabolite concentrations were reasonably well correlated with the degree of exposure, averaging about 90–100 mg/L at p-dichlorobenzene air concentrations of 33 ppm. 2,5-Dichlorophenol urine concentrations reach a maximum at the end of an exposure, decline rapidly at first and then more slowly, with excretion continuing for a period of some weeks after a single exposure (Pagnotto and Walkley, 1965).

Adipose concentrations of p-dichlorobenzene in 34 Tokyo residents averaged 2.3 mg/kg, with a range of 0.2–11.7 mg/kg (Morita and Ohi, 1975).

p-dichlorobenzene   p-dichlorophenol

Toxicity. p-Dichlorobenzene causes eye and nose irritation at air concentrations of 80–160 ppm, and only slight skin irritation upon dermal contact (Hollingsworth et al., 1956). Exposure to higher concentrations has caused headache, nausea, malaise, jaundice, anemia and hepatic necrosis and cirrhosis (Cotter, 1953).

Analysis. Intact p-dichlorobenzene has been measured in blood and tissue specimens by electron-capture gas chromatography (Morita and Ohi, 1975). 2,5-Dichlorophenol, a major metabolite, has been determined in urine by colorimetry, but this method is subject to interference by other phenolic substances (Pagnotto and Walkley, 1965). More specific procedures have involved gas chromatography with either flame-ionization (Van Roosmalen et al., 1980) or electron-capture detection (McKinney et al., 1970).

References

W.M. Azouz, D.V. Parke and R.T. Williams. The metabolism of halogenobenzenes. Ortho- and para-dichlorobenzenes. Biochem. J. 59: 410–415, 1955.

L.H. Cotter. Paradichlorobenzene poisoning from insecticides. N.Y. State J. Med. 53: 1690–1692, 1953.

D.R. Hawkins, L.F. Chasseaud, R.N. Woodhouse and D.G. Cresswell. The distribution, excretion and biotransformation of p-dichloro(14C)benzene in rats after repeated inhalation, oral and subcutaneous doses. Xenobiotica 10: 81–95, 1980.

R.L. Hollingsworth, V.K. Rowe, F. Oyen et al. Toxicity of paradichlorobenzene. Arch. Hyg. Occ. Med. 14: 138–147, 1956.

J.D. McKinney, L. Fishbein, C.E. Fletcher and W.F. Barthel. The electron-capture gas chromatography of paradichlorobenzene metabolites as a measure of exposure. Bull. Env. Cont. Tox. 5: 354–361, 1970.

M. Morita and G. Ohi. Para-dichlorobenzene in human tissue and atmosphere in Tokyo metropolitan area. Env. Pollut. 8: 269–274, 1975.

L.D. Pagnotto and J.E. Walkley. Urinary dichlorophenol as an index of para-dichlorobenzene exposure. Am. Ind. Hyg. Asso. J. 26: 137–142, 1965.

P.B. Van Roosmalen, A.L. Klein and I. Drummond. Simultaneous determination by gas chromatography of phenol, 2-chlorophenol, 2,4- and 2,6-dichlorophenol, 2,4,6-trichlorophenol, and 2,3,5,6-tetrachlorophenol in the urine of industrially exposed workers. Int. Arch. Occ. Env. Health 45: 57–62, 1980.

Dichloromethane

T½: 40 min $\qquad$ CH_2Cl_2
Vd: ?
Fb: ?

Occurrence and Usage. Dichloromethane (methylene chloride) is commonly employed commercially and industrially as a paint remover, degreaser, aerosol propellant and solvent. Prior to 1972 it was thought that the major toxic effect of the chemical in normal usage was narcosis, and the threshold limit value was accordingly set at 500 ppm. It is now recognized that dichloromethane inhalation at this level may lead to accumulation of dangerous quantities of carbon monoxide, and an atmospheric concentration of 50 ppm (174 mg/m³) has been adopted for industrial purposes. This chemical is listed as a suspected human carcinogen.

Blood Concentrations. Subjects exposed to 200 ppm of dichloromethane vapors for 2 hours achieved maximal blood concentrations of approximately 2 mg/L; the blood levels declined with a half-life of 40 minutes after the cessation of the exposure (DiVincenzo et al., 1972). Average blood concentrations of 3.1 and 12.5 mg/L were achieved by subjects exposed to 500 ppm of the vapor for 30 minutes during rest and heavy physical exertion, respectively (Astrand et al., 1975).

Carboxyhemoglobin (COHb) saturation levels averaged about 3% in sedentary non-smokers after an 8 hour exposure to 100 ppm of dichloromethane (DiVincenzo and Kaplan, 1981). Carboxyhemoglobin saturation levels of 7% and 10% were observed in volunteers exposed to dichloromethane at concentrations of 250 and 500 ppm, respectively, for 7.5 hours (Peterson, 1978). The COHb saturation in 3 subjects exposed to 986 ppm of the vapor for 2 hours ranged from 7–15% at one hour post-exposure, with a mean value of 10% (Stewart et al., 1972).

Metabolism and Excretion. DiVincenzo et al. (1972) have estimated that as much as 40% of an absorbed dose of dichloromethane is not eliminated in the expired air. A portion of this retained amount is known to be metabolized to carbon monoxide; the half-life of excretion of the CO so produced is approximately 13 hours, or 2.5 times that of inhaled carbon monoxide. This effect may be due to the continued metabolism of accumulated dichloromethane (Ratney et al., 1974). Only a small fraction of a dose is excreted unchanged in the urine; an average of 0.022 mg was eliminated in the 24 hour urine following a 2 hour exposure to 100 ppm of the chemical (DiVincenzo et al., 1972). Rats metabolize only 7% of an administered dose of dichloromethane, as much as 5% being converted to carbon monoxide, and excrete 92% unchanged in the breath (DiVincenzo and Hamilton, 1975). Workers exposed to an average of 50 mg/m³ dichloromethane in workplace air for 4 hours had urine dichloromethane levels averaging 191 µg/L (range, 4–788) (Ghittori et al., 1993).

Toxicity. Toxic reactions to dichloromethane have been limited for the most part to acute exposures, and have resulted from either its direct central nervous system depressant effects, its *in vivo* conversion to carbon monoxide, or its oxidation to phosgene in an open flame (Gerritsen and Buschmann, 1960). This latter property is shared with many other chlorinated hydrocarbons. The use of dichloromethane as a paint remover has produced carboxyhemoglobin levels of 26 and 40% in 2 healthy persons (Langehennig et al., 1976) and death in a person with a history of coronary disease (Stewart and Hake, 1976).

The narcotic effects of this chemical have been held accountable for several fatalities, 6 of which were industrial accidents; postmortem blood dichloromethane concentrations averaging 364 mg/L (range, 95–601) were reported in 5 cases (Moskowitz and Shapiro, 1952; Baselt, 1978; Winek et al., 1981; Franc, 1983; Forrest, 1990; Manno et al., 1992). Chemical findings for a death by inhalation following home usage of a paint remover are presented below (Bonventre et al., 1977):

Dichloromethane Concentrations in a Fatal Case (mg/L or mg/kg)

Blood	Brain	Liver	Blood COHb
510	248	144	3%

Analysis. Dichloromethane is conveniently assayed in biologic media with headspace sampling techniques by flame-ionization gas chromatography (DiVincenzo et al., 1971; Bonventre et al., 1977) or gas chromatography-mass spectrometry (Ghittori et al., 1993). Procedures for carboxyhemoglobin determination are cited in the section on carbon monoxide.

References

I. Astrand, P. Ovrum and A. Carlsson. Exposure to methylene chloride. Scand. J. Work Env. Health 1: 78–94, 1975.

R.C. Baselt. Unpublished results, 1978.

J. Bonventre, O. Brennan, D. Jason et al. Two deaths following accidental inhalation of dichloromethane and 1,1,1-trichloroethane. J. Anal. Tox. 1: 158–160, 1977.

G.D. DiVincenzo, F.J. Yanno and B.D. Astill. Human and canine exposures to methylene chloride vapor. Am. Ind. Hyg. Asso. J. 33: 125–135, 1972.

G.D. DiVincenzo and M.L. Hamilton. Fate and disposition of (14C)methylene chloride in the rat. Tox. Appl. Pharm. 32: 385–393, 1975.

G.D. DiVincenzo and C.J. Kaplan. Uptake, metabolism, and elimination of methylene chloride vapor by humans. Tox. Appl. Pharm. 59: 130–140, 1981.

A.R.W. Forrest. Personal communication, 1990.

A. Franc. Personal communication, 1983.

W.B. Gerritsen and C.H. Buschmann. Phosgene poisoning caused by the use of chemical paint removers containing methylene chloride in ill-ventilated rooms heated by kerosene stoves. Brit. J. Ind. Med. 17: 187–189, 1960.

S. Ghittori, P. Marraccini, G. Franco and M. Imbriani. Methylene chloride exposure in industrial workers. Am. Ind. Hyg. Asso. J. 54: 27–31, 1993.

P.L. Langehennig, R.A. Seeler and E. Berman. Paint removers and carboxyhemoglobin. New Eng. J. Med. 295: 1137, 1976.

M. Manno, M. Rugge and V. Cocheo. Double fatal inhalation of dichloromethane. Hum. Exp. Tox. 11: 540–545, 1992.

S. Moskowitz and H. Shapiro. Fatal exposure to methylene chloride vapor. Arch. Ind. Hyg. Occ. Med. 6: 116–123, 1952.

J.E. Peterson. Modeling the uptake, metabolism and excretion of dichloromethane by man. Am. Ind. Hyg. Asso. J. 39: 41–47, 1978.

R.S. Ratney, D.H. Wegman and H.B. Elkins. In vivo conversion of methylene chloride to carbon monoxide. Arch. Env. Health 28: 223–226, 1974.

R.D. Stewart, T.N. Fisher, M.J. Hosko et al. Carboxyhemoglobin elevation after exposure to dichloromethane. Science 176: 295–296, 1972.

R.D. Stewart and C.L. Hake. Paint-remover hazard. J. Am. Med. Asso. 235: 398–401, 1976.

C.L. Winek, W.D. Collom and F. Esposito. Accidental methylene chloride fatality. For. Sci. Int. 18: 165–168, 1981.

2,4-Dichlorophenoxyacetic Acid

T½: 4–140 hr (urine pH-dependent)
Vd: 0.1 L/kg
Fb: ?
pKa: 3.3

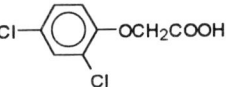

Occurrence and Usage. The chlorinated phenoxyacid derivatives, 2,4-dichlorophenoxyacetic acid (2,4-D) and its congener, 2,4,5-trichlorophenoxyacetic acid (2,4,5-T), have been used increasingly as herbicides over the last 30 years. The two compounds are often found combined in commercial preparations, which may contain up to 50% of active ingredients, in the form of the dimethylamine salts or various alkyl esters. These hormonal agents produce their effects by overstimulating plant growth. Dioxin (2,3,7,8-tetrachlorodibenzodioxin), a contaminant in some preparations of 2,4-D and 2,4,5-T, is one of the most potent teratogenic agents known. The current threshold limit value for both 2,4-D and 2,4,5-T is 10 mg/m³.

Blood Concentrations. Plasma 2,4-D concentrations did not exceed 0.2 mg/L in workers exposed to 2,4-D ester at an atmospheric concentration of 0.1–0.2 mg/m³; no accumulation was noted during the working week (Kolmodin-Hedman et al., 1980). The oral ingestion of 5 mg/kg (350 mg/70 kg) of 2,4-D by 6 healthy subjects resulted in an average peak plasma concentration of about 35 mg/L at 12 hours; the average plasma half-life in these asymptomatic volunteers was 33 hours (Kohli et al., 1974).

Metabolism and Excretion. Metabolites of 2,4-D other than conjugates have not been detected in human urine. An average of 77% of a dose was eliminated unchanged in the urine during the 4 days following a single oral dose (Kohli et al., 1974). About 13% of a dose is present as an acid-labile conjugate of 2,4-D in the urine (Sauerhoff et al., 1976).

Asymptomatic workers involved in the application of 2,4-D were found to have urine 2,4-D concentrations of 0.2–1.0 mg/L in one study (Shafik et al., 1971) and 0.04–8.2 mg/L (average, 1.4) in another (Libich et al., 1984). Similar workers exposed to 2,4-D ester at an atmospheric concentration of 0.1–0.2 mg/m³ developed 2,4-D urine concentrations of 3–14 mg/L after a day of exposure (Kolmodin-Hedman et al., 1980).

Toxicity. Instances of neuritis and peripheral neuropathy with incomplete recovery have been reported following dermal exposure to the agent (Goldstein et al., 1959; Berkley and Magee., 1963). A terminally ill coccidioidomycosis patient received a total of 16.3 g of the sodium salt of 2,4-D by intravenous injection over a period of a month; injection of as much as 2.0 g had no apparent effects, but an infusion of 3.6 g over a period of 2 hours produced fibrillary twitching, stupor and hyporeflexia (Seabury, 1963). One person has survived the gastritis, hyperthermia and respiratory muscle paralysis associated with the accidental ingestion of 7.2 g of 2,4-D (Berwick, 1970). Another nonfatal case, which involved intentional ingestion and absorption of about 7 g of the amine salt of 2,4-D, included treatment with forced alkaline diuresis. An initial 2,4-D plasma concentration of 400 mg/L was noted to decline with a half-life of 220 hours, but the enhancement of renal elimination brought about by urinary alkalinization reduced the plasma half-life to 4.7 hours (Park et al., 1977). Maximal concentrations of 1031 mg/L in serum and 1900 mg/L in urine were observed during the first and third days, respectively, of a nonfatal overdosage with 2,4-D (Rivers et al., 1970). Treatment of 2,4-D intoxication with forced alkaline diuresis is recommended if the patient has not developed renal dysfunction (Prescott et al., 1979; Wells et al., 1981; Flanagan et al., 1990). Hemodialysis has been used successfully to treat 4 patients who ingested from 40–200 g of the chemical and had admission serum 2,4-D levels of 370–1770 mg/L (Durakovic et al., 1992).

The mean lethal dose of 2,4-D in man is estimated to be 28 g. The following tissue concentrations were observed in 5 adults who died within 1–6 days after the intentional ingestion of large amounts of the chemical (Curry, 1962; Nielsen et al., 1965; Dudley and Thapar, 1972; Coutselinis et al., 1977; Ryall, 1978; Osterloh et al., 1983; Fraser et al., 1984; Smith and Lewis, 1987):

2,4-D Concentrations in Fatal Cases (mg/L or mg/kg)

	Blood	Brain	Liver	Kidney	Urine
Average	464	103	237	143	314
(Range)	(58–826)	(13–299)	(21–540)	(62–315)	(111–670)

Analysis. Toxic concentrations of 2,4-D in body fluids are often measured by ultraviolet spectrophotometry at the absorption maximum of 282 nm. A more specific and sensitive determination of 2,4-D and related compounds in biological specimens may be conveniently performed by flame-ionization or electron-capture gas chromatography after methylation (Park et al., 1977; Smith and Hayden, 1979; Vural and Burgaz, 1984) or ethylation (Kohli et al., 1974).

References

M.C. Berkley and K.R. Magee. Neuropathy following exposure to dimethylamine salt of 2,4-D. Arch. Int. Med. 111: 351–352, 1963.

P. Berwick. 2,4-Dichlorophenoxyacetic acid poisoning in man. J. Am. Med. Asso. 214: 1114–1117, 1970.

A. Coutselinis, R. Kentarchou and D. Boukis. Concentration levels of 2,4-D and 2,4,5-T in forensic material. For. Sci. 10: 203–204, 1977.

A.S. Curry. Twenty-one uncommon cases of poisoning. Brit. Med. J. 1: 687–689, 1962.

A.W. Dudley, Jr. and N.T. Thapar. Fatal human ingestion of 2,4-D, a common herbicide. Arch. Path. 94: 270–275, 1972.

Z. Durakovic, A. Durakovic, S. Durakovic and D. Ivanovic. Poisoning with 2,4-dichlorophenoxyacetic acid treated by hemodialysis. Arch. Tox. 66: 518–521, 1992.

R.J. Flanagan, T.J. Meredith, M. Ruprah et al. Alkaline diuresis for acute poisoning with chlorophenoxy herbicides and ioxynil. Lancet 335: 454–458, 1990.

A.D. Fraser, A.F. Isner and R.A. Perry. Toxicologic studies in a fatal overdose of 2,4-D, mecoprop, and dicamba. J. For. Sci. 29: 1237–1241, 1984.

N.P. Goldstein, P.H. Jones and J.R. Brown. Peripheral neuropathy after exposure to an ester of dichlorophenoxyacetic acid. J. Am. Med. Asso. 171: 1306–1309, 1959.

J.D. Kohli, R.N. Khanna, B.N. Gupta et al. Absorption and excretion of 2,4-dichlorophenoxyacetic acid in man. Xenobiotica 4: 97–100, 1974.

B. Kolmodin-Hedman, E. Erne and M. Akerblom. Field application of phenoxy acid herbicides. In *Field Worker Exposure During Pesticide Application* (W.F. Tordoir and E.A.H. van Heemstra, eds.), Elsevier, New York, 1980, pp. 73–77.

S. Libich, J.C. To, R. Frank and G.J. Sirons. Occupational exposure of herbicide applicators to herbicides used along electric power transmission line right-of-way. Am. Ind. Hyg. Asso. J. 45: 56–62, 1984.

K. Nielsen, B. Kaempe and J. Jensen-Holm. Fatal poisoning in man by 2,4-dichlorophenoxyacetic acid (2,4-D): determination of the agent in forensic materials. Acta Pharm. Tox. 22: 224–234, 1965.

J. Osterloh, M. Lott: and S.M. Pond. Toxicologic studies in a fatal overdose of 2,4-D, MCPP, and chlorpyrifos. J. Anal. Tox. 7: 125–129, 1983.

J. Park, I. Darrien and L.F. Prescott. Pharmacokinetic studies in severe intoxication with 2,4-D and mecoprop. Proc. Eur. Soc. Tox. 18: 154–155, 1977.

L.F. Prescott, J. Park and I. Darrien. Treatment of severe 2,4-D and mecoprop intoxication with alkaline diuresis. Brit. J. Clin. Pharm. 7: 111–116, 1979.

J.B. Rivers, W.L. Yauger and H.W. Klemmer. Simultaneous gas chromatographic determination of 2,4-D and dicamba in human blood and urine. J. Chrom. 50: 334–337, 1970.

J.E. Ryall. Personal communication, 1978.

M.W. Sauerhoff, W.H. Braun, G.E. Blau and J.E. LeBeau. The fate of 2,4-dichlorophenoxyacetic acid (2,4-D) following oral administration. Tox. Appl. Pharm. 37: 136–137, 1976.

J.H. Seabury. Toxicity of 2,4-dichlorophenoxyacetic acid for man and dog. Arch. Env. Health 7: 202–209, 1963.

M.T. Shafik, H.C. Sullivan and H.F. Enos. A method for determination of low levels of exposure to 2,4-D and 2,4,5-T. Int. J. Env. Anal. Chem. 1: 23–33, 1971.

A.E. Smith and B.J. Hayden. Method for the determination of 2,4-dichlorophenoxyacetic acid residues in urine. J. Chrom. 171: 482–485, 1979.

R.A. Smith and D. Lewis. Suicide by ingestion of 2,4-D: a case history demonstrating the prudence of using GC/MS as an investigative rather than a confirmatory tool. Vet. Hum. Tox. 29: 259–261, 1987.

N. Vural and S. Burgaz. A gas chromatographic method for determination of 2,4-D residues in urine after occupational exposure. Bull. Env. Cont. Tox. 33: 518–524, 1984.

W.D.E. Wells, N. Wright and W.B. Yeoman. Clinical features and management of poisoning with 2,4-D and mecoprop. Clin. Tox. 18: 273–276, 1981.

Diclofenac

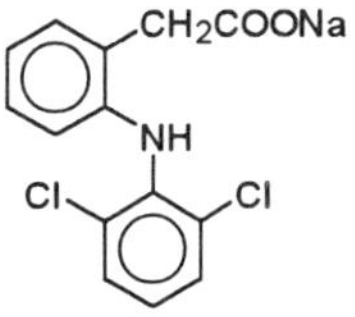

T½: 1–2 hr
Vd: 0.55 L/kg
FB: 0.99
pKa: 4.0

Occurrence and Usage. Diclofenac (Voltaren) is a phenylacetic acid derivative marketed as a nonsteroidal anti-inflammatory drug. It has analgesic, antipyretic and anti-inflammatory activities and is used in the treatment of rheumatic diseases and for the relief of pain. Diclofenac is available as the sodium salt tablets containing 25–75 mg for oral administration. The usual dosage is 100–200 mg/day in divided doses.

Blood Concentrations. Following a single 50 mg oral dose of diclofenac to 12 fasting subjects, an average peak plasma concentration of 1.3 mg/L (range, 0.75–2.0) was attained in approximately 2 hours (Willis et al., 1981). Following 50 mg oral doses given 3 times daily to 4 volunteers, peak plasma concentrations averaged 0.8 mg/L (range, 0.1–2.2) for diclofenac and 1.2 mg/L (range, 0.3–2.0) for 4'-hydroxydiclofenac (Fowler et al., 1983).

Metabolism and Excretion. Diclofenac is almost completely metabolized in man by hydroxylation of one or both of the aromatic rings or by conjugation of the carboxyl group (Stierlin et al., 1979a,

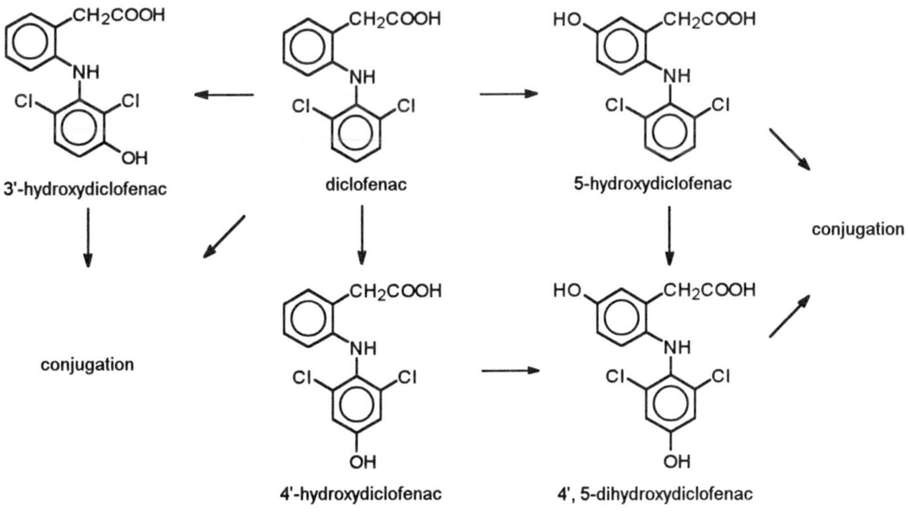

1979b). After oral administration of diclofenac, 35–65% of the dose is recovered in the urine and 15–45% in feces, largely as conjugated metabolites (Riess et al., 1978; John, 1979; Crook et al., 1982; Lansdorp et al., 1990a). The primary urinary metabolite is 4'-hydroxydiclofenac; little or no unchanged drug is excreted (Lansdorp et al., 1990a).

Toxicity. Adverse reactions to diclofenac include abdominal pain, headache and dizziness. Overdose may cause nausea, vomiting, drowsiness and reversible nephrotoxicity. No fatalities have been reported and an adult has ingested up to 2.0 g acutely and remained asymptomatic. Following ingestion of 1.5 g of diclofenac by an adult male who experienced temporary renal dysfunction, a plasma concentration of 60 mg/L was measured some 6 hours post-ingestion, dropping to 0.2 mg/L by 15 hours (Netter et al., 1984).

Analysis. Diclofenac has been determined in biological specimens by gas chromatography (Geiger et al., 1975; Schneider and Degan, 1987) and gas chromatography-mass spectrometry (DelPuppo et al., 1991; Sioufi et al., 1991). Liquid chromatography has also been employed (Chan et al., 1982; El-Sayed et al., 1988; Lansdorp et al., 1990b; Zecca et al., 1991; Blagbrough et al., 1992; Moncrieff, 1992).

References

I.S. Blagbrough, M.M. Daykin, M. Doherty et al. High-performance liquid chromatographic determination of naproxen, ibuprofen, and diclofenac in plasma and synovial fluid in man. J. Chrom. 578: 251–258, 1992.

K.K.H. Chan, K.H. Vyas and K. Wnuck. A rapid and sensitive method for the determination of diclofenac sodium in plasma by high-performance liquid chromatography. Anal. Letters 15: 1649–1663, 1982.

P.R. Crook, J.V. Willis, M.J. Kendall et al. The pharmacokinetics of diclofenac sodium in patients with active rheumatoid disease. Eur. J. Clin. Pharm. 21: 331–334, 1982.

M. DelPuppo, G. Cighetti, M.G. Kienle et al. Determination of diclofenac in human plasma by selected ion monitoring. Biol. Mass Spec. 20: 426–430, 1991.

Y.M. El-Sayed, M.E. Abdel-Hameed, M.S. Suleiman and N.M. Najib. A rapid and sensitive high-performance liquid chromatographic method for the determination of diclofenac sodium in serum and its use in pharmacokinetic studies. J. Pharm. Pharmac. 40: 727–729, 1988.

P.D. Fowler, M.F. Shadforth, P.R. Crook and V.A. John. Plasma and synovial fluid concentrations of diclofenac sodium and its major hydroxylated metabolites during long-term treatment of rheumatoid arthritis. Eur. J. Clin. Pharm. 25: 389–394, 1983.

U.P. Geiger, P.H. Degen and A. Sioufi. Quantitative assay of diclofenac in biological material by gas-liquid chromatography. J. Chrom. 111: 293–298, 1975.

V.A. John. The pharmacokinetics and metabolism of diclofenac sodium (Voltarol) in animals and man. Rheum. Rehab. 2 (Suppl.): 22–35, 1979.

D. Lansdorp, T.B. Vree, T.J. Janssen and P.J.M. Guelen. Pharmacokinetics of rectal diclofenac and its hydroxy metabolites in man. Int. J. Clin. Pharm. Ther. Tox. 28: 298–302, 1990a.

D. Lansdorp, T.J. Janssen, P.J.M. Guelen and T.B. Vree. High-performance liquid chromatographic method for the determination of diclofenac and its hydroxy metabolites in human plasma and urine. J. Chrom. 528: 487–494, 1990b.

J. Moncrieff. Extractionless determination of diclofenac sodium in serum using reversed-phase high-performance liquid chromatography with fluorimetric detection. J. Chrom. 577: 185–189, 1992.

P. Netter, H. Lamberg, A. Larcan et al. Diclofenac sodium—clormezanone poisoning. Eur. J. Clin. Pharm. 26: 535–536, 1984.

W. Riess, H. Stierlin, P. Degen et al. Pharmacokinetics and metabolism of the anti-inflammatory agent Voltaren. Scand. J. Rheum. 22 (Suppl.): 17–29, 1978.

W. Schneider and P.H. Degen. Simultaneous determination of diclofenac sodium and its metabolites in plasma by capillary column gas chromatography with electron-capture detection. J. Chrom. 383: 412–415, 1987.

A. Sioufi, F. Pommier and J. Godbillon. Determination of diclofenac in plasma and urine by capillary gas chromatography-mass spectrometry with possible simultaneous determination of deuterium-labelled diclofenac. J. Chrom. 571: 87–100, 1991.

H. Stierlin, J.W. Faigle, A. Sallmann et al. Biotransformation of diclofenac sodium (Voltaren) in animals and in man. Xenobiotica 9: 601–610, 1979a.

H. Stierlin and J.W. Faigle. Biotransformation of diclofenac sodium (Voltaren) in animals and in man. Xenobiotica 9: 611–621, 1979b.

J.V. Willis, M.J. Kendall and D.B. Jack. The influence of food on the absorption of diclofenac after single and multiple oral dose. Eur. J. Clin. Pharm. 19: 33–37, 1981.

L. Zecca, P. Ferrario and P. Costi. Determination of diclofenac and its metabolites in plasma and cerebrospinal fluid by high-performance liquid chromatography with electrochemical detection. J. Chrom. 567: 425–432, 1991.

Dicumarol

T½: 7–100 hr (genetically determined and dose-dependent)
Vd: 0.14 L/kg
Fb: 0.99
pKa: 5.7

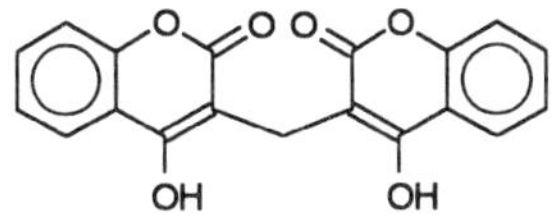

Occurrence and Usage. Dicumarol (bishydroxycoumarin) is a naturally-occurring vitamin K antagonist in widespread use as an anticoagulant. It is formed in spoiled sweet clover from the decomposition of coumarin and is responsible for sweet clover disease in cattle. The compound was first isolated and synthesized in 1934, and is currently available as the free acid for oral administration in doses of 25–200 mg daily.

Blood Concentrations. A single oral dose of 150 mg given to 4 subjects produced an average plasma concentration of about 17 mg/L at 10 hours, with an average half-life of 21 hours (Solomon and Schrogie, 1966). Concentrations of the drug in the plasma of 3 subjects who received chronic oral doses of 2 mg/kg (140 mg/70 kg) averaged 38 mg/L (range, 32–42) and 53 mg/L (range, 44–59) on days 5 and 6, respectively; it was found that the rate of disappearance from the plasma is a function of genetic differences as well as of dose, since increasing the dose from 2 mg/kg to 4 mg/kg resulted in a doubling of the half-life, from 24 to 48 hours (Vesell and Page, 1968). Plasma concentrations of 8–30 mg/L have been shown effective during sustained therapy with dicumarol (Weiner et al., 1950). No direct relationship could be established between concentrations of the drug in plasma and inhibition of prothrombin complex activity, although drug concentrations were shown to be inversely proportional to the rate of synthesis of the prothrombin complex (O'Reilly and Levy, 1970).

Metabolism and Excretion. Dicumarol undergoes slow and extensive metabolism in man to unknown biotransformation products. Less than 1% of a dose is excreted unchanged in the urine (Weiner et al., 1950).

Toxicity. Overdosage with dicumarol causes hematuria, epistaxis, generalized ecchymoses, gingival bleeding, and severe anemia. Patients with unexplained hemorrhagic diathesis should be evaluated for possible surreptitious ingestion of dicumarol or other anticoagulant drugs, especially if psychiatric problems are evident. Several reports of accidental or intentional dicumarol intoxication have appeared in which plasma concentrations of 22–192 mg/L and half-lives of up to 96 hours were measured; the patients were treated successfully by administration of vitamin K or a synthetic analogue (O'Reilly et al., 1962; Bowie et al., 1965; O'Reilly and Aggeler, 1966; Cole and Bachman, 1976).

Analysis. Determination of dicumarol in biological fluids has been accomplished by solvent extraction from aqueous acid solution with spectrophotometric measurement at 315 nm; thiopental and salicylate are known to interfere with this procedure (Axelrod et al., 1949).

References

J. Axelrod, J.R. Cooper and B.B. Brodie. Estimation of dicumarol, 3,3'-methylenebis (4-hydroxycoumarin) in biological fluids. Proc. Soc. Exp. Biol. Med. 70: 693–695, 1949.

E.J.W. Bowie, M. Todd, J.H. Thompson, Jr. et al. Anticoagulant malingerers (the "dicumarol-eaters"). Am. J. Med. 39: 855–864, 1965.

E.R. Cole and F. Bachman. Spectrophotometric assays for warfarin sodium and dicumarol. Arch. Int. Med. 136: 474–479, 1976.

R.A. O'Reilly, P.M. Aggeler and J.O. Gibbs. Hemorrhagic state due to surreptitious ingestion of bishydroxycoumarin. New Eng. J. Med. 267: 19–24, 1962.

R.A. O'Reilly and P.M. Aggeler. Surreptitious ingestion of coumarin anticoagulant drugs. Ann. Int. Med. 64: 1034–1041, 1966.

R.A. O'Reilly and G. Levy. Kinetics of the anticoagulant effect of bishydroxycoumarin in man. Clin. Pharm. Ther. 11: 378–384, 1970.

H.M. Solomon and J.J. Schrogie. The effect of phenyramidol on the metabolism of bishydroxycoumarin. J. Pharm. Exp. Ther. 154: 660–666, 1966.

E.S. Vesell and J.G. Page. Genetic control of dicumarol levels in man. J. Clin. Invest. 47: 2657–2663, 1968.

M. Weiner, S. Shapiro, J. Axelrod et al. The physiological disposition of dicumarol in man. J. Pharm. Exp. Ther. 99: 409–421, 1950.

Dicyclomine

T½: 5 hr
Vd: ?
Fb: ?
pKa: ?

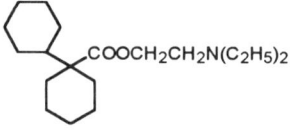

Occurrence and Usage. Dicyclomine (Bentyl) is an antispasmodic and anticholinergic agent used for control of irritable colon, spastic colitis, mucous colitis, pylorospasm and biliary dyskinesia. It is available as the hydrochloride in 10 or 20 mg tablets, a syrup containing 10 mg/5 mL and in ampules for intramuscular injection. The usual dose for adults is 10–40 mg taken 3 or 4 times daily.

Blood Concentrations. A peak plasma dicyclomine concentration of about 0.02 mg/L was observed in a single subject 1.5 hours after a single 20 mg oral dose; the same subject achieved a peak plasma concentration of approximately 0.08 mg/L 2 hours after oral administration of a single 40 mg sustained-release tablet (Meffin et al., 1973). Blood samples taken from a volunteer 1, 2 and 3 hours after three hourly 20 mg liquid doses of dicyclomine resulted in dicyclomine blood concentrations of 0.02, 0.02 and 0.06 mg/L, respectively (Garriott et al., 1984).

Metabolism and Excretion. Dicyclomine is rapidly absorbed after oral administration. Approximately 80% of a dose is eliminated in the urine and 10% in the feces (Moffat et al., 1986). No information has been reported on its metabolism in man.

Toxicity. Adverse effects attributed to dicyclomine include dizziness, nausea, vomiting, dilated pupils, central nervous system stimulation and difficulty in swallowing. Several reports of dicyclomine intoxication in infants describe symptoms of shallow respiration, apnea and, in some cases, convulsions (Edwards, 1984; Williams and Watkin-Jones, 1984). In the case of a 2.5 year old infant found in coma and pronounced dead soon after admission to hospital, the blood dicyclomine concentration was 0.50 mg/L, bile, 0.64 mg/L and vitreous humor, 0.08 mg/L. In another case in which resuscitation attempts were unsuccessful, a 2.5 month old infant had a postmortem blood dicyclomine concentration of 0.22 mg/L (Garriott et al., 1984).

Analysis. Dicyclomine has been determined in biological specimens employing gas chromatography with either nitrogen-selective (Meffin et al., 1973; Beretta and Vanazzi, 1984; Walker et al., 1987) or flame-ionization detection (Randall et al., 1986).

References

E. Beretta and G. Vanazzi. Determination of nanogram amounts of dicyclomine with gas chromatography and nitrogen-selective detection. J. Chrom. 308: 341–344, 1984.

J.C. Garriott, R. Rodriguez and L.E. Norton. Two cases of deaths involving dicyclomine in infants: measurements of therapeutic and toxic concentrations in blood. Clin. Tox. 22: 455–462, 1984.

P.D.L. Edwards. Dicyclomine in babies. Brit. Med. J. 288: 1230, 1984.

P.J. Meffin, G. Morre and J. Thomas. Determination of dicyclomine in plasma by gas chromatography. Anal. Chem. 45: 1964–1966, 1973.

A.C. Moffat, J.V. Jackson, M.S. Moss and B. Widdop (eds.). *Clarke's Isolation and Identification of Drugs,* 2nd ed., Pharmaceutical Press, London, 1986, p. 536.

B. Randall, G. Gerry and F. Rance. Dicyclomine in the sudden infant death syndrome (SIDS)—a cause of death or an incidental finding? J. For. Sci. 31: 1470–1474, 1986.

B.J. Walker, J.F. Land and R.A. Okerholm. Quantitative analysis of dicyclomine in human plasma by capillary gas chromatography and nitrogen-selective detection. J. Chrom. 416: 150–153, 1987.

J. Williams and R. Watkin-Jones. Dicyclomine: worrying symptoms associated with its use in some small babies. Brit. Med. J. 288: 901, 1984.

Dieldrin

T½: 2–12 months
Vd: 13–69 L/kg
Fb: ?

Occurrence and Usage. The epoxide of aldrin is known as dieldrin (HEOD), an organochlorine insecticide that has seen widespread usage since its development nearly 30 years ago. Technical grades of the chemical contain at least 85% dieldrin and are available in the form of powders, solutions and bait granules. Dieldrin, a stereoisomer of endrin, has been banned from most uses in the United States due to its persistence and accumulation in the environment and its chronic toxicity potential. The threshold limit value is currently 0.25 mg/m^3 for industrial exposure to dieldrin, which is known to be well-absorbed after inhalation or dermal contact.

Blood Concentrations. Blood concentrations of dieldrin resulting from dietary intake in some United States residents were found to average 0.0015 mg/L; approximately 25% of whole blood dieldrin was present in erythrocytes (Radomski et al., 1971). The same value for whole blood dieldrin was reported by Dale and co-workers (1966), who also determined that plasma dieldrin concentrations in persons occupationally exposed to varying amounts of the chemical averaged 0.0094–0.0270 mg/L. Adults who were orally administered either 0.050 or 0.211 mg of dieldrin daily for 24 months developed steady-state blood levels averaging 0.007 and 0.020 mg/L, respectively; these concentrations had no apparent effect on the subjects and the levels declined with an average half-life of 1 year upon termination of dieldrin intake (Hunter et al., 1969). Half-lives of 50 and 97 days have also been reported (Brown et al., 1964; Garrettson and Curley, 1969).

Metabolism and Excretion. Dieldrin is not thought to undergo appreciable metabolic degradation in man, but this has not been definitely established. A major fecal detoxification product in rats has been identified as 9-hydroxydieldrin, which bears a hydroxyl group on the carbon of the methylene bridge (Baldwin et al., 1970), whereas the major urinary metabolite is 2-ketodieldrin, a product of oxidative dechlorination (McKinney et al., 1972).

Adipose tissue is a major body depot for dieldrin storage; the average fat concentration in the general population of southern England was found to be 0.21 mg/kg (Hunter et al., 1963), while the mean value for United States residents was 0.14 mg/kg (Hoffman et al., 1967). Fat concentrations of dieldrin in subjects ingesting 0.050 or 0.211 mg of the chemical daily for 24 months reached maximum levels of 1.59 and 4.94 mg/kg, respectively (Hunter et al., 1969). Industrially exposed asymptomatic workers had an average fat concentration of 6.12 mg/kg (Hayes and Curley, 1968). Only negligible amounts of unchanged dieldrin, if any, are excreted in human urine (Cueto and Hayes, 1962).

Toxicity. The acute lethal dose of dieldrin in man is on the order of 1.5–5 g. Clinical signs of poisoning, including headache, dizziness, nausea, sweating, myoclonic limb movements and convulsive seizures, may be evident when the blood dieldrin concentration exceeds 0.15–0.20 mg/L (Brown et al., 1964). A 4 year old boy who survived the ingestion of dieldrin was found to have concentrations of 0.27 mg/L in serum and 47 mg/kg in fat 3 days after the incident (Garrettson and Curley, 1969). A 21 year old man ingested 9 g of dieldrin in toluene and did not regain consciousness for 5 days; a peak serum dieldrin concentration of 1.16 mg/L was achieved on the first, and a peak fat concentration of about 80 mg/kg was measured on the fourth day (Black, 1974).

Several dieldrin fatalities have occurred, in both children and adults, although chemical determinations on tissue specimens were not performed (Conley, 1960; Pribilla, 1963; Weinig et al., 1966; Garrettson and Curley, 1969). Liver dieldrin concentrations of 4–25 mg/kg were observed in 3 fatal cases (Black, 1974), and blood and liver concentrations of 0.5 mg/L and 29 mg/kg, respectively, were reported in the case of a man who intentionally ingested a large amount of dieldrin (Steentoft, 1979).

Analysis. Dieldrin concentrations in biologic specimens may be estimated using electron-capture gas chromatographic techniques developed for the organochlorine pesticides as a class (Dale et al., 1966; Richardson et al., 1967; Radomski et al., 1971).

References

M.K. Baldwin, J. Robinson and R.A.G. Carrington. Metabolism of HEOD (dieldrin) in the rat: examination of the major faecal metabolites. Chem. Ind.: 595–597, 1970.

A.M.S. Black. Self poisoning with dieldrin: a case report and pharmacokinetic discussion. Anaesth. Int. Care 4: 369–374, 1974.

V.K.H. Brown, C.G. Hunter and A. Richardson. A blood test diagnostic of exposure to aldrin and dieldrin. Brit. J. Ind. Med. 21: 283–286, 1964.

B.E. Conley. Occupational dieldrin poisoning. J. Am. Med. Asso. 172: 2077–2080, 1960.

C. Cueto, Jr. and W.J. Hayes, Jr. The detection of dieldrin metabolites in human urine. J. Agr. Food Chem. 10: 366–369, 1962.

W.E. Dale, A. Curley and C. Cueto, Jr. Hexane extractable chlorinated insecticides. Life Sci. 5: 47–54, 1966.

L.K. Garrettson and A. Curley. Dieldrin. Studies in a poisoned child. Arch. Env. Health 19: 814–822, 1969.

W.J. Hayes, Jr. and C. Curley. Storage and excretion of dieldrin and related compounds. Arch. Env. Health 16: 155–162, 1968.

W.S. Hoffman, H. Adler, W.I. Fishbein and F.C. Bauer. Relation of pesticide concentrations in fat to pathological changes in tissues. Arch. Env. Health 15: 758–765, 1967.

C.G. Hunter, J. Robinson and A. Richardson. Chlorinated insecticide content of human body fat in southern England. Brit. Med. J. 1: 221–224, 1963.

C.G. Hunter, J. Robinson and M. Roberts. Pharmacodynamics of dieldrin (HEOD). Arch. Env. Health 18: 12–21, 1969.

J.D. McKinney, H.B. Matthews and L. Fishbein. Major fecal metabolite of dieldrin in rat. Structure and chemistry. J. Agr. Food Chem. 20: 597–602, 1972.

O. Pribilla. Akute toedliche Dieldrinvergiftung. Arch. Tox. 20: 61–71, 1963.

J.L. Radomski, W.B. Deichmann, A.A. Rey and T. Merkin. Human pesticide blood levels as a measure of body burden and pesticide exposure. Tox. Appl. Pharm. 20: 175–185, 1971.

A. Richardson, J. Robinson, B. Bush and J.M. Davies. Determination of dieldrin (HEOD) in blood. Arch. Env. Health 14: 703–708, 1967.

A. Steentoft. A case of fatal dieldrin poisoning. Med. Sci. Law 19: 268–269, 1979.

W. Weinig, G. Machbert and P. Zink. Ueber den Nachweis des Dieldrins bei einer Dieldrinvergiftung. Arch. Tox. 22: 115–124, 1966.

Diethylpropion

T½: ?
Vd: ?
Fb: ?
pKa: ?

Occurrence and Usage. Diethylpropion (Tenuate) is a phenethylamine derivative synthesized in 1928 and used clinically as an anorectic agent since 1962. It is available as the hydrochloride salt in tablets of 25 mg (normal-release) or 75 mg (sustained-release); the usual adult dose is 75 mg per day. It has been determined that the compound is only half as effective when given parenterally, and thus it is likely that the numerous active metabolites contribute significantly to the overall effect of this agent.

Blood Concentrations. Following a 75 mg oral dose, plasma diethylpropion concentrations averaged 0.007 mg/L at 0.5 hours and declined to 0.003 mg/L by 2 hours; the concentrations of nordiethylpropion and dinordiethylpropion together reached an average peak of 0.185 mg/L at 2 hours and declined to only 0.104 mg/L by 8 hours. At higher doses, significant concentrations of the reduction products, mono- and di-ethylnorephedrine, were detected in plasma (Wright et al., 1975).

Metabolism and Excretion. Diethylpropion undergoes extensive biotransformation primarily to active metabolites. The metabolism involves de-ethylation to nordiethylpropion and dinordiethylpropion, and reduction of the parent and these 2 metabolites to the corresponding aminopropanol derivatives, with creation of a second asymmetric center (Testa and Beckett, 1973). The 6 resulting compounds undergo p-hydroxylation and conjugation to some extent; deamination occurs with formation of a benzoic acid conjugate (Schreiber et al., 1968). As much as 87% of a

diethylpropion → nordiethylpropion → dinordiethylpropion

N,N-diethylnorephedrine — N-ethylnorephedrine — norephedrine

p-hydroxylation, deamination and conjugation

dose has been accounted for in the 30 hour urine (under acidic conditions) as unchanged diethylpropion (1.8%), nordiethylpropion (26.5%), dinordiethylpropion (2.6%), N,N-diethylnorephedrine (15.8%), N-ethylnorephedrine (14.1%) and norephedrine (26.2%) (Testa and Beckett, 1973). The remainder of the dose may largely represent deaminated products (Milhailova et al., 1974).

Toxicity. Adverse reactions to diethylpropion may include anxiety, blurred vision, tremor and insomnia. Psychosis with paranoid or manic features has been reported with chronic use or abuse (Carney, 1988).

Overdosage with diethylpropion results in a clinical picture very similar to that of amphetamine intoxication. The following tissue concentrations were determined in the case of a 35 year old man who died after self-administering an intravenous injection of the drug (Fysh, 1978):

Diethylpropion Concentrations in a Fatal Case (mg/L or mg/kg)

Blood	Liver	Bile	Kidney	Injection Site
5.4	0.9	14	0.9	43

Analysis. Determination of diethylpropion and its metabolites in biofluids has been accomplished by gas chromatography with detection by flame-ionization (Testa and Beckett, 1972) or mass spectrometry (Wright et al., 1975). The metabolites may be converted to their N-acetyl derivatives for ease in chromatographing, and p-chlorodiethylpropion has been used as an internal standard.

References

M.W.P. Carney. Diethylpropion and psychosis. Clin. Neuropharm. 11: 183–188, 1988.

R.R. Fysh. Personal communication., 1978.

M. Mihailova, A. Rosen, B. Testa and A.H. Beckett. A pharmacokinetic investigation of the distribution and elimination of diethylpropion and its metabolites in man. J. Pharm. Pharmac. 26: 711–721, 1974.

E.C. Schreiber, B.H. Min, A.V. Zeiger and J.F. Lang. Metabolism of diethylpropion-1-C^{14} hydrochloride by the human. J. Pharm. Exp. Ther. 159: 372–378, 1968.

B. Testa and A.H. Beckett. Studies on the metabolism of diethylpropion. I. Analytical procedure. J. Chrom. 71: 39–51, 1972.

B. Testa and A.H. Beckett. Metabolism and excretion of diethylpropion in man under acidic urine conditions. J. Pharm. Pharmac. 25: 119–124, 1973.

G.J. Wright, J.F. Lang, R.E. Lemieux and M.J. Goodfriend, Jr. The objective and timing of drug disposition studies, appendix III. Diethylpropion and its metabolites in the blood plasma of the human after subcutaneous and oral administration. Drug Met. Rev. 4: 267–276, 1975.

Diflunisal

T½: 5–20 hr (dose-related)
Vd: 0.1–0.2 L/kg
Fb: 0.99
pKa: ?

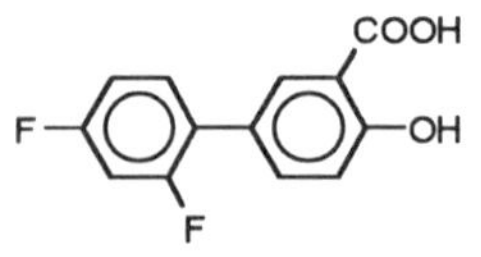

Occurrence and Usage. Diflunisal (Dolobid), a difluorophenyl derivative of salicylic acid, is commonly used as an analgesic and anti-inflammatory agent in the treatment of arthritis. The drug is available as the free acid in tablets of 250 and 500 mg. For osteoarthritis and rheumatoid arthritis, the suggested dosage range is 500–1000 mg daily in divided doses; maintenance doses higher than 1500 mg/day are not recommended.

Blood Concentrations. Peak plasma concentrations of diflunisal ranging from 6.8–95 mg/L (average, 62) have been reported following a single 500 mg dose (Nuernberg et al., 1991). Following a single 750 mg oral dose in 2 healthy volunteers, an average peak plasma concentration of 99 mg/L occurred in 3.5–4.0 hours (Ray and Day, 1983).

Trough steady-state plasma concentrations ranged from 85–90 mg/L following a 500 mg dose every 12 hours (Steelman et al., 1978). Steady-state plasma concentrations ranged from 66–130 mg/L following oral administration of 500 mg twice daily to healthy subjects (Wahlin-Boll et al., 1981).

Metabolism and Excretion. Approximately 14% of a single oral dose of diflunisal is excreted as unchanged drug, with another 80% present as either the phenolic or acyl glucuronide. A sulfate conjugate is believed to be a minor urinary metabolite (Tocco et al., 1975; Loewen et al., 1986; Hansen-Moller et al., 1987).

Toxicity. Symptoms of diflunisal overdosage include drowsiness, vomiting, diarrhea, hyperventilation, tachycardia, sweating, tinnitus, disorientation, stupor and coma. Two adults who died after acute ingestion of large amounts of the drug had postmortem blood diflunisal concentrations of 370 and 580 mg/L (Warren and Sharp, 1993). Postmortem studies on a 38 year old male who died soon after ingestion of 18 diflunisal tablets showed the following concentrations (Levine et al., 1987):

Diflunisal Concentrations in a Fatal Case (mg/L or mg/kg)

Blood	Liver	Kidney	Urine	Gastric
260	400	350	78	34 mg

Analysis. Diflunisal may be determined in biological specimens by many of the commercially available techniques intended for salicylate that rely on colorimetry or immunoassay (Adelman et al., 1991). Liquid chromatography is able to distinguish between salicylate and diflunisal and is often the method of choice (Wahlin-Boll et al., 1981; Ray and Day, 1983; Schwartz et al., 1986; Kazemifard and Moore, 1991; Warren and Sharp, 1993).

References

H.M. Adelman, P.M. Wallach and M.T. Flannery. Inability to interpret toxic salicylate levels in patients taking aspirin and diflunisal. J. Rheum. 18: 522–523, 1991.

J. Hansen-Moller, L. Dalgaard and S.H. Hansen. Reversed-phase high-performance liquid chromatographic assay for the simultaneous determination of diflunisal and its glucuronides in serum and urine. J. Chrom. 420: 99–110, 1987.

A.G. Kazemifard and D.E. Moore. Liquid chromatography with amperometric detection for the determination of non-steroidal and anti-inflammatory drugs in plasma. J. Chrom. 533: 125–132, 1990.

B. Levine, D.F. Smyth and Y.H. Caplan. A diflunisal related fatality: a case report. For. Sci. Int. 35: 45–50, 1987.

G.R. Loewen, G. McKay and R.K. Verbeeck. Isolation and identification of new major metabolite of diflunisal in man. Drug Met. Disp. 14: 127–131, 1986.

B. Nuernberg, G. Koehler and K. Brune. Pharmacokinetics of diflunisal in patients. Clin. Pharmacokin. 20: 81–89, 1991.

J.E. Ray and R.O. Day. High-performance liquid chromatographic analysis of diflunisal in plasma and urine: application to pharmacokinetic studies in two normal volunteers. J. Pharm. Sci. 72: 1403–1405, 1983.

M. Schwartz, R. Chiou, R.J. Stubbs and W.F. Bayne. Determination of diflunisal in human plasma and urine by fast high-performance liquid chromatography. J. Chrom. 380: 420–424, 1986.

S.L. Steelman, K.F. Tempero and V.F. Cirillo. The chemistry, pharmacology, toxicology and clinical pharmacology of diflunisal. Clin. Ther. 1 (Suppl. A): 1–9, 1978.

D.J. Tocco, G.O. Breault, A.G. Zacchei et al. Physiological disposition and metabolism of 5-(2',4'-difluorophenyl) salicylic acid, a new salicylate. Drug Met. Disp. 3: 453–466, 1975.

E. Wahlin-Boll, B. Brantmark, A. Hanson et al. High-pressure liquid chromatographic determination of acetyl salicylic acid, salicylic acid, diflunisal, indomethacin, indoprofen and indobufen. Eur. J. Clin. Pharm. 20: 375–378, 1981.

R.J. Warren and M.E. Sharp. Diflunisal overdose: a report of two cases. Can. Soc. For. Sci. J. 26: 33–35, 1993.

Digitoxin

T½: 4–10 days
Vd: 41 L/kg
Fb: 0.97

(digitoxose)₃O

Occurrence and Usage. Digitoxin (Crystodigin, Lanatoxin) is one of a group of naturally-occurring plant glycosides that are used for their cardiotonic action in the treatment of congestive heart failure. The drug is derived from the leaves of *Digitalis purpurea* and *Digatalis lanata*, in which it is found in amounts of up to 0.4% in combination with glucose. Upon acid hydrolysis, digitoxin yields the aglycone, digitoxigenin, which retains the activity of glycoside, and 3 molecules of a sugar, digitoxose. The compound is available in the form of ampules (0.2 mg/mL) and tablets (0.05–0.20 mg) and may be administered by intravenous or intramuscular injection or orally in daily maintenance doses of 0.05–0.3 mg; loading doses of 1.2–1.6 mg are sometimes given when initiating therapy.

Blood Concentrations. Serum concentrations of digitoxin in 52 patients who were maintained on daily doses of 0.05–0.3 mg (average, 0.11) and who showed no signs of toxicity ranged from 3–39 μg/L (average, 17) in samples drawn 6–12 hours after the last dose (Smith, 1970). A linear relationship was found between daily dose and steady-state plasma concentration of the drug, and it was noted that only 2% of the whole blood digitoxin is contained in erythrocytes (Lukas and Peterson, 1966). The compound exhibits plasma protein binding of 97% (Storstein, 1976b) and an elimination half-life of 6.1 days (range, 3.7–9.6) (Rasmussen et al., 1971). A single intravenous injection of 0.6 mg in 5 subjects produced a mean serum drug concentration of 51 μg/L after 2–5 minutes and this declined with a distribution half-life of 71 minutes until, after 2 hours, the concentration fell below 20 μg/L and the elimination phase began (Storstein, 1974).

Metabolism and Excretion. The biotransformation of digitoxin in man is complex; at least 24 metabolites have been postulated and many of these identified. Hydrolytic cleavage of the digitoxose molecules occurs in a stepwise fashion, and each of the successive metabolites as well as the parent may be hydroxylated at the 12-position to form the corresponding digoxin analogue. Each of the above compounds is cardioactive and each may be inactivated by glucuronide or sulfate conjugation. After a single dose, digoxin is the major serum and urine metabolite, but during chronic therapy it constitutes less than 1% of the active serum constituents and is a minor urinary metabolite. Patients on chronic therapy excrete 90% of a daily dose in about equal amounts in the 24 hour urine and feces; unchanged digitoxin constitutes 90% of the cardioactive serum substances and 87% of the active urine substances. About 32% of the dose is present in the urine as active drug or metabolites and 12% as inactive conjugates (Lukas, 1971; Storstein, 1977). The absorption of orally administered digitoxin is complete (Beermann et al., 1971).

Toxicity. Digitoxin toxicity is manifested by nausea, vomiting, diarrhea, blurred vision, and cardiac disturbances such as tachycardia, premature contractions, atrial fibrillation and atrioventricular block. Six patients exhibiting these toxic signs had serum digitoxin concentrations of 26–43 µg/L (average, 34) on daily doses of 0.07–0.20 mg (average, 0.12) (Smith, 1970). A woman who ingested 10 mg of digitoxin achieved a plasma concentration of 150 µg/L after 12 hours; the plasma half-life of the drug was reduced to 20 hours through charcoal hemoperfusion, compared to a half-life of 145 hours when the same patient was studied under therapeutic drug administration 3 weeks later (Gilfrich et al., 1979). Six of seven patients survived the acute ingestion of 3–20 mg of digitoxin after developing maximal plasma concentrations of 38–181 µg/L (average, 112); the survivors were discharged 6–43 days after admission (Hansteen et al., 1981).

A series of 91 acute digitoxin intoxications was reported that included 24 deaths. Doses ranged from 2–25 mg and plasma digitoxin concentrations were as high as 800 µg/L. A positive correlation was found between serum potassium concentration measured within 3–18 hours of drug ingestion and mortality; serum potassium concentrations averaged 4.2 mmol/L in the patients who recovered and 6.2 mmol/L in those who died (Bismuth et al., 1973). One subject who acutely ingested 15 mg of the drug developed a plasma concentration of 320 µg/L after 4 hours and died 10 hours later (Mercier, 1971). Digitoxin was identified by bioassay in the skeletal muscle of 9 out of 14 victims, dead for 17–40 months, suspected of having accidentally received digitoxin in place of estradiol (Thomas et al., 1979).

Analysis. Methods for the determination of therapeutic concentrations of digitoxin in biologic specimens have included an ATP-ase inhibition assay (Bentley et al., 1970), a double-isotope dilution derivative technique (Lukas and Peterson, 1966) and a red cell Rb-86 uptake inhibition method (Gjerdrum, 1970). This latter procedure has been coupled with thin-layer chromatography to provide a specific means of analyzing the drug and its numerous metabolites in blood and urine (Storstein, 1976a). Radioimmunoassay systems are now commercially available and, as they are highly sensitive, specific and rapid (Smith, 1970), are most frequently employed in the clinical measurement of this drug. Although most systems cross-react with digoxin, therapeutic serum digoxin concentrations are very low compared to those of digitoxin and thus do not cause significant error in the measurement. Liquid chromatography combined with radioimmunoassay has also been described (Santos et al., 1987).

References

B. Beermann, K. Hellstrom and A. Rosen. Fate of orally administered ³H-digitoxin in man with special reference to the absorption. Circulation 43: 852–861, 1971.

J.D. Bentley, G.H. Burnett, R.L. Conklin and R.H. Wasserburger. Clinical application of serum digitoxin levels. Circulation 41: 67–75, 1970.

C. Bismuth, M. Gaultier, F. Conso and M.L. Efthymiou. Hyperkalemia in acute digitalis poisoning: prognostic significance and therapeutic implications. Clin. Tox. 6: 153–162, 1973.

H.J. Gilfrich, W. Kasper, T. Meinertz et al. Successful treatment of massive digitoxin overdose by charcoal hemoperfusion. Vet. Hum. Tox. 21: 18–19, 1979.

K. Gjerdrum. Determination of ditigalis in blood. Acta Med. Scand. 187: 371–379, 1970.

V. Hansteen, D. Jacobsen, K. Knudsen et al. Acute, massive poisoning with digitoxin: report of seven cases and discussion of treatment. Clin. Tox. 18: 679–692, 1981.

D.S. Lukas and R.E. Peterson. Double isotope dilution derivative assay of digitoxin in plasma, urine, and stool of patients maintained on the drug. J. Clin. Invest. 45: 782–795, 1966.

D.S. Lukas. Some aspects of the distribution and disposition of digitoxin in man. Ann. N.Y. Acad. Sci. 179: 338–361, 1971.

M. Mercier. Personal communication, 1971.

K. Rasmussen, J. Jervell and O. Storstein. Clinical use of bio-assay of serum digitoxin activity. Eur. J. Clin. Pharm. 3: 236–242, 1971.

S.R.C.J. Santos, W. Kirch and E.E. Ohnhaus. Simultaneous analysis of digitoxin and its clinically relevant metabolites using high-performance liquid chromatography and radioimmunoassay. J. Chrom. 419: 155–164, 1987.

T.W. Smith. Radioimmunoassay for serum digitoxin concentration: methodology and clinical experience. J. Pharm. Exp. Ther. 175: 352–360, 1970.

L. Storstein. Studies on digitalis. I. Renal excretion of digitoxin and its cardioactive metabolites. Clin. Pharm. Ther. 16: 14–24, 1974.

L. Storstein. Studies on digitalis. IV. A method for thin-layer chromatographic separation and determination of digitoxin and cardioactive metabolites in human blood and urine. J. Chrom. 117: 87–96, 1976a.

L. Storstein. Studies on digitalis. VII. Influence of nephrotic syndrome on protein binding, pharmacokinetics, and renal excretion of digitoxin and cardioactive metabolites. Clin. Pharm. Ther. 20: 158–166, 1976b.

L. Storstein. Studies on digitalis. VIII. Digitoxin metabolism on a maintenance regimen and after a single dose. Clin. Pharm. Ther. 21: 125–140, 1977.

F. Thomas, J. La Barre, J. Renaux and E. Draux. A therapeutic catastrophe, entailing 16 exhumations, following the administration of digitoxin instead of oestradiol benzoate to prostatic cancer patients: identification of the poison. Med. Sci. Law 19 : 8–18, 1979.

Digoxin

T½: 30–45 hr
Vd: 5.1–7.4 L/kg
Fb: 0.20

(digitoxose)$_3$O

Occurrence and Usage. Digoxin (Lanoxin) is a cardiotonic plant glycoside that occurs in *Digitalis lanata* in combination with glucose and acetic acid. It is the 12-hydroxy analogue of digitoxin and is a major metabolite of that compound in man. In the treatment of congestive heart failure, digoxin is commonly given in daily oral maintenance doses of 0.25–0.75 mg; when initiating therapy, loading doses of 0.75–1.5 mg by intravenous or intramuscular injection or 2–3 mg orally may be administered. It is supplied in tablets of 0.125–0.5 mg and ampules containing 0.25 mg/mL.

Blood Concentrations. A single oral 0.25 mg digoxin dose administered to 6 fasting normal subjects resulted in serum concentrations that peaked at 1.13 µg/L at 1 hour and declined to 0.32 µg/L by 6 hours (Panisset et al., 1973). Peak plasma concentrations following a single 0.5 mg oral dose in 5 subjects averaged 1.4 µg/L at 2 hours on a full stomach, and 2.4 µg/L at 1 hour when fasting (White et al., 1971). Serum concentrations after a single intravenous 0.75 mg dose are initially as high as 13 µg/L at 10 minutes after injection but decline rapidly (Koup et al., 1975). Serum digoxin concentrations in 131 controlled patients receiving an average daily oral dose of 0.31 mg (range, 0.0625–1.0) averaged 1.4 µg/L (range, 0.3–3.0) (Smith and Haber, 1970). Blood for serum digoxin analysis should be drawn at least 6 hours after the last dose to avoid erroneously high values (Murphy et al., 1985).

Digoxin, unlike digitoxin, exhibits negligible binding to plasma proteins (Doherty et al., 1971) and distributes nearly equally between erythrocytes and plasma (Abshagen et al., 1971). The average elimination half-life in normal subjects is 37 hours (Huffman et al., 1974). The bioavailability of oral preparations ranges from 67% for tablets to 100% for an encapsulated elixir (Aronson, 1980). Recent data strongly suggests that digoxin follows nonlinear kinetics (Wagner et al., 1981).

Serum digoxin concentrations are effectively doubled during the co-administration of quinidine or quinine; this may result from a reduction in the binding of digoxin to skeletal muscle (Chen and Friedman, 1980; Leahey et al., 1980; Wandell et al., 1980; Schenck-Gustafsson et al., 1981).

Metabolism and Excretion. Digoxin is biotransformed to only a small degree in man. The metabolites are largely products of hydrolytic cleavage of the digitoxose group and of sulfate and glucuronide conjugation (Okita, 1964). An average of 59% of a single dose is excreted in the urine over a 7 day period, of which 95–98% is unchanged drug; an average of 15% is excreted in the feces over the same period (Marcus et al., 1964; Doherty et al., 1970). In a 5 day period, 2% of a dose is eliminated as digoxigenin-bis-digitoxoside, 0.8% as digoxigenin-mono-digitoxoside, 0.3% as digoxigenin, and 0.3% as dihydrodigoxin (Gault et al., 1979). During chronic oral therapy, an average of 57% of a dose appears in the daily urine as apparently unchanged drug and urine concentrations are on the order of 25–125 µg/L (Huffman et al., 1974).

Myocardial/serum digoxin concentration ratios average 149 in infants and 28 in adults during therapy (Park et al., 1982). The following tissue distribution of the drug was determined from 17 adult patients who had been maintained on a mean daily dose of 0.005 mg/kg digoxin and who had not exhibited signs of toxicity prior to death (Andersson et al., 1975):

Digoxin Tissue Distribution During Therapy (µg/kg)*

	Brain	Atrial Myocardium	Ventricular Myocardium	Liver	Kidney	Skeletal Muscle	Fat
Average	32	65	133	72	128	30	10
(Range)	(3–74)	(27–129)	(50–296)	(29–186)	(56–253)	(13–56)	(4–23)

* By ^{86}Rb uptake inhibition after dichloromethane extraction

Toxicity. Digoxin toxicity is manifested by the same clinical signs as seen with digitoxin. Psychosis with vivid hallucinations has been described (Carney et al., 1985). Serum concentrations averaged 3.7 µg/L (range, 1.6–13.7) in 48 patients exhibiting toxic signs who were being maintained on a mean dose of 0.36 mg (range, 0.125–1.0) daily (Smith and Haber, 1970). A series of clinical reports of nonfatal and fatal digoxin poisoning have described cases of oral overdosage with 2.5–25 mg of the drug in which serum concentrations of 11–42 µg/L and elimination half-lives of 5–48 hours were observed (Smith and Willerson, 1971; Hobson and Zettner, 1973; Watanabe et al., 1977; Pearce et al., 1980). One subject who self-administered 200 mg of digoxin intravenously developed a maximum serum concentration of 52 µg/L after 4 hours and died after 6 hours (Reza et al., 1974). Antidotal treatment of a case of ingestion of 22.5 mg was successfully accomplished by the intravenous administration of digoxin-specific antibodies (Smith et al., 1976). Several authors have obtained benefit with charcoal hemoperfusion (Smiley et al., 1978; Marbury et al., 1979), while others do not recommend its use (Warren and Fanestil, 1979; Rowett, 1980); orally-administered charcoal has been reported to markedly shorten the elimination half-life (Boldy et al., 1985). Atropine and phenytoin have been found to completely reverse digoxin-induced arrhythmias (Ekins and Watanabe, 1978).

Reported postmortem blood concentrations for persons on therapy with digoxin vary considerably depending on the analytical method used and the anatomical origin of the blood specimen. Concentrations averaged 1.3 µg/L (range, 0.5–2.1) in 18 specimens of serum obtained from the right heart, but these values may be falsely low due to the effect of hemolysis on the ^{3}H-radioimmunoassay used (DiMaio et al., 1975). At the other end of the postmortem "therapeutic" range, Karjalainen et al. (1974) found an average of 4.6 µg/L (range, 1.3–8.2) in 13 samples of blood obtained from an unidentified source using an extraction-radioimmunoassay procedure. Probably the best defined study is that of Holt and Benstead (1975), who determined that complete hemolysis of a blood sample causes a decline of only 12% in the digoxin value relative to plasma; that serum taken from the right heart of 10 patients contained an average of 2.3 µg/L (range, 1.3–3.9) digoxin compared to an average of 1.4 µg/L (range, 0.7–2.9) in serum from the femoral vein of the same subjects; and that equivalent results were obtained for samples analyzed directly with either the ^{3}H or ^{125}I-radioimmunoassay, if correction for color quench was made when using the tritium label. It has been determined that serum digoxin levels nearly always increase after death due to leaching from muscle, with an average postmortem/antemortem ratio ranging from 1.42 for femoral vein blood specimens to 1.96 for heart blood specimens (Vorpahl and Coe, 1978). Fletcher et al. (1979)

suggested that postmortem blood samples for digoxin assay be taken from the peripheral circulation within a few hours after death, that they be completely hemolyzed by freezing and thawing several times, and centrifuged before analysis; the analytical value may then be multiplied by 1.3 to estimate the serum digoxin concentration at the moment of death.

At least 30 digoxin fatalities have been reported in which postmortem blood or serum concentrations were determined; the values range from 3.5–200 µg/L (average, 25) and represent both accidental and intentional overdoses (Iisalo and Nuutila, 1973; Moffat, 1974; Phillips, 1974a; DiMaio et al., 1975; Holt and Benstead, 1975; Ma, 1976; Dickson and Blazey, 1977; Selesky et al., 1977). In 2 digoxin fatalities, concentrations of 200 and 283 µg/L were measured in the left ventricular myocardium (Iisalo and Nuutila, 1973); these concentrations exceed the average therapeutic level for this tissue but are still within the normal range according to the above table. Aderjan et al. (1979) recommended that kidney concentrations be measured in the investigation of fatal digoxin poisoning, since this tissue appears to be dramatically elevated in such cases over normal values (140 ± 35 µg/kg). These authors found the following concentrations in a case of suicide by digoxin:

Digoxin Concentrations in a Fatal Case (µg/L or µg/kg)

Blood	Brain	Heart	Lung	Liver	Kidney
22	9.7	43	53	81	1400

Analysis. Digoxin has been successfully quantitated in body fluids by an ATP-ase inhibition technique (Burnett and Conklin, 1971) and by ^{86}Rb uptake inhibition assay (Gjerdrum, 1970). The latter method has been combined with solvent extraction in order to accommodate solid tissues (Andersson et al., 1975). The most frequently used technique for the determination of digoxin is radioimmunoassay (Smith et al., 1969). Certain of the commercially available radioimmunoassay systems are prone to errors from hemolysis, bilirubinemia or abnormal albumin levels (Cerceo and Elloso, 1972); removal of the digoxin from the specimen by extraction or dialysis improves the accuracy of the ^{3}H-radioimmunoassay (Phillips, 1974b), although the development of ^{125}I-systems has circumvented most of the problems associated with earlier assays. The commercial digoxin radioimmunoassay kits exhibit from 0.6–25% cross-reactivity with digitoxin, and many of the digoxin metabolites react to the same degree as digoxin itself (Stoll et al., 1972); on average, only 64% (range, 35–80) of serum digoxin as measured by radioimmunoassay is actually parent drug (Gault et al., 1984). Digoxin-like immunoreactivity has been reported present in the body fluids of individuals not receiving the drug (Balzan et al., 1984; Spiehler et al., 1985); this may be avoided by increasing incubation time during radioimmunoassay or by ultrafiltration of the specimen (Graves et al., 1986; Dasgupta et al., 1990). Thin-layer chromatography (Aderjan et al., 1979), liquid chromatography (Fletcher et al., 1980; Loo et al., 1981; Stone and Soldin, 1988) and solvent extraction (Picotte et al., 1991) have been used prior to immunoassay to provide additional specificity. Liquid chromatography with formation of a fluorescent derivative has been reported (Kwong and McErlane, 1986; Shepard et al., 1986).

References

U. Abshagen, H. Kewitz and N. Reitbrock. Distribution of digoxin, digitoxin and ouabain between plasma and erythrocytes in various species. N.-S. Arch. Exp. Path. Pharm. 270: 105–116, 1971.

A. Aderjan, H. Buhr and G. Schmidt. Investigation of cardiac glycoside levels in human post mortem blood and tissues determined by a special radioimmunoassay procedure. Arch. Tox. 42: 107–114, 1979.

K.E. Andersson, A. Bertler and G. Wettrell. Post-mortem distribution and tissue concentrations of digoxin in infants and adults. Acta Paediat. Scand. 64: 497–504, 1975.

J.K. Aronson. Clinical pharmacokinetics of digoxin 1980. Clin. Pharm. 5: 137–149, 1980.

S. Balzan, A. Clerico, M.G. del Chicca et al. Digoxin-like immunoreactivity in normal human plasma and urine, as detected by a solid-phase radioimmunoassay. Clin. Chem. 30: 450–451, 1984.

D.A.R. Boldy, V. Smart and J.A. Vale. Multiple doses of charcoal in digoxin poisoning. Lancet 2: 1076–1077, 1985.

G.H. Burnett and R.L. Conklin. Enzymatic assay of plasma digoxin. J. Lab. Clin. Med. 78: 779–784, 1971.

M.W.P. Carney, S. Rapp and K. Pearce. Digoxin toxicity presenting with psychosis in a patient with chronic phobic anxiety. Clin. Neuropsych. 8: 193–195, 1985.

E. Cerceo and C.A. Elloso. Factors affecting the radioimmunoassay of digoxin. Clin. Chem. 18: 539–543, 1972.

T.S. Chen and H.S. Friedman. Alteration of digoxin pharmacokinetics by a single dose of quinidine. J. Am. Med. Asso. 244: 669–672, 1980.

A. Dasgupta, S. Saldana and P. Heimann. Monitoring free digoxin instead of total digoxin in patients with congestive heart failure. Clin. Chem. 36: 2121–2123, 1990.

S.J. Dickson and N.D. Blazey. Post-mortem digoxin levels—two unusual case reports. For. Sci. 9: 145–150, 1977.

V.J.M. DiMaio, J.C. Garriott and R. Putnam. Digoxin concentrations in postmortem specimens after overdose and therapeutic use. J. For. Sci. 20: 340–347, 1975.

J.E. Doherty, W.J. Flanigan, M.L. Murphy et al. Tritiated digoxin. XIV. Enterohepatic circulation, absorption, and excretion studies in human volunteers. Circulation 42: 867–873, 1970.

J.E. Doherty, W.H. Hall, J. Sherwood et al. Tritiated digoxin. XV. Serum protein binding in human subjects. Am. J. Cardiol. 28: 326–330, 1971.

B.R. Ekins and A.S. Watanabe. Acute digoxin poisonings: review of therapy. Am. J. Hosp. Pharm. 35: 268–277, 1978.

S.M. Fletcher, G. Lawson and A.C. Moffat. Radioimmunoassay of cardiac glycosides in haemolysed blood: derivation of serum levels. J. For. Sci. Soc. 19: 183–188, 1979.

S.M. Fletcher, G. Lawson, B. Law and A.C. Moffat. Identification of cardiac glycosides in human body fluids by a combination of high-performance liquid chromatography and radioimmunoassay. J. For. Sci. Soc. 20: 203–209, 1980.

M.H. Gault, D. Sugden, C. Maloney et al. Biotransformation and elimination of digoxin with normal and minimal renal function. Clin. Pharm. Ther. 25: 499–513, 1979.

M.H. Gault, L.L. Longerich, J.C.K. Loo et al. Digoxin biotransformation. Clin. Pharm. Ther. 35: 74–82, 1984.

K. Gjerdrum. Determination of digitalis in blood. Acta Med. Scand. 187: 371–379, 1970.

S.W. Graves, K. Sharma and A.B. Chandler. Methods for eliminating interferences in digoxin immunoassays caused by digoxin-like factors. Clin. Chem. 32: 1506–1509, 1986.

J.D. Hobson and A. Zettner. Digoxin serum half-life following suicidal digoxin poisoning. J. Am. Med. Asso. 223: 147–149, 1973.

D.W. Holt and J.G. Benstead. Postmortem assay of digoxin by radioimmunoassay. J. Clin. Path. 28: 483–486, 1975.

D.H. Huffman, C.V. Manion and D.L. Azarnoff. Absorption of digoxin from different oral preparations in normal subjects during steady state. Clin. Pharm. Ther. 16: 310–317, 1974.

E. Iisalo and M. Nuutila. Myocardial digoxin concentrations in fatal intoxications. Lancet 1: 257, 1973.

J. Karjalainen, K. Ojala and P. Reissell. Tissue concentrations of digoxin in an autopsy material. Acta Pharm. Tox. 34: 385–390, 1974.

J.R. Koup, D.J. Greenblatt, W.J. Jusko et al. Pharmacokinetics of digoxin in normal subjects after intravenous bolus and infusion doses. J. Pharm. Biopharm. 3: 181–192, 1975.

E. Kwong and K.M. McErlane. Analysis of digoxin at therapeutic concentrations using high-performance liquid chromatography with post-column derivatization. J. Chrom. 381: 357–363, 1986.

E.B. Leahey, Jr., J.A. Reiffel, E.V. Giardina and J.T. Bigger, Jr. The effect of quinidine and other oral antiarrhythmic drugs on serum digoxin. Ann. Int. Med. 92: 605–608, 1980.

J.C.K. Loo, I.J. McGilveray and N. Jordan. The estimation of serum digoxin by combined HPLC separation and radioimmunological assay. J. Liq. Chrom. 4: 879–886, 1981.

C. Ma. Personal communication, 1976.

T. Marbury, J. Mahoney, L. Juncos et al. Advanced digoxin toxicity in renal failure: treatment with charcoal hemoperfusion. South. Med. J. 72: 279–281, 1979.

F.I. Marcus, G.J. Kapadia and G.G. Kapadia. The metabolism of digoxin in normal subjects. J. Pharm. Exp. Ther. 145: 203–209, 1964.

A.C. Moffat. Interpretation of post mortem serum levels of cardiac glycosides after suspected overdosage. Acta Pharm. Tox. 35: 386–394, 1974.

J.E. Murphy, E.S. Ward and M.L. Job. Avoiding erroneous serum digoxin concentrations. Am. J. Hosp. Pharm. 42: 2418–2420, 1985.

G.T. Okita. Metabolism of radioactive cardiac glycosides. Pharmacologist 6: 45, 1964.

J.C. Panisset, P. Biron, G. Tremblay et al. Comparative bioavailability of two oral preparations of digoxin in healthy volunteers. Can. Med. Asso. J. 109: 700–702, 1973.

M.K. Park, T. Ludden, K.V. Arom et al. Myocardial vs serum digoxin concentrations in infants and adults. Am. J. Dis. Child. 136: 418–420, 1982.

G. Pearce, N. Buchanan and J. Uther. Massive digoxin ingestion in a child. Med. J. Aust. 2: 277–280, 1980.

A.P. Phillips. Case experience with digoxin analysis of postmortem blood. J. For. Sci. Soc. 14: 137–140, 1974a.

A.P. Phillips. A radioimmunoassay technique for digoxin in postmortem blood. J. For. Sci. 19: 900–912, 1974b.

P. Picotte, C. Peclet, M. Gaudet and J.J. Rousseau. Interpretation des concentrations sanguines post-mortem de digoxine. Can. Soc. For. Sci. J. 24: 97–101, 1991.

M.J. Reza, R.B. Kovick, K.L. Shine and M.L. Pearce. Massive intravenous digoxin overdosage. New Eng. J. Med. 291: 777–778, 1974.

D.A. Rowett. Failure of hemoperfusion in digoxin overdose. J. Am. Med. Asso. 244: 1558, 1980.

K. Schenck-Gustafsson, T. Jogestrand, R. Nordlander and R. Dahlqvist. Effect of quinidine on digoxin concentrations in skeletal muscle and serum in patients with atrial fibrillation. New Eng. J. Med. 305: 209–211, 1981.

M. Selesky, V. Spiehler, R.H. Cravey and H.W. Elliot. Digoxin concentrations in fatal cases. J. For. Sci. 22: 409–417, 1977.

T.A. Shepard, J. Hui, A. Chandrasekaran et al. Digoxin and metabolites in urine and feces: a fluorescence derivatization-high performance liquid chromatographic technique. J. Chrom. 380: 89–98, 1986.

J.W. Smiley, N.M. March and E.T. Del Guercio. Hemoperfusion in the management of digoxin toxicity. J. Am. Med. Asso. 240: 2736–2737, 1978.

T.W. Smith, V.P. Butler, Jr. and E. Haber. Determination of therapeutic and toxic serum digoxin concentrations by radioimmunoassay. New Eng. J. Med. 281: 1212–1216, 1969.

T.W. Smith and E. Haber. Digoxin intoxication: relationship of clinical presentation to serum digoxin concentration. J. Clin. Invest. 49: 2377–2386, 1970.

T.W. Smith and J.T. Willerson. Suicidal and accidental digoxin ingestion. Circulation 44: 29–36, 1971.

T.W. Smith, E. Haber, L. Yeatman and V.P. Butler, Jr. Reversal of advanced digoxin intoxication with Fab fragments of digoxin-specific antibodies. New Eng. J. Med. 294: 797–800, 1976.

V.R. Spiehler, W.R. Fischer and R.G. Richards. Digoxin-like immunoreactive substance in postmortem blood of infants and children. J. For. Sci. 30: 86–91, 1985.

R.G. Stoll, M.S. Christensen, E. Sakmar and J.G. Wagner. The specificity of the digoxin radioimmunoassay procedure. Res. Comm. Chem. Path. Pharm. 4: 503–510, 1972.

J.A. Stone and S.J. Soldin. Improved liquid chromatographic/immunoassay of digoxin in serum. Clin. Chem. 34: 2547–2551, 1988.

T.E. Vorpahl and J.I. Coe. Correlation of antemortem and postmortem digoxin levels. J. For. Sci. 23: 329–334, 1978.

J.G. Wagner, K.D. Popat, S.K. Das et al. Evidence of nonlinearity in digoxin pharmacokinetics. J. Pharm. Biopharm. 9: 147–166, 1981.

M. Wandell, J.R. Powell, W.D. Hager et al. Effect of quinine on digoxin kinetics. Clin. Pharm. Ther. 28: 425–430, 1980.

S.E. Warren and D.D. Fanestil. Digoxin overdose. Limitations of hemoperfusion-hemodialysis treatment. J. Am. Med. Asso. 242: 2100–2101, 1979.

A.S. Watanabe, B.R. Ekins, J.C. Veltri and A.R. Temple. Acute digoxin poisoning: case report and determination of elimination half-life. In *Management of the Poisoned Patient* (B.H. Rumack and A.R. Temple, eds.), Science Press, Princeton, 1977, pp. 115–124.

R.J. White, D.A. Chamberlain, M. Howard and T.W. Smith. Plasma concentrations of digoxin after oral administration in the fasting and postprandial state. Brit. Med. J. 1: 380–381, 1971.

Dihydrocodeine

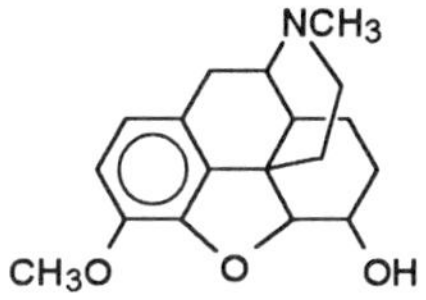

T½: 3.4–4.5 hr
Vd: 1.0–1.3 L/kg
Fb: ?
pKa: 8.8

Occurrence and Usage. Dihydrocodeine (drocode, DHCplus, Synalgos-DC) is a semisynthetic narcotic analgesic, prepared by the hydrogenation of codeine. It is supplied as the bitartrate salt in 16 mg tablets or capsules for oral administration. Single doses of 16–32 mg may be taken every 4 hours, with a maximum recommended daily limit of 192 mg.

Blood Concentrations. Following a single oral dose of 30 or 60 mg in 7 adult volunteers, peak plasma dihydrocodeine concentrations averaged 0.07 and 0.15 mg/L, respectively, at 1.6 and 1.8 hours post-dose (Rowell et al., 1983).

Metabolism and Excretion. Dihydrocodeine is believed to undergo the same series of biotransformation steps as codeine, i.e., N- and O-dealkylation, and glucuronide or sulfate conjugation at the 3- and 6-hydroxy positions. Conjugated metabolites reach plasma concentrations several times those of the parent drug even after a single dose (Rowell et al., 1983). Two urinary metabolites have been isolated, with chromatographic properties suggestive of dihydronorcodeine and dihydromorphine (Peat and Sengupta, 1977).

Toxicity. Adverse reactions to dihydrocodeine include dizziness, drowiness, lightheadedness, nausea and constipation. Overdosage may result in respiratory depression, coma, convulsions, cardiovascular collapse, and death.

Four persons who died following acute intentional overdosage had postmortem blood dihydrocodeine levels of 7.2–12 mg/L (average, 9.0) (Paterson, 1985).

Analysis. The analytical methods described for codeine are generally applicable to the determination of dihydrocodeine. A liquid chromatographic technique for the drug and its major metabolites has been reported (Ohno et al., 1994).

References

M. Ohno, Y. Shiono and M. Konishi. Simultaneous determination of dihydrocodeine and its metabolites in dog plasma by hplc with electrochemical and ultraviolet detection. J. Chrom. 654: 213–219, 1994.

S.C. Paterson. Drug levels found in cases of fatal self-poisoning. For. Sci. 27: 129–133, 1985.

M.A. Peat and A. Sengupta. Toxicological investigations of cases of death involving codeine and dihydrocodeine. For. Sci. 9: 21–32, 1977.

F.J. Rowell, R.A. Seymour and M.D. Rawlins. Pharmacokinetics of intravenous and oral dihydrocodeine and its acid metabolites. Eur. J. Clin. Pharm. 25: 419–424, 1983.

Diltiazem

T½: 5.1 hr
Vd: 3–13 L/kg
Fb: 0.85–0.98
pKa: 7.7

Occurrence and Usage. Diltiazem (Cardizem) is a calcium channel blocker effective in the treatment of angina pectoris, hypertension and supraventricular arrhythmias. Diltiazem is available for oral administration in tablets and capsules containing from 30–300 mg of the hydrochloride salt. It is also available in injectable form as a 5 mg/mL solution.

Blood Concentrations. Following a single 90 mg oral dose of diltiazem to 4 volunteers, the maximum plasma concentration ranged from 86–188 μg/L (average, 130) 3–4 hours post-administration (Yeung et al., 1989). Following a single oral dose of 120 mg of diltiazem to 6 healthy men, the peak plasma concentration ranged from 98–304 μg/L (average, 174) and occurred 1.5–4.3 hours after the dose; peak concentrations of nordiltiazem and deacetyldiltiazem averaged 43 and 15 μg/L, respectively, and occurred from 1.5–6 hours after the dose (Boyd et al., 1989).

Twelve healthy volunteers, aged 21–26 and weighing from 59–90 kg, were given either 240 mg of diltiazem or 320 mg as a slow-release tablet in divided daily doses until they reached steady-state serum concentrations of 100–200 μg/L (Gordin et al., 1986). Morselli et al. (1979) found that plasma concentrations 4 hours after diltiazem administration were between 100 and 200 μg/L in patients who "responded", but were usually below 100 μg/L in those who did not.

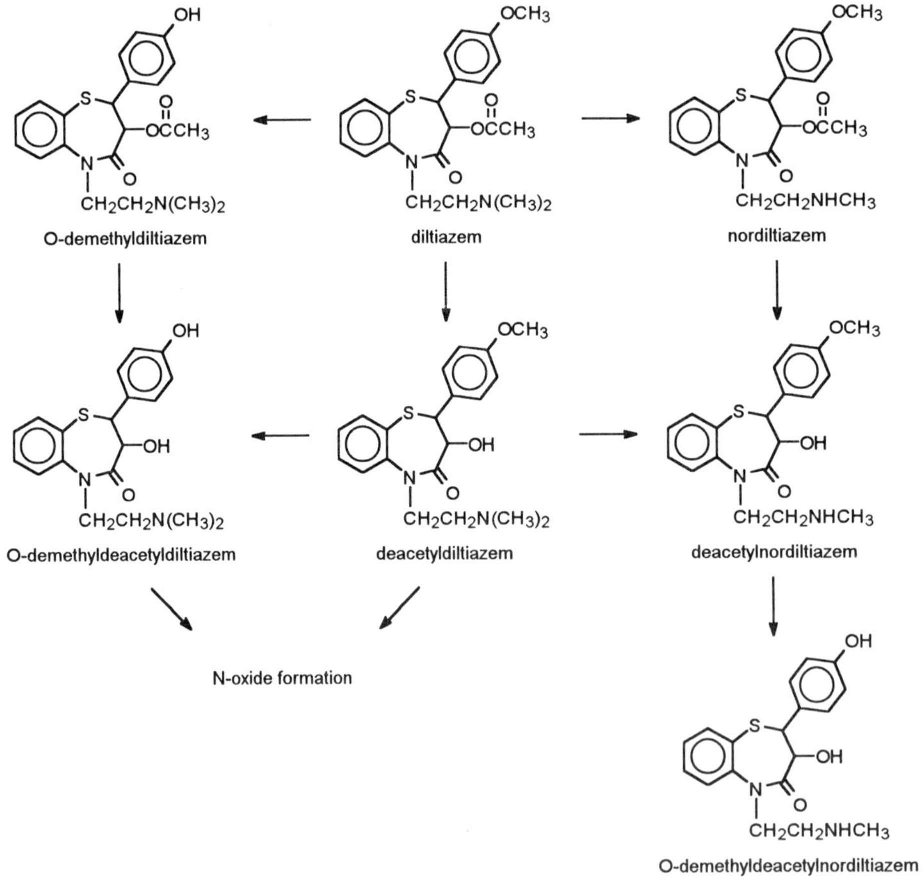

Metabolism and Excretion. Diltiazem is extensively metabolized by N- and O-demethylation, deacetylation, N-oxide formation and conjugation. About 73% of a labelled dose is excreted within 4 days in the urine, with another 18% in the feces. The parent drug in free form accounts for about 1% of a dose in the 8 hour urine; its presence is eclipsed by its numerous metabolites, largely in conjugated form. The major urinary species are deacetyldiltiazem-N-oxide and O-demethyldeacetylnordiltiazem, accounting for 21% and 13% of a dose, respectively (Clozel et al., 1984; Hoglund and Nilsson, 1989).

Deacetyldiltiazem and nordiltiazem, both of which are present in plasma, exhibit about 45% and 20%, respectively, of the parent drug's vasodilatory potency (Rovei et al., 1980; Yabana et al., 1985).

Toxicity. The most common adverse reactions for diltiazem include weakness, edema, dizziness, nausea, vomiting and rash. In overdose situations, bradycardia, hypotension, cardiac failure and death may occur. A 38 year old female who ingested 900 mg of diltiazem and displayed hypotension and bradycardia was successfully treated in a hospital; she was found to have a maximum plasma diltiazem concentration of 1.7 mg/L 7 hours following ingestion (Roberts et al., 1991).

A 25 year old female who ingested an unknown quantity of diltiazem and metoclopramide exhibited a peak serum concentration of diltiazem of 8.5 mg/L 2 hours post-dose, at which time she was minimally responsive, hypotensive, bradycardic and acidotic; she later suffered cardiorespiratory arrest and was pronounced dead after 4 days (Beno and Nemeth, 1991). In 5 apparent adult suicides, the following diltiazem concentrations were reported at autopsy (Holzbecher and Hutton, 1988; Wiese et al., 1988; Picotte, 1991; Kaliciak et al., 1992; Cravey, 1992):

Diltiazem Concentrations in Fatalities (mg/L or mg/kg)

	Blood	Brain	Liver	Urine	Gastric
Average	16	76	63	33	630 mg
(Range)	(6.7–33)	(76)	(41–79)	(5.4–60)	(1–1800)

Analysis. The stability of diltiazem and its metabolites is of concern. Whole blood kept at room temperature for about 1 hour between sampling and centrifugation showed an average loss of 14% of the parent compound and a loss of 24% for nordiltiazem; the concentrations of the other metabolites did not change significantly. Plasma samples immediately frozen at -80° C. can be stored for up to 5 weeks before analysis (Dube et al., 1988; Caille et al., 1989; Bonnefous et al., 1992).

Diltiazem and its metabolites have been determined by gas chromatography (Rovei et al., 1977; Alebic-Kolbah and Plavsics, 1990) and liquid chromatography (Montamat et al., 1987; Dube et al., 1988; Caille et al., 1989; Yeung et al., 1989; Boulieu et al., 1990; Johnson and Pieper, 1990; Hussain et al., 1992; Rutledge et al., 1993).

References

T. Alebic-Kolbah and F. Plavsics. Determination of serum diltiazem concentrations in a pharmacokinetic study using gas chromatography with electron capture detection. J. Pharm. Biomed. Anal. 8: 915–918, 1990.

J.M. Beno and D.R. Nemeth. Diltiazem and metoclopramide overdose. J. Anal. Tox. 15: 285–287, 1991.

J.L. Bonnefous, R. Boulieu and C. Lahet. Stability of diltiazem and its metabolites in human blood samples. J. Pharm. Sci. 81: 341–344, 1992.

R. Boulieu, J.L. Bonnefous and S. Ferry. Determination of diltiazem and its metabolites in plasma by high performance liquid chromatography. J. Liq. Chrom. 13: 291–302, 1990.

R.A. Boyd, S.K. Chin, O. Don-Pedro et al. The pharmacokinetics and pharmacodynamics of diltiazem and its metabolites in healthy adults after a single oral dose. Clin. Pharm. Ther. 46: 408–419, 1989.

G. Caille, L.M. Dube, Y. Theoret et al. Stability study of diltiazem and two of its metabolites using a high performance liquid chromatographic method. Biopharm. Drug Disp. 10: 107–114, 1989.

J.P. Clozel, G. Caille, Y. Taeymans et al. High-performance liquid chromatographic determination of diltiazem and six of its metabolites in human urine. J. Pharm. Sci. 73: 771–773, 1984.

R.H. Cravey. Unpublished results, 1992.

L.M. Dube, N. Mousseau and I.J. Mcgilveray. High-performance liquid chromatographic determination of diltiazem and four of its metabolites in plasma. J. Chrom. 430: 103–111, 1988.

A. Gordin, P. Pohto, S. Sundberg et al. Pharmacokinetics of slow-release diltiazem and its effect on atrioventricular conduction in healthy volunteers. Eur. J. Clin. Pharm. 31: 423–426, 1986.

P. Hoglund and L.G. Nilsson. Pharmacokinetics of diltiazem and its metabolites after repeated multiple-dose treatments in healthy volunteers. Ther. Drug Mon. 11: 543–550, 1989.

M.D. Holzbecher and C.J. Hutton. A fatal case involving diltiazem. Can. Soc. For. Sci. J. 21: 135–137, 1988.

M.D. Hussain, Y.K. Tam, B.A. Finegan et al. Simple and sensitive high-performance liquid chromatographic method for the determination of diltiazem and 6 of its metabolites in human plasma. J. Chrom. 582: 203–210, 1992.

K.E. Johnson and J.A. Pieper. An HPLC method for the determination of diltiazem and three of its metabolites in serum J. Liq. Chrom. 13: 951–960, 1990.

H.A. Kaliciak, S.N. Huckin and W.S. Cave. A death attributed solely to diltiazem. J. Anal. Tox. 16: 102–103, 1992.

S.C. Montamat, D.R. Abernethy and J.R. Mitchell. High-performance liquid chromatographic determination of diltiazem and its major metabolites, N-monodemethyldiltiazem and desacetyldiltiazem, in plasma. J. Chrom. 415: 203–207, 1987.

P.L. Morselli, V. Rovei, M. Mitchard et al. Pharmacokinetics and metabolism of diltiazem in man (observations on healthy volunteers and angina pectoris patients). In *New Drug Therapy with a Calcium Antagonist* (R.J. Bing, ed.), Excerpta Medica, Amsterdam, 1979.

P. Picotte. Personal communication, 1991.

D. Roberts, N. Honcharik, D.S. Sitar and M. Tenenbein. Diltiazem overdose: pharmacokinetics of diltiazem and its metabolites and effect of multiple dose charcoal therapy. Clin. Tox. 29: 45–52, 1991.

V. Rovei, M. Mitchard and P. Morselli. Simple, sensitive, and specific gas chromatographic method for the quantitation of diltiazem in human body fluids. J. Chrom. 138: 391, 1977.

V. Rovei, R. Gomeni, M. Mitchard et al. Pharmacokinetics and metabolism of diltiazem in man. Acta Cardiol. 35: 35–45, 1980.

D.R. Rutledge, A.H. Abadi, L.M. Lopez and C.A. Beaudreau. High-performance liquid chromatographic determination of diltiazem and 2 of its metabolites in plasma using a short akyl chain silanol deactivated column. J. Chrom. 615: 111–116, 1993.

J. Wiese, E. Klug, V. Schneider et al. Todliche Diltiazemvergiftung. Z. Rechtsmed. 100: 271–276, 1988.

H. Yabana, T. Nagao and M. Sato. Cardiovascular effects of the metabolites of diltiazem in dogs. J. Cardiovasc. Pharm. 7: 152–157, 1985.

P.K.F. Yeung, T.J. Montague, B. Tsui and C. McGregor. High-performance liquid chromatographic assay of diltiazem and six of its metabolites in plasma: application to a pharmacokinetic study in healthy volunteers. J. Pharm. Sci. 78: 592–597, 1989.

Dimethylformamide

T½: 2–6 hr (whole blood)
Vd: ? $HCON(CH_3)_2$
Fb: ?

Occurrence and Usage. Dimethylformamide (DMF) is a common laboratory and industrial solvent that is readily absorbed following inhalation of the vapor or skin contact with the liquid. A metabolite, methylformamide, has been investigated as an anticancer drug in humans. The current threshold limit value for occupational exposure to DMF is 10 ppm (30 mg/m³) in the industrial atmosphere.

Blood Concentrations. Dimethylformamide reached an average level of 2.8 mg/L in the blood of subjects exposed to 21 ppm of the vapor for 4 hours, and was undetectable at 4 hours after the exposure; the metabolite, methylformamide, averaged between 1 and 2 mg/L in the blood and this level was maintained for at least 4 hours after exposure. Maximal blood levels of about 14 mg/L and 8 mg/L were observed for dimethylformamide and methylformamide, respectively, at 0 and 3 hours after a 4 hour exposure to 87 ppm of the vapor. Repeated daily exposures to 21 ppm of dimethylformamide did not result in accumulation of the chemical or its metabolite in blood (Kimmerle and Eben, 1975b).

Metabolism and Excretion. It is believed that dimethylformamide is metabolized in man by se-quential N-demethylation to methylformamide and formamide, both of which may undergo conju-gation with glutathione. Hydroxymethyl derivatives have also been identified. All of the metabo-lites are present in urine to some extent, but dimethylformamide is only detectable in urine after acute exposure to higher concentrations of the chemical (Kimmerle and Eben, 1975b; Mraz, 1988; Santoni et al., 1992). Although quantitative data have not been obtained, it is likely that a substan-tial portion of an absorbed dose of dimethylformamide is excreted unchanged in the expired breath.

Alveolar air concentrations of dimethylformamide in workers have been found to correlate with environmental air concentrations of the chemical (Brugnone et al., 1980). After a 4 hour exposure to 26 ppm of dimethylformamide, methylformamide and formamide excretion in the 24 hour urine of 4 persons averaged 24 and 6.9 mg, respectively. The corresponding values for an 87 ppm expo-sure were 97 and 17 mg, respectively (Kimmerle and Eben, 1975b). The urinary concentration of methylformamide has proved to be the best index of worker exposure to dimethylformamide (Maxfield et al., 1975; Krivanek et al., 1978; Lauwerys et al., 1980; Yonemoto and Suzuki, 1980).

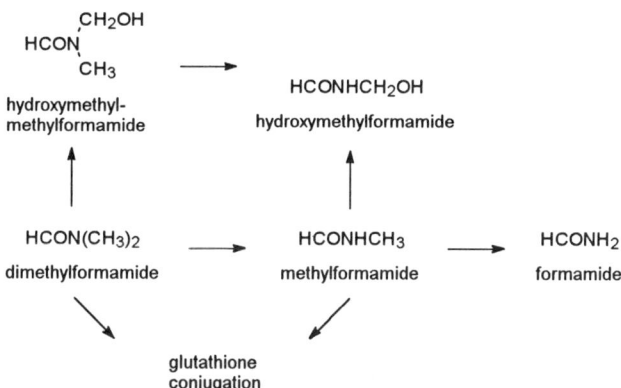

Toxicity. Exposure to dimethylformamide by inhalation, dermal contact or ingestion can produce nausea and vomiting at lower levels of exposure, and severe abdominal pain, hepatomegaly and hepatic necrosis at higher levels. Liver and kidney damage are frequently observed in animal toxic-ity testing (Massmann, 1956; Clayton et al., 1963; Potter, 1973). Reinl and Urban (1965) presented data on 13 industrial workers who showed signs of acute or chronic intoxication due to dimethylformamide exposure; 5 individuals demonstrated laboratory or clinical evidence of liver toxicity.

The ingestion of alcohol during or after an exposure to dimethylformamide can produce a disulfiram-like reaction, resulting in facial flushing, dizziness, sweating, nausea, palpitation, breath-lessness, and loss of consciousness; this is believed due to the inhibition of acetaldehyde (an ethanol metabolite) metabolism by methylformamide (Lyle et al., 1979).

Analysis. Dimethylformamide and methylformamide in blood have been measured after extraction into ethanol by nitrogen-selective gas chromatography (Kimmerle and Eben, 1975a). Methylformamide concentrations in urine may be determined by gas chromatography (Barnes and Henry, 1974; Lauwerys et al., 1980; Mraz, 1988) or liquid chromatography (Santoni et al., 1992).

References

J.R. Barnes and N.W. Henry. The determination of N-methylformamide and N-methylacetamide in urine. Am. Ind. Hyg. Asso. J. 35: 84–87, 1974.

F. Brugnone, L. Perbellini and E. Gaffuri. N,N-dimethylformamide concentration in environmental and alveolar air in an artificial leather factory. Brit. J. Ind. Med. 37: 185–188, 1980.

J.W. Clayton, Jr., J.R. Barnes, D.B. Hood and G.W.H. Schepers. The inhalation toxicity of dimethylformamide. Am. Ind. Hyg. Asso. J. 24: 144–154, 1963.

G. Kimmerle and A. Eben. Metabolism studies of N,N-dimethylformamide. Int. Arch. Arbeitsmed. 34: 109–126, 1975a.

G. Kimmerle and A. Eben. Metabolism studies of N,N-dimethylformamide. Int. Arch. Arbeitsmed. 34: 127–136, 1975b.

N.D. Krivanek, M. McLaughlin and W.E. Fayerweather. Monomethylformamide levels in human urine after repetitive exposure to dimethylformamide vapor. J. Occ. Med. 20: 179–182, 1978.

R.R. Lauwerys, A. Kivits, M. Lhoir et al. Biological surveillance of workers exposed to dimethylformamide and the influence of skin protection on its percutaneous absorption. Int. Arch. Occ. Env. Health 45: 189–203, 1980.

W.H. Lyle, T.W.M. Spence, W.M. McKinneley and K. Duckers. Dimethylformamide and alcohol intolerance. Brit. J. Ind. Med. 36: 63–66, 1979.

W. Massmann. Toxicological investigations on dimethylformamide. Brit. J. Ind. Med. 13: 51–54, 1956.

M.E. Maxfield, J.R. Barnes, A. Azar and H.T. Trochimowicz. Urinary excretion of metabolite following experimental human exposures to DMF or to DMAC. J. Occ. Med. 17: 506–511, 1975.

J. Mraz. Gas chromatographic method for the determination of N-acetyl-S-(N-methylcarbamoyl)cysteine, a metabolite of N,N-dimethylformamide and N-methylformamide, in human urine. J. Chrom. 431: 361–368, 1988.

H.P. Potter. Dimethylformamide-induced abdominal pain and liver injury. Arch. Env. Health. 27: 340–341, 1973.

W. Reinl and H.J. Urban. Erkrankungen durch Dimethylformamid. Int. Arch. Gewerbepath. Gewerbehyg. 21: 333–346, 1965.

G. Santoni, P. Bavazzano, A. Perico et al. High-performance liquid chromatographic determination of N-methylformamide and N-methyl-N-(hydroxymethyl)-formamide in human urine. J. Chrom. 581: 287–292, 1992.

J. Yonemoto and S. Suzuki. Relation of exposure to dimethylformamide vapor and the metabolite, methylformamide, in urine of workers. Int. Arch. Occ. Env. Health 46: 159–165, 1980.

Dimethylsulfoxide

T½: 11–14 hr
Vd: ?
Fb: ?

$$CH_3\overset{\overset{\displaystyle O}{\|}}{S}CH_3$$

Occurrence and Usage. Dimethylsulfoxide (DMSO, Rimso-50) is a synthetic chemical used industrially as a solvent. At room temperature the chemical is a clear, water-miscible liquid with a specific gravity of 1.10. Its original pharmaceutical use was as a vehicle for drugs intended for dermal application. However, DMSO itself has been found effective in the treatment of musculo skeletal inflammation and injury and interstitial cystitis. It is applied topically as a 90% solution in single doses of 2–5 mL, with a daily maximum of 10–20 mL, or by instillation into the urinary bladder of 50 mL of a 50% solution. The chemical has also been the subject of clinical studies to determine its effectiveness in reducing intracranial pressure in trauma victims; intravenous doses of 1 g/kg have been administered for this purpose.

Blood Concentrations. Dermal application of 1 g/kg (64 mL/70 kg) produced maximal serum DMSO concentrations of 504–560 mg/L in 2 subjects within 4–8 hours; by 48 hours only traces of the chemical were detectable, the levels having declined with a half-life of 11–14 hours. Concentrations of dimethylsulfone, a metabolite, reached peak levels of 333 and 514 mg/L within 36–72 hours and declined with a half-life of 60–70 hours. An equivalent oral dose given to 6 subjects resulted in peak serum DMSO concentrations of 1029–3380 mg/L after 1–4 hours; peak dimethylsulfone concentrations of 263–596 mg/L were measured at 48–96 hours. Daily oral administration of 0.5 g/kg (32 mL/70 kg) for 14 days produced peak serum levels of 1850 mg/L for DMSO and 1040 mg/L for dimethylsulfone on the eighth day in one subject (Hucker et al., 1967).

Metabolism and Excretion. DMSO is well-absorbed after either dermal or oral administration. It does not concentrate in particular tissues, but is evenly distributed throughout the body water (Hucker et al., 1966). Urinary excretion accounts for 13% of a dermal dose as unchanged DMSO within 48 hours, and 18% as dimethylsulfone over a period of 19 days. Oral administration increases urinary excretion of these 2 compounds to an average of 51% and 22%, respectively (Hucker et al., 1967). Up to 3% of a dose is excreted in the breath within 24 hours as dimethylsulfide (Kolb et al., 1967).

$$CH_3SCH_3 \longleftarrow CH_3\overset{O}{\underset{\|}{S}}CH_3 \longrightarrow CH_3\overset{O}{\underset{\underset{O}{\|}}{\overset{\|}{S}}}CH_3$$

dimethylsulfide   dimethylsulfoxide   dimethylsulfone

Toxicity. Side-effects of DMSO administration include local dermatitis, nausea, headache, loss of taste, and garlic odor of the breath (John and Laudahn, 1967). The intravenous administration of 100 g of 20% DMSO on several occasions produced vomiting and drowsiness in 2 elderly arthritis patients; laboratory tests showed evidence of hemolysis, liver damage, and decreased renal function. Both patients recovered after 5 days (Yellowlees et al., 1980). Another elderly patient, who became moribund after 3 weeks of daily intravenous DMSO therapy, had serum DMSO and dimethylsulfone levels of 1600 and 3000 mg/L, respectively, at 4 days after the last dose (Bond et al., 1988).

Analysis. DMSO and dimethylsulfone have been measured in biological fluids by flame-ionization or electron-capture gas chromatography after solvent extraction (Hucker et al., 1967; Wong et al., 1971) or protein precipitation (Garretson and Aitchison, 1982; Mehta et al., 1986). Dimethylsulfide has been analyzed by headspace gas chromatography-mass spectrometry (Terazawa et al., 1991). Osmometry has been suggested as a means of estimating serum concentrations of DMSO (Runckel and Swanson, 1980).

References

R. Bond, D. Dahl and S. Curry. Acute mental deterioration associated with intravenous dimethylsulfoxide. Vet. Hum. Tox. 30: 350, 1988.

S.E. Garretson and J.P. Aitchison. Determination of dimethyl sulfoxide in serum and other body fluids by gas chromatography. J. Anal. Tox. 6: 76–81, 1982.

H.B. Hucker, P.M. Ahmad and E.A. Miller. Absorption, distribution and metabolism of dimethylsulfoxide in the rat, rabbit and guinea pig. J. Pharm. Exp. Ther. 154: 176–184, 1966.

H.B. Hucker, J.K. Miller, A. Hochberg et al. Studies on the absorption, excretion and metabolism of dimethylsulfoxide (DMSO) in man. J. Pharm. Exp. Ther. 155: 309–317, 1967.

H. John and G. Laudahn. Clinical experiences with the topical application of DMSO in orthopedic diseases: evaluation of 4180 cases. Ann. N.Y. Acad. Sci. 141: 506–516, 1967.

K.H. Kolb, G. Jaenicke, M. Kramer and P.E. Schulze. Absorption, distribution and elimination of labeled dimethyl sulfoxide in man and animals. Ann. N.Y. Acad. Sci. 141: 85–95, 1967.

A.C. Mehta, S. Peaker, C. Acomb and R.T. Calvert. Rapid gas chromatographic determination of dimethyl sulphoxide and its metabolite dimethyl sulphone in plasma and urine. J. Chrom. 383: 400–404, 1986.

D.N. Runckel and J.R. Swanson. Effect of dimethyl sulfoxide on serum osmolality. Clin. Chem. 26: 1745–1747, 1980.

K. Terazawa, K. Mizukami, B. Wu and T. Takatori. Fatality due to inhalation of dimethyl sulfide in a confined space. Int. J. Leg. Med. 104: 141–144, 1991.

K.K. Wong, G.M. Wang, J. Dreyfuss and E.C. Schreiber. Absorption, excretion, and biotransformation of dimethyl sulfoxide in man and miniature pigs after topical application as an 80% gel. J. Invest. Dermatol. 56: 44–48, 1971.

P. Yellowlees, C. Greenfield and N. McIntyre. Dimethylsulphoxide-induced toxicity. Lancet 2: 1004–1006, 1980.

Dimethyltryptamine

T½: 30 min
Vd: ?
Fb: ?
pKa: ?

$CH_2CH_2N(CH_3)_2$

Occurrence and Usage. Dimethyltryptamine (DMT) is a short-acting hallucinogenic indole derivative that is structurally related to serotonin (5-hydroxytryptamine), a neurotransmitter. DMT occurs naturally in certain South American plants and was first prepared synthetically in 1954. Since the compound is believed to be produced endogenously in small amounts as the result of serotonin biotransformation, its possible role in the etiology of schizophrenia has been the subject for much speculation. As a drug of abuse, dimethyltryptamine is commonly applied to tobacco, marijuana or other plant leaves and smoked; doses of 50–150 mg are typical. It is commonly synthesized from indole and dimethylamine, in a manner similar to that of its homologues diethyltryptamine and dipropyltryptamine, both of which have been identified in seizures of illicit drugs.

Blood Concentrations. Plasma concentrations of endogenous DMT in both normal subjects and schizophrenic patients have been found to be generally less than 0.001 mg/L using a specific gas chromatographic-mass spectrometric method (Walker et al., 1973; Wyatt et al., 1973). Using the same technique, blood concentrations of DMT after a single intramuscular injection of 0.7 mg/kg (49 mg/70 kg) reached an average peak of 0.10 mg/L in 10 minutes and declined to 0.03 mg/L by 30 minutes (Kaplan et al., 1974).

Metabolism and Excretion. DMT is rapidly and extensively metabolized in man; the primary metabolite is 3-indoleacetic acid, which may be formed via N-demethylation and oxidative deamination. N-oxidation and 6-hydroxylation are also suspected pathways of DMT biotransformation. About 33% of a dose is excreted in the 6 hour urine as free and conjugated (probably with glycine) 3-indoleacetic acid. An average of 0.07% of a dose is excreted unchanged in the 24 hour urine (Szara, 1956; Szara and Axelrod, 1959; Kaplan et al., 1974).

$CH_2CH_2N(CH_3)_2$ $\longrightarrow$ CH_2COOH $\longrightarrow$ conjugation

dimethyltryptamine   3-indoleacetic acid

Toxicity. The effects of DMT administration include hallucinations, anxiety, perceptual distortions, pupillary dilation, and elevated blood pressure (Rosenberg et al., 1963).

Analysis. Analytical procedures for the determination of dimethyltryptamine in biologic fluids have relied on fluorimetry (Gross and Franzen, 1965), gas chromatography (Narasimhachari et al.,

1971) and gas chromatography-mass spectrometry (Walker et al., 1973). Liquid chromatography with fluorescence detection has been used in the analysis of the drug and its metabolites in tissues (Sitaram et al., 1987).

References

V.H. Gross and F. Franzen. Zur Bestimmung koerpereigener Amine in biologischen Substraten. Z. Klin. Chem. 3: 99–102, 1965.

J. Kaplan, L.R. Mandel, R. Stillman et al. Blood and urine levels of N,N-dimethyltryptamine following administration of psychoactive dosages in human subjects. Psychopharmacologia 38: 239–245, 1974.

N. Narasimhachari, B. Heller, J. Spaide et al. N,N-dimethylated indoleamines in blood. Biol. Psych. 3: 21–23, 1971.

D.E. Rosenberg, H. Isbell and E.J. Miner. Comparison of a placebo, N-dimethyltryptamine, and 6-hydroxy-N-dimethyltryptamine in man. Psychopharmacologia 4: 39–42, 1963.

B.R. Sitaram, L. Lockett, M. McLeish et al. Gas chromatographic-mass spectroscopic characterisation of the psychotomimetic indolealkylamines and their *in vivo* metabolites. J. Chrom. 422: 13–23, 1987.

S.T. Szara. Dimethyltryptamin: its metabolism in man; the relation of its psychotic effect to the serotonin metabolism. Experientia 12: 441–442, 1956.

S. Szara and J. Axelrod. Hydroxylation and N-demethylation of N,N-dimethyltryptamine. Experientia 15: 216–217, 1959.

R.W. Walker, H.S. Ahn, G. Albers-Schonberg et al. Gas chromatographic-mass spectrometric isotope dilution assay for N,N-dimethyltryptamine in human plasma. Biochem. Med. 8: 105–113, 1973.

R.J. Wyatt, L.R. Mandel, H.S. Ahn et al. Gas chromatographic-mass spectrometric isotope dilution determination of N,N-dimethyltryptamine concentrations in normal and psychiatric patients. Psychopharmacologia 31: 265–270, 1973.

Dinitro-o-Cresol

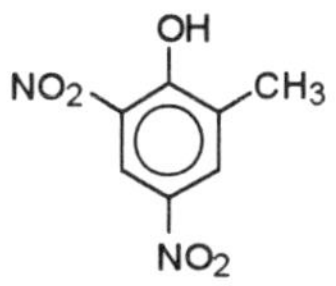

T½: 5–6 days
Vd: ?
Fb: ?
pKa: ?

Occurrence and Usage. Dinitro-o-cresol (DNOC) is used primarily as a blossom-thinning agent and as a fungicide and insecticide on fruit trees. Occupational exposure generally is a result of inhalation or skin contact with the aerosol. The current threshold limit value is 0.2 mg/m^3 in the environmental air.

Blood Concentrations. Plasma levels of DNOC measured 1 day after exposure in asymptomatic workers exposed to 0.2 mg/m^3 of the chemical for periods of 5–48 hours ranged from 1.4–4.3 mg/L (Batchelor et al., 1956). Volunteers given 75 mg of DNOC orally once daily for 5 days exhibited accumulation of the substance in the blood, with no symptoms of toxicity apparent until the third or fourth day when the blood concentrations had risen to a level of 15–20 mg/L. The chemical was still detectable in the blood at a level of about 1 mg/L 40 days after the experiment (Harvey et al., 1951).

Metabolism and Excretion. The metabolism of DNOC has not been investigated in man, but it is known that about 2% of an ingested dose is excreted unchanged in the 24 hour urine (Harvey et al., 1951), and that the urinary concentration of the substance is a poor index of the blood concentrations (Bidstrup et al., 1952).

In sheep, about 34% of an intraperitoneal dose is eliminated in the 72 hour urine as free DNOC (4%), conjugated DNOC (7%), conjugated 6-amino-4-nitro-o-cresol (23%) and traces of 4,6-diamino-o-cresol (Jegatheeswaran and Harvey, 1970).

Toxicity. DNOC is known to have a mild corrosive effect on skin, to cause moderate CNS stimulation and to cause severe systemic poisoning by uncoupling oxidative phosphorylation. In volunteers administered daily oral doses of the chemical, a sense of well-being appeared at blood DNOC levels of 20 mg/L, while symptoms of headache, malaise and yellow coloration of the sclera developed at levels around 40 mg/L (Harvey et al., 1951). Blood concentrations of 44–60 mg/L have produced serious intoxication in exposed workers, and a level of 75 mg/L caused death in 1 subject (Bidstrup et al., 1952). A number of deaths have occurred as a result of occupational exposure, preceded by hyperthermia, rapid respiration and coma. Rigor mortis sets in rapidly after death, and autopsy findings include pulmonary edema and liver and kidney congestion (Bidstrup and Payne, 1951).

Analysis. DNOC may be conveniently analyzed in blood specimens by a colorimetric procedure (Smith et al., 1978).

References

G.S. Batchelor, K.C. Walker and J.W. Elliot. Dinitroorthocresol exposure from apple-thinning sprays. Arch. Ind. Health 13: 593–596, 1956.

P.L. Bidstrup and D.J.H. Payne. Poisoning by dinitro-ortho-cresol. Brit. Med. J. 2: 16–19, 1951.

P.L. Bidstrup, J.A.L. Bonnell and D.G. Harvey. Prevention of acute dinitro-ortho-cresol (D.N.O.C.) poisoning. Lancet 1: 794–795, 1952.

D.G. Harvey, P.L. Bidstrup and J.A.L. Bonnell. Poisoning by dinitro-ortho-cresol. Some observations on the effects of dinitro-ortho-cresol administered by mouth to human volunteers. Brit. Med. J. 2: 13–16, 1951.

T. Jegatheeswaran and D.G. Harvey. The metabolism of DNOC in sheep. Vet. Rec. 87: 19–20, 1970.

D.L. Smith, J.R. May, R.A. Rhoden et al. *Criteria for a Recommended Standard—Occupational Exposure to Dinitro-ortho-Cresol,* U.S. Dept. of HEW (NIOSH) Pub. No. 78–131, 1978.

Dioxane

T½: 1 hr
Vd: ?
Fb: ?

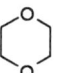

Occurrence and Usage. Dioxane (dioxan, p-dioxane, 1,4-dioxane) is a widely used laboratory and industrial solvent that is well-absorbed following inhalation and skin contact. The current threshold limit value is 25 ppm (90 mg/m^3).

Blood Concentrations. Subjects exposed to 50 ppm of dioxane for a period of 6 hours developed an average steady-state plasma dioxane concentration of 12 mg/L; at the end of exposure this level declined with a half-life of 1 hour and it was predicted that no accumulation of dioxane would occur with repeated daily exposure. A dioxane metabolite, beta-hydroxyethoxyacetic acid, attained a peak plasma level of about 10 mg/L at 1 hour after the end of the exposure, declining with a half-life of about 3 hours (Young et al., 1977).

Metabolism and Excretion. Dioxane is metabolized in man by oxidation to beta-hydroxyethoxyacetic acid (HEAA), which accumulates in blood and is extensively excreted in urine. The total elimination of dioxane from the human body has not been studied, and it is probable that a substantial portion of a dose is eliminated unchanged in the expired breath; however, of that portion eliminated as known metabolites in urine, the vast majority is HEAA and only a fraction is found as unchanged dioxane.

The highest urinary concentrations of both dioxane and HEAA occur during the latter portion of an exposure period. Workers exposed to dioxane vapor for 7.5 hours at a level of 1.6 ppm had end-of-shift urine concentrations that averaged 0.3 mg/L for dioxane and 50 mg/L for HEAA; these concentrations were estimated at 8 mg/L and 813 mg/L, respectively, in subjects exposed to 50 ppm of dioxane for 6 hours (Young et al., 1976; Young et al., 1977).

In the rat, between 40 and 60% of a labeled dose of dioxane is eliminated in the 48 hour urine. About 11% of the dose was found as unchanged dioxane in the urine and 33% as p-dioxane-2-one; the latter compound is the lactone of HEAA and is the form that Woo et al. (1977) believe predominates in urine, probably due to the spontaneous arrangement of HEAA.

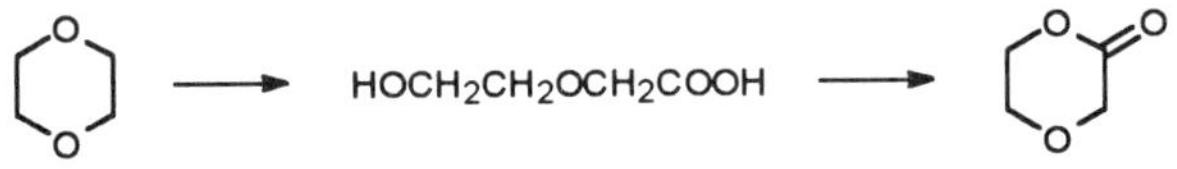

dioxane $HOCH_2CH_2OCH_2COOH$ dioxane-2-one

HEAA

Toxicity. Dioxane is irritating to the eyes, nose and throat at an air concentration of 300 ppm, and to the skin upon contact. Prolonged exposure to high concentrations of the vapor may produce severe intoxication characterized by anorexia, nausea, vomiting, abdominal pain, convulsions and unconsciousness; autopsy of several victims has shown evidence of cerebral edema, bronchopneumonia and necrosis of the liver and kidneys (Barber, 1934; Johnstone, 1959).

Studies in animals have shown that dioxane can cause malignant tumors of the lung, liver, kidney and nasal cavity.

Analysis. Dioxane in plasma or urine may be analyzed by the gas chromatographic methods described in the section on benzene. A method for the determination of HEAA in urine has been described that involves flame-ionization gas chromatography (Braun, 1977).

References

H. Barber. Haemorrhagic nephritis and necrosis of the liver from dioxan poisoning. Guys Hosp. Report 84: 267–280, 1934.

W.H. Braun. Rapid method for the simultaneous determination of 1,4-dioxan and its major metabolite, beta-hydroxyethoxyacetic acid, concentrations in plasma and urine. J. Chrom. 113: 263–266, 1977.

R.T. Johnstone. Death due to dioxane? Arch. Ind. Health 20: 445–447, 1959.

T. Woo, J.C. Arcos, M.F. Argus et al. Structural identification of p-dioxane-2-one as the major urinary metabolite of p-dioxane. Arch. Pharm. 299: 283–287, 1977.

J.D. Young, W.H. Braun, P.J. Gehring et al. 1,4-Dioxane and beta-hydroxyethoxyacetic acid excretion in urine of humans exposed to dioxane vapors. Tox. Appl. Pharm. 38: 643–646, 1976.

J.D. Young, W.H. Braun, L.W. Braun et al. Pharmacokinetics of 1,4-dioxane in humans. J. Tox. Env. Health 3: 507–520, 1977.

Dioxin

T½: 5.8–9.6 years
Vd: ?
Fb: >0.80

Occurrence and Usage. Dioxin (2,3,7,8-tetrachlorodibenzo-p-dioxin, TCDD) is one of the most potentially toxic synthetic chemicals yet discovered. It arises as a byproduct in the manufacture of trichlorophenol, the industrial precursor of hexachlorophene and 2,4,5-T. The rate of formation of dioxin is enhanced when the reaction temperature is allowed to exceed 160 ° C. Early formulations of 2,4,5-T (Agent Orange), widely used in Vietnam as a defoliant, contained up to 30 ppm of dioxin, although recent preparations are reported to contain less than 0.1 ppm. Dioxin has been found to be extremely stable and persistent in the environment; the average human daily intake is estimated at 0.05 ng, 98% of which is obtained from dietary sources.

Blood Concentrations. Serum dioxin concentrations in 50 Missouri citizens averaged 0.5 ng/L (range, 0–8.3) (Patterson et al., 1988). In 1987, serum dioxin concentrations averaged 4.1 ng/L (range, 0–15) in 97 Army veterans with no Vietnam duty and 4.2 ng/L (range, 0–45) in 646 veterans with Vietnam duty during 1967–1968 (CDC, 1988). The serum elimination half-life for dioxin has been found to average 7.1 years (Pirkle et al., 1989).

Metabolism and Excretion. Dioxin is highly lipid-soluble and tends to accumulate in body fat. High concentrations are also found in the pancreas, and secondarily in the liver. The chemical is not known to be metabolized in man. The major route of excretion is the feces. The whole body half-life of dioxin in rats is about 30 days (Reggiani, 1979). Human milk, taken from women living in areas of the U.S. where 2,4,5-T is used as a herbicide, has not been found to contain dioxin using a method with a detectability limit of less than 1 ng/L (Shadoff, 1980). Adipose tissue in 57 members of the general U.S. population contained from 1.9–20 µg/kg (average, 7.4) of dioxin, versus 2.8–750 µg/kg (average, 80) in 39 exposed persons (Petterson et al., 1986a).

Toxicity. Three scientists working with dioxin in a chemical laboratory developed chloracne about 2 months after the time of greatest exposure to the poison. The rash gradually subsided over the next year and a half. Two years after the original episode, without further exposure to dioxin, 2 of the scientists developed a variety of unusual symptoms. These included abdominal pains, extreme fatigue, irritability, headaches, blurring of vision, and difficulty with muscular and mental processes. Also, excessive hair growth appeared on the shoulders, upper back, eyebrows and the backs of the hands. Although all other blood chemistries were normal, all 3 men had a definite elevation of serum cholesterol (Oliver, 1975).

The July 10, 1976, explosion of a chemical reactor in Seveso, Italy, released an estimated several kilograms of dioxin into the atmosphere. Numerous animals died, but the incident caused no human deaths; however, at least 134 cases of chloracne, a severe and disfiguring rash, have been confirmed, primarily in children (Walsh, 1977). The rates of spontaneous abortions or birth malformations did not increase significantly in the first year after the accident (Reggiani, 1978). The only human analytical data arising from this accident were obtained from a 55 year old Seveso woman who died of pancreatic cancer (not believed related to TCDD) 7 months after the dioxin incident. She lived in an area close to the factory and was not evacuated from the area until 16 days after the explosion. She did not develop signs of toxicity, although 2 children living with her developed severe chloracne (Montagna et al., 1979):

Dioxin Concentrations in an Exposed Individual (µg/kg)

Blood	Brain	Lung	Liver	Pancreas	Kidney	Fat
0.006	0.06	0.06	0.15	1.04	0.04	1.84

Two other industrial accidents that occurred during the 1960s have been reported. One resulted only in chloracne in 79 individuals (May, 1973), while the second also involved metabolic, hepatic and neurological disturbances in many of the 80 exposed workers (Pazderova-Vejlupkova et al., 1981). A residential exposure of 154 persons in Missouri in 1971 did not result in any clinical manifestations of disease but may have caused depression of immune function (Hoffman et al., 1986; Stehr et al., 1986).

During the U.S. involvement in South Vietnam, an estimated 368 pounds of dioxin were released into the atmosphere during the years 1962–1971 as a contaminant of the defoliant used there (Agent Orange). This release of toxic chemical has been linked to liver cancer, numbness, chloracne and behavior changes in Vietnam veterans and birth defects in their children. A preliminary study by the Veterans Administration of dioxin in adipose tissue of veterans found positive results in 13 of 20 individual specimens, with dioxin concentrations ranging from 3–99 μg/kg (Holden, 1979; New York Times News Service, 1979; Wade, 1980; Gross et al., 1984).

Before the Agent Orange defoliation program in South Vietnam, liver cancer was the eighth most common form of cancer in that country, accounting for 2.9% of all cancers. As of 1979, liver cancer was the second most prevalent form of cancer, accounting for 10% of all cancers. By contrast, liver cancer rates in Hanoi, North Vietnam (which did not receive direct spraying), have not changed significantly. Liver cancer is one of the effects of chronic low-level exposure to dioxin in animals (Reggiani, 1978; New York Times News Service, 1979).

Analysis. Dioxin levels in biological specimens are extremely low, and require a very sensitive and specific method of analysis. The only successfully applied method thus far has been gas chromatography-mass spectrometry (Harless and Oswald, 1978; diDomenico et al., 1979; Haas and Friesen, 1979; Harless et al., 1980; Langhorst and Shadoff, 1980; Raisanen et al., 1981; Patterson et al., 1986b).

References

Centers for Disease Control. Serum 2,3,7,8-tetrachlordibenzo-p-dioxin levels in US Army Vietnam-era veterans. J. Am. Med. Asso. 260: 1249–1254, 1988.

L. diDomenico, F. Marli, L. Boniforti et al. Analytical techniques for 2,3,7,8-tetrachlorodibenzo-p-dioxin detection in environmental samples after the industrial accident at Seveso. Anal. Chem. 51: 735–740, 1979.

M.L. Gross, J.O. Lay, P.A. Lyon et al. 2,3,7,8-Tetrachlorodibenzo-p-dioxin levels in adipose tissue of Vietnam veterans. Env. Res. 33: 261–268, 1984.

J.R. Haas and M.D. Friessen. Qualitative and quantitative methods for dioxin analysis. Ann. N.Y. Acad. Sci. 320: 28–42, 1979.

R.L. Harless and E.O. Oswald. Low- and high-resolution gas chromatography-mass spectrometry (GC-MS) method of analysis for the presence of 2,3,7,8-tetrachlorodibenzo-p-dioxin (TCDD) in environmental samples. In *Dioxin: Toxicological and Chemical Aspects* (F. Chattabeni, A. Cavallaro and G. Galli, eds.), Halstead Press, New York, 1978, pp. 51–57.

R.L. Harless, E.O. Oswald, M.K. Wilkinson et al. Sample preparation and gas chromatography-mass spectrometry determination of 2,3,7,8-tetrachlorodibenzo-p-dioxin. Anal. Chem. 52: 1239–1245, 1980.

R.E. Hoffman, P.A. Stehr-Green, K.B. Webb et al. Health effects of long-term exposure to 2,3,7,8-tetrachlorodibenzo-p-dioxin. J. Am. Med. Asso. 255: 2031–2038, 1986.

C. Holden. Agent Orange furor continues to build. Science 205: 770–772, 1979.

M.L. Langhorst and L.A. Shadoff. Determination of parts-per-trillion concentrations of tetra-, hexa-, hepta-, and octachlorodibenzo-p-dioxins in human milk. Anal. Chem. 52: 2037–2044, 1980.

G. May. Chloracne from the accidental production of tetrachlorodibenzodioxin. Brit. J. Ind. Med. 30: 276–283, 1973.

M. Montagna, A. Fornari and S. Facchetti. Analysis of autopsy samples for the detection of 2,3,7,8-tetrachlorodibenzo-p-dioxin by high resolution GC-MS. In *Forensic Toxicology* (J.S. Oliver, ed.), Croom Helm, London, 1979, pp. 78–85.

New York Times News Service. High Vietnam cancer rate linked to dioxin. The New York Times, May 6, 1979.

R.M. Oliver. Toxic effects of 2,3,7,8-tetrachloro-1,4-dioxin in laboratory workers. Brit. J. Ind. Med. 32: 49–53, 1975.

D.G. Patterson, R.E. Hoffman, L.L. Needham et al. 2,3,7,8-Tetrachlorodibenzo-p-dioxin levels in adipose tissue of exposed and control persons in Missouri. J. Am. Med. Asso. 256: 2683–1686, 1986a.

D.G. Patterson, J.S. Holler, C.R. Lapeza et al. High-resolution gas chromatographic/high-resolution mass spectrometric analysis of human adipose tissue for 2,3,7,8-tetrachlorodibenzo-p-dioxin. Anal. Chem. 58: 705–713, 1986b.

D.G. Patterson, L.L. Needham, J.L. Pirkle et al. Correlation between serum and adipose tissue levels of 2,3,7,8-tetrachlorodibenzo-p-dioxin in 50 persons from Missouri. Arch. Env. Cont. Tox. 17: 139–143, 1988.

J. Pazderova-Vejlupkova, M. Nemcova, J. Pickova et al. The development and prognosis of chronic intoxication by tetrachlordibenzo-p-dioxin in men. Arch. Env. Health 36: 5–11, 1981.

J.L. Pirkle, W.H. Wolfe, D.G. Patterson et al. Estimates of the half-life of 2,3,7,8-tetrachlorodibenzo-p-dioxin in Vietnam veterans of Operation Ranch Hand. J. Tox. Env. Health 27: 165–171, 1989.

S. Raisanen, R. Hiltunen, A.U. Arstila and T. Sipilainen. Determination of 2,3,7,8-tetrachlorodibenzo-p-dioxin in goat milk and tissues by glass capillary gas chromatography and medium resolution mass fragmentography. J. Chrom. 208: 323–330, 1981.

G. Reggiani. Medical problems raised by the TCDD contamination in Seveso, Italy. Arch. Tox. 40: 161–188, 1978.

G. Reggiani. Estimation of the TCDD toxic potential in the light of the Seveso accident. Arch. Tox. Suppl. 2: 291–302, 1979.

L.A. Shadoff. The determination of 2,3,7,8-tetrachlorodibenzo-p-dioxin in human milk. In *Pesticide Analytical Methodology* (J. Harvey, Jr. and G. Zweig, eds.), American Chemical Society, Washington, D.C., 1980, pp. 277–285.

P.A. Stehr, G. Stein, H. Falk et al. A pilot epidemiological study of possible health effects associated with 2,3,7,8-tetrachlorodibenzo-p-dioxin contaminations in Missouri. Arch. Env. Health 41: 16–22, 1986.

N. Wade. Agent Orange again. Science 207: 41, 1980.

J. Walsh. Seveso: the questions persist where dioxin created a wasteland. Science 197: 1064–1067, 1977.

Diphenhydramine

T½: 3–14 hr
Vd: 3–4 L/kg
Fb: 0.98
pKa: 8.3

$OCH_2CH_2N(CH_3)_2$

Occurrence and Usage. Diphenhydramine (Benadryl) was one of the first effective antihistamine agents discovered, its properties having been described in 1946. The compound is also used for its sedative and antiemetic effects. The hydrochloride salt is available as the sole agent for oral use in doses of 50–100 mg and for intravenous or intramuscular use in doses of 10–50 mg. The 8-chlorotheophyllinate salt is a nonprescription drug known as dimenhydrinate (Dramamine) and is a popular remedy for motion sickness.

Blood Concentrations. A single 50 mg oral dose resulted in average plasma concentrations of 0.083 mg/L at 3 hours, 0.049 mg/L at 6 hours and 0.009 mg/L by 24 hours (Bilzer and Gundert-Remy, 1973). A 50 mg oral dose in 10 adults produced an average peak plasma diphenhydramine concentration of 0.066 mg/L at 2.3 hours and an average peak nordiphenhydramine concentration of 0.017 mg/L at 3.9 hours (Blyden et al., 1986). Following a 100 mg oral dose, plasma levels averaged 0.112 mg/L at 2 hours and declined to 0.014 mg/L by 24 hours; half-lives of 5.4–7.9 hours were determined in 4 subjects (Glazko et al., 1974). Plasma half-lives averaging 5.4, 9.2 and 13.5 hours have been observed for children, adults and elderly subjects, respectively (Simons et al., 1990).

The administration of 50 mg of the hydrochloride in a 2 hour intravenous infusion produced maximal plasma drug levels of 0.179 and 0.258 mg/L in 2 subjects at the end of the infusion. A blood/plasma concentration ratio of 0.82 was measured for the drug (Albert et al., 1975).

Metabolism and Excretion. Diphenhydramine is believed to undergo extensive oxidative metabolic transformation to nor- and dinordiphenhydramine and diphenylmethoxyacetic acid. The latter metabolite is a product of deamination and is probably excreted as a glycine or glutamine conjugate. No quantitative descriptions of this metabolic pattern have appeared (Chang et al., 1974). An average of 64% of a dose is eliminated as metabolites in the 96 hour urine (Glazko et al., 1974), with the unchanged drug accounting for only about 1% (Albert et al., 1975). Urine concentrations of intact diphenhydramine were found to range from 0.1–3.5 mg/L during the first 24 hours after ingestion of 100 mg of the drug by 4 volunteers (Wallace et al., 1966).

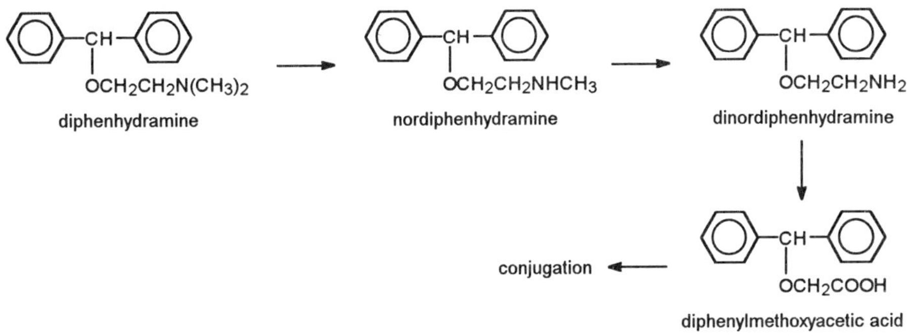

Toxicity. Diphenhydramine is often considered to be a relatively nontoxic drug, although a number of cases of intoxication due to overdosage have been described. These have usually involved infants who ingested 100–500 mg of the drug and who exhibited muscle tremors, anxiety, disorientation, hallucinations, loss of consciousness, seizures, fever, respiratory arrest, and cardiac arrhythmia (Weil, 1947; Judge and Dumars, 1953; Hestand and Teske, 1977). A series of 29 intentional overdoses in adults was described in which plasma diphenhydramine levels ranged from 0.1–4.7 mg/L, with only one death (Koppel et al., 1987). A 9 year old boy developed agitation, confusion, hallucinations and a serum diphenhydramine concentration of 1.4 mg/L after excessive dermal application of the drug to treat skin eruptions (Filloux, 1986). A case of diphenhydramine dependence was reported in which a 34 year old man was taking as much as 1600 mg of the drug daily with no apparent physical effects (Feldman and Behar, 1986).

A 2 year old child died in hyperpyrexic coma 13 hours after ingesting 474 mg of diphenhydramine (Davis and Hunt, 1949). Siek (1974) reported a fatal case that involved the ingestion of 24 g of dimenhydrinate and in which the following postmortem specimen concentrations of diphenhydramine were found: blood, 5 mg/L; liver, 34 mg/kg; urine, 41 mg/L. The following values were obtained in 11 fatalities due to acute diphenhydramine ingestion (Backer et al., 1977; Baselt and Cravey, 1977; Peclet, 1981; Rousseau, 1983; Hausmann et al., 1983; Shkrum et al., 1990; Sidebotham, 1991):

Diphenhydramine Concentrations in Fatal Cases (mg/L or mg/kg)

	Blood	Brain	Liver	Kidney	Urine
Average	16	34	34	32	52
(Range)	(8–31)	(8–77)	(23–47)	(13–51)	(40–64)

Diphenhydramine is subject to postmortem redistribution; heart blood/peripheral blood concentration ratios averaged 2.4 (range, 0.4–6.0) in 7 reported cases (Anderson and Prouty, 1989; Roettger, 1990).

Analysis. Diphenhydramine has been determined in biological fluids by a variety of methods, including ultraviolet spectrophotometry of an oxidation product (Wallace et al., 1966) and a fluorescence dye technique (Glazko et al., 1974). Specific gas chromatographic procedures have relied on flame-ionization detection (Albert et al., 1974; Backer et al., 1977) or nitrogen-selective detection (Bilzer and Gundert-Remy, 1973; Abernethy and Greenblatt, 1983; Yoo et al., 1986).

References

D.R. Abernethy and D.J. Greenblatt. Diphenhydramine determination in human plasma by gas-liquid chromatography using nitrogen-phosphorus detection: application to single low-dose pharmacokinetic studies. J. Pharm. Sci. 72: 941–943, 1983.

K.S. Albert, E. Sakmar, J.A. Morais et al. Determination of diphenhydramine in plasma by gas chromatography. Res. Comm. Chem. Path. Pharm. 7: 95-103, 1974.

K.S. Albert, M.R. Hallmark, E. Sakmar et al. Pharmacokinetics of diphenhydramine in man. J. Pharm. Biopharm. 3: 159–169, 1975.

W.H. Anderson and R.W. Prouty. Postmortem redistribution of drugs. In *Advances in Analytical Toxicology* (R.C. Baselt, ed.), Vol. 2, Yearbook Medical, Chicago, 1989.

R.C. Backer, R.V. Pisano and I.M. Sopher. Diphenhydramine suicide—case report. J. Anal. Tox. 1: 227–228, 1977.

R.C. Baselt and R.H. Cravey. A compendium of therapeutic and toxic concentrations of toxicologically significant drugs in human biofluids. J. Anal. Tox. 1: 81–103, 1977.

W. Bilzer and U. Gundert-Remy. Determination of nanogram quantities of diphenhydramine and orphenadrine in human plasma using gas-liquid chromatography. Eur. J. Clin. Pharm. 6: 268–270, 1973.

G.T. Blyden, D.J. Greenblatt, J.M. Scavone and R.I. Shader. Pharmacokinetics of diphenhydramine and a demethylated metabolite following intravenous and oral administration. J. Clin. Pharm. 26: 529–533, 1986.

S.G. Carruthers, D.W. Shoeman, C.E. Hignite and D.L. Azarnoff. Correlation between plasma diphenhydramine level and sedative and antihistamine effects. Clin. Pharm. Ther. 23: 375–382, 1978.

T. Chang, R.A. Okerholm and A.J. Glazko. Identification of diphenhydramine (Benadryl) metabolites in human subjects. Res. Comm. Chem. Path. Pharm. 9: 391–404, 1974.

J.H. Davis and H.H. Hunt. Accidental Benadryl poisoning: report of a fatal case. J. Pediat. 34: 358–361, 1949.

M.D. Feldman and M. Behar. A case of massive diphenhydramine abuse and withdrawal from use of the drug. J. Am. Med. Asso. 255: 3119–3120, 1986.

F. Filloux. Toxic encephalopathy caused by topically applied diphenhydramine. J. Pediat. 108: 1018–1020, 1986.

A.J. Glazko, W.A. Dill, R.M. Young et al. Metabolic disposition of diphenhydramine. Clin. Pharm. Ther. 16: 1066–1076, 1974.

E. Hausmann, H. Wewer, H.H. Wellhoner and J.P. Weller. Lethal intoxication with diphenhydramine. Arch. Tox. 53: 33–39, 1983.

H.E. Hestand and D.W. Teske. Diphenhydramine hydrochloride intoxication. J. Pediat. 90: 1017–1018, 1977.

D.J. Judge and K.W. Dumars, Jr. Diphenhydramine (Benadryl) and tripelennamine (Pyribenzamine) intoxication in children. Am. J. Dis. Child. 85: 545–550, 1953.

C. Koppel, K. Ibe and J. Tenczer. Clinical sympatomatology of diphenhydramine overdose: an evaluation of 136 cases in 1982 to 1985. Clin. Tox. 25: 53–70, 1987.

C. Peclet. Personal communication, 1981.

J.R. Roettger. The importance of blood collection site for the determination of basic drugs. J. Anal. Tox. 14: 191–192, 1990.

M.G. Rousseau. Personal communication, 1983.

M.J. Shkrum, A.E.D. Hall and S.G. Tallon. Deaths due to diphenhydramine. Can. Soc. For. Sci. J. 23: 1–8, 1990.

C. Sidebotham. Personal communication, 1991.

T.J. Siek. Personal communication, 1974.

K.J. Simons, W.T.A. Watson, T.J. Martin et al. Diphenhydramine: pharmacokinetics and pharmacodynamics in elderly adults, young adults, and children. J. Clin. Pharm. 30: 665–671, 1990.

R. Spector, A.K. Choudhury, C. Chiang et al. Diphenhydramine in Orientals and Caucasians. Clin. Pharm. Ther. 28: 229–234, 1980.

J.E. Wallace, J.D. Biggs and E.V. Dahl. Determination of diphenhydramine and certain related compounds by ultraviolet spectrophotometry. Anal. Chem. 38: 831–834, 1966.

H.R. Weil. Unusual side effect from Benadryl. J. Am. Med. Asso. 133: 393–394, 1947.

S.D. Yoo, J.E. Axelson and D.W. Rurak. Determination of diphenhydramine in biological fluids by capillary gas chromatography using nitrogen-phosphorus detection. J. Chrom. 378: 385–393, 1986.

Diphenoxylate

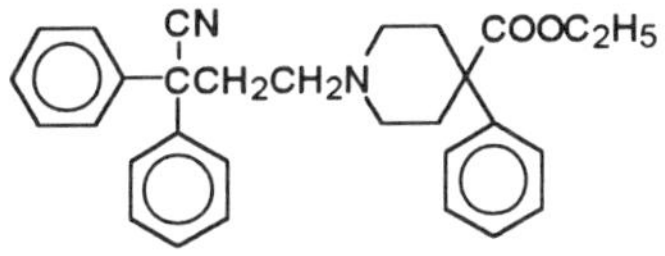

T½: 2.5 hr
Vd: 3.8 L/kg
Fb: ?
pKa: 7.1

Occurrence and Usage. Diphenoxylate (Lomotil) is used as an antidiarrheal agent, generally as a tablet or liquid in doses of 2.5 mg of the hydrochloride salt. It is always found in combination with subtherapeutic amounts of atropine, which is added in order to discourage abuse of the drug. At higher than therapeutic dosages diphenoxylate produces typical morphine-like effects.

Blood Concentrations. Pharmacokinetic analysis with C-14 labeled diphenoxylate shows that the compound is rapidly absorbed, resulting in a peak plasma concentration of 0.01 mg/L at 2 hours after oral administration of 5 mg, and is rapidly cleared with a half-life of 2.5 hours. The major metabolite, diphenoxylic acid (difenoxine), a product of hydrolysis of the ester group in diphenoxylate, is 5 times as active as an antidiarrheal agent and has a plasma half-life of 4.4 hours. Diphenoxylic acid plasma concentrations also peaked at 2 hours, reaching a concentration of 0.04 mg/L in the study described above (Karim et al., 1972). In another study involving oral administration of 10 mg of the drug to 6 volunteers, a peak diphenoxylic acid concentration of approximately 0.08 mg/L was observed at 2 hours (Ford et al., 1976).

Metabolism and Excretion. Less than 0.1% of the administered dose is excreted in the urine as unchanged drug and only 0.8% as diphenoxylic acid. These compounds, together with other products of hydroxylation and conjugation, accounted for a total of 63% of the administered dose in the 96 hour urine (13.7%) and feces (49.2%) (Karim et al., 1972). Other investigators have indicated that as much as 8% of a single dose of diphenoxylate may be excreted unchanged in the 96 hour urine (Haskins et al., 1978).

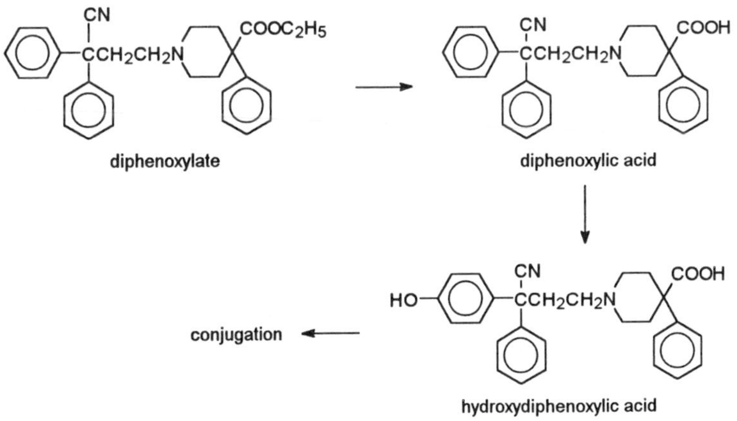

Toxicity. One case of massive abuse of diphenoxylate was reported; the subject was not adversely affected by the atropine present in the formulation when taking up to 140 tablets at one time

(Rubenstein, 1979). Numerous cases of accidental pediatric poisoning with doses of up to 100 mg of diphenoxylate have been reported, with several fatalities. The first phase of intoxication, due to atropine, is manifested by sudden high fever, a flushed appearance, and rapid breathing. The second phase, due to diphenoxylate, includes progressive central nervous system depression, pinpoint pupils, cyanosis, severe respiratory depression, seizures, and coma. Gastric lavage and naloxone administration are recommended in the treatment of diphenoxylate overdose (Ament, 1969; Ginsburg and Angle, 1969; Rumack and Temple, 1974; Wasserman et al., 1975; Curtis and Goel, 1979).

In one case of fatal pediatric poisoning, a liver diphenoxylate concentration of 0.096 mg/kg was determined (Pascucci, 1981). A 3.5 year old girl who died 43 hours after ingesting an unknown quantity of diphenoxylate had a postmortem blood concentration of 0.34 mg/L; the drug was undetectable in urine (Al Ragheb et al., 1982).

Analysis. A mass spectrometric method with a sensitivity of 0.02 mg/L has been used to measure therapeutic concentrations of diphenoxylic acid in plasma (Ford et al., 1976) and urine (Haskins et al., 1978). Methods for the analysis of intact diphenoxylate in biological specimens have not been reported.

References

S.A. Al Ragheb, B.M. Dajani, A.A. Salhab et al. A case of fatal Lomotil overdosage. Med. Sci. Law 22: 210–214, 1982.

M.E. Ament. Diphenoxylate poisoning in children. J. Pediat. 74: 462–464, 1969.

J.A. Curtis and K.M. Goel. Lomotil poisoning in children. Arch. Dis. Child. 54: 222–225, 1979.

G.C. Ford, N.J. Haskins, R.F. Palmer et al. The measurement of diphenoxylic acid in plasma following administration of diphenoxylate. Biomed. Mass Spec. 3: 45–47, 1976.

C.M. Ginsburg and C.R. Angle. Diphenoxylate-atropine (Lomotil) poisoning. Clin. Tox. 2: 377–382, 1969.

N.J. Haskins, G.C. Ford, S.J.W. Grigson and K.A. Waddell. An assay for diphenoxylic acid in urine using an automated gas chromatograph mass spectrometer system. In *Quantitative Mass Spectrometry in Life Sciences II* (A.P. de Leenheer, R.R. Rancucci and C. van Peteghem, eds.), Elsevier, New York, 1978, pp. 287–293.

A. Karim, R.E. Ranney, K.L. Evensen and M.L. Clark. Pharmacokinetics and metabolism of diphenoxylate in man. Clin. Pharm. Ther. 13: 407–419, 1972.

R. Pascucci. Personal communication, 1981.

J.S. Rubinstein. Deliberate abuse of diphenoxylate hydrochloride, a schedule V narcotic. West. J. Med. 131: 148–150, 1979.

B.H. Rumack and A.R. Temple. Lomotil poisoning. Pediatrics 53: 495–500, 1974.

G.S. Wasserman, V.A. Green and G.W. Wise. Lomotil ingestions in children. Am. Fam. Phys. 11(6): 93–97, 1975.

Diquat

T½: ?
Vd: ?
Fb: ?

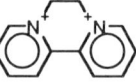

Occurrence and Usage. Diquat (1,1'-ethylene-2,2'-dipyridylium ion, Reglone) is a less toxic analogue of paraquat, both compounds being widely used as herbicides. Diquat is usually supplied as the dibromide in a 20% concentrate for spraying.

Blood Concentrations. Blood concentrations of diquat in asymptomatic exposed persons have not been reported.

Metabolism and Excretion. The fate of diquat in man has not been studied. In rats, less than 10% of an oral dose is absorbed, the unabsorbed portion being excreted in the feces. If the substance is administered by subcutaneous injection, over 90% of the dose is eliminated unchanged in the 24 hour urine. No metabolites of diquat are known (Daniel and Gage, 1966).

Toxicity. Contact with diquat can lead to cracking of the fingernails, inflammation and bleeding of the nasal mucosa, and eye damage. Inhalation or ingestion of large amounts of diquat has produced local necrosis, muscle stiffness, confusion, cough, fever, and pulmonary consolidation (Oreopoulos and McEvoy, 1969; Wood et al., 1976). Diquat apparently does not cause the progressive pulmonary fibrosis characteristic of paraquat. An adult survived an accidental aerosol exposure after developing abdominal pain, blurred vision, renal dysfunction and a peak plasma diquat level of 0.56 mg/L (Williams et al., 1986).

In 5 fatalities involving the ingestion of 20–50 mL of a 20% diquat solution, the victims first experienced a symptomless period of several hours to 2 days. Acute circulatory shock followed, accompanied by progressive renal failure, coma, and cardiorespiratory arrest. Death occurred within 2–7 days of diquat ingestion. Initial serum diquat concentrations ranged from 0.4–4.5 mg/L; hemodialysis was judged effective for reducing serum levels in one case but ineffective in another (Schoenborn et al., 1971; Okonek and Hofmann, 1975; VanHolder et al., 1981; Pond et al., 1983). Liver and kidney concentrations of 5.2 and 10 mg/L, respectively, were observed in a woman who died 16 hours after ingesting an undetermined amount of diquat (Pannell, 1982). The following postmortem tissue concentrations were measured in a patient who died 7 days after ingestion (Schoenborn et al., 1971):

Diquat Concentrations in a Fatal Case (mg/L or mg/kg)

Blood	Lung	Liver	Kidney
0.60	0.56	0.33	1.19

Analysis. Diquat may be analyzed in biological specimens by most of the procedures described for paraquat. The diquat reduction product produced by treatment with sodium dithionite in the colorimetric technique has a maximum absorbance at 379 nm in the visible region. Diquat may be differentially extracted from biological specimens in the presence of paraquat using n-butanol (Minakata et al., 1990).

References

J.W. Daniel and J.C. Gage. Absorption and excretion of diquat and paraquat in rats. Brit. J. Ind. Med. 23: 133–136, 1966.

K. Minakata, O. Suzuki and M. Asano. Extraction of diquat with l-butanol from biological materials. For. Sci. Int. 44: 27–35, 1990.

S. Okonek and A. Hofmann. On the question of extracorporeal hemodialysis in diquat intoxication. Arch. Tox. 33: 251–257, 1975.

D.G. Orepoulos and J. McEvoy. Diquat poisoning. Postgrad. Med. J. 45: 635–637, 1969.

L.K. Pannell. Personal communication, 1982.

S.M. Pond, D. Powell and T.B. Allen. Fatal pontine infarction in a child who ingested diquat. Vet. Hum. Tox. 25 (Suppl. 1): 41–43, 1983.

H. Schoenborn, H.P. Schuster and F.K. Kossling. Klinik und Morphologie der akuten peroralen Diquatintoxikation (Reglone). Arch. Tox. 27: 204–216, 1971.

R. VanHolder, F. Colardyn, J. De Reuck et al. Diquat intoxication. Am. J. Med. 70: 1267–1271, 1981.

P.F. Williams, D.R. Jarvie and A.P. Whitehead. Diquat intoxication: treatment by charcoal haemoperfusion and description of a new method of diquat measurement in plasma. Clin. Tox. 24: 11–20, 1986.

T.E. Wood, H. Edgar and J. Salcedo. Recovery from inhalation of diquat aerosol. Chest 70: 774–775, 1976.

Disopyramide

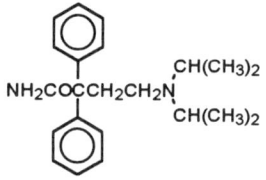

T½: 3–11 hr (dose-dependent)
Vd: 0.6–1.3 L/kg
Fb: 0.35–0.95 (concentration-dependent)
pKa: 8.4

Occurrence and Usage. Disopyramide (Norpace, Rythmodan) was synthesized in 1955 and has been in clinical use as an antiarrhythmic agent since about 1970. The compound is available for oral administration as the phosphate salt of the racemic mixture, in capsules of 100 and 150 mg (expressed as the free base). The usual adult dose is 400–800 mg daily. In Europe, disopyramide is also available for intravenous administration.

Blood Concentrations. Following oral administration of a single 150 mg tablet to 10 subjects, average peak plasma concentrations of 1.7–1.8 mg/L were attained at 1–3 hours and declined subsequently with a half-life of 5–6 hours. After a single oral dose of 6 mg/kg of the phosphate salt (300 mg/70 kg as the free base), an average peak plasma concentration of 3.0 mg/L was reached at 1.5 hours. Concentrations of 2–4 mg/L are associated with desirable antiarrhythmic activity (Karim, 1975; Aitio, 1981). Plasma concentrations of nordisopyramide normally average one-third of the disopyramide value in patients on chronic therapy, but may reach equivalent concentrations in those patients co-administered enzyme-inducing drugs such as phenytoin (Aitio, 1981). Binding to plasma protein and the elimination half-life of disopyramide are dose-dependent, both decreasing as the dose is increased; the half-life has been found to range from 3–11 hours in healthy subjects, and up to 54 hours in patients with reduced cardiac or renal function (Bryson et al., 1978; Dubetz et al., 1978; Meffin et al., 1979; Ilett et al., 1979; Landmark et al., 1981).

Metabolism and Excretion. Disopyramide is metabolized largely by mono-N-dealkylation. The metabolite, nordisopyramide, is about one-half as active as its parent. Nearly the entire dose is eliminated over a 5 day period in the urine (80%) and feces (15%). About 57% of the dose is present in the urine as unchanged drug and 23% as nordisopyramide; no other metabolites have been identified (Ranney et al., 1971; Karim et al., 1972; Karim, 1975).

$$NH_2COCCH_2CH_2N\begin{matrix}CH(CH_3)_2\\CH(CH_3)_2\end{matrix} \longrightarrow NH_2COCCH_2CH_2NHCH(CH_3)_2$$

disopyramide   nordisopyramide

Toxicity. Side effects of disopyramide therapy include urinary retention, dry mouth, constipation, blurred vision, hypotension, nausea, and fatigue. Congestive heart failure occurred in 13 of 38 patients receiving long-term therapy with the drug; the average serum disopyramide level in these 13 patients was 3.1 mg/L, compared to 3.6 mg/L in the other 25 (Podrid et al., 1980). A 16 year old female ingested 2 g of drug and experienced cardiorespiratory arrest, but survived with treatment; blood taken 4 hours post-ingestion contained 11 mg/L disopyramide and 1.8 mg/L nordisopyramide (Accornero et al., 1993). A 21 year old man who ingested 20 g of the drug and developed a plasma level of 16.6 mg/L after 2 hours suffered sudden circulatory collapse; he recovered with supportive treatment (O'Keefe et al., 1980).

A 19 year old girl ingested 3.75 g of disopyramide; 1 hour later when her plasma drug level was 29 mg/L she became hypotensive, apneic, convulsed, and lost consciousness. She reawoke and complained of a dry mouth, but soon again became apneic and died in ventricular fibrillation about 5 hours after ingestion (Powell et al., 1978). Blood concentrations in 10 fatal cases averaged 51 mg/L and ranged from 2.1 mg/L, in a 2 year old who ingested 600 mg and died after 12 hours, to 146 mg/L, in a 31 year old who ingested an unknown quantity of drug (Donkin, 1977; Hayler et al., 1978; Orloff, 1980; Michalek et al., 1982; Sathyavagiswaran, 1987). The following tissue distribution was noted in a 44 year old woman who died after ingesting an unknown amount of drug (Anderson et al., 1980):

Drug Concentrations in a Disopyramide Fatality (mg/L or mg/kg)

Drug	Blood	Liver	Bile	Kidney
Disopyramide	27	36	349	147
Nordisopyramide	6	11	145	7

Analysis. Disopyramide may be assayed in biological specimens using fluorometry (Ranney et al., 1971) or ultraviolet spectrophotometry (Martin et al., 1978), both of which may be subject to interference by nordisopyramide. Gas chromatographic techniques have utilized flame-ionization (Hutsell and Stachelski, 1975; Doedens and Forney, 1978; Hayler and Flanagan, 1978; Johnston and McHaffie, 1978; Foster and Reid, 1979) and nitrogen-selective detection (Duchateau et al., 1975; Aitio, 1979; Vasiliades et al., 1979a; Bredesen, 1980; Gal et al., 1980). Since disopyramide and its metabolite are thermally labile, liquid chromatographic methods of determination are often preferred (Lagerstrom and Persson, 1978; Broussard and Frings, 1979; Lima, 1979; Nygard et al., 1979; Vasiliades et al., 1979b; Charette et al., 1983; Angelo et al., 1986). A commercial enzyme immunoassay is also available for the parent drug.

References

F. Accornero, A. Pellanda, C. Rufini et al. Prolonged cardiopulmonary resuscitation during acute disopyramide poisoning. Vet. Hum. Tox. 35: 231–232, 1993.

M. Aitio. Simultaneous determination of disopyramide and its mono-N-dealkylated metabolite in plasma by gas-liquid chromatography. J. Chrom. 164: 515–520, 1979.

M. Aitio. Plasma concentrations and protein binding of disopyramide and mono-N-dealkyldisopyramide during chronic oral disopyramide therapy. Brit. J. Clin. Pharm. 11: 369–376, 1981.

W.H. Anderson, D.T. Stafford and J.S. Bell. Disopyramide (Norpace) distribution at autopsy of an overdose case. J. For. Sci. 25: 33–39, 1980.

H.R. Angelo, J. Bonde, J.P. Kampmann et al. A HPLC method for the simultaneous determination of disopyramide, lidocaine, and their monodealkylated metabolites. Scand. J. Clin. Lab. Invest. 46: 623–627, 1986.

J.E. Bredesen. Gas-chromatographic determination of disopyramide and its mono-N-dealkylated metabolite in serum with use of a nitrogen-selective detector. Clin. Chem. 26: 638–640, 1980.

L.A. Broussard and C.S. Frings. Quantitative high-performance liquid-chromatographic method for determining disopyramide (Norpace) in serum. Clin. Tox. 14: 579–586, 1979.

S.M. Bryson, B. Whiting and J.R. Lawrence. Disopyramide serum and pharmacologic effect kinetics applied to the assessment of bioavailability. Brit. J. Clin. Pharm. 6: 409–419, 1978.

C. Charette, I.J. McGilveray and C. Mainville. Simultaneous determination of disopyramide and its mono-N-dealkyl metabolite in plasma and urine by high-performance liquid chromatography. J. Chrom. 274: 219–230, 1983.

D.J. Doedens and R.B. Forney. Gas chromatographic analysis of disopyramide. J. Chrom. 161: 337–339, 1978.

P. Donkin. Personal communication, 1977.

D.K. Dubetz, N.N. Brown, W.D. Hooper et al. Disopyramide pharmacokinetics and bioavailability. Brit. J. Clin. Pharm. 6: 279–281, 1978.

A.M.J.A. Duchateau, F.W.H.M. Merkus and F. Schobben. Rapid gas chromatographic determination of disopyramide in serum using a nitrogen detector. J. Chrom. 109: 432–435, 1975.

E.N. Foster and P.R. Reid. Simplified method for the measurement of disopyramide in plasma. J. Chrom. 178: 571–574, 1979.

J. Gal, J.T. Brady and J. Kett. Gas-chromatographic determination of diospyramide with nitrogen detection. J. Anal. Tox. 4: 15–19, 1980.

A.M. Hayler and R.J. Flanagan. Simple gas-liquid chromatographic method for the measurement of disopyramide in blood-plasma or serum and in urine. J. Chrom. 153: 461–471, 1978.

A.M. Hayler, D.W. Holt and G.N. Volans. Fatal overdosage with disopyramide. Lancet 1: 968–969, 1978.

T.C. Hutsell and S.J. Stachelski. Determination of disopyramide and its mono-N-dealkylated metabolite in blood serum and urine. J. Chrom. 106: 151–158, 1975.

K.F. Ilett, B.W. Madsen, and J.D. Woods. Disopyramide kinetics in patients with acute myocardial infarction. Clin. Pharm. Ther. 26: 1–7, 1979.

A. Johnston and D. McHaffie. Gas-liquid chromatographic method for the routine estimation of disopyramide in plasma or serum. J. Chrom. 152: 501–506, 1978.

A. Karim, R.E. Ranney and S. Kraychy. Species differences in the biotransformation of a new antiarrhythmic agent: disopyramide phosphate. J. Pharm. Sci. 61: 888–893, 1972.

A. Karim. The pharmacokinetis of Norpace. Angiology 26: 85–96, 1975.

P. Lagerstrom and B. Persson. Liquid chromatography in the monitoring of plasma levels of antiarrhythmic drugs. J. Chrom. 149: 331–340, 1978.

S. Lakshmanan. Two cases of fatal Norpace (disopyramide) intoxication from suicidal overdose. Presented at the annual meeting of the American Academy of Forensic Sciences, Las Vegas, Nevada, February 15, 1985.

K. Landmark, J.E. Bredesen, E. Thaulow et al. Pharmacokinetics of disopyramide in patients with imminent to moderate cardiac failure. Eur. J. Clin. Pharm. 19: 187–192, 1981.

J.J. Lima. Liquid chromatographic analysis of disopyramide and its mono-N-dealkylated metabolite. Clin. Chem. 25: 405–408, 1979.

D. Martin, L. Burke, W. Nordin and S. Chen. A simple spectrophotometric method for disopyramide phosphate (Norpace) measurement in biological fluids. Clin. Chem. 24: 991, 1978.

P.J. Meffin, E.W. Robert, R.A. Winkle et al. Role of concentration-dependent plasma protein binding in disopyramide disposition. J. Pharm. Biopharm. 7: 29–46, 1979.

R.W. Michalek, T.A. Rejent and R.A. Spencer. Disopyramide fatality: case report and GC/FID analysis. J. Anal. Tox. 6: 255, 1982.

G. Nygard, W.H. Shelver and S.K.W. Khalil. Sensitive high-pressure liquid chromatographic determination of disopyramide and mono-N-dealkyldisopyramide. J. Pharm. Sci. 68: 1318–1320, 1979.

D.B. O'Keefe, D.W. Holt, A.M. Hayler and R.K. Medd. The toxicology and treatment of disopyramide poisoning. Presented at the IX Congress of the European Association of Poison Control Centers, Thessaloniki, Greece, August, 1980.

K.G. Orloff. Personal communication, 1980.

P.J. Podrid, A. Schoeneberger and B. Lown. Congestive heart failure caused by oral disopyramide. New Eng. J. Med. 302: 614–617, 1980.

F. Powell, O. Carey and P. Smith. Fatal disopyramide overdose. J. Irish Med. Asso. 71: 552, 1978.

R.E. Ranney, R.R. Dean, A. Karim and F.M. Radzialowski. Disopyramide phosphate: pharmacokinetic and pharmacologic relationships of a new antiarrhythmic agent. Arch. Int. Pharm. 191: 162–188, 1971.

L. Sathyavagiswaran. Fatal disopyramide intoxication from suicidal/accidental overdose. J. For. Sci. 32: 1813–1818, 1987.

J. Vasiliades, C. Owens and D. Pirkle. Gas-chromatographic determination of disopyramide in serum, with use of a nitrogen-selective detector. Clin. Chem. 25: 311–313, 1979a.

Disulfiram

T½: 7.3 hr
Vd: ?
Fb: ?

$$(C_2H_5)_2N\overset{\overset{S}{\|}}{C}S S\overset{\overset{S}{\|}}{C}N(C_2H_5)_2$$

Occurrence and Usage. Disulfiram (tetraethylthiuram disulfide, Antabuse) was synthesized in 1881 and has been used industrially in the vulcanization of rubber. It was introduced into clinical medicine in the 1930's as a scabiescide and vermicide on the basis of its ability to chelate copper, necessary to the respiratory enzymes of lower life forms. After investigators noted an unusual interaction between alcohol and disulfiram in 1948, it was proposed for use in aversion therapy for alcoholism. Disulfiram is known to inhibit the oxidative metabolism of a large number of drugs and chemicals, including ethanol. It is supplied for oral use in 250 and 500 mg tablets; daily doses of 125–500 mg are recommended for maintenance therapy.

Blood Concentrations. Disulfiram and 4 of its metabolites, diethyldithiocarbamate (dithiocarb), methyldiethyldithiocarbamate, carbon disulfide, and diethylamine, appear in blood after oral disulfiram administration, but the concentrations produced and their duration are highly variable between subjects. Average half-lives for these 5 substances have been reported as 7.3, 15.5, 22.1, 8.9 and 13.9 hours, respectively (Faiman et al., 1984). A single 500 mg dose in one subject produced a peak disulfiram concentration of about 0.38 mg/L at 5 hours; a peak diethyldithiocarbamate level of about 1.2 mg/L at 8 hours; a peak methyldiethyldithiocarbamate level of about 0.40 mg/L at 8 hours; a peak carbon disulfide level of about 14 mg/L at 3 hours; and a peak diethylamine level of about 0.7 mg/L at 1.5 hours. The carbon disulfide value remained fairly constant over the ensuing 24 hours, whereas the levels of the other moieties declined to about 10–20% of their peak concentrations (Jensen and Faiman, 1980). In patients receiving 200 mg of disulfiram daily, blood taken approximately 12 hours after the single daily dose contained from 0.27–1.43 mg/L diethyldithiocarbamate and 0.02–0.31 mg/L carbon disulfide (Sauter and von Wartburg, 1977).

Metabolism and Excretion. About 90% of an oral dose of disulfiram is absorbed. The drug is highly lipid soluble and, in animals, tends to accumulate in fatty tissues. Disulfiram is completely reduced to diethyldithiocarbamate (DDC) within 4 minutes after addition to human blood or plasma. Diethyldithiocarbamate, an excellent chelator of numerous metal ions, has an *in vitro* half-life of approximately 70 minutes in either blood or plasma, being nonenzymatically degraded (especially in an acid medium) to carbon disulfide and diethylamine. Diethyldithiocarbamate is considered by some investigators to represent the pharmacologically active principle of disulfiram; it is further metabolized by methylation to methyldiethyldithiocarbamate or by glucuronide conjugation. Within 6 days of a single oral dose of disulfiram, 63% is excreted in the urine as sulfate ion, 6% as organic sulfur, and 4% as ethereal sulfate (Eldjarn, 1950; Gessner and Jakubowski, 1972; Cobby et al., 1977a; 1977b). The measurement of both the pulmonary elimination of carbon disulfide (Rogers et al., 1978; Phillips et al., 1986) and the urinary excretion of diethylamine (Neiderhiser et al., 1976) have been proposed for use in monitoring disulfiram compliance.

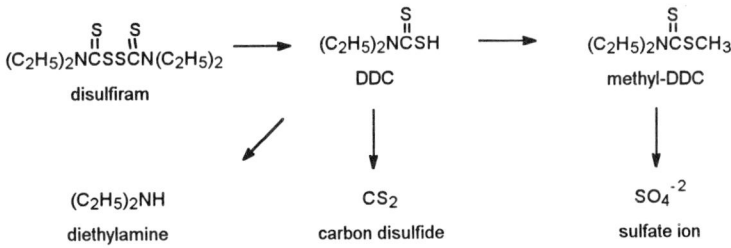

Toxicity. The side-effects of disulfiram administration include skin rash, drowsiness, headache, polyneuritis, and an occasional psychotic reaction. Several episodes of moderate to severe hepatotoxicity have been reported (Keeffe and Smith, 1974; Eisen and Ginsberg, 1975; Nassberger, 1984). The neurotoxic and psychotomimetic effects of the drug have been ascribed in large part to its metabolite carbon disulfide (Kane, 1970; Rainey, 1977).

The disulfiram-ethanol interaction is characterized by flushing of the face, tachycardia, severe headache, apprehension, rapid breathing, hypotension, dizziness, nausea, vomiting, and fainting. These symptoms may begin to appear in a patient receiving disulfiram therapy at a blood ethanol concentration of 0.01 g/dL, are fully developed at a concentration of 0.05 g/dL, and lead to unconsciousness at levels of 0.12–0.15 g/dL. An individual with a blood ethanol concentration of 0.18 g/dL who intentionally ingested 7 g of disulfiram became comatose and hypotensive after 11–16 hours; he recovered 12 hours later with supportive therapy (Woolley and Devenyi, 1980).

A 2 year old boy who accidentally ingested an unknown amount of disulfiram developed fever, vomiting, drowsiness and coma over a 3 day period. Blood disulfiram concentrations (probably representing diethyldithiocarbamate) of 17.4 and 6.5 mg/L were measured 9 and 17 days after admission, respectively. Consciousness gradually returned over a 25 day period, but the child was unable to stand; over a 3 year period he recovered most of his motor functions although was found to be mentally retarded (Reichelderfer, 1969).

Two deaths involving the simultaneous use of alcohol and disulfiram have been reported in which analytical results were available. One victim had postmortem blood diethyldithiocarbamate and ethanol concentrations of 8 mg/L and 0.96 g/dL, respectively (Heyndrickx, 1975); the other had corresponding concentrations of 120 mg/L and 0.27 g/dL (Gottschalk and Cravey, 1980).

Analysis. Several spectrophotometric procedures based on the chelation of copper by diethyldithiocarbamate have been reported for measuring "disulfiram" in blood and urine (Linderholm and Berg, 1951; Divatia et al., 1952; Tompsett, 1964). This technique has been made more specific by first degrading disulfiram and diethyldithiocarbamate to carbon disulfide, with subsequent conversion back to DDC and formation of the DDC-copper complex (Sauter et al., 1976; Rogers et al., 1978). Similarly, copper or zinc chelates with DDC may be analyzed by atomic absorption spectrometry (Kovatsis, 1978; Martens and Heyndrickx, 1978). Gas chromatographic methods have been developed for unchanged disulfiram (Davidson and Wilson, 1979), diethyldithiocarbamate (Cobby et al., 1977a; Martens and Heyndrickx, 1978), methyldiethyldithiocarbamate (Cobby et al., 1977a), and carbon disulfide (Sauter and von Wartburg, 1977; see also section on carbon disulfide) in blood. Liquid chromatographic methods are available for the step-wise (Jensen and Faiman, 1980) or simultaneous (Masso and Kramer, 1981; Johansson, 1986; Irth et al., 1988) determination of each of these substances. Diethylamine in urine has been assayed by a spectrophotometric procedure following thin-layer chromatographic separation (Neiderhiser et al., 1976) and by liquid chromatography (Neiderhiser and Fuller, 1982). A simple colorimetric breath test for carbon disulfide has been recommended for monitoring compliance with disulfiram therapy (Kraml, 1973; Paulson et al., 1977).

References

J. Cobby, M. Mayersohn and S. Selliah. The rapid reduction of disulfiram in blood and plasma. J. Pharm. Exp. Ther. 202: 724–731, 1977a.

J. Cobby, M. Mayersohn and S. Selliah. Methyl diethyldithiocarbamate, a metabolite of disulfiram in man. Life Sci. 21: 937–942, 1977b.

W.J. Davidson and A. Wilson. Determination of nanogram quantities of disulfiram in human and rat plasma by gas-liquid chromatography. J. Stud. Alc. 40: 1073–1077, 1979.

K.J. Divatia, C.H. Hine and T.N. Burbridge. A simple method for the determination of tetraethylthiuramdisulfide (Antabus) and blood levels obtained experimentally in animals and clinically in man. J. Lab. Clin. Med. 39: 974–982, 1952.

H.J. Eisen and A.L. Ginsberg. Disulfiram hepatotoxicity. Ann. Int. Med. 83: 673–675, 1975.

L. Eldjarn. The metabolism of tetraethyl thiuramdisulphide (Antabus, Aversan) in man, investigated by means of radioactive sulphur. Scand. J. Clin. Lab. Invest. 2: 202–208, 1950.

M.D. Faiman, J.C. Jensen and R.B. Lacoursiere. Elimination kinetics of disulfiram in alcoholics after single and repeated doses. Clin. Pharm. Ther. 36: 520–526, 1984.

T. Gessner and M. Jakubowski. Diethyldithiocarbamic acid methyl ester—a metabolite of disulfiram. Biochem. Pharm. 21: 219–230, 1972.

L.A. Gottschalk and R.H. Cravey. *Toxicological and Pathological Studies on Psychoactive Drug-Involved Deaths*, Biomedical Publications, Davis, California, 1980, p. 178.

A. Heyndrickx. Personal communication, 1980.

H. Irth, G.J. deJong, V.A.T. Brinkman and R.W. Frei. Determination of disulfiram and two of its metabolites in urine by reversed-phase liquid chromatography. J. Chrom. 424: 95–102, 1988.

J.C. Jensen and M.D. Faiman. Determination of disulfiram and metabolites from biological fluids by high-performance liquid chromatography. J. Chrom. 181: 407–416, 1980.

B. Johansson. Rapid and sensitive on-line precolumn purification and high-performance liquid chromatographic assay for disulfiram and its metabolites. J. Chrom. 378: 419–429, 1986.

F.J. Kane, Jr. Carbon disulfide intoxication from overdosage of disulfiram. Am. J. Psych. 127: 690–694, 1970.

E.B. Keeffe and F.W. Smith. Disulfiram hypersensitivity hepatitis. J. Am. Med. Asso. 230: 435–436, 1974.

A.V. Kovatsis. Progress in indirect atomic absorption spectroscopy. In *Human Toxicology* (A. Heyndrickx, ed.), European Press, Ghent, 1978, pp. 47–61.

M. Kraml. A rapid test for Antabuse ingestion. Can. Med. Asso. J. 109: 578, 1973.

H. Linderholm and K. Berg. A method for the determination of tetraethylthiuram disulphide (Antabus, Abstinyl) and diethyldithiocarbamate in blood and urine. Some studies on the metabolism of tetraethylthiuram disulphide. Scand. J. Clin. Lab. Invest. 3: 96–102, 1951.

F.K. Martens and A. Heyndrickx. Analysis of sodium diethyldithiocarbamate (NaDEDC), a metabolite of tetraethylthiuramdisulfide (TETD) in human serum and urine. J. Anal. Tox. 2: 269–274, 1978.

P.D. Masso and P.A. Kramer. Simultaneous determination of disulfiram and two of its dithiocarbamate metabolites in human plasma by reversed-phase liquid chromatography. J. Chrom. 224: 457–464, 1981.

L. Nassberger. Hepatotoxicity due to disulfiram. Clin. Tox. 22: 403–408, 1984.

D.H. Neiderhiser, R.K. Fuller, L.J. Hejduk and H.P. Roth. Method for the detection of diethylamine, a metabolite of disulfiram, in urine. J. Chrom. 117: 187–192, 1976.

D.H. Neiderhiser and R.K. Fuller. High-performance liquid chromatographic method for the determination of diethylamine, a metabolite of disulfiram, in urine. J. Chrom. 229: 470–474, 1982.

S.M. Paulson, S. Krause and F.L. Iber. Development and evaluation of a compliance test for patients taking disulfiram. Johns Hopkins Med. J. 141: 119–125, 1977.

M. Phillips, J. Greenberg and V. Martinez. Measurement of breath carbon disulfide during disulfiram therapy by gas chromatography with flame photometric detection. J. Chrom. 381: 164–167, 1986.

J.M. Rainey, Jr. Disulfiram toxicity and carbon disulfide poisoning. Am. J. Psych. 134: 371–378, 1977.

T.E. Reichelderfer. Acute disulfiram poisoning in a child. Quart. J. Stud. Alc. 30: 724–728, 1969.

W.K. Rogers, K.M. Wilson and C.E. Becker. Methods for detecting disulfiram in biologic fluids: application in studies of compliance and effect of divalent cations on bioavailability. Alcoholism: Clin. Exp. Res. 2: 375–380, 1978.

A.M. Sauter, W. Wiegrebe and J.P. von Wartburg. Determination of disulfiram and its metabolites in human blood. Arz. Forsch. 26: 173–177, 1976.

A.M. Sauter and J.P. von Wartburg. Quantitative analysis of disulfiram and its metabolites in human blood by gas-liquid chromatography. J. Chrom. 133: 167–172, 1977.

S.L. Tompsett. The determination of disulfiram (Antabuse tetraethyl thiuramdisulphide) in blood and urine. Acta Pharm. Tox. 21: 20–22, 1964.

B. Woolley and P. Devenyi. Acute disulfiram overdose. J. Stud. Alc. 41: 740–743, 1980.

Dothiepin

T½: 11–32 hr
Vd: 20–92 L/kg
Fb: ?
pKa: ?

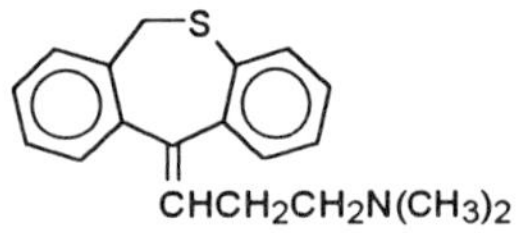

Occurrence and Usage. Dothiepin (Prothiaden) is a tricyclic antidepressant structurally related to amitriptyline and doxepin. Single oral doses of 25–100 mg are administered as the hydrochloride; daily doses may range from 75–300 mg.

Blood Concentrations. A single 75 mg oral dose of dothiepin given to 6 subjects produced an average peak plasma concentration of 0.062 mg/L (range, 0.025–0.095) at 3 hours; an average elimination half-life of 24 hours was observed (Crampton et al., 1980). Dothiepin sulfoxide peak blood levels in 7 volunteers after a single 75 mg oral dose averaged 0.081 mg/L at 5 hours, declining with a half-life of 19 hours; peak nordothiepin (northiaden) levels averaged 0.011 mg/L at 6 hours, and declined with a half-life of 83 hours. An average blood/plasma concentration ratio of 0.7 was noted for the parent drug (Maguire et al., 1981a). Steady-state plasma dothiepin concentrations averaging 0.106 mg/L (range, 0.020–0.420) were measured in 16 patients on chronic therapy with 150 mg daily (Crampton et al., 1980).

Metabolism and Excretion. Dothiepin is known to be metabolized in man by N-demethylation and sulfoxidation; hydroxylation and conjugation are also believed to occur. From 49–62% of a labeled dose is excreted in urine and 15–41% in feces in a 24 hour period, largely as metabolites (Crampton et al., 1978). Only 0.3% and 0.1% of a dose are excreted as dothiepin and nordothiepin, respectively, in the 72 hour urine; 11% and 0.7%, respectively, are excreted as conjugates of these 2 substances (Kawahara et al., 1986).

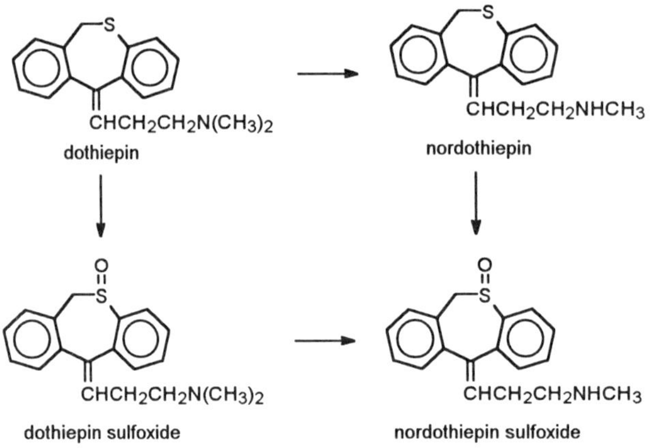

dothiepin

nordothiepin

dothiepin sulfoxide

nordothiepin sulfoxide

Toxicity. Eight victims of overdoage whose manifestations included confusion, drowsiness, coma, seizures and tachycardia survived with treatment after developing plasma dothiepin and nordothiepin levels of 0.82–3.9 mg/L and 0.09–0.42 mg/L, respectively (Ilett et al., 1991).

Seven cases of fatal dothiepin overdosage have been reported; postmortem blood concentrations averaged 1.5 mg/L (range, 0.3–2.5), liver, 8.0 mg/kg (range, 2.0–14), and urine, 3.2 mg/L (range, 0.4–5.1) (Robinson et al., 1974, 1979).

Analysis. Dothiepin and its metabolites have been analyzed in biological specimens by nitrogen-selective gas chromatography (Gifford et al., 1975), gas chromatography-mass spectrometry (Maguire et al., 1981b), and liquid chromatography (Brodie et al., 1977; Kawahara et al., 1987; Taylor et al., 1992).

References

R.R. Brodie, L.F. Chasseaud, E.L. Crampton et al. High performance liquid chromatographic determination of dothiepin and northiaden in human plasma and serum. J. Int. Med. Res. 5: 387–390, 1977.

E.L. Crampton, W. Dickinson, G. Haran et al. The metabolism of dothiepin hydrochloride *in vivo* and *in vitro*. Brit. J. Pharm. 64: 405P, 1978.

E.L. Crampton, R.C. Glass, B. Marchant and J.A. Rees. Chemical ionisation mass fragmentographic measurement of dothiepin plasma concentrations following a single oral dose in man. J. Chrom. 183: 141–148, 1980.

L.A. Gifford, P. Turner and C.M.B. Pare. Sensitive method for the routine determination of tricyclic antidepressants in plasma using a specific nitrogen detector. J. Chrom. 105: 107–113, 1975.

K.F. Ilett, L.P. Hackett, L.J. Dusci and J.W. Paterson. Disposition of dothiepin after overdose. Ther. Drug Mon. 13: 485–498, 1991.

K. Kawahara, T. Awaji, K. Uda et al. Urinary excretion of conjugates of dothiepin and northiaden (mono-N-demethyl-dothiepin) after an oral dose of dothiepin to humans. Eur. J. Drug Met. Pharmacokin. 11: 29–32, 1986.

K. Kawahara, T. Awaji, K. Uda and Y. Sakai. Determination of four metabolites of dothiepin in urine by high-performance liquid chromatography. J. Pharm. Biomed. Anal. 5: 183–189, 1987.

K.P. Maguire, G.D. Burrows, T.R. Norman and B.A. Scoggins. Metabolism and pharmacokinetics of dothiepin. Brit. J. Clin. Pharm. 12: 405–409, 1981a.

K.P. Maguire, T.R. Norman and G.D. Burrows. Simultaneous measurement of dothiepin and its major metabolites in plasma and whole blood by gas chromatography-mass fragmentography. J. Chrom. 222: 399–408, 1981b.

A.E. Robinson, A.I. Coffer and R.D. McDowall. Toxicology of some autopsy cases involving tricyclic antidepressant drugs. Z. Rechtsmed. 74: 261–266, 1974.

A.E. Robinson, R.D. McDowall, H. Sattar et al. Tricyclic and tetracyclic antidepressant drugs: forensic toxicology of some autopsy cases. J. Anal. Tox. 3: 3–13, 1979.

P.J. Taylor, B.G. Charles, R. Norris et al. Measurement of dothiepin and its major metabolites in plasma by high-performance liquid chromatography. J. Chrom. 581: 152–155, 1992.

Doxapram

T½: 6–9 hr
Vd: 1.5 L/kg
Fb: ?
pKa: ?

Occurrence and Usage. Doxapram (Dopram) is a peripherally- and centrally-acting respiratory stimulant that has been in clinical use since 1966. It is available as the hydrochloride in a 20 mg/mL solution for intravenous administration. Single doses of 0.5–2.0 mg/kg are given to alleviate respiratory insufficiency or to reverse drug-induced respiratory depression; the daily dose is not to exceed 3000 mg.

Blood Concentrations. An intravenous injection of 1.5 mg/kg (105 mg/70 kg) in 6 subjects produced an average peak plasma doxapram concentration of about 3 mg/L, declining to less than 2 mg/L by 1 hour. A 2 hour intravenous infusion of 7.0 mg/kg (490 mg/70 kg) resulted in an average peak level of 4.0 mg/L (range, 2.7–5.2) in 4 subjects at the end of the infusion, dropping rapidly to 0.5 mg/L by 4 hours later and exhibiting an elimination half-life of 7.4 hours. The infusion had to be terminated in 1 volunteer at 1.5 hours due to extreme agitation. The plasma concentrations of a metabolite, 2-ketodoxapram, achieved an average peak level of about 1.6 mg/L by 2 hours after the termination of the infusion and declined with a half-life of 6.5 hours (Robson and Prescott, 1978).

Metabolism and Excretion. An average of 1.2% of a single intravenous dose of doxapram is excreted unchanged in the 24 hour urine. A metabolite, 2-ketodoxapram (AHR-5955), is present in plasma at levels of about 40% of the parent drug (Robson and Prescott, 1978). Two other urinary metabolites, products of morpholine ring cleavage, have been tentatively identified (Nichol et al., 1980).

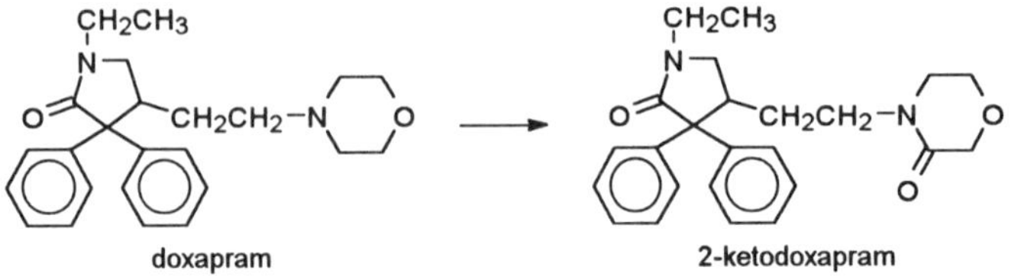

doxapram   2-ketodoxapram

Toxicity. Toxic effects of doxapram include dizziness, headache, agitation, fever, sweating, tachycardia, and convulsive seizures.

Analysis. Doxapram and its known metabolites have been analyzed in blood or urine by gas chromatography with nitrogen-selective (Robson and Prescott, 1977; Torok-Both et al., 1985), flame-ionization, and mass spectrometric detection (Nichol et al., 1980). Liquid chromatography has also been used (Aranda et al., 1988).

References

J.V. Aranda, K. Beharry, J. Rex et al. High pressure liquid chromatographic microassay for simultaneous measurement of doxapram and its metabolites in premature newborn infants. J. Liq. Chrom. 11: 2983–2991, 1988.
H. Nichol, J. Vine, J. Thomas and R.G. Moore. Quantitation of doxapram in blood, plasma and urine. J. Chrom. 182: 191–200, 1980.
R.H. Robson and L.F. Prescott. Rapid gas-liquid chromatographic estimation of doxapram in plasma. J. Chrom. 143: 527–529, 1977.
R.H. Robson and L.F. Prescott. A pharmacokinetic study of doxapram in patients and volunteers. Brit. J. Clin. Pharm. 7: 81–87, 1978.
G.A. Torok-Both, R.T. Coutts, F. Jamali et al. Sensitive nitrogen-phosphorus capillary gas chromatographic assay for doxapram in premature infants. J. Chrom. 344: 372–377, 1985.

Doxepin

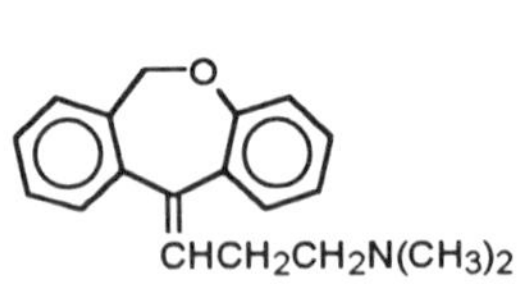

T½: 8–25 hr
Vd: 9–33 L/kg
Fb: 0.76
pKa: 8.0

CHCH2CH2N(CH3)2

Occurrence and Usage. Doxepin (Sinequan, Adapin) is a dibenzoxepin analogue of amitriptyline that is supplied as an isomeric mixture with a cis:trans distribution of approximately 15:85. It was first synthesized in 1962 and was evaluated clinically as early as 1963. The drug is administered as the hydrochloride in oral doses of 75–150 mg daily, with some patients receiving 300 mg/day.

Blood Concentrations. Administration of a 75 mg oral dose to 7 subjects produced an average peak doxepin plasma concentration of 0.024 mg/L at 2 hours; plasma nordoxepin levels averaged 0.009 mg/L at 6 hours. The levels of the 2 substances declined with average half-lives of 15 and 45 hours, respectively (Ziegler et al., 1978). Patients receiving an average daily dose of 113 mg of doxepin for several weeks exhibited average plasma concentrations of 0.023 mg/L (range, 0.005–0.115) for doxepin and 0.021 mg/L (range, 0–0.082) for nordoxepin (Norman et al., 1980).

Metabolism and Excretion. The metabolism of doxepin in man has not been fully described. Nordoxepin, which has pharmacologic and toxicologic properties comparable to its parent, is known to be a primary metabolite and doxepin-N-oxide has been presumptively identified in human tissues (de Groot et al., 1978b). The existence of dinordoxepin and phenolic metabolites has been postulated on the basis of animal studies (Hobbs, 1969). An average of 0.4% of a 50 mg oral dose of doxepin is eliminated unchanged in the 24 hour urine; concentrations of the drug in urine during this period ranged from 0.01–1.12 mg/L (Dusci and Hackett, 1971). An N-glucuronide conjugate of the parent drug has been shown to constitute 18–23% of a dose in the 24 hour urine (Luo et al., 1991).

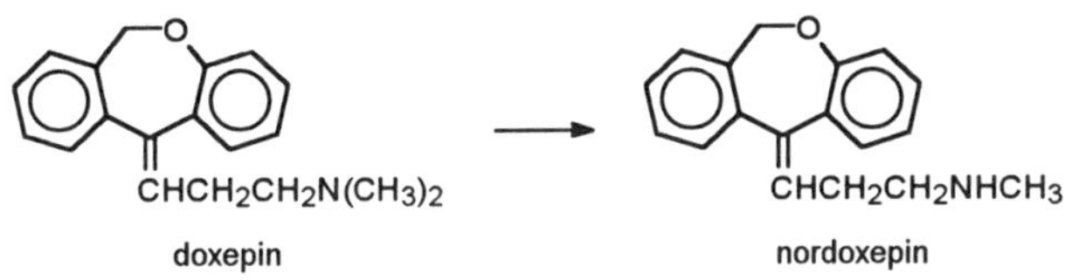

doxepin $\longrightarrow$ nordoxepin

$CHCH_2CH_2N(CH_3)_2$　　　$CHCH_2CH_2NHCH_3$

Toxicity. Agitation, hallucinations, drowsiness, tachycardia, and hypertension occurred in an individual who ingested 600 mg of doxepin and developed a blood concentration of 0.14 mg/L; he was successfully treated with physostigmine (Janson et al., 1977). Doxepin serum concentrations of 0.112–0.431 mg/L were determined in 4 other poisoned patients who exhibited symptoms ranging from dizziness to coma (Vasiliades et al., 1979). Overdosage resulted in a plasma concentration of 2.1 mg/L in a patient who survived the episode (Biggs et al., 1977).

At least 18 fatalities due to the drug have been reported; blood concentrations in these cases averaged 13 mg/L (range, 2–26) and liver concentrations, 131 mg/kg (range, 64–320) (Frank, 1973; Lachambre, 1973; Norheim, 1973; Oliver and Watson, 1974; Baselt and Cravey, 1977; Gottschalk and Cravey, 1980; Cordonnier et al., 1983). The following distribution of doxepin and its active metabolite was observed in 4 fatalities (de Groot et al., 1978b):

Drug Concentrations in Doxepin Fatalities (mg/L or mg/kg)

	Blood	Brain	Liver	Bile	Kidney	Urine
Doxepin						
Average	9.3	14	32	95	12	7.5
(Range)	(0.7–29)	(9–21)	(22–38)	(38–195)	(3.3–19)	(2.1–12)
Nordoxepin						
Average	1.7	7.2	7.5	7.1	3.0	2.8
(Range)	(0.1–6.2)	(1.5–22)	(1.2–20)	(1.0–19)	(0.5–9.0)	(0.7–6.4)

Doxepin may be subject to postmortem redistribution; heart blood/femoral blood concentration ratios in 8 cases averaged 3.1 and ranged from 0.8–7.6 (Anderson and Prouty, 1989).

Analysis. Analytical procedures specific for doxepin and nordoxepin have relied on gas chromatographic separation and involve flame-ionization (O'Brien and Hinsvark, 1976), nitrogen-phosphorus (Vasiliades et al., 1979), electron-capture (Wallace et al., 1978), or mass spectrometric detection (Frigerio et al., 1977; Wilson et al., 1977; de Groot et al., 1978a; Davis et al., 1983). Liquid chromatography has also been described (Park et al., 1986; Emm et al., 1987).

References

W.H. Anderson and R.W. Prouty. Postmortem redistribution of drugs. In *Advances in Analytical Toxicology* (R.C. Baselt, ed.), Vol. 2, YearBook Medical, Chicago, 1989, pp. 70–102.

R.C. Baselt and R.H. Cravey. A compendium of therapeutic and toxic concentrations of toxicologically significant drugs in human biofluids. J. Anal. Tox. 1: 81–103, 1977.

J.T. Biggs, D.G. Spiker, J.M. Petit and V.E. Ziegler. Tricyclic antidepressant overdose. J. Am. Med. Asso. 237: 135–138, 1977.

J. Cordonnier, A. Heyndrickx, L. Jordaens et al. A fatal intoxication due to doxepin. J. Anal. Tox. 7: 161–164, 1983.

T.P. Davis, S.K. Veggeberg, S.R. Hameroff and K.L. Watts. Sensitive and quantitative determination of plasma doxepin and desmethyldoxepin in chronic pain patients by gas chromatography and mass spectrometry. J. Chrom. 273: 436–441, 1983.

G. de Groot, J.G. Leferink and R.A.A. Maes. Toxicological determination in biological material of doxepin by gas chromatography and some of its metabolites by mass fragmentography. J. Anal. Tox. 2: 13–17, 1978a.

G. de Groot, R.A.A. Maes, C.N. Hodnett et al. Four cases of fatal doxepin poisoning. J. Anal. Tox. 2: 18–20, 1978b.

L.J. Dusci and L.P. Hackett. Gas chromatographic determination of doxepin in human urine following therapeutic doses. J. Chrom. 61: 231–236, 1971.

T. Emm, L.J. Lesko and M.B. Perkal. Simultaneous determination of doxepin and nordoxepin in serum using high-performance liquid chromatography. J. Chrom. 419: 445–451, 1987.

L. Frank. Personal communication, 1973.

A. Frigerio, C. Pantarotto, R. Franco et al. Quantitative determination of doxepin and desmethyldoxepin in rat plasma by means of gas-liquid chromatography-mass fragmentography. J. Chrom. 130: 354–360, 1977.

L.A. Gottschalk and R.H. Cravey. *Toxicological and Pathological Studies on Psychoactive Drug-Involved Deaths,* Biomedical Publications, Davis, California, 1980.

D.C. Hobbs. Distribution and metabolism of doxepin. Biochem. Pharm. 18: 1941–1954, 1969.

P.A. Janson, J.B. Watt and J.A. Hermos. Doxepin overdose. J. Am. Med. Asso. 237: 2632–2633, 1977.

P. Lachambre. Personal communication, 1973.

H. Luo, E.M. Hawes, G. McKay et al. The quaternary ammonium-linked glucuronide of doxepin. Drug Met. Disp. 19: 722–724, 1991.

G. Norheim. Determination of doxepin in autopsy material. Arch. Tox. 31: 7–12, 1973.

T.R. Norman, G.D. Burrows and G.N. Bianchi. Doxepin plasma levels and anxiolytic response. Int. Pharmacopsych. 15: 247–252, 1980.

J.E. O'Brien and O.N. Hinsvark. GLC determination of doxepin plasma levels. J. Pharm. Sci. 65: 1068–1069, 1976.

J.S. Oliver and A.A. Watson. Doxepin poisoning. Med. Sci. Law 14: 280–283, 1974.

Y.H. Park, C. Goshorn and O.N. Hinsvark. Quantitative determination of doxepin and nordoxepin in urine by high-performance liquid chromatography. J. Chrom. 375: 202–206, 1986.

J. Vasiliades, T.M. Sahawneh and C. Owens. Determination of therapeutic and toxic concentrations of doxepin and loxapine using gas-liquid chromatography with a nitrogen-sensitive detector, and gas chromatography-mass spectrometry of loxapine. J. Chrom. 164: 457–470, 1979.

J.E. Wallace, H.E. Hamilton, R. Olivares and S.C. Harris. Determination of doxepin by electron-capture gas chromatography. J. Anal. Tox. 2: 44–49, 1978.

J.M. Wilson, L.J. Williamson and V.A. Raisys. Simultaneous measurement of secondary and tertiary tricyclic antidepressants by GC/MS chemical ionization mass fragmentography. Clin. Chem. 23: 1012–1017, 1977.

V.E. Ziegler, J.T. Biggs, L.T. Wylie et al. Doxepin kinetics. Clin. Pharm. Ther. 23: 573–579, 1978.

Doxylamine

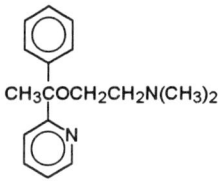

T½: 10 hr
Vd: 2.7 L/kg
Fb: ?
pKa: 9.2

Occurrence and Usage. Doxylamine (Unisom, Bendectin) is an antihistamine of the ethanolamine class first introduced in 1948. The drug is used primarily as a sleep-inducing agent. It is available in tablets containing 25 mg of the succinate salt or in liquids containing 7.5 mg per dose. The production of Bendectin, used as an antinauseant in pregnancy, was halted in 1983 due to public concern over the possible teratogenic effects of the drug.

Blood Concentrations. Following an overnight fast, 16 healthy men aged 19–28 years and weighing 61–81 kg were given a 25 mg tablet of doxylamine succinate with 240 mL of water. Peak plasma concentrations occurred 1–4 hours after drug ingestion and ranged from 69–138 µg/L (average, 99). At 24 hours post-dose, the average plasma concentration was 21 µg/L. The elimination half-life averaged 10.1 hours (Friedman and Greenblatt, 1985). In another study, a healthy adult male was given 25 mg orally after an overnight fast. A peak plasma concentration of 150 µg/L was measured 2 hours post-administration. This declined to 28 µg/L at 24 hours and 10 µg/L at 36 hours (Kohlhof et al., 1983).

Metabolism and Excretion. The biotransformation of doxylamine has been little studied in man. The drug is known to be excreted in the urine as unchanged doxylamine, nordoxylamine and dinordoxylamine (Gielsdorf and Schubert, 1981).

CH₃COCH₂CH₂N(CH₃)₂ $\longrightarrow$ CH₃COCH₂CH₂NHCH₃ $\longrightarrow$ CH₃COCH₂CH₂NH₂

doxylamine   nordoxylamine   dinordoxylamine

Toxicity. Doxylamine in overdosage causes sedation, anticholinergic effects, respiratory depression and coma. Twenty-three acutely poisoned patients who were successfully treated had admission plasma doxylamine levels of 0.2–5.0 mg/L (Koppel et al., 1987).

Three fatalities have occurred that involved the following postmortem drug concentrations (Bayley et al., 1975; Wu Chen et al., 1983; Siek and Dunn, 1993):

Doxylamine Concentrations in Fatalities (mg/L or mg/kg)

	Blood	Liver	Urine
Average	4.6	14	17
(Range)	(0.7–12)	(14)	(16–17)

Analysis. Doxylamine has been analyzed in biological specimens by gas chromatography using flame-ionization (Fortan et al., 1963) and nitrogen-phosphorus detection (Thompson et al., 1982; Holder et al., 1984; Friedman and Greenblatt, 1985; Watts and Simonick, 1986). Liquid chromatography has been used in the determination of the drug in plasma and serum (Kohlhof et al., 1983;

Holder et al., 1984; Slikker et al., 1986; Thompson et al., 1986; Siek and Dunn, 1993). A sensitive and specific means of detection and quantitation is offered with gas chromatography-mass spectrometry (Wu Chen et al., 1983; Slikker et al., 1986).

References

M. Bayley, F.M. Walsh and M.J. Valaske. Fatal overdose from Bendectin. Clin. Pediat. 14: 507–509, 1975.

C.R. Fortan, W.C. Smith and P.L. Kirk. Gas chromatography of the antihistamines. Anal. Chem. 35: 591–595, 1963.

H. Friedman and D.J. Greenblatt. The pharmacokinetics of doxylamine: use of automated gas chromatography with nitrogen-phosphorus detection. J. Clin. Pharm. 25: 448–451, 1985.

W. Gielsdorf and K. Schubert. Biotransformation of doxylamine: isolation, identification and synthesis of some metabolites. J. Clin. Biochem. 19: 485–490, 1981.

C.L. Holder, H.C. Thompson, Jr. and W. Slikker, Jr. Trace level determination of doxylamine in nonhuman primate plasma and urine by GC/NPD and HPLC. J. Anal. Tox. 8: 46–50, 1984.

K.J. Kohlhof, D. Stump and J.A. Zizzamia. Analysis of doxylamine in plasma by high-performance liquid chromatography. J. Pharm. Sci. 72: 961–962, 1983.

C. Koppel. J. Tenczer and K. Ibe. Poisoning with over-the-counter doxylamine preparations. Hum. Tox. 6: 355–359, 1987.

T.J. Siek and W.A. Dunn. Documentation of a doxylamine overdose death. J. For. Sci. 38: 713–720, 1993.

W. Slikker, Jr., C.L. Holder, G.W. Lipe et al. Metabolism of ^{14}C-labeled doxylamine succinate (Bendectin) in the Rhesus monkey (*Macaca mulatta*). J. Anal. Tox. 10: 87– 92, 1986.

H.C. Thompson, Jr., C.L. Holder and M.C. Bowman. Trace analysis of doxylamine succinate in animal feed, human urine, and wastewater by GC using a rubidium-sensitized nitrogen detector. J. Chrom. Sci. 20: 373–380, 1982.

H.C. Thompson, Jr., A.B. Gosnell, C.L. Holder et al. Metabolism of doxylamine succinate in Fischer 344 rats Part 1: distribution and excretion. J. Anal. Tox. 10: 18– 23, 1986.

V.W. Watts and T.F. Simonick. Screening of basic drugs in biological samples using dual column capillary chromatography and nitrogen-phosphorus detectors. J. Anal. Tox. 10: 198– 204, 1986.

N.B. Wu Chen, M.I. Schaffer, R.L. Lin et al. The general toxicology unknown II. A case report: doxylamine and pyrilamine intoxication. J. For. Sci. 28: 398– 403, 1983.

Dyphylline

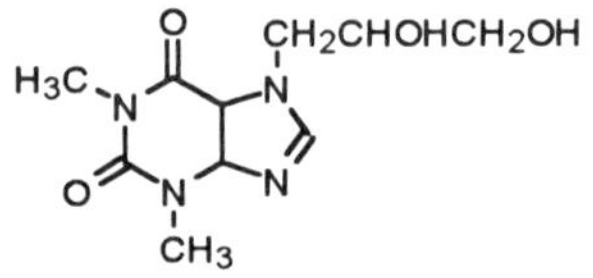

T½: 1.7– 2.7 hr
Vd: 0.6– 1.1 L/kg
Fb: less than 0.03
pKa: ?

Occurrence and Usage. Dyphylline (7-dihydroxypropyltheophylline, glyphylline, Lufylin, Neothylline) is a synthetic theophylline derivative first prepared and introduced as a bronchodilator in 1946. It is supplied as the free acid in tablets or syrup for oral usage in amounts of 100–400 mg, often in combination with ephedrine, guaifenesin, and phenobarbital. A solution containing 250 mg/mL is available for intramuscular injection. Single doses of 250–500 mg by injection or 100–1000 mg orally may be given every 6 hours. Dyphylline is much more water-soluble than theophylline and is considered significantly less potent as a bronchodilator.

Blood Concentrations. A 5 mg/kg (350 mg/70 kg) dose of dyphylline given to 7 subjects produced an average peak serum concentration of 6.5 mg/L when administered as an oral tablet and 8.8 mg/L as an intramuscular injection; both peak levels occurred at approximately 1 hour. A 10 mg/kg dose (700 mg/70 kg) resulted in peak levels of 14.3 mg/L and 12.3 mg/L after oral and intramuscular administration, respectively. The levels declined with an average half-life of 2.1 hours (Simons et al., 1975a). A 15 mg/kg (1050 mg/70 kg) oral dose given to 7 subjects produced an average serum concentration of 12.1 mg/L at 0.6 hours, declining to 10.6 mg/L at 1.0 hours; the investigators concluded that 12 mg/L represents the lower end of the therapeutic serum concentration range for dyphylline (Simons et al., 1975b). A 40 mg/kg (2800 mg/70 kg) dose given as a sustained-release tablet resulted in an average peak serum level of 12.2 mg/L at 3 hours, declining to 7.9 mg/L by 6 hours and 3.1 mg/L by 12 hours (Simons et al., 1977). Half-lives of 10.6 and 13.2 hours were measured in uremic patients receiving dyphylline (Lee et al., 1981); the average dyphylline half-life was increased from 2.6 to 4.9 hours in 12 subjects by the simultaneous administration of probenecid (May and Jarboe, 1983).

Metabolism and Excretion. Metabolites of dyphylline have not been identified in man. An average of 83% of a dose is excreted in the 24 hour urine (Gisclon et al., 1979a; Simons and Simons, 1979).

Toxicity. Dyphylline is capable of producing headache, nervousness, insomnia, nausea, vomiting, tachycardia, hypotension, convulsions, and circulatory failure in overdosage. Single doses of up to 27 mg/kg (1890 mg/70 kg), resulting in peak serum concentrations of 19–24 mg/L, have been tolerated without adverse effect. One subject developed a severe headache at a serum dyphylline concentration of 36.4 mg/L following a 28 mg/kg (1960 mg/70 kg) oral dose (Simons and Simons, 1979).

Analysis. Dyphylline may be assayed in biological fluids by many of the procedures cited for theophylline. Specific methods for the drug have included flame-ionization gas chromatography after trimethylsilyl derivatization (Butts et al., 1974; Shihabi and Dave, 1977) and liquid chromatography (Maijub and Stafford, 1976; Gisclon et al., 1979b; Valia et al., 1980; Paterson, 1982; Kester et al., 1987).

References

W.C. Butts, V.A. Raisys, M.A. Kenny and C.W. Bierman. A specific gas chromatographic method for the determination of dyphylline in serum. J. Lab. Clin. Med. 84: 451–458, 1974.

L.G. Gisclon, J.W. Ayres and G.H. Ewing. Pharmacokinetics of orally administered dyphylline. Am. J. Hosp. Pharm. 36: 1179–1184, 1979a.

L. Gisclon, K. Rowse and J. Ayres. Saliva, urine and plasma analysis of dyphylline via HPLC. Res. Comm. Chem. Path. Pharm. 23: 523–531, 1979b.

M.B. Kester, C.L. Saccar and H.C. Mansmann. Microassay for the simultaneous determination of theophylline and dyphylline in serum by high-performance liquid chromatography. J. Chrom. 416: 91–97, 1987.

C.C. Lee, L.H. Wang, B.L. Majeske and T.C. Marbury. Pharmacokinetics of dyphylline elimination by uremic patients. J. Pharm. Exp. Ther. 217: 340–344, 1981.

A.G. Maijub and D.T. Stafford. Theophylline and dyphylline levels in serum by liquid chromatography. J. Chrom. Sci. 14: 521–525, 1976.

D.C. May and C.H. Jarboe. Effect of probenecid on dyphylline elimination. Clin. Pharm. Ther. 33: 822–825, 1983.

N. Paterson. High-performance liquid chromatographic method for the determination of diprophylline in human serum. J. Chrom. 232: 450–455, 1982.

Z.K. Shihabi and R.P. Dave. Gas chromatographic determination of dyphylline in serum and saliva. Clin. Chem. 23: 942–943, 1977.

F.E.R. Simons, K.J. Simons and C.W. Bierman. The pharmacokinetics of dihydroxypropyltheophylline: a basis for rational therapy. J. Allergy Clin. Immunol. 56: 347–355, 1975a.

F.E.R. Simons, C.W. Bierman, A.C. Sprenkle and K.J. Simons. Efficacy of dyphylline (dihydroxypropyltheophylline) in exercise-induced bronchospasm. Pediatrics 56: 916–918, 1975b.

K.J. Simons, F.E.R. Simons and C.W. Bierman. Bioavailability of a sustained-release dyphylline formulation. J. Clin. Pharm. 17: 237–242, 1977.

K.J. Simons and F.E.R. Simons. Urinary excretion of dyphylline in humans. J. Pharm. Sci. 68: 1327–1329, 1979.

K.H. Valia, C.A. Hartman, N. Kucharczyk and R.D. Sofia. Simultaneous determination of dyphylline and theophylline in human plasma by high-performance liquid chromatography. J. Chrom. 221: 170–175, 1980.

Emetine

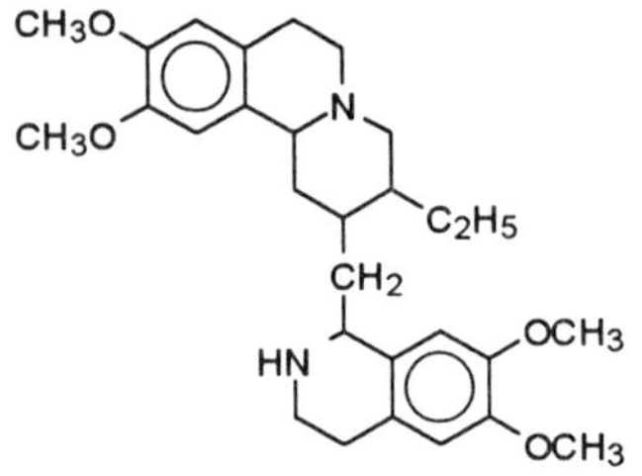

T½: ?
Vd: ?
Fb: ?
pKa: 7.4, 8.3

Occurrence and Usage. Emetine is an alkaloid present in the roots of *Cephaelis ipecacuanha* and *Cephaelis acumenata*. The only medically approved use of emetine in the United States is as an emetic, although it has been found to be parenterally effective in controlling intestinal amoebiasis and amoebic abscesses of the liver. The usual dose of syrup of ipecac to induce vomiting is 15 mL, repeated after 20 minutes if emesis has not occurred. Ipecac syrup contains approximately 0.7 mg/mL of emetine and is available without a prescription in 30 mL bottles.

Blood Concentrations. Blood concentrations of emetine were measureable in only 6 of 10 emergency room adult patients who received 30 mL of ipecac syrup for treatment of drug or chemical overdose; the levels varied from 5–75 µg/L within 2 hours of administration (Moran et al., 1983).

Metabolism and Excretion. Emetine is absorbed after oral administration, although vomiting may remove from 10% to nearly 100% of a dose (Crouch et al., 1984). Because of its slow hepatic and renal excretion, multiple small doses may accumulate in body tissues, thereby exerting the same or even greater toxic effect as a single large dose (Leibly, 1930; Manno and Manno, 1977; Adler et al., 1980). Emetine is excreted very slowly in the urine and detectable concentrations may be found up to 60 days following treatment (Moffat et al., 1986). An estimated 3% of a single dose is eliminated in the 24 hour urine (Moran et al., 1983).

Toxicity. Toxic effects from emetine include tachycardia, EKG abnormalities, cardiac arrest, gastrointestinal disorders (including stenosis of the lumen of the esophagus, bloody diarrhea, and protracted vomiting) and neuromuscular weakness. Several reports have described children presenting with protracted vomiting and diarrhea who were the victims of chronic intentional emetine poisoning; in one such case, a serum emetine level of 0.50 mg/L was measured (McClung et al., 1988; Day et al., 1989).

Several deaths following overdosage of emetine have been reported in which tissue concentrations have been measured; case 1 involved a 26 year old woman who drank syrup of ipecac to induce vomiting for weight reduction (Adler et al., 1980) and case 2, a 22 year old male who was inadvertently given 60 mL of ipecac liquid extract instead of 30 mL of syrup of ipecac and who died after 6 days (Verma, 1982):

Emetine Concentrations in Fatal Cases (mg/L or mg/kg)

	Blood	Liver	Bile	Kidney	Heart
Case 1	2.4	14	1.9	7.4	
Case 2	0	30		5.0	2.5

Analysis. Early methods for the determination of emetine in biological specimens included radiometry and spectrofluorometry (Schwartz and Herrero, 1965). Liquid chromatography with fluorescence detection appears to be the current method of choice (Bannister et al., 1979; Crouch et al., 1984).

References

A.G. Adler, P. Walinsky, R.A. Krall et al. Death resulting from ipecac syrup poisoning. J. Am. Med. Asso. 243: 1927–1928, 1980.

S.J. Bannister, J. Stevens, D. Mussun et al. High performance liquid chromatographic analysis of emetine after oxidative activation to a fluorescent product. J. Chrom. 176: 381–390, 1979.

D.J. Crouch, D.M. Moran, B.S. Finkle et al. Quantitative analysis of emetine and cephaeline by reversed-phase high performance liquid chromatography with fluorescence detection. J. Anal. Tox. 8: 63–65, 1984.

L. Day, C. Kelly, G. Reed et al. Fatal cardiomyopathy: suspected child abuse by chronic ipecac administration. Vet. Hum. Tox. 31: 255–257, 1989.

B.S. Leibly. Fatal emetine poisoning due to cumulative action in amoebic dysentery. Am. J. Med. Sci. 179: 834–839, 1930.

B. Manno and J. Manno. Toxicology of ipecac. Clin. Tox. 10: 221–242, 1977.

H.J. McClung, R. Murray, N.J. Braden et al. Intentional ipecac poisoning in children. Am. J. Dis. Child. 142: 637–639, 1988.

A.C. Moffat, J.V. Jackson, M.S. Moss and B. Widdop (eds). *Clarke's Isolation and Identification of Drugs*, 2nd ed., Pharmaceutical Press, London, 1986, pp. 581–582.

D.M. Moran, D.C. Crouch, B.S. Finkle and D.E. Rollins. Absorption of ipecac alkaloids in emergency room patients. Vet. Hum. Tox. 25: 286, 1983.

D.E. Schwartz and J. Herroro. Comparative pharmacokinetic studies of dehydroemetine and emetine in guinea pigs using spectrofluorometric and radiometric methods. Am. J. Trop. Med. 14: 78–83, 1965.

S.C.L. Verma. Personal communication, 1982.

Encainide

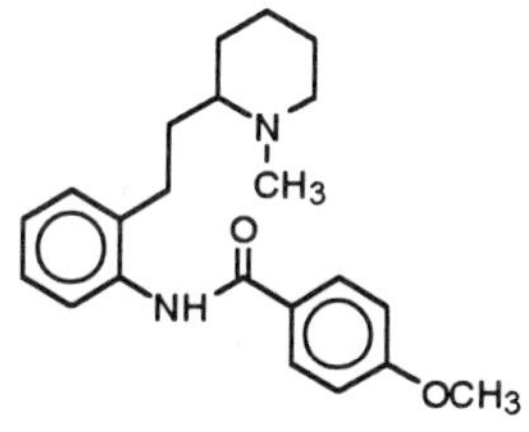

T½: 2.3 hr (normal metabolizers)
    11 hr (slow metabolizers)
Vd: 2.7–4.3 L/kg
Fb: 0.75–0.85
pKa: ?

Occurrence and Usage. Encainide (EnKaid) is a potent antiarrhythmic compound with class 1c activity, synthesized in 1969 but only recently introduced to the American market. It is used primarily for the treatment of life-threatening ventricular arrhythmias. The drug is available in capsules containing 25, 35 or 50 mg of the hydrochloride salt for oral administration. The initial dose is 25 mg every 8 hours with a gradual increase, if necessary, to a maximum dose of 150 mg/day.

Blood Concentrations. Steady-state plasma concentrations in a group of normal metabolizers receiving 150 mg encainide orally per day averaged 18 µg/L for the parent drug, 118 µg/L for O-demethylencainide and 94 µg/L for 3 methoxy-O-demethylencainide; the same therapy in slow metabolizers produced steady-state values of 450, 12 and 0 µg/L, respectively (Wang et al., 1984). The average elimination half-life of encainide in normal metabolizers is 2.3 hours, while that of slow metabolizers is 11.3 hours (Roden and Woosley, 1988).

Metabolism and Excretion. Encainide is metabolized by O- and N-demethylation, methoxylation of the terminal phenyl group, and conjugation. The extent of metabolism to O-demethylencainde (ODE) and 3-methoxy-0-demethylencainide (MODE) is genetically determined (Roden et al., 1980; Wang et al., 1984; McAllister et al., 1986). About 93% of the Caucasian population of North America extensively metabolizes encainide to ODE and MODE, and they are referred to as having the extensive metabolizer phenotype. The other 7% functionally lacks the enzyme responsible for the formation of ODE and MODE and are characterized as having poor metabolizer phenotype (Roden and Woosley, 1988; Selinger and Crawhall, 1989). In extensive metabolizers, 70% of a radioactive dose of encainide is recovered in the 96 hour urine, with 11% of a dose present as parent drug; in poor metabolizers, the corresponding figures are 85% and 59%, respectively (Turgeon and Roden, 1989).

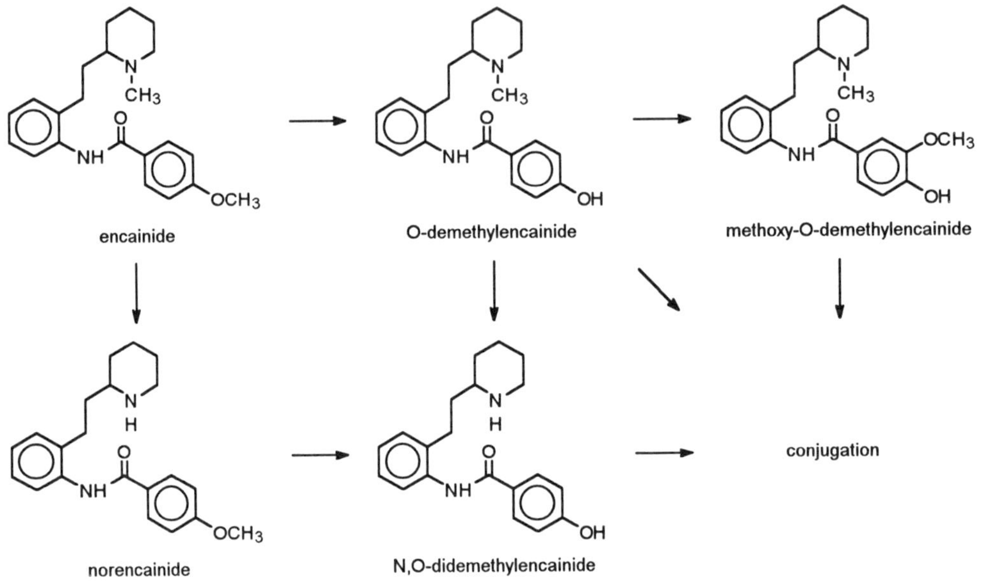

Toxicity. Encainide can cause new or worsened arrhythmias. Fifteen hundred post-infarction patients in clinical trials showed a death rate 2.5 times that of patients on placebo (Echt et al., 1991).

Analysis. Encainide and its metabolites can be determined in biological specimens by liquid chromatography (Bartek et al., 1988; Kazierad et al., 1989; Selinger and Crawhall, 1989; Turgeon et al., 1989; Dasgupta et al., 1990; Jajoo et al., 1990; Poirier et al., 1990) and by gas chromatography-mass spectrometry (Jajoo et al., 1990).

References

M.J. Bartek, R.F. Mayol, M.P. Boarman et al. Analysis of encainide and metabolites in plasma and urine by high-performance liquid chromatography. Ther. Drug Mon. 10: 446–452, 1988.

A. Dasgupta, I.B. Rosenzweig, J. Turgeon and V.A. Raisys. Encainide and metabolites analysis in serum or plasma using a reversed-phase high-performance liquid chromatographic technique. J. Chrom. 526: 260–265, 1990.

D.S. Echt, P.R. Liebson, L.B. Mitchell et al. Mortality and morbidity in patients receiving encainide, flecainide or placebo. The cardiac arrhythmia suppression trial. New Eng. J. Med. 324: 781–788, 1991.

H.K. Jajoo, R.F. Mauol, J.A. LaBudde and I.A. Blair. Structural characterization of urinary metabolites of the antiarrhythmic drug encainide in human subjects. Drug Met. Disp. 18: 28–35, 1990.

D.J. Kazierad, T.J. Hoon and M.B. Buttorff. A high-performance liquid chromatographic method for the deter- mination of encainide and its major metabolites in urine and serum using solid-phase extraction. Ther. Drug Mon. 11: 327–331, 1989.

C.B. McAllister, H.T. Wolfenden, W. Aslanian et al. Oxidative metabolism of encainide: polymorphism, phar- macokinetics and clinical considerations. Xenobiotica 16: 483–490, 1986.

J.M. Poirier, M. Lebot and G. Cheymol. Analysis of encainide and its three major metabolites in plasma by column liquid chromatography. J. Chrom. 534: 223–227, 1990.

D.M. Roden, S.B. Reele, S.B. Higgins et al. Total suppression of ventricular arrhythmias by encainide: phar- macokinetic and electrocardiographic characteristics. New Eng. J. Med. 302: 877–882, 1980.

D.M. Roden and R.L. Woosley. Clinical pharmacokinetics of encainide. Clin. Pharmacokin. 14: 141–147, 1988.

K. Selinger and J.C. Crawhall. Determination of encainide and its metabolites by high-performance liquid chromatography. J. Pharm. Biomed. Anal. 7: 355–359, 1989.

J. Turgeon, C. Funck-Brentano, H.T. Gray and D.M. Roden. Improved high-performance liquid chromato- graphic assay for encainide and its metabolites in human body `luids. J. Chrom. 490: 165–174, 1989.

T. Wang, D.M. Roden, H.T. Wolfenden et al. Influence of genetic polymorphism on the metabolism and disposition of encainide in man. J. Pharm. Exp. Ther. 228: 605–611, 1984.

Endrin

T½: ?
Vd: ?
Fb: ?

Occurrence and Usage. Endrin, a stereoisomer of dieldrin, is considered one of the most toxic of the chlorinated hydrocarbon insecticides. It has seen widespread usage in agriculture against soil and foliage pests since 1950, although its use has been recently curtailed in some countries due to its environmental persistence. Industrial exposure is generally via inhalation or dermal absorption. The current threshold limit value is 0.1 mg/m^3 in the occupational environment.

Blood Concentrations. Endrin was not found present in plasma, fat or urine of members of the general population or of occupationally exposed workers in amounts measurable by a technique with detectability limits of 0.003, 0.03 and 0.002 mg/L, respectively (Hayes and Curley, 1968).

Metabolism and Excretion. The disposition of endrin in man has not been investigated, although it is likely handled in a manner similar to that of dieldrin. In rats, endrin is oxidized on the meth- ylene bridge carbon atom to 9-hydroxyendrin, the major fecal metabolite, which undergoes further oxidation to 9-ketoendrin, the major urinary excretion product (Baldwin et al., 1970). Urine from workers at an endrin manufacturing plant was found to contain 0.01–0.14 mg/L hydroxyendrin as a glucuronide conjugate (Baldwin and Hutson, 1980).

Toxicity. The contamination of foodstuffs by endrin has resulted in several mass poisonings, with multiple fatalities; the onset of symptoms, which included vomiting, convulsions and unconscious- ness, ranged from 0.5–10 hours after ingestion of the poison (Davies and Lewis, 1956; Weeks, 1967). Death often occurs within 1–2 hours after ingestion of 6 g of endrin (Reddy et al., 1966). One subject who ate endrin-contaminated bread and suffered a convulsion exhibited a serum endrin concentration of 0.053 mg/L within 30 minutes of the convulsion; this concentration fell to 0.038 mg/L after 20 hours, while a urine concentration of only 0.020 mg/L was observed for the first 24 hour specimen. A serum concentration of 0.004 mg/L was determined for the patient's husband, who had also eaten the bread but failed to develop symptoms (Coble et al., 1967). In the surviving victims of several mass endrin poisoning, blood concentrations of 0.007–0.032 mg/L and urine concentrations of less than 0.004 to 0.007 mg/L were measured on the day of onset of symptoms;

samples of blood and urine taken 29–31 days after the outbreak of poisoning were uniformly negative for endrin. Concentrations of 0.685 mg/kg in liver and 0.116 mg/kg in kidney were found in one fatal case (Curley et al., 1970). Blood endrin concentrations of 0.450, 0.086 and 0.071 mg/L were measured 4 hours, 6 and 11 days, respectively, after ingestion of 12 g of the chemical by an adult male who died on the 11th day; postmortem tissue concentrations were generally less than 1 mg/kg except for adipose, which contained 90 mg/kg (Runhaar et al., 1985).

Analysis. Endrin is measured in biological specimens using electron-capture gas chromatography techniques developed for the organochlorine insecticides as a class (Dale et al., 1966; Cueto and Biros, 1967).

References

M.K. Baldwin, J. Robinson and D.V. Parke. Metabolism of endrin in the rat. J. Agr. Food Chem. 18: 1117–1123, 1970.

M.K. Baldwin and D.H. Hutson. Analysis of human urine for a metabolite of endrin by chemical oxidation and gas-liquid chromatography as an indicator of exposure to endrin. Analyst 105: 60–65, 1980.

Y. Coble, P. Hildebrandt, J. Davis et al. Acute endrin poisoning. J. Am. Med. Asso. 202: 489–493, 1967.

C. Cueto, Jr. and F.J. Biros. Chlorinated insecticides and related materials in human urine. Tox. Appl. Pharm. 10: 261–269, 1967.

A. Curley, R.W. Jennings, H.T. Mann and V. Sedlak. Measurement of endrin following epidemics of poisoning. Bull. Env. Cont. Tox. 5: 24–29, 1970.

W.E. Dale, A. Curley and C. Cueto, Jr. Hexane extractable chlorinated insecticides in human blood. Life Sci. 5: 47–54, 1966.

G.M. Davies and I. Lewis. Outbreak of food-poisoning from bread made of chemically contaminated flour. Brit. Med. J. 2: 393–398, 1956.

W.J. Hayes, Jr., and C. Curley. Storage and excretion of dieldrin and related compounds. Arch. Env. Health 16: 155–162, 1968.

D.B. Reddy, V.D. Edward, G.J.S. Abraham and K.V. Rao. Fatal endrin poisoning. J. Ind. Med. Asso. 46: 121–124, 1966.

E.A. Runhaar, B. Sangster, P.A. Greve and M. Voortman. A case of fatal endrin poisoning. Hum. Tox. 4: 241–247, 1987.

D.E. Weeks. Endrin food-poisoning. Bull. W.H.O. 37: 499–512, 1967.

Enflurane

T½: 36 hr
Vd: ?
Fb: ?

CHF_2-O-CF_2CHClF

Occurrence and Usage. Enflurane (Ethrane) is a nonflammable halogenated methyl ethyl ether. It was introduced in 1973 as an alternative to other halogenated anesthetics such as halothane and methoxyflurane, whose biotransformation products have been implicated in hepatic and renal damage in man. The extent of metabolism of enflurane is less than for other related agents, due possibly to its higher stability and lower blood:gas (1.9) and fat:blood (37) partition coefficients.

Blood Concentrations. In 20 surgical patients receiving 0.5–2.5% enflurane, venous blood enflurane concentrations reached an average maximum of 95 mg/L after 30 minutes of anesthesia, and declined to less than 0.5 mg/L by 90 minutes after the discontinuance of the agent (Corall et al., 1977). The elimination of enflurane follows a 3 term exponential decay, with half-lives of 18 minutes (17% of the absorbed dose, located in the central compartment), 3.2 hours (41%, from the muscle tissue compartment), and 36 hours (42%, from the fat compartment) (Chase et al., 1971).

Metabolism and Excretion. An average of 82.7% of an administered dose of enflurane (1.5% constant alveolar concentration for up to 197 min) is exhaled unchanged over a 5 day period, with 50% exhaled during the first 18 hours. The total amount of enflurane absorbed by these patients during surgical anesthesia ranged from 12–32 g. Only 2.4% of the dose could be accounted for as non-volatile urinary metabolites in the 10 day postoperative period (Chase et al., 1971). Difluoromethoxydifluoroacetic acid, a product of oxidative dehalogenation, has been identified as a human urinary metabolite of enflurane (Miller and Gandolfi, 1980; Burke et al., 1981).

In a study of 102 patients receiving enflurane anesthesia, it was found that the mean serum inorganic fluoride concentration reached a maximum of 17 μmol/L at 3 hours after the initiation of exposure, and that the maximum individual concentration of 80 μmol/L was short-lived. It was concluded that enflurane was unlikely to produce renal failure as a result of the release of inorganic fluoride (Maduska, 1974). Renal fluoride excretion is urinary pH-dependent; enflurane patients with acid urine had an average maximal plasma fluoride concentration of 26 μmol/L as opposed to 14 μmol/L for those with alkaline urine (Jarnberg et al., 1981).

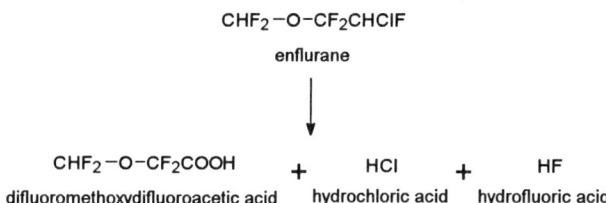

Toxicity. Several cases of severe acute hepatotoxicity after enflurane use have been reported, including two fatalities (Denlinger et al., 1974; van der Reis, 1974; Danilewitz et al., 1980; Ona et al., 1980; Paull and Fortune, 1987). Renal toxicity is not considered to be a hazard with this agent, although an occasional patient may develop a plasma fluoride concentration that exceeds the proposed nephrotoxic threshold level of 50 μmol/L (Cousins et al., 1976).

Two cases of fatal enflurane abuse by adult males have been reported; one individual had a postmortem blood enflurane concentration of 710 mg/L and the other had blood and brain concentrations of 130 mg/L and 350 mg/kg, respectively (Jacob et al., 1989; Walker and Morano, 1990).

Analysis. Enflurane has been determined in blood by gas chromatography with flame-ionization (Toner et al., 1977; Miller and Gandolfi, 1979; Jacob et al., 1989) or mass spectrometric detection (Urich et al., 1977).

References

T.R. Burke, Jr., R.V. Branchflower, D.E. Lees and L.R. Pohl. Mechanism of defluorination of enflurane. Drug Met. Disp. 9: 19–24, 1981.

R.E. Chase, D.A. Holaday, V. Fiserova-Bergerova et al. The biotransformation of Ethrane in man. Anesthesiology 35: 262–267, 1971.

I.M. Corall, K.M. Knights and L. Strunin. Enflurane (Ethrane) anesthesia in man. Brit. J. Anaesth. 49: 881–885, 1977.

M.J. Cousins, L.R. Greenstein, B.A. Hitt and R.I. Mazze. Metabolism and renal effects of enflurane in man. Anesthesiology 44: 44–53, 1976.

M.D. Danilewitz, B.M. Braude, H.M. Bloch et al. Acute hepatitis following enflurane anaesthesia. Brit. J. Anaesth. 52: 1151–1153, 1980.

J.K. Denlinger, J.H. Lecky and M.L. Nahrwold. Hepatocellular dysfunction without jaundice after enflurane anesthesia. Anesthesiology 41: 86–87, 1974.

B. Jacob, C. Heller, T. Daldrup et al. Fatal accidental enflurane intoxication. J. For. Sci. 34: 1408–1412, 1989.

P.O. Jarnberg, J. Ekstrand and L. Irestedt. Renal fluoride excretion and plasma fluoride levels during and after enflurane anesthesia are dependent on urinary pH. Anesthesiology 54: 48–52, 1981.

A.L. Maduska. Serum inorganic fluoride levels in patients receiving enflurane anesthesia. Anesth. Anal. 53: 351–353, 1974.

M.S. Miller and A.J. Gandolfi. A rapid, sensitive method for quantifying enflurane in whole blood. Anesthesiology 51: 542–544, 1979.

M.S. Miller and A.J. Gandolfi. Enflurane biotransformation in humans. Life Sci. 27: 1465–1468, 1980.

F.V. Ona, H. Patanella and A. Ayub. Hepatitis associated with enflurane anesthesia. Anesth. Anal. 59: 146–149, 1980.

J.D. Paull and D.W. Fortune. Hepatotoxicity and death following two enflurane anaesthetics. Anaesthesia 42: 1191–1196, 1987.

W. Toner, P.J. Howard, M.G. Scott et al. Estimation of blood enflurane concentrations by gas-liquid chromatography. Brit. J. Anaesth. 49: 871–873, 1977.

R.W. Urich, D.L. Bowerman, P.H. Wittenberg et al. Head space mass spectrometric analysis for volatiles in biological specimens. J. Anal. Tox. 1: 195–199, 1977.

L. van der Reis, S.J. Askin, G.N. Frecker and W.J. Fitzgerald. Hepatic necrosis after enflurane anesthesia. J. Am. Med. Asso. 227: 76, 1974.

F.B. Walker and R.A. Morano. Fatal recreational inhalation of enflurane. J. For. Sci. 35: 197–198, 1990.

Ephedrine

T½: 5.0– 7.5 hr
Vd: ?
Fb: ?
pKa: 9.6

Occurrence and Usage. Ephedrine, as the l-isomer, is a naturally-occurring sympathomimetic amine that has pronounced peripheral actions and a mild central stimulant effect. It is used as a nasal decongestant, bronchodilator and pressor agent, and may be administered orally or by parenteral injection in doses of 10–50 mg as the hydrochloride or sulfate salt.

Blood Concentrations. A single 24 mg oral dose of ephedrine given to a volunteer resulted in a peak plasma concentration slightly exceeding 0.100 mg/L after 1 hour, declining to about 0.068 mg/L by 3 hours (Midha et al., 1979). A patient receiving chronic daily oral therapy with 45 mg of ephedrine in 3 divided doses achieved plasma concentrations of 0.095 and 0.065 mg/L at 4 and 6 hours after one 15 mg dose (Pickup and Paterson, 1974). The elimination half-life of the drug averages 5.7 hours (Welling et al., 1971).

Metabolism and Excretion. Ephedrine is metabolized in man primarily by N-demethylation to norephedrine and probably to a minor extent by p-hydroxylation and conjugation. In normal subjects, from 70–80% of a dose is eliminated unchanged in the 48 hour urine and about 4% is present as norephedrine. Acidification of the urine increases these values only slightly, whereas alkalinization results in the excretion of less ephedrine (22–35%) and more norephedrine (11–24%) (Beckett and Wilkinson, 1965a; Wilkinson and Beckett, 1968; Welling et al., 1971). A 14 mg intranasal dose in 8 adults gave rise to urinary ephedrine concentrations of 0.9–17 mg/L over the next 10 hours (Lefebvre et al., 1992).

ephedrine → norephedrine

Toxicity. The effects of overdosage with ephedrine are similar to those of amphetamine. At least 5 cases of psychosis due to chronic abuse of the drug have been reported; symptoms included paranoid delusions, hallucinations, and hostile behavior (Herridge and A'Brook, 1968; Roxanas and Spalding, 1977). A 20 year old woman survived the ingestion of 7.5 g of ephedrine after developing agitation, anxiety, tremors, tachycardia and emesis; her peak serum ephedrine concentration at 1.5 hours post-ingestion was 23 mg/L (Snook et al. 1992).

A young woman who died several hours after ingesting 2.1 g ephedrine and 7.0 g caffeine had postmortem ephedrine levels of 5 mg/L in blood, 15 mg/kg in liver and 547 mg/L in urine (Ryall, 1984).

Analysis. Ephedrine has been assayed in biological specimens by ultraviolet spectrophotometry after periodate oxidation (Wallace, 1969). Gas chromatographic techniques for the determination of ephedrine in plasma (Pickup and Paterson, 1974) and of the parent and norephedrine in urine (Beckett and Wilkinson, 1965b; Welling et al., 1971) have relied on flame-ionization detection of the underivatized compounds, or electron-capture detection of a halogenated derivative (Midha et al., 1979). Liquid chromatography has also been described (Lefebvre et al., 1992).

References

A.H. Beckett and G.R. Wilkinson. Urinary excretion of (-)-methylephedrine, (-)-ephedrine and (-)-norephedrine in man. J. Pharm. Pharmac. 17: 107S–108S, 1965a.

A.H. Beckett and G.R. Wilkinson. Identification and determination of ephedrine and its congeners in urine by gas chromatography. J. Pharm. Pharmac. 17: 104S–106S, 1965b.

C.F. Herridge and M.F. A'Brook. Ephedrine psychosis. Brit. Med. J. 2: 160, 1968.

R.A. Lefebvre, F. Surmont, J. Bouckaert and E. Moerman. Urinary excretion of ephedrine after nasal application in healthy volunteers. J. Pharm. Pharmacol. 44: 672–675, 1992.

K.K. Midha, J.K. Cooper and I.J. McGilveray. Simple and specific electron-capture GLC assay for plasma and urine ephedrine concentrations following single doses. J. Pharm. Sci. 68: 557–560, 1979.

M.E. Pickup and J.W. Paterson. The determination of ephedrine plasma levels by a gas chromatographic method. J. Pharm. Pharmac. 26: 561–562, 1974.

M.G. Roxanas and J. Spalding. Ephedrine abuse psychosis. Med. J. Aust. 2: 639–640, 1977.

J.E. Ryall. Personal communication, 1984.

C. Snook, M. Otten and M. Hassan. Massive ephedrine overdose. Vet. Hum. Tox. 34: 335, 1992.

J.E. Wallace. Determination of phenethanolamine drugs in biologic specimens by ultraviolet spectrophotometry. J. Pharm. Sci. 58: 1489–1492, 1969.

P.G. Welling, K.P. Lee, J.A. Patel et al. Urinary excretion of ephedrine in man without pH control following oral administration of three commercial ephedrine sulfate preparations. J. Pharm. Sci. 60: 1629–1634, 1971.

G.R. Wilkinson and A.H. Beckett. Absorption, metabolism and excretion of the ephedrine in man. I. The influence of urinary pH and urine volume output. J. Pharm. Exp. Ther. 162: 139–147, 1968.

Estazolam

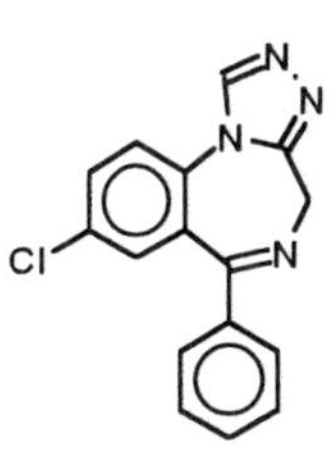

T½: 10–24 hr
Vd: ?
Fb: 0.93
pKa: ?

Occurrence and Usage. Estazolam (Prosom) is a triazolobenzodiazepine derivative that is similar structurally to alprazolam and triazolam. Estazolam has been classified as an intermediate-acting benzodiazepine hypnotic, indicated for the short-term management of insomnia. It is available for oral use in tablets containing 1–2 mg of the free base.

Blood Concentrations. A single 1 mg oral dose of estazolam to 17 healthy male volunteers weighing 61–81 kg produced an average maximum plasma concentration of 55 µg/L (range, 42–70) within 2 hours; a 2 mg dose to the same group gave a maximum plasma concentration of 98 µg/L (range, 75–137) (Gustavson and Carrigan, 1990).

Metabolism and Excretion. Only 2 metabolites, 1-oxoestazolam and 4-hydroxyestazolam, are detectable in human plasma up to 18 hours after dosage; both metabolites have some pharmacologic activity, but their low potencies and low concentrations argue against significant contribution to the hypnotic effect of estazolam. After 5 days, 87% of a single dose was recovered in human urine while fecal excretion accounted for 4%. The parent drug in the urine accounted for less than 4% of the administered dose (Kanai, 1974; Machinist et al., 1986).

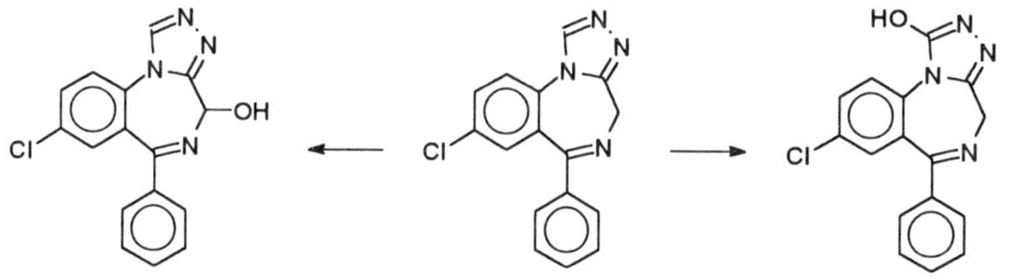

4-OH-estazolam   estazolam   1-oxoestazolam

Toxicity. Manifestations of overdosage with estazolam include somnolence, respiratory depression, confusion, impaired coordination, slurred speech and coma. Following ingestion of approximately 60 mg of estazolam in an unsuccessful suicide attempt, a woman exhibited drowsiness, confusion and agitation; blood collected 2 days later contained 1250 µg/L estazolam (di Tella et al., 1986).

Analysis. Estazolam has been determined in biological specimens by gas chromatography with electron-capture detection (Allen et al., 1979; Cailleux and Turcant, 1981). Liquid chromatography has also been employed (di Tella et al., 1986; Machinist et al., 1986; Boukhabza et al., 1991).

References

M.D. Allen, D. Greenblatt and J.D. Arnold. Single and multiple dose kinetics of estazolam, a triazolo-benzodiazepine. Psychopharmacologia 66: 267–274, 1979.

A. Boukhabza, A.A.J. Lugnier, P. Kintz and P. Mangin. Simultaneous HPLC analysis of the hypnotic benzodiazepines nitrazepam, estazolam, flunitrazepam, and triazolam in plasma. J. Anal. Tox. 15: 319–322, 1991.

A.S. di Tella, P. Ricci, C. Di Nunzio and P. Cassandro. A new method for the determination in blood and urine of a novel triazolobenzodiazepine (estazolam) by HPLC. J. Anal. Tox. 10: 65–67, 1986.

L.E. Gustavson and P.J. Carrigan. The clinical pharmacokinetics of single doses of estazolam. Am. J. Med. 88: 2S–5S, 1990.

Y. Kanai. The biotransformation of 8-chloro-6-phenyl-4H-s-triazolo(4,3a)(1,4)benzodiazepine (D-40 TA), a new central depressant in man, dog and rats. Xenobiotica 4: 441–456, 1974.

J.M. Machinist, B.A. Bopp, D.J. Anderson et al. Metabolism of ^{14}C-estazolam in dogs and humans. Xenobiotica 16: 11–20, 1986.

Ethanol

T½: 2–14 hr (zero-order)
Vd: 0.53 L/kg
Fb: 0

CH_3CH_2OH

Occurrence and Usage. Like caffeine and nicotine, ethanol (ethyl alcohol, alcohol) is primarily a social drug and is used only rarely in therapeutics. It is present to the extent of 3–6% by volume in naturally fermented beers and ales, 10–12% in wines, and 20–60% in distilled beverages. The compound is also found in many elixirs, mouthwashes, and other medicinal liquids in appreciable amounts. Ethanol is widely encountered as a manufactured product and as a solvent in industry, where many employees are exposed to the compound by inhalation of the vapor. The current threshold limit value for industrial exposure is 1000 ppm (1900 mg/m^3). Therapeutically, ethanol may be administered intravenously to patients poisoned by methanol or ethylene glycol to prevent their conversion to toxic metabolites.

Blood Concentrations. Because ethanol distributes evenly throughout the body water, its concentration in blood following a known dose may be estimated on the basis of the subject's sex, body weight and degree of adiposity. Ethanol is present as an endogenous substance in the blood of man, probably produced in the intestinal tract, at an average level of 0.00015 g/dL (Lester, 1962). Resting subjects developed blood ethanol concentrations of less than 0.01 g/dL when exposed to vapor concentrations of 7500–8500 ppm for 3 hours, while an exercising subject developed a blood level of 0.05 g/dL under the same conditions (Lester and Greenberg, 1951). A single oral dose of 0.5 mL/kg (35 mL/70 kg) of pure ethanol given to 4 fasting men produced an average maximal blood concentration of about 0.04 g/dL at 2 hours; a dose of 1.4 mL/kg (98 mL/70 kg) produced a level of 0.12 g/dL at 1 hour; and 2.0 mL/kg (140 mL/70 kg), a level of 0.20 g/dL at 1 hour. The levels declined at a mean rate for the 21 subjects of 0.0189 g/dL per hour (Sidell and Pless, 1971). The presence of food in the stomach may cause up to 70% reduction in the peak blood ethanol concentration attained after a measured oral dose; this effect is due to a reduction in both the efficiency and rate of absorption of the ethanol (Lin et al., 1976; Wilkinson et al., 1977).

Metabolism and Excretion. The metabolism of alcohol proceeds at a rate that has been assumed to be essentially independent of the dose (zero-order); this is a valid approximation at higher concentrations, but at concentrations less than 0.02 g/dL the kinetics of elimination become first-order and therefore non-linear (Wagner et al., 1976). There is evidence that first-order kinetics also apply at very high blood ethanol concentrations (Hammond et al., 1973; Bogusz et al., 1977). Ethanol is biotransformed to acetaldehyde and then to acetic acid by liver enzymes; these enzymes are induced during chronic ethanol administration, which may result in an increase of up to 72% in the rate of ethanol disappearance from the blood of naive subjects (Misra et al., 1971). Other authors have found that this effect is not consistent in all subjects (Vesell et al., 1971). Acetaldehyde accumulates to a slight extent in the blood of normal persons after ethanol administration, and to a greater extent in alcoholic subjects; these concentrations are on the order of a thousandth of the ethanol levels (Korsten et al., 1975). About 95% of a dose undergoes metabolism and the remainder is excreted unchanged in the breath, urine, sweat and feces.

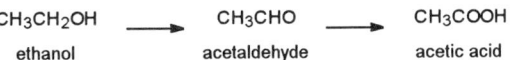

At equilibrium, the concentration of ethanol in any tissue or fluid is a function of the water content of that specimen. It has been determined that the plasma/whole blood ratio varies from 1.10–1.35 with an average of 1.18 (Payne et al., 1968). Urine concentrations of alcohol are often used to estimate blood concentrations; during the elimination phase the urine/blood ratio of 1.3

applies and provides a valid estimate in most cases (Heise, 1967). The blood/breath ratio during the elimination phase averages 2180, with a range of 1837–2863 (Jones, 1978). The mean alcohol content of other tissues expressed as a ratio to blood is as follows (Committee on Medicolegal Problems, 1970):

Tissue/Blood Ethanol Distribution Ratios

Brain	Blood Clot	Fat	Liver	Saliva
0.65–0.94	0.77	0.02	0.91	1.12

Toxicity. A blood alcohol concentration of 0.53 g/dL was determined in a 45 year old man who was involved in an automobile accident and who was unable to stand without assistance (Pons, 1976). A 23 year old female patient in light coma was found to have a blood ethanol level of 0.78 g/dL; after 3 hours this had fallen to 0.52 g/dL and the woman was able to provide a medical history (Hammond et al., 1973). Lindblad and Olsson (1976) reported on 16 intoxicated patients with serum alcohol concentrations of 0.52–0.78 g/dL who demonstrated only mild to moderate central nervous system depression. A 55 year old man achieved a blood alcohol concentration of 1.13 g/dL during a suicide attempt, but survived the incident with supportive treatment (Berild and Hasselbalch, 1981).

The range of blood alcohol concentrations in 94 acute fatal ethanol intoxications was 0.18–0.60 g/dL; the blood concentrations were found to vary inversely with the length of the survival period, and it was estimated that antemortem concentrations in these cases had at one time ranged from 0.50–0.60 g/dL (Kaye and Haag, 1957). Christopoulos et al. (1973) reported on 10 such cases involving unusually high concentrations that demonstrated the following body distribution:

Ethanol Concentrations in Acute Fatal Cases (g/dL or g/100 g)

	Blood	Brain	CSF	Liver	Kidney	Urine
Average	0.74	0.44	0.58	0.45	0.48	0.62
(Range)	(0.42–1.77)	(0.31–0.91)	(0.40–0.82)	(0.25–1.16)	(0.29–1.04)	(0.49–0.94)

Analysis. Since ethanol is both formed and destroyed in biological specimens *in vitro*, the proper preservation of these specimens is important for analytical purposes. The formation of alcohol by microorganisms is inhibited by fluoride, mercuric ion and cold storage; ethanol loss occurs by volatilization and destruction by microorganisms, both of which are retarded by the above conditions, and by hemoglobin oxidation, which may be inhibited by sodium azide (Bradford, 1966; Brown et al., 1973; Christopoulos et al., 1973; Smalldon and Brown, 1973; Corry, 1978). Blood alcohol produced by postmortem decomposition rarely exceeds 0.05 g/dL in concentration (Winek, 1975).

Chemical, enzymatic and instrumental methods for the determination of ethanol in biologic specimens have been reviewed by Jain and Cravey (1972a; 1972b). Flame-ionization gas chromatographic techniques are in use in most laboratories and usually involve direct sample injection (Parker et al., 1962; Jain, 1971; Cooper, 1971; Manno and Manno, 1978) or headspace analysis (Wallace and Dahl, 1966; Wilkinson et al., 1975; Anthony et al., 1980; Penton, 1985). Recently, mass fragmentography procedures have been proposed that are sensitive and highly specific (Bonnichsen et al., 1972; Pereira et al., 1974). Ethanol causes an increase in the serum osmolality ("osmolal gap") in proportion to its serum concentration, providing a convenient means of estimating ethanol levels in clinical situations (Pappas et al., 1981).

References

R.A. Anthony, C.A. Sutheimer and I. Sunshine. Acetaldehyde, methanol, and ethanol analysis by headspace gas chromatography. J. Anal. Tox. 4: 43–45, 1980.

D. Berild and H. Hasselbalch. Survival after a blood alcohol of 1127 mg/dL. Lancet 2: 363, 1981.

M. Bogusz, J. Pach and W. Stasko. Comparative studies on the rate of ethanol elimination in acute poisoning and in controlled conditions. J. For. Sci. 22: 446–451, 1977.

R. Bonnichsen, B. Hedfjall and R. Ryhage. Determination of ethyl alcohol by computerized mass chromatography. Z. Rechtsmed. 71: 134–138, 1972.

L.W. Bradford. Preservation of blood samples containing alcohol. J. For. Sci. 11: 214–216, 1966.

G.A. Brown, D. Neylan, W.J. Reynolds and K.W. Smalldon. The stability of ethanol in stored blood. Anal. Chim. Acta 66: 271–283, 1973.

G. Christopoulos, E.R. Kirch and J.E. Gearien. Determination of ethanol in fresh and putrefied post mortem tissues. J. Chrom. 87: 455–472, 1973.

Committee on Medicolegal Problems. *Alcohol and the Impaired Driver*, American Medical Association, Chicago, 1970, pp. 18–19.

J.D.H. Cooper. Determination of blood ethanol by gas chromatography. Clin. Chim. Acta 33: 483–485, 1971.

J.E.L. Corry. Possible sources of ethanol ante- and post-mortem: its relationship to the biochemistry and microbiology of decomposition. J. Appl. Bacteriol. 44: 1–56, 1978.

K.B. Hammond, B.H. Rumack and D.O. Rodgerson. Blood ethanol. J. Am. Med. Asso. 226: 63–64, 1973.

H.A. Heise. Concentrations of alcohol in samples of blood and urine taken at the same time. J. For. Sci. 12: 454–462, 1967.

N.C. Jain. Direct blood-injection method for gas chromatographic determination of alcohols and other volatile compounds. Clin. Chem. 17: 82–85, 1971.

N.C. Jain and R.H. Cravey. Analysis of alcohol. I. A review of chemical and infrared methods. J. Chrom. Sci. 10: 257–262, 1972a.

N.C. Jain and R.H. Cravey. Analysis of alcohol. II. A review of gas chromatographic methods. J. Chrom. Sci. 10: 263–267, 1972b.

A.W. Jones. Variability of the blood:breath alcohol ratio in vivo. J. Stud. Alc. 39: 1931–1933, 1978.

S. Kaye and H.B. Haag. Terminal blood alcohol concentrations in ninety-four fatal cases of acute alcoholism. J. Am. Med. Asso. 165: 451–452, 1957.

M.A. Korsten, S. Matsuzaki, L. Feinman and C.S. Leiber. High blood acetaldehyde levels after ethanol administration. New Eng. J. Med. 292: 386–389, 1975.

D. Lester. The concentration of apparent endogenous ethanol. Quart. J. Stud. Alc. 23: 17–25, 1962.

D. Lester and L.A. Greenberg. The inhalation of ethyl alcohol by man. Quart. J. Stud. Alc. 12: 167–178, 1951.

Y.J. Lin, D.J. Weidler, D.C. Garg and J.G. Wagner. Effects of solid food on blood levels of alcohol in man. Res. Comm. Chem. Path. Pharm. 13: 713–722, 1976.

B. Lindblad and R. Olsson. Unusually high levels of blood alcohol. J. Am. Med. Asso. 236: 1600–1602, 1976.

B.R. Manno and J.E. Manno. A simple approach to gas chromatographic microanalysis of alcohols in blood and urine by a direct-injection technique. J. Anal. Tox. 2: 257–261, 1978.

P.S. Misra, A. LeFevre, H. Ishii et al. Increase of ethanol, meprobamate and pentobarbital metabolism after chronic ethanol administration in man and in rats. Am. J. Med. 51: 346–351, 1971.

A.A. Pappas, R.H. Gadsden, Jr., R.H. Gadsden, Sr. and W.E. Groves. Osmolality, blood ethanol compared. Clin. Chem. News, July, 1981, p. 46.

K.D. Parker, C.R. Fontan, J.L. Yee and P.L. Kirk. Gas chromatographic determination of ethyl alcohol in blood for medicolegal purposes. Anal. Chem. 34: 1234–1236, 1962.

J.P. Payne, D.W. Hill and D.G.L. Wood. Distribution of ethanol between plasma and erythrocytes in whole blood. Nature 217: 963–964, 1968.

Z. Penton. Headspace measurement of ethanol in blood by gas chromatography with a modified autosampler. Clin. Chem. 31: 439–441, 1985.

W.E. Pereira, R.E. Summons, T.C. Rindfleisch and A.M. Duffield. The determination of ethanol in blood and urine by mass fragmentography. Clin. Chim. Acta 51: 109–112, 1974.

C. Pons. Personal communication, 1976.

F.R. Sidell and J.E. Pless. Ethyl alcohol: blood levels and performance decrements after oral administration to man. Psychopharmacologia 19: 246–261, 1971.

K.W. Smalldon and G.A. Brown. The stability of ethanol in stored blood. Part II. The mechanism of ethanol oxidation. Anal. Chim. Acta 66: 285–290, 1973.

E.S. Vesell, J.G. Page and G.T. Passananti. Genetic and environmental factors affecting ethanol metabolism in man. Clin. Pharm. Ther. 12: 192–201, 1971.

J.G. Wagner, P.K. Wilkinson, A.J. Sedman et al. Elimination of alcohol from human blood. J. Pharm. Sci. 65: 152–154, 1976.

J.E. Wallace and E.V. Dahl. Rapid vapor phase method for determining ethanol in blood and urine by gas chromatography. Am. J. Clin. Path. 46: 152–154, 1966.

P.K. Wilkinson, J.G. Wagner and A.J. Sedman. Sensitive head-space gas chromatographic method for the determination of ethanol utilizing capillary blood samples. Anal. Chem. 47: 1506–1510, 1975.

P.K. Wilkinson, A.J. Sedman, E. Sakmar et al. Fasting and nonfasting blood ethanol concentrations following repeated oral administration of ethanol to one adult male subject. J. Pharm. Biopharm. 5: 41–52, 1977.

C.L. Winek. Reliability of 22-hour postmortem blood and gastric alcohol samples. J. Am. Med. Asso. 233: 912, 1975.

Ethchlorvynol

T½: 19–32 hr
Vd: 2.4–3.2 L/kg
Fb: 0.62

$$CH_3CH_2\overset{\overset{\displaystyle C\equiv CH}{|}}{\underset{\underset{\displaystyle OH}{|}}{C}}CH\text{--}CHCl$$

Occurrence and Usage. Ethchlorvynol (Placidyl) is an acetylenic alcohol first released for use as a sedative and hypnotic agent in 1955. The compound is an aromatic liquid at room temperature that darkens on exposure to air. It is available in oral dosage forms of 100–500 mg and up to 1000 mg may be administered in a single dose.

Blood Concentrations. A single oral 200 mg dose of ethchlorvynol produced an average peak blood concentration of 1.2 mg/L (range, 0.6–1.8) in 6 subjects at 1 hour after ingestion (Maes et al., 1969). After a 500 mg oral dose given to 8 subjects, serum concentrations of the drug averaged 6.5 mg/L at 1 hour, 2.0 mg/L at 6 hours and 0.5 mg/L at 48 hours. The peak concentration after a 750 mg dose was 8.0 mg/L at 1 hour and the terminal serum half-life averaged 23 hours (Cummins et al., 1971). The blood/plasma concentration ratio for ethchlorvynol averages 0.88 (Benowitz et al., 1980).

Metabolism and Excretion. Very little is known regarding the metabolic fate of ethchlorvynol. Only 0.025% of a dose is excreted in the 25 hour urine as the unchanged drug or a conjugate. Urine concentrations of intact drug during this period are generally less than 2 mg/L (Cummins et al., 1971; Maes et al., 1969). The compound is known to localize in adipose tissue and is probably slowly released from these depots to be metabolized and excreted over a period of many days. A metabolite, hydroxyethchlorvynol, has been isolated from human tissues (Horwitz et al., 1980).

$$CH_3CH_2\overset{\overset{\displaystyle C\equiv CH}{|}}{\underset{\underset{\displaystyle OH}{|}}{C}}CH=CHCl \longrightarrow CH_3CHOH\overset{\overset{\displaystyle C\equiv CH}{|}}{\underset{\underset{\displaystyle OH}{|}}{C}}CH=CHCl$$

ethchlorvynol   hydroxyethchlorvynol

Toxicity. A number of clinical reports have appeared regarding patients with severe ethchlorvynol intoxication who have survived the prolonged deep coma that is a common feature of overdosage with this drug. Maximal serum or plasma ethchlorvynol concentrations in these persons have ranged from 111–280 mg/L after the ingestion of up to 50 g; estimates of the half-life of ethchlorvynol ranged from 21–105 hours, and in many instances hemodialysis or resin hemoperfusion significantly enhanced the clearance of the agent. Using nonspecific analytical methods to measure urine ethchlorvynol concentrations, the renal clearance of unchanged drug appears significant; however, with gas chromatographic techniques it was found that unchanged drug represented only 2% of the drug-related urinary excretion products (Schultz et al., 1966; Teehan et al., 1970; Gibson and Wright, 1972; Welch et al., 1972; Tozer et al., 1974; Pochopien, 1975; Benowitz et al., 1980; Hull et al., 1980).

While chronic abusers of ethchlorvynol have been known to consume up to 4 g of the drug daily for many months and to attain steady-state serum concentrations of up to 37 mg/L, one adult has died after the acute ingestion of 2.5 g (Millhouse et al., 1966; Flemenbaum and Gunby, 1971). In 13 deaths due to overdosage with ethchlorvynol, postmortem blood concentrations averaged 119 mg/L (range, 14–400) (Rehling, 1967). The following tissue concentrations were determined in 8 acute ethchlorvynol fatalities (Cravey and Baselt, 1968; Poklis, 1974; Finkle, 1975; Gottschalk and Cravey, 1980; Winek et al., 1981; Winek et al., 1989):

Ethchlorvynol Concentrations in Fatal Cases (mg/L or mg/kg)

	Blood	Brain	Liver	Kidney	Fat
Average	98	147	401	284	591
(Range)	(22–213)	(57–285)	(60–1600)	(54–860)	(142–1040)

Analysis. Several spectrophotometric procedures for the determination of ethchlorvynol in biologic media have been found to be convenient and sensitive, but somewhat non-specific, especially when the organs of excretion or their products are analyzed. These techniques have employed phloroglucinol (Algeri et al., 1962), diphenylamine (Andryauskis et al., 1967; Frings and Cohen, 1970; Haux, 1973) or formation of an oxidation product (Wallace et al., 1964). The latter method has been modified to improve upon its specificity (Wallace et al., 1974). The published gas chromatographic procedures involve solvent extraction of the specimen with detection by flame-ionization (Robinson, 1968; Maes et al., 1969; Gibson and Wright, 1972; Evenson and Poquette, 1974; Flanagan and Lee, 1977; McCurdy, 1977) or electron-capture (Cummins et al., 1971). Preliminary results pertaining to a high-pressure liquid chromatographic method that requires synthesis of a semicarbazone derivative have appeared (Needham and Kochhar, 1975). Winek et al. (1981) have noted substantial losses (13–90%) of ethchlorvynol from biological specimens after 3 months of refrigeration.

References

E.J. Algeri, G.G. Katsas and M.A. Luongo. Determination of ethchlorvynol in biologic mediums, and report of two fatal cases. Am. J. Clin. Path. 38: 125–130, 1962.

S. Andryauskis, W. Matusiak, J.R. Broich et al. Ethchlorvynol in toxicological analysis. Int. Microfilm J. Leg. Med. 2: Card 4, 1967.

N. Benowitz, C. Abolin, T. Tozer et al. Resin hemoperfusion in ethchlorvynol overdose. Clin. Pharm. Ther. 27: 236–242, 1980.

R.H. Cravey and R.C. Baselt. Studies of the body distribution of ethchlorvynol. J. For. Sci. 13: 532–536, 1968.

L.M. Cummins, Y.C. Martin and E.E. Scherfling. Serum and urine levels of ethchlorvynol in man. J. Pharm. Sci. 60: 261–263, 1971.

M.A. Evenson and M.A. Poquette. Rapid gas chromatographic method for quantitation of ethchlorvynol ("Placidyl") in serum. Clin. Chem. 20: 212–216, 1974.

B. Finkle. Personal communication, 1975.

R.J. Flanagan and T.J. Lee. Rapid micro-method for the measurement of ethchlorvynol in blood plasma and in urine by gas-liquid chromatography. J. Chrom. 137: 119–126, 1977.

A. Flemenbaum and B. Gunby. Ethchlorvynol (Placidyl) abuse and withdrawal. Dis. Nerv. Sys. 32: 188–192, 1971.

C.S. Frings and P.S. Cohen. Rapid colorimetric method for the quantitative determination of ethchlorvynol (Placidyl) in serum and urine. Am. J. Clin. Path. 54: 833–836, 1970.

P.F. Gibson and N. Wright. Ethchlorvynol in biological fluids: specificity of assay methods. J. Pharm. Sci. 169–171, 1972.

L.A. Gottschalk and R.H. Cravey. *Toxicological and Pathological Studies on Psychoactive Drug-Involved Deaths*, Biomedical Publications, Davis, California, 1980, pp. 220–227.

P. Haux. Ethchlorvynol (Placidyl) estimation in urine and serum. Clin. Chim. Acta 43: 139–141, 1973.

J.P. Horwitz, W. Brukwinski, J. Treisman et al. Ethchlorvynol: potential of metabolites for adverse effects in man. Drug Met. Disp. 8: 77–83, 1980.

J.D. Hull, K.J. Tabor, D.P. Hays et al. Resin hemoperfusion for ethchlorvynol (Placidyl) intoxication. Vet. Hum. Tox. 22 (Suppl. 2): 31–34, 1980.

R. Maes, N. Hodnett, H. Landesman et al. The gas chromatographic determination of selected sedatives (ethchlorvynol, paraldehyde, meprobamate, and carisoprodol) in biological material. J. For. Sci. 14: 235–254, 1969.

H.H. McCurdy. Quantitation of ethchlorvynol by gas chromatography. J. Anal. Tox. 1: 164–165, 1977.

J. Millhouse, D.M. Davies and S.R. Wraith. Chronic ethchlorvynol intoxication. Lancet 2: 1251–1252, 1966.

L.L. Needham and M.M. Kochhar. Determination of ethchlorvynol by high-pressure liquid chromatography. J. Chrom. 111: 422–425, 1975.

D.J. Pochopien. Rate of decrease in serum ethchlorvynol concentrations after extreme overdosage—a case study. Clin. Chem. 21: 894–895, 1975.

A. Poklis. Personal communication, 1974.

C.J. Rehling. Poison residues in human tissues. In *Progress in Chemical Toxicology*, Vol. 3 (A. Stolman, ed.), Academic Press, New York, 1967, pp. 363–386.

D.W. Robinson. Method for determining ethchlorvynol in urine and serum by gas chromatography. J. Pharm. Sci. 57: 185–186, 1968.

J.C. Schultz, D.G. Crowder and W.S. Medart. Excretion studies in ethchlorvynol (Placidyl) intoxication. Arch. Int. Med. 117: 409–411, 1966.

B.P. Teehan, J.F. Maher, J.J.H. Carey et al. Acute ethchlorvynol (Placidyl) intoxication. Ann. Int. Med. 72: 875–882, 1970.

T.N. Tozer, L.D. Witt, L. Gee et al. Evaluation of hemodialysis for ethchlorvynol (Placidyl) overdosage. Am. J. Hosp. Pharm. 31: 986–989, 1974.

J.E. Wallace, W.J. Wilson, Jr. and E.V. Dahl. A rapid and specific method for determining ethchlorvynol. J. For. Sci. 9: 342–352, 1964.

J.E. Wallace, H.E. Hamilton, J.A. Riloff and K. Blum. Spectrophotometric determination of ethchlorvynol in biological specimens. Clin. Chem. 20: 159–162, 1974.

L.T. Welch, J.D. Bower, C.E. Ott and A.S. Hume. Oil dialysis for ethchlorvynol intoxication. Clin. Pharm. Ther. 13: 745–749, 1972.

C.L. Winek, J.D. Bricker and F.M. Esposito. A death due to ethchlorvynol abuse. A case report. For. Sci. Int. 17: 219–224, 1981.

C.L. Winek, W.W. Wahba and C.L. Winek, Jr. Body distribution of ethchlorvynol. J. For. Sci. 34: 687–690, 1989.

Ether

T½: ?

Vd: ? $CH_3CH_2OCH_2CH_3$

Fb: ?

Occurrence and Usage. Ether (diethyl ether, ethyl ether) is a volatile and flammable liquid that is utilized primarily as a solvent in the manufacture of synthetic dyes and plastics. Although it was the first successful surgical anesthetic agent, due to its flammability and irritating odor it is rarely used today. Also, its high solubility in body fluids and tissues results in a slow induction of anesthesia and a lengthy recovery. For this reason, induction is often performed at ether concentrations of 10–15% in the inspired air and the concentration is gradually reduced to approximately 5% as the desired level of anesthesia is attained. The current threshold limit value for occupational exposure is 400 ppm (1210 mg/m^3) in the workroom air.

Blood Concentrations. Blood ether concentrations in workers exposed at the current TLV have been estimated to reach 18 mg/L (ACGIH, 1971). Subanesthetic doses of ether, which produce analgesia but not unconsciousness, result in arterial blood concentrations of 100–500 mg/L. During surgical anesthesia these concentrations vary between 500 and 1500 mg/L, with an average deep surgical anesthesia concentration of 1200 mg/L in arterial blood (Faulconer, 1952).

Metabolism and Excretion. Over 90% of a dose of ether is exhaled unchanged after exposure ceases; a small amount is excreted in urine and there is a minor degree of biotransformation via oxidation to water and carbon dioxide (Price, 1975). Acetaldehyde is believed to be a minor metabolite of ether in man (Aune et al., 1978). The following partition coefficients are exhibited by ether at normal body temperature (Wollman and Smith, 1975):

Blood:Gas	Brain:Blood	Liver:Blood	Kidney:Blood	Fat:Blood
12	1.0–1.1	0.9	0.8	4.2

Toxicity. Inhalation of ether at the TLV may cause nose and throat irritation. Exposure to higher concentrations produces central nervous system depression, with nausea, irregular respiration, and lowering of body temperature and pulse rate. Concentrations of 2000 ppm are known to cause dizziness in some individuals and are associated with a blood ether concentration of about 90 mg/L; a level of 100,000 ppm may be rapidly fatal. Reports of toxicity due to chronic exposure to ether indicate that symptoms include loss of appetite, headache, exhaustion and psychic disturbances (ACGIH, 1971).

Relatively little data are available regarding tissue concentrations of ether in overdosage, although persons have died following the intentional ingestion of as little as 30 mL of the liquid. The following information on ether distribution was obtained on 3 surgical patients who died within 2.5 hours of cessation of ether administration (Campbell, 1960):

Tissue Distribution of Ether in Surgical Deaths (mg/L or mg/kg)

Blood	Brain	Lungs	Liver	Urine
600	700	200	400	
2880	2720	210	260	
3750	610	1580	1280	340

Analysis. While gas chromatography is used most frequently in the analysis of ether in biological specimens (Noehren and Cudmore, 1961; Northington and Owens, 1964; Rackow et al., 1966; Yokota et al., 1967), other techniques such as mass spectrometry (Jones et al., 1950) and infrared spectrophotometry (Feldstein, 1965) have also been investigated. Ether may co-elute with acetone in gas chromatographic systems designed for analysis of common volatiles in blood.

References

ACGIH. *Documentation of the Threshold Limit Values*, American Conference of Governmental Industrial Hygienists, Cincinnati, Ohio, 1971, p. 106.

H. Aune, H. Renck, A. Bessesen and J. Morland. Metabolism of diethyl ether to acetaldehyde in man. Lancet 2: 97, 1978.

J.E. Campbell. Deaths associated with anesthesia. J. For. Sci. 5: 501–549, 1960.

A. Faulconer, Jr. Correlation of concentrations of ether in arterial blood with electron-encephalographic patterns occurring during ether-oxygen and during nitrous oxide, oxygen and ether anesthesia of human surgical patients. Anesthesiology 13: 361–369, 1952.

M. Feldstein. Analysis of toxic gases in blood by infrared spectroscopy. J. For. Sci. 10: 207–216, 1965.

C.S. Jones, E.J. Baldes and A. Faulconer, Jr. Ether concentrations in gas and blood samples obtained during anesthesia in man and analyzed by mass spectrometry. Fed. Proc. 9: 68, 1950.

T.H. Noehren and J.W. Cudmore. Ethyl ether content in blood as determined by gas chromatography. Anesthesiology 22: 519–524, 1961.

M.S. Northington and G. Owens. Determination of blood ether levels by gas-liquid chromatography. Anal. Biochem. 9: 48–53, 1964.

H.L. Price. General anesthetics. In *The Pharmacological Basis of Therapeutics*, 5th ed. (L.S. Goodman and A. Gilman, eds.), MacMillan, New York, 1975, pp. 89–96.

H. Rackow, E. Salanitre and G.L. Wolf. Quantitative analysis of diethyl ether in blood. Anesthesiology 27: 829–834, 1966.

H. Wollman and T.C. Smith. Uptake, distribution, elimination and administration of inhalational anesthetics. In *The Pharmacological Basis of Therapeutics*, 5th ed. (L.S. Goodman and A. Gilman, eds.), MacMillan, New York, 1975, pp. 71–80.

Y. Yokota, Y. Hitomi, K. Ohta and F. Kosaka. Direct injection method for gas chromatographic measurement of inhalation anesthetics in whole blood and tissues. Anesthesiology 28: 1064–1073, 1967.

Ethinamate

T$\frac{1}{2}$: 2.3 hr
Vd: ?
Fb: ?

Occurrence and Usage. Ethinamate (1-ethynylcyclohexyl carbamate, Valmid) is an acetylenic carbamate that was synthesized in 1953 and introduced into clinical usage in 1955. It receives occasional use as a hypnotic and is administered in single oral doses of 500–1000 mg.

Blood Concentrations. An oral dose of 1000 mg given to 8 volunteers resulted in an average peak plasma concentration of 5.9 mg/L (range, 3.5–11.7) at 1 hour, declining to 3.6 mg/L by 3 hours and 1.2 mg/L by 6 hours. The mean half-life of the drug was determined to be 2.3 hours (Clifford et al., 1974).

Metabolism and Excretion. Ethinamate is known to be transformed *in vivo* by hydroxylation of the cyclohexyl ring to 4-hydroxyethinamate (McMahon, 1958; McMahon, 1959), which exists as stereoisomers and is excreted largely as a glucuronide. The presence of 3- and 2-hydroxyethinamate has also been demonstrated in human urine (Preuss and Willig, 1963).

Toxicity. One case of fatal overdosage involving the ingestion of at least 15 g of ethinamate has been described, whereas another patient survived following a dose of 28 g (Davis et al., 1959). Two adults who died of ethinamate overdosage had postmortem blood concentrations of 100 and 200 mg/L (Gottschalk and Cravey, 1980).

Analysis. Ethinamate has been included in a general scheme for the analysis of sedative drugs by gas chromatography (Proelss and Lohmann, 1971).

References

J.M. Clifford, J.H. Cookson and P.E. Wickham. Absorption and clearance of secobarbital, heptabarbital, methaqualone, and ethinamate. Clin. Pharm. Ther. 16: 376–389, 1974.

R.P. Davis, W.B. Blythe, M. Newton and L.G. Welt. The treatment of intoxication with ethynyl-cyclohexyl carbamate (Valmid) by extracorporeal hemodialysis: a case report. Yale J. Biol. Med. 32: 192–196, 1959.

L.A. Gottschalk and R.H. Cravey. *Toxicological and Pathological Studies on Psychoactive Drug-Involved Deaths*, Biomedical Publications, Davis, California, 1980, pp. 232–233.

R.E. McMahon. The *in vivo* hydroxylation of 1-ethynylcyclohexyl carbamate. J. Am. Chem. Soc. 80: 411–414, 1958.

R.E. McMahon. In vivo hydroxylation of 1-ethynylcyclohexyl carbamate. II. The orientation of hydroxylation. J. Org. Chem. 24: 1834–1837, 1959.

F.R. Preuss and G. Willig. Die Struktur einiger renaler Ausscheidungsprodukte des 1-Athinyl-cyclohexylcarbamat-(1). Arz. Forsch. 13: 234–237, 1963.

H.F. Proelss and H.J. Lohman. Profile of sedatives and tranquilizers in serum, as measured by gas-liquid chromatography. Clin. Chem. 17: 222–228, 1971.

Ethosuximide

T½: 48–60 hr
Vd: 0.9 L/kg
Fb: 0
pKa: 9.3

Occurrence and Usage. Ethosuximide (2-ethyl-2-methylsuccinimide, Zarontin), is one of several succinimide derivatives found effective as anticonvulsant drugs. The compound was first described for the treatment of petit mal epilepsy in 1958 and is still considered the drug of choice for this condition, which is usually associated with childhood. It is applied as the free acid in 250 mg tablets or a 250 mg/5 mL syrup. Daily oral doses of 1000 mg are usual, often in combination with other agents, and it requires 5–8 days to achieve a steady-state plasma level.

Blood Concentrations. A single 500 mg oral dose of ethosuximide given to 20 subjects produced an average peak plasma concentration of 9.4 mg/L at 3 hours, declining to 6.9 mg/L by 24 hours; the elimination half-life averaged 54 hours in these 20 healthy adults (Goulet et al., 1976).

Nine pediatric patients on a chronic daily dosage of 11–40 mg/kg of ethosuximide developed an average steady-state plasma concentration of 50 mg/L (range, 28–83), with a mean half-life of 29 hours (Buchanan et al., 1976). In 5 young adults receiving a daily maintenance dosage of 1000 mg, an average plasma concentration of 49 mg/L (range, 31–68) was observed (Solow and Green, 1971). Browne et al. (1975) have found that a linear relationship exists between dosage of ethosuximide and plasma concentration, with an increase of about 3 mg/L in the plasma level for every additional 1 mg/kg increase in dosage. Most authors agree that effective ethosuximide plasma concentrations lie within the range of 40–100 mg/L.

Metabolism and Excretion. Ethosuximide is metabolized largely by oxidation of the 2-ethyl group to a hydroxyl derivative, a ketone, and a carboxylic acid. The hydroxyethyl metabolite (as diastereoisomers) is excreted in the 24 hour urine to the extent of 25% of the dose as the glucuronide and

14% unconjugated. An additional 18% is eliminated as unchanged ethosuximide over a 9 day period (Buchanan et al., 1969; Chang et al., 1972; Pettersen, 1978). None of the metabolites has been found present in plasma, and it is likely that they are devoid of anticonvulsant activity. An additional product of oxidation, 3-hydroxyethosuximide, has been isolated in urine in amounts approximately equal to those of the hydroxyethyl metabolite (Preste et al., 1974).

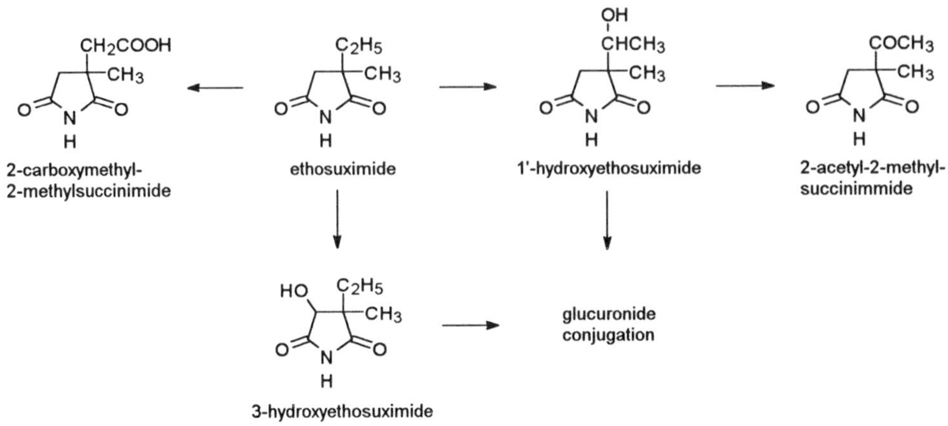

Toxicity. The incidence of toxic reactions to ethosuximide is relatively low, and attempts at correlating plasma concentrations with toxic symptoms have not been particularly successful. Fatal cases of pancytopenia as a result of the drug have been reported (Buchanan, 1972). The following concentrations were determined in the postmortem tissues of an 18 year old male who committed suicide with ethosuximide (Rousseau, 1980):

Ethosuximide Concentrations in a Fatal Case (mg/L or mg/kg)

Blood	Liver	Urine	Gastric
250	280	120	400 mg

Analysis. Ethosuximide has been analyzed by flame-ionization or nitrogen-selective gas chromatography of the underivatized drug (Glazko and Dill, 1972; van der Kleijn et al., 1973; Bonitati, 1976; Fellenberg and Pollard, 1978), or of the methyl (Solow et al., 1978), ethyl (Solow and Green, 1971), or butyl (Least et al., 1975; Menyharth et al., 1977) derivatives. Electron-capture detection of a halogenated derivative has been reported (Wallace et al., 1979), and commercial enzyme immunoassays are also available. Underivatized ethosuximide is relatively volatile and losses may occur when evaporating organic solvent extracts of the drug to dryness.

References

J. Bonitati. Gas-chromatographic analysis of succinimide anticonvulsants in serum: macro- and micro-scale methods. Clin. Chem. 22: 341–345, 1976.

T.R. Browne, F.E. Dreifuss, P.R. Dyken et al. Ethosuximide and the treatment of absence (petit mal) seizures. Neurology 25: 515–524, 1975.

R.A. Buchanan, L. Fernandez and A.W. Kinkel. Absorption and elimination of ethosuximide in children. J. Clin. Pharm. 9: 393–398, 1969.

R.A. Buchanan. Ethosuximide—toxicity. In *Antiepileptic Drugs* (D.M. Woodbury, J.K. Penry and R.P. Schmidt, eds.), Raven Press, New York, 1972, pp. 449–454.

R.A. Buchanan, A.W. Kinkel, J.L. Turner and J.C. Heffelfinger. Ethosuximide dosage regimens. Clin. Pharm. Ther. 19: 143–147, 1976.

T. Chang, A.R. Burkett and A.J. Glazko. Ethosuximide—biotransformation. In *Antiepileptic Drugs* (D.M. Woodbury, J.K. Penry and R.P. Schmidt. eds.), Raven Press, New York, 1972, pp. 425–429.

A.J. Fellenberg and A.C. Pollard. Gas-liquid chromatographic microdetermination of underivatized ethosuximide (<N>-ethyl-<N>-methyl succinimide) in plasma or serum. Clin. Chem. 24: 1821–1823, 1978.

A.J. Glazko and W.A. Dill. Ethosuximide—chemistry and methods for determination. In *Antiepileptic Drugs* (D.M. Woodbury, J.K. Penry and R.P. Schmidt, eds.), Raven Press, New York, 1972, pp. 413–415.

J.R. Goulet, A.W. Kinkel and T.C. Smith. Metabolism of ethosuximide. Clin. Pharm. Ther. 20: 213–218, 1976.

C.J. Least, G.F. Johnson and H.M. Solomon. A quantitative gas chromatographic determination of ethosuximide based on N-butylation. Clin. Chim. Acta 60: 285–292, 1975.

P. Menyharth, D.P. Lehane and A.L. Levy. Rapid gas-chromatographic method for the determination of ethosuximide in serum. Clin. Chem. 23: 1795–1796, 1977.

J.E. Pettersen. Urinary metabolites of 2-ethyl-2-methylsuccinimide (ethosuximide) studied by combined gas chromatography mass spectrometry. Biomed. Mass Spec. 5: 601–603, 1978.

P.G. Preste, C.E. Westerman, N.P. Das et al. Identification of 2-ethyl-2-methyl-3-hydroxysuccinimide as a major metabolite of ethosuximide in humans. J. Pharm. Sci. 63: 467–469, 1974.

M. Rousseau. Personal communication, 1980.

E.B. Solow and J.B. Green. The determination of ethosuximide in serum by gas chromatography. Clin. Chim. Acta 33: 87–90, 1971.

E.B. Solow, N.L. Tupper and C.P. Kenfield. An alternative internal standard for analysis of ethosuximide by on-column methylation and gas chromatography. J. Anal. Tox. 2: 39–40, 1978.

E. van der Kleijn, P. Collste, B. Norlander et al. Gas chromatographic determination of ethosuximide and phensuximide in plasma and urine of man. J. Pharm. Pharmac. 25: 324–327, 1973.

J.E. Wallace, H.A. Schwertner, H.E. Hamilton et al. Electron-capture gas-liquid chromatographic determination of ethosuximide and desmethylmethsuximide in plasma and serum. Clin. Chem. 25: 252–255, 1979.

Ethotoin

T½: 3–11 hr (dose-dependent)
Vd: ?
Fb: ?
pKa: ?

Occurrence and Usage. Ethotoin (3-ethyl-5-phenylhydantoin, Peganone) is a hydantoin derivative that has been in clinical use as an anticonvulsant since 1956. It is less widely used than its relatives, phenytoin and mephenytoin. The drug is supplied for oral administration as the free acid in 250 mg tablets; daily doses of 1000–3000 mg are recommended.

Blood Concentrations. Steady-state plasma ethotoin concentrations ranged from 5–14 mg/L in patients receiving chronic daily oral therapy with 30 mg/kg (2100 mg/70 kg) of the drug, and 14–50 mg/L in those receiving 60 mg/kg (4200 mg/70 kg). Dose-dependent kinetics were observed at ethotoin plasma concentrations exceeding 8 mg/L (Sjo et al., 1975).

Metabolism and Excretion. Ethotoin is rapidly and extensively metabolized in man by oxidation. In patients on chronic therapy with the drug, from 0.2–1.9% is excreted in the daily urine as unchanged drug, 5–14% as norethotoin, 17–34% as 5-hydroxynorethotoin, 14–32% as conjugated p-hydroxyethotoin, and minor amounts of other phenyl-substituted oxidation products (Naestoft and Larsen, 1977; Bius et al., 1980). Saturation of the N-deethylation and p-hydroxylation pathways are believed to occur with increasing doses (Naestoft et al., 1976). The presence of norethotoin in plasma has not yet been reported.

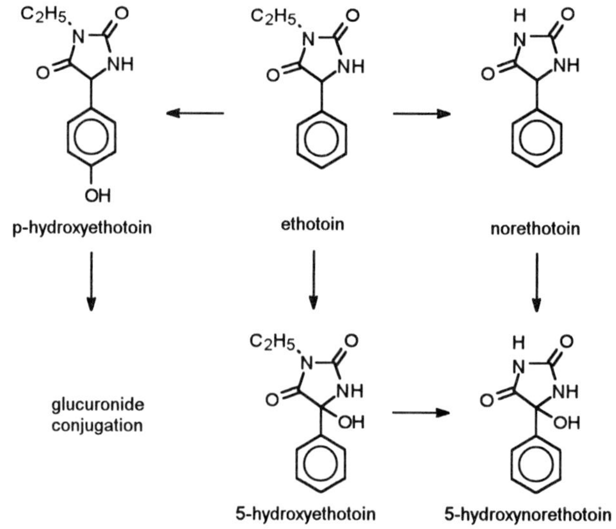

p-hydroxyethotoin   ethotoin   norethotoin

glucuronide
conjugation

5-hydroxyethotoin   5-hydroxynorethotoin

Toxicity. Adverse reactions to ethotoin have included dizziness, nausea, vomiting, headache, diplopia, skin rash, fever, diarrhea, and blood dyscrasias.

Analysis. Ethotoin has been analyzed in serum by flame-ionization gas chromatography of the underivatized drug (Larsen and Naestoft, 1974). It has also been included in a general procedure for anticonvulsant drugs using liquid chromatography (Kabra et al., 1978).

References

D.L. Bius, W.D. Yonekawa, H.J. Kupferberg et al. Gas chromatographic-mass spectrometric studies on the metabolic fate of ethotoin in man. Drug Met. Disp. 8: 223–229, 1980.

P.M. Kabra, D.M. McDonald and L.J. Marton. A simultaneous high-performance liquid chromatographic analysis of the most common anticonvulsants and their metabolites in the serum. J. Anal. Tox. 2: 127–133, 1978.

N.E. Larsen and J. Naestoft. Quantitative determination of ethotoin in serum by gas chromatography. J. Chrom. 92: 157–161, 1974.

J. Naestoft, E.F. Hvidberg and O. Sjo. Saturable metabolic pathways for ethotoin in man. Clin. Exp. Pharm. Physiol. 3: 453–459, 1976.

J. Naestoft and N.E. Larsen. Mass fragmentographic quantitation of ethotoin and some of its metabolites in human urine. J. Chrom. 143: 161–169, 1977.

O. Sjo, E.F. Hvidberg, N.E. Larsen et al. Dose-dependent kinetics of ethotoin in man. Clin. Exp. Pharm. Physiol. 2: 185–192, 1975.

Ethylbenzene

T½: ?
Vd: ?
Fb: ?

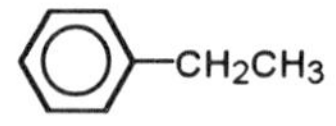

Occurrence and Usage. Ethylbenzene is employed commercially as a solvent, fuel additive and chemical intermediate in the production of styrene. It is readily absorbed by the pulmonary route and after direct application to the skin. The current threshold limit value for ethylbenzene in the industrial atmosphere is 100 ppm (434 mg/m^3).

Blood Concentrations. Ethylbenzene has not been measured in the blood of exposed workers.

Metabolism and Excretion. Ethylbenzene is metabolized in man by oxidation of the side-chain to methylphenylcarbinol, which accounts for about 5% of a dose as a urinary glucuronide conjugate. Further oxidation of this first metabolite produces mandelic acid and phenylglyoxylic acid, which are also major metabolites of styrene and which represent 64 and 25% of a dose of ethylbenzene as urinary excretion products. Mandelic acid is an endogenous urinary substance found in normal urine at levels of up to 5 mg/L (Van Roosmalen and Drummond, 1978). Only a minor portion of a dose is eliminated unchanged in the expired breath and urine (Bardodej and Bardodejova, 1970).

The urinary excretion of mandelic acid reaches a maximum during the last 2 hours of an 8 hour exposure, and then declines with a half-life of 4–7 hours following the termination of exposure. Mandelic acid concentrations in the urine of resting subjects exposed to 92 ppm of ethylbenzene for 8 hours average about 900 mg/L (Piotrowski, 1977).

Toxicity. Exposure to ethylbenzene at an air concentration of 1000 ppm causes eye and nose irritation. Concentrations of 2000 ppm may produce lacrimation and dizziness, while higher levels cause increasing degrees of central nervous system depression.

Analysis. Mandelic acid may be analyzed in urine by a gas chromatographic procedure, which is also applicable to the determination of phenylglyoxylic acid, hippuric acid, and m- and p-methylhippuric acid (Van Roosmalen and Drummond, 1978). Phenylglyoxylic acid is unstable in urine unless the specimen is frozen.

References

Z. Bardodej and E. Bardodejova. Biotransformation of ethyl benzene, styrene, and alpha-methylstyrene in man. Am. Ind. Hyg. Asso. J. 31: 206–209, 1970.

J.K. Piotrowski. *Exposure Tests for Organic Compounds in Industrial Toxicology*, U.S. Government Printing Office, Washington, D.C., 1977, pp. 58–59.

P.B. Van Roosmalen and I. Drummond. Simultaneous determination by gas chromatography of the major metabolites in urine of toluene, xylenes and styrene. Brit. J. Ind. Med. 35: 56–60, 1978.

Ethyl Chloride

T½: ?
Vd: ?
Fb: ?

C_2H_5Cl

Occurrence and Usage. Ethyl chloride (chloroethane, Ethyl Gaz, Kelene) is a flammable gas (b.p., 12° C.) that has been used as a refrigerant, solvent and chemical intermediate. It is employed therapeutically as a topical anesthetic spray for the control of pain associated with minor surgical procedures, athletic injuries, and muscle spasm. The chemical has also become a popular substance of abuse, and can be purchased at various retail shops, ostensibly for use as an electronic cleaner or aromatic spray. The current TLV for occupational exposure is 1000 ppm (2640 mg/m³).

Blood Concentrations. Blood or plasma concentrations associated with therapeutic or industrial usage have not been reported.

Metabolism and Excretion. The metabolic fate of the chemical in man has not been investigated.

Toxicity. Over-application of ethyl chloride as a topical spray can cause freezing and tissue necrosis. Inhalation of the vapor can result in dizziness, euphoria, confusion, incoordination and narcosis. Overexposure can produce ventricular arrhythmia, coma and death. Chronic exposure in animals is known to cause liver and kidney damage, while chronic abuse by humans has caused severe but reversible neurological impairment (Nordin et al., 1988).

A young adult who was found unresponsive following recreational abuse of ethyl chloride had a 200 mg/L serum concentration of the chemical during hospital treatment; he was declared dead after 1 hour of resuscitative efforts, and postmortem blood contained 650 mg/L ethyl chloride (Yacoub et al., 1993).

Analysis. Ethyl chloride has been determined in biological specimens by gas chromatographic techniques designed for blood alcohol testing (Yacoub et al., 1993). It may be mistaken for ethanol during routine analysis for common volatiles (Laferty, 1994).

References

P.I. Laferty. Ethyl chloride: possible misidentification as ethanol. J. For. Sci. 39: 261–265, 1994.
C. Nordin, M. Rosenquist and C. Hollstedt. Sniffing of ethyl chloride. Int. J. Addictions 23: 623–627, 1988.
I. Yacoub, C.A. Robinson, G.T. Simmons and M. Hall. Death attributed to ethyl chloride. J. Anal. Tox. 17: 384–385, 1993.

Ethylene Glycol

T½: 3–5 hr
Vd: 0.5–0.8 L/kg   HOCH₂CH₂OH
Fb: ?

Occurrence and Usage. Ethylene glycol is a relatively nonvolatile liquid (b.p. 197° C.) used as a principal component of many automotive antifreeze solutions. It may be considered a derivative of ethanol; its physical properties (clear, odorless liquid, miscible with water) and its soporific effects in man have led to its occasional use as a beverage by persons unfamiliar with its toxicity. The current threshold limit value for occupational exposure to ethylene glycol vapor is 50 ppm (127 mg/m³).

Blood Concentrations. Ethylene glycol has not been measured in human blood except in toxic situations. In rats, the substance disappeared from the bloodstream with an initial half-life of 2.9–4.9 hours (dose-dependent) and a terminal half-life of 60 hours (Marshall et al., 1980).

Metabolism and Excretion. The metabolism of ethylene glycol has not been investigated experimentally in man, although oxalic acid is known to be a metabolite on the basis of clinical experience (Zarembski and Hodgkinson, 1967). In laboratory animals, it is apparent that the compound undergoes extensive oxidation in a manner analogous to that of ethanol, with the formation of glyoxal, glycolic acid, glyoxylic acid and formic acid. Oxalic acid is a relatively minor metabolite in most species, but it was found that ethylene glycol was most toxic to those species that formed the most oxalate. At lower dosage levels, the rabbit excretes about 60% of a dose as carbon dioxide in the expired air within 3 days and 20% unchanged in the urine, with only traces of oxalic acid present; with higher doses, up to 50% is eliminated unchanged in urine (Gessner et al., 1961). Less than 1% of a dose is believed to be converted to oxalic acid in man (von Oettingen, 1943).

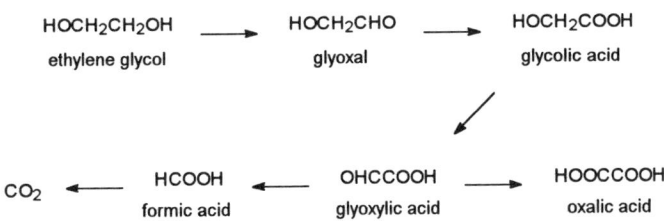

Toxicity. An oral dose of 100 mL of ethylene glycol is believed to be fatal to most adults. Over 200 fatal cases have been reported, and it is estimated that the chemical causes the death of 40–60 persons annually. Those who survive the early toxic period of central nervous system depression with severe metabolic acidosis and seizures almost always develop acute renal failure (Friedman et al., 1962). Renal tubular oxalate crystal deposition is a common finding in such persons (Raekallio et al., 1967), who may die after a period of some days. Each of the acidic ethylene glycol metabolites is more toxic than the parent compound and it is felt that renal failure may be a result of cytotoxicity due to these metabolites (Bove, 1966). The administration of ethanol to competitively inhibit the biotransformation of ethylene glycol has been proven effective in clinical use (Wacker et al., 1965). In one case, ethanol administration increased the plasma half-life of ethylene glycol from 3–17 hours. Hemodialysis is recommended to more rapidly clear the unmetabolized chemical from the bloodstream (Peterson et al., 1981); this technique is also effective in reducing the levels of glycolic acid, the metabolite present in highest concentration in serum during poisoning and believed to be largely responsible for the severe acidosis (Hewlett et al., 1986). Intentional poisoning of a child with ethylene glycol has been misdiagnosed as an inherited metabolic disorder (Wolf et al., 1992); the reverse situation has also occurred (Shoemaker et al., 1992). Ethylene glycol concentrations in 5 persons who survived massive poisoning were initially as high as 900–9050 mg/L in serum and 1000–9500 mg/L in urine (Underwood and Bennett, 1973; Parry and Wallach, 1974; Stokes and Aueron, 1980; Peterson et al., 1981; Cheng et al., 1987; Curtin et al., 1992).

Serum ethylene glycol concentrations of 500–7750 mg/L have been measured 6–24 hours after ingestion in 4 patients who later died of ethylene glycol poisoning (Bowen et al., 1978; Godolphin et al., 1980; Cadnapaphornchai et al., 1981; Gordon and Hunter, 1982). A liver oxalic acid concentration of 245 mg/kg was found in a man who died of ethylene glycol poisoning; control livers contained less than 3 mg/kg (Zarembski and Hodgkinson, 1967). The following ethylene glycol concentrations were noted in the tissues of 9 persons who died within 6–48 hours of ingesting unknown amounts of the substance (Harger and Forney, 1959; Klendshoj and Rejent, 1966; Winek, 1975):

Ethylene Glycol Concentrations in Fatal cases (g/L or g/kg)

	Blood	Brain	Liver	Kidney	Urine
Average	2.4	2.0	6.7	4.6	5.7
(Range)	(0.3–4.3)	(0.3–3.9)	(0.2–15.1)	(0.2–11.3)	(0.6–10.8)

Analysis. Serum osmolality measurements can yield a useful approximation of the ethylene glycol level (Cheng et al., 1987). Ethylene glycol may be determined in tissues by a colorimetric method after oxidation to formaldehyde (Harger and Forney, 1959). More specific fluorometric (Meola et al., 1980) and enzymatic (Hansson and Masson, 1989) methods have been reported. Gas chromatographic procedures have utilized flame-ionization detection of ethylene glycol itself (Brown et al., 1968; Baselt, 1980; Bost and Sunshine, 1980; Cummings and Jatlow, 1982; Jonsson et al., 1989; Edinboro et al., 1993) or of a derivative (Peterson and Rodgerson, 1974; Robinson and Reive, 1981; McCurdy and Solomons, 1982; Porter and Avansakul, 1982; Balikova and Kohlicek, 1988; Houze et al., 1993). Liquid chromatography of a derivative has also been accomplished for ethylene glycol (Gupta et al., 1982) and for glycolic acid (Hewlett et al., 1983). It has been observed that ethylene glycol concentrations in postmortem tissue specimens decline rapidly during refrigerator storage when measured with a colorimetric method (Harger and Forney, 1959), but not with a gas chromatographic procedure (Winek et al., 1978). Some colorimetric and chromatographic methods may exhibit positive interference by propylene glycol in pharmaceuticals (Robinson et al., 1982), 2,3-butanediol in alcoholics (Jones et al., 1991), ketoacids in diabetics (Bjellerup and Kollind, 1994) and propionic acid in a patient with methylmalonic acidemia (Shoemaker et al., 1992). Glycolic acid analysis has been recommended to avoid the potential interferences associated with ethylene glycol determination (Fraser and MacNeil, 1993). Techniques for oxalate determination in fluids and tissues are cited in the section on oxalic acid. The four acidic metabolites of ethylene glycol have been measured simultaneously by isotachophoresis (Ovrebo et al., 1987).

References

M. Balikova and J. Kohlicek. Rapid determination of ethylene glycol at toxic levels in serum and urine. J. Chrom. 434: 469–474, 1988.

R.C. Baselt. *Analytical Procedures for Therapeutic Drug Monitoring and Emergency Toxicology*, Biomedical Publications, Davis, California, 1980, pp. 114–115.

P. Bjellerup and M. Kollind. GLC determination of serum-ethylene glycol, interferences in ketotic patients. Ciln. Tox. 32: 85–87, 1994.

R.O. Bost and I. Sunshine. Ethylene glycol analysis by gas chromatography. J. Anal. Tox. 4: 102–103, 1980.

K.E. Bove. Ethylene glycol toxicity. Am. J. Clin. Path. 45: 46–50, 1966.

D.A.L. Bowen, P.S.B. Minty and A. Sengupta. Two fatal cases of ethylene glycol poisoning. Med. Sci. Law 18: 102–107, 1978.

D.J. Brown, N.C. Jain, R.B. Forney et al. Gas chromatographic assay of glycol-ethanol combinations in biological materials. J. For. Sci. 13: 537–543, 1968.

P. Cadnapaphornchai, S. Taher, D. Bhathena et al. Ethylene glycol poisoning: diagnosis based on high osmolal and anion gaps and crystalluria. Ann. Emer. Med. 10: 94–97, 1981.

J.T. Cheng, T.D. Beysolow, B. Kaul et al. Clearance of ethylene glycol by kidneys and hemodialysis. Clin. Tox. 25: 95–108, 1987.

K.C. Cummings and P.I. Jatlow. Sample preparation by ultrafiltration for direct gas chromatographic analysis of ethylene glycol in plasma. J. Anal. Tox. 6: 324–326, 1982.

L. Curtin, J. Kraner, H. Wine et al. Complete recovery after massive ethylene glycol ingestion. Arch. Int. Med. 152: 1311–1313, 1992.

L.E. Edinboro, C.R. Nanco, D.M. Soghoian and A. Poklis. Determination of ethylene glycol in serum utilizing direct injection on a wide-bore capillary column. Ther. Drug. Mon. 15: 220–223, 1993.

A.D. Fraser and W. MacNeil. Colorimetric and gas chromatographic procedures for glycolic acid in serum. Clin. Tox. 31: 397–405, 1993.

E.A. Friedman, J.B. Greenberg, J.P. Merrill and G.J. Dammin. Consequences of ethylene glycol poisoning. Am. J. Med. 32: 891–902, 1962.

P.K. Gessner, D.V. Parke and R.T. Williams. Studies in detoxication. 86. The metabolism of ^{14}C-labelled ethylene glycol. Biochem. J. 79: 482–489, 1961.

W. Godolphin, E.P. Meagher, H.D. Sanders and J. Frohlich. Unusual calcium oxalate crystals in ethylene glycol poisoning. Clin. Tox. 16: 479–486, 1980.

H.L. Gordon and J.M. Hunter. Ethylene glycol poisoning. Anaesthesia 37: 332–338, 1982.

R.N. Gupta, F. Eng and M.L. Gupta. Liquid-chromatographic determination of ethylene glycol in plasma. Clin. Chem. 28: 32–33, 1982.

P. Hansson and P. Masson. Simple enzymatic screening assay for ethylene glycol (ethane-1,2-diol) in serum. Clin. Chim. Acta 182: 95–102, 1989.

R.N. Harger and R.B. Forney. A simple method for detecting and estimating ethylene glycol in body materials; analytical results in six fatal cases. J. For. Sci. 4: 136–143, 1959.

T.P. Hewlett, A.C. Ray and J.C. Reagor. Diagnosis of ethylene glycol (antifreeze) intoxication in dogs by determination of glycolic acid in serum and urine with high pressure liquid chromatography and gas chromatography-mass spectrometry. J. Asso. Off. Anal. Chem. 66: 276–283, 1983.

T.P. Hewlett, K.E. McMartin, A.J. Lauro and F.A. Ragan. Ethylene glycol poisoning. The value of glycolic acid determinations for diagnosis and treatment. Clin. Tox. 24: 389–402, 1986.

P. Houze, J. Chaussaud, P. Harry and M. Pays. Simultaneous determination of ethylene glycol, propylene glycol, 1,3-butylene glycol and 2,3-butylene glycol in human serum and urine. J. Chrom. 619: 251–257, 1993.

A.W. Jones, L. Nilsson, S.A. Gladh et al. 2,3-Butanediol in plasma from an alcoholic mistakenly identified as ethylene glycol. Clin. Chem. 37: 1453–1455, 1991.

J.A. Jonsson, A. Eklund and L. Molin. Determination of ethylene glycol in postmortem blood by capillary gas chromatography. J. Anal. Tox. 13: 25–26, 1989.

N.C. Klendshoj and T.A. Rejent. Tissue levels of some poisoning agents less frequently encountered. J. For. Sci. 11: 75–80, 1966.

T.C. Marshall, C.R. Clark and R.O. McClellan. Pharmacokinetics of ethylene glycol in the rat following intravenous administration. Presented at the 19th annual Society of Toxicology meeting, Washington, D.C., March 9–13, 1980.

H.H. McCurdy and E.T. Solomons. An improved procedure for the determination of ethylene glycol in blood. J. Anal. Tox. 6: 253–254, 1982.

J.M. Meola, T.G. Rosano and T.A. Swift. Fluorometry of ethylene glycol in serum. Clin. Chem. 26: 1709, 1980.

S. Ovrebo, D. Jacobsen and O.M. Sejersted. Determination of ionic metabolites from ethylene glycol in human blood by isotachophoresis. J. Chrom. 416: 111–117, 1987.

M.F. Parry and R. Wallach. Ethylene glycol poisoning. Am. J. Med. 57: 143– 150, 1974.

C.D. Peterson, A.J. Collins, J.M. Himes et al. Ethylene glycol poisoning. New Eng. J. Med. 304: 21–23, 1981.

R.L. Peterson and D.O. Rodgerson. Gas-chromatographic determination of ethylene glycol in serum. Clin. Chem. 20: 820–824, 1974.

W.H. Porter and A. Avansakul. Gas-chromatographic determination of ethylene glycol in serum. Clin. Chem. 28: 75–78, 1982.

J. Raekallio, A.J. Jaaskelainen and P.L. Makinen. The simple demonstration of calcium oxalate crystals in kidneys of victims of ethylene glycol poisoning. J. For. Sci. 12: 238–140, 1967.

D.W. Robinson and D.S. Reive. A gas chromatographic procedure for quantitation of ethylene glycol in postmortem blood. J. Anal. Tox. 5: 69–72, 1981.

C.A. Robinson, J.W. Scott and C. Ketchum. Propylene glycol interference with ethylene glycol procedures. Clin. Chem. 28: 727, 1982.

J.D. Shoemaker, R.E. Lynch, J.W. Hoffman and W.S. Sly. Misidentification of propionic acid as ethylene glycol in a patient with methylmalonic acidemia. J. Pediat. 120: 417–421, 1992.

J.B. Stokes and F. Aueron. Prevention of organ damage in massive ethylene glycol ingestion. J. Am. Med. Asso. 243: 2065–2066, 1980.

F. Underwood and W.M. Bennett. Ethylene glycol intoxication. J. Am. Med. Asso. 226: 1453–1454, 1973.

V.F. von Oettingen. Ethylene glycol. U.S. Public Health Bull. 281: 166–174, 1943.

W.E.C. Wacker, H. Haynes, R. Druyan et al. Treatment of ethylene glycol poisoning with ethyl alcohol. J. Am. Med. Asso. 194: 1231–1233, 1965.

C. Winek. Ethylene glycol poisoning. Presented at the 27th annual meeting of the American Academy of Forensic Sciences, Chicago, February 19, 1975.

C.L. Winek, D.P. Shingleton and S.P. Shanor. Ethylene and diethylene glycol toxicity. Clin. Tox. 13: 297–324, 1978.

A.D. Woolf, A. Wynshaw-Boris, P. Rinaldo and H.L. Levy. Intentional infantile ethylene glycol poisoning presenting as an inherited metabolic disorder. J. Pediat. 120: 421–424, 1992.

P.M. Zarembski and A. Hodgkinson. Plasma oxalic acid and calcium levels in oxalate poisoning. J. Clin. Path. 20: 283–285, 1967.

Ethylene Oxide

T½: ?
Vd: ?
Fb: ?

$$\underset{CH_2CH_2}{\overset{O}{\triangle}}$$

Occurrence and Usage. Ethylene oxide is a colorless, sweet-smelling gas that is widely used in industrial facilities for the sterilization of surgical equipment and in industry as an agricultural fumigant and fungicide for clothing and foodstuffs. The odor threshold for the compound is about 700 ppm, while eye and nose irritation begin at about 600 ppm. The threshold limit value (TLV) for industrial exposure was set at 50 ppm as recently as 1979, but has since been lowered to 1 ppm (1.8 mg/m³) in recognition of its mutagenic and carcinogenic effects in animals.

Blood Concentrations. Blood ethylene oxide concentrations in workers employed in a hospital sterilizer unit ranged from 0–104 μg/L, averaging 10–61 μg/L at various times during the workshift; during this study, the environmental air concentrations of ethylene oxide ranged from 0.4–23 mg/m³, averaging 3.8–17 mg/m³ (Brugnone et al., 1986).

Metabolism and Excretion. The metabolism of ethylene oxide has not been specifically studied in man. The chemical is a highly reactive alkylating agent and probably undergoes rapid chemical changes in all tissues of the body.

In rats administered ethylene oxide by intravenous injection, 35% of the dose is eliminated in the 24 hour urine as 2-hydroxyethylmercapturic acid (Gerin and Tardif, 1986). In dogs, from 7–24% of a dose is excreted as ethylene glycol in the 24 hour urine (Martis et al., 1982).

Alveolar breath concentrations of ethylene oxide in workers average between 20–36% of the environmental air level (Brugnone et al., 1986).

Toxicity. Severe skin burns, neurotoxicity, chromosomal damage, and leukemia have been identified as effects of ethylene oxide exposure in man. Acute exposure to high concentrations of the gas may cause nausea, vomiting, weakness, headache, shortness of breath, pulmonary edema, convulsions and death due to respiratory failure.

A number of large chemical spills have occurred in which liquid ethylene oxide was accidentally released from tank cars or storage tanks at medical or industrial facilities. The liquid quickly vaporizes and forms a gaseous cloud that lingers, unless dissipated by wind or ventilating devices. Ethylene oxide gas is heavier than air, so it tends to remain at ground level. The gas is highly flammable, so presents an explosion hazard at high concentrations. An ethylene oxide leak at a medical laboratory in 1982 resulted in hospitalization of 27 individuals for respiratory problems. Protracted nausea and vomiting also occur in this type of exposure, but usually do not appear until 2–4 hours later (Dodson and Jarlson, 1982).

Neurotoxicity has been reported in a number of individuals working as operators of ethylene oxide sterilizers for medical equipment. The victims have been primarily young (17–33 years) men who first developed symptoms within 3 weeks to 4 years after beginning employment. Symptoms commonly included headache, numbness of the extremities, muscular weakness, impaired gait, staggering, and increased fatigability. These cases were diagnosed as peripheral neuropathy due to ethylene oxide. At least 1 individual developed encephalopathy, with convulsions, fever and coma lasting for 2 days. In most cases, the neurologic symptoms cleared spontaneously within several months (Gross et al., 1979; Finelli et al., 1983; Kuzuhara et al., 1983).

An outbreak of very serious dermal burns in 19 hospital patients was attributed to the use of ethylene oxide for the sterilization of operating room gowns and sheets. The levels of residual ethylene oxide found in the items, 3600–10,800 ppm, were 16 to 50 times the level considered safe for skin contact, 200 ppm (Biro et al., 1974).

Three individuals, out of a group of 30 similarly exposed, developed leukemia after 6–9 years of exposure to ethylene oxide at estimated levels of 10–30 ppm. The solution used in this work, involving the sterilization of hospital equipment, consisted of 50% ethylene oxide and 50% methyl formate. Being less volatile and less toxic, the methyl formate was not considered to have contributed significantly to the disease process. Two of the patients died, while one went into remission after chemotherapy (Hogstedt et al., 1979).

Analysis. Ethylene oxide in blood or breath may be measured by flame-ionization gas chromatography (Brugnone et al., 1986).

References

L. Biro, A.A. Fisher and E. Price. Ethylene oxide burns. Arch. Dermatol. 110: 924–925, 1974.

F. Brugnone, L. Perbellini, G.B. Faccini et al. Ethylene oxide exposure. Int. Arch. Occ. Env. Health 58: 105–112, 1986.

M. Dodson and G. Jarlson. *Los Angeles Times*, November 14, 1982.

P.F. Finelli, T.F. Morgan, I. Yaar and C.V. Granger. Ethylene oxide-induced polyneuropathy. Arch. Neurol. 40: 419–421, 1983.

M. Gerin and R. Tardif. Urinary N-acetyl-S-2-hydroxyethyl-L-cysteine in rats as biological indicator of ethylene oxide exposure. Fund. Appl. Tox. 7: 419–423, 1986.

J.A. Gross, M.L. Hass and T.R. Swift. Ethylene oxide neurotoxicity: report of four cases and review of the literature. Neurology 29: 978–983, 1979.

C. Hogstedt, N. Malmqvist and B. Wadman. Leukemia in workers exposed to ethylene oxide. J. Am. Med. Asso. 241: 1132–1133, 1979.

S. Kuzuhara, I. Kanazawa, T. Nakanish and T. Egashira. Ethylene oxide polyneuropathy. Neurology 33: 377–380, 1983.

L. Martis, R. Kroes, T.D. Darby and E.F. Woods. Disposition kinetics of ethylene oxide, ethylene glycol, and 2-chloroethanol in the dog. J. Tox. Env. Health 10: 847–856, 1982.

Etidocaine

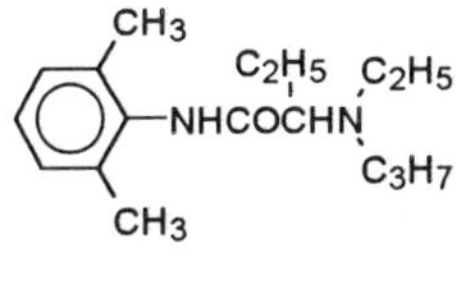

T½: 2.7 hr
Vd: 1.9 L/kg
Fb: 0.94
pKa: 7.7

Occurrence and Usage. Etidocaine (Duranest) is an amide-type local anesthetic that is closely related to lidocaine, but is of considerably higher lipid solubility. The drug is supplied as 0.5–1.5% solutions of the hydrochloride, with or without epinephrine, for epidural, caudal, peripheral nerve, and infiltration anesthesia. Single doses should not exceed 300 mg without epinephrine and 400 mg with epinephrine.

Blood Concentrations. Pregnant women who received an average dose of 160 mg of etidocaine for epidural anesthesia demonstrated peak plasma concentrations of 0.5–1.5 mg/L between 5 and 30 minutes after administration. Both of the mono-N-dealkylated metabolites were measurable in plasma within minutes of administration (Morgan et al., 1977a).

Metabolism and Excretion. Etidocaine is extensively metabolized in man by N-dealkylation, hydrolysis, and ring hydroxylation. Less than 0.3% of a dose is excreted in the 48 hour urine; other metabolites, many in conjugated form, include N-desethyletidocaine (0.3%), N-despropyletidocaine (0.5%), dinoretidocaine (9.5%), 2,6-xylidine (0.5%), and 4-hydroxy-2,6-xylidine (8.3%). Three cyclic metabolites, designated I, II and X, account for 7.3, 5.0 and 10% of a dose, respectively. Meta- or para-hydroxylation of each metabolite occurs, with the hydroxylated metabolites representing about 10% of a dose. About half of a dose is yet unaccounted for (Thomas et al., 1976; Morgan et al., 1977b; Vine et al., 1978).

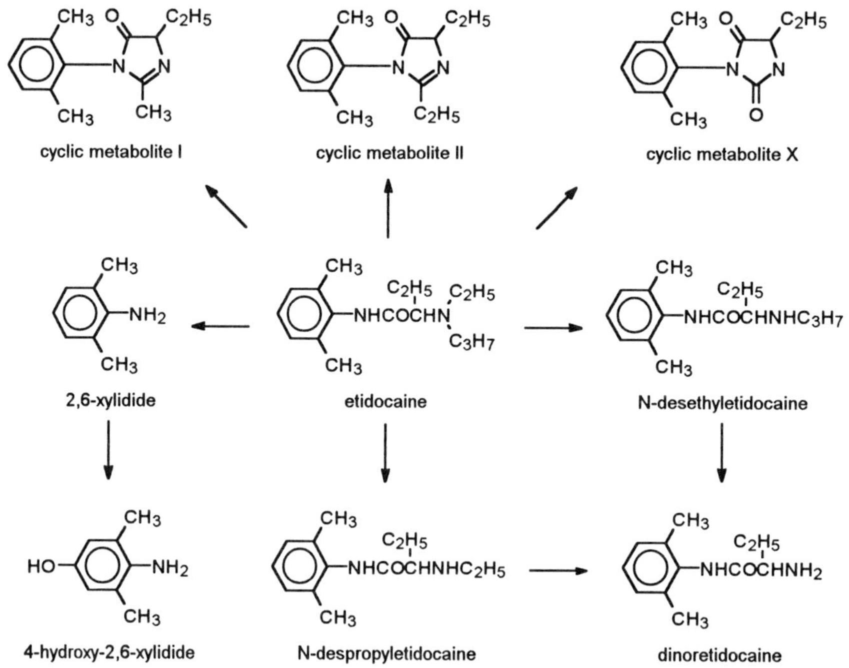

Toxicity. Adverse effects of etidocaine administration may include nervousness or drowsiness, blurred vision, tremors, convulsions, hypotension, bradycardia, unconsciousness, and respiratory and cardiac arrest.

Analysis. Etidocaine and its N-dealkylated metabolites may be assayed in plasma or urine by gas chromatography with flame-ionization detection (Morgan et al., 1977a).

References

D.J. Morgan, M.J. Cousins, D. McQuillan and J. Thomas. Disposition and placental transfer of etidocaine in pregnancy. Eur. J. Clin. Pharm. 12: 359–365, 1977a.

D.J. Morgan, M.P. Smyth, J. Thomas and J. Vine. Cyclic metabolites of etidocaine in humans. Xenobiotica 7: 365–375, 1977b.

J. Thomas, D. Morgan and J. Vine. Metabolism of etidocaine in man. Xenobiotica 6: 39–48, 1976.

J. Vine, D. Morgan and J. Thomas. The identification of eight hydroxylated metabolites of etidocaine by chemical ionization mass spectrometry. Xenobiotica 8: 509–513, 1978.

Etodolac

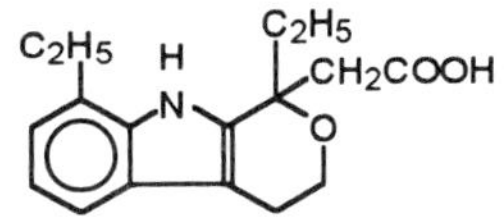

T½: 7.3 hr
Vd: 0.4 L/kg
Fb: 0.99
pKa: 4.7

Occurrence and Usage. Etodolac (Lodine) is a nonsteroidal anti-inflammatory drug that also exhibits analgesic and antipyretic activity in man. The drug is available in capsules of 200 or 300 mg as the free acid. The usual dose for acute pain is 200–400 mg every 6–8 hours, with a maximum recommended daily dose of 1200 mg.

Blood Concentrations. Peak plasma etodolac concentrations of 12–16 mg/L are attained within 1–2 hours after oral administration of a single 200 mg dose in healthy adults (Ferdinandi et al., 1986; Lasseter et al., 1988; Brater and Lasseter, 1989). The average peak plasma concentration of etodolac in 18 subjects following a 400 mg dose was 21 mg/L (Kraml et al., 1984).

Metabolism and Excretion. After a single administration of etodolac, 73% of the dose is recovered in the urine and 14% in the feces in 7 days; glucuronide conjugates of etodolac and 3 hydroxylated metabolites represent more than 60% of the dose. Less than 1.2% is excreted unchanged in the urine (Ferdinandi et al., 1986). The metabolites of etodolac apparently have no pharmacological activity (Balfour and Buckley, 1991).

Toxicity. Symptoms following etodolac overdose include lethargy, drowsiness, nausea, vomiting and epigastric pain. An adult female ingested from 3–9 g of the drug and developed a plasma etodolac level of 22 mg/L within 5 hours, but remained asymptomatic (Boldy et al., 1988).

Analysis. Etodolac and its metabolites have been determined in biological specimens by liquid chromatography (Cosyns et al., 1983).

References

J.A. Balfour and M.M.T. Buckley. Etodolac—a reappraisal of its pharmacology and therapeutic use in rheumatic diseases and pain states. Drugs 42: 274–299, 1991.

D.A.R. Boldy, K.A. Hale and J.A. Vale. Etodolac overdose. Hum. Tox. 7: 203–204, 1988.

D.C. Brater and K.C. Lasseter. Profile of etodolac: pharmacokinetic evaluation in special populations. Clin. Rheum. 8: 25–35, 1989.

L. Cosyns, M. Spain and M. Kraml. Sensitive high-performance liquid chromatographic method for the determination of etodolac in serum. J. Pharm. Sci. 72: 275–277, 1983.

E.S. Ferdinandi, S.N. Schgal, C.A. Demerson et al. Disposition and biotransformation of ^{14}C-etodolac in man. Xenobiotica 16: 153–166, 1986.

M. Kraml, L. Cosyns, D.R. Hicks et al. Bioavailability studies with etodolac in dogs and man. Biopharm. Drug Disp. 5: 63–74, 1984.

K. Lasseter, E. Shamblen, A. Murdoch et al. Pharmacokinetics of etodolac in patients with hepatic cirrhosis. J. Clin. Pharm. 28: 933–935, 1988.

Etorphine

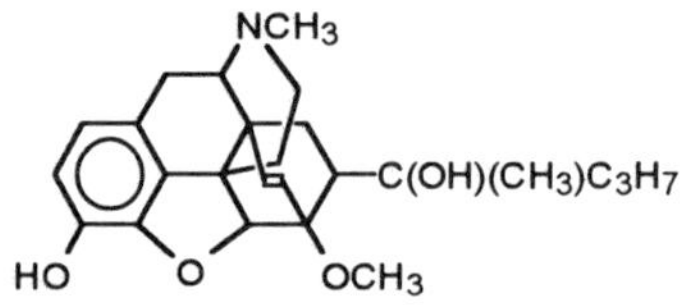

T½: ?
Vd: ?
Fb: ?
pKa: ?

$$NCH_3$$

$$C(OH)(CH_3)C_3H_7$$

HO   O   OCH₃

Occurrence and Usage. Etorphine (M99, Oripavine, ingredient of Immobilon) is a synthetic narcotic analgesic used in veterinary medicine that was originally prepared from thebaine in the early 1960's. The drug is used for the immobilization of large animals and is administered by intravenous injection or on the tip of a dart fired from a gun. Its potency is estimated at 400–1000 times that of morphine. Etorphine is supplied as the hydrochloride salt in solutions that range from 0.07–2.5 mg/mL, often in combination with a phenothiazine tranquilizer.

Blood Concentrations. Blood concentrations of etorphine in man have not been reported.

Metabolism and Excretion. Although no human metabolic studies of etorphine have been performed, etorphine-3-glucuronide has been reported as a metabolite of etorphine in the rat (Dobbs and Hall, 1969). Following a single subcutaneous injection of 100 μg of etorphine in 7 prisoner volunteers, urine collected over a 3 day period analyzed both before and after acid hydrolysis failed to show the presence of the parent drug or metabolites using thin-layer chromatography or gas chromatography with flame-ionization detection (Gorodetzky and Kullberg, 1975).

Toxicity. The effects of etorphine have been reported as indistinguishable from those of morphine, except for more rapid onset and significantly shorter duration of action. It is considered to have a very high potential for abuse (Jasinski et al., 1975).

Analysis. Etorphine may be analyzed in urine using a commercially available radioimmunoassay (Woods et al., 1986) or by gas chromatography-mass spectrometry (Jindal and Vestergaard, 1978; Jindal et al., 1979; Bonnaire et al., 1989).

References

Y. Bonnaire, P. Plou, N. Pages et al. GC/MS confirmatory method for etorphine in horse urine. J. Anal. Tox. 13: 193–196, 1989.

H.E. Dobbs and J.M. Hall. Metabolism and biliary excretion of etorphine (M99-Reckitt)—an extremely potent morphine-like drug. Proc. Eur. Soc. Stud. Drug Tox. 10: 77–86, 1969.

C.W. Gorodetky and M.P. Kullberg. Etorphine in man. II. Detectability in urine by common screening methods. Clin. Pharm. Ther. 17: 273–276, 1975.

D.R. Jasinski, J.D. Griffin and C.B. Carr. Etorphine in man. I. Subjective effects and suppression of morphine abstinence. Clin. Pharm. Ther. 17: 267–272, 1975.

S.P. Jindal and P. Vestergaard. Quantitation of etorphine in urine by selective ion monitoring using tritiated etorphine as an internal standard. J. Pharm. Sci. 67: 260–261, 1978.

S.P. Jindal, T. Lutz and P. Vestergaard. Gas chromatographic-mass spectrometric determination of etorphine with stable isotope labeled internal standard. Anal. Chem. 51: 269–271, 1979.

C.J. Polson, M.A. Green and M.R. Lee (eds.). *Clinical Toxicology*, 3rd ed., J.B. Lippincott Co., Philadelphia, 1983, p. 64.

W.E. Woods, T. Weckman, T. Wood et al. Radioimmunoassay for etorphine in racing horses. Res. Comm. Chem. Path. Pharm. 52: 237–249, 1986.

Felbamate

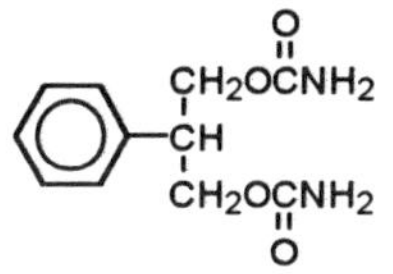

T½: 11–23 hr
Vd: 0.7–1.0 L/kg
Fb: 0.25

Occurrence and Usage. Felbamate (W-554, Felbatol) is a neutral dicarbamate, related to meprobamate, that is used as an anticonvulsant in the treatment of epilepsy. It is available in 400 and 600 mg tablets or a 600 mg/5 mL suspension for oral administration; daily doses in adults may range from 1200–3600 mg.

Blood Concentrations. A single 200 mg oral dose in 8 adult patients produced an average peak serum felbamate concentration of 3.0 mg/L (range, 2.7–4.1) at 1–3 hours; the elimination half-life in this study averaged 13 hours (range, 11–16). Eight patients receiving 800 mg daily for 36 days had average steady-state peak and trough serum levels of 31 and 24 mg/L, respectively (Wilensky et al., 1985). Patients receiving an average daily oral dose of 2300 mg had steady-state trough plasma felbamate concentrations averaging 33 mg/L (range, 18–52) (Leppik et al., 1991).

Metabolism and Excretion. A single labeled oral dose of felbamate is eliminated in the urine (90%) and feces (less than 5%), with parent drug representing 40–49% of the total urinary activity (Shumaker et al., 1990). The compound is metabolized by oxidation and hydrolysis to p-hydroxyfelbamate (pOHF), 2-hydroxyfelbamate (2OHF), 2-phenyl-1,3-propanediol carbamate (MCF) and 3-carbamoyloxy-2-phenyl propionic acid (CPPA). These products appear in both plasma and urine in free and conjugated form, but none has significant anticonvulsant properties (Leppik and Graves, 1989; Shumaker et al., 1990; Romanyshyn et al., 1994).

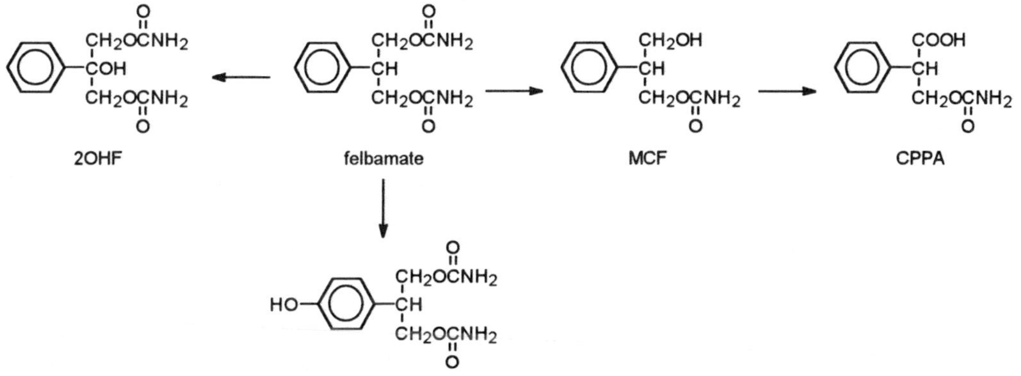

Toxicity. Adverse reactions to felbamate therapy include nausea, vomiting, headache, dizziness, blurred vision and ataxia. The drug is relatively free of sedative effects, but it can inhibit the metabolism of other concurrently-administered agents, such as phenytoin and valproate (Leppik and Graves, 1989; Leppik et al., 1991).

Analysis. Felbamate may be analyzed in biological fluids by flame-ionization gas chromatography (Rifai et al., 1994). Felbamate and its polar metabolites may be determined using liquid chromatographic techniques (Clark et al., 1992; Romanyshyn et al., 1994).

References

L.A. Clark, J.K. Wickmann, N. Kucharczyk and R.D. Sofia. Detection of the anticonvulsant felbamate in beagle dog plasma by hplc. J. Chrom. 573: 113–119, 1992.

I.E. Leppik and N.M. Graves. Felbamate. In *Antiepileptic Drugs* (R. Levy, R. Mattson, B. Meldrum et al., eds.), Raven Press, New York, 1989, pp. 983–990.

I.E. Leppik, F.E. Dreifuss, G.W. Pledger et al. Felbamate for partial seizures. Neurology 41: 1785–1789, 1991.

N. Rifai, D. Fuller, T. Lar and M. Mikati. Measurement of felbamate by wide-bore capillary gas chromatography and flame ionization detection. Clin. Chem. 40: 745–748, 1994.

L.A. Romanyshyn, J.K. Wichmann, N. Kucharczyk and R.D. Sofia. Simultaneous detection of felbamate and three metabolites in human plasma by hplc. Ther. Drug Mon. 16: 83–89, 1994.

R.C. Shumaker, C. Fantel, E. Kelton et al. Evaluation of the elimination of (^{14}C) felbamate in healthy men. Epilepsia 31: 642, 1990.

A.J. Wilensky, P.N. Friel, L.M. Ojemann et al. Pharmacokinetics of W-554 (ADD 03055) in epileptic patients. Epilepsia 26: 602–606, 1985.

Fenfluramine

T½: 13–30 hr (urine pH-dependent)
Vd: 12–16 L/kg
Fb: 0.34
pKa: 9.9

Occurrence and Usage. Fenfluramine (Ponderax, Pondimin) was synthesized in 1963 for use as an anorectic agent. It is reported to produce less central stimulation than amphetamine while retaining the pharmacological properties necessary for appetite suppression. The compound is administered orally as the hydrochloride of the racemic mixture, in single doses of 20 mg and daily doses of up to 160 mg.

Blood Concentrations. Following a single oral dosage of 60 mg, peak plasma fenfluramine concentrations of 0.05–0.07 mg/L were observed at 3 hours with a slow decline to 0.03 mg/L by 24 hours; plasma norfenfluramine concentrations reached 0.02 mg/L by 4 hours and remained at that level for at least 24 hours (Campbell, 1970). In 39 subjects receiving an average of 142 mg (range, 60–160) of the drug daily, steady-state plasma concentrations averaged 0.158 mg/L (range, 0.035–0.299) for fenfluramine and 0.072 mg/L (range, 0.022–0.144) for norfenfluramine. The most significant weight loss was effected in those subjects whose plasma fenfluramine concentrations exceeded 0.200 mg/L (Innes et al., 1977).

Metabolism and Excretion. Fenfluramine is primarily metabolized by N-dealkylation to norfenfluramine in man, and the pharmacologic activity of this metabolite has led to the supposition that it contributes significantly to the efficacy of its parent (Broekkamp et al., 1975). Over a 48 hour period, during conditions of acid urine, approximately 23% of a dose is eliminated in the urine as unchanged drug and 19% as norfenfluramine (Beckett and Salmon, 1972). Under normal pH conditions only 7% of a dose is excreted unchanged and 3–7% as norfenfluramine in the 48 hour urine; the remainder of a dose is deaminated to a benzoic acid derivative, excreted as a glycine conjugate in urine, and to several alcoholic derivatives (Beckett and Brookes, 1967; Bruce and Maynard, 1968; Midha et al., 1983).

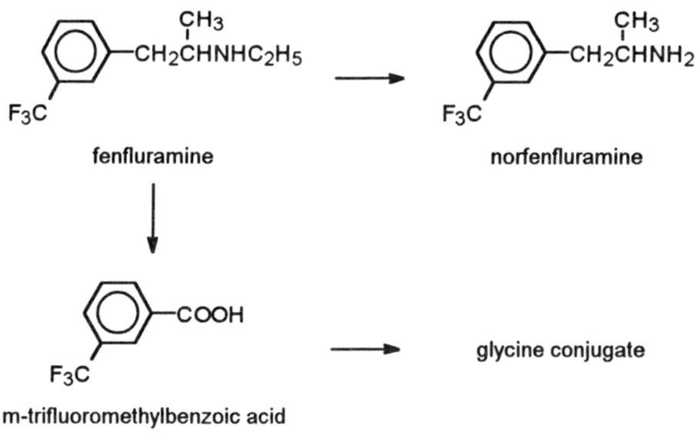

fenfluramine → norfenfluramine

m-trifluoromethylbenzoic acid → glycine conjugate

Toxicity. A number of instances of serious intoxication due to fenfluramine overdosage have been described, some with fatal outcome. An adult has survived the acute ingestion of 1600 mg of the drug after attaining fenfluramine concentrations of 0.85 mg/L in plasma and 103 mg/L in urine (Richards, 1969). A 2.5 year old child who ingested 440 mg and survived was admitted to a hospital in a semi-conscious agitated state with a rapid pulse rate; plasma levels of 0.78 mg/L fenfluramine and 0.17 mg/L norfenfluramine were found (Campbell and Moore, 1969).

In the deaths of 3 children aged 2–6 who ingested up to 1200 mg of the drug, postmortem concentrations of fenfluramine ranged from 6.5–16 mg/L in blood and 24–136 mg/kg in liver (Gold et al., 1969; Simpson and McKinlay, 1975). A 36 year old woman who was found dead after ingesting an overdose had postmortem blood and liver fenfluramine concentrations of 7.5 mg/L and 155 mg/kg, respectively (Kintz and Mangin, 1992). The following distribution was noted in the tissues of a 13 year old who died 3.5 hours after ingestion of 2000 mg of fenfluramine (Fleisher and Campbell, 1969):

Drug Concentrations in a Fenfluramine Fatality (mg/L or mg/kg)

Drug	Blood	Brain	Liver	Bile	Kidney	Urine
Fenfluramine	6.5	42	49	65	27	89
Norfenfluramine	0.8	5.3	8.5	10	1.5	10

Analysis. Fenfluramine and norfenfluramine may be determined in biologic media by gas chromatography with flame-ionization (Beckett and Brookes, 1967; Campbell, 1970), electron-capture (Bruce and Maynard, 1968; Caccia and Jori, 1977; Midha et al., 1979) or nitrogen-selective detection (Morris and Reece, 1983; Krebs et al., 1984).

References

A.H. Beckett and L.G. Brookes. The absorption and urinary excretion in man of fenfluramine and its main metabolite. J. Pharm. Pharmac. 19: 42S–52S, 1967.

A.H. Beckett and J.A. Salmon. Pharmacokinetics of absorption, distribution and elimination of fenfluramine and its main metabolite in man. J. Pharm. Pharmac. 24: 108–114, 1972.

C.L.E. Broekkamp, A.J.M. Weemaes and J.M. van Rossum. Does fenfluramine act via norfenfluramine? J. Pharm. Pharmac. 27: 129–130, 1975.

R.B. Bruce and W.R. Maynard, Jr. Fenfluramine metabolism. J. Pharm. Sci. 57: 1173–1176, 1968.

S. Caccia and J. Jori. Gas-liquid chromatographic determination of the optical isomers of fenfluramine and norfenfluramine in biological samples. J. Chrom. 144: 127–131, 1977.

D.B. Campbell and B.W.R. Moore. Fenfluramine overdosage. Lancet 2: 1306, 1969.

D.B. Campbell. Gas chromatographic measurement of levels of fenfluramine and norfenfluramine in human plasma, red cells and urine following therapeutic doses. J. Chrom. 49: 442–447, 1970.

M.R. Fleisher and D.B. Campbell. Fenfluramine overdosage. Lancet 2: 1306, 1969.

R.G. Gold, H.E. Gordon, R.W.D. Da Costa et al. Fenfluramine overdosage. Lancet 2: 1306, 1969.

J.A. Innes, M.L. Watson, M.J. Ford et al. Plasma fenfluramine levels, weight loss, and side effects. Brit. Med. J. 2: 1322–1325, 1977.

P. Kintz and P. Mangin. Toxicological findings after fatal fenfluramine self-poisoning. Hum. Exp. Tox. 11: 51–52, 1992.

H.A. Krebs, L.K. Cheng and G.J. Wright. Determination of fenfluramine and norfenfluramine in plasma using a nitrogen-sensitive detector. J. Chrom. 310: 412–417, 1984.

K.K. Midha, I.J. McGilveray and J.K. Cooper. A GLC-ECD assay for simultaneous determination of fenfluramine and norfenfluramine in human plasma and urine. Can. J. Pharm. Sci. 14: 18–21, 1979.

K.K. Midha, E.M. Hawes, J.K. Cooper et al. The identification of two new urinary metabolites of fenfluramine in man. Xenobiotica 13: 31–38, 1983.

R.G. Morris and P.A. Reece. Improved gas-liquid chromatographic method for measuring fenfluramine and norfenfluramine in heparinised plasma. J. Chrom. 278: 434–438, 1983.

A.J. Richards. Fenfluramine overdosage. Lancet 2: 1367, 1969.

H. Simpson and I. McKinlay. Poisoning with slow-release fenfluramine. Brit. Med. J. 4: 462–463, 1975.

Fenoprofen

T½: 1.5–3.0 hr
Vd: 0.08–0.10 L/kg
Fb: 0.99
pKa: 4.5

Occurrence and Usage. Fenoprofen (Nalfon) was first prepared in 1970 and was shown in 1971 to exhibit anti-inflammatory and analgesic effects in man. It is available as the calcium dihydrate salt of the racemic mixture, in capsules or tablets containing 200–600 mg as the free acid. The drug is administered orally for the treatment of rheumatoid arthritis in amounts of 1200–3200 mg daily.

Blood Concentrations. A single oral 250 mg dose of fenoprofen given to 4 subjects produced peak plasma concentrations at 0.5–2 hours that averaged 27 mg/L (range, 23–31); the levels declined with a mean half-life of 2.5 hours and averaged 1.5 mg/L after 12 hours (Rubin et al., 1971). A single oral dose of 600 mg given to 12 subjects resulted in an average peak plasma level of about 50 mg/L after 1–2 hours. With oral doses of 600 mg every 6 hours (2400 mg/day), plasma concentrations generally range from a minimum of 25 mg/L to a maximum of 65 mg/L (Waife et al., 1975).

Metabolism and Excretion. Fenoprofen is biotransformed in man primarily by 4'-hydroxylation, with extensive glucuronide conjugation of both the parent and the major metabolite, 4'-hydroxyfenoprofen. The unchanged drug is highly bound (99%) to plasma proteins and no metabolites have been detected in plasma. A single dose is eliminated nearly quantitatively in the 24 hour urine as intact drug (1%), fenoprofen glucuronide (41–43%), 4'-hydroxyfenoprofen (2–3%) and its glucuronide (43–51%), and as unidentified conjugated metabolites (5–12%) (Rubin et al., 1972a, 1972b).

fenoprofen

4'-OH-fenoprofen

glucuronide conjugation

Toxicity. Adverse reactions to fenoprofen include nausea, vomiting, constipation, loss of appetite, dizziness, headache, drowsiness, tremor and confusion.

Analysis. Fenoprofen may be assayed in biological fluids by flame-ionization gas chromatography of the trimethylsilyl derivative (Nash et al., 1971). Analysis of 4'-hydroxyfenoprofen in urine has been accomplished in a similar manner after acid or enzymatic hydrolysis (Rubin et al., 1972a). Liquid chromatography is well suited to the analysis of fenoprofen in serum (Dusci and Hackett, 1979; Miceli et al., 1980; Bopp et al., 1981; Katogi et al., 1983).

References

R.J. Bopp, K.Z. Farid and J.F. Nash. High-performance liquid chromatographic assay for fenoprofen in human plasma. J. Pharm. Sci. 70: 507–509, 1981.

L.J. Dusci and L.P. Hackett. Determination of some anti-inflam ratory drugs in serum by high-performance liquid chromatography. J. Chrom. 172: 516–519, 1979.

Y. Katogi, T. Ohmura and M. Adachi. Simple and rapid determination of fenoprofen in plasma using high-performance liquid chromatography. J. Chrom. 278: 475–477, 1983.

J.N. Miceli, D.M. Ryan and A.K. Done. High-performance liquid column chromatography of fenoprofen in serum. J. Chrom. 183: 250–254, 1980.

J.F. Nash, R.J. Bopp and A. Rubin. GLC determination of dl-2-(3-phenoxyphenyl) propionic acid (fenoprofen) in human plasma. J. Pharm. Sci. 60: 1062–1064, 1971.

A. Rubin, B.E. Rodda, P. Warrick et al. Physiological disposition of fenoprofen in man I: pharmacokinetic comparison of calcium and sodium salts administered orally. J. Pharm. Sci. 60: 1797–1801, 1971.

A. Rubin, B.E. Rodda, P. Warrick et al. Physiological disposition of fenoprofen in man II: plasma and urine pharmacokinetics after oral and intravenous administration. J. Pharm. Sci. 61: 739–745, 1972a.

A. Rubin, P. Warrick, R.L. Wolen et al. Physiological disposition of fenoprofen in man III. Metabolism and protein binding of fenoprofen. J. Pharm. Exp. Ther. 183: 449–457, 1972b.

S.O. Waife, C.M. Gruber, Jr., B.E. Rodda and J.F. Nash. Problems and solutions to single-dose testing of analgesics: comparison of propoxyphene, codeine, and fenoprofen. Int. J. Clin. Pharm. 12: 301–304, 1975.

Fentanyl

T½: 3–12 hr
Vd: 3–8 L/kg
Fb: 0.79
pKa: 8.4

Occurrence and Usage. Fentanyl (Sublimaze, Duragesic, ingredient of Innovar) is a synthetic narcotic analgesic of high potency and short duration of action. It is closely related to methylfentanyl, a street drug (see separate section), and to alfentanil and sufentanil, which are marketed as narcotic analgesics. Fentanyl has been in clinical use since 1963 as an adjunct to surgical anesthesia, often in combination with nitrous oxide or droperidol. The drug is available as the citrate salt in an injectable solution containing 50 µg/mL; single doses of 25–100 µg are administered intravenously or intramuscularly as needed. Transdermal patches are also available that contain 2.5–10 mg fentanyl and provide a dose of 25–100 µg/hr for 72 hours for management of chronic pain.

Blood Concentrations. Serum fentanyl concentrations after a single 2 µg/kg (140 µg/70 kg) intravenous dose to 4 volunteers were initially as high as 11 µg/L, but declined to about 1 µg/L after 1 hour (Fung and Eisele, 1980). A 6.4 µg/kg (448 µg/70 kg) intravenous dose given to 5 volunteers produced an initial plasma level of 18 µg/L, which declined to less than 1 µg/L by 1.5 hours

(McClain and Hug, 1980). A 60 µg/kg (4200 µg/70 kg) intravenous injection resulted in initial plasma concentrations exceeding 100 µg/L, declining to about 10 µg/L after 1 hour (Bovill and Sebel, 1980). Lunn et al. (1979) noted that patients lost consciousness at an average plasma fentanyl concentration of 34 µg/L when plasma levels were brought to a peak of about 50 µg/L by the intravenous infusion of 75 µg/kg (5250 µg/70 kg) over a 15 minute period. The whole blood/plasma ratio for fentanyl is 1.0 (Bower, 1982). The elimination half-life is increased to as much as 16 hours in neonates (Koehntop et al., 1986) or the elderly (Bentley et al., 1982), but apparently is not influenced significantly by either hepatic or renal disease (Haberer et al., 1982; Koren et al., 1984). Serum fentanyl concentrations attain a range of 0.3–1.2 µg/L within 24 hours after application of a 25 µg/hr transdermal patch; the ranges for the 50, 75 and 100 µg/hr patches are 0.6–1.8, 1.1–2.6 and 1.9–3.8 µg/L, respectively (PDR, 1994).

Metabolism and Excretion. Up to 85% of a labeled dose of fentanyl is excreted in the urine over a 3–4 day period, with from 0.4–6% eliminated as unchanged drug; 26–55% is excreted as norfentanyl, together with unknown amounts of hydroxyfentanyl and hydroxynorfentanyl (Hess et al., 1972; McClain and Hug, 1980; Goromaru et al., 1984). Norfentanyl and despropionylfentanyl have been found in human plasma at levels similar to that of the parent drug (van Rooy et al., 1981). Norfentanyl was detectable for up to 72 hours at concentrations of 0.2–1.3 µg/L in urine of patients receiving a single 50–100 µg fentanyl dose; fentanyl was detectable for 24 hours in just 3 of 7 patients, and despropionylfentanyl was not found in any urine specimens (Silverstein et al., 1993).

Toxicity. Fentanyl is capable of producing severe respiratory depression, muscle rigidity, seizures, coma, and hypotension. Occasional patients exhibit delayed central nervous system and respiratory depression several hours after apparent recovery from surgical anesthesia (Adams and Pybus, 1978). Plasma fentanyl levels have been found to rebound at about 1 hour after an intravenous dose in some patients (Stoeckel et al., 1979; van Rooy et al., 1981).

An individual who died after smoking the contents of a transdermal fentanyl patch had postmortem blood and liver concentrations of 6.1 µg/L and 122 µg/kg, respectively (Marquardt and Tharratt, 1994). Fentanyl concentrations in a large series of intravenous abuse fatalities averaged 3.0 µg/L in blood and 3.9 µg/L in urine (Henderson, 1991). In another series of 30 abuse deaths, blood fentanyl concentrations averaged 18 µg/L (range, 2.2–100) (Smialek et al., 1994). The following tissue concentrations were noted in 7 adults who died after self-administered intravenous injections of fentanyl (Garriott et al., 1984; Levine et al., 1987; Pare et al., 1987; Felgate, 1988; Matejczyk, 1988; Levine et al., 1989; Chaturvedi et al., 1990):

Fentanyl Concentrations in Fatal Cases (µg/L or µg/kg)

	Blood	Brain	Liver	Kidney	Urine
Average	8.3	20	37	18	28
(Range)	(3.0–28)	(9.2–30)	(5.9–78)	(6.1–42)	(5.0–93)

Analysis. Fentanyl has been measured in biological fluids by radioimmunoassay (Michiels et al., 1977), which is now available commercially. Gas chromatographic methods have utilized nitrogen-phosphorus (Gillespie et al., 1981; van Rooy et al., 1981; Phipps et al., 1983; Kowalski et al., 1987; Kintz et al., 1989) and mass spectrometric detection (Watts and Caplan, 1988). Liquid chromatography has also been described (Kumar et al., 1987).

References

A.P. Adams and D.A. Pybus. Delayed respiratory depression after use of fentanyl during anaesthesia. Brit. Med. J. 1: 278–279, 1978.

J.B. Bentley, J.D. Borel, R.E. Nenad and T.J. Gillespie. Age and fentanyl pharmacokinetics. Anesth. Anal. 61: 968–971, 1982.

J.G. Bovill and P.S. Sebel. Pharmacokinetics of high-dose fentanyl. Brit. J. Anaesth. 52: 795–801, 1980.

S. Bower. The uptake of fentanyl by erythrocytes. J. Pharm. Pharmac. 34: 181–185, 1982.

A.K. Chaturvedi, N.G.S. Rao and J.R. Baird. A death due to self-administered fentanyl. J. Anal. Tox. 14: 385–387, 1990.

H.E. Felgate. Personal communication, 1988.

D.L. Fung and J.H. Eisele. Fentanyl pharmacokinetics in awake volunteers. J. Clin. Pharm. 27: 652–658, 1980.

J.C. Garriott, R. Rodriguez and V.J.M. DiMaio. A death from fentanyl overdose. J. Anal. Tox. 8: 288–289, 1984.

T.J. Gillespie, A.J. Gandolfi, R.M. Maiorino and R.W. Vaughan. Gas chromatographic determination of fentanyl and its analogues in human plasma. J. Anal. Tox. 5: 133–137, 1981.

T. Goromaru, H. Matsuura, N. Yoshimura et al. Identification and quantitative determination of fentanyl metabolites by gas chromatography-mass spectrometry. Anesthesiology 61: 73–77, 1984.

J.P. Haberer, P. Schoeffler, E. Couderc and P. Duvaldestin. Fentanyl pharmacokinetics in anaesthetized patients with cirrhosis. Brit. J. Anaesth. 54: 1267–1270, 1982.

G.L. Henderson. Fentanyl-related deaths: demographics, circumstances, and toxicology of 112 cases. J. For. Sci. 37: 422–433, 1991.

R. Hess, G. Stiebler and A. Herz. Pharmacokinetics of fentanyl in man and the rabbit. Eur. J. Clin. Pharm. 4: 137–141, 1972.

P. Kintz, P. Mangin, A.A. Lugnier and A.J. Chaumont. Simultaneous determination of fentanyl and its major metabolites and fentanyl analogues using gas chromatography and nitrogen-selective detection. J. Chrom. 489: 459–461, 1989.

D.E. Koehntop, J.H. Rodman, D.M. Brundage et al. Pharmacokinetics of fentanyl in neonates. Anesth. Anal. 65: 227–232, 1986.

G. Koren, P. Crean, G.V. Goresky et al. Pharmacokinetics of fentanyl in children with renal disease. Res. Comm. Chem. Path. Pharm. 46: 371–379, 1984.

S.R. Kowalski, G.K. Gourlay, D.A. Cherry and C.J. McLean. Sensitive gas liquid chromatography method for the determination of fentanyl concentrations in blood. J. Pharm. Meth. 18: 347–355, 1987.

K. Kumar, D.J. Morgan and D.P. Crankshaw. Determination of fentanyl and alfentanil in plasma by high-performance liquid chromatography with ultraviolet detection. J. Chrom. 419: 464–468, 1987.

B. Levine, G. Kauffman and Y.H. Caplan. The determination and distribution of fentanyl in a postmortem case. Presented at the annual meeting of the American Academy of Forensic Sciences, San Diego, February 19, 1987.

B. Levine, J.C. Goodin and Y.H. Caplan. A fentanyl fatality involving midazolam. Presented at the annual meeting of the Society of Forensic Toxicologists, Chicago, October 20, 1989.

J.K. Lunn, T.H. Stanley, J. Eisele et al. High dose fentanyl anesthesia for coronary artery surgery: plasma fentanyl concentrations and influence of nitrous oxide on cardiovascular responses. Anesth. Anal. 58: 390–395, 1979.

K.A. Marquardt and R.S. Tharratt. Inhalation abuse of fentanyl patch. Clin. Tox. 32: 75–78, 1994.

R.J. Matejczyk. Fentanyl related overdose. J. Anal. Tox. 12: 236–238, 1988.

D.A. McClain and C.C. Hug, Jr. Intravenous fentanyl kinetics. Clin. Pharm. Ther. 28: 106–114, 1980.

M. Michiels, R. Hendriks and J. Heykants. A sensitive radioimmunoassay for fentanyl. Eur. J. Clin. Pharm. 12: 153–158, 1977.

E.M. Pare, J.R. Monforte, R. Gault and H. Mirchandani. A death involving fentanyl. J. Anal. Tox. 11: 272–275, 1987.

J.A. Phipps, M.A. Sabourin, W. Buckingham and L. Strunin. Detection of picogram concentrations of fentanyl in plasma by gas-liquid chromatography. J. Chrom. 272: 392–395, 1983.

Physicians' Desk Reference, Medical Economics Company, Montvale, New Jersey, 1994, pp. 1083–1086.

J.H. Silverstein, M.F Rieders, M. McMullin et al. An analysis of the duration of fentanyl and its metabolites in urine and saliva. Anesth. Anal. 76: 618–621, 1993.

J.E. Smialek, B. Levine, L. Chin et al. A fentanyl epidemic in Maryland 1992. J. For. Sci. 39: 159–164, 1994.

H. Stoeckel, J.H. Hengstmann and J. Schuttler. Pharmacokinetics of fentanyl as a possible explanation for recurrence of respiratory depression. Brit. J. Anaesth. 51: 741–745, 1979.

H.H. van Rooy, N.P.E. Vermeulen and J.B. Bovill. The assay of fentanyl and its metabolites in plasma of patients using gas chromatography with alkali flame ionisation detection and gas chromatography-mass spectrometry. J. Chrom. 223: 85–93, 1981.

V. Watts and Y. Caplan. Determination of fentanyl in whole blood at subnanogram concentrations. J. Anal. Tox. 12: 246–254, 1988.

Flecainide

T½: 12–27 hr
Vd: 9–10 L/kg
Fb: 0.40
pKa: 9.3

Occurrence and Usage. Flecainide (Tambocor) is a class IC antiarrhythmic drug used in the treatment of ventricular tachycardia and premature ventricular contractions when other treatment is ineffective. It is available for oral administration as the acetate salt in tablets containing from 100–200 mg. The initial dose is usually 100 mg every 12 hours, increasing by 50 mg twice a day every 4 days if needed and tolerated.

Blood Concentrations. Following a single 200 mg dose of flecainide in 4 healthy fasting subjects, peak plasma concentrations occurred at 2–3 hours postdose and ranged from 214–281 µg/L (average, 251) (McQuinn et al., 1984).

Twenty adult patients with impaired kidney function received 100 mg flecainide orally every 12–24 hours for 10 days; peak plasma concentrations ranged from 174–1883 µg/L (average, 687) (Forland et al., 1988). In cardiac patients receiving chronic daily oral flecainide doses of 200, 300 or 400 mg, steady-state plasma concentrations averaged 411, 595 and 764 µg/L, respectively (Plomp et al., 1988). Nappi and Anderson (1985) established that the optimal effect of flecainide occurs when its "trough" plasma concentration is maintained at 200–1000 µg/L; they suggested a therapeutic range of approximately 400–1000 µg/L for patients without advanced renal failure or congestive heart failure.

Metabolism and Excretion. Flecainide undergoes biotransformation via O-dealkylation to m-O-dealkylflecainide (MODF); this compound may be conjugated or may first undergo oxidation of the piperidine ring to form a lactam, which then is conjugated. Neither of the metabolites exhibits significant antiarrhythmic activity. About 50% of a single oral dose is excreted in the 24 hour urine, with the parent drug representing approximately 10% of the dose (McQuinn et al., 1984).

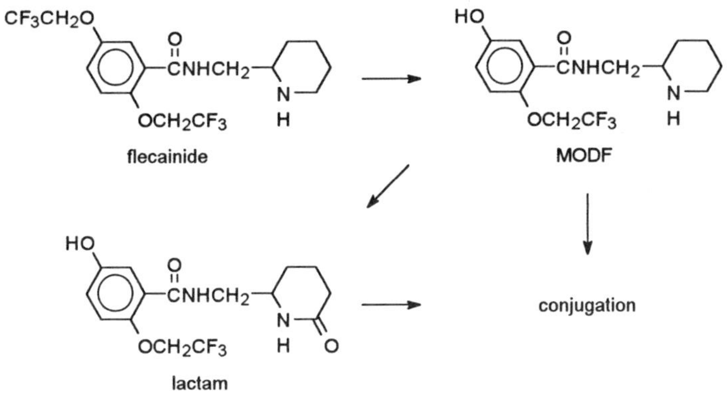

CF₃CH₂O — represented as structural formula

flecainide → MODF

lactam → conjugation

Toxicity. Flecainide can cause new or worsened arrhythmias, while other adverse effects include edema, tremors, confusion, stupor, convulsions and death. The most common manifestations of nonfatal overdosage are nausea and vomiting, bradycardia and hypotension (Koppel et al., 1990).

The following concentrations were found in 4 fatal cases attributed to flecainide overdose (Levine et al., 1990; Forrest et al., 1991; Cravey, 1991; Rogers et al., 1993):

Flecainide Concentrations in Fatal Cases (mg/L or mg/kg)

	Blood	Brain	Liver	Kidney	Urine
Average	44	33	330	74	68
(Range)	(13–94)	(33)	(111–550)	(74)	(54–82)

Analysis. The most commonly used method for flecainide determination in biological specimens is liquid chromatography with ultraviolet (Grgurinovich, 1988; Kramer et al., 1988) or fluorescence detection (Chang et al., 1984; Plomp et al., 1986; Annesley and Matz, 1988; Welscher et al., 1988; Munafo and Biollaz, 1989; Woollard, 1989). Flecainide and its metabolites may also be analyzed by gas chromatography-mass spectrometry (Taylor et al., 1987).

References

T. Annesley and K. Matz. Liquid chromatographic analysis for flecainide with use of a microbore column and small sample volume. J. Liq. Chrom. 11: 1041–1049, 1988.

S.F. Chang, A.M. Miller, J.M. Fox and T.M. Welscher. Determination of flecainide in human plasma by high performance liquid chromatography with fluorescence detection. J. Liq. Chrom. 7: 167–176, 1984.

R.H. Cravey. Unpublished data, 1991.

S.C. Forland, R.E. Cutler, R.L. McQuinn et al. Flecainide pharmacokinetics after multiple dosing in patients with impaired renal function. J. Clin. Pharm. 28: 727–735, 1988.

A.R.W. Forrest, I. Marsh and J.H. Galloway. Rapidly fatal overdose with flecainide. J. Anal. Tox. 15: 41–43, 1991.

N. Grgurinovich. A simple high-performance liquid chromatography method for the routine measurement of flecainide in plasma. J. Anal. Tox. 12: 38–41, 1988.

C. Koppel, U. Oberdisse and G. Heinemeyer. Clinical course and outcome in class IC antiarrhythmic overdose. Clin. Tox. 28: 433–444, 1990.

B.K. Kramer, F. Mayer, H.M. Liebich et al. Rapid and inexpensive high-performance liquid chromatographic method for the quantification of flecainide in serum. J. Chrom. 427: 351–358, 1988.

B. Levine, D. Chute and Y.H. Caplan. Flecainide intoxication. J. Anal. Tox. 14: 335–336, 1990.

R.L. McQuinn, G.J. Quarfoth, J.D. Johnson et al. Biotransformation and elimination of ¹⁴C-flecainide acetate in humans. Drug Met. Disp. 12: 414–420, 1984.

A. Munafo and J. Biollaz. High-performance liquid chromatography assay with fluorometric detection for flecainide and its major metabolites in urine and serum. J. Chrom. 490: 450–457, 1989.

J.M. Nappi and J.L. Anderson. Flecainide: a new prototype antiarrhythmic agent. Pharmacotherapy 5: 209–221, 1985.

T.A. Plomp, H.T. Boom and R.A.A. Maes. Measurement of flecainide plasma concentrations by high performance liquid chromatography with fluorescence detection. J. Anal. Tox. 10: 102–106, 1986.

C. Rogers, D.T. Anderson, J.K. Ribe and L. Sathyavagiswaran. Fatal flecainide intoxication. J. Anal. Tox. 17: 434–435, 1993.

E.H. Taylor, E.E. Kennedy and A.S. Pappas. Determination of flecainide by gas chromatography-mass spectrometry. J. Chrom. 416: 365–369, 1987.

T.M. Welscher, R.L. McQuinn and S.F. Chang. High-performance liquid chromatographic procedure with fluorescence detection for the m-O-dealkylated lactam metabolite of flecainide acetate in human plasma. J. Chrom. 431: 438–443, 1988.

G.A. Woollard. Therapeutic drug monitoring of flecainide using high-performance liquid chromatography and comparison with fluorescence polarisation immunoassay. J. Chrom. 487: 409–420, 1989.

Flumazenil

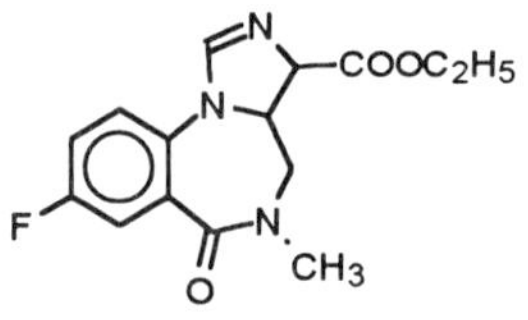

T½: 41–79 min
Vd: 0.8–1.6 L/kg
Fb: 0.55
pKa: ?

Occurrence and Usage. Flumazenil (Mazicon, Romazicon), an imidazobenzodiazepine derivative, is a specific antagonist used when the central effects of a benzodiazepine need to be attenuated or terminated. It was first marketed in European countries in 1987 and in the United States in 1992. Single intravenous doses range from 0.2–2 mg; the maximum recommended cumulative dose is 3 mg per hour or 5 mg total. Flumazenil is available in 5 mL vials containing 0.1 mg/mL of the free base in acidified solution.

Blood Concentrations. In 18 healthy subjects who received a loading dose of 0.5, 1 or 3 mg of flumazenil followed by an infusion of the same dose hourly, steady-state plasma concentrations were attained in 1.5 hours and were 6, 13 and 39 µg/L, respectively. Clinical studies suggest that plasma flumazenil concentrations of 10–20 µg/L for 1–2 hours reverse benzodiazepine-induced central nervous system depression (Klotz et al., 1984, 1985).

Metabolism and Excretion. Flumazenil is metabolized primarily by hydrolysis to a carboxylic acid derivative, which then undergoes glucuronide conjugation (Amrein and Hetzel, 1990). Elimination of a single radioactive dose is essentially complete within 72 hours, with up to 95% of the radioactivity appearing in urine and 5–10% in the feces (Klotz et al., 1984; Roncari et al., 1986).

Toxicity. The most commonly reported adverse effects in patients receiving flumazenil following general anesthesia are nausea, vomiting, agitation and mild depressive mood. Convulsions, ventricular tachycardia and complete heart block have also been reported, with one fatality occurring (Short et al., 1988; Burr et al., 1989; Marchant et al., 1989; Herd and Clarke, 1991).

Analysis. Flumazenil has been determined in biological fluids by gas chromatography with nitrogen-phosphorus (Abernethy et al., 1983; Zell and Timm, 1986) or mass spectrometric detection (Fukuda et al., 1989; Kintz and Mangin, 1991). The drug and its metabolites have also been measured using liquid chromatography (Timm and Zell, 1983; Bun et al., 1989; Vletter et al., 1990; Chan and Jones, 1993).

References

D.R. Abernethy, R. Arend, P. Lauven and D. Greenblatt. Determination of Ro15-1788 a benzodiazepine antagonist in human plasma by gas-liquid chromatography with nitrogen phosphorus detection. Pharmacology 26: 285–289, 1983.

R. Amrein and W. Hetzel. Pharmacology of Dormicum (midazolam) and Anexate (flumazenil). Acta Anaesth. Scand. 34 (Suppl. 92): 6–15, 1990.

H. Bun, V. Duplan, P. Crevat-Pisano et al. Rapid determination of the benzodiazepine antagonist flumazenil, Ro 15-1788, by high-performance liquid chromatography. Biomed. Chem. 3: 269–271, 1989.

W. Burr, P. Sandham and A. Judd. Death after flumazenil. Brit. Med. J. 298: 1713, 1989.

K. Chan and R.D.M. Jones. Simultaneous determination of flumazenil, midazolam and metabolites in human biological fluids by liquid chromatography. J. Chrom. 619: 154–160, 1993.

E.K. Fukuda, N. Choma and P.P. David. Quantitation of the benzodiazepine flumazenil in human plasma by gas chromatography-mass spectrometry. J. Chrom. 491: 97–106, 1989.

B. Herd and F. Clarke. Complete heart block after flumazenil. Hum. Exp. Tox. 10: 289, 1991.

P. Kintz and P. Mangin. Plasma determination of flumazenil, a benzodiazepine antagonist, by immunotoxicology and by capillary gas chromatography/mass spectrometry. J. Anal. Tox. 15: 202–203, 1991.

U. Klotz, G. Ziegler and I.W. Reimann. Pharmacokinetics of the selective benzodiazepine antagonist Ro 15-1788 in man. Eur. J. Clin. Pharm. 27: 115–117, 1984.

U. Klotz, G. Ziegler, L. Ludwig and I.W. Reinmann. Pharmacodynamic interaction between midazolam and a specific benzodiazepine antagonist in humans. J. Clin. Pharm. 25: 400–406, 1985.

B. Marchant, R. Wray, A. Leach and M. Nama. Flumazenil causing convulsions and ventricular tachycardia. Brit. Med. J. 29: 860, 1989.

G. Roncari, W.H. Ziegler and T.W. Guentert. Pharmacokinetics of the new benzodiazepine antagonist Ro 15-1788 in man following intravenous and oral administration. Brit. J. Clin. Pharm. 22: 421–428, 1986.

T.G. Short, T. Maling and D.C. Galletly. Ventricular arrhythmia precipitated by flumazenil. Brit. Med. J. 296: 1070–1071, 1988.

U. Timm and M. Zell. Determination of the benzodiazepine antagonist Ro 15-1788 in plasma by high-performance liquid chromatography with UV detection. Arz. Forsch. 33: 358–362, 1983.

A.A. Vletter, A.G.L. Burm, L.T.M. Breimer and J. Spierdijk. High-performance liquid chromatographic assay to determine midazolam and flumazenil simultaneously in human plasma. J. Chrom. 530: 177–185, 1990.

M. Zell and U. Timm. Highly sensitive assay of a benzodiazepine antagonist in plasma by capillary gas chromatography with nitrogen-selective detection. J. Chrom. 382: 175–188, 1986.

Flunitrazepam

T½: 9–25 hr
Vd: 3.4–5.5 L/kg
Fb: ?
pKa: 1.8

Occurrence and Usage. Flunitrazepam (Rohypnol) is the N-methyl-2'-fluoro analogue of nitrazepam. It is available in a number of western European countries for use as a hypnotic and anesthetic induction agent and is administered orally or by intravenous injection in doses of 2 mg.

Blood Concentrations. After a single 2 mg dose given orally to 1 subject, a peak flunitrazepam blood concentration of 0.006 mg/L was observed at 2 hours, declining to 0.003 mg/L by 4 hours (deSilva and Bekersky, 1974). Immediately following intravenous administration of 2 mg of flunitrazepam to 2 subjects, peak plasma concentrations of 0.028–0.052 mg/L were measured; the concentrations fell below 0.010 mg/L within 10 minutes (Cano et al., 1977). Maximal plasma concentrations in subjects receiving a chronic dose of 2 mg daily ranged from 0.010–0.020 mg/L within 5 hours of administration and declined with an average half-life of 19 hours (Boxenbaum et al., 1978; Wickstrom et al., 1980). During chronic frequent intravenous administration, plasma concentrations of 7-aminoflunitrazepam closely parallel those of the parent drug; lesser amounts of norflunitrazepam and 7-aminonorflunitrazepam are present (Sumirtapura et al., 1982).

Metabolism and Excretion. Flunitrazepam undergoes biotransformation via N-demethylation, 3-hydroxylation and glucuronidation, and reduction of the nitro group to an amine with subsequent acetylation. Over a 7 day period, an average of 84% of a labeled dose is eliminated in urine and 11% in feces. At least 11 metabolites are present in urine; the major ones include 7-aminoflunitrazepam (10% of a dose), 3-hydroxyflunitrazepam (3.5%), 7-acetamidonorflunitrazepam (2.6%), and 3-hydroxy-7-acetamidoflunitrazepam (2.0%). Less than 0.2% is excreted unchanged. Both norflunitrazepam and 7-aminoflunitrazepam are present in plasma at concentrations of 0.002–0.004 mg/L for up to 24 hours after a single dose of flunitrazepam (Wendt, 1976).

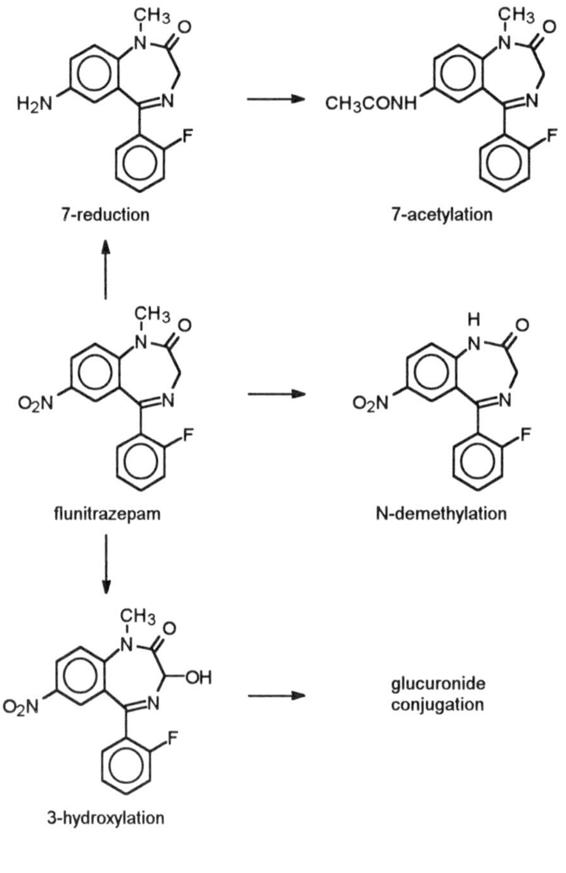

7-reduction

7-acetylation

flunitrazepam

N-demethylation

3-hydroxylation

glucuronide conjugation

Toxicity. Mignee et al. (1980) reviewed 706 cases of overdosage with flunitrazepam and concluded that the predominant symptoms of ataxia, drowsiness, hypotension, respiratory depression and coma could be controlled successfully with supportive therapy.

In a fatality resulting from ingestion of 28 mg of drug, kidney levels of flunitrazepam and the 7-amino metabolite were each 0.5 mg/kg (Heyndrickx, 1987).

Analysis. Determination of the drug and its N-demethyl metabolite has been accomplished by electron-capture gas chromatography, either after acid hydrolysis (deSilva et al., 1974; Cano et al., 1977) or as the intact drugs (deSilva and Bekersky, 1974; Faber et al., 1977). Liquid chromatographic methods have also been reported (Vree et al., 1977; Sumirtapura et al., 1982).

References

H.G. Boxenbaum, H.N. Posmanter, T. Macasieb et al. Pharmacokinetics of flunitrazepam following single- and multiple-dose oral administration to healthy human subjects. J. Pharm. Biopharm. 6: 283–293, 1978.

J.P. Cano, J. Guintrand, C. Aubert et al. Determination of flunitrazepam, desmethylflunitrazepam and clonazepam in plasma by gas liquid chromatography with an internal standard. Arz. Forsch. 27: 338–342, 1977.

J.A.F. deSilva, C.V. Puglisi and N. Munno. Determination of clonazepam and flunitrazepam in blood and urine by electron-capture GLC. J. Pharm. Sci. 63: 520–527, 1974.

J.A.F. deSilva and I. Bekersky. Determination of clonazepam and flunitrazepam in blood by electron-capture gas-liquid chromatography. J. Chrom. 99: 447–460, 1974.

D.B. Faber, R.M. Kok and E.N. Rempt-Van Dijk. Quantitative gas chromatographic analysis of flunitrazepam in human serum with electron capture detection. J. Chrom. 133: 319–326, 1977.

B. Heyndrickx. Fatal intoxication due to flunitrazepam. J. Anal. Tox. 11: 278, 1987.

C. Mignee, R. Garnier, F. Conso et al. Intoxication aigue par le flunitrazepam. Therapie 35: 581–589, 1980.

Y.C. Sumirtapura, C. Aubert, P. Coassolo and J.P. Cano. Determination of 7-amino-flunitrazepam (Ro 20-1815) and 7-amino-desmethylflunitrazepam (Ro 5-4650) in plasma by high-performance liquid chromatography and fluorescence detection. J. Chrom. 232: 111–118, 1982.

T.B. Vree, B. Lenselink, E. van der Kleijn and G.M.M. Nijhuis. Determination of flunitrazepam in body fluids by means of high-performance liquid chromatography. J. Chrom. 143: 530–534, 1977.

G. Wendt. Schicksal des Hypnotikums Flunitrazepam im menschlichen Organismus. In *Bisherige Erfahrungen mit Rohypnol (Flunitrazepam) in der Anasthesiologie und Intensivtherapie* (W. Huegin, G. Hossli and M. Gemperle, eds.), Hoffmann-LaRoche, Basel, 1976, pp. 27–38.

W. Wickstrom, R. Amrein, P. Haefelfinger and D. Hartmann. Pharmacokinetic and clinical observations on prolonged administration of flunitrazepam. Eur. J. Clin. Pharm. 17: 189–196, 1980.

Fluoride

T½: 2–9 hr
Vd: 0.5–0.7 L/kg
Fb: 0

F^-

Occurrence and Usage. Hydrogen fluoride and its inorganic salts find wide application in industry. Sodium fluoride, sodium fluosilicate (Na_2SiF_6) and cryolite (Na_3AlF_6) are employed as insecticides, rodenticides and delousing powders. Fluoride is an excellent enzyme inhibitor, and is commonly used as an anticoagulant and preservative in biological specimens. The presence of fluoride in drinking water promotes resistance to tooth decay in children, and thus in many geographic areas where water supplies are lacking in this anion, it is added at a recommended level of 1 ppm. It is also incorporated into some dentrifices as stannous fluoride (SnF_2), is often applied topically to the teeth in dental treatment programs, and may be administered to children in daily oral doses of 2.2 mg of sodium fluoride on a chronic basis. Since fluoride increases the density and calcification of bone, its use for patients with osteoporosis has been recommended, in a daily dose of 33–220 mg as the sodium salt. The average daily dietary fluoride intake for an adult ranges from 0.5–5 mg as the anion. Industrial exposure to fluoride is generally the result of inhalation of dust produced during the processing of fluoride-containing minerals in many different industries. The current threshold limit value for fluoride in air is 2.5 mg/m^3 (expressed as F).

Blood Concentrations. Background plasma fluoride concentrations in 3 subjects on a low fluoride diet (<0.4 mg F/day) were on the order of 0.010 mg/L. Workers in an aluminum plant with an environmental air fluoride level averaging 0.9 mg/m^3 had pre-shift plasma fluoride concentrations that averaged 0.023 mg/L and post-shift concentrations that averaged 0.048 mg/L (range, 0.014–0.151) (Ehrnebo and Ekstrand, 1986). Following single oral doses of 1.5–10 mg of fluoride (3.3–22 mg as NaF) given to healthy subjects, plasma fluoride concentrations reached peaks of 0.06–0.4

mg/L within 30 minutes of administration and declined with half-lives of 2.0–9.0 hours. Plasma contains about 72% of whole blood fluoride (Carlson et al., 1960); fluoride occurs as a free ion in plasma and is not protein bound (Ekstrand et al., 1977).

Metabolism and Excretion. In both healthy and osteoporotic subjects, about half of the ingested fluoride is excreted unchanged in the daily urine, about 6–10% in the feces, and from 13–23% in sweat. Retention in bone probably accounts for much of the balance, and this percentage is relatively unaffected by the extent of daily intake (McClure et al., 1945; Spencer et al., 1975; Ekstrand et al., 1977).

Urine concentrations of fluoride in normal subjects have been found to range from 0.2–3.2 mg/L, being largely dependent on the dietary intake. Urine fluoride concentrations in a group of asymptomatic workers averaged 4.5 mg/L (range, 2.1–14.7) during chronic exposure to air fluoride levels averaging 2.65 mg/m^3 (Derryberry et al., 1963). The normal fluoride content of brain, lung, liver and kidney ranges from 0.2–0.8 mg/kg, whereas that of bone and teeth ranges from 112–310 mg/kg (Gettler and Ellerbrook, 1939).

Toxicity. Low-level exposure to airborne fluoride is first expressed as irritation of mucous membranes of the eyes, nose and throat. Continued exposure may produce symptoms of early fluoride toxicity that include respiratory distress, neurological abnormalities, gastrointestinal pain and muscular fibrillation. The daily absorption of 10–80 mg of fluoride over a period of years can lead to a condition known as crippling skeletal fluorosis, in which excessive calcification of bone results in stiffening of ligaments and fusion of joints (Hodge and Smith, 1977; Waldbott, 1979).

Numerous instances of acute fluoride poisoning have occurred as a result of the accidental or intentional ingestion or inhalation of fluorides. One mass poisoning involved 263 persons, 47 of whom died, following the inadvertent addition of sodium fluoride to food (Lidbeck et al., 1943). The victims often exhibit nausea, vomiting, salivation, tetanic contractions, coma, respiratory arrest, and ventricular arrhythmias. Treatment includes intravenous administration of calcium to correct hypocalcemia and diuresis to hasten fluoride excretion. Contaminated drinking water caused poisoning in 296 persons, one of who died; the most seriously affected survivor had a serum fluoride concentration of 9.1 mg/L (Gessner et al., 1994). Hospitalized individuals have survived the acute ingestion of up to 120 g of sodium fluoride and serum fluoride levels as high as 14 mg/L (Abukurah et al., 1972; Yolken et al., 1976; Saady and Rose, 1988).

The acute ingestion of 1.5 g of hydrofluoric acid has caused death in an adult (Curry, 1962), while it is felt that 5–10 g represents a minimal lethal dose of sodium fluoride. The following tissue distribution of fluoride was compiled from 14 fatal cases resulting from both ingestion and inhalation (Gettler and Ellerbrook, 1939; Curry, 1962; Greendyke and Hodge, 1964; Cranston and Bastos, 1975; Speaker, 1976; Menchel and Dunn, 1984; Kaa et al., 1986; Poklis and Mackell, 1989):

Fluoride Concentrations in Fatal Cases (mg/L or mg/kg)

	Blood	Brain	Liver	Kidney	Urine
Average	15	2.1	16	17	211
(Range)	(2.6–56)	(1.2–3.4)	(1.7–81)	(2.1–68)	(17–320)

Analysis. Inorganic fluoride is frequently isolated from biological specimens by microdiffusion, and then measured by a colorimetric technique (Sunshine and Finkle, 1975) or by a fluoride-specific electrode (Griffith and Barnes, 1975; Speaker, 1976). Direct measurements with this electrode in plasma and urine are also possible (Sun, 1969; Cernik et al., 1970; Neefus et al., 1970; Ekstrand, 1977; Singer and Ophaug, 1979). A gas chromatographic procedure has been developed that requires conversion of fluoride ion to an organofluorine derivative (Fresen et al., 1968).

References

A.R. Abukurah, A.M. Moser, Jr., C.L. Baird et al. Acute sodium fluoride poisoning. J. Am. Med. Asso. 222: 816–817, 1972.

C.H. Carlson, W.D. Armstrong and L. Singer. Distribution and excretion of radiofluoride in the human. Proc. Soc. Exp. Biol. Med. 104: 235–239, 1960.

A.A. Cernik, J.A. Cooke and R.J. Hall. Specific ion electrode in the determination of urinary fluoride. Nature 227: 1260–1261, 1970.

D. Cranston and M.L. Bastos. Personal communication, 1975.

A.S. Curry. Twenty-one uncommon cases of poisoning. Brit. Med. J. 1: 687–689, 1962.

O.M. Derryberry, M.D. Bartholomew and R.B.L. Fleming. Fluoride exposure and worker health. Arch. Env. Health 6: 503–511, 1963.

M. Ehrnebo and J. Ekstrand. Occupational fluoride exposure and plasma fluoride levels in man. Int. Arch. Occ. Env. Health 58: 179–190, 1986.

J. Ekstrand. A micromethod for the determination of fluoride in blood plasma and saliva. Calc. Tiss. Res. 23: 225–228, 1977.

J. Ekstrand, G. Alvan, L.O. Boreus and A. Norlin. Pharmacokinetics of fluoride in man after single and multiple oral doses. Eur. J. Clin. Pharm. 12: 311–317, 1977.

J.A. Fresen, F.H. Cox and M.J. Witter. The determination of fluoride in biological materials by means of gas chromatography. Pharm. Weekblad. 103: 909–914, 1968.

B.D. Gessner, M. Beller, J.P. Middaugh and G.M. Whitford. Acute fluoride poisoning from a public water system. New Eng. J. Med. 330: 95–99, 1994.

A.O. Gettler and L. Ellerbrook. Toxicology of fluorides. Am. J. Med. Sci. 197: 625–638, 1939.

R.M. Greendyke and H.C. Hodge. Accidental death due to hydrofluoric acid. J. For. Sci. 9: 383–390, 1964.

F.D. Griffith and J.R. Barnes. Fluoride, type C procedure. In *Methodology for Analytical Toxicology* (I. Sunshine, ed.), CRC Press, Cleveland, 1975, pp. 170–172.

H.C. Hodge and F.A. Smith. Occupational fluoride exposure. J. Occ. Med. 19: 12–39, 1977.

E. Kaa, K. Selvig, H. Dybdahl and A. Siboni. A case of fluoride poisoning. Am. J. For. Med. Path. 7: 266–267, 1986.

W.L. Lidbeck, I.B. Hill and J.A. Beeman. Acute sodium fluoride poisoning. J. Am. Med. Asso. 121: 826–827, 1943.

F.J. McClure, H.H. Mitchell, T.S. Hamilton and C.A. Kinser. Balances of fluorine ingested from various sources in food and water by five young men. J. Ind. Hyg. Tox. 27: 159–170, 1945.

S.M. Menchel and W.A. Dunn. Hydrofluoric acid poisoning. Am. J. For. Med. Path. 5: 245–248, 1984.

J.D. Neefus, J. Cholak and B.E. Saltzman. The determination of fluoride in urine using a fluoride-specific ion electrode. Am. Ind. Hyg. Asso. J. 31: 96–99, 1970.

A. Poklis and M.A. Mackell. Disposition of fluoride in a fatal case of unsuspected sodium fluoride poisoning. For. Sci. Int. 41: 55–59, 1989.

J.J. Saady and C.S. Rose. A case of nonfatal sodium fluoride ingestion. J. Anal Tox. 12: 270–271, 1988.

L. Singer and R.H. Ophaug. Concentrations of ionic, total, and bound fluoride in plasma. Clin. Chem. 25: 523–525, 1979.

J.H. Speaker. Determination of fluoride by specific ion electrode and report of a fatal case of fluoride poisoning. J. For. Sci. 21: 121–126, 1976.

H. Spencer, D. Osis and E. Waitrowski. Retention of fluoride with time in man. Clin. Chem. 21: 613–618, 1975.

M.W. Sun. Fluoride ion activity electrode for determination of urinary fluoride. Am. Ind. Hyg. Asso. J. 30: 133–136, 1969.

I. Sunshine and B.S. Finkle. Fluoride, type B procedure. In *Methodology for Analytical Toxicology* (I. Sunshine, ed.), CRC Press, Cleveland, 1975, pp. 168–170.

G.L. Waldbott. Preskeletal fluorosis near an Ohio enamel factory: a preliminary report. Vet. Hum. Tox. 21: 4–8, 1979.

R. Yolken, P. Konecny and P. McCarthy. Acute fluoride poisoning. Pediatrics 58: 90–93, 1976.

Fluoroacetate

T½: ?
Vd: ?   FCH₂COOH
Fb: ?
pKa: 2.6

Occurrence and Usage. Sodium fluoroacetate (compound 1080) and fluoroacetamide (compound 1081) are highly toxic chemicals used primarily as insecticides and rodenticides. Fluoroacetate ion produces inhibition of oxidative cellular metabolism by entering the citric acid cycle and, after conversion to fluorocitrate, by poisoning the enzyme aconitase. Fluoroacetic acid was identified in 1944 as the main toxic constituent of a very poisonous South African plant, *Dichapetalum cymosum*.

Blood Concentrations. Normal human body fluids and tissues contain no detectable amounts of fluoroacetate. Note should be taken of normal fluoride or citrate levels, however, in the event these substances are measured as an indication of fluoroacetate exposure.

Metabolism and Excretion. The metabolism of fluoroacetate has been investigated only superficially in animals and not at all in man. It is known to be activated by oxidation to fluorocitrate (Peters, 1952), but has not been found to undergo detoxification via further metabolism (Peters, 1957). Only 1% of an oral dose is excreted in urine and feces of rats by 5 hours and 12% by 48 hours (Hagan et al., 1950).

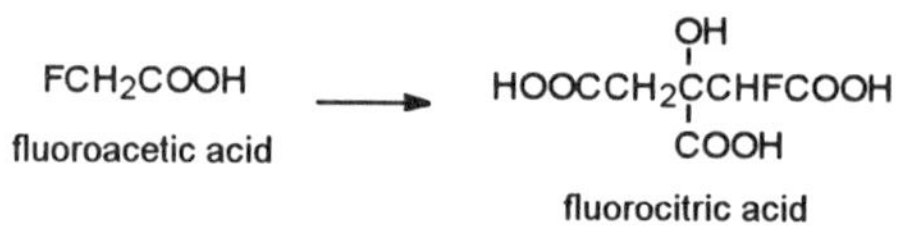

$$FCH_2COOH \longrightarrow HOOCCH_2 \overset{\overset{\displaystyle OH}{|}}{\underset{\underset{\displaystyle COOH}{|}}{C}} CHFCOOH$$

fluoroacetic acid   fluorocitric acid

Toxicity. As of 1955 there had been 23 known cases of fluoroacetate poisoning in man, 17 of which were fatal (Brockmann et al., 1955). The mean lethal dose for an adult has been estimated at 2–10 mg/kg (140–700 mg/70 kg) for sodium fluoroacetate. The onset of toxicity is delayed, pending biotransformation to fluorocitrate, and death due to cardiac or respiratory arrest may follow as much as 5 days after the ingestion of large amounts of the poison. Interference with acetate metabolism causes a marked increase in tissue citrate levels, and this effect has been used as an aid in the diagnosis of fluoroacetate poisoning (Allcroft et al., 1969). Survivors often develop acute renal failure (Chung, 1984). Fluoroacetate has been detected in liver and kidney of poisoned animals in concentrations of 2.5–17 mg/kg; fluorocitrate has also been found present but was not quantitated (Stahr et al., 1974; Stevens et al., 1976). In a case of fatal human poisoning due to the ingestion of at least 465 mg of sodium fluoroacetate, organ concentrations of fluorine were measured and expressed as fluoroacetate (Harrisson et al., 1952):

Fluoroacetate Concentrations in a Fatal Case (mg/L or mg/kg)

Brain	Liver	Kidney	Urine	Gastric
76	58	65	368	12 mg

Analysis. The total fluoride in tissues may be measured using a fluoride-specific electrode after liberation of organic fluorine in an oxygen combustion flask (Peters and Baxter, 1974; Egezeke and Oehme, 1979). Specific gas chromatographic procedures for the identification of fluoroacetate in biological specimens have relied on flame-ionization, electron-capture or mass spectrometric detection of a derivative (Stahr et al., 1974; Peterson, 1975; Stevens et al., 1976; Hoogenboom and

Rammell, 1987; Allender, 1990). Citric acid concentrations may also be estimated by gas chromatography of the methyl ester (Rumsey and Noller, 1966). A liquid chromatographic method for fluoroacetate in gastric contents has been reported (Ray et al., 1981).

References

R. Allcroft, R.A. Peters and M. Shorthouse. Fluoroacetamide poisoning—part II. Toxicity in dairy cattle: a confirmation of diagnosis. Vet. Rec. 84: 403–409, 1969.

W.J. Allender. Determination of sodium fluoroacetate (compound 1080) in biological tissues. J. Anal. Tox. 14: 45–49, 1990.

J.L. Brockmann, A.V. McDowell and W.G. Leeds. Fatal poisoning with sodium fluoroacetate. J. Am. Med. Asso. 159: 1529–1532, 1955.

H.M. Chung. Acute renal failure caused by acute monofluoroacetate poisoning. Vet. Hum. Tox. 26 (Suppl. 2): 29–32, 1984.

J.O. Egekeze and F.W. Oehme. Determination of sodium monofluoroacetate (compound 1080) in biological tissues using oxygen combustion and a fluoride selective membrane electrode. Tox. Letters 4: 461–467, 1979.

E.C. Hagan, L.L. Ramsey and G. Woodard. Absorption, distribution, and excretion of sodium fluoroacetate (1080) in rats. J. Pharm. Exp. Ther. 99: 432–434, 1950.

J.W.E. Harrisson, J.L. Ambrus, C.M. Ambrus et al. Acute poisoning with sodium fluoroacetate (compound 1080). J. Am. Med. Asso. 149: 1520–1522, 1952.

J.J.L. Hoogenboom and C.G. Rammell. Determination of sodium monofluoroacetate (compound 1080) in tissues and baits as its benzyl ester by reaction-capillary gas chromatography. J. Anal. Tox. 11: 140–143, 1987.

J.A. Peters and K.J. Baxter. Analytical determination of compound 1080 (sodium fluoroacetate) residues in biological materials. Bull. Env. Cont. Tox. 11: 177–183, 1974.

R.A. Peters. Lethal synthesis. Proc. Roy. Soc. Lond. 139: 143–170, 1952.

R.A. Peters. Mechanism of the toxicity of the active constituent of Dichapetalum cymosum and related compounds. Adv. Enzymol. 18: 113–159, 1957.

J.E. Peterson. A gas chromatographic method for sodium fluoroacetate (compound 1080) in biological materials. Bull. Env. Cont. Tox. 13: 751–757, 1975.

A.C. Ray, L.O. Post and J.C. Reagor. High pressure liquid chromatographic determination of sodium fluoroacetate (compound 1080) in canine gastric contents. J. Asso. Off. Anal. Chem. 64: 19–24, 1981.

T.S. Rumsey and C.H. Noller. A study of the quantitative measurement of certain metabolic acids by gas-liquid chromatography. J. Chrom. 24: 325–334, 1966.

H.M. Stahr, W.B. Buck and P.F. Ross. Gas-liquid chromatographic determination of sodium fluoroacetate. J. Asso. Off. Anal. Chem. 57: 405–407, 1974.

H.M. Stevens, A.C. Moffat and J.V. Drayton. The recovery and identification of fluoroacetamide and fluoroacetic acid from tissues. For. Sci. 8: 131–137, 1976.

Fluorocarbons

T½: 1.5 hr (FC-11)
Vd: ?
Fb: 0

Occurrence and Usage. The fluorocarbons comprise a group of synthetic halogen-substituted methane and ethane derivatives, primarily, which find extensive commercial application as aerosol propellants and refrigerants. Though they were shown many years ago to have a very low order of toxicity in laboratory animals, it has become evident that the fluorocarbons are capable of producing rapid death in persons abusing the chemicals for their euphoric effects. The structures of the most common examples of this class are as follows:

CCl_3F	CCl_2F_2	$CHClF_2$	CCl_2FCClF_2	$CClF_2CClF_2$
FC-11	FC-12	FC-22	FC-113	FC-114
b.p., 24° C.	b.p., -30° C.	b.p., -41° C.	b.p., 47° C.	b.p., 4° C.

Fluorocarbons 11 and 12, especially, have been commonly used as propellants in hundreds of household products and pharmaceutical preparations; these materials have been largely withdrawn from the United States market as a result of their potential effect on ozone concentrations in the upper atmosphere (Wofsy et al., 1975). The current industrial threshold limit value for either FC-11 or FC-12 is 1000 ppm.

Blood Concentrations. Peak arterial blood concentrations in asthmatic patients 10–20 seconds after 2 puffs from a bronchodilator inhaler (delivering 25 mg FC-11 and 65 mg FC-12 per puff) ranged from 0.5–4.5 mg/L for FC-11 and 0.2–4.7 mg/L for FC-12; the distribution half-lives were 18–38 seconds and 12–24 seconds, respectively (Dollery et al., 1974). Venous blood concentrations of 0.3–2.6 mg/L were observed for FC-11 in 5 asthmatic patients 30–90 seconds after 2 puffs from an inhaler (25 mg per puff); after 10 minutes, the blood concentrations were all less than 0.06 mg/L (Paterson et al., 1971). Three volunteers exposed for approximately 3 hours to an FC-11 air concentration of 657 ppm developed venous blood concentrations of 2.7–2.9 mg/L during the exposure (Angerer et al., 1985). It has been calculated that constant exposure to fluorocarbons at air concentrations of 1000 ppm would produce equilibrium venous blood levels of 4.9 and 1.2 mg/L for FC-11 and FC-12, respectively (Adir et al., 1975). An elimination half-life of 1.5 hours has been estimated for FC-11 (Chiou, 1974).

FC-22 blood concentrations reached an average peak level of 1.4 mg/L in 3 volunteers exposed to 518 ppm of the vapor for 4 hours; the levels declined with a terminal half-life of 2.6 hours (Woollen et al., 1992). FC-113 blood concentrations reached an average peak of 3.1 mg/L in 7 volunteers exposed to 1004 ppm of the vapor for 4 hours; the levels declined with a terminal half-life of 29 hours (Woollen et al., 1990).

Metabolism and Excretion. About 92 and 35% of administered doses of FC-11 and FC-12, respectively, is absorbed. Of the absorbed amount, an average of 89 and 99%, respectively, is exhaled unchanged within 1 hour. Less than 0.2% of each compound is excreted as carbon dioxide in the 1 hour breath and as unidentified metabolites in the 72 hour urine (Mergner et al., 1975). Less than 0.01% of a dose of FC-11 is excreted unchanged in the urine (Angerer et al., 1985).

Toxicity. The first reported death due to intentional inhalation of fluorocarbons occurred in 1967 and involved a 15 year old boy (Baselt and Cravey, 1968). In 1970, Bass published a study of 110 sudden deaths attributed to deliberate sniffing of fluorocarbons and other solvents. It is believed that these materials sensitize the myocardium to circulating catecholamines, producing ventricular arrhythmia and cardiac arrest under certain circumstances (Taylor and Harris, 1970; Reinhardt et al., 1971; Flowers and Horan, 1972). Venous blood concentrations found to produce cardiac sensitization in the dog averaged 20 mg/L for FC-11 and 23 mg/L for FC-12; it required a tenfold difference in the inspired air concentration for FC-11 (0.5%) and FC-12 (5%) to produce these levels (Azar et al., 1973). Fluorocarbon concentrations in tissues from human victims and animals exposed to lethal concentrations of the vapor are remarkably comparable; additionally, there is little change in concentrations of FC-22 in the intact animal body over a 3 day period (Morita et al., 1977). Significant fluorocarbon losses may be incurred during specimen handling and storage, however, unless precautions are taken. From the analytical results in 7 fatalities attributed to the intentional inhalation of a combination of FC-11 and FC-12, it may be seen that FC-11 concentrations nearly always exceed those of FC-12, despite a nearly 1:1 ratio of the agents in most of the products involved), and that the lung is generally the tissue with the highest concentrations of those studied (Baselt and Cravey, 1968; Christopoulos and Kirch, 1974; Bednarczyk, 1975; Poklis, 1975; Standefer, 1975):

Fluorocarbon Concentrations in Fatal Cases (mg/L or mg/kg)

	Blood	Brain	Lung	Liver	Kidney
FC-11					
Average	12	30	43	21	18
(Range)	(1.2–32)	(0.4–64)	(5.8–94)	(5–45)	(5.4–26)
FC-12					
Average	3.0	4.3	33	4.7	1.3
(Range)	(0.6–12)	(0.5–9.7)	(0.9–134)	(1–10)	(0.7–1.8)

Additionally, the deaths of 3 adults following exposure to FC-22 were investigated; much higher concentrations and a somewhat different tissue distribution were observed (Bidanset, 1973; Morita et al., 1977):

Fluorocarbon-22 Concentrations in Fatal Cases (mg/L or mgkg)

	Blood	Brain	Lung	Liver	Kidney
Average	371	715	248	358	83
(Range)	(286–538)	(282–1450)	(75–590)	(294–400)	(33–140)

At least 5 deaths due to accidental industrial exposure to FC-113 have been reported; postmortem lung concentrations of 0.05–1.0 mg/kg were determined in 4 of the cases, while brain and liver concentrations of 111 and 5.6 mg/kg, respectively, were found in the fifth case (May and Blotzer, 1984; Clark et al., 1985).

Analysis. The fluorocarbons are conveniently assayed in biological tissues by flame-ionization or electron-capture gas chromatography with headspace sampling (Baselt and Cravey, 1968; Chiou and Niazi, 1973; Standefer, 1975; Woollen et al., 1992) or solvent extraction techniques (Terrill, 1972; Christopoulos and Kirch, 1974; Dollery et al., 1974; Woollen et al., 1990). Gas chromatography-mass spectrometry has also been described (Hamill and Kee, 1991; Fitzgerald et al., 1993).

References

J. Adir, D.A. Blake and G.M. Mergner. Pharmacokinetics of fluorocarbon 11 and 12 in dogs and humans. J. Clin. Pharm. 15: 760–770, 1975.

J. Angerer, B. Schroeder and R. Heinrich. Exposure to fluorotrichloromethane (R-11). Int. Arch. Occ. Env. Health 56: 67–72, 1985.

A. Azar, H.J. Trochimowicz, J.B. Terrill and L.S. Mullin. Blood levels of fluorocarbon related to cardiac sensitization. Am. Ind. Hyg. Asso. J. 34: 102–109, 1973.

R.C. Baselt and R.H. Cravey. A fatal case involving trichloromonofluoromethane and dichlorodifluoromethane. J. For. Sci. 13: 407–410, 1968.

M. Bass. Sudden sniffing death. J. Am. Med. Asso. 212: 2075–2079, 1970.

L.R. Bednarczyk. Personal communication, 1975.

J. Bidanset. Unusual volatile compounds encountered in six years experience with gas chromatographic head space technique. Presented at the 25th Annual Meeting of the American Academy of Forensic Sciences, Las Vegas, February 22, 1973.

W.L. Chiou. Aerosol propellants: cardiac toxicity and long biological half-life. J. Am. Med. Asso. 227: 658, 1974.

W.L. Chiou and S. Niazi. A simple and ultra-sensitive head-space gas chromatographic method for the assay of fluorocarbon propellants in blood. Res. Comm. Chem. Path. Pharm. 6: 481–498, 1973.

G.N. Christopoulos and E.R. Kirch. Estimation of fluoroalkane propellants. J. For. Sci. 19: 168–171, 1974.

M.A. Clark, J.W. Jones, J.J. Robinson and J.T. Lord. Multiple deaths resulting from shipboard exposure to trichlorotrifluoroethane. J. For. Sci. 30: 1256–1259, 1985.

C.T. Dollery, F.M. Williams, G.H. Draffan et al. Arterial blood levels of fluorocarbons in asthmatic patients following use of pressurized aerosols. Clin. Pharm. Ther. 15: 59–66, 1974.

R.L. Fitzgerald, C.E. Fishel and L.L.E. Bush. Fatality due to recreational use of chlorodifluoromethane and chloropentafluoroethane. J. For. Sci. 38: 476–482, 1993.

N.C. Flowers and L.G. Horan. Nonanoxic aerosol arrhythmias. J. Am. Med. Asso. 219: 33–37, 1972.

J. Hamill and T.G. Kee. The detection of aerosol propellants in body fluids and tissues by gas chromatography-mass spectrometry. J. For. Sci. Soc. 31: 301–307, 1991.

D.C. May and M.J. Blotzer. A report of occupational deaths attributed to fluorocarbon-113. Arch. Env. Health 39: 352–354, 1984.

G.W. Mergner, D.A. Blake and M. Helrich. Biotransformation and elimination of ^{14}C-trichlorofluoromethane (FC-11) and ^{14}C-dichlorofluoromethane (FC-12) in man. Anesthesiology 42: 345–351, 1975.

M. Morita, A. Miki, H. Kazama and M. Sakata. Case report of deaths caused by Freon gas. For. Sci. 10: 253–260, 1977.

J.W. Paterson, M.F. Sudlow and S.R. Walker. Blood-levels of fluorinated hydrocarbons in asthmatic patients after inhalation of pressurized aerosols. Lancet 2: 565–568, 1971.

A. Poklis. Determination of fluorocarbon 11 and fluorocarbon 12 in post-mortem tissues: a case report. For. Sci. 5: 53–59, 1975.

C.F. Reinhardt, A. Azar, M.E. Maxfield et al. Cardiac arrhythmias and aerosol "sniffing." Arch. Env. Health 22: 265–279, 1971.

J.C. Standefer. Death associated with fluorocarbon inhalation: a report of a case. J. For. Sci. 20: 548–551, 1975.

G.J. Taylor and W.S. Harris. Cardiac toxicity of aerosol propellants. J. Am. Med. Asso. 214: 81–85, 1970.

J.B. Terrill. Determination of fluorocarbon propellants in blood and animal tissue. Am. Ind. Hyg. Asso. J. 33: 736–744, 1972.

S.C. Wofsy, M.B. McElroy and N.D. Sze. Freon consumption: implications for atmosphere ozone. Science 187: 535–537, 1975.

B.H. Woollen, E.A. Guest, W. Howe et al. Human inhalation pharmacokinetics of 1,1,2-trichloro-1,2,2-trifluoroethane (FC113). Int. Arch. Occ. Env. Health 62: 73–78, 1990.

B.H. Woollen, J.R. Marsh, J.D. Mahler et al. Human inhalation pharmacokinetics of chlorodifluoromethane (HCFC22). Int. Arch. Occ. Env. Health 64: 383–387, 1992.

5-Fluorouracil

T½: 11 hr
Vd: 0.25 L/kg
Fb: 0.08–0.12
pKa: 8.0, 13.0

Occurrence and Usage. 5-Fluorouracil (5-FU, Efudex, Fluoroplex) is an antineoplastic antimetabolite used in the treatment of certain types of cancer in patients who are considered incurable by surgery or other means. It is available in ampules containing 50 mg/mL as the sodium salt for intravenous administration. The usual adult dose is up to 800 mg daily, or 400 mg daily in poor risk patients. The drug is usually not administered orally since absorption is unpredictable and incomplete. Fluorouracil is also available as a 1% topical cream or 1–5% topical solution for dermatological use. The cream or solution is applied once or twice daily in an amount sufficient to cover the lesions; usage is continued for 3–12 weeks.

Blood Concentrations. In 5 adult patients who received intravenous fluorouracil at a dose of 3.3–4.5 mg/kg (average, 3.7), the average peak plasma concentration was 13 mg/L (range, 6.4–30). In 6 adult patients who received oral fluorouracil in doses ranging from 5.6–9.1 mg/kg (average, 7.6), peak plasma concentrations ranged from 4.4–12 mg/L (average, 7.8) and occurred within 15–20 minutes after dosing (Phillips et al., 1980).

Metabolism and Excretion. Following intravenous injection, no intact drug can be detected in the plasma after 3 hours, and 60–80% of the dose is excreted as expired carbon dioxide in 8–12 hours.

The metabolic pathway generating the various urinary metabolites of 5-fluorouracil is not fully understood. The urinary excretion products include unchanged drug, 5,6-dihydro-5-fluorouracil ($5FUH_2$), alpha-fluoro-beta-ureidopropionic acid (FUPA), alpha-fluoro-beta-alanine (FBAL), and fluoride ion. The fluoride ion is thought to come from the metabolic degradation of FBAL. FBAL accounts for about 80% of the total urinary excretion products, with unchanged drug, FUPA and fluoride accounting for 10.8%, 7.9% and 2%, respectively. The proportion excreted as $5FUH_2$ is less than 0.5% (Myers, 1981; Bernadou et al., 1985; Martino et al., 1985).

Toxicity. Stomatitis, esophagopharyngitis, diarrhea, anorexia, nausea and emesis are common adverse reactions to the drug. Others are leukopenia, thrombocytopenia, dermatitis and alopecia.

Analysis. Over a 24 hour period of storage at room temperature, losses of 94% in whole blood and 52% in plasma were observed for the parent drug; storage at 0° C. reduced the losses to 30% and 10%, respectively (Murphy et al., 1987). 5-Fluorouracil has been determined in blood, plasma, serum and urine using gas chromatography (Cohen and Brennan, 1973; van den Berg et al., 1978; Driessen et al., 1979; De Leenheer and Cosyn-Duyck, 1979). Liquid chromatography has also been used to measure both the parent compound and its metabolites (Cohen and Brown, 1978; Au et al., 1982; Samson et al., 1982; Stetson et al., 1985; Lacreta and Williams, 1987; Jager et al., 1990; Barberi-Heyob et al., 1992). Gas chromatography-mass spectrometry offers a more specific means of determining 5-fluorouracil and its metabolites in biological samples (Kok et al., 1985; Min et al., 1985).

References

J.L.S. Au, M.G. Wientjes, C.M. Luccioni and Y.M. Rustum. Reversed-phase ion-pair high-performance liquid chromatographic assay of 5-fluorouracil, 5'-deoxy-5-fluorouridine, their nucleosides, mono-, di-, and triphosphate nucleotides with a mixture of quaternary ammonium ions. J. Chrom. 228: 245–256, 1982.

M. Barberi-Heyob, J.L. Merlin and B. Weber. Determination of 5-fluorouracil and its main metabolites in plasma by high-performance liquid chromatography. J. Chrom. 573: 247–252, 1992.

J. Bernadou, J.P. Armand, A. Lopez et al. Complete urinary excretion profile of 5-fluorouracil during a six-day chemotherapeutic schedule, as resolved by ^{19}F nuclear magnetic resonance. Clin. Chem. 31: 846–848, 1985.

A. Buur and H. Bundgaard. Prodrugs of 5-fluorouracil. 1-Alkoxycarbonyl derivatives as potential forms for improved rectal or oral delivery of 5-fluorouracil. J. Pharm. Sci. 75: 522–527, 1986.

J.L. Cohen and P.B. Brennan. GLC assay for 5-fluorouracil in biological fluids. J. Pharm. Sci. 62: 572–575, 1973.

J.L. Cohen and R.E. Brown. High performance liquid chromatographic analysis of 5-fluorouracil in plasma. J. Chrom. 151: 237–240, 1978.

A.P. De Leenheer and M.I. Cosyns-Duyck. Flame-ionization GLC assay for fluorouracil in plasma of cancer patients. J. Pharm. Sci. 68: 1174–1177, 1979.

O. Driessen, D. De Vos and P.J. Timmermans. Sensitive gas-liquid chromatographic assay of underivatized 5-fluorouracil in plasma. J. Chrom. 162: 451–456, 1979.

M. Iwamato, S. Yoshida and S. Hirose. Fluorescence determination of 5-fluorouracil and 1-(tetrahydro-2-furanyl)-5-fluorouracil in blood serum by high-performance liquid chromatography. J. Chrom. 310: 151–158, 1984.

W. Jager, M.J. Czejka, J. Schuller et al. Rapid and simple high-performance liquid chromatographic assay for 5'-fluorouracil in plasma for bioavailability studies. J. Chrom. 532: 411–417, 1990.

R.M. Kok, A.P.J.M. de Jong, C.J. van Groeningen et al. Highly sensitive determination of 5-fluorouracil in human plasma by capillary gas chromatography and negative ion chemical ionization mass spectrometry. J. Chrom. 343: 59–66, 1985.

F.P. Lacreta and W.M. Williams. High-performance liquid chromatographic analysis of fluoropyrimidine nucleosides and fluorouracil in plasma. J. Chrom. 414: 197–201, 1987.

R. Martino, A. Lopez, M.C. Malet-Martino et al. Release of fluoride ion from 5-fluorouridine, an antineoplastic fluoropyrimidine, in humans. Drug Met. Disp. 13: 116–118, 1985.

B.H. Min, W.A. Garland and T.M. Lewinson. Comparison of gas chromatographic/mass spectrometric and microbiological assays for 5-fluorouracil in plasma. Biomed. Mass Spec. 12: 238–240, 1985.

R.F. Murphy, F.M. Balis and D.G. Poplack. Stability of 5-fluorouracil in whole blood and plasma. Clin. Chem. 33: 2299–2300, 1987.

C.E. Myers. The pharmacology of the fluoropyrimidines. Pharm. Rev. 33: 1–15, 1981.

G.J. Peters, I. Fraal, E. Laurensse et al. Separation of 5-fluorouracil and uracil by ion-pair reversed-phase high-performance liquid chromatography on a column with porous polymeric packing. J. Chrom. 307: 464–468, 1984.

T.A. Phillips, A. Howell, R.J. Grieve and P.G. Welling. Pharmacokinetics of oral and intravenous fluorouracil in humans. J. Pharm. Sci. 69: 1428–1431, 1980.

E.J. Quebbeman, N.E. Hoffman, A.A.R. Hamid and R.K. Ausman. An HPLC method for measuring 5-fluorouracil in plasma. J. Liq. Chrom. 7: 1489–1494, 1984.

D.C. Sampson, R.M. Fox, M.H.N. Tattersall and W.J. Hensley. A rapid high-performance liquid chromatographic method for quantitation of 5-fluorouracil in plasma after continuous intravenous infusion. Ann. Clin. Biochem. 19: 125–128, 1982.

P.L. Stetson, U.A. Shukla and W.D. Ensminger. Sensitive high-performance liquid chromatographic method for the determination of 5-fluorouracil in plasma. J. Chrom. 344: 385–390, 1985.

H.W. Van Den Berg, R.F. Murphy, R. Hunter and D.T. Elmore. An improved gas-liquid chromatographic assay for 5-fluorouracil in plasma. J. Chrom. 145: 311–314, 1978.

Fluoxetine

T½: 1–3 days
Vd: 26 L/kg
Fb: 0.94
pKa: ?

F_3C—⬡—$OCHCH_2CH_2NHCH_3$

Occurrence and Usage. Fluoxetine (Prozac) is an atypical antidepressant with blockade of serotonin reuptake as the proposed mechanism of action. The drug has structural similarities to methamphetamine and fenfluramine and has been used for the management of depression in the United States since 1987. Fluoxetine is available as the hydrochloride salt in capsules containing 20 mg and as a liquid containing 20 mg/5 mL for oral administration. The recommended initial dose is 20 mg/day administered in the morning; if no clinical improvement is observed after several weeks, the dose may be increased to a maximum of 80 mg/day.

Blood Concentrations. A single oral 40 mg dose in adults produces peak plasma fluoxetine levels of 15–55 µg/L within 6–8 hours (PDR, 1993).

Twenty-four patients receiving 20–60 mg of the drug daily developed steady-state serum concentrations that averaged 109 µg/L (range, 25–473) for fluoxetine and 130 µg/L (range, 18–466) for norfluoxetine (Orsulak et al., 1988). A similar study of 13 patients receiving 20–60 mg daily produced steady-state serum levels of 60–453 µg/L (range, 231) for fluoxetine and 54–362 µg/L (average, 231) for norfluoxetine (Kelly et al., 1981).

Plasma elimination half-lives of 1–3 days for fluoxetine and 7–15 days for norfluoxetine have been reported in single-dose studies (Lemberger et al., 1985), but half-lives averaging 8 days for fluoxetine and 19 days for norfluoxetine have been observed in patients following discontinuation of long-term therapy (Pato et al., 1991). The blood/plasma concentration ratios for the drug and its metabolite average 1.04 and 1.12, respectively (Amitai et al., 1993).

Metabolism and Excretion. Fluoxetine is biotransformed to the active metabolite, norfluoxetine; both compounds may undergo O-dealkylation, with release of p-trifluoromethylphenol (Benfield et al., 1986). Less than 10% of the parent drug is excreted unchanged in the urine (Lemberger et al., 1985).

Brain concentrations of fluoxetine plus norfluoxetine in patients on chronic therapy with the drug averaged 2.6 times that of plasma (Renshaw et al., 1992).

Toxicity. Adverse reactions to fluoxetine therapy include nausea, insomnia, anxiety and headache. Less frequently, manic behavior and suicidal ideation have been reported; encephalopathy with seizures may occur if the drug is used in combination with lithium, tranylcypromine or the tricyclic antidepressants (Noveske et al., 1989; Spiller et al., 1990; Stoll et al., 1991). Acute overdosage with up to 1500 mg of fluoxetine often results in relatively benign symptoms, including lethargy, tachycardia and hypertension (Borys et al., 1990).

Six fatalities have been reported in adults who ingested from 1–2 g of fluoxetine and, in 4 of the cases, at least one other drug (codeine, meperidine, clozapine or diphenhydramine); the following tissue concentrations reflect postmortem findings (Cravey, 1989; Kincaid et al., 1990; Roetger, 1990; Fraser, 1991; Osciewicz, 1992; PDR, 1993):

Drug Concentrations in Fluoxetine Fatilities (mg/L or mg/kg)

	Blood	Brain	Liver	Urine	Gastric
Fluoxetine					
Average	3.8	71	70	12	153
(Range)	(1.3–6.8)	(71)	(29–128)	(5.5–19)	(0.3–270)
Norfluoxetine					
Average	2.1	12	17	3	0
(Range)	(0.9–5.0)	(12)	(17)	(3)	(0)

Fluoxetine is apparently subject to postmortem redistribution; heart blood/femoral blood concentration ratios of 3.5 and 4.5 were observed in 2 cases of fatal overdosage (Rohrig and Prouty, 1989; Roettger, 1990).

Analysis. Gas chromatography with electron-capture detection has been used for the determination of fluoxetine in biological specimens (Nash et al., 1982; Dixit et al., 1991; Torokboth et al., 1992; Lantz et al., 1993). Liquid chromatography has been employed in the analysis of both fluoxetine and norfluoxetine (Orsulak et al., 1988; Kelly et al., 1989; Gupta and Steiner, 1990; Thomare et al., 1992; Elmaanni et al., 1993).

References

Y. Amitai, E. Kennedy, P. DeSandre et al. Red cell and plasma concentrations of fluoxetine and norfluoxetine. Vet. Hum. Tox. 35: 134–136, 1993.

P. Benfield, R.C. Heel and S.P. Lewis. Fluoxetine: a review of its pharmacodynamic and pharmacokinetic properties, and therapeutic efficacy in depressive illness. Drugs 32: 481–508, 1986.

D.J. Borys, S.C. Setzer, L.J. Ling et al. The effects of fluoxetine in the overdose patient. Clin. Tox. 28: 331–340, 1990.

R.H. Cravey. Unpublished data, 1989.

V. Dixit, H. Nguyen and V.M. Dixit. Solid-phase extraction of fluoxetine and norfluoxetine from serum with gas-chromatography electron-capture detection. J. Chrom. 563: 379–384, 1991.

A. Elmaanni, I. Combourieu, M. Bonini and E.E. Creppy. Fluoxetine, an anti-depressant, and norfluoxetine, its metabolite, determined by HPLC with a C-8 column and ultraviolet detection. Clin. Chem. 39: 1749, 1993.

A.D. Fraser. Personal communication, 1991.

R.N. Gupta and M. Steiner. Determination of fluoxetine and norfluoxetine in serum by liquid chromatography with fluorescence detection. J. Liq. Chrom. 13: 3785–3798, 1990.

M.W. Kelly, P.J. Perry, S.G. Holstad and M.J. Garvey. Serum fluoxetine and norfluoxetine concentrations and antidepressant response. Ther. Drug Mon. 11: 165–170, 1989.

R.L. Kincaid, M.M. McMullin, S.B. Crookham and F. Rieders. Report of a fluoxetine fatality. J. Anal. Tox. 14: 327–329, 1990.

R.J. Lantz, K.Z. Farid, J. Koons et al. Determination of fluoxetine and norfluoxetine in human plasma by capillary gas chromatography with electron-capture detection. J. Chrom. 614: 175–179, 1993.

L. Lemberger, R.F. Bergstrom, R.L. Wolen et al. Fluoxetine: clinical pharmacology and physiologic disposition. J. Clin. Psych. 46: 14–19, 1985.

J.F. Nash, R.J. Bopp, R.H. Carmichael et al. Determination of fluoxetine and norfluoxetine in plasma by gas chromatography with electron-capture detection. Clin. Chem. 28: 2100–2102, 1982.

F.G. Noveske, K.R. Hahn and R.J. Flynn. Possible toxicity of combined fluoxetine and lithium. Am. J. Psych. 146: 1515, 1989.

P.J. Orsulak, J.T. Kenney, J.R. Debus et al. Determination of the antidepressant fluoxetine and its metabolite norfluoxetine in serum by reversed-phase HPLC with ultraviolet detection. Clin. Chem. 34: 1875–1878, 1988.

R. Osiewicz. Personal communication, 1992.

M.T. Pato, D.L. Murphy and C.L. DeVane. Sustained plasma concentrations of fluoxetine and/or norfluoxetine four and eight weeks after fluoxetine discontinuation. J. Clin. Psychopharm. 11: 224–225, 1991.

Physicians' Desk Reference, Medical Economics Company, Montvale, New Jersey, 1993, pp. 943–946.

P.F. Renshaw, A.R. Guimaraes, M. Fava et al. Accumulation of fluoxetine and norfluoxetine in human brain during therapeutic administration. Am. J. Psych. 149: 1592–1594, 1992.

J.R. Roettger. The importance of blood collection site for the determination of basic drugs: a case with fluoxetine and diphenhydramine overdose. J. Anal. Tox. 14: 191–192, 1990.

T.P. Rohrig and R.W. Prouty. Fluoxetine overdose: a case report. J. Anal. Tox. 13: 305–307, 1989.

H.A. Spiller, S. Morse and C. Muir. Fluoxetine ingestion: a one year retrospective study. Vet. Hum. Tox. 32: 153–155, 1990.

A.L. Stoll, H.G. Pope and S.L. McElroy. High-dose fluoxetine: safety and efficacy in 27 cases. J. Clin. Psychopharm. 11: 225–226, 1991.

P. Thomare, K. Wang, V. Vandermeerschmougeot and B. Diquet. Sensitive micromethod for column liquid chromatographic determination of fluoxetine and norfluoxetine in human plasma. J. Chrom. 583: 217–222, 1992.

G.A. Torokboth, G.B. Baker, R.T. Coutts et al. Simultaneous determination of fluoxetine and norfluoxetine enantiomers in biological samples by gas chromatography with electron-capture detection. J. Chrom. 579: 99–106, 1992.

Fluphenazine

T½: 13–58 hr (hydrochloride)
   3–4 days (enanthate)
   5–12 days (decanoate)
Vd: 220 L/kg
Fb: 0.99
pKa: 3.9, 8.1

Occurrence and Usage. Fluphenazine (Prolixin, Permitil) is a phenothiazine derivative, chemically related to perphenazine and trifluoperazine, that has been in clinical use since 1968 in the treatment of psychotic disorders. It is available as the hydrochloride in 1–10 mg tablets or a 2.5 mg/5 mL syrup for oral use, and a 2.5 mg/mL solution for intramuscular injection. Daily doses of the hydrochloride range from 2.5–20 mg. Fluphenazine is also available as long-acting decanoate and enanthate esters in 25 mg/mL oil solutions for subcutaneous or intramuscular injection. Doses of 12.5–100 mg are administered once every 1–3 weeks.

Blood Concentrations. Six volunteers given a single 5 mg oral dose of fluphenazine hydrochloride developed peak plasma concentrations of 0.26–1.1 µg/L at an average time of 2.8 hours; the levels declined with an average half-life of 33 hours (Midha et al., 1983). A single 25 mg oral dose of the hydrochloride produced a peak plasma concentration in 1 subject of 1.7 µg/L at 0.5 hours; the same dose by intramuscular administration resulted in peak levels of 13.0 and 22.6 µg/L at 1.5–2.0 hours in 2 subjects. Plasma levels declined in both situations with an average half-life of 15 hours. A 25 mg intramuscular dose of fluphenazine enanthate produced peak plasma levels of 1.1 and 1.5 µg/L in 2 subjects after 48 hours, and declined with a half-life of 3.7 days. The same dose of the decanoate ester resulted in high initial plasma concentrations (2–20 µg/L) that dropped to 0.5 µg/L by 12–24 hours and then declined with a half-life of 7–10 days (Curry et al., 1979).

Steady-state plasma fluphenazine concentrations in patients receiving an intramuscular injection of the decanoate ester every 1–2 weeks ranged from 0.9–3.5 µg/L at a dose of 12.5 mg, 4.7–7.3 µg/L at 25 mg, and 5.1–16.8 µg/L at 50 mg (Wiles and Gelder, 1979). Plasma concentrations of fluphenazine sulfoxide, 7-hydroxyfluphenazine and fluphenazine-N-oxide were approximately 320%, 210% and 90%, respectively, of the parent drug in patients maintained on oral fluphenazine hydrochloride; the metabolite concentrations averaged 68%, 23% and 9%, respectively, in patients maintained on depot fluphenazine decanoate (Mardet et al., 1989).

Metabolism and Excretion. The human disposition of fluphenazine has not been quantitatively studied. Fluphenazine, 7-hydroxyfluphenazine and fluphenazine sulfoxide have been identified as urinary excretion products in both free and conjugated form (Breyer et al., 1974; Curry et al., 1979) and fluphenazine-N-oxide has been identified as an important plasma species (Marder et al., 1989). All 3 of these metabolites are believed to exhibit significant pharmacological activity (Aravagiri et al., 1994). After a single oral dose of the hydrochloride, monkeys eliminated 12–19% in the urine and 56–69% in the feces, largely as metabolites (Dreyfuss et al., 1971).

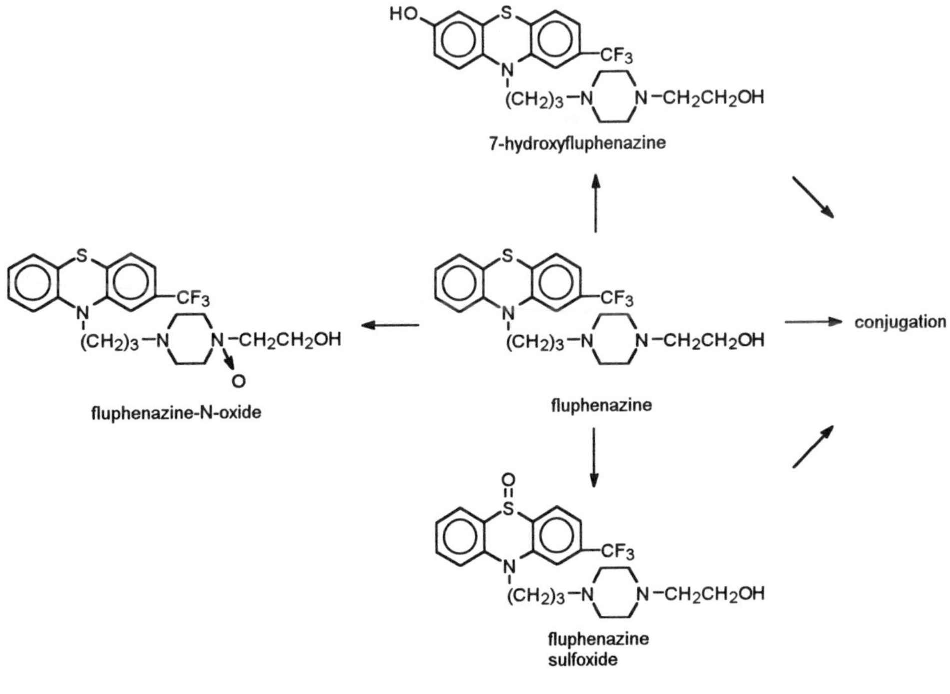

7-hydroxyfluphenazine

fluphenazine-N-oxide

fluphenazine

conjugation

fluphenazine
sulfoxide

Toxicity. Patients refractory to normal treatment regimens have been placed on very high dose fluphenazine therapy without apparent adverse effects. Doses of 300–1200 mg per day as the hydrochloride (Rifkin et al., 1971) and 250 mg per week as the decanoate (McClelland et al., 1976) have been used successfully. However, extrapyramidal symptoms, catatonia, severe hypotension, convulsive seizures, and aspiration of gastric contents have occurred at lower doses than these in occasional patients. An adult patient accidentally received 1050 mg of fluphenazine decanoate by intramuscular injection over a 6 day period; 3 weeks later she developed toxic effects that lasted 1 month and included hypothermia, tachycardia, salivation and extrapyramidal symptoms (Cheung and Yu, 1983).

A 33 year old male suffering an acute psychotic reaction was given a total of 55 mg of fluphenazine hydrochloride orally over a 24 hour period; he died either of aspiration or suffocation during a terminal struggle. Autopsy revealed pulmonary edema, aspiration pneumonitis, and the following fluphenazine concentrations: blood, undetectable; liver, 5 mg/kg; gastric contents, 1.2 mg (Baselt, 1976). A second adult male was an institutional patient receiving daily oral doses of 120 mg fluphenazine hydrochloride and 2000 mg chlorprothixene, in addition to 150 mg of fluphenazine decanoate subcutaneously every 2 weeks. He suffered several convulsive seizures with loss of consciousness in the days prior to his death, and the decision was made to lower his drug dosages; however, he died the next day during another seizure episode. Autopsy revealed pulmonary edema, aspiration of gastric contents, and the following drug concentrations (Baselt, 1981):

Drug Concentrations in a Psychotic Patient (mg/L or mg/kg)

Drug	Blood*	Liver	Gastric
Fluphenazine	neg	23	neg
Chlorprothixene	1.4	8.7	neg

* Also lithium, 0.4 mmol/L

Analysis. Fluphenazine has been assayed in plasma by fluorometry (Smulevitch et al., 1973) and radioimmunoassay (Wiles and Franklin, 1978; Midha et al., 1980), but these methods suffer from metabolite interference. Gas chromatographic methods for urine have utilized flame-ionization detection (Kelsey et al., 1973), while those for plasma involved nitrogen-selective (Franklin et al., 1978; Javaid et al., 1980), electron-capture (Larsen and Naestoft, 1973; Rivera-Calimlim and Siracusa, 1977), or mass spectrometric detection (McKay et al., 1983; Jemal et al., 1987); all have required derivatization of fluphenazine prior to chromatography. Liquid chromatographic techniques have also been described (Johansson et al., 1976; Tjaden et al., 1976; Hoffman et al., 1987; Cooper et al., 1989).

References

M. Aravagiri, S.R. Marder, T. Van Putten et al. Radioimmunoassay for 7-hydroxy metabolite of fluphenazine. Ther. Drug Mon. 16: 21–29, 1994.

R.C. Baselt. Unpublished results, 1976.

R.C. Baselt. Unpublished results, 1981.

U. Breyer, H.J. Gaertner and A. Prox. Formation of identical metabolites from piperazine—and dimethylamino-substituted phenothiazine drugs in man, rat and dog. Biochem. Pharm. 23: 313–322, 1974.

H.K. Cheung and E.C.S. Yu. Effect of 1050 mg fluphenazine decanoate given intramuscularly over six days. Brit. Med. J. 286: 1016–1017, 1983.

J.K. Cooper, E.M. Hawes, J.W. Hubbard et al. An ultrasensitive method for the measurement of fluphenazine in plasma. Ther. Drug Mon. 11: 354–360, 1989.

S.H. Curry, R. Whelpton, P.J. de Schepper et al. Kinetics of fluphenazine after fluphenazine dihydrochloride, enanthate and decanoate administration to man. Brit. J. Clin. Pharm. 7: 325–331, 1979.

J. Dreyfuss, J.J. Ross, Jr., and E.C. Schreiber. Biological disposition and metabolic fate of fluphenazine-^{14}C in the dog and rhesus monkey. J. Pharm. Sci. 60: 821–825, 1971.

M. Franklin, D.H. Wiles and D.J. Harvey. Sensitive gas-chromatographic determination of fluphenazine in human plasma. Clin. Chem. 24: 41–44, 1978.

D.W. Hoffman, R.D. Edkins, S.D. Shillcutt and A. Salama. New high-performance liquid chromatographic method for fluphenazine and metabolites in human plasma. J. Chrom. 414: 504–509, 1987.

J.I. Javaid, H. Dekirmenjian, M. Dysken and J.M. Davis. Measurement of fluphenazine by gas chromatography in human plasma and red blood cells. In *Long-Term Effects of Neuroleptics* (F. Cattabeni, G. Racagni, P.F. Spano and E. Costa, eds.), Raven Press, New York, 1980, pp. 585–589.

M. Jemal, E. Ivashkiv, D. Both et al. Picogram level determination of fluphenazine in human plasma by automated gas chromatography/mass selective detection. Biomed. Env. Mass Spec. 14: 699–704, 1987.

R. Johansson, K.O. Borg and M. Gabrielsson. Determination of fluphenazine in plasma by ion-pair partition chromatography. Acta Pharm. Sci. 13: 193–200, 1976.

M.I. Kelsey, A. Keskiner and E.A. Moscatelli. Gas-liquid chromatographic analysis of fluphenazine and fluphenazine sulfoxide in the urine of chronic schizophrenic patients. J. Chrom. 75: 294–297, 1973.

N.E. Larsen and J. Naestoft. Determination of perphenazine and fluphenazine in whole blood by gas chromatography. Med. Lab. Tech. 30: 129–132, 1973.

S.R. Marder, T. Van Putten, M. Aravagiri et al. Plasma levels of parent drug and metabolites in patients receiving oral and depot fluphenazine. Psychopharm. Bull. 25: 479–482, 1989.

G. McKay, K. Hall, R. Edom et al. Subnanogram determination of fluphenazine in human plasma by gas chromatography mass spectrometry. Biomed. Mass Spec. 10: 550–555, 1983.

H.A. McClelland, R.G. Farquharson, P. Leyburn et al. Very high dose fluphenazine decanoate. Arch. Gen. Psych. 33: 1435–1439, 1976.

K.K. Midha, J.K. Cooper and J.W. Hubbard. Radioimmunoassay for fluphenazine in human plasma. Comm. Psychopharm. 4: 107–114, 1980.

K.K. Midha, G. McKay, R. Edom et al. Kinetics of oral fluphenazine disposition in humans by GC-MS. Eur. J. Clin. Pharm. 25: 709–711, 1983.

A. Rifkin, F. Quitkin, C. Carrillo and D.F. Klein. Very high dosage fluphenazine for nonchronic treatment-refractory patients. Arch. Gen. Psych. 25: 398–403, 1971.

L. Rivera-Calimlim and A. Siracusa. Plasma assay of fluphenazine. Comm. Psychopharm. 1: 233–242, 1977.

A.B. Smulevitch, E.I. Minsker, N.A. Mazayeva et al. The problem of clinical activity of long-acting neuroleptics. Comp. Psych. 14: 227–233, 1973.

U.R. Tjaden, J. Lankelma, H. Poppe and R.G. Muusze. Determination of blood levels of perphenazine and fluphenazine. J. Chrom. 125: 275–286, 1976.

D.H. Wiles and M. Franklin. Radioimmunoassay for fluphenazine in human plasma. Brit. J. Clin. Pharm. 5: 265–268, 1978.

D.H. Wiles and M.G. Gelder. Plasma fluphenazine levels by radioimmunoassay in schizophrenic patients treated with depot injections of fluphenazine decanoate. Brit. J. Clin. Pharm. 8: 565–570, 1979.

Flurazepam

T½: 1–3 hr; 47–100 hr for N-1-desalkylflurazepam
Vd: 3.4–5.5 L/kg
Fb: 0.97
pKa: 1.9, 8.2

Occurrence and Usage. Flurazepam (Dalmane) was introduced in 1970 as a benzodiazepine derivative with hypnotic efficacy. It is administered orally as the dihydrochloride salt in doses of 15–30 mg and appears to have a higher therapeutic index than other commonly used hypnotics.

Blood Concentrations. In 2 adult subjects given a 15 mg oral dose, plasma flurazepam concentrations of <2.0 µg/L were detectable only during the first 30 minutes; plasma concentrations of N-1-hydroxyethylflurazepam, flurazepam aldehyde and N-1-desalkylflurazepam peaked at 6.0, 9.1 and 18 µg/L at 1.0, 1.5 and 12 hours, respectively (Burstein et al., 1988). After a 30 mg oral dose in 9 adults, plasma concentrations reached average peak levels of 2.1 µg/L for flurazepam at 1.0 hour, 12 µg/L for desethylflurazepam at 1.5 hours, 19 µg/L for didesethylflurazepam at 1.8 hours, 18 µg/L for N-1-hydroxyethylflurazepam at 1.0 hour and 23 µg/L for N-1-desalkylflurazepam at 12 hours; elimination half-lives for these 5 plasma species averaged 1.3, 3.0, 18, 1.6 and 68 hours, respectively (Selinger et al., 1989). At 1 hour following the unusually high single oral dose of 90 mg, blood concentrations of flurazepam averaged 13 µg/L, of N-1-hydroxyethylflurazepam, 70 µg/L, and of N-1-desalkylflurazepam, 50 µg/L (deSilva and Strojny, 1971).

During chronic daily administration of 30 mg of the drug, steady-state blood concentrations of N-1-desalkylflurazepam ranged from 33–114 µg/L, with a half-life of 47–100 hours; N-1-hydroxyethylflurazepam was measurable only during the first few post-dose hours (half-life about 2 hours), always at concentrations less than 17 µg/L; and flurazepam was present at concentrations below the sensitivity limit of the assay (Kaplan et al., 1973). The predominant plasma metabolites are pharmacologically active and may be responsible for much of flurazepam's effect (Randall and Kappell, 1973; Garland et al., 1983).

Metabolism and Excretion. Metabolism of flurazepam proceeds via oxidative loss of the diethylaminoethyl group on the ring nitrogen, with production of flurazepam aldehyde, which is further oxidized to N-1-hydroxyethylflurazepam and N-1-desalkylflurazepam; this latter compound accumulates in blood and is slowly metabolized by 3-hydroxylation. The resulting N-1-desalkyl-3-hydroxyflurazepam is pharmacologically active but is not a major blood component, being rapidly conjugated and excreted. Flurazepam also is metabolized by N-deethylation to desethyl- and didesethylflurazepam. Up to 60% of a dose is excreted in the urine within 48 hours, and eventually urinary excretion accounts for all but the 8–9% that is eliminated in the feces. The major urinary metabolite is a conjugate of N-1-hydroxyethylflurazepam, representing 29–55% of the dose; about 1–2% is excreted as conjugated N-1-desalkyl-3-hydroxyflurazepam, and only trace amounts of intact flurazepam and the unconjugated metabolites are found (Schwartz and Postma, 1970; deSilva and Strojny, 1971; deSilva et al., 1974a; Hasegawa and Matsubara, 1975; Garland et al., 1983).

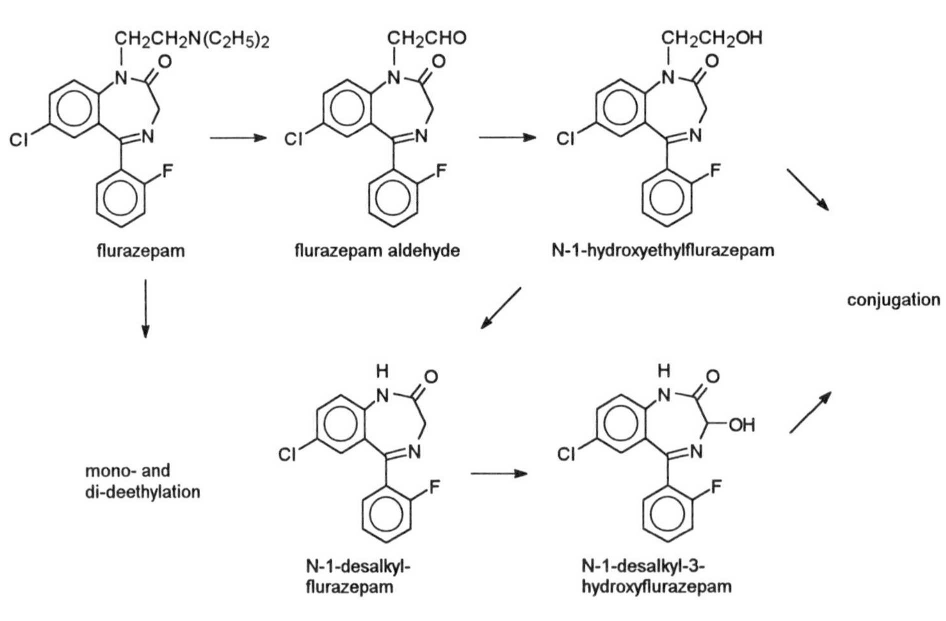

flurazepam   flurazepam aldehyde   N-1-hydroxyethylflurazepam

conjugation

mono- and di-deethylation

N-1-desalkyl-flurazepam   N-1-desalkyl-3-hydroxyflurazepam

Toxicity. Ingestion of 15 mg of flurazepam at bedtime has been shown to produce driving impairment the next morning (Betts and Birtle, 1982). Withdrawal symptoms have occurred upon abrupt cessation of chronic use (Berlin and Conell, 1983). Overdosage may cause nausea, vomiting, respiratory depression, coma, and death. In contrast with therapeutic situations, overdosage with flurazepam usually produces relatively high blood concentrations of the intact drug and lower levels of the metabolites. Four fatal cases that involved flurazepam and at least one other agent showed blood flurazepam concentrations by gas chromatography of 0.5–4.0 mg/L and liver concentrations of 2–17 mg/kg (Finkle, 1974; Morano and Niles, 1976; Baselt, 1977; Cravey, 1977). Blood flurazepam concentrations of 0.5 and 1.8 mg/L were detected in two deaths due solely to this drug (Baselt and Cravey, 1977; Aderjan and Mattern, 1979). The following tissue distribution of flurazepam and its metabolites was obtained in the case of a 5 year old girl who ingested an overdose of the drug; therapeutic levels of phenobarbital and subtherapeutic levels of phenytoin were also present (Ferrara et al., 1979):

Drug Concentrations in a Flurazepam Death (mg/L or mg/kg)

	Blood	Brain	Liver	Kidney
Flurazepam	3.2	0.8	2.7	0.9
Desalkylflurazepam	1.8	0.7	3.1	0.6
Hydroxyethylflurazepam	2.5	0.7	3.5	1.1

Analysis. Flurazepam and its metabolites have been assayed in body fluids by fluorometry (deSilva and Strojny, 1971) and fluorodensitometry (deSilva et al., 1974b) of the hydrolysis products. Gas chromatographic procedures have involved flame-ionization (Baselt et al., 1977), nitrogen-selective (Ferrara et al., 1979), electron-capture (deSilva et al., 1974a; Hasegawa and Matsubara, 1975; Riva et al., 1981; Cooper and Drolet, 1982; Burstein et al., 1988; Salama et al., 1988) and mass spectrometric detection (Clatworthy et al., 1977). Liquid chromatography has also been employed (Weinfeld and Miller, 1981; Dadgar et al., 1983; Lau et al., 1987; Selinger et al., 1989).

References

R. Aderjan and R. Mattern. Eine toedlich verlaufene Monointoxikation mit Flurazepam (Dalmadorm). Arch. Tox. 43: 69–75, 1979.

R.C. Baselt. Unpublished results, 1977.

R.C. Baselt, C.B. Stewart and S.J. Franch. Toxicological determination of benzodiazepines in biological fluids and tissues by flame-ionization gas chromatography. J. Anal. Tox. 1: 10–13, 1977.

R.C. Baselt and R.H. Cravey. A compendium of therapeutic and toxic concentrations of toxicologically significant drugs in human biofluids. J. Anal. Tox. 1: 81–103, 1977.

R.M. Berlin and L.J. Conell. Withdrawal symptoms after long-term treatment with therapeutic doses of flurazepam: a case report. Am. J. Psych. 140: 488–490, 1983.

T.A. Betts and J. Birtle. Effect of two hypnotic drugs on actual driving performance next morning. Brit. Med. J. 285: 852, 1982.

E.S. Burstein, H. Friedman, D.J. Greenblatt et al. Quantitation of flurazepam and three metabolites by electron capture gas liquid chromatography. J. Anal. Tox. 12: 122–125, 1988.

A.J. Clatworthy, L.V. Jones and M.J. Whitehouse. The gas chromatography mass spectrometry of the major metabolites of flurazepam. Biomed. Mass Spec. 4: 248–254, 1977.

S.F. Cooper and D. Drolet. Gas-liquid chromatographic determination of flurazepam and its major metabolites in plasma with electron capture detection. J. Chrom. 231: 321–331, 1982.

R.H. Cravey. Personal communication, 1977.

D. Dadgar, W.F. Smyth and H. Hojabri. High-performance liquid chromatographic determination of flurazepam and its metabolites in human blood plasma. Anal. Chim. Acta 147: 381–385, 1983.

J.A.F. deSilva and N. Strojny. Determination of flurazepam and its major biotransformation products in blood and urine by spectrophotofluorometry and spectrophotometry. J. Pharm. Sci. 60: 1303–1314, 1971.

J.A.F. deSilva, C.V. Puglisi, M.A. Brooks and M.R. Hackman. Determination of flurazepam (Dalmane) and its major metabolites in blood by electron-capture gas-liquid chromatography and in urine by differential pulse polarography. J. Chrom. 99: 461–483, 1974a.

J.A.F. deSilva, I. Bekersky and C.V. Puglisi. Spectrofluorodensitometric determination of flurazepam and its major metabolites in blood. J. Pharm. Sci. 63: 1837–1841, 1974b.

S.D. Ferrara, L. Tedeschi, M. Marigo and F. Castagna. Concentrations of phenobarbital, flurazepam, and flurazepam metabolites in autopsy cases. J. For. Sci. 24: 61–69, 1979.

B. Finkle. Personal communication, 1974.

W.A. Garland, B.J. Miwa, W. Dairman et al. Identification of 7-chloro-5-(2'-fluorophenyl)-2,3-dihydro-2-oxo-1H-1,4-benzodiazepine-1-acetaldehyde, a new metabolite of flurazepam in man. Drug Met. Disp. 11: 70–72, 1983.

M. Hasegawa and I. Matsubara. Metabolic fates of flurazepam. I. Gas chromatographic determination of flurazepam and its metabolites in human urine and blood using electron capture detector. Chem. Pharm. Bull. 23: 1826–1833, 1975.

S. Kaplan, J.A.F. deSilva, M.L. Jack et al. Blood level profile in man following chronic oral administration of flurazepam hydrochloride. J. Pharm. Sci. 62: 1932–1935, 1973.

C.E. Lau, J.L. Falk, S. Dolan and M. Tang. Simultaneous determination of flurazepam and five metabolites in serum. J. Chrom. 423: 251–259, 1987.

R.A. Morano. Personal communication, 1976.

L.O. Randall and B. Kappell. Pharmacological activity of some benzodiazepines and their metabolites. In *The Benzodiazepines* (S. Garattini, E. Mussini and L.O. Randall, eds.), Raven Press, New York, 1973, pp. 27–51.

R. Riva, M. De Anna, F. Albani and A. Baruzzi. Rapid quantitation of flurazepam and its major metabolite, N-desalkylflurazepam, in human plasma by gas-liquid chromatography with electron-capture detection. J. Chrom. 222: 491–495, 1981.

Z. Salama, B. Schraufstetter and H. Jaeger. Determination of flurazepam and its major metabolites in plasma by capillary gas chromatography. Arz. Forsch. 38: 400–403, 1988.

M.A. Schwartz and E. Postma. Metabolism of flurazepam, a benzodiazepine, in man and dog. J. Pharm. Sci. 59: 1800–1806, 1970.

K. Selinger, D. Lessard and H.M. Hill. Simultaneous determination of flurazepam and its metabolites in human plasma by high-performance liquid chromatography. J. Chrom. 494: 247–256, 1989.

R.E. Weinfeld and K.F. Miller. Determination of the major urinary metabolites of flurazepam in man by high-performance liquid chromatography. J. Chrom. 223: 123–130, 1981.

Flurbiprofen

T½: 2–6 hr
Vd: 0.1 L/kg
Fb: 0.99
pKa: 4.2

Occurrence and Usage. Flurbiprofen (Ansaid) is a potent nonsteroidal anti-inflammatory drug of the arylacetic acid class that is used for the acute and chronic treatment of rheumatoid arthritis, osteo-arthritis and acute gouty arthritis. Flurbiprofen is a prescription drug available for oral administration in tablets containing 50–100 mg. The recommended starting dose is 100 mg per day in divided doses; daily doses exceeding 300 mg are not recommended.

Blood Concentrations. Following the oral administration of a single 50 mg dose of flurbiprofen to 2 adult subjects, peak serum concentrations ranging from 8.0–9.4 mg/L were measured in 2–4 hours (Albert et al., 1984). A solution containing 68 mg of flurbiprofen given to 12 healthy, fasting young men produced an average maximum plasma flurbiprofen concentration of 11 mg/L at 0.5 hour post-ingestion (Gonzalez-Younes et al., 1991). The average plasma concentration following the last of 4 oral 100 mg doses of flurbiprofen in 15 male volunteers was 11 mg/L at 2 hours, 4.9 mg/L at 6 hours and 0.05 mg/L at 48 hours (Szpunar et al., 1987).

A mean maximum steady-state plasma flurbiprofen concentration of 14 mg/L was attained in 12 adult arthritic patients following a 100 mg twice a day regimen; in older patients, aged 65–83, following the same dose regimen, the average concentration was 16 mg/L (Kean et al., 1992).

Metabolism and Excretion. Flurbiprofen is metabolized either by formation of glucuronide or sulfate conjugates or by oxidation to 4'-hydroxyflurbiprofen, 3'-hydroxyflurbiprofen and 3',4'-dihydroxyflurbiprofen. The oxidative metabolites may also undergo conjugation before appearing in the urine (Risdall et al., 1978; Kaiser et al., 1986; Szpunar et al., 1987). Studies of patient urine at steady-state showed the presence of conjugates representing 16% of the dose as parent drug, 44% as 4'-hydroxyflurbiprofen, 7.8% as 3'-hydroxyflurbiprofen, and 2.2% as 3',4'-dihydroxyflurbiprofen (Kean et al., 1992).

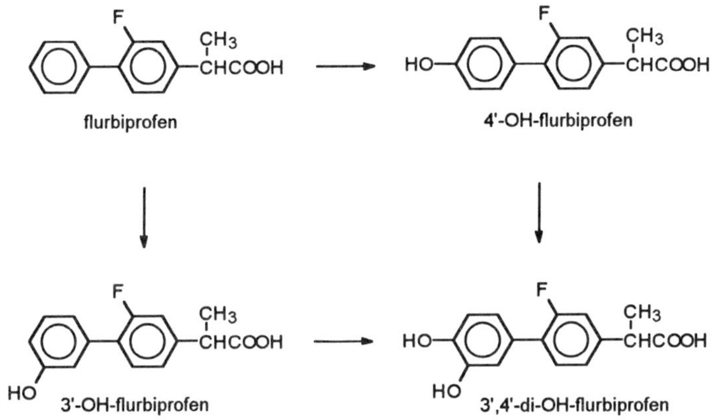

Toxicity. In overdose, dizziness, drowsiness, disorientation, epigastric pain, coma and respiratory depression may occur.

Analysis. Flurbiprofen has been determined in biological samples by gas chromatography following derivatization (Kaiser et al., 1974) and by liquid chromatography (Albert et al., 1984; Babhair, 1988).

References

K.S. Albert, W.R. Gillespie, A. Raabe and M. Garry. Determination of flurbiprofen in human serum by reverse-phase high-performance liquid chromatography with fluorescence detection. J. Pharm. Sci. 73: 1823–1825, 1984.

S.A. Babhair. Determination of flurbiprofen in dosage form and in biological fluids by high performance liquid chromatography. J. Liq. Chrom. 11: 463–474, 1988.

I. Gonzalez-Younes, J.G. Wagner, D.A. Gaines et al. Absorption through human buccal mucosa. J. Pharm. Sci. 80: 820–823, 1991.

D.G. Kaiser, S.R. Shaw and G.J. Vangiessen. GLC determination of dl-2-(2-fluoro-4-biphenylyl)propionic acid (flurbiprofen) in plasma. J. Pharm. Sci. 63: 567–570, 1974.

W.F. Kean, E.J. Antal, E.M. Grace et al. The pharmacokinetics of flurbiprofen in younger and elderly patients with rheumatoid arthritis. J. Clin. Pharm. 32: 41–48, 1992.

P.C. Risdall, S.S. Adams, E.L. Crampton and B. Marchant. The disposition and metabolism of flurbiprofen in several species including man. Xenobiotica 8: 691–704, 1978.

G.J. Szpunar, K.S. Albert, G.G. Bole et al. Pharmacokinetics of flurbiprofen in man. I. Area/dose relationships. Biopharm. Drug Disp. 8: 273–283, 1987.

Formaldehyde

T½: ?
Vd: ?   HCHO
Fb: ?

Occurrence and Usage. Formaldehyde is a gas at room temperature, but is commonly used in the laboratory as a 37% aqueous solution known as formalin. As much as 15% methanol may be added to this solution to prevent polymerization of the chemical. Formaldehyde is employed in the manufacture of synthetic resins, fabrics, paper, wood products, preservatives and disinfectants. Occupational exposure is usually by inhalation of the gas or direct contact with the liquid. Significant residential exposures have occurred as a result of the release of formaldehyde fumes from synthetic foam insulation used in exterior walls. The current threshold limit value for occupational exposure is 0.3 ppm in air (0.4 mg/m³), which is below the odor threshold for the compound. Formaldehyde is suspected of having carcinogenic potential in man.

Blood Concentrations. Six adult volunteers exposed to 1.9 ppm of formaldehyde in air for 40 minutes had blood formaldehyde concentrations that averaged 2.6 mg/L prior to exposure and 2.8 mg/L just after the exposure (Heck et al., 1985). Workers exposed to formaldehyde at a concentration of 7 mg/m³ developed blood levels of 0.6–4.0 mg/L (Piotrowski, 1977). Formic acid concentrations in the blood of over 100 unexposed persons averaged 6 mg/L (range, 0–12), while concentrations in 10 individuals believed to be exposed to formaldehyde averaged 100 mg/L (range, 22–326) (Schweda, 1985).

   In animals administered 35 mg/kg of formaldehyde by intravenous infusion, a blood formaldehyde concentration of about 25 mg/L was produced, which declined to about 1 mg/L by 1 hour after the end of the infusion. About 4 times as much formaldehyde was found in erythrocytes as in plasma. The peak plasma concentration of formic acid, a metabolite, was 144 mg/L at the end of the infusion, and this level declined with a half-life of 1.5 hours (Malorny et al., 1965).

Metabolism and Excretion. Formaldehyde is a highly reactive substance that probably combines rapidly with cellular constituents in all exposed tissues, including the mucous membranes of the respiratory tract. It is known to be oxidized to formic acid in erythrocytes and in the liver, and this metabolite is further oxidized to carbon dioxide and water (Malorny et al., 1965). A portion of the formic acid produced by the metabolism of formaldehyde is excreted in urine. Formic acid is also an endogenous substance, being formed by the degradation of glycine, and its concentration in the urine of normal unexposed subjects averages 17–19 mg/L (range, 0–27) (Triebig et al., 1978; Schweda, 1985). In 11 persons believed to be exposed to formaldehyde, urine formic acid concentrations averaged 101 mg/L (range, 33–384) (Schweda, 1985).

Toxicity. Formaldehyde vapor causes mild irritation of the mucous membranes of the eyes and respiratory passages at a level of 2–3 ppm, while levels of 10–20 ppm result in moderate to severe irritation after only a few minutes. Lacrimation, cough, inflammation of the bronchi, pulmonary edema and death have resulted from exposure to very high concentrations of the chemical. Direct contact with formalin may produce dermatitis, with sensitization occurring in some persons upon repeated exposure.

   Persons with pre-existing lung disease may react more adversely to the presence of formaldehyde in the environment. Certain individuals may develop bronchial sensitization as a result of chronic exposure to even moderately elevated formaldehyde levels; once this occurs, any degree of exposure may trigger a response (Bernstein et al., 1984).

   The ingestion of formalin has caused several deaths, preceded by severe corrosive damage to the stomach and small intestine, circulatory collapse and kidney damage (Gosselin et al., 1976). A middle-aged female drank about 120 mL of 10% formaldehyde and immediately developed severe abdominal pains and went into shock. She was treated at home with milk and emetics and recovered. However, she suffered episodes of epigastric distress, nausea and vomiting over the next 3 months. Her discomfort made surgery necessary, and at that time diffuse ulceration, fibrosis and contracture of the stomach, causing almost complete obstruction, was found. A total gastrectomy was performed and the patient recovered (Bartone et al., 1968).

A 41 year old woman ingested 120 mL of 37% formaldehyde solution (containing 12.5% methanol), complained of severe abdominal pain, and lost consciousness. Blood formaldehyde concentrations were initially as high as 4.8 mg/L, but dropped rapidly and remained within a range of 1–2 mg/L over the next 15 hours; blood formic acid concentrations rose and fell within a range of 250–500 mg/L. Efforts were made to control the hypotension, apnea, and acidosis that developed, but the patient became anuric 7 hours after admission and died 21 hours later (Eells et al., 1981). In a similar case involving a 57 year old male who ingested 120 mL of formalin, peak serum formaldehyde and formic acid levels of 11 and 1360 mg/L, respectively, were observed at 5.5 hours post-ingestion, with death occurring at 12 hours (Burkhart et al., 1990). After the ingestion of an unknown quantity of formaldehyde solution containing 11% methanol and 35% formaldehyde, a 58 year old female was found dead. At autopsy, her blood was found to contain 0.04% (400 mg/L) methanol and only a trace amount of formaldehyde. The gastric contents contained a total of 900 mg of methanol and 4500 mg of formaldehyde (Finkle, 1975). Two renal dialysis patients developed dyspnea and died after dialysis on a machine that had been disinfected with formalin (Erkrath et al., 1981).

Analysis. Formic acid may be determined in blood and urine by oxidimetric titration (Bastrup, 1947), colorimetry (Rietbrock and Hinrichs, 1964), gas chromatography after derivatization (Doms, 1975; Angerer, 1976; Bricknell and Finegold, 1978; Triebig et al., 1978; Abolin et al., 1980), or by a specific enzymatic method (Makar et al., 1975; Shahangian et al., 1984; Grady and Osterloh, 1986). Intact formaldehyde is measurable in toxic amounts by most of the gas chromatographic procedures cited in the section on ethanol.

References

C. Abolin, J.D. McRae, T.N. Tozer and S. Takki. Gas chromatographic head-space assay of formic acid as methyl formate in biologic fluids: potential application to methanol poisoning. Biochem. Med. 23: 209–218, 1980.

J. Angerer. Gaschromatographische Bestimmung von Ameisensaeure im Harn in Form von Kohlenmonoxid. J. Clin. Chem. Clin. Biochem. 14: 73–77, 1976.

N.F. Bartone, R.V. Grieco and B.S. Henn, Jr. Corrosive gastritis due to ingestion of formaldehyde. J. Am. Med. Asso. 203: 50–51, 1968.

J.T. Bastrup. Method for the determination of formic acid in urine. Acta Pharm. 3: 303–311, 1947.

R.S. Bernstein, L.T. Stayner, L.J. Elliott et al. Inhalation exposure to formaldehyde: an overview of its toxicology, epidemiology, monitoring, and control. Am. Ind. Hyg. Asso. J. 45: 778–785, 1984.

K.S. Bricknell and S.M. Finegold. Improved method for assay of formic acid by gas-liquid chromatography. J. Chrom. 151: 374–378, 1978.

K.K. Burkhart, K.W. Kulig and K.E. McMartin. Formate levels following a formalin ingestion. Vet. Hum. Tox. 32: 135–137, 1990.

E.K. Doms. Gaschromatographische Bestimmung der Ameisensaeure als Benzylester unter Verwendung von Phenyldiazomethan als Benzylierungsmittel. J. Chrom. 105: 79–88, 1975.

J.T. Eells, K.E. McMartin, K. Black et al. Formaldehyde poisoning. J. Am. Med. Asso. 246: 1237–1238, 1981.

K.D. Erkrath, G. Adebahr and A. Kloppel. Todliche Formalin-Vergiftung bei Dialyse-Behandlung. Z. Rechtsmed. 87: 233–236, 1981.

B.S. Finkle. Personal communication, 1975.

R.E. Gosselin, H.C. Hodge, R.P. Smith and M.N. Gleason. *Clinical Toxicology of Commercial Products*, 4th ed., Williams and Wilkins, Baltimore, 1976, pp. 166–168 (Section III).

L.M. Gottschling, H.J. Beaulieu and W.W. Melvin. Monitoring of formic acid in urine of humans exposed to low levels of formaldehyde. Am. Ind. Hyg. Asso. J. 45: 19–23, 1984.

S. Grady and J. Osterloh. Improved enzymic assay for serum formate with colorimetric end point. J. Anal. Tox. 10: 1–5, 1986.

H.D. Heck, M. Casanova-Schmitz, P.B. Dodd et al. Formaldehyde (CH_2O) concentrations in the blood of humans and Fischer-344 rats exposed to CH_2O under controlled conditions. Am. Ind. Hyg. Asso. J. 46: 1–3, 1985.

A.B. Makar, K.E. McMartin, M. Palese and T.R. Tephly. Formate assay in body fluids: application in methanol poisoning. Biochem. Med. 13: 117–126, 1975.

G. Malorny, N. Rietbrock and M. Schneider. Die Oxydation des Formaldehyds zu Ameisensaeure im Blut, ein Beitrag zum Stoffwechsel des Formaldehyds. Naunyn-Schmiedebergs Arch. Exp. Path. Pharm. 250: 419–436, 1965.

J.K. Piotrowski. *Exposure Tests for Organic Compounds in Industrial Toxicology,* U.S. Government Printing Office, Washington, D.C., 1977, p. 122.

N. Rietbrock and W.D. Hinrichs. Eine einfache Methode zum quantitativen Nachweis der Ameisensaeure in Harn und Blut des Menschen. Klin. Wochenschr. 42: 981–985, 1964.

P. Schweda. Formic acid levels in body fluids as index of formaldehyde exposure. In *Proceedings of the 21st International Meeting,* September 13–17, Brighton, UK (N. Dunnet and K.J. Kimber, eds.), International Association of Forensic Toxicologists, 1985.

S. Shahangian, K.O. Ash and D.E. Rollins. An enzymatic method for the analysis of formate in human plasma. J. Anal. Tox. 8: 273–276, 1984.

G. Triebig, K.H. Schaller and K. Gobler. Eine einfache und zuverlaessige gas-chromatographische Bestimmung von Ameisensaeure im Urin. Fresenius Z. Anal. Chem. 290: 114, 1978.

Gamma-Hydroxybutyrate

T½: 0.3–1.0 hr
Vd: 0.4 L/kg
Fb: 0 $HOCH_2CH_2CH_2COOH$
pKa: ?

Occurrence and Usage. Gamma-hydroxybutyrate (4-hydroxybutyrate, sodium oxybate, GHB) is an endogenous metabolite, present in most mammalian tissues at nanomolar concentrations, that has been hypothesized to have a role as a cerebral neurotransmitter. It has been employed clinically since 1960 as an anesthetic and hypnotic agent, but its current availability in the United States is limited to investigational use only. Oral or intravenous doses of 10 mg/kg in humans cause amnesia and hypotonia; doses of 20–30 mg/kg are sleep-inducing; and doses of 50 mg/kg or higher produce anesthesia. The sodium salt has been marketed illicitly for the past several years at gymnasiums and health food stores, where it is promoted as a steroid alternative for body-building and as a tryptophan replacement for weight control and sedation. Illicit use of GHB often involves oral doses of one teaspoon (2.5 g or 35 mg/kg in a 70 kg adult) of the powder dissolved in water.

Blood Concentrations. A 25 mg/kg (1.75 g/70 kg) oral dose caused dizziness or drowsiness in 8 adult subjects and an average peak plasma GHB level of 80 mg/L at 0.5 hours (Palatini et al., 1993). A 75 mg/kg (5.25 g/70 kg) oral dose given to 4 adults prior to bedtime produced peak plasma GHB concentrations averaging 90 mg/L at 2 hours, with a decline to 9 mg/L by 6 hours (Hoes et al., 1980). An intravenous dose of 50 mg/kg (3.5 g/70 kg) in an adult produced a peak blood GHB level of approximately 170 mg/L within 15 minutes. The authors found in a series of patients that blood GHB concentrations exceeding 260 mg/L were associated with deep sleep, levels of 156–260 mg/L with moderate sleep, levels of 52–156 mg/L with light sleep, and levels of less than 52 mg/L with wakefulness (Helrich et al., 1964).

Metabolism and Excretion. GHB is believed to be extensively metabolized by alcohol dehydrogenase to unknown oxidation products. Peak urine GHB concentrations on the order of 1100 mg/L are observed within the first 4 hours after a 100 mg/kg (7 g/70 kg) oral dose, but the drug is undetectable in urine by 12 hours. Less than 5% of an oral dose is eliminated unchanged in urine (Hoes et al., 1980).

Toxicity. Effects of GHB including drowsiness, euphoria, dizziness, nausea, visual disturbances and unconsciousness are usually manifested by 15 minutes after administration and persist for about 3 hours on average (Luby et al., 1992). Serious adverse reactions have included hypotension, bradycardia, respiratory depression, seizures and coma (Dyer et al., 1991; Nightingale, 1991).

A 42 year old man ingested a white powder that he believed was an "amino acid" to aid in muscular development and an hour later was found behind the steering wheel of his car, stopped in a traffic lane, apparently asleep; he was noted to have severe ataxia, nystagmus, mental confusion and a urine GHB concentration of 1975 mg/L (Stephens and Baselt, 1994). An emergency room patient was treated for coma of 3 hours duration after ingesting GHB at a nightclub; serum and urine collected 1 hour post-ingestion contained 101 and 141,000 mg/L GHB, respectively (Dyer et al., 1994).

Analysis. GHB determination in biological specimens has been accomplished with gas chromatography employing flame-ionization (Roth and Giarman, 1970; Vree et al., 1976), electron-capture (Doherty et al., 1975) or mass spectrometric detection (Eli and Cattabeni, 1983). Some extraction protocols include an acid hydrolysis step to convert GHB to gamma-butyrolactone, which is more amenable to gas chromatographic analysis.

References

J.D. Doherty, O.C. Snead and R.H. Roth. A sensitive method for quantitation of α-hydroxybutyric acid and α-butyrolactone in brain by electron capture gas chromatography. Anal. Biochem. 69: 268–277, 1975.

J.E. Dyer, R. Kreutzer, A. Quattrone et al. Multistate outbreak of poisonings associated with illicit use of gamma hydroxy butyrate. J. Am. Med. Asso. 265: 447–448, 1991.

J.E. Dyer, S.M. Isaacs and K.H. Keller. Gamma hydroxybutyrate (GHB)-induced coma with serum and urine drug levels. Vet. Hum. Tox. 36: 348, 1994.

M. Eli and F. Cattabeni. Endogenous α-hydroxybutyrate in rat brain areas: postmortem changes and effects of drugs interfering with α-aminobutyric acid metabolism. J. Neurochem. 41: 524–530, 1983.

M. Helrich, T.C. McAslan, S. Skolnick and S.P. Bessman. Correlation of blood levels of 4-hydroxybutyrate with state of consciousness. Anesthesiology 25: 771–775, 1964.

M.J.A.J.M. Hoes, T.B. Vree and P.J.M. Guelen. Gamma-hydroxybutyric acid as hypnotic. L'Encephale 6: 93–99, 1980.

S. Luby, J. Jones and A. Zalewski. GHB use in South Carolina. Am. J. Pub. Health 82: 128, 1992.

S.L. Nightingale. Warning about GHB. J. Am. Med. Asso. 265: 1802, 1991.

P. Palatini, L. Tedeschi, G. Frison et al. Dose-dependent absorption and elimination of gamma-hydroxybutyric acid in healthy volunteers. Eur. J. Clin. Pharm. 45: 353–356, 1993.

R.H. Roth and N.J. Giarman. Natural occurrence of gamma-hydroxybutyric acid in mammalian brain. Biochem. Pharm. 19: 1087–1093, 1970.

B. Stephens and R.C. Baselt. Driving under the influence of GHB? J. Anal. Tox. 18: 357-358, 1994.

T.B. Vree, E. van der Kleijn and H.J. Knop. Rapid determination of 4-hydroxybutyric acid (Gamma OH) and 2-propyl pentanoate (Depakine) in human plasma by means of gas-liquid chromatography. J. Chrom. 121: 150–152, 1976.

Gasoline

T½: 17 hr
Vd: ?
Fb: 0

Occurrence and Usage. Gasoline (petrol) is a flammable liquid produced from the light distillates obtained during petroleum fractionation. It consists largely of a mixture of C_4 to C_{12} saturated aliphatic hydrocarbons, but also contains aromatics, olefins, paraffins and naphthenes. Gasoline is widely used as a fuel, solvent for rubber adhesives, extractant or diluent for essential oils, and finishing agent for artificial leathers. The current threshold limit value for occupational exposure is 300 ppm (890 mg/m³).

Blood Concentrations. Gasoline has not been measured in the blood of asymptomatic or occupationally-exposed individuals.

Metabolism and Excretion. Gasoline is absorbed slowly from the stomach after ingestion (Machle, 1941). Excretion is primarily by the lungs and kidneys.

Toxicity. Although gasoline grades vary with octane number and engine requirements, toxic effects do not differ significantly, except to some extent with volatility and lead content (see tetraethyllead) (Sandmeyer, 1981). Exposure to fumes may cause flushing of the face, ataxia, mental confusion, slurred speech and difficulty in swallowing. Delirium, coma, convulsions, and respiratory and cardiac arrest may occur (Ainsworth, 1960). In adults, ingestion of 20 to 50 g of gasoline may produce severe symptoms of poisoning (Sandmeyer, 1981).

Two fatalities have occurred as a result of exposure to gasoline fumes in confined spaces; in one case, a postmortem brain gasoline concentration of 400 mg/kg was measured and in another, liver and lung concentrations of 700 and 400 mg/kg were reported (Nelms et al., 1970). Blood xylene concentrations of 3 and 20 mg/L were measured in two adults who died as a result of intentional ingestion of gasoline (Bonnichsen et al., 1966). A peak blood gasoline concentration of 247 mg/L was observed in a man who eventually died of gasoline vapor inhalation (Matsumoto et al., 1992). Carnevale et al. (1983) reported a case of accidental oral ingestion of gasoline in a 25 year old man who vomited and aspirated gastric contents; his postmortem tissue concentrations (calculated as 2-methylpentane) were as follows:

Gasoline Concentrations in a Fatal Case (mg/L or mg/kg)

Blood	Brain	Lung	Liver	Kidney	Urine
52	44	457	663	52	0

Analysis. Gasoline has been measured in tissues by gas chromatography with detection by thermal-conductivity (Schunegger, 1967), flame-ionization (Nelms et al., 1970; Shankels et al., 1982) or mass spectrometry (Ikebuchi et al., 1986; Kimura et al., 1988; Matsumoto et al., 1992).

References

R.W. Ainsworth. Petrol-vapour poisoning. Brit. Med. J. 1: 1547–1548, 1960.

R. Bonnichsen, A.C. Maehly and M. Moeller. Poisoning by volatile compounds. I. Aromatic compounds. J. For. Sci. 11: 186–204, 1966.

A. Carnevale, M. Chiarotti and N. De Giovanni. Accidental death by gasoline ingestion. Am. J. For. Med. Path. 4: 153–157, 1983.

J. Ikebuchi, S. Kotoku, M. Yashiki et al. Gas chromatographic and gas chromatographic-mass spectrometric determination of gasoline in a case of gasoline vapor and alcohol poisoning. Am. J. For. Med. Path. 7: 146–150, 1986.

K. Kimura, T. Nagata, K. Hara and M. Kageura. Gasoline and kerosene components in blood—a forensic analysis. Hum. Tox. 7: 299–305, 1988.

W. Machle. Gasoline intoxication. J. Am. Med. Asso. 117: 1965–1971, 1941.

T. Matsumoto, M. Koga, T. Sata et al. The changes of gasoline compounds in blood in a case of gasoline intoxication. Clin. Tox. 30: 653–662, 1992.

R.J. Nelms, Jr., R.L. Davis and J. Bond. Verification of fatal gasoline intoxication in confined spaces utilizing gas-liquid chromatography. Am. J. Clin. Path. 53: 641–646, 1970.

E.E. Sandmeyer. Aromatic hydrocarbons. In *Patty's Industrial Hygiene and Toxiciology*, Vol. 2B, *Toxicology*, 3rd ed. (G.D. Clayton and F.E. Clayton, eds.), Wiley-Interscience, New York, 1981, pp. 3384–3387.

U.P. Schlunegger. Gaschromatographischer nachweis von Benzinintoxikationen im Blut von Ratten. Arch. Tox. 22: 252–254, 1967.

B. Shankles, S.B. Weinberg and L.A. Dal Cortivo. Detection and identification of gasoline in tissues by capillary GC using pattern recognition techniques. J. Anal. Tox. 6: 241–243, 1982.

Gentamicin

T½: 1–3 hr
Vd: 0.28 L/kg
Fb: less than 0.10
pKa: 8.2

R = $CH_3CHNHCH_3$
CH_3CHNH_2 or
CH_2NH_2

Occurrence and Usage. Gentamicin (Garamycin) is an aminoglycoside antibiotic isolated in 1963 and used since 1969 in the treatment of gram-negative bacterial infections. It exists as a complex of 3 major (and several minor) chemically similar components that have comparable antimicrobial activity. The drug is available for parenteral administration as the sulfate in injectable solutions of 2, 10, or 40 mg/mL. It is administered by intramuscular or intravenous injection in doses of 1–2 mg/kg at 8 hour intervals, or by intrathecal injection of 4–8 mg once daily.

Blood Concentrations. A 30 minute intravenous infusion of 1.5 mg/kg gentamicin to 17 adults produced an average peak serum concentration of 4.7 mg/L measured 30 minutes after the end of infusion. The levels declined with an average half-life of 1.3 hours and were largely below 1.0 mg/L by 7.5 hours after the end of infusion (Siber et al., 1975). The serum half-life correlates directly with the serum creatinine concentration in patients with renal failure, and may be estimated by multiplying the creatinine value (in mg/dL) by 4 (Cutler et al., 1972). Optimal peak serum concentrations of gentamicin have been suggested to lie between 8–12 mg/L (Noone et al., 1974).

Metabolism and Excretion. In subjects with normal renal function, from 42–65% of a single labeled gentamicin dose is excreted in the urine, apparently as unchanged drug. By the tenth consecutive administration, nearly the entire dose is excreted in the daily urine (Wilson et al., 1973). With chronic dosing, about 8% of the total administered dose remains in the body, sequestered largely in skeletal muscle, kidney, and bone. It has been shown that this accumulation occurs independently of renal function, and that the true elimination half-life of the drug is on the order of 6 days (French et al., 1981).

Urine gentamicin concentrations in patients receiving 1.5 mg/kg/day ranged from 16–125 mg/L (Riff and Jackson, 1971). Kidney concentrations of gentamicin in patients who died during therapy (average, 4.4 days) ranged from 140–540 mg/kg in the cortex and 128–230 mg/kg in the medulla; these levels were 16–89 times the antemortem plasma concentration (Edwards et al., 1976).

Toxicity. Ototoxicity and renal damage are common in patients treated chronically with gentamicin. Ototoxicity was observed in 25% of patients who received larger than recommended doses and who exhibited peak serum gentamicin levels of 4–32 mg/L (Meyers, 1970). Of 21 patients with trough gentamicin levels greater than 2 mg/L, 36% developed increased serum creatinine concentrations (Dahlgren et al., 1975). Sixteen of 29 patients (55%) who received 2–5 mg/kg/day of the drug for 7 days exhibited at least one-third reduction in renal function (Kumin, 1980). Nephrotoxicity is reversible and recovery is complete in 1–2 months in most patients (Gary et al., 1976).

Analysis. Microbiological assays for gentamicin and other aminoglycoside antibiotics have largely been supplanted by more sensitive and specific tests such as enzyme immunoassay, radioimmunoassay, and enzymatic radiochemical assay (Maitra et al., 1979). Fluorometry (Csiba, 1979; Habbal, 1979), gas chromatography (Mayhew and Gorbach, 1978), and high-pressure liquid chromatography (Anhalt, 1977; Maitra et al., 1977; Peng et al., 1977; Larsen et al., 1980; Barends et al., 1981; Walker and Coates, 1981; D'Souza and Ogilvie, 1982) are also utilized. Serum specimens for gentamicin analysis from patients receiving concurrent therapy with carbenicillin or ticarcillin should be refrigerated or frozen, if not analyzed immediately, due to *in vivo* and *in vitro* inactivation of the drug by these beta-lactam antibiotics (Davies et al., 1975).

References

J.P. Anhalt. Assay of gentamicin in serum by high-pressure liquid chromatography. Antimicrob. Agents Chemother. 11: 651–665, 1977.

D.M. Barends, C.L. Zwaan and A. Hulshoff. Improved microdetermination of gentamicin and sisomicin in serum by high-performance liquid chromatography with ultraviolet detection. J. Chrom. 222: 316–323, 1981.

A. Csiba. Spectrofluorimetric method for aminoglycoside antibiotics. J. Pharm. Pharmac. 31: 115–116, 1979.

R.E. Cutler, A.M. Gyselynck, P. Fleet and A.W. Forrey. Correlation of serum creatinine concentration and gentamicin half-life. J. Am. Med. Asso. 219: 1037–1041, 1972.

J.G. Dahlgren, E.T. Anderson and W.L. Hewitt. Gentamicin blood levels: a guide to nephrotoxicity. Antimicrob. Agents Chemother. 8: 58–62, 1975.

M. Davies, J.R. Morgan and C. Anand. Interactions of carbenicillin and ticarcillin with gentamicin. Antimicrob. Agents Chemother. 7: 431–434, 1975.

J. D'Souza and R.I. Ogilvie. Determination of gentamicin components C_{1a}, C_2 and C_1 in plasma and urine by high-performance liquid chromatography. J. Chrom. 232: 212–218, 1982.

C.Q. Edwards, C.R. Smith, K.L. Baughman et al. Concentrations of gentamicin and amikacin in human kidneys. Antimicrob. Agents Chemother. 9: 925–927, 1976.

M.A. French, F.B. Cerra, M.E. Plaut and J.J. Schentag. Amikacin and gentamicin accumulation pharmacokinetics and nephrotoxicity in critically ill patients. Antimicrob. Agents Chemother. 19: 147–152, 1981.

N.E. Gary, L. Buzzeo, J. Salaki and R.P. Eisinger. Gentamicin-associated acute renal failure. Arch. Int. Med. 136: 1101–1104, 1976.

Z.M. Habbal. Spectrofluorometric assay of gentamicin in serum. Clin. Chim. Acta 95: 301–309, 1979.

G.D. Kumin. Clinical nephrotoxicity of tobramycin and gentamicin. J. Am. Med. Asso. 244: 1808–1810, 1980.

N.E. Larsen, K. Marinelli and A.M. Heilesen. Determination of gentamicin in serum using liquid column chromatography. J. Chrom. 221: 182–187, 1980.

S.K. Maitra, T.T. Yoshikawa, J.L. Hansen et al. Serum gentamicin assay by high-pressure liquid chromatography. Clin. Chem. 23: 2275–2278, 1977.

S.K. Maitra, T.T. Yoshikawa, L.B. Guze and M.C. Schotz. Determination of aminoglycoside antibiotics in biological fluids: a review. Clin. Chem. 25: 1361–1367, 1979.

J.W. Mayhew and S.L. Gorbach. Gas-liquid chromatographic method for the assay of aminoglycoside antibiotics in serum. J. Chrom. 151: 133–146, 1978.

R.M. Meyers. Ototoxic effects of gentamicin. Arch. Otolarygn. 92: 160–162, 1970.

P. Noone, T.M.C. Parsons, J.R. Pattison et al. Experience in monitoring gentamicin therapy during treatment of serious gram-negative sepsis. Brit. Med. J. 1: 477–481, 1974.

G.W. Peng, M.A.F. Gadalla, A. Peng et al. High-pressure liquid-chromatographic method for determination of gentamicin in plasma. Clin. Chem. 23: 1838–1844, 1977.

L.J. Riff and G.G. Jackson. Pharmacology of gentamicin in man. J. Infect. Dis. 124: S98–S105, 1971.

G.R. Siber, P. Echeverria, A.L. Smith et al. Pharmacokinetics of gentamicin in children and adults. J. Infect. Dis. 132: 637–651, 1975.

S.E. Walker and P.E. Coates. High-performance liquid chromatographic method for determination of gentamicin in biological fluids. J. Chrom. 223: 131–138, 1981.

T.W. Wilson, W.A. Mahon, T. Inaba et al. Elimination of tritiated gentamicin in normal human subjects and in patients with severely impaired renal function. Clin. Pharm. Ther. 14: 815–822, 1973.

Glutethimide

T½: 5–22 hr
Vd: 2.7 L/kg
Fb: 0.54
pKa: 9.2

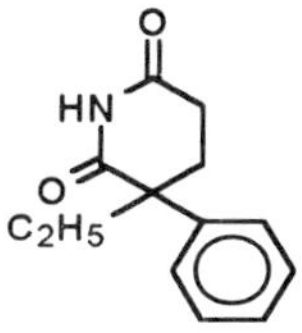

Occurrence and Usage. Glutethimide (2-ethyl-2-phenylglutarimide, Doriden) is a piperidinedione derivative related to phenobarbital that was first synthesized in 1952 and introduced clinically in 1954. It has been widely used as a sedative and hypnotic, being quite similar to the barbiturates in regard to its pharmacological effects. The compound behaves as a neutral or slightly acidic substance, and is available as the racemic mixture for oral use in single doses of 125–1000 mg.

Blood Concentrations. A single oral dose of 500 mg given to 6 subjects produced a mean peak plasma glutethimide concentration of 4.3 mg/L (range, 2.9–7.1) at a mean time of 2.2 hours (range, 1–6). The levels exhibited a biphasic decline, with an initial half-life of 3.9 hours and a terminal half-life of 12 hours (Curry et al., 1971). This was confirmed by other investigators, who found an average elimination half-life of 14 hours (range, 8.1–18) for the drug (Kadar et al., 1973). A maximal blood concentration of 6.2 mg/L was observed in 1 subject at 2 hours after a 1000 mg oral dose, with a decline to 4.2 mg/L by 5 hours and 1.3 mg/L by 48 hours (Algeri and Katsas, 1960). Following the administration of 2000 mg of the drug over a 1.5 hour period to 5 subjects, blood concentrations averaged 10 mg/L (range, 6.3–12) at 2 hours, 6.4 mg/L at 6 hours and 3.1 mg/L at 19.5 hours (Parker et al., 1970). Plasma concentrations of 4-hydroxyglutethimide, an active metabolite, reached peak levels of 4–6 mg/L at 24 hours after a single oral 13.5 mg/kg (945 mg/70 kg) dose of glutethimide in 3 volunteers (Kennedy and Fischer, 1979).

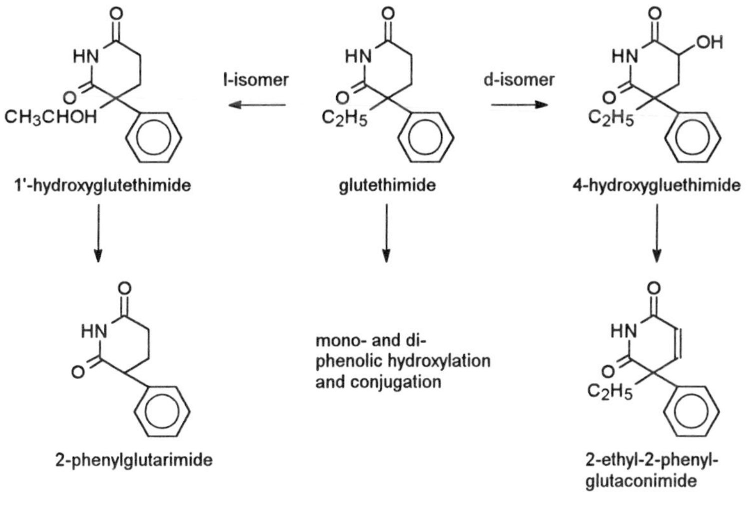

Metabolism and Excretion. Glutethimide exhibits a complex pattern of biotransformation that has been extensively investigated. There is apparently a differential metabolism of the stereoisomers, primarily by hydroxylation of the glutarimide ring and the ethyl and phenyl side groups (Buetikofer et al., 1962). Certain of the metabolites, especially 4-hydroxyglutethimide and 2-phenylglutarimide, have been shown to possess significant pharmacological activity. The former compound may contribute to the central depression observed in victims of glutethimide overdosage (Ambre and Fischer, 1972; Ambre and Fischer, 1974; Hansen and Fischer, 1974; Hansen et al., 1975), but is probably not important during therapeutic administration (Crow et al., 1977). Numerous other mono- and dihydroxyphenyl metabolites have been isolated from human urine (Stillwell, 1975; Andresen et al., 1975; Andresen et al., 1976), and recently alpha-phenyl-gamma-butyrolactone was identified and found to possess pharmacological activity (Andresen et al., 1977).

Less than 2% of a dose of glutethimide is excreted unchanged in the 24 hour urine (Curry et al., 1971); urine concentrations of the drug ranged from 2.1–7.3 mg/L during the 21 hour period following a 2000 mg oral dose, and represented only 0.2% of the total drug (Parker et al., 1970). 2-Phenylglutarimide and 2-ethyl-2-phenylglutaconimide each account for about 2–4% of a dose as urinary excretion products, and the remainder consists largely of glucuronide conjugates of the hydroxylated metabolites (Buetikofer et al., 1962; Kennedy and Fischer, 1979).

Toxicity. Numerous cases of nonfatal and fatal overdosage with glutethimide have been recorded, with the minimum lethal dose for an adult estimated at 5 g. Chazan and Garella (1971) reported on a large series of intoxicated patients and found that those with mild intoxication had blood concentrations of 5–56 mg/L (average, 27), those with moderate intoxication, 22–78 mg/L (average, 45) and those suffering from severe intoxication, 15–120 mg/L (average, 50). The coma seen with glutethimide is often of long duration and sometimes recurs as the patient appears to be recovering (Maher et al., 1962; Decker et al., 1970); subjects often regain consciousness when their plasma level falls below 10–20 mg/L (Maher et al., 1962; Sunshine et al., 1968; Gold et al., 1973). In one intoxicated patient, plasma glutethimide concentrations declined slowly from 12–3.8 mg/L over an 11.5 hour period, during which the 4-hydroxyglutethimide concentration increased from 17–21 mg/L (Hansen and Fischer, 1974). Concentrations of this active metabolite in the plasma of other patients have exceeded 50 mg/L at a time when the glutethimide concentrations were less than 10 mg/L (Ambre and Fischer, 1972). Although hemodialysis has been shown to reduce the half-life of glutethimide in poisoned patients from an average of 40–15 hours (Maher, 1970), most investigators have concluded that its use does not significantly alter the course of intoxication (Wright and Roscoe, 1970; Chazan and Garella, 1971).

In 11 fatal cases, blood concentrations have ranged from 10–97 mg/L (average, 45) and liver concentrations, 63–141 mg/kg (average, 89) (Baselt and Cravey, 1977). Concentrations of glutethimide and 4-hydroxyglutethimide in 2 fatalities averaged 17 and 18 mg/L, respectively, in blood, and 101 and 61 mg/kg in liver (Hansen et al., 1975). The following distribution was observed in 2 deaths and is demonstrative of the lipid solubility of glutethimide (Goldbaum et al., 1962):

Glutethimide Concentrations in Fatalities (mg/L or mg/kg)

	Serum	Brain	Liver	Kidney	Fat
Case I	23	61	75	31	200
Case 2	10		28	13	60

Analysis. Spectrophotometric methods for the analysis of glutethimide in biological specimens have made use of the gradual hydrolysis of the glutarimide ring in alkaline solution and the resulting decline in absorbance with time (Goldbaum et al., 1957; Goldbaum et al., 1962; Knowlton and Goldbaum, 1969). This method is unable to differentially measure the parent drug and its metabolites and thus chromatographic procedures are generally preferable. Flame-ionization gas chromatography has been used for the analysis of the parent drug (Finkle, 1967; Sunshine et al., 1968; Kadar and Kalow, 1972) and for the simultaneous assay of the parent and its active metabolites (Fischer and Ambre, 1973; Hansen and Fischer, 1974; Evans et al., 1977). A gas chromatographic-mass spectrometric method has been described for glutethimide and 6 of its metabolites in blood and urine (Kennedy et al., 1978). Liquid chromatography has also been used to determine glutethimide in serum (Van Veldhuizen and Hartman, 1981).

References

E.J. Algeri and G.G. Katsas. Toxicology of glutethimide. J. For. Sci. 5: 217–225, 1960.

J.J. Ambre and L.J. Fischer. Glutethimide intoxication: plasma levels of glutethimide and a metabolite in humans, dogs and rats. Res. Comm. Chem. Path. Pharm. 4: 307–326, 1972.

J.J. Ambre and L.J. Fischer. Identification and activity of the hydroxy metabolite that accumulates in the plasma of humans intoxicated with glutethimide. Drug Met. Disp. 2: 151–158, 1974.

B.D. Andresen, J.L. Templeton, R.H. Hammer et al. Definitive characterization of the para-hydroxyphenyl metabolite of glutethimide in human urine. Res. Comm. Chem. Path. Pharm. 12: 627–634, 1975.

B.D. Andresen, J.L. Templeton, R.H. Hammer et al. Identification of a methylated catechol metabolite of glutethimide (Doriden) in human urine. Res. Comm. Chem. Path. Pharm. 13: 193–201, 1976.

B.D. Andresen, F.T. Davis, J.L. Templeton et al. Toxicity of alpha-phenyl-gamma-butyrolactone, a metabolite of glutethimide in human urine. Res. Comm. Chem. Path. Pharm. 18: 439–451, 1977.

R.C. Baselt and R.H. Cravey. A compendium of therapeutic and toxic concentrations of toxicologically significant drugs in human biofluids. J. Anal. Tox. 1: 81–103, 1977.

E. Buetikofer, P. Cottier, P. Imhof et al. Ueber die Eliminierungsgeschwindigkeit von Glutethimid (Doriden) und die Natur der Ausscheidungsprodukte beim Menschen. Arch. Exp. Path. Pharm. 244: 97–108, 1962.

J.A. Chazan and S. Garella. Glutethimide intoxication. Arch. Int. Med. 128: 215–219, 1971.

J.W. Crow, P. Lain, F. Bochner et al. Glutethimide and 4-OH glutethimide: pharmacokinetics and effect on performance in man. Clin. Pharm. Ther. 22: 458–464, 1977.

S.H. Curry, D. Riddall, J.S. Gordon et al. Disposition of glutethimide in man. Clin. Pharm. Ther. 12: 849–857, 1971.

W.J. Decker, H.L. Thompson and L.A. Arneson. Glutethimide rebound. Lancet 1: 778–779, 1970.

M.A. Evans, A.S. Nies, J.T. Watson and R.D. Harbison. Confirmation of the identity of an active metabolite in glutethimide intoxication. J. Anal. Tox. 1: 229–232, 1977.

B.S. Finkle. The identification, quantitative determination and distribution of meprobamate and glutethimide in biological material. J. For. Sci. 12: 509–528, 1967.

L.J. Fischer and J.J. Ambre. Possible interference by a metabolite in gas chromatographic assays for glutethimide which employ certain non-selective liquid phases. J. Chrom. 87: 379–386, 1973.

M. Gold, E. Tassoni and M. Etzl. Comparison of glutethimide concentration in the serum and cerebrospinal fluid of humans in drug overdose. Clin. Chem. 19: 1158–1161, 1973.

L.R. Goldbaum, M. Williams and T. Koppanyi. Determination of Doriden. Fed. Proc. 16: 300, 1957.

L.R. Goldbaum, M. Williams and E.H. Johnston. Determination and distribution of Doriden. J. For. Sci. 7: 499–503, 1962.

A.R. Hansen and L.J. Fischer. Gas-chromatographic simultaneous analysis for glutethimide and an active hydroxylated metabolite in tissues, plasma, and urine. Clin. Chem. 20: 236–242, 1974.

A.R. Hansen, K.A. Kennedy, J.J. Ambre and L.J. Fischer. Glutethimide poisoning. New. Eng. J. Med. 292: 250–252, 1975.

D. Kadar and W. Kalow. A method for measuring glutethimide (Doriden) in human serum after intake of therapeutic doses. J. Chrom. 72: 21–27, 1972.

D. Kadar, T. Inaba, L. Endrenyi et al. Comparative drug elimination capacity in man—glutethimide, amobarbital, antipyrine, and sulfinpyrazone. Clin. Pharm. Ther. 14: 552–560, 1973.

K.A. Kennedy, J.J. Ambre and L.J. Fischer. A selected ion monitoring method for glutethimide and six metabolites: application to blood and urine from humans intoxicated with glutethimide. Biomed. Mass Spec. 5: 679–685, 1978.

K.A. Kennedy and L.J. Fischer. Quantitative and stereochemical aspects of glutethimide metabolism in humans. Drug Met. Disp. 7: 319–324, 1979.

M. Knowlton and L.R. Goldbaum. An improved rapid method for the determination of glutethimide (Doriden) in blood. J. For. Sci. 14: 129–135, 1969.

J.F. Maher, G.E. Schreiner and F.B. Westervelt. Acute glutethimide intoxication. Am. J. Med. 33: 70–82, 1962.

J.F. Maher. Determinants of serum half-life of glutethimide in intoxicated patients. J. Pharm. Exp. Ther. 174: 450–455, 1970.

K.D. Parker, H.W. Elliott, J.A. Wright et al. Blood and urine concentrations of subjects receiving barbiturates, meprobamate, glutethimide, or diphenylhydantoin. Clin. Tox. 3: 131–145, 1970.

W.G. Stillwell. Metabolism of glutethimide in the human. Res. Comm. Chem. Path. Pharm. 12: 25–41, 1975.

I. Sunshine, R. Maes and R. Faracci. Determination of glutethimide (Doriden) and its metabolites in biologic specimens. Clin. Chem. 14: 595–609, 1968.

J.E. Van Veldhuizen and A.E. Hartmann. Hypnotic-sedative screen by high performance liquid chromatography. J. Liq. Chrom. 4: 501–514, 1981.

N. Wright and P. Roscoe. Acute glutethimide poisoning. J. Am. Med. Asso. 214: 1704–1706, 1970.

Gold

T½: 5–16 days
Vd: 0.1 L/kg   Au
Fb: 0.95

Occurrence and Usage. Monovalent gold compounds have been used in the treatment of rheumatoid arthritis for many years. Among the most commonly used agents are aurothioglucose (Solganal) and sodium aurothiomalate (Myochrysine), both of which are water-soluble, contain 50% gold by weight and are usually administered by intramuscular injection. Treatment schedules vary, but often involve a single 10–50 mg injection of one of these drugs every 1–4 weeks.

Blood Concentrations. Serum gold concentrations reached peak levels of 6.0–8.0 mg/L 2–6 hours after intramuscular administration of 50 mg of aurothiomalate, declining to 4.0–6.0 mg/L by 2 days and 2.5–3.5 mg/L by 7 days (Gottlieb and Gray, 1978). During chronic administration of 25 mg of gold (as sodium aurothiomalate) once weekly by intramuscular injection, plasma gold concentrations averaged 5.7 mg/L (range, 3.2–8.0) on the day after the injection and declined to an average of 3.1 mg/L by the seventh day (Krusius et al., 1970). Optimal results have been achieved when serum gold levels are maintained in excess of 3 mg/L (Lorber, 1977). A mean serum half-life of 5.5 days has been determined for aurothiomalate (Gerber et al., 1974). Gold is restricted to the serum in most patients, but is found in significant quantitites in the red cells of other patients (Smith et al., 1973).

Metabolism and Excretion. Within 7 days of a single injection of aurothiomalate, about 13% of a dose is eliminated in the urine and 3% in feces (Gerber et al., 1974). During therapy about 30% is found in the weekly urine and 10% in feces, representing gold from both recent and prior injections (Gottlieb et al., 1972). The remainder is very slowly excreted; gold has been found in the tissues of persons who had not received the drug for at least 20 years (Grahame et al., 1974). Urine gold concentrations of 1–5 mg/L are commonly observed in patients on chrysotherapy (Harth, 1974).

Toxicity. Toxic side-effects of gold therapy afflict up to 50% of patients, and include dermatitis and nephrotic syndrome (Gottlieb et al., 1972). Several cases of gold-induced thrombocytopenia have been successfully treated by dimercaprol (BAL) chelation therapy (Lockie et al., 1947; Hazlett and Yendt, 1958; Stafford and Crosby, 1978).

One subject who died 6 days after the intramuscular injection of 400 mg of sodium aurothiomalate was found to exhibit the following tissue distribution (Leung, 1975):

Gold Concentrations in a Fatal Case (mg/L or mg/kg)

Blood	Liver	Spleen	Kidney Cortex	Kidney Medulla
0.4	2.6	0.7	15.7	11.0

Analysis. Gold is frequently determined in biologic specimens by atomic absorption spectrophotometry after sample digestion or chelation and solvent extraction (Balazs et al., 1972; Harth et al., 1973; Sharma, 1982); some authors suggest that solvent extraction is unpredictable and that direct analysis of the entire specimen is preferred (Lorber et al., 1968; Dunckley, 1971; Barrett et al., 1978; Dunckley et al., 1979).

References

N.D.H. Balazs, D.J. Pole and J.R. Masarei. Determination of gold in body fluids by atomic absorption spectrophotometry. Clin. Chim. Acta 40: 213–218, 1972.

M.J. Barrett, R. DeFries and W.M. Henderson. Rapid determination of gold in whole blood of arthritis patients using flameless atomic absorption spectrophotometry. J. Pharm. Sci. 67: 1332–1334, 1978.

J.V. Dunckley. Estimation of gold in serum by atomic absorption spectroscopy. Clin. Chem. 17: 992–993,
1971.

J.V. Dunckley, D.M. Grennan and D.G. Palmer. The estimation of serum and urinary gold by atomic absorption spectroscopy in rheumatoid patients receiving gold therapy. J. Anal. Tox. 3: 242–245, 1979.

R.C. Gerber, H.E. Paulus, R.I. Jennrich et al. Gold kinetics following aurothiomalate therapy: use of a whole-
body radiation counter. J. Lab. Clin. Med. 83: 778–789, 1974.

N.L. Gottlieb, P.M. Smith and E.M. Smith. Gold excretion correlated with clinical course during chrysotherapy
in rheumatoid arthritis. Arth. Rheum. 15: 582–592, 1972.

N.L. Gottlieb and R.G. Gray. Diagnosis and management of adverse reactions from gold compounds. J. Anal.
Tox. 2: 173–184, 1978.

R. Grahame, R. Billings, M. Laurence et al. Tissue gold levels after chrysotherapy. Ann. Rheum. Dis. 33: 536–
539, 1974.

M. Harth, D.S.M. Haines and D.C. Bondy. A simple method for the determination of gold in serum, blood, and
urine by atomic absorption spectroscopy. Am. J. Clin. Path. 59: 423–428, 1973.

M. Harth. Serum gold levels during chrysotherapy with relation to urinary and fecal excretion. Clin. Pharm.
Ther. 15: 354–360, 1974.

B.E. Hazlett and E.R. Yendt. Thrombocytopenia following gold therapy with successful treatment. Can. Med.
Asso. J. 79: 31–33, 1958.

F.E. Krusius, A. Markkanen and P. Peltola. Plasma levels and urinary excretion of gold during routine treatment of rheumatoid arthritis. Ann. Rheum. Dis. 29: 232–235, 1970.

S.C. Leung. Personal communication, 1975.

L.M. Lockie, B.M. Norcross and C.W. George. Treatment of two reactions due to gold. J. Am. Med. Asso. 133:
754–755, 1947.

A. Lorber, R.L. Cohen, C.C. Chang and H.E. Anderson. Gold determination in biological fluids by atomic
absorption spectrophotometry. Arth. Rheum. 11: 170–177, 1968.

A. Lorber. Monitoring gold plasma levels in rheumatoid arthritis. Clin. Pharmacokin. 2: 127–146, 1977.

R.P. Sharma. A microanalytical method for the analysis of gold in biological media by flameless atomic
absorption spectrometry. Ther. Drug Mon. 4: 219–224, 1982.

P.M. Smith, E.M. Smith and N.L. Gottlieb. Gold distribution in whole blood during chrysotherapy. J. Lab.
Clin. Med. 82: 930–937, 1973.

B.T. Stafford and W.H. Crosby. Late onset of gold-induced thrombocytopenia. J. Am. Med. Asso. 239: 50–51,
1978.

Guaifenesin

T½: 1.4–5.3 hr
Vd: 1.0 L/kg
Fb: ?

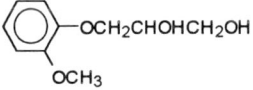

Occurrence and Usage. Guaifenesin (guaiphenesin, glyceryl guaiacolate, guaiacol glyceryl ether)
is a guaicol derivative that is extensively used as an expectorant and veterinary muscle relaxant. It
is chemically related to methocarbamol, the carbamate of guaifenesin, and to mephenesin, a desoxy
analogue. Guaifenesin is available in numerous over-the-counter and prescription tablets and syrups, usually in combination with antihistamines, antitussives, or decongestants. Single oral doses
of 50–200 mg and daily doses of up to 1200 mg are commonly used.

Blood Concentrations. A single 600 mg oral dose given to 3 subjects resulted in peak blood concentrations of approximately 1.4 mg/L after 15 minutes; by 2 hours, the average level had declined to about 0.3 mg/L, and by 8 hours guaifenesin was no longer detectable in the blood (Maynard and Bruce, 1970). An individual who ingested ten 240 mg oral doses of guaifenesin within a 24 hour period had a blood concentration of 1.0 mg/L at 1 hour after the last dose; this declined to 0.4 mg/L 8 hours later (Cravey, 1981). The elimination half-life averages 2.9 hours (Aluri and Stavchansky, 1993).

Metabolism and Excretion. Guaifenesin is known to be metabolized in man by oxidation to beta-(2-methoxyphenoxy)lactic acid, which accounts for about 40% of a single dose in the 3 hour urine. Unchanged drug has not been detected in urine (Vandenheuvel et al., 1972).

guaifenesin   β-(2-methoxyphenoxy)lactic acid

Toxicity. Guaifenesin causes central nervous system depression at the higher dose levels. In horses, an intravenous dose of 130 mg/kg caused collapse and complete muscle relaxation within a few minutes. Movement was first observed when the plasma guaifenesin concentration declined to an average of 238 mg/L, and the righting reflex returned at a level of 210 mg/L (Davis and Wolff, 1970). A 76 year old woman died after intentionally ingesting a bottle of Hycotuss cough syrup; her postmortem blood contained 3.0 mg/L hydrocodone and 14 mg/L guaifenesin (Cravey, 1981).

Analysis. Guaifenesin may be determined in biological fluids by a chromotropic acid colorimetric procedure (Morgan et al., 1957) or electron-capture gas chromatography of a halogenated derivative (Maynard and Bruce, 1970). Liquid chromatography has also been employed (Ketelaars and Peters, 1981; Aluri and Stavchansky, 1993).

References

J.B. Aluri and S. Stavchansky. Determination of guaifenesin in human plasma by liquid chromatography in the presence of pseudoephedrine. J. Pharm. Biomed. Anal. 11: 803–808, 1993.

R.H. Cravey. Personal communication, 1981.

L.E. Davis and W.A. Wolff. Pharmacokinetics and metabolism of glyceryl guaiacolate in ponies. Am. J. Vet. Res. 31: 469–473, 1970.

H.C.J. Ketelaars and J.G.P. Peters. Determination of guaiphenesin and its metabolite, beta-(2-methoxyphenoxy)-lactic acid, in plasma by high-performance liquid chromatography. J. Chrom. 224: 144–148, 1981.

W.R. Maynard, Jr. and R.B. Bruce. GLC determination of guaiacol glyceryl ether in blood. J. Pharm. Sci. 59: 1346–1348, 1970.

A.M. Morgan, E.B. Truitt, Jr. and J.M. Little. Plasma levels of mephenesin, mephenesin carbamate, guaiacol glyceryl ether, and methocarbamol (AHR-85) after oral and intravenous administration in the dog. J. Am. Pharm. Asso. Sci. Ed. 46: 374–377, 1957.

W.J.A. Vandenheuvel, J.L. Smith and R.H. Silber. β-(2-Methoxyphenoxy)lactic acid, the major urinary metabolite of glyceryl guaiacolate in man. J. Pharm. Sci. 61: 1997–1998, 1972.

Halazepam

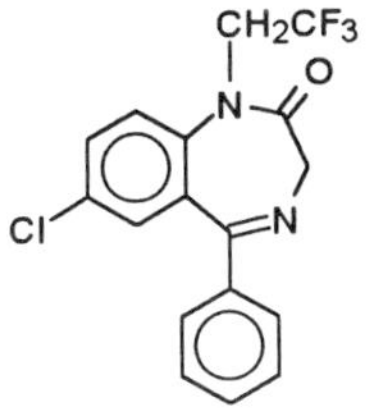

T½: 14–16 hr
Vd: 1.0 L/kg
Fb: ?
pKa: ?

Occurrence and Usage. Halazepam (Paxipam) is a 1,4-benzodiazepine derivative used for the management of anxiety disorders or the short term relief of the symptoms of anxiety. It is available for oral use in tablets containing 20 or 40 mg as the free base. The usual adult dose is 20–40 mg taken 3 or 4 times daily.

Blood Concentrations. A healthy adult subject ingested a single 40 mg oral dose of halazepam in the fasting state and attained a peak plasma concentration of 37 µg/L after 1 hour; thereafter, halazepam disappeared rapidly from plasma, falling to less than 4 µg/L by 10 hours postdose. The peak plasma nordiazepam concentration of 146 µg/L was achieved 2.5 hours after dosage; the metabolite disappeared with a half-life of 50 hours, and could still be detected in plasma after 14 days (Greenblatt et al., 1983).

In a study to determine steady-state kinetics, 11 healthy men ranging in age from 19–35 years and weighing 63–82 kg (average, 71) were given oral doses of 40 mg every 8 hours (120 mg/day) for 14 days; peak plasma concentrations of halazepam were as high as 125 µg/L about 2 hours after each dose. The average steady-state plasma concentration of halazepam was approximately 77 µg/L, with steady-state being reached by the seventh dose on the third day; peak plasma concentrations of nordiazepam ranged from 1404–1657 µg/L on day 13, with steady-state for the metabolite being reached on day 11 (Chung et al., 1984).

Metabolism and Excretion. The major plasma metabolite of halazepam is nordiazepam, which is formed rapidly but eliminated slowly with a half-life of 50–100 hours (Allen et al., 1980; Greenblatt et al., 1981; Greenblatt et al., 1983). Less than 1% of a dose is eliminated as unchanged drug; the major urinary metabolite is conjugated 3-hydroxyhalazepam. Presumably, the nordiazepam that is formed is further oxidized to oxazepam and excreted as a glucuronide.

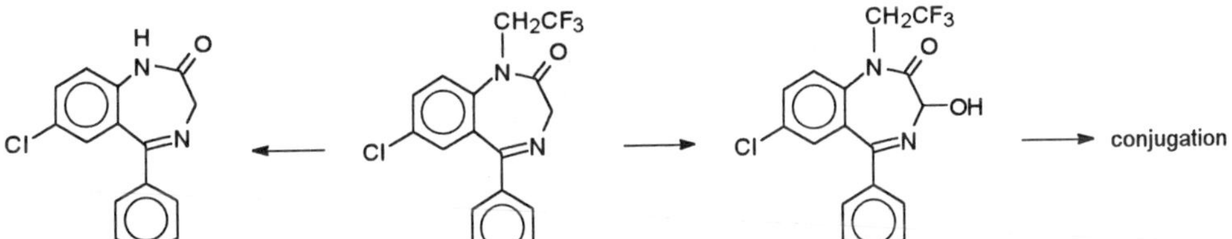

nordiazepam   halazepam   3-hydroxyhalazepam   conjugation

Toxicity. In overdose, halazepam may cause confusion, somnolence, impaired coordination, diminished reflexes and coma. Withdrawal symptoms may appear upon abrupt cessation after long use. One subject received 1120 mg of halazepam within a 24 hour period through a medication error and apparently suffered no ill effects acutely or in follow-up (Fann et al., 1983).

Analysis. Gas chromatography with electron-capture detection has been used for the quantitation of halazepam and its major metabolite, nordiazepam, in plasma (Greenblatt et al., 1983). Methods described for diazepam, flurazepam and other benzodiazepines may be used for the analysis. Liquid chromatography has also been described (Gupta and Ellinwood, 1990).

References

M.D. Allen, D.J. Greenblatt, J.S. Harmatz et al. Desmethyldiazepam kinetics in the elderly after oral prazepam. Clin. Pharm. Ther. 28: 196–202, 1980.

M. Chung, J.M. Hilbert, R.P. Gural et al. Multiple-dose halazepam kinetics. Clin. Pharm. Ther. 35: 838–842, 1984.

W.E. Fann, J. Garcia and B.W. Richman. High-dose benzodiazepine therapy in hospitalized anxious patients. J. Clin. Pharm. 23: 100–105, 1983.

D.J. Greenblatt, R.I. Shader, M. Divoll et al. Benzodiazepines: a summary of pharmacokinetic properties. Brit. J. Clin. Pharm. 11: 11s–16s, 1981.

D.J. Greenblatt, A. Locniskar and R.I. Shader. Halazepam as a precursor of desmethyldiazepam: quantitation by electron-capture gas-liquid chromatography. Psychopharmacology 80: 178–180, 1983.

S.K. Gupta and E.H. Ellinwood. Liquid chromatographic assay and pharmacokinetics of halazepam and its metabolite in humans. J. Pharm. Sci. 79: 822–825, 1990.

Haloperidol

T½: 14–41 hr
Vd: 18–30 L/kg
Fb: 0.90
pKa: 8.3

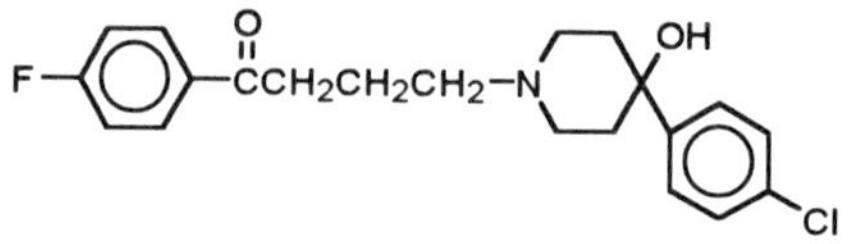

Occurrence and Usage. Haloperidol (Haldol) is a butyrophenone derivative that was synthesized in 1958 and first marketed in the United States in 1967. It is an effective antipsychotic agent often used interchangeably with the phenothiazines. It is administered orally or by intramuscular injection as the lactate in single doses of 0.5–5 mg and daily doses of up to 100 mg or more.

Blood Concentrations. A single 10 mg oral dose of haloperidol given to 7 subjects resulted in an average peak serum concentration of 3 µg/L at 5 hours (Forsman and Ohman, 1976). Intramuscular injection of 2 mg produced plasma concentrations in 12 subjects that averaged 5 µg/L after 20 minutes and 1 µg/L after 3 hours (Cressman et al., 1974).

In patients receiving an average daily dose of 5.7 mg (range, 1–90) of haloperidol, the mean steady-state serum concentration was 6 µg/L (range, 0.5–121). The half-life of the drug was observed to range from 14–41 hours (Forsman and Ohman, 1977). Concentrations of the drug in the serum of patients who received 20–200 mg daily ranged proportionately from 6–245 µg/L (Clark et al., 1977). In 5 patients receiving chronic daily doses of 0.5–1.5 mg/kg (35–105 mg/70 kg), plasma levels ranged from 14–98 µg/L for haloperidol and 10–319 µg/L for reduced haloperidol; the individual ratios for metabolite/parent plasma concentration ranged from 0.19–4.68 (Ereshefsky et al., 1984). A once monthly intramuscular injection of 100 mg of haloperidol decanoate is capable of maintaining a steady-state plasma haloperidol level of 4 µg/L in adult patients (Reyntjens et al., 1982). The blood/plasma ratio for the drug averages 0.79 (Cheng et al., 1987). Various studies have reported optimal patient response at plasma haloperidol levels ranging from 5–50 µg/L (Volavka et al., 1992).

Metabolism and Excretion. Haloperidol is extensively biotransformed to inactive metabolites. The compound is cleaved at the N-C bond with resultant urinary excretion of 4-fluorobenzoylpropionic acid and 4-fluorophenylacetic acid. Less than 1% of a dose is excreted unchanged, and no evidence was found for the formation of haloperidol glucuronide. The urinary excretion of metabolites has not been quantitatively studied (Forsman et al., 1977). A reduced form of haloperidol, less active than its parent, has been found at comparable concentrations in plasma of patients on therapy

(Forsman and Larsson, 1978; Pape, 1981) and is believed to be formed by erythrocytes both *in vivo* and *in vitro* (Eyles et al., 1992).

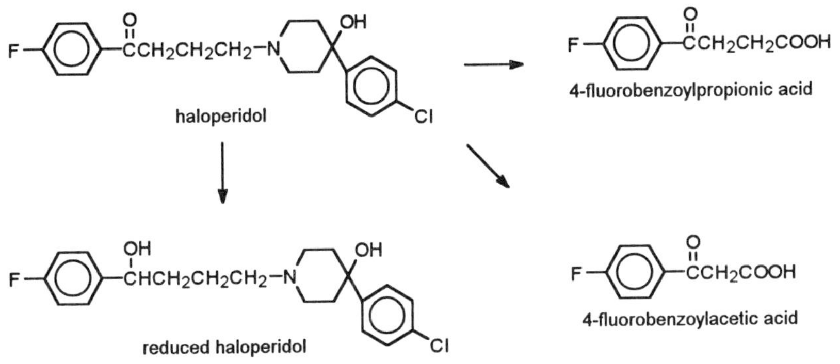

haloperidol

4-fluorobenzoylpropionic acid

reduced haloperidol

4-fluorobenzoylacetic acid

Toxicity. Adverse reactions to haloperidol include drowsiness, blurred vision, extrapyramidal effects, tardive dyskinesia, tachycardia, hypotension, and muscular rigidity. In pediatric patients, these side effects were present in 75% of those with plasma haloperidol concentrations between 6 and 9 μg/L, and in 90% of those with concentrations greater than 10 μg/L (Morselli et al., 1979). The major effects seen with high-dose use (100 mg/day) are drowsiness and increased serum enzyme levels (McCreadie and MacDonald, 1977).

Two children ages 4 and 5, accidentally given haloperidol doses of 2 and 5 mg orally, developed acute muscle rigidity that persisted for some 30 hours; peak serum levels of 6 and 23 μg/L were observed (Tsujimoto et al., 1982). Several children who became acutely poisoned after ingesting haloperidol were successfully treated by administration of an anticholinergic agent, biperiden (Sinaniotis et al., 1978). In 2 similar cases, the patients exhibited bradycardia, hypothermia, sinus arrhythmia, neuromuscular rigidity, tremors, and coma; the symptoms were partially relieved with intravenous diphenhydramine (Scialli and Thornton, 1978). Two young children (body weights of 16 and 17.8 kg) who accidentally ingested as much as 12–20 mg of haloperidol and became comatose developed blood concentrations of 42 and 68 mg/L, respectively, at 2 hours; the concentrations fell to 18 and 31 mg/L, respectively, after 24 hours and were negative by 72 hours (Coutselinis et al., 1977). These concentrations appear vastly overestimated; the units probably should read μg/L rather than mg/L.

At least 6 patients on haloperidol therapy have died suddenly, possibly due to laryngeal spasm (Ketai et al., 1979; Baden et al., 1981; Modestin et al., 1981). Postmortem blood concentrations of 1.0 mg/L have been reported in 2 adults who died following intentional overdose with the drug; in 1 case, the level represents haloperidol while in the other it represents reduced haloperidol (Lewellen, 1983; Rousseau, 1983). The following concentrations were measured in an adult male who died after ingesting as many as 120 haloperidol tablets (Levine et al., 1991):

Haloperidol Concentrations in a Fatality (mg/L or mg/kg)

Drug	Blood	Liver	Bile	Urine	Gastric
Haloperidol	1.9	44	3.4	6.6	67 mg
Reduced haloperidol	1.4	43	1.6	5.7	0

Analysis. Haloperidol has been assayed in biological fluids by radioimmunoassay (Clark et al., 1977). Gas chromatographic procedures have involved nitrogen-phosphorus detection (Bianchetti and Morselli, 1978; Franklin, 1980; Abernethy et al., 1984), electron-capture detection (Zingales, 1971; Forsman et al., 1974), and mass spectrometry (Hornbeck et al., 1979; Moulin et al., 1979; Haring et al., 1987). Liquid chromatography has also been employed (Miyazaki et al., 1981; Korpi et al., 1983; Dhar and Kutt, 1984; Susanto et al., 1985; Miller and DeVane, 1986; Vatassery et al., 1988; Park et al., 1991; Eyles et al., 1992). Eyles et al. (1992) recommend either freezing of blood specimens or immediate centrifugation of plasma specimens to minimize changes in the concentrations of haloperidol and reduced haloperidol.

References

D.R. Abernethy, D.J. Greenblatt, H.R. Ochs et al. Haloperidol determination in serum and cerebrospinal fluid using gas-liquid chromatography with nitrogen-phosphorus detection: application to pharmacokinetic studies. J. Chrom. 307: 194–199, 1984.

M.M. Baden, A. Blaustein, L.R. Ferraro et al. Sudden death after haloperidol. Can. Soc. For. Sci. J. 14: 70–72, 1981.

G. Bianchetti and P.L. Morselli. Rapid and sensitive method for determination of haloperidol in human samples using nitrogen-phosphorus selective detection. J. Chrom. 153: 203–209, 1978.

Y.F. Cheng, L.K. Paalzow, U. Bondesson et al. Pharmacokinetics of haloperidol in psychotic patients. Psychopharmacology 91: 410–414, 1987.

B.R. Clark, B.B. Tower and R.T. Rubin. Radioimmunoassay of haloperidol in human serum. Life Sci. 20: 319–325, 1977.

A. Coutselinis, D. Boukis and P. Kentarchon. Haloperidol concentrations in blood and cases of acute intoxication. Clin. Chem. 23: 900, 1977.

W.A. Cressman, J.R. Bianchine, V.B. Slotnick et al. Plasma level profile of haloperidol in man following intramuscular administration. Eur. J. Clin. Pharm. 7: 99–103, 1974.

A.K. Dhar and H. Kutt. Improved liquid-chromatographic determination of haloperidol in plasma. Clin. Chem. 30: 1228–1230, 1984.

L. Ereshefsky, C.M. Davis, C.A. Harrington et al. Haloperidol and reduced haloperidol plasma levels in selected schizophrenic patients. J. Clin. Psychopharm. 4: 138–142, 1984.

D.W. Eyles, H.A. Whiteford, T.J. Stedman and S.M. Pond. Determination of haloperidol and reduced haloperidol in the plasma and blood of patients on depot haloperidol. Psychopharmacology 106: 268–274, 1992.

A. Forsman, E. Martensson, G. Nyberg and R. Ohman. A gas chromatographic method for determining haloperidol. Arch. Pharm. 286: 113–124, 1974.

A. Forsman and R. Ohman. Pharmacokinetic studies on haloperidol in man. Curr. Ther. Res. 20: 319–336, 1976.

A. Forsman and R. Ohman. Applied pharmacokinetics of haloperidol in man. Curr. Ther. Res. 21: 396–410, 1977.

A. Forsman, G. Folsch, M. Larsson and R. Ohman. On the metabolism of haloperidol in man. Curr. Ther. Res. 21: 606–616, 1977.

A. Forsman and M. Larsson. Metabolism of haloperidol. Curr. Ther. Res. 24: 567–568, 1978.

M. Franklin. Gas-chromatographic measurement of haloperidol in plasma. Clin. Chem. 26: 1367–1368, 1980.

H. Haring, Z. Salama, L. Todesko and H. Jaeger. Gas chromatographic-mass spectrometric determination of haloperidol in plasma. Arz. Forsch. 37: 1402–1404, 1987.

C.L. Hornbeck, J.C. Griffiths, R.J. Neborsky and M.A. Faulkner. A gas chromatographic mass spectrometric chemical ionization assay for haloperidol with selected ion monitoring. Biomed. Mass Spec. 6: 427–430, 1979.

R. Ketai, J. Matthews and J.J. Mozdzen, Jr. Sudden death in a patient taking haloperidol. Am. J. Psych. 136: 112–113, 1979.

E.R. Korpi, B.H. Phelps, H. Granger et al. Simultaneous determination of haloperidol and its reduced metabolite in serum and plasma by isocratic liquid chromatography with electrochemical detection. Clin. Chem. 29: 624–628, 1983.

B.S. Levine, S.C. Wu, B.A. Goldberger and Y.H. Caplan. Two fatalities involving haloperidol. J. Anal. Tox. 15: 282–284, 1991.

L.J. Lewellen. Personal communication, 1983.

R.G. McCreadie and I.M. MacDonald. High dosage haloperidol in chronic schizophrenia. Brit. J. Psych. 131: 310–316, 1977.

R.L. Miller and C.L. DeVane. Measurement of haloperidol and reduced haloperidol in human plasma using reversed-phase high-performance liquid chromatography. J. Chrom. 374: 405–408, 1986.

K. Miyazaki, T. Arita, I. Oka et al. High-performance liquid chromatographic determination of haloperidol in plasma. J. Chrom. 223: 449–453, 1981.

J. Modestin, R. Krapf and W. Boker. A fatality during haloperidol treatment: mechanism of sudden death. Am. J. Psych. 138: 1616–1617, 1981.

P.L. Morselli, G. Bianchetti, G. Durand et al. Haloperidol plasma level monitoring in pediatric patients. Ther. Drug Mon. 1: 35–46, 1979.

M.A. Moulin, R. Camsonne, J.P. Davy et al. Gas chromatography-electron-impact and chemical-ionization mass spectrometry of haloperidol and its chlorinated homologue. J. Chrom. 178: 324–329, 1979.

B.E. Pape. Isolation and identification of a metabolite of haloperidol. J. Anal. Tox. 5: 113–117, 1981.

K.H. Park, M.H. Lee and M.G. Lee. Simultaneous determination of haloperidol and its metabolite, reduced haloperidol. J. Chrom. 572: 259–267, 1991.

A.J.M. Reyntjens, J.J.P. Heykants, R.J.H. Woestenborghs et al. Pharmacokinetics of haloperidol decanoate. Int. Pharmacopsych. 17: 238–246, 1982.

M. Rousseau. Personal communication, 1983.

J.V.K. Scialli and W.E. Thornton. Toxic reactions from a haloperidol overdose in two children. J. Am. Med. Asso. 239: 48–49, 1978.

C.A. Sinaniotis, P. Spyrides, P. Vlachos and C. Papadatos. Acute haloperidol poisoning in children. J. Pediat. 93: 1038–1039, 1978.

F. Susanto, S. Humfeld and A. Neumann. Simple plasma treatment for the quantitative determination of haloperidol by HPLC. Fres. Z. Anal. Chem. 321: 177–179, 1985.

A. Tsujimoto, G. Tsujimoto, T. Ishizaki et al. Toxic haloperidol reactions with observation of serum haloperidol concentration in two children. Dev. Pharm. Ther. 4: 12–17, 1982.

G.T. Vatassery, L.A. Herzan and M.W. Dysken. Simultaneous determination of very low concentrations of haloperidol and reduced haloperidol in human serum by a liquid chromatographic method. J. Chrom. 433: 312–317, 1988.

J. Volavka, T. Cooper, P. Czobor et al. Haloperidol blood levels and clinical effects. Arch. Gen. Psych. 49: 354–361, 1992.

I. Zingales. A gas chromatographic method for the determination of haloperidol in human plasma. J. Chrom. 54: 15–24, 1971.

Halothane

T½: 43 hr
Vd: 1 L/kg
Fb: ?

$CF_3CHBrCl$

Occurrence and Usage. Since 1956, halothane (Fluothane) has received widespread usage as the first of the modern halogenated nonflammable anesthetics. Since it is a poor analgesic, it is commonly used at concentrations of 0.5–3% in conjunction with other drugs such as nitrous oxide and neuromuscular blocking agents. Halothane is suspected of producing hepatotoxicity in man, due possibly to the products of its biotransformation.

Blood Concentrations. During surgical anesthesia (plane II of stage III), arterial blood levels of halothane ranged from 80–260 mg/L; after anesthesia the patients were able to respond to verbal commands when arterial concentrations were 30 mg/L or less; and all were ambulatory at concentrations of 1–20 mg/L. Venous blood concentrations were found to lag behind arterial concentrations during induction, and to decline less rapidly during recovery, so that ambulatory venous concentrations were on the order of 25–50 mg/L (Ardoin et al., 1966). The average uptake of halothane by patients is 3–5 mL of the liquid per hour, and most of this is eliminated during the 9 hour post-anesthetic period (Duncan and Raventos, 1959). The drug exhibits elimination half-lives of 9 minutes from the central compartment, 1.4 hours from muscle tissue and 43 hours from the fat (Yasuda et al., 1991).

Metabolism and Excretion. Halothane is one of the more soluble anesthetic agents, requiring a long period for induction and recovery, and at normal body temperature it distributes in the following pattern (Wollman and Smith, 1975):

Partition Coefficients for Halothane

Blood:Gas	Brain:Blood	Liver:Blood	Kidney:Blood	Fat:Blood
2.4	2.1–3.3	2.5	1.5	65

Approximately 64% of a dose of halothane is excreted unchanged via the lungs (Yasuda et al., 1991). Most of the remainder has been accounted for as metabolites, making the compound one of the most extensively metabolized of the volatile anesthetic agents. Apparently defluorination of the compound does occur to a limited extent, but the major pathway involves both debromination and dechlorination. The product of these reactions is trifluoroacetic acid, which is excreted in the urine and which represents about 12% of the administered dose (Rehder et al., 1967). Concentrations of free trifluoroacetic acid in the urine of anesthetized patients reached maximum levels of 130–300 mg/L about 2 days after halothane administration and were still detectable for up to 12 days (Witte et al., 1977).

The bromide ion that is released is slowly excreted by the kidney. The peak plasma bromide concentrations that occurred in surgical patients 2–3 days after anesthesia ranged from 52–180 mg/L in one study (Tinker et al., 1976) and 192–336 mg/L in another (Johnstone et al., 1975). Serum bromide concentrations of 250 mg/L or higher undoubtedly produce a sedative effect on the individual.

Two volatile metabolites, chlorotrifluoroethane and chlorodifluoroethylene, have been identified in breath (Sharp et al., 1979) and other conjugated halothane metabolites have been found in the urine, implying conversion of the drug to reactive intermediates that may be linked to the hepatic toxicity of halothane (Cohen et al., 1975).

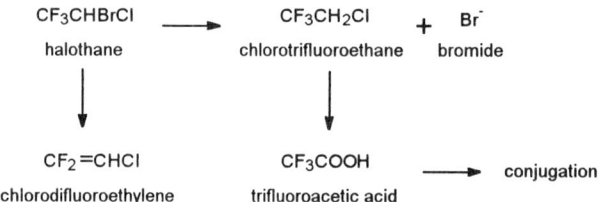

Toxicity. A number of instances of halothane-induced hepatotoxicity ("halothane hepatitis") in surgical patients have been reported, characterized by fever, jaundice, increased serum enzyme levels, and occasional death. The incidence is especially high in obese women aged 40 or more who undergo lengthy abdominal surgery (Carney and Van Dyke, 1972; Hoft et al., 1981). Hepatitis may also occur in persons with occupational exposure to halothane (Sutherland and Smith, 1992). The volatile metabolites of halothane are known to be highly hepatotoxic and may account for the clinical toxicity of the agent (Sharp et al., 1979).

An adult patient who was administered excessive amounts of halothane during surgery developed an antemortem blood concentration of 720 mg/L and was eventually declared brain dead (Randall and Corbett, 1982). Several documented fatalities involving halothane have occurred as a result of abuse in non-medical situations or ingestion with suicidal intention (Spencer and Green, 1968; Bidanset, 1973; Wright, 1975):

Tissue Concentrations of Halothane in Fatal Cases (mg/L or mg/kg)*

Route	Blood	Brain	Lung	Liver	Bile	Kidney	Urine	Gastric
Ingestion	45	30	38		15		8	20 mg
Ingestion	60	450	50	160		110		trace
Inhalation	33			295				
Inhalation	650	1560	500	880			20	96 mg

* By headspace gas chromatography

Analysis. Analysis of halothane in biological specimens is most often performed by gas chromatography with either direct sample injection (Cole et al., 1975) or headspace analysis (Fink and Morikawa, 1970; Koupil et al., 1988). A mass spectrometric procedure that relies on headspace analysis has also been described (Urich et al., 1977).

The volatile metabolites of halothane have been analyzed by headspace flame-ionization gas chromatography (Maiorino et al., 1979), while the nonvolatile metabolites, trifluoroacetic acid and bromide, have been determined in a similar manner after methylation (Maiorino et al., 1980). Other techniques for inorganic bromide determination are cited in the section on bromide.

References

D. Ardoin, R.A. Hingson, A.J. Tomaro and W.W. Fike. Chromatographic blood-gas studies of halothane in ambulatory oral surgical anesthesia. Anesth. Anal. 45: 275–281, 1966.

J. Bidanset. Personal communication, 1973.

F.M.T. Carney and R.A. Van Dyke. Halothane hepatitis: a critical review. Anesth. Anal. 51: 135–160, 1972.

E.N. Cohen, J.R. Trudell, H.N. Edmunds and E. Watson. Urinary metabolites of halothane in man. Anesthesiology 43: 392–401, 1975.

W.J. Cole, R.F. Salamonsen and K.J. Fish. A method for the gas chromatographic analysis of inhalation anesthetics in whole blood by direct injection into a simple precolumn device. Brit. J. Anaesth. 47: 1043–1047, 1975.

W.A.M. Duncan and J. Raventos. The pharmacokinetics of halothane (Fluothane) anaesthesia. Brit. J. Anaesth. 31: 302–315, 1959.

B.R. Fink and K. Morikawa. A simplified method for the measurement of volatile anesthetics in blood by gas chromatography. Anesthesiology 32: 451–455, 1970.

R.H. Hoft, J.P. Bunker, H.I. Goodman and P.B. Gregory. Halothane hepatitis in three pairs of closely related women. New Eng. J. Med. 304: 1023–1024, 1981.

R.E. Johnstone, E.M. Kennell, M.G. Behar et al. Increased serum bromide concentration after halothane anesthesia in man. Anesthesiology 42: 598–601, 1975.

P. Koupil, J. Novak and J. Drozd. Comparison of the absolute calibration method with the method of standard addition for the determination of halothane in blood. J. Chrom. 425: 99–105, 1988.

R.M. Maiorino, I.G. Sipes, A.J. Gandolfi and B.R. Brown, Jr. Quantitative analysis of volatile halothane metabolites in biological tissues by gas chromatography. J. Chrom. 164: 63–72, 1979.

R.M. Maiorino, A.J. Gandolfi and I.G. Sipes. Gas-chromatographic method for the halothane metabolites, trifluoroacetic acid and bromide, in biological fluids. J. Anal. Tox. 4: 250–254, 1980.

B. Randall and B. Corbett. Fatal halothane poisoning during anesthesia with other agents. J. For. Sci. 27: 225–230, 1982.

K. Rehder, J. Forbes, H. Alter et al. Halothane biotransformation in man: a quantitative study. Anesthesiology 28: 711–715, 1967.

J.H. Sharp, J.R. Trudell and E.N. Cohen. Volatile metabolites and decomposition products of halothane in man. Anesthesiology 50: 2–8, 1979.

J.A.E. Spencer and N.M. Green. Suicide by ingestion of halothane. J. Am. Med. Asso. 205: 112–113, 1968.

D.E. Sutherland and W.A. Smith. Chemical hepatitis associated with occupational exposure to halothane in a research laboratory. Vet. Hum. Tox. 34: 423–424, 1992.

J.H. Tinker, A.J. Gandolfi and R.A. Van Dyke. Elevation of plasma bromide levels in patients following halothane anesthesia. Anesthesiology 44: 194–196, 1976.

R.W. Urich, D.L. Bowerman, P.H. Wittenberg et al. Head space mass spectrometric analysis for volatiles in biological specimens. J. Anal. Tox. 1: 195–199, 1977.

L. Witte, H. Nau, J.H. Fuhrhop et al. Quantitative analysis of trifluoroacetic acid in body fluids of patients treated with halothane. J. Chrom. 143: 329–334, 1977.

H. Wollman and T.C. Smith. Uptake, distribution, elimination and administration of inhalational anesthetics. In *The Pharmacological Basis of Therapeutics*, 5th ed. (L.S. Goodman and A. Gilman, eds.), MacMillan, New York, 1975, pp. 71–80.

J. Wright. Personal communication, 1975.

N. Yasuda, S.H. Lockhart, E.I. Eger et al. Kinetics of desflurane, isoflurane, and halothane in humans. Anesthesiology 74: 489–498, 1991.

Heroin

T½: 60–90 min
Vd: 25 L/kg
Fb: 0.40
pKa: 7.6

$$NCH_3$$

$$CH_3COO \qquad O \qquad OOCCH_3$$

Occurrence and Usage. Heroin (diacetylmorphine, diamorphine) was first synthesized from morphine in 1874 and is currently a Schedule I substance (no currently accepted medical use) in the United States. A national epidemic of heroin usage and overdose fatalities swept through major cities in the early 1970s, but has subsided significantly since then. The average street-grade heroin is 2–6% pure and each dosage packet may contain from 3–16 mg of heroin (Greene et al., 1974). The drug is usually administered as the hydrochloride salt by intravenous or subcutaneous injection or by nasal insufflation, in daily doses of up to 200 mg.

Blood Concentrations. A single 5 mg intravenous heroin injection produced a plasma morphine concentration of 0.035 mg/L after 25 minutes. A 13 mg intravenous injection resulted in an increase of 0.082 mg/L in the plasma morphine concentration in a heroin-dependent subject (Tress et al., 1978). Nasal insufflation of 12 mg by 6 adults produced plasma levels averaging 0.016 mg/L heroin at 0.08 hours, 0.014 mg/L 6-acetylmorphine at 0.08–0.17 hours, and 0.019 mg/L morphine at 0.08–1.5 hours; elimination half-lives averaged 0.07, 0.22 and 2.8 hours, respectively (Cone et al., 1993). Serum morphine concentrations increased by an average of 0.031 mg/L for every 10 mg of orally administered heroin in patients receiving the drug every 4 hours for several weeks (Aherne et al., 1979). Plasma morphine levels as high as 0.300 mg/L were observed in addicts self-administering intravenous heroin doses of 150–200 mg (Bolelli et al., 1979). Although heroin is known to be rapidly hydrolyzed in blood or plasma *in vitro*, its terminal half-life averages about 1 hour, probably representing release of heroin that had distributed to esterase-free tissues (Garrett and Gurkan, 1980).

Metabolism and Excretion. It is known from animal or *in vitro* experiments that heroin is rapidly deacetylated in whole blood to 6-acetylmorphine (half-life, 9 min), and that 6-acetylmorphine is further hydrolyzed to morphine at a somewhat slower rate (half-life, 38 min). The first reaction is catalyzed by blood esterases and is inhibited by the addition of sodium fluoride or tetraethyl pyrophosphate, while the second presumably occurs in the liver. Spontaneous hydrolysis of the drug in pH 7.4 buffer or cerebrospinal fluid occurs with a half-life of 144 minutes (Nakamura et al., 1975; Garrett and Gurkan, 1979).

The percentage uptake for heroin by brain tissue following a single intra-arterial injection in rats was found to be 68%, significantly higher than for methadone or codeine (Oldendorf et al., 1972). Heroin *per se* only persists in brain for a few minutes, however, with higher concentrations of 6-acetylmorphine and substantial amounts of morphine present for up to 30 minutes (Way et al., 1960). Heroin has very little affinity for the opiate receptor in brain tissue, and it is believed that 6-acetylmorphine and morphine account for all or most of the narcotic activity of heroin (Inturrisi et al., 1983). Morphine-6-glucuronide may also contribute to the effects of heroin, especially with chronic usage (Pasternak et al., 1987).

Following intravenous infusion of 70 mg of heroin to volunteers approximately 45% of the dose was recovered as urinary metabolites over a 40 hour period: 4.2% morphine, 38.3% conjugated morphine, 1.3% 6-acetylmorphine and 0.1% unchanged heroin. Unconjugated morphine was excreted primarily in the early hours of the study and very little was found after 12 hours had elapsed. Maximum urine concentrations of total morphine averaged 116 mg/L between 5.6 and 8.6 hours following the start of the 7 hour infusion (Elliot et al., 1971). 6-Acetylmorphine is present in urine in 64–73% of all heroin users studied, averaging approximately 0.8 mg/L and ranging up to 10 mg/L (Fehn and Megges, 1985; Derks et al., 1986). Urinary elimination half-lives averaged 0.6, 4.4 and 7.9 hours for 6-acetylmorphine, morphine and conjugated morphine, respectively, in 6 volunteers given a single 6 mg intramuscular heroin dose (Cone et al., 1991). Normorphine has also been reported as a minor urinary metabolite of heroin (Yeh et al., 1976; Yeh et al., 1977). It should be noted that the small amounts of codeine often found in specimens from heroin overdose victims are the result of codeine being present in heroin as an impurity, and are not due to metabolism.

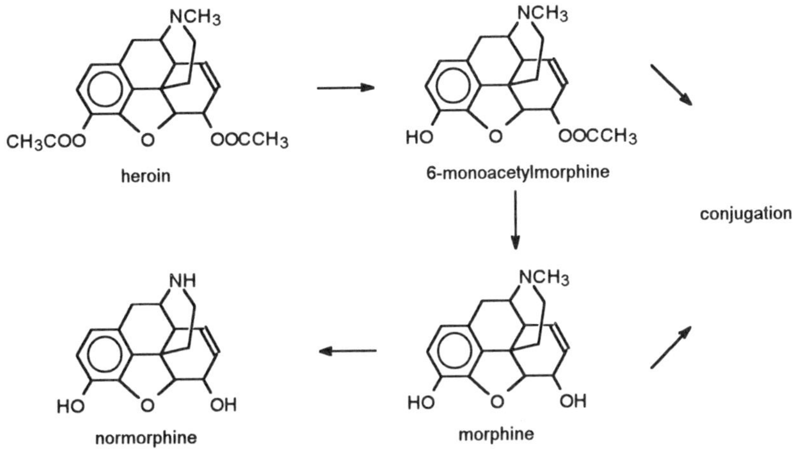

Toxicity. Complications of chronic intravenous heroin usage include liver disease (Edland, 1972; Stimmel et al., 1972; Force and Millar, 1974), pulmonary hypertension (Kurtzman, 1970) and peripheral nerve lesions (Richter et al., 1973). Plasma concentrations of free and total morphine averaged 0.088 and 0.277 mg/L, respectively, in 54 persons treated for acute heroin overdose; the degree of intoxication correlated better with total than with free morphine levels (Gutierrez-Cebollada et al., 1991).

Postmortem fluid and tissue concentrations of morphine in victims of heroin overdosage can vary considerably depending on the prior narcotic history of the subject. Liver, bile, kidney and urine concentrations (usually expressed as total morphine) may be more representative of past exposure to the drug, while blood concentrations (usually expressed as free morphine) are probably the best guide to very recent usage. For instance, a comparison of bile and urine morphine concentration in documented heroin fatalities from San Francisco and Connecticut, in which no other drugs were involved, indicates that the typical San Francisco victim was an established addict, while those in Connecticut were either newcomers to the practice or had returned after a period of withdrawal. The blood concentrations, however, are more nearly comparable and are consistent with the idea that death from heroin injection is the result of true pharmacologic overdosage (Baselt, 1978):

Morphine Concentrations (mg/L) in Heroin Fatalities

	No. of Cases	Blood	Bile	Urine
San Francisco	27			
Average		0.43	32	18
(Range)		(0.05–3.0)	(3.2–119)	(0.7–86)
Connecticut	15			
Average		0.30	4.4	5.1
(Range)		(0.01–1.1)	(0.01–33)	(0.07–15)

Determination of the clinical effects of heroin administration from absolute postmortem blood morphine concentrations may present a problem, though, since concentrations in addicts dying from traumatic causes (gunshot wounds, vehicular accidents) have been shown to equal or exceed those found in actual overdose situations (Baselt et al., 1975). In a limited series of well-investigated cases it has been possible to establish that blood morphine concentrations vary inversely with survival time of victims up to 24 hours (Garriott and Sturner, 1973). Blood concentrations of free morphine and 6-acetylmorphine averaged 0.360 and 0.019 mg/L, respectively, in 8 persons who died within 15 minutes of injecting heroin intravenously, and 0.104 and 0.007 mg/L in 7 persons who lived for several hours after administration (Goldberger et al., 1994). Free morphine in blood averaged 0.78 mg/L (range, 0.05–2.1) and represented 76% of total blood morphine in 42 persons who died rapidly after heroin injection, while free morphine averaged 0.34 mg/L (range, 0.05–0.50) and represented 31% of the total morphine in 8 persons who survived for a period of time (Straub et al., 1990). Blood morphine concentrations as high as 120 mg/L have been reported in fatalities involving heroin body packers (Connet, 1985; Joynt and Mikhael, 1985). Brain morphine concentrations appear to correlate very well with blood concentration in a large number of cases reported by Richards et al. (1976) and thus brain should be considered an indicator of recent heroin usage when blood is not available. Cerebellum/blood morphine concentration ratios were found to average 1.0 when death occurred rapidly (less than 1 hour after administration) and 3.5 when death occurred within 2–48 hours (Spiehler et al., 1978).

Two cases of suicide by heroin were reported in which body distribution studies of total morphine by radioimmunoassay were performed (Reed et al., 1977). This data appears representative of acute heroin overdosage with no recent prior heroin usage:

Morphine Concentrations (mg/L or mg/kg) in Heroin Suicides

	Blood	Brain	Lung	Liver	Kidney	Urine
Case 1	0.41	0.35	0.97	0.66	1.51	0.10
Case 2	0.38	0.25	0.14	0.35	0.70	0.49

Analysis. The quantitative assay of heroin metabolites in biological specimens may be performed by gas chromatography with flame-ionization (Jain et al., 1975; Nakamura and Way, 1975; Yeh and McQuinn, 1975), nitrogen-phosphorus (Lee and Lee, 1991), electron-capture (Yeh, 1973; Wallace et al., 1974; Kogan and Chedekel, 1976; Felby, 1979) or mass spectrometric detection (Wu Chen et al., 1982; Jones et al., 1984; Bowie and Kirkpatrick, 1989; Fuller and Anderson, 1992). In many instances biological specimens are subjected to acid or enzyme hydrolysis before analysis in order to liberate morphine from its conjugated form (Predmore et al., 1978), especially when the specimens represent excretory organs or their products (liver, bile, kidney, urine). Morphine immunoassays have found acceptance in many clinical and forensic laboratories, although it should be noted that most of these exhibit significant cross-reactivity with morphine glucuronide and codeine. Recently, liquid chromatographic techniques have appeared for heroin metabolites, several of which allow the simultaneous determination of conjugated metabolites (Svensson et al., 1982; Umans et al., 1982; Posey and Kimble, 1983; Hepler et al., 1984; Derks et al., 1986; Barrett et al., 1991; Hanisch and Meyer, 1993).

References

G.W. Aherne, E.M. Piall and R.G. Twycross. Serum morphine concentration after oral administration of diamorphine hydrochloride and morphine sulphate. Brit. J. Clin. Pharm. 8: 577–580, 1979.

D.A. Barrett, P.N. Shaw and S.S. Davis. Determination of morphine and 6-acetylmorphine in plasma by high-performance liquid chromatography with fluorescence detection. J. Chrom. 566: 135–145, 1991.

R.C. Baselt, D.J. Allison, J.A. Wright et al. Acute heroin fatalities in San Francisco—demographic and toxicologic characteristics. West. J. Med. 122: 455–458, 1975.

R.C. Baselt. Unpublished results, 1978.

G. Bolelli, S. Lafisca, C. Flamigni et al. Heroin addiction: relationship between the plasma levels of testosterone, dihydrotestosterone, androstenedione, LH, FSH, and the plasma concentration of heroin. Toxicology 15: 19–29, 1979.

L.J. Bowie and P.B. Kirkpatrick. Simultaneous determination of monoacetylmorphine, morphine, codeine and other opiates by GC/MS. J. Anal. Tox. 13: 326–329, 1989.

E.J. Cone, P. Welch, J.M. Mitchell and B.D. Paul. Forensic drug testing for opiates: I. J. Anal. Tox. 15: 1–7, 1991.

E.J. Cone, B.A. Holicky, T.M. Grant et al. Pharmacokinetics and pharmacodynamics of intranasal "snorted" heroin. J. Anal. Tox. 17: 327–337, 1993.

B.E. Connett. A human drug capsule. In *Proceedings of the 21st International Meeting*, International Association of Forensic Toxicologists, Brighton, England, September 13–17, 1985.

H.J.G.M. Derks, K. Van Twillert, D.P.K.H. Pereboom-de Fauw et al. Determination of the heroin metabolite 6-acetylmorphine by high-performance liquid chromatography using automated pre-column derivatization and fluorescence detection. J. Chrom. 370: 173–178, 1986.

J.F. Edland. Liver disease in heroin addicts. Hum. Path. 3: 75–84, 1972.

H.W. Elliot, K.D. Parker, J.A. Wright et al. Actions and metabolism of heroin administered by continuous intravenous infusion to man. Clin. Pharm. Ther. 12: 806–814, 1971.

J. Fehn and G. Megges. Detection of 0_6-monoacetylmorphine in urine samples by GC/MS as evidence for heroin use. J. Anal. Tox. 9: 134–138, 1985.

S. Felby. Morphine: its quantitative determination in nanogram amounts in small samples of whole blood by electron-capture gas chromatography. For. Sci. Int. 13: 145–150, 1979.

E.E. Force and J.W. Millar. Liver disease in fatal narcotism. Arch. Path. 97: 166–170, 1974.

D.C. Fuller and W.H. Anderson. A simplified procedure for the determination of free codeine, free morphine, and 6-acetylmorphine in urine. J. Anal. Tox. 16: 315–318, 1992.

E.R. Garrett and T. Gurkan. Pharmacokinetics of morphine and its surrogates II: methods of separation of stabilized heroin and its metabolites from hydrolyzing biological fluids and applications to protein binding and red blood cell partition studies. J. Pharm. Sci. 68: 26–32, 1979.

E.R. Garrett and T. Gurkan. Pharmacokinetics of morphine and its surrogates IV: pharmacokinetics of heroin and its derived metabolites in dogs. J. Pharm. Sci. 69: 1116–1134, 1980.

J.C. Garriott and W.Q. Sturner. Morphine concentrations and survival periods in acute heroin fatalities. New Eng. J. Med. 289: 1276–1278, 1973.

B.A. Goldberger, E.J. Cone, T.M. Grant et al. Disposition of heroin and its metabolites in heroin-related deaths. J. Anal. Tox. 18: 22–28, 1994.

M.H. Greene, J.L. Luke, R.L. Dupont. Opiate "overdose" deaths in the District of Columbia 1. Heroin related fatalities. Med. Ann. Dist. Col. 43: 175–181, 1974.

J. Gutierrez-Cebollada, J. Cami and R. de la Torre. Heroin intoxication: the relation between plasma morphine concentration and clinical state at admission. Eur. J. Clin. Pharm. 401: 635, 1991.

W. Hanisch and L.V. Meyer. Determination of the heroin metabolite 6-monoacetylmorphine in urine. J. Anal. Tox. 17: 48–50, 1993.

B.R. Hepler, C. Sutheimer, I. Sunshine and G.F. Sebrosky. Combined enzyme immunoassay-LCEC method for the identification, confirmation, and quantitation of opiates in biological fluids. J. Anal. Tox. 8: 78–90, 1984.

C.E. Inturrisi, M. Schultz, S. Shin et al. Evidence from opiate binding studies that heroin acts through its metabolites. Life Sci. 33 (Suppl. 1): 773–776, 1983.

N.C. Jain, T.C. Sneath, R.D. Budd et al. Gas chromatographic/thin-layer chromatographic analysis of acetylated codeine and morphine in urine. Clin. Chem. 21: 1486–1489, 1975.

A.W. Jones, Y. Blom, U. Bondesson and E. Anggard. Determination of morphine in biological samples by gas chromatography-mass spectrometry. J. Chrom. 309: 73–80, 1984.

B.P. Joynt and N.Z. Mikhael. Sudden death of a heroin body packer. J. Anal. Tox. 9: 238–240, 1985.

M.J. Kogan and M.A. Chedekel. Rapid GLC method for the separation of picogram quantities of morphine and codeine. J. Pharm. Pharmac. 28: 261, 1976.

R.S. Kurtzman. Complications of narcotic addiction. Radiology 96: 23–30, 1970.

H.M. Lee and C.W. Lee. Determination of morphine and codeine in blood and bile by gas chromatography with a derivatization procedure. J. Anal. Tox. 15: 182–187, 1991.

G.R. Nakamura, J.I. Thornton and T.T. Noguchi. Kinetics of heroin deacylation in aqueous alkaline solution and in human serum and whole blood. J. Chrom. 110: 81–89, 1975.

G.R. Nakamura and E.L. Way. Determination of morphine and codeine in postmortem specimens. Anal. Chem. 47: 775–778, 1975.

W.H. Oldendorf, S. Hyman, L. Braun et al. Blood-brain barrier: penetration of morphine, codeine, heroin, and methadone after carotid injection. Science 178: 984–986, 1972.

G.W. Pasternak, R.J. Bodnar, J.A. Clark and C.E. Inturrisi. Morhine-6-glucuronide, a potent mu agonist. Life Sci. 41: 2845–2849, 1987.

B.L. Posey and S.N. Kimble. Simultaneous determination of codeine and morphine in urine and blood by HPLC. J. Anal. Tox. 7: 241–245, 1983.

D.B. Predmore, G.D. Christian and T.A. Loomis. Recovery of morphine from biological samples by hydrolysis and solvent extraction. J. For. Sci. 23: 481–489, 1978.

D. Reed, V.R. Spiehler and R.H. Cravey. Two cases of heroin-related suicide. For. Sci. 9: 49–52, 1977.

R.G. Richards, D. Reed and R.H. Cravey. Death from intravenously administered narcotics: a study of 114 cases. J. For. Sci. 21: 467–482, 1976.

R.W. Richter, J. Pearson and B. Bruun. Neurological complications of addiction to heroin. Bull. N.Y. Acad. Med. 49: 3–21, 1973.

V.R. Spiehler, R.H. Cravey, R.G. Richards and H.W. Elliott. The distribution of morphine in the brain in fatal cases due to the intravenous administration of heroin. J. Anal. Tox. 2: 62–67, 1978.

C. Staub, R. Jeanmonod and O. Frye. Morphine in postmortem blood. Int. J. Leg. Med. 104: 39–42, 1990.

B. Stimmell, S. Vernace and H. Tobias. Hepatic dysfunction in heroin addicts. J. Am. Med. Asso. 222: 811–812, 1972.

J.O. Svensson, A. Rane, J. Sawe and F. Sjoquist. Determination of morphine, morphine-3-glucuronide and (tentatively) morphine-6-glucuronide in plasma and urine using ion-pair high-performance liquid chromatography. J. Chrom. 230: 427–432, 1982.

K.H. Tress, A.A. El-Sobky, W. Aherne and E. Piall. Degree of tolerance and the relationship between plasma morphine concentration and pupil diameter following intravenous heroin in man. Brit. J. Clin. Pharm. 5: 299–303, 1978.

J.G. Umans, T.S.K. Chiu, R.A. Lipman et al. Determination of heroin and its metabolites by high-performance liquid chromatography. J. Chrom. 233: 213–225, 1982.

J.E. Wallace, H.E. Hamilton, K. Blaum and C. Petty. Determination of morphine in biological fluids by electron capture gas-liquid chromatography. Anal. Chem. 46: 2107–2110, 1974.

E.L. Way, J.W. Kemp, J.M. Young et al. The pharmacologic effects of heroin in relationship to its rate of biotransformation. J. Pharm. Exp. Ther. 129: 144–154, 1960.

N.B. Wu Chen, M.I. Schaffer, R.I. Lin and R.J. Stein. Simultaneous quantitation of morphine and codeine in biological samples by electron impact mass fragmentography. J. Anal. Tox. 6: 231–234, 1982.

S.Y. Yeh. Separation and identification of morphine and its metabolites and congeners. J. Pharm. Sci. 62: 1827–1829, 1973.

S.Y. Yeh and R.L. McQuinn. GLC determination of heroin and its metabolites in human urine. J. Pharm. Sci. 64: 1237–1239, 1975.

S.Y. Yeh, C.W. Gorodetzky and R.L. McQuinn. Urinary excretion of heroin and its metabolites in man. J. Pharm. Exp. Ther. 196: 249–256, 1976.

S.Y. Yeh, R.L. McQuinn and C.W. Gorodetzky. Identification of diacetylmorphine metabolites in humans. J. Pharm. Sci. 66: 201–204, 1977.

Hexachlorobenzene

T½: 60 days
Vd: ?
Fb: ?

Occurrence and Usage. Hexachlorobenzene (HCB, Bunt-Cure) is used as a fungicide for the control of smut diseases in cereal grains, primarily seed wheat. The chemical is an aromatic benzene derivative, and is not to be confused with benzene hexachloride (lindane, hexachlorocyclohexane), which is actually a cyclohexane derivative. Occupational exposure to HCB occurs during manufacturing, application and transport of chemical wastes. Environmental exposure occurs as a result of dietary intake of contaminated food or water; at one time the feeding of HCB-treated seed grain to livestock or its incorporation into bread was a common practice in certain areas of the world. HCB has no assigned threshold limit value.

Blood Concentrations. Hexachlorobenzene concentrations in the whole blood of German children were found to range from 2.6–78 µg/L in 1975 (Richter and Schmid, 1976). In New Zealand adults with no known occupational exposure, these values ranged from 0–95 µg/L and averaged 22 µg/L, whereas a group of occupationally exposed but asymptomatic subjects showed whole blood values of 0–410 µg/L with an average of 56 µg/L (Siyali, 1972). Some otherwise unexposed United States citizens living near a chemical factory had background plasma HCB concentrations of 0–1.8 µg/L (average, 0.5) (Burns and Miller, 1975), while a group of vegetable spraymen using an HCB-contaminated herbicide developed plasma HCB levels that averaged 40 µg/L and ranged from 0–310 µg/L (Burns et al., 1974). A group of chemical workers in the U.S. had blood concentrations that decreased on average from 311 to 170 µg/L over the period 1974–1977 due to improved industrial hygiene practices; individual blood concentrations were related to the duration of exposure (Currier et al., 1980).

Metabolism and Excretion. Very little information regarding the disposition of HCB in humans is available. It is known to be stored in body fat, and has been found in amounts from a trace to 8.2 mg/kg (average, 1.3) in the fat of residents of Australia, where the feeding of HCB-contaminated grain to livestock was once practiced (Brady and Siyali, 1972). The half-life of HCB in adipose tissue of sheep is approximately 16 weeks (Avrahami, 1972).

In rats, about 7% of a single dose is eliminated in urine and 27% in feces as metabolites over a 4 week period. Known metabolites include pentachlorophenol, pentachlorobenzene, tetrachlorohydroquinone, tetrachlorophenol, and trichlorophenol (Courtney, 1979).

Toxicity. Several eposides of mass poisoning have occurred due to the chronic ingestion of HCB-contaminated food, with an estimated daily intake of 50–200 mg of the compound continuing for some months before the onset of symptoms. The primary toxic effect is cutaneous porphyria, involving blistering and epidermolysis of the face and hands (Schmid, 1960; De Matteis et al., 1961; Cam and Nigogosyan, 1963). Peters (1976) reported on the successful treatment of this condition with sodium calcium EDTA. A chemical worker in Argentina with cutaneous lesions of the hands and face and increased urinary porphyrins had a hexachlorobenzene blood level of 383 µg/L; one year later, after leaving his job, the blood level had declined to 268 µg/L and the lesions had cleared (Courtney, 1979).

Analysis. Hexachlorobenzene may be determined in biological specimens by the general procedure for chlorinated hydrocarbon pesticides cited in the section on aldrin. HCB elutes in this electron-capture gas chromatographic assay at about the same retention time as alpha-benzene hexachloride, which has not been detected in blood specimens and is only infrequently encountered in fat. A special procedure for HCB in fat, with a confirmation step, has been described (Watts et al., 1980) and gas chromatography-mass spectrometry has also been utilized (Yost et al., 1984).

References

M. Avrahami. Hexachlorobenzene. New Zealand J. Agr. Res. 15: 476–481, 1972.

M.N. Brady and D.S. Siyali. Hexachlorobenzene in human body fat. Med. J. Aust. 1: 158–161, 1972.

J.E. Burns, F.M. Miller, E.D. Gomes and R.A. Albert. Hexachlorobenzene exposure from contaminated DCPA in vegetable spraymen. Arch. Env. Health 29: 192–194, 1974.

J.E. Burns and F.M. Miller. Hexachlorobenzene contamination: its effects in a Louisiana population. Arch. Env. Health 30: 44–48, 1975.

C. Cam and G. Nigogosyan. Acquired toxic porphyria cutanea tarda due to hexachlorobenzene. J. Am. Med. Asso. 183: 90–93, 1963.

K.D. Courtney. Hexachlorobenzene (HCB): a review. Env. Res. 20: 225–266, 1979.

M.F. Currier, C.D. McClimans and G. Barna-Lloyd. Hexachlorobenzene blood levels and the health status of men employed in the manufacture of chlorinated solvents. J. Tox. Env. Health 6: 367–377, 1980.

F. De Matteis, B.E. Prior and C. Rimington. Nervous and biochemical disturbances following hexachlorobenzene intoxication. Nature 191: 363–366, 1961.

H.A. Peters. Hexachlorobenzene poisoning in Turkey. Fed. Proc. 35: 2400–2403, 1976.

E. Richter and A. Schmid. Hexachlorbenzolgehalt im Vollblut von Kindern. Arch. Tox. 35: 141–147, 1976.

R. Schmid. Cutaneous porphyria in Turkey. New Eng. J. Med. 263: 397–398, 1960.

D.S. Siyali. Hexachlorobenzene and other organochloride pesticides in human blood. Med. J. Aust. 2: 1063–1066, 1972.

R.R. Watts, D.W. Hodgson, H.L. Crist and R.F. Moseman. Improved method for hexachlorobenzene and mirex determination with hexachlorobenzene confirmation in adipose tissue: collaborative study. J. Asso. Off. Anal. Chem. 63: 1128–1134, 1980.

R.A. Yost, D.D. Fetterholf, J.R. Hass et al. Comparison of mass spectrometric methods for trace level screening of hexachlorobenzene and trichlorophenol in human blood serum and urine. Anal. Chem. 56: 2223–2228, 1984.

Hexachlorophene

T½: 24 hr
Vd: ?
Fb: ?
pKa: ?

Occurrence and Usage. Hexachlorophene (hexachlorophane, pHisoHex) is an antibacterial agent that was first synthesized in 1939 and has been used extensively in various commercial hygienic products. It has been found in concentrations of up to 0.2% in cosmetics, up to 0.5% in mouthwashes and up to 3% in soaps and antiseptic solutions. Many of these products have been withdrawn from the United States market due to accumulation of the agent in users. Hexachlorophene does not have an assigned threshold limit value. Occupational exposure may be via dermal absorption, inhalation or ingestion.

Blood Concentrations. Blood concentrations of hexachlorophene in 50 infants averaged 0.022 mg/L (range, 0.003–0.182) at birth and 0.109 mg/L (range, 0.009–0.646) upon discharge from the hospital, after 1–11 days of daily washing with diluted 3% hexachlorophene solution. The baseline blood levels of hexachlorophene in normal adults averaged 0.028 mg/L (range, 0–0.089) (Curley et al., 1971). Adults who used mouthwash containing 0.5% hexachlorophene once daily for 3 weeks developed blood concentrations that averaged 0.06 mg/L; those who performed whole body washings once daily for 3–6 weeks with a 3% soap attained concentrations that averaged 0.24 mg/L (range, 0.10–0.38) (Ulsamer et al., 1973). Other workers have reported mean blood values as high as 0.655 mg/L after similar whole body washing by adults (Calesnick et al., 1975). The use of hexachlorophene as a vaginal disinfectant during labor produced serum levels as high as 0.942 mg/L in the mothers and 0.617 mg/L in the neonates (Strickland et al., 1983).

Metabolism and Excretion. The disposition of hexachlorophene in man has not been studied. A brief report indicated that up to 10% of a single oral 20 mg/kg dose is eliminated in the urine over a 4–5 day period (Chung et al., 1963). Concentrations of the chemical in human milk have been found to range from trace amounts to 0.009 mg/L (West et al., 1975) and in adult adipose tissue, from 0.00–0.05 mg/kg (Ulsamer et al., 1973). In rats, 74% of a dose is excreted in feces and 5% in urine over a 7 day period, largely as a glucuronide conjugate (Black et al., 1974).

Toxicity. Repeated exposure of newborns to high concentrations of hexachlorophene is associated with vacuolar encephalopathy of the brainstem reticular formation (Shuman et al., 1974). Premature infants and patients with burned or abraded skin are highly susceptible to dermal use of the compound. An increased incidence of congenital malformations has been observed in neonates born to mothers who used hexachlorophene-containing soaps (Halling, 1979).

Levels of 24–74 mg/L have been observed in the serum of 5 adult burn patients whose wounds were washed with 3% hexachlorophene; 3 of these patients exhibited symptoms of toxicity such as diplopia, irritability, vomiting and seizures, and 2 were asymptomatic (Larson, 1968). Two infants who survived the ingestion of large amounts of the chemical developed maximal plasma concentrations of 40 and 88 mg/L (Boehm and Czaja, 1979; Herskowitz and Rosman, 1979).

A 10 year old boy with first and second degree burns was given multiple daily baths with hexachlorophene for 2 weeks and developed seizures, irrational behavior and coma; he died after attaining a blood concentration of 2.2 mg/L (Plueckhahn, 1973). Serum hexachlorophene concentrations of 3 and 16 mg/L were observed several days after hospital admission in children who died after cutaneous exposure to talc contaminated with 6% hexachlorophene (Goutieres and Aicardi, 1977). A number of fatalities have occurred after accidental ingestion of this chemical, with a blood hexachlorophene concentration of 35 mg/L being observed in one adult at autopsy and a blood level of 40 mg/L in a child several days prior to death (Wear et al., 1962; Lustig, 1963; Pilapil, 1966; DiMaio et al., 1973; Martinez et al., 1974). The acutely lethal dose in humans has been estimated at 250 mg/kg (17.5 g/70 kg) (Kimbrough, 1971).

Analysis. Hexachlorophene is usually analyzed in blood or plasma by electron-capture gas chromatography of a silyl (Porcaro et al., 1969), methyl (Ferry and McQueen, 1973) or acetyl derivative (Pleuckhahn, 1973; Calesnick et al., 1975; Dodson et al., 1977).

References

J.G. Black, W.E. Sprott, D. Howes and T. Rutherford. Percutaneous absorption of hexachlorophene. Toxicology 2: 127–139, 1974.

R.M. Boehm, Jr. and P.A. Czaja. Hexachlorophene poisoning and the ineffectiveness of peritoneal dialysis. Clin. Tox. 14: 257–262, 1979.

B. Calesnick, C.H. Costello, J.P. Ryan and C.G. DiGregorio. Percutaneous absorption of hexachlorophene following daily body washings. Tox. Appl. Pharm. 32: 204–211, 1975.

H. Chung, W. Ts'ao, H. Hsu et al. Hexachlorophene (G-11) as a new specific drug against *Clonorchiasis sinensis*. Chin. Med. J. 82: 691–701, 1963.

A. Curley, R.E. Hawk, R.D. Kimbrough et al. Dermal absorption of hexachlorophene in infants. Lancet 2: 296–297, 1971.

V.J.M. DiMaio, F.G. Mullick and L.D. Henry. Hexachlorophene poisoning. J. For. Sci. 18: 303–308, 1973.

W.E. Dodson, E.E. Tyrala and R.E. Hillman. Micromethod for measuring hexachlorophene in whole blood by gas-liquid chromatography. Clin. Chem. 23: 944–947, 1977.

D.G. Ferry and E.G. McQueen. Hexachlorophene analysis in blood by electron capture gas chromatography. J. Chrom. 76: 233–235, 1973.

F. Goutieres and J. Aicardi. Accidental percutaneous hexachlorophane intoxication in children. Brit. Med. J. 2: 663–665, 1977.

H. Halling. Suspected link between exposure to hexachlorophene and malformed infants. Ann. N.Y. Acad. Sci. 320: 426–435, 1979.

J. Herskowitz and N.P. Rosman. Acute hexachlorophene poisoning by mouth in neonate. J. Pediat. 94: 495–496, 1979.

R.D. Kimbrough. Review of the toxicity of hexachlorophene. Arch. Env. Health 23: 119–122, 1971.

D.L. Larson. Studies show hexachlorophene causes burn syndrome. Hospitals 42 (Dec.): 63–64, 1968.

F.W. Lustig. A fatal case of hexachlorophane ("pHisoHex") poisoning. Med. J. Aust. 1: 737, 1963.

A.J. Martinez, R. Boehm and M.G. Hadfield. Acute hexachlorophene encephalopathy: clinico-neuropathological correlation. Acta Neuropath. 28: 93–103, 1974.

V.R. Pilapil. Hexachlorophene toxicity in an infant. Am. J. Dis. Child. 111: 333–336, 1966.

V.D. Plueckhahn. Infant antiseptic skin care and hexachlorophene. Med. J. Aust. 1: 93–100, 1973.

P.J. Porcaro, P. Shubiak and M. Manowitz. Determination of hexachlorophene in whole blood. J. Pharm. Sci. 58: 251–252, 1969.

R.M. Shuman, R.W. Leech and E.C. Alvord, Jr. Neurotoxicity of hexachlorophene in the human: I. A clinicopathologic study of 248 children. Pediatrics 54: 689–695, 1974.

D.M. Strickland, R.G Leonard, S. Stavchansky et al. Vaginal absorption of hexachlorophene during labor. Am. J. Obs. Gyn. 147: 769–772, 1983.

A.G. Ulsamer, F.N. Marzulli and R.W. Coen. Hexachlorophene concentrations in blood associated with the use of products containing hexachlorophene. Food Cos. Tox. 11: 625–633, 1973.

J.B. Wear, Jr., R. Shanahan and R.K. Ratliff. Toxicity of ingested hexachlorophene. J. Am. Med. Asso. 181: 587–589, 1962.

R.W. West, D.J. Wilson and W. Schaffner. Hexachlorophene concentrations in human milk. Bull. Env. Cont. Tox. 13: 167–169, 1975.

Hexane

T½: 1.5–2.0 hr

Vd: ? $CH_3CH_2CH_2CH_2CH_2CH_3$

Fb: ?

Occurrence and Usage. Hexane (n-hexane) is widely used as a solvent in numerous industries. Technical grades contain only about 40% n-hexane, together with various amounts of isomers and related compounds such as 2-methylpentane, 3-methylpentane, 2,3-dimethylbutane, and cyclohexane. The current threshold limit value for industrial exposure is 50 ppm (176 mg/m³).

Blood Concentrations. Hexane concentrations averaged 0.6 µg/L (range, 0.02–7.7) in the blood of 90 unexposed adults (Brugnone et al., 1991). Blood hexane concentrations averaged 207 and 368 µg/L in volunteers exposed to air concentrations of 100 and 200 ppm, respectively, for 3.3 hours; the blood levels fell relatively rapidly after the end of exposure, declining with a half-life of 1.5–2.0 hours (Veulemans et al., 1982). Workers in a leather factory exhibited blood hexane concentrations that averaged 376 µg/L and ranged from 105–833 µg/L; the blood levels were highly correlated with environmental hexane concentrations, which ranged from 43–396 ppm (Brugnone et al., 1978).

Metabolism and Excretion. Approximately 20% of an absorbed dose of hexane is exhaled unchanged in the expired air (Filser et al., 1987). A small percentage of an absorbed dose of hexane is excreted in the urine as products of metabolic oxidation. 2-Hexanol (as a glucuronide), 2,5-hexanedione, 2,5-dimethylfuran, and gamma-valerolactone have been identified as urinary metabolites of n-hexane, while 2-methyl-2-pentanol and 3-methyl-2-pentanol are metabolites of 2-methylpentane and 3-methylpentane, respectively, components of technical hexane (Perbellini et al., 1980). Hexane itself was present in urine at an average of 6 µg/L for workers exposed to an average air hexane level of 69 mg/m³ for 4 hours; hexane was not present in urine collected prior to beginning work (Imbriani et al., 1984). However, hexane was found in 50 out of 64 urine specimens from unexposed persons at an average concentration of 1.4 µg/L (Brugnone et al., 1991).

In the urine of workers exposed to an average n-hexane air concentration of 182 mg/m³ for a normal working day, concentrations averaged 5.4 mg/L (range, 0.4–22) for 2,5-hexanedione, 3.7 mg/L for 2,5-dimethylfuran, 3.3 mg/L for gamma-valerolactone, and 0.2 mg/L (range, 0.1–1.2) for 2-hexanol. Concentrations of 2-hexanol and 2,5-hexanedione correlated best with atmospheric n-hexane concentrations (Perbellini et al., 1981a). Iwata et al. (1983) failed to find 2-hexanol in workers' urine, although the air concentrations of hexane studied (average, 16 ppm) were substantially lower than those employed by Perbellini. 2,.5-Hexanedione is excreted in the urine with a half-life of 13–14 hours; hexane tends to accumulate in fat with repeated exposure and its concentration in fat declines with an average half-life of 64 hours (Perbellini et al., 1986). Fedtke and Bolt (1987) observed that approximately 80% of the 2,5-hexanedione reported in human urine originates as 4,5-dihydroxy-2-hexanone and is converted to the former substance by the acid hydrolysis procedures routinely used to hydrolyze conjugated metabolites.

$CH_3CH_2CH_2CH_2CH_2CH_3$ → $CH_3CHCH_2CH_2CH_2CH_3$ → $CH_3CCH_2CH_2CCH_3$

hexane   2-hexanol   2,5-hexanedione

2,5-dimethylfuran   γ-valerolactone

Toxicity. Acute exposure to hexane causes central nervous system depression. Chronic exposure to an average air concentration of 450–650 ppm for as little as 2 months may result in peripheral neuropathy, characterized by muscular weakness, loss of sensation, and impaired gait (Herskowitz et al., 1971; Ruff et al., 1981; Scelsi et al., 1981). 2,5-Hexanedione, a major metabolite of n-hexane, is believed to be primarily responsible for the neurotoxic effects. This compound is also a metabolite of methyl-n-butyl ketone (Krasavage et al., 1980).

Analysis. Hexane may be assayed in blood by headspace flame-ionization gas chromatography (Brugnone et al., 1978). The urinary metabolites of hexane and its isomers have been measured by flame-ionization gas chromatography with acid hydrolysis (Perbellini et al., 1981b; Perbellini et al., 1990; Saito et al., 1991) or without acid hydrolysis (Kawai et al., 1990; Vohra and Gaind, 1992).

References

F. Brugnone, L. Perbellini, L. Grigolini and P. Apostoli. Solvent exposure in a shoe upper factory. Int. Arch. Occ. Env. Health 42: 51–62, 1978.

F. Brugnone, G. Maranelli, L. Romeo et al. Ubiquitous pollution by n-hexane and reference biological levels in the general population. Int. Arch. Occ. Env. Health 63: 157–160, 1991.

N. Fedtke and H.M. Bolt. The relevance of 4,5-dihydroxy-2-hexanone in the excretion kinetics of n-hexane metabolites in rat or man. Arch. Tox. 61: 131–137, 1987.

J.G. Filser, H. Peter, H.M. Bolt and N. Fedtke. Pharmacokinetics of the neurotoxin n-hexane in rat and man. Arch. Tox. 60: 77–80, 1987.

A. Herskowitz, N. Ishh and H. Schaumburg. n-Hexane neuropathy. New Eng. J. Med. 285: 82–85, 1971.

M. Imbriani, S. Ghittori, G. Pezzagno and E. Capodaglio. n-Hexane urine elimination and weighted exposure concentration. Int. Arch. Occ. Env. Health 55: 33–41, 1984.

M. Iwata, Y. Takeuchi, N. Hisanaga and Y. Ono. A study on biological monitoring of n-hexane exposure. Int. Arch. Occ. Env. Health 51: 253–260, 1983.

T. Kawai, K. Mizunuma, T. Yasugi et al. The method of choice for the determination of 2,5-hexanedione as an indicator of occupational exposure to hexane. Int. Arch. Occ. Env. Health 62: 403–408, 1990.

W.J. Krasavage, J.L. O'Donoghue, G.D. DiVincenzo and C.J. Terhaar. The relative neurotoxicity of methyl-n-butyl ketone, n-hexane and their metabolites. Tox. Appl. Pharm. 52: 433–441, 1980.

L. Perbellini, F. Brugnone and I. Pavan. Identification of the metabolites of n-hexane, cyclohexane, and their isomers in men's urine. Tox. Appl. Pharm. 53: 220–229, 1980.

L. Perbellini, F. Brugnone and G. Faggionato. Urinary excretion of the metabolites of n-hexane and its isomers during occupational exposure. Brit. J. Ind. Med. 38: 20–26, 1981a.

L. Perbellini, F. Brugnone, R. Silvestri and E. Gaffuri. Measurement of the urinary metabolites of n-hexane, cyclohexane and their isomers by gas chromatography. Int. Arch. Occ. Env. Health 48: 99–106, 1981b.

L. Perbellini, P. Mozzo, F. Brugnone and A. Zedde. Physiologicomathematical model for studying human exposure to organic solvents. Brit. J. Ind. Med. 43: 760–768, 1986.

L. Perbellini, D.M. Amoros, A.C. Llorens et al. An improved method of analysing 2,5-hexanedione in urine. Brit. J. Ind. Med. 47: 421–424, 1990.

R.L. Ruff, C.K. Petito and L.S. Acheson. Neuropathy associated with chronic low level exposure to n-hexane. Clin. Tox. 18: 515–519, 1981.

I. Saito, E. Shibata, J. Huang et al. Determination of urinary 2,5-hexanedione concentration by an improved analytical method as an index of exposure to n-hexane. Brit. J. Ind. Med. 48: 568–574, 1991.

R. Scelsi, P. Poggi, L. Fera and G. Gonella. Industrial neuropathy due to n-hexane. Clin. Tox. 18: 1387–1393, 1981.

H. Veulemans, E. Van Vlem, H. Janssens et al. Experimental human exposure to n-hexane. Int. Arch. Occ. Env. Health 49: 251–263, 1982.

K. Vohra and V.S. Gaind. Gas chromatographic determination of 2,5-hexanedione in urine as an indicator of exposure to n-hexane. J. Anal. Tox. 16: 176–178, 1992.

Hydralazine

T½: 2–8 hr
Vd: 1.6 L/kg
Fb: 0.90
pKa: 7.1

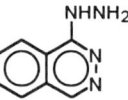

Occurrence and Usage. The synthesis and the pharmacological effects of hydralazine (1-hydrazinophthalazine, Apresoline) were first reported in 1950. The compound is a peripherally-acting vasodilator used in the treatment of essential hypertension. It is available as the hydrochloride salt and may be administered by intravenous or intramuscular injection of 20–40 mg or orally in daily doses of 40–300 mg. Oral dosage forms often contain hydrochlorothiazide and/or reserpine.

Blood Concentrations. A single oral 50 mg dose resulted in a maximal plasma concentration of 0.27 mg/L at 0.5 hours, which declined to 0.12 mg/L by 3 hours (Jack et al., 1975). An average peak plasma level of 0.91 mg/L was observed in 3 subjects at 1 hour postadministration of 100 mg of the drug by mouth; intramuscular administration of 20 mg to 3 subjects produced peak plasma concentrations of 0.16–0.61 mg/L within 1 hour. After oral administration of labeled hydralazine, only about 40% of the plasma radioactivity was unchanged drug; estimates of the plasma half-life have ranged from 2–8 hours in different subjects (Zak et al., 1974a). During chronic oral therapy with 1.5 mg/kg (105 mg/70 kg) of hydralazine, plasma concentrations measured 1–2 hours after the last dose averaged 0.3 mg/L in fast acetylators and 0.5 mg/L in slow acetylators (Zacest and Koch-Weser, 1972). No statistical difference in the elimination half-life for the drug has been noted between fast and slow acetylators (Reece et al., 1980a; Shepherd et al., 1980).

Metabolism and Excretion. Hydralazine is metabolized in man by oxidation to phthalazinone (PZ) and by N-acetylation. The N-acetyl metabolite rearranges to 3-methyltriazolophthalazine (MTP) or is oxidized to acetylhydrazinophthalazinone (AHP). MTP is subsequently hydroxylated to 3-hydroxy-MTP and 9-hydroxy-MTP, which are conjugated or, in the case of 3-hydroxy-MTP, further metabolized to triazolophthalazine (TP). MTP is known to be highly protein bound and may accumulate in plasma (Israili and Dayton, 1977). Hydralazine pyruvate hydrazone (HPH), a conjugate with pyruvic acid, is the major plasma metabolite (Reece et al., 1980a). Hydrazine, present at trace levels in the plasma of some patients receiving hydralazine, may be a chemical degradation product (Blair et al., 1985).

Up to 81% of a dose is excreted in the 72 hour urine and 12% in the feces (Zak et al., 1974a). The urinary excretion products include unchanged drug (7%), PZ (2%), MTP (6–9%), AHP (15%), TP (2%), HPH (4%), conjugated 3-hydroxy-MTP (45%), and conjugated 9-hydroxy-MTP (7%) (Zak et al., 1974b; Wagner et al., 1977). Hydralazine is known to degrade rapidly upon standing in serum (Talseth, 1976a; Reece et al., 1980b) or urine (Talseth, 1976b).

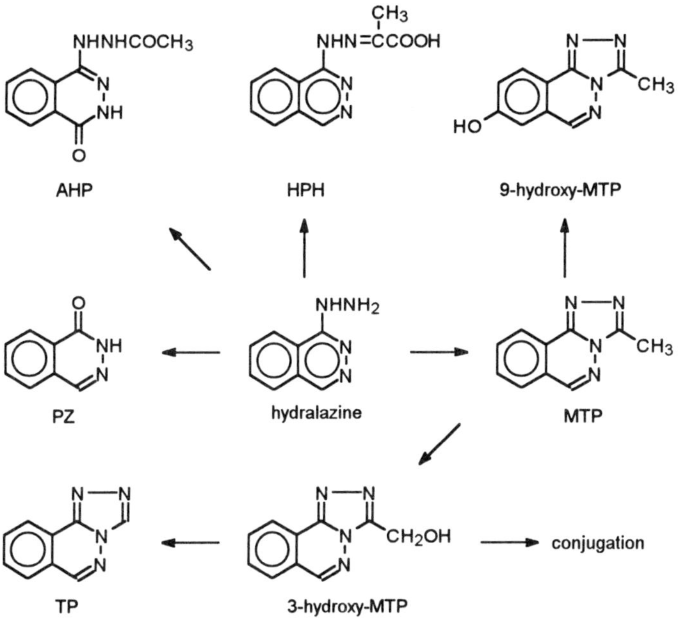

Toxicity. Of 371 patients treated with hydralazine for hypertension, 44 developed moderate to serious toxic reactions to the drug. The signs and symptoms of toxicity included mild to severe joint pain simulating rheumatoid arthritis, malaise, chest pain, loss of sensation, weakness, fever, hepatomegaly, splenomegaly, adenopathy, skin rash typical of lupus erythematosus, and anemia. All symptoms of toxicity disappeared within 6 months of discontinuance of hydralazine except hyperglobulinemia, which persisted in 2 patients for up to 30 months, and antinuclear antibodies (ANA), which were found consistently up to 10 years after drug withdrawal. It was concluded that hydralazine toxicity results from a combination of drug hypersensitivity and drug-induced lupus erythematosus (Perry, 1973).

A 72 year old woman died of massive intestinal bleeding after 2 years of hydralazine therapy at a dose of 100 mg per day. Autopsy revealed fibrinoid degeneration and a proliferative necrotizing process affecting all blood vessels, consistent with disseminated lupus erythematosus (Bendersky and Ramirez, 1960).

Analysis. Direct solvent extraction of hydralazine from biologic specimens has not been successful due to the instability of the compound under alkaline conditions, and thus methods for its determination have relied on derivatization prior to extraction. Colorimetric procedures have involved condensation with p-hydroxybenzaldehyde (Schulert, 1961) or p-methoxybenzaldehyde (Zak et al., 1974a); the latter method has proven relatively specific for the unchanged drug (Zak et al., 1977). Gas chromatographic procedures have involved electron-capture detection (Jack et al., 1975) or nitrogen-phosphorus detection (Degen, 1979; Angelo et al., 1980) of the derivatized drug. Hydralazine and several of its metabolites may be analyzed by liquid chromatography (Ludden et al., 1979; Proveaux et al., 1979; Reece et al., 1980b; Ludden et al., 1983).

References

H.R. Angelo, J.M. Christensen, M. Christensen and A. McNair. Gas chromatographic method for the simultaneous determination of hydralazine and its acetylated metabolite in serum using a nitrogen-selective detector. J. Chrom. 183: 159–166, 1980.

G. Bendersky and C. Ramirez. Hydralazine poisoning. J. Am. Med. Asso. 173: 1789–1794, 1960.

I.A. Blair, R.M. Tinoco, M.J. Brodie et al. Plasma hydrazine concentrations in man after isoniazid and hydralazine administration. Hum. Tox. 4: 195–202, 1985.

P.H. Degen. Determination of unchanged hydralazine in plasma by gas-liquid chromatography using nitrogen-specific detection. J. Chrom. 176: 375–380, 1979.

Z.H. Israili and P.G. Dayton. Metabolism of hydralazine. Drug Met. Rev. 6: 283–305, 1977.

D.B. Jack, S. Brechbuehler, P.H. Degen et al. The determination of hydralazine in plasma by gas-liquid chromatography. J. Chrom. 115: 87–92, 1975.

T.M. Ludden, L.K. Goggin, J.L. McNay, Jr. et al. High-pressure liquid chromatographic assay for hydralazine in human plasma. J. Pharm. Sci. 68: 1423–1425, 1979.

T.M. Ludden, L.K. Ludden, K.E. Wade and S.R.B. Allerheiligen. Determination of hydralazine in human whole blood. J. Pharm. Sci. 72: 693–695, 1983.

H.M. Perry, Jr. Late toxicity to hydralazine resembling systemic lupus erythematosus or rheumatoid arthritis. Am. J. Med. 54: 58–72, 1973.

W.J. Proveaux, J.P. O'Donnell and J.K.M. Ma. Liquid chromatographic analysis of hydralazine and metabolites in plasma. J. Chrom. 176: 480–484, 1979.

P.A. Reece, I. Cozamanis and R. Zacest. Kinetics of hydralazine and its main metabolites in slow and fast acetylators. Clin. Pharm. Ther. 28: 769–778, 1980a.

P.A. Reece, I. Cozamanis and R. Zacest. Selective high-performance liquid chromatographic assays for hydralazine and its metabolites in plasma of man. J. Chrom. 181: 427–440, 1980b.

A.R. Schulert. Physiological disposition of hydralazine (1-hydrazinophthalazine) and a method for its determination in biological fluids. Arch. Int. Pharm. Ther. 132: 1–15, 1961.

A.M.M. Shepherd, T.M. Ludden, J.L. McNay and M.S. Lin. Hydralazine kinetics after single and repeated oral doses. Clin. Pharm. Ther. 28: 804–811, 1980.

T. Talseth. Studies on hydralazine. I. Serum concentrations of hydralazine in man after a single dose and at steady-state. Eur. J. Clin. Pharm. 10: 183–187, 1976a.

T. Talseth. Studies on hydralazine. II. Elimination rate and steady-state concentration in patients with impaired renal function. Eur. J. Clin. Pharm. 10: 311–317, 1976b.

J. Wagner, J.W. Faigle, P. Imhof and G. Liehr. Metabolism of hydralazine in man. Arz. Forsch. 27: 2388–2395, 1977.

R. Zacest and J. Koch-Weser. Relation of hydralazine plasma concentration to dosage and hypotension action. Clin. Pharm. Ther. 13: 420–425, 1972.

S.B. Zak, M.F. Bartlett, W.E. Wagner et al. Disposition of hydralazine in man and a specific method for its determination in biological fluids. J. Pharm. Sci. 63: 225–229, 1974a.

S. Zak, T.G. Gilleran, J. Karliner and G. Lukas. Identification of two new metabolites of hydralazine from human urine. J. Med. Chem. 17: 381–382, 1974b.

S.B. Zak, G. Lukas and T.G. Gilleran. Plasma levels of real and "apparent" hydralazine in man and rat. Drug Met. Disp. 5: 116–121, 1977.

Hydrochlorothiazide

T½: 6–15 hr
Vd: 3 L/kg
Fb: 0.40
pKa: 7.9, 9.2

Occurrence and Usage. Hydrochlorothiazide (Hydrodiuril) is a thiazide derivative used as a diuretic and antihypertensive agent since 1957. It is a weakly acidic substance and a close structural analogue of the less potent chlorothiazide. The drug is available in 25–100 mg tablets, often in combination with other diuretics or antihypertensive drugs. Daily oral doses range from 25–200 mg in adults.

Blood Concentrations. Plasma concentrations of hydrochlorothiazide in 8 volunteers reached average peak levels of 0.142, 0.260, and 0.376 mg/L within 1.5–5 hours of oral doses of 25, 50 or 75 mg, respectively. There was a biphasic decline in plasma levels, with the terminal elimination half-life averaging 9.5 hours and ranging from 6–15 hours (Beermann and Groschinsky-Grind, 1977). Plasma concentrations in patients on chronic daily oral therapy with 25 or 75 mg of the drug averaged 0.017 and 0.034 mg/L, respectively, just prior to the next dose and 0.076 and 0.202 mg/L at 5 hours after the dose. No correlation was evident between plasma hydrochlorothiazide concentration and blood pressure (Beermann and Groschinsky-Grind, 1978). The erythrocyte/plasma concentration ratio for the drug averages 3.5 (Beermann et al., 1976).

Metabolism and Excretion. From 65–72% of an oral dose of hydrochlorothiazide is excreted unchanged in the urine within 48 hours. The drug is not known to be metabolized in man, and up to 95% of a dose is eventually eliminated by the kidneys. The oral bioavailability is about 65% on an empty stomach and is increased to 75% when taken with a meal (Beermann and Groschinsky-Grind, 1980).

Toxicity. Adverse reactions to hydrochlorothiazide include nausea, vomiting, dizziness, headache, hematologic disorders, hypotension, weakness, and various hypersensitivity manifestations. The drug may cause azotemia in patients with renal disease, and all persons receiving it should be monitored for possible fluid or electrolyte depletion.

Analysis. Hydrochlorothiazide may be assayed in urine by a somewhat nonspecific colorimetric method (Sheppard et al., 1960; Suria, 1978). Gas chromatographic methods for its determination in plasma have utilized electron-capture detection of a methyl derivative (Lindstrom et al., 1975; Vandenheuvel et al., 1975; Redalieu et al., 1978). Liquid chromatographic procedures have appeared that are applicable to both plasma and urine (Robinson and Cosyns, 1978; Soldin et al., 1979; Henion and Maylin, 1980; Tisdall et al., 1980; Barbhaiya et al., 1981; Koopmans et al., 1984; Alton et al., 1986).

References

K.B. Alton, D. Desrivieres and J.E. Patrick. High-performance liquid chromatographic assay for hydrochlorothiazide in human urine. J. Chrom. 374: 103–110, 1986.

R.H. Barbhaiya, T.A. Phillips and P.G. Welling. High-pressure liquid chromatographic determination of chlorothiazide and hydrochlorothiazide in plasma and urine: preliminary results of clinical studies. J. Pharm. Sci. 70: 291–295, 1981.

B. Beermann, M. Groschinsky-Grind and A. Rosen. Absorption, metabolism, and excretion of hydrochlorothiazide. Clin. Pharm. Ther. 19: 531–537, 1976.

B. Beermann and M. Groschinsky-Grind. Pharmacokinetics of hydrochlorothiazide in man. Eur. J. Clin. Pharm. 12: 297–303, 1977.

B. Beermann and M. Groschinsky-Grind. Antihypertensive effect of various doses of hydrochlorothiazide and its relation to the plasma level of the drug. Eur. J. Clin. Pharm. 13: 195–201, 1978.

B. Beermann and M. Groschinsky-Grind. Clinical pharmacokinetics of diuretics. Clin. Pharmacokin. 5: 221–245, 1980.

J.D. Henion and G.A. Maylin. Qualitative and quantitative analysis of hydrochlorothiazide in equine plasma and urine by high-performance liquid chromatography. J. Anal. Tox. 4: 185–191, 1980.

P.P. Koopmans, Y. Tan, C.A.M. Van Ginneken and F.W.J. Gribnau. High-performance liquid chromatographic determination of hydrochlorothiazide in plasma and urine. J. Chrom. 307: 445–450, 1984.

B. Lindstrom, M. Molander and M. Groschinsky-Grind. Gas chromatographic determination of hydrochlorothiazide in plasma, blood corpuscles and urine using extractive alkylation technique. J. Chrom. 114: 459–462, 1975.

E. Redalieu, V.V. Tipnis and W.E. Wagner, Jr. Determination of plasma hydrochlorothiazide levels in humans. J. Pharm. Sci. 67: 726–728, 1978.

W.T. Robinson and L. Cosyns. A sensitive method for the determination of hydrochlorothiazide in serum by high pressure liquid chromatography. Clin. Biochem. 11: 172–174, 1978.

H. Sheppard, T.F. Mowles and A.J. Plummer. Determination of hydrochlorothiazide in urine. J. Am. Pharm. Asso. Sci. Ed. 49: 722–723, 1960.

S.J. Soldin, E. Hach, A. Pollard and A.G. Logan. High performance liquid chromatographic analysis of hydrochlorothiazide in serum and urine. Ther. Drug Mon. 1: 399–408, 1979.

D. Suria. Quantitative determination of thiazides in urine by a sensitive colorimetric method. Clin. Biochem. 11: 222–224, 1978.

P.A. Tisdall, T.P. Moyer and J.P. Anhalt. Liquid-chromatographic detection of thiazide diuretics in urine. Clin. Chem. 26: 702–706, 1980.

W.J.A. Vandenheuvel, V.F. Gruber, R.W. Walker and F.J. Wolf. GLC analysis of hydrochlorothiazide in blood and plasma. J. Pharm. Sci. 64: 1309–1312, 1975.

Hydrocodone

T½: 3.4–8.8 hr
Vd: 3.3–4.7 L/kg
Fb: ?
pKa: 8.9

Occurrence and Usage. Hydrocodone (dihydrocodeinone, Anexsia, Damason-P, Hycodan, Lortab, Panacet, Vicodin) is a semisynthetic narcotic analgesic prepared from codeine. It is widely used as an antitussive in cough syrups and tablets (2.5–5 mg) and as an analgesic in tablets and capsules (5–10 mg), usually as the bitartrate salt. Oral doses may be taken every 4–6 hours, with a maximum recommended daily limit of 45 mg. Hydrocodone is considered to have approximately 6 times the analgesic potency of codeine.

Blood Concentrations. A maximal serum hydrocodone concentration of 0.011 mg/L was observed in a volunteer 1.5 hours after oral ingestion of 5 mg of the bitartrate; this level declined to 0.002 mg/L by 9 hours (Hoffman et al., 1983). Peak serum concentrations averaging 0.024 mg/L were found at 1.5 hours after oral administration of 10 mg of the bitartrate to 5 volunteers, declining to 0.007 mg/L by 8 hours. The terminal serum half-life of the drug was determined to be 3.8 hours (Barnhart and Caldwell, 1977). The elimination half-life averaged 4.2 hours in rapid metabolizers and 6.2 hours in slow metabolizers (Otton et al., 1993).

Metabolism and Excretion. Hydrocodone is metabolized in man by O- and N-demethylation and reduction of the 6-keto group. About 26% of a single dose is eliminated in the 72 hour urine as unchanged drug (12%), norhydrocodone (5%), conjugated hydromorphone (4%), 6-hydrocodol (3%), and conjugated 6-hydromorphol (0.1%). Hydrocodol and hydromorphol exist as stereoisomers. Each of the unconjugated metabolites is believed to contribute to the pharmacological activity of hydrocodone (Cone and Darwin, 1978; Cone et al., 1978). Rapid metabolizers excrete significantly more of a dose as conjugated hydromorphone than poor metabolizers (5.9% versus 1.0%) in the 48 hour urine (Otton et al., 1993).

Toxicity. Hydrocodone is more toxic than codeine (minimum adult lethal dose, 100 mg) and has a greater addiction liability. Adverse or toxic effects include stupor, muscle flaccidity, respiratory depression, hypotension, cold and clammy skin and coma. Two individuals, stopped for erratic driving and believed to have been chronically abusing hydrocodone, had blood levels of 0.13 and 0.19 mg/L (Baselt, 1994).

Eleven persons who died after accidental or intentional oral overdosage with hydrocodone had postmortem blood concentrations of 0.13–7.0 mg/L (average, 1.4); in 8 of the cases, blood levels ranged from 0.13–0.60 mg/L (Vivian, 1979; Cravey, 1980; Gottschalk and Cravey, 1980; Cravey, 1981; Park et al., 1982; Janssens, 1986; Morrow and Faris, 1987; Sidebotham, 1991).

Analysis. Hydrocodone may be estimated in plasma using a commercially available radioimmunoassay designed for morphine (Honigberg and Stewart, 1980). Gas chromatographic methods have employed nitrogen-phosphorus (Hoffman et al., 1983), electron-capture (Barnhart and Caldwell, 1977) and mass spectrometric detection (Cone and Darwin, 1978). Liquid chromatography has also been described (Otton et al., 1993).

References

J.W. Barnhart and W.J. Caldwell. Gas chromatographic determination of hydrocodone in serum. J. Chrom. 130: 243–249, 1977.

R.C. Baselt. Unpublished results, 1994.

E.J. Cone and W.D. Darwin. Simultaneous determination of hydromorphone, hydrocodone and their 6α- and 6β-hydroxy metabolites in urine using selected ion recording with methane chemical ionization. Biomed. Mass Spec. 5: 291–295, 1978.

E.J. Cone, W.D. Darwin, C.W. Gorodetzky and T. Tan. Comparative metabolism of hydrocodone in man, rat, guinea pig, rabbit, and dog. Drug Met. Disp. 6: 488–493, 1978.

R.H. Cravey. Personal communication, 1980.

R.H. Cravey. Personal communication, 1981.

L.A. Gottschalk and R.H. Cravey. *Toxicological and Pathological Studies on Psychoactive Drug-Involved Deaths*, Biomedical Publications, Davis, California, 1980, pp. 246–247.

D.J. Hoffman, M.J. Leveque and T. Thomson. Capillary GLC assay for carbinoxamine and hydrocodone in human serum using nitrogen-sensitive detection. J. Pharm. Sci. 72: 1342–1344, 1983.

I.L. Honigberg and J.T. Stewart. Radioimmunoassay of hydromorphone and hydrocodone in human plasma. J. Pharm. Sci. 1171–1173, 1980.

J. Janssens. Personal communication, 1986.

P.L. Morrow and E.C. Faris. Death associated with inadvertent hydrocodone overdose in a child with a respiratory tract infection. Am. J. For. Med. Path. 8: 60–63, 1987.

S.V. Otton, M. Schadel, S.W. Cheung et al. CYP2D6 phenotype determines the metabolic conversion of hydrocodone to hydromorphone. Clin. Pharm. Ther. 54: 463–472, 1993.

J.I. Park, G.R. Nakamura, E.C. Griesemer and T.T. Noguchi. Hydromorphone detected in bile following hydrocodone ingestion. J. For. Sci. 27: 223–224, 1982.

C. Sidebotham. Personal communication, 1991.

D. Vivian. Three deaths due to hydrocodone in a resin-complex cough mixture. Drug Int. Clin. Pharm. 13: 445–446, 1979.

Hydrogen Sulfide

T½: ?
Vd: ?   s⁻²
Fb: ?
pKa: 8.1, 14.9

Occurrence and Usage. Although organic and inorganic sulfide compounds have many industrial applications, the most common source of sulfide in episodes of human poisoning is gaseous hydrogen sulfide, a product of organic decomposition. The gas is easily detected by its offensive odor in concentrations as low as 0.03 ppm, but in higher concentrations (150 ppm) it produces paralysis of the olfactory nerves and is therefore dangerous. Hydrogen sulfide is similar to hydrogen cyanide in both its acute effects and its apparent lack of chronic toxicity. The current threshold limit value for hydrogen sulfide in industry is 10 ppm (14 mg/m³).

Blood Concentrations. Inorganic sulfide is not normally present in biological fluids *in vivo* in significant quantities. The sulfide concentration of whole blood from normal subjects is less than 0.05 mg/L (McAnalley et al., 1979).

Metabolism and Excretion. Exogenous sulfide is partially oxidized both by hemoglobin and by liver enzymes to thiosulfate; a portion may also be excreted unchanged by the lungs as hydrogen sulfide (Sorbo, 1960; Evans, 1967). A small but distinct fraction of normal blood exists as sulfhemoglobin, due to the metabolism of endogenous sulfur, but sulfhemoglobin is not produced during acute exposure to hydrogen sulfide (Adelson and Sunshine, 1966).

Normal human postmortem tissue specimens of blood, brain, lung and thigh muscle did not contain detectable sulfide when the body was stored at a temperature of less than 20° C. prior to autopsy, but these tissues contained from 0.02–5.7 mg/kg sulfide when the storage temperature exceeded 20° C.; liver, kidney and abdominal muscle contained 0.02–7.4 mg/kg sulfide regardless of storage temperature (Nagata et al., 1990). In another study, postmortem brain specimens from 45 normal persons contained 0.54–0.73 mg/kg sulfide (Goodwin et al., 1989).

Toxicity. Sulfide is thought to produce its systemic toxicity by inhibition of cytochrome oxidase, as with cyanide. Air concentrations of hydrogen sulfide of up to 200 ppm cause primarily local tissue irritation, while concentrations of 1000–2000 ppm may result in rapid death. Experimental evidence indicates that methemoglobin induction by nitrite administration protects against sulfide poisoning by complexing hydrosulfide as inactive sulfmethemoglobin (Smith et al., 1976). Persons who survive acute poisoning with the gas often require a several month recuperation period, characterized by fatigue, headache, lack of initiative, irritability, loss of memory and loss of equilibrium (Ahlborg, 1951; Kemper, 1966). Six persons who experienced nausea or momentary loss of consciousness following exposure to hydrogen sulfide for 1–8 minutes exhibited blood sulfide levels of 0.04–0.11 mg/L within 0.5–2 hours (Jappinen and Tenhunen, 1990).

Numerous instances of acute intoxication have been reported, with many fatalities known to have occurred (Freireich, 1946; Breysse, 1961; Milby, 1962; Kleinfeld et al., 1964; Adelson and Sunshine, 1966; Poda, 1966; Thoman, 1969; Simson and Simpson, 1971; Stine et al., 1976). Following the accidental fatal exposure of 6 workers to hydrogen sulfide in industrial situations, postmortem blood sulfide concentrations of 0.9–3.8 mg/L (average, 2.4) were observed (Winek et al., 1968; McAnalley et al., 1979). In one of these cases, involving the fatal exposure of a workman to hydrogen sulfide in a tank containing up to 6100 ppm of the gas, the following tissue levels were determined (Winek et al., 1968):

Sulfide Concentrations in a Fatal Case (mg/L or mg/kg)

Blood	Brain	Liver	Kidney
0.92	1.06	0.38	0.34

Analysis. Sulfide may be demonstrated in biological specimens by microdiffusion isolation with determination by colorimetry (Feldstein and Klendshoj, 1957; Debevere and Voets, 1972) or ion-specific electrode (McAnalley et al., 1979). Gas chromatography with electron-capture has also been used (Kage et al., 1988; Chen et al., 1994). Several investigators have stressed the need for promptness in analyzing specimens, due to the rapid loss of sulfide from biological materials. Also, significant quantities of sulfide may be produced during *in vitro* storage of tissues at temperatures exceeding 20° C. (Goodwin et al., 1989).

References

L. Adelson and I. Sunshine. Fatal hydrogen sulfide intoxication. Arch. Path. 81: 375–380, 1966.

G. Ahlborg. Hydrogen sulfide poisoning in shale oil industry. Arch. Ind. Hyg. Occ. Med. 3: 247–266, 1951.

P.A. Breysse. Hydrogen sulfide fatality in a poultry feather fertilizer plant. Am. Ind. Hyg. Asso. J. 22: 220–222, 1961.

S. Chen, S.M. Wu, H.S. Kou and H.L. Wu. Electron-capture gas chromatographic determination of cyanide, iodide, nitrite and thiocyanate anions. J. Anal. Tox. 18: 81–85, 1994.

J.M. Debevere and J.P. Voets. A rapid microdiffusion method for the determination of sulphides in biological fluids. Lab. Prac. 21: 713–714, 1972.

C.L. Evans. The toxicity of hydrogen sulphide and other sulphides. Quart. J. Exp. Physiol. 52: 231–248, 1967.

M. Feldstein and N.C. Klendshoj. The determination of volatile substances by microdiffusion analysis. J. For. Sci. 2: 39–58, 1957.

A.W. Freireich. Hydrogen sulfide poisoning. Report of two cases, one with fatal outcome, from associated mechanical asphyxia. Am. J. Path. 22: 147–150, 1946.

L.R. Goodwin, D. Francom, F.P. Dieken et al. Determination of sulfide in brain tissue by gas dialysis/ion chromatography. J. Anal. Tox. 13: 105–109, 1989.

P. Jappinen and R. Tenhunen. Hydrogen sulphide poisoning. Brit. J. Ind. Med. 47: 283–285, 1990.

S. Kage, T. Nagata, K. Kumura and K. Kudo. Extractive alkylation and gas chromatographic analysis of sulfide. J. For. Sci. 33: 217–222, 1988.

F.D. Kemper. A near-fatal case of hydrogen sulfide poisoning. Can. Med. Asso. J. 94: 1130–1131, 1966.

M. Kleinfeld, C. Giel and A. Rosso. Acute hydrogen sulfide intoxication; an unusual source of exposure. Ind. Med. Surg. 33: 656–660, 1964.

B.H. McAnalley, W.T. Lowry, R.D. Oliver and J.C. Garriott. Determination of inorganic sulfide and cyanide in blood using specific ion electrodes: application to the investigation of hydrogen sulfide and cyanide poisoning. J. Anal. Tox. 3: 111–114, 1979.

T.H. Milby. Hydrogen sulfide intoxication. J. Occ. Med. 4: 431–437, 1962.

T. Nagata, S. Kage, K. Kimura et al. Sulfide concentrations in postmortem mammalian tissues. J. For. Sci. 35: 706–712, 1990.

G.A. Poda. Hydrogen sulfide can be handled safely. Arch. Env. Health 12: 795–800, 1966.

R.E. Simson and G.R. Simpson. Fatal hydrogen sulphide poisoning associated with industrial waste exposure. Med. J. Aust. 1: 331–334, 1971.

R.P. Smith, R. Kruszyna and H. Kruszyna. Management of acute sulfide poisoning. Arch. Env. Health 22: 166–169, 1976.

B. Sorbo. On the mechanism of sulfide oxidation in biological systems. Biochim. Biophys. Acta 38: 349–351, 1960.

R.J. Stine, B. Slosberg and B.E. Beacham. Hydrogen sulfide intoxication. Ann. Int. Med. 85: 756–758, 1976.

M. Thoman. Sewer gas: hydrogen sulfide intoxication. Clin. Tox. 2: 383–386, 1969.

C.L. Winek, W.D. Collom and C.H. Wecht. Death from hydrogen-sulphide fumes. Lancet 1: 1096, 1968.

Hydromorphone

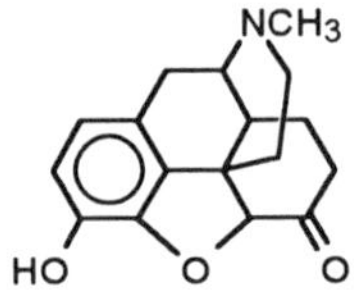

T½: 1.5–3.8 hr
Vd: 2.9 L/kg
Fb: 0.19
pKa: 8.2

Occurrence and Usage. Hydromorphone (dihydromorphinone, Dilaudid) is a semisynthetic narcotic analgesic that is available in a variety of forms for oral, parenteral and rectal administration in
doses of 1–4 mg every 4–6 hours as the hydrochloride. The compound is prescribed both as an
antitussive and analgesic, and has achieved popularity as a drug of abuse. Its addiction liability is
similar to that of morphine and it is reportedly 7–10 times more potent.

Blood Concentrations. Plasma concentrations reached an average peak of 0.022 mg/L (range,
0.018–0.027) in 6 volunteers at 0.8–1.5 hours after a single 4 mg oral dose, and declined with an
average half-life of 2.5 hours (Vallner et al., 1981). Plasma hydromorphone concentrations averaged 0.242 mg/L at 3 minutes after an intravenous 2 mg dose in 8 subjects, but dropped to approximately 0.020 mg/L by 15 minutes and 0.009 mg/L by 30 minutes (Parab et al., 1988). Plasma
concentrations of 0.001–0.049 mg/L have been reported in patients with severe pain receiving
analgesic doses (Honigberg et al., 1977; Reidenberg et al., 1988). The oral and rectal bioavailability
were found to be 51% and 36%, respectively. The blood/plasma concentration ratio for the drug
averages 1.35 (Parab et al., 1988).

Metabolism and Excretion. An average of 6% of a dose is excreted as free and 30% as conjugated
hydromorphone in the 24 hour urine; only traces of the conjugated 6-alpha- and 6-beta-hydroxy
reduction products were present (Cone et al., 1977; Cone and Darwin, 1978).

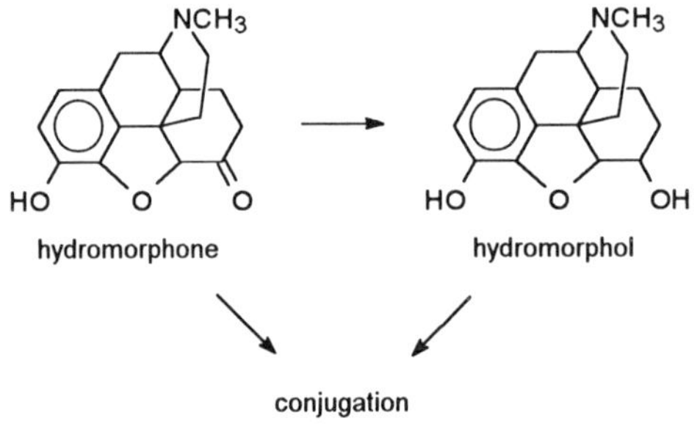

hydromorphone   hydromorphol

conjugation

Toxicity. Adverse or toxic reactions to hydromorphone include stupor, hypotension, respiratory
depression, cold and clammy skin, muscle flaccidity and coma. Patients have occasionally experienced toxic reactions when hydromorphone was used interchangably with morphine on either a
dose or dosing frequency basis. One person survived the accidental epidural injection of 5 mg
hydromorphone with minimal untoward effects (Moon and Clements, 1985). Eight deaths due to
oral or intravenous hydromorphone overdosage have been reported, several involving other drugs.
The following tissue concentrations were noted (Walls, 1976; Garriott and Baselt, 1978; Levine et
al., 1984; Manning, 1984):

Hydromorphone Concentrations in Fatal Cases (mg/L or mg/kg)

	Blood	Liver	Bile	Kidney	Urine
Average	0.3	1.4	9.2	1.2	8.6
(Range)	(0.02–1.2)	(0.07–7.7)	(1–20)	(0.1–5.2)	(1–29)

Analysis. Hydromorphone will cross-react to a limited extent (10–15% of the morphine value) with either the EMIT opiate assay or the Roche morphine radioimmunoassay, and thus these techniques may be used quantitatively when other opiates are not present (Honigberg et al., 1977; Honigberg and Stewart, 1980). The drug will form the usual silyl and acetyl derivatives and may be included in general gas chromatographic schemes for opiate analysis (see heroin). Liquid chromatographic methods have also been reported (Wetzelsberger et al., 1986; Reidenberg et al., 1988; Bouquillon et al., 1992).

References

A.I. Bouquillon, D. Freeman and D.E. Moulin. Simultaneous solid-phase extraction and chromatographic analysis of morphine and hydromorphone in plasma. J. Chrom. 577: 354–357, 1992.

E.J. Cone, B.A. Phelps and C.W. Gorodetzky. Urinary excretion of hydromorphone and metabolites in humans, rats, dogs, guinea pigs, and rabbits. J. Pharm. Sci. 66: 1709–1713, 1977.

E.J. Cone and W.D. Darwin. Simultaneous determination of hydromorphone, hydrocodone and their 6α- and 6β-hydroxy metabolites in urine using selected ion recording with methane chemical ionization. Biomed. Mass Spec. 5: 291–295, 1978.

J.C. Garriott and R.C. Baselt. Deaths involving hydromorphone (Dilaudid). For. Sci. Gaz. 9 (3): 1–2, 1978.

I.L. Honigberg, J.T. Stewart, W.J. Brown et al. Radioimmunoassay of hydromorphone in plasma. J. Anal. Tox. 1: 70–72, 1977.

I.L. Honigberg and J.T. Stewart. Radioimmunoassay of hydromorphone and hydrocodone in human plasma. J. Pharm. Sci. 69: 1171–1173, 1980.

B. Levine, J. Saady, M. Fierro and J. Valentour. A hydromorphone and ethanol fatality. J. For. Sci. 29: 655–659, 1984.

T. Manning. Personal communication, 1984.

R.E. Moon and F.M. Clements. Accidental epidural overdose of hydromorphone. Anesthesiology 63: 238–239, 1985.

P.V. Parab, W.A. Ritschel, D.E. Coyle et al. Pharmacokinetics of hydromorphone after intravenous, peroral and rectal administration to human subjects. Biopharm. Drug Disp. 9: 187–199, 1988.

M.M. Reidenberg, H. Goodman, H. Erle et al. Hydromorphone levels and pain control in patients with severe chronic pain. Clin. Pharm. Ther. 44: 376–382, 1988.

J.J. Vallner, J.T. Stewart, J.A. Kotzan et al. Pharmacokinetics and bioavailability of hydromorphone following intravenous and oral administration to human subjects. J. Clin. Pharm. 21: 152–156, 1981.

H.C. Walls. Personal communication, 1976.

N. Wetzelsberger, P.W. Lucker and W. Erking. High-pressure liquid chromatographic method for the determination of hydromorphone in human plasma with electrochemical detection. Arz. Forsch. 36: 1707–1710, 1986.

Hydroxychloroquine

T½: 16–36 days (plasma)
    32–56 days (whole blood)
Vd: 580–815 L/kg
Fb: 0.40–0.45
pKa: ?

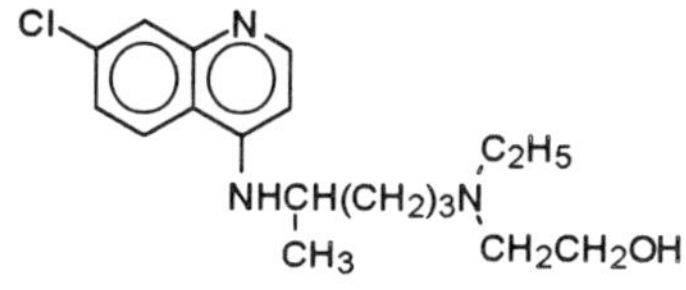

Occurrence and Usage. Hydroxychloroquine (Plaquenil) is an aminoquinoline derivative, closely related to chloroquine, that is used in the treatment of malaria, lupus erythematosus, and rheumatoid arthritis. It is available as the sulfate in 200 mg tablets. Oral doses range from as little as 400 mg per week for suppressive therapy to as much as 1200 mg in a single day for acute malarial attacks. Daily doses of 200–600 mg are used for lupus and rheumatoid diseases.

Blood Concentrations. Plasma concentrations in volunteers after single oral doses of 400 or 800 mg of hydroxychloroquine sulfate averaged 0.082 and 0.210 mg/L, respectively, at 3 hours, and 0.019 and 0.056 mg/L by 24 hours. In subjects receiving 400 mg once a week for several weeks, plasma concentrations averaged 0.121 mg/L (range, 0.106–0.140) at 3 hours after the dose, 0.062 mg/L (range, 0.045–0.077) at 24 hours, and 0.015 mg/L (range, 0.011–0.024) at 96 hours. Plasma concentrations in excess of 0.010 mg/L were considered by the investigators to be effective in the suppressive treatment of malaria (McChesney et al., 1962). Blood elimination half-lives exceeded those of plasma and averaged 48, 130 and 217 days for hydroxychloroquine, desethylhydroxychloroquine and desethylchloroquine, respectively. The blood/plasma concentration ratio for chloroquine averaged 7.2 (range, 1–21) (Tett et al., 1988).

Metabolism and Excretion. In patients on daily therapy with hydroxychloroquine, only 13% of a dose is excreted in the daily urine as identifiable products. About 8% is eliminated as unchanged drug, 2% as desethylchloroquine, 2% as desethylhydroxychloroquine, and 0.5% as didesethylchloroquine (McChesney et al., 1966). By the fourth week of once weekly oral dosing with 400 mg of the drug, 2 subjects exhibited urine hydroxychloroquine concentrations of 2–10 mg/L during the first 24 hours post-dose; the concentrations of the three desethyl metabolites remained below 1 mg/L (Williams et al., 1988).

Cl —[quinoline ring]— $NHCH(CH_2)_3N(C_2H_5)(CH_2CH_2OH)$ with CH_3 substituent
hydroxychloroquine

$\longrightarrow$

Cl —[quinoline ring]— $NHCH(CH_2)_3NHC_2H_5$ with CH_3 substituent
desethylchloroquine

$\downarrow$

Cl —[quinoline ring]— $NHCH(CH_2)_3NHCH_2CH_2OH$ with CH_3 substituent
desethylhydroxychloroquine

$\longrightarrow$

Cl —[quinoline ring]— $NHCH(CH_2)_3NH_2$ with CH_3 substituent
didesethylchloroquine

Toxicity. The effects of overdosage with hydroxychloroquine include headache, drowsiness, visual disturbances, convulsions, cardiovascular collapse, and respiratory arrest. An adult who ingested 36 tablets of the drug became moribund and vomited, but responded to supportive therapy; his plasma hydroxychloroquine level of 6.1 mg/L on admission declined to 2.7 mg/L after 2 days (Graham, 1960). An adult female ingested 12 g of the drug and survived; she exhibited cardiac arrhythmias and an admission plasma hydroxychloroquine level of 3.0 mg/L (Villalobos, 1991).

A diabetic woman who believed she was pregnant attempted chemical abortion with the drug and died; her liver was found to contain 180 mg/kg hydroxychloroquine (Bonnichsen and Maehly, 1965). Blood, liver and urine concentrations of 61 mg/L, 71 mg/kg, and 970 mg/L were observed postmortem in the case of a 16 year old boy who ingested an overdose of hydroxychloroquine and died within a short time thereafter (Dalley and Hainsworth, 1965). A 2.5 year old child accidentally ingested 12 g of drug and suffered seizures and cardiorespiratory arrest; postmortem blood and liver hydroxychloroquine concentrations of 104 mg/L and 500 mg/kg, respectively, were reported (Kemmenoe, 1990).

Analysis. Hydroxychloroquine may be analyzed in biological specimens at therapeutic levels by fluorometry (McChesney et al., 1962) or at toxic levels by ultraviolet spectrophotometry (Bonnichsen and Maehly, 1965). Desalkyl metabolites of the drug are believed to interfere in both of these procedures. Liquid chromatographic techniques are available that can separately quantitate the parent drug and its principal metabolites (Morris, 1985; Tett et al., 1985; Brown et al., 1986; Williams et al., 1988).

References

R. Bonnichsen and A.C. Maehly. Two fatal poisonings by chloroquine and by hydroxychloroquine. J. For. Sci. Soc. 5: 201–202, 1965.

R.R. Brown, R.M. Stroshane and D.P. Benziger. High-performance liquid chromatographic assay for hydroxychloroquine and three of its major metabolites, desethylhydroxychloroquine, desethylchloroquine and bidesethylchloroquine, in human plasma. J. Chrom. 377: 454–459, 1986.

R.A. Dalley and D. Hainsworth. Fatal Plaquenil poisoning. J. For. Sci. Soc. 5: 99–101, 1965.

J.D.P. Graham. An overdose of "Plaquenil". Brit. Med. J. 1: 1256, 1960.

A.V. Kemmenoe. An infant fatality due to hydroxychloroquine poisoning. J. Anal. Tox. 14: 186–188, 1990.

E.W. McChesney, W.F. Banks, Jr. and J.P. McAuliff. Laboratory studies on the 4-aminoquinoline antimalarials: II. Plasma levels of chloroquine and hydroxychloroquine in man after various oral dosage regimens. Antibiot. Chemother. 12: 583–594, 1962.

E.W. McChesney, W.D. Conway, W.F. Banks, Jr. et al. Studies of the metabolism of some compounds of the 4-amino-7-chloroquinoline series. J. Pharm. Exp. Ther. 151: 482–493, 1966.

R.G. Morris. Estimation of plasma hydroxychloroquine by high-performance liquid chromatography with ultraviolet detection. J. Chrom. 338: 422–427, 1985.

S.E. Tett, D.J. Cutler and K.F. Brown. High-performance liquid chromatographic assay for hydroxychloroquine and metabolites in blood and plasma. J. Chrom. 344: 241–248, 1985.

S.E. Tett, D.J. Cutler, R.O. Day and K.F. Brown. A dose-ranging study of the pharmacokinetics of hydroxychloroquine following intravenous administration to healthy adults. Brit. J. Clin. Pharm. 26: 303–313, 1988.

D. Villalobos. Plaquenil (hydroxychloroquine) plasmapheresis in an overdose. Vet. Hum. Tox. 33: 364, 1991.

S.B. Williams, L.C. Patchen and F.C. Churchill. Analysis of blood and urine samples for hydroxychloroquine and three major metabolites by high-performance liquid chromatography with fluorescence detection. J. Chrom. 433: 197–206, 1988.

Hydroxyzine

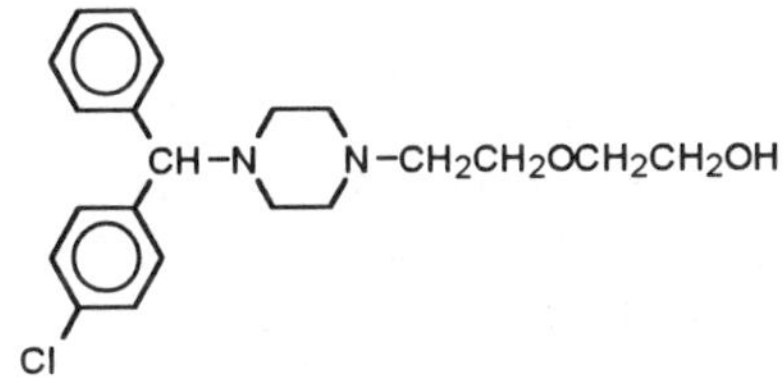

T½: 13–27 hr
Vd: 13–31 L/kg
Fb: ?
pKa: 2.1, 7.1

Occurrence and Usage. Hydroxyzine (Atarax, Vistaril) is an antihistaminic agent with sedative properties, closely related to chlorcyclizine and meclizine, that is used in the control of anxiety and emesis. It is also frequently administered parenterally in concert with meperidine to augment the analgesic effects of that drug. Hydroxyzine is available as the hydrochloride or pamoate salt for oral or intramuscular injection. Certain combination formulations may contain a decongestant, anticholinergic or vasodilator. Tablets of 10–100 mg, syrups of 10 mg/5 mL, and injectable solutions containing 25–50 mg/mL are in common use. Single doses of 25–100 mg and daily doses of up to 400 mg may be administered by either route.

Blood Concentrations. Serum hydroxyzine concentrations in 7 adults given a 0.7 mg/kg (49 mg/70 kg) oral dose averaged 0.070 mg/L at 2 hours, 0.039 mg/L at 6 hours and 0.022 mg/L at 12 hours (Simons et al., 1984). Plasma concentrations in 4 subjects after a single oral 100 mg dose reached an average peak level of 0.078 mg/L (range, 0.065–0.089) at 4 hours and declined to 0.035 mg/L (range, 0.031–0.038) by 8 hours (Fouda et al., 1979). The elimination half-life in young adults averages 20 hours for hydroxyzine and 11 hours for cetirizine, an active metabolite; peak serum levels for cetirizine after a single oral hydroxyzine dose occur at about 4 hours and average 5 times those of the parent drug (Simons et al., 1989).

Metabolism and Excretion. The metabolism of hydroxyzine has not been studied in humans. In rats, the compound is extensively metabolized, with 15% of a labeled dose eliminated in urine and 35% in feces over a 5 day period. The metabolites are products of N-dealkylation (norhydroxyzine or norchlorcyclizine), oxidative removal of the piperazine ring (p-chlorobenzhydrol and p-chloro-benzophenone), and p-hydroxylation of the benzene ring (p'-hydroxy-p-chlorobenzophenone). No unchanged drug was found in urine (Pong and Huang, 1974). The presence of norhydroxyzine in human urine has been reported (Kageura et al., 1986). Cetirizine, a carboxylic acid metabolite, accumulates in serum and has significant antihistaminic activity, but is apparently devoid of sedative effects (Gengo et al., 1987).

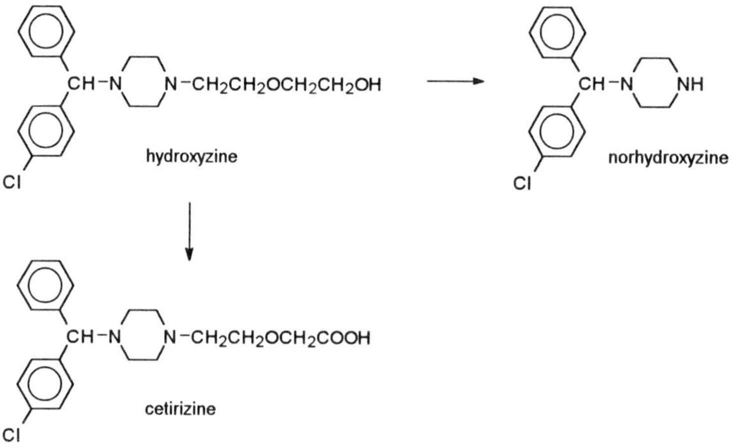

Toxicity. Side effects of hydroxyzine administration include dry mouth, drowsiness, and tremor. Overdosage produces central nervous system depression. A 1 year old child accidentally ingested up to 625 mg of the drug and developed seizures and tachycardia; a plasma hydroxyzine concentration of 103 mg/L was measured after 8.5 hours (Magera et al., 1981).

Only hydroxyzine was found in the body of an alcoholic woman who died unattended; concentrations of 1.1 mg/L in blood and 16 mg/kg in liver were reported (Spiehler and Fukumoto, 1984). An 18 year old female found dead after apparently ingesting an acute overdose had postmortem blood and urine hydroxyzine levels of 4.2 and 1.4 mg/L, respectively (Kintz et al., 1990). The following tissue concentrations were determined in the case of a 43 year old woman who committed suicide with hydroxyzine (Johnson, 1982):

Hydroxyzine Concentrations in a Fatal Case (mg/L or mg/kg)

Blood	Brain	Liver	Bile	Urine	Gastric
39	163	414	122	19	487 mg

Analysis. Hydroxyzine may be assayed in biological fluids by electron-capture gas chromatography after conversion to a benzophenone (Hartvig and Handl, 1975) or by gas chromatography-mass spectrometry of the acetyl derivative (Fouda et al., 1979). Liquid chromatography has also been described (Simons et al., 1984).

References

H.G. Fouda, D.C. Hobbs and J.E. Stambaugh. Sensitive assay for determination of hydroxyzine in plasma and its human pharmacokinetics. J. Pharm. Sci. 68: 1456–1458, 1979.

F.M. Gengo, J. Dabronzo, A. Yurchak et al. The relative antihistaminic and psychomotor effects of hydroxyzine and cetirizine. Clin. Pharm. Ther. 42: 265–272, 1987.

P. Hartvig and W. Handl. Gas chromatography and electron capture detection of benzophenones. Acta Pharm. Suec. 12: 349–360, 1975.

G.R. Johnson. A fatal case involving hydroxyzine. J. Anal. Tox. 6: 69–70, 1982.

M. Kageura, M. Kataoka, K. Hara and T. Nagata. Changed compounds of hydroxyzine in a human urine. For. Sci. Int. 32: 229–235, 1986.

P. Kintz, B. Godelar and P. Mangin. Gas chromatographic identification and quantitation of hydroxyzine. For. Sci. Int. 48: 139–143, 1990.

B.E. Magera, C.J. Betlach, A.P. Sweatt and C.W. Derrick, Jr. Hydroxyzine intoxication in a 13-month-old child. Pediatrics 67: 280–283, 1981.

S.F. Pong and C.L. Huang. Comparative studies on distribution, excretion, and metabolism of hydroxyzine-^{3}H and its methiodide-^{14}C in rats. J. Pharm. Sci. 63: 1527–1532, 1974.

V.R. Spiehler and R.I. Fukumoto. Another fatal case involving hydroxyzine. J. Anal. Tox. 8: 242–243, 1984.

F.E.R. Simons, K.J. Simons and E.M. Frith. The pharmacokinetics and antihistaminic of the H1 receptor antagonist hydroxyzine. J. Allergy Clin. Immun. 73: 69–75, 1984.

F.E.R. Simons, W.T.A. Watson, X.Y. Chen et al. The pharmacokinetics and pharmacodynamics of hydroxyzine in patients with primary biliary cirrhosis. J. Clin. Pharm. 29: 809–815, 1989.

Ibuprofen

T½: 0.9–2.5 hr
Vd: 0.14 L/kg
Fb: 0.99
pKa: 4.4

$(CH_3)_2CHCH_2$—⟨O⟩—$CHCOOH$ with CH_3

Occurrence and Usage. Ibuprofen (Advil, Motrin, Nuprin) is a nonnarcotic analgesic and antiinflammatory agent, chemically related to fenoprofen and ketoprofen, that has been available as a prescription drug since 1968 and as a nonprescription drug since 1984. It is available as the free acid in tablets of 300–600 mg for oral administration in daily doses of 900–2400 mg. Arthritic patients may require several weeks of high-dose therapy before beneficial effects are apparent.

Blood Concentrations. A single 200 mg oral dose in a volunteer produced a peak plasma ibuprofen concentration of 26 mg/L at 1.5 hours (Rustum, 1991). A single 400 mg oral dose of ibuprofen resulted in an average peak plasma concentration of 28 mg/L (range, 17–36) at 1.0–1.3 hours after ingestion; the levels declined with a mean half-life of 1.9 hours (Collier et al., 1978). After an 800 mg oral dose, peak plasma concentrations averaged 49 mg/L at 1 hour; the 2 optimal isomers of ibuprofen were in approximately equal amounts, but the d-isomer was found to have a slightly longer half-life (Vangiessen and Kaiser, 1975). No accumulation of ibuprofen in plasma was noted after 14 days of thrice daily dosing with 200 mg per dose (Mills et al., 1973).

Metabolism and Excretion. Ibuprofen is known to be extensively metabolized in man by oxidation of the isobutyl group. No unchanged drug, in either free or conjugated form, was found in the 24 hour urine after a 600 mg dose. 2-Carboxyibuprofen accounted for 16% of the dose in free and 19% in bound form, while 2-hydroxyibuprofen accounted for 9% and 17% in free and conjugated form, respectively. These 2 metabolites were found in low levels (0.3–3.0 mg/L) in plasma during chronic dosing with the drug (Mills et al., 1973). Other investigators have found that up to 9% of a dose may be eliminated unchanged in the 24 hour urine (Vangiessen and Kaiser, 1975).

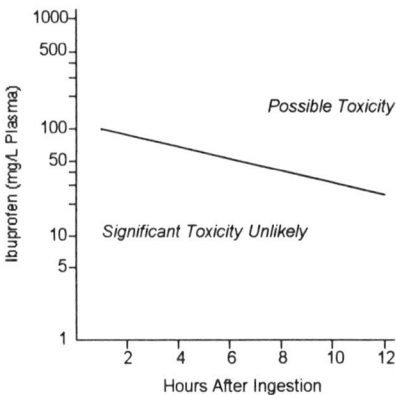

Toxicity. Side effects of ibuprofen usage include nausea, epigastric pain, diarrhea, vomiting, dizziness, blurred vision and edema. Single doses have caused severe anaphylactic reactions in persons with allergic hypersensitivity to ibuprofen. A 19 year old who ingested 8000 mg of the drug exhibited only dizziness and nystagmus. A 10 kg child ingested 1200 mg and developed a blood ibuprofen concentration of 700 mg/L after 1.5 hours, but was asymptomatic. A 19 month old child ingested up to 4000 mg and became apneic and unresponsive; the blood concentration 8.5 hours after ingestion was 103 mg/L, and the child completely recovered several hours later with only supportive therapy (PDR, 1981). A 2.5 year old child ingested up to 12,000 mg, vomited and became unresponsive; about 4 hours after ingestion, during maximum sedation, his blood concentration was 84 mg/L and it declined with a half-life of 2 hours (Garrettson et al., 1981). Several patients developed coma, metabolic acidosis and renal failure after ibuprofen overdosage, while exhibiting serum levels of 185–680 mg/L (Lee and Finkler, 1986; Linden and Townsend, 1986). The following nomogram was devised to assist in relating plasma drug concentration, time since ingestion, and the possibility of renal toxicity in overdosed patients (Hall et al., 1992):

The following concentrations were noted in an adult who died after ingesting large amounts of ibuprofen and acetaminophen (Steinmetz et al., 1987):

Drug Concentrations in a Fatal Case (mg/L or mg/kg)

Drug	Blood	Liver	Kidney
Ibuprofen	81	238	622
Carboxyibuprofen	101	225	385
Hydroxyibuprofen	43	115	160

Analysis. Gas chromatographic procedures for the determination of ibuprofen in biological fluids have relied on flame-ionization detection of the free drug (Hoffman, 1977; Hackett and Dusci, 1978; Heikkinen, 1984) or its methyl ester (Kaiser and Vangiessen, 1974; Midha et al., 1977) or electron-capture detection of a halogenated derivative (Kaiser and Martin, 1978). A number of convenient liquid chromatographic techniques have been reported (Pitre and Grandi, 1979; Shimek et al., 1981; Lockwood and Wagner, 1982; Aravind et al., 1984; Shah and Jung, 1986; Minkler and Hoppel, 1988; Rustum, 1991).

References

M.K. Aravind, J.N. Miceli and R.E. Kauffman. Determination of ibuprofen by high-performance liquid chromatography. J. Chrom. 308: 350–353, 1984.

P.S. Collier, P.F. D'Arcy, D.W.G. Harron and N. Morrow. Pharmacokinetic modelling of ibuprofen. Brit. J. Clin. Pharm. 5: 528–530, 1978.

L.K. Garrettson, J.M. Goplerud and J.J. Saady. Ibuprofen overdose with sedation. Vet. Hum. Tox. 23: 350, 1981.

L.P. Hackett and L.J. Dusci. Gas-liquid chromatographic determination of ibuprofen in human plasma. Clin. Chim. Acta 87: 301–303, 1978.

A.H. Hall, S.C. Smolinske, B. Stover et al. Ibuprofen overdose in adults. Clin. Tox. 30: 23–37, 1992.

L. Heikkinen. Silica capillary gas chromatographic determination of ibuprofen in serum. J. Chrom. 307: 206–209, 1984.

D.J. Hoffman. Rapid GLC determination of ibuprofen in serum. J. Pharm. Sci. 66: 749–750, 1977.

D.G. Kaiser and G.J. Vangiessen. GLC determination of ibuprofen ((±)-2-(p-isobutylphenyl)propionic acid) in plasma. J. Pharm. Sci. 63: 219–221, 1974.

D.G. Kaiser and R.S. Martin. Electron-capture GLC determination of ibuprofen in serum. J. Pharm. Sci. 67: 627–630, 1978.

C.Y. Lee and A. Finkler. Acute intoxication due to ibuprofen. Arch. Path. Lab. Med. 110: 747–749, 1986.

C.H. Linden and P.L. Townsend. Metabolic acidosis following ibuprofen overdose. Vet. Hum. Tox. 28: 483, 1986.

G.F. Lockwood and J.G. Wagner. High-performance liquid chromatographic determination of ibuprofen and its major metabolites in biological fluids. J. Chrom. 232: 335–343, 1982.

K.K. Midha, J.K. Cooper, J.W. Hubbard and I.J. McGilveray. A rapid and simple GLC procedure for determinations of plasma concentrations of ibuprofen. Can. J. Pharm. Sci. 12: 29–31, 1977.

R.F.N. Mills, S.S. Adams, E.E. Cliffe et al. The metabolism of ibuprofen. Xenobiotica 3: 589–598, 1973.

P.E. Minkler and C.L. Hoppel. Determination of ibuprofen in human plasma by high-performance liquid chromatography. J. Chrom. 428: 388–394, 1988.

Physicians' Desk Reference, Medical Economics Co., Oradell, New Jersey, 1981, pp. 1831–1833.

D. Pitre and M. Grandi. Rapid determination of ibuprofen in plasma by high-performance liquid chromatography. J. Chrom. 170: 278–281, 1979.

A.M. Rustum. Assay of ibuprofen in human plasma by rapid and sensitive reversed-phase high-performance liquid chromatography. J. Chrom. Sci. 29: 16–20, 1991.

A. Shah and D. Jung. Rapid and simple determination of the major metabolites of ibuprofen in biological fluids by high-performance liquid chromatography. J. Chrom. 378: 232–236, 1986.

J.L. Shimek, N.G.S. Rao and S.K.W. Khalil. High-pressure liquid chromatographic determination of ibuprofen in plasma. J. Pharm. Sci. 70: 514–516, 1981.

J.C. Steinmetz, C.Y. Lee and A. Wu. Tissue levels of ibuprofen after fatal overdosage of ibuprofen and acetaminophen. Vet. Hum. Tox. 29: 381–383, 1987.

G.J. Vangiessen and D.G. Kaiser. GLC determination of ibuprofen (dl-2-(p-isobutylphenyl)propionic acid) enantiomers in biological specimens. J. Pharm. Sci. 64: 798–801, 1975.

Imipramine

T½: 6–20 hr
Vd: 20–40 L/kg
Fb: 0.80–0.95
pKa: 9.5

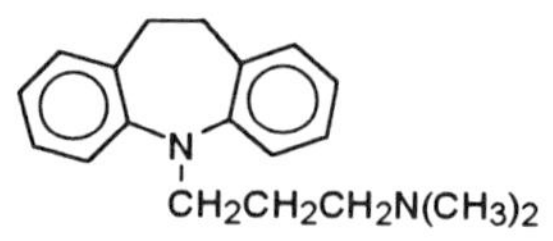

Occurrence and Usage. Imipramine (Tofranil) is the prototype of the tricyclic antidepressant drugs, which now exceed 10 in number and are among the most frequently used agents for the treatment of depression. They bear a close chemical relationship to the phenothiazines (imipramine is a promazine analogue) and yet have certain distinct pharmacological effects. Imipramine was first synthesized in 1948 and its antidepressant effects in human first recognized in 1958. It is available as the hydrochloride salt in 10–50 mg tablets and in 25 mg/2 mL ampules, or as the pamoate salt in 75–150 mg capsules. The compound is administered orally or by intramuscular injection as the hydrochloride in daily doses of 75–300 mg.

Blood Concentrations. Following a single 75 mg oral dose, plasma concentrations reached an average peak of 0.037 mg/L (range, 0.008–0.084) of imipramine at 4 hours and 0.011 mg/L (range, 0.002–0.029) of desipramine at 8 hours (Cooper et al., 1975). During chronic therapy with 150 mg of the drug daily, steady-state plasma concentrations of imipramine averaged 0.052 mg/L (range 0.008–0.105) and of desipramine, 0.132 mg/L (range, 0.016–0.567) (Nagy and Treiber, 1973). The average plasma half-lives of imipramine and its active metabolite have been estimated at 14 hours and 30 hours, respectively (Nagy and Johansson, 1975). The best clinical response was observed in patients whose combined imipramine and desipramine plasma concentrations fell into the range of 0.150–0.240 mg/L (Perel et al., 1978). In patients on chronic therapy, 2-hydroxyimipramine plasma concentrations ranged from 0.010–0.070 mg/L and 2-hydroxydesipramine concentrations from 0.010–0.120 mg/L; these metabolites are believed to be psychoactive (Suckow and Cooper, 1981). The blood/plasma concentration ratio for imipramine averages 1.1–1.2 (Maguire et al., 1980).

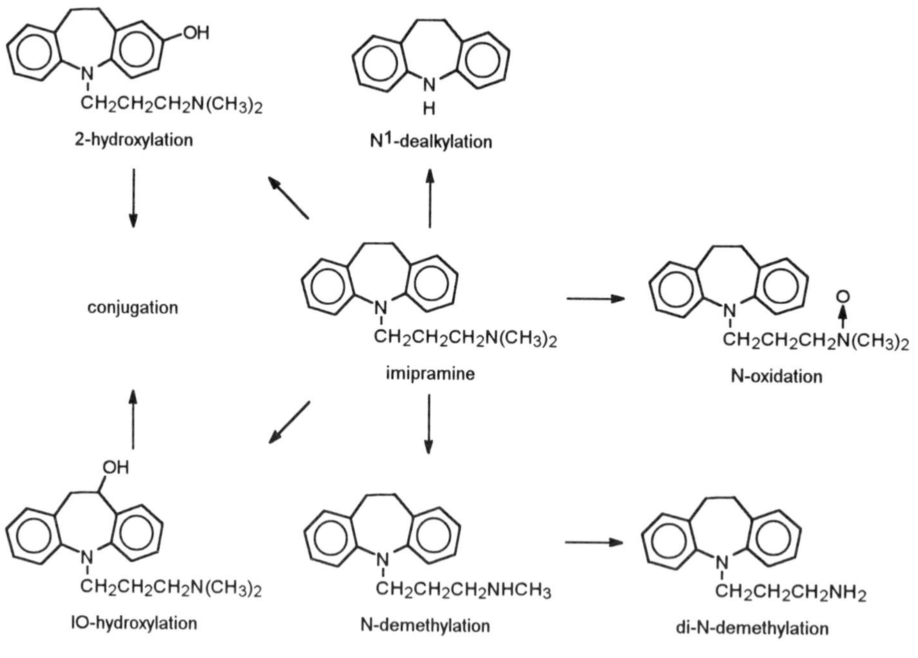

Metabolism and Excretion. Imipramine has as its primary active metabolite desipramine, which accumulates in plasma and which may account for much of the therapeutic effectiveness of the drug. Imipramine is further metabolized extensively by N-demethylation, N-oxidation, N-dealkylation, 2- and 10-hydroxylation and conjugation of the hydroxy-metabolites. At least 20 metabolites are possible and most of these have been isolated. An average of 70% of a dose is excreted in the urine and up to 22% in feces over a 3 day period, largely as free and conjugated hydroxy-metabolites. The major urinary metabolites, in both free and conjugated form, are 2-hydroxydesipramine, 2-hydroxyimipramine and 2-hydroxyiminodibenzyl. Less than 0.3% of a dose is excreted unchanged, although this figure is elevated somewhat during conditions of acid urine (Crammer and Scott, 1966; Crammer et al., 1968; Crammer et al., 1969; Gram et al., 1971; Bickel, 1975; Gram and Christiansen, 1975). A similar portion of a dose is eliminated as desipramine.

Toxicity. Imipramine toxicity is characterized by hyperactivity, seizures, respiratory depression, hypertension, cardiac arrhythmias, hyperpyrexia, tachycardia, urinary retention, coma, circulatory collapse and death. Numerous instances of imipramine intoxication have occurred with at least 40 fatalities recorded in the literature. Death may result after ingestion of as little as 625 mg of the drug by an adult, and survival has been reported after ingestion of as much as 5375 mg (Bickel, 1975). Plasma concentrations as high as 0.410 and 0.720 mg/L of imipramine and desipramine, respectively, were observed in a patient who survived an overdose of imipramine (Spiker et al., 1975).

Imipramine concentrations in fatal cases have ranged from 0.3–30 mg/L in blood and from 5–317 mg/kg in liver (Baselt and Cravey, 1977; Oliver and Smith, 1977). Using a colorimetric assay, Curry (1964) found that liver concentrations of imipramine in 3 persons on therapy with the drug averaged 13 mg/kg (range, 5–21), while the following levels were observed in the tissues from 4 fatal cases:

Imipramine Concentrations in Fatalities (mg/L or mg/kg)

	Blood	Brain	Liver	Kidney
Average	5.3	52	167	47
(Range)	(2.8–7.0)	(30–74)	(86–250)	(38–56)

The following distribution was noted in the cases of 4 individuals who died after ingesting unknown quantities of imipramine (Baselt, 1978; Gottschalk and Cravey, 1980):

Drug Concentrations in Imipramine Fatalities (mg/L or mg/kg)

	Blood	Brain	Liver	Bile	Kidney	Urine	Gastric
Imipramine							
Average	7.3	31	166	56	73	20	1044 mg
(Range)	(6–8.5)	(27–35)	(33–301)	(30–80)	(40–151)	(0.6–54)	(390–2360)
Desipramine							
Average	2.8	15	98	12	29	20	0
(Range)	(0.5–7.8)	(5.6–25)	(35–200)	(2.6–18)	(17–50)	(0.4–55)	(0–0)

Postmortem blood concentrations of imipramine, desipramine, and 2-hydroxyimipramine in a woman who ingested an imipramine overdose were 9.0, 1.1, and 3.9 mg/L, respectively (Fraser et al., 1987). Imipramine may exhibit postmortem redistribution; heart blood/femoral blood concentration ratios averaged 2.2 (range, 1.3–3.0) in 6 cases (Prouty and Anderson, 1990).

Analysis. Imipramine and its primary metabolite have been estimated in biological specimens using colorimetry (Dal Cortivo et al., 1963; Wallace and Biggs, 1969), fluorimetry (Dingell et al., 1964), thin-layer densitometry (Nagy and Treiber, 1973) and gas chromatography with either flame-ionization detection (Nyberg and Martensson, 1977), nitrogen-selective detection (Cooper et al., 1975; Bailey and Jatlow, 1976; Witts and Turner, 1977; Midha et al., 1980) or mass spectrometric detection (Belvedere et al., 1975; Wilson et al., 1977; Alkalay et al., 1979). Liquid chromatography has also received attention as a means of analysis of imipramine and its metabolites in plasma and urine (Watson and Stewart, 1977; Sutfin and Jusko, 1979; Suckow and Cooper, 1981; Kobayashi et al., 1984).

References

D. Alkalay, J. Volk and S. Carlsen. A sensitive method for the simultaneous determination in biological fluids of imipramine and desipramine or clomipramine and N-desmethylclomipramine by gas chromatography mass spectrometry. Biomed. Mass Spec. 6: 200–204, 1979.

D.N. Bailey and P.I. Jatlow. Gas-chromatographic analysis of therapeutic concentrations of imipramine and desipramine in plasma, with use of a nitrogen detector. Clin. Chem. 22: 1697–1701, 1976.

R.C. Baselt. Unpublished results, 1978.

R.C. Baselt and R.H. Cravey. A compendium of therapeutic and toxic concentrations of toxicologically significant drugs in human biofluids. J. Anal. Tox. 1: 81–103, 1977.

G. Belvedere, L. Burti, A. Frigerio and C. Pantarotto. Gas chromatographic-mass fragmentographic determination of "steady-state" plasma levels of imipramine and desipramine in chronically treated patients. J. Chrom. 111: 313–321, 1975.

M.H. Bickel. Poisoning by tricyclic antidepressant drugs. Int. J. Clin. Pharm. 11: 145–176, 1975.

T.B. Cooper, D. Allen and G.M. Simpson. A sensitive method for determination of imipramine and desmethylimipramine using a nitrogen detector. Psychopharm. Comm. 1: 445–454, 1975.

J.L. Crammer and B. Scott. New metabolites of imipramine. Psychopharmacologia 8: 461–468, 1966.

J.L. Crammer, B. Scott, H. Woods and B. Rolfe. Metabolism of ^{14}C-imipramine. I. Excretion in the rat and in man. Psychopharmacologia 12: 263–277, 1968.

J.L. Crammer, B. Scott and B. Rolfe. Metabolism of ^{14}C-imipramine: II. Urinary metabolites in man. Psychopharmacologia 15: 207–225, 1969.

A.S. Curry. Seven fatal cases involving imipramine in man. J. Pharm. Pharmac. 16: 265–267, 1964.

L.A. Dal Cortivo, P. Giaquinta and C.J. Umberger. The determination of imipramine in biologic material. J. For. Sci. 8: 526–534, 1963.

J.V. Dingell, F. Sulser and J.R. Gillette. Species differences in the metabolism of imipramine and desmethylimipramine (DMI). J. Pharm. Exp. Ther. 143: 14–22, 1964.

A.D. Fraser, E. Susnik and A.F. Isner. Analysis of 2-hydroxyimipramine in an imipramine-related fatality. J. For. Sci. 32: 543–549, 1987.

L.A. Gottschalk and R.H. Cravey. *Toxicological and Pathological Studies on Psychoactive Drug-Involved Deaths*, Biomedical Publications, Davis, California, 1980, pp. 247–253.

L.F. Gram, B. Kofod, J. Christiansen and O.J. Rafaelson. Imipramine metabolism: pH-dependent distribution and urinary excretion. Clin. Pharm. Ther. 12: 239–244, 1971.

L.F. Gram and J. Christiansen. First-pass metabolism of imipramine in man. Clin. Pharm. Ther. 17: 555–563, 1975.

A. Kobayashi, S. Sugita and K. Nakazawa. High-performance liquid chromatographic determination of imipramine and desipramine in human serum. J. Chrom. 336: 410–414, 1984.

K.P. Maguire, G.D. Burrows, T.R. Norman and B.A. Scoggins. Blood/plasma distribution ratios of psychotropic drugs. Clin. Chem. 26: 1624–1625, 1980.

K.K. Midha, C. Charette, J.K. Cooper and I.J. McGilveray. Comparison of a new GLC-AFID method with a GLC-MS selected ion monitoring technique and a radioimmunoassay for the determination of plasma concentrations of imipramine and desipramine. J. Anal. Tox. 4: 237–243, 1980.

A. Nagy and R. Johansson. Plasma levels of imipramine and desipramine in man after different routes of administration. Arch. Pharm. 290: 145–160, 1975.

A. Nagy and L. Treiber. Quantitative determination of imipramine and desipramine in human blood plasma by direct densitometry of thin-layer chromatograms. J. Pharm. Pharmac. 25: 599–603, 1973.

G. Nyberg and E. Martensson. Quantitative analysis of tricyclic antidepressants in serum from psychiatric patients. J. Chrom. 143: 491–497, 1977.

J.S. Oliver and H. Smith. A case of fatal imipramine poisoning in an infant. Med. Sci. Law 17: 193–194, 1977.

J.M. Perel, R.L. Stiller and A.H. Glassman. Studies on plasma level/effect relationships in imipramine therapy. Comm. Psychopharm. 2: 429–439, 1978.

R.W. Prouty and W.H. Anderson. The forensic science implications of site and temporal influences on post-mortem blood-drug concentrations. J. For. Sci. 35: 243–270, 1990.

D.G. Spiker, A.N. Weiss, S.S. Chang et al. Tricyclic antidepressant overdose: clinical presentation and plasma levels. Clin. Pharm. Ther. 18: 539–546, 1975.

R.F. Suckow and T.B. Cooper. Simultaneous determination of imipramine, desipramine, and their 2-hydroxy metabolites in plasma by ion-pair reversed-phase high-performance liquid chromatography with amperometric detection. J. Pharm. Sci. 70: 257–261, 1981.

T.A. Sutfin and W.J. Jusko. High-performance liquid chromatographic assay for imipramine, desipramine, and their 2-hydroxylated metabolites. J. Pharm. Sci. 68: 703–705, 1979.

J.E. Wallace and J.D. Biggs. Colorimetric determination of imipramine in biologic specimens. J. For. Sci. 14: 528–537, 1969.

I.D. Watson and M.J. Stewart. Assay of tricyclic structured drugs and their metabolites in urine by high-performance liquid chromatography. J. Chrom. 134: 182–186, 1977.

J.M. Wilson, L.J. Williamson and V.A. Raisys. Simultaneous measurement of secondary and tertiary tricyclic antidepressants by GC/MS chemical ionization mass fragmentography. Clin. Chem. 23: 1012–1017, 1977.

D.J. Witts and P. Turner. A single comprehensive gas chromatographic assay for tricyclic antidepressant drugs and their major metabolites in plasma. Brit. J. Clin. Pharm. 4: 249–252, 1977.

Indomethacin

T½: 1–16 hr (adults)
  10–33 hr (neonates)
Vd: 0.33–0.40 L/kg
Fb: 0.98
pKa: 4.5

Occurrence and Usage. Indomethacin (Indocin) is a potent nonsteroidal anti-inflammatory drug used in the treatment of arthritis and other inflammatory diseases. The drug is available as the free acid in tablets of 25 or 50 mg, as a 25 mg/5 mL syrup, and as a 50 mg suppository. The sodium salt is available in a 1 mg ampule for intravenous injection. Adult doses may range from 50–200 mg daily.

Blood Concentrations. After intramuscular injection of 50 mg to patients, plasma indomethacin concentrations ranged from 0.8–2.6 mg/L at 0.5 hour, from 0.4–0.6 mg/L at 3 hours and from 0.1–0.7 mg/L at 12 hours (Bannwarth et al., 1990). Following the rectal administration of a 100 mg indomethacin suppository to 12 healthy adult volunteers, an average plasma concentration of 4.0 mg/L was achieved at 1.8 hours (Taggert et al., 1987). A 250 mg oral dose given to 15 adult volunteers produced an average peak plasma concentration of 2.7 mg/L at 1 hour, declining to 1.0 mg/L by 3 hours and 0.3 mg/L by 6 hours (Settlage et al., 1983).

Metabolism and Excretion. Indomethacin and its desmethyl, desbenzoyl and desmethyldesbenzoyl metabolites, all in the unconjugated form, can be found in the plasma. The drug is excreted in the urine intact and as a glucuronide conjugate. Other metabolites have been identified as O-desmethyl-indomethacin (DMI), N-deschlorobenzoylindomethacin (DBI), and N-deschlorobenzoyl-O-desmethylindomethacin (DMBI), which are eliminated both in free form and as glucuronide conjugates (Duggan et al., 1972; Stubbs et al., 1986; Vree et al., 1993).

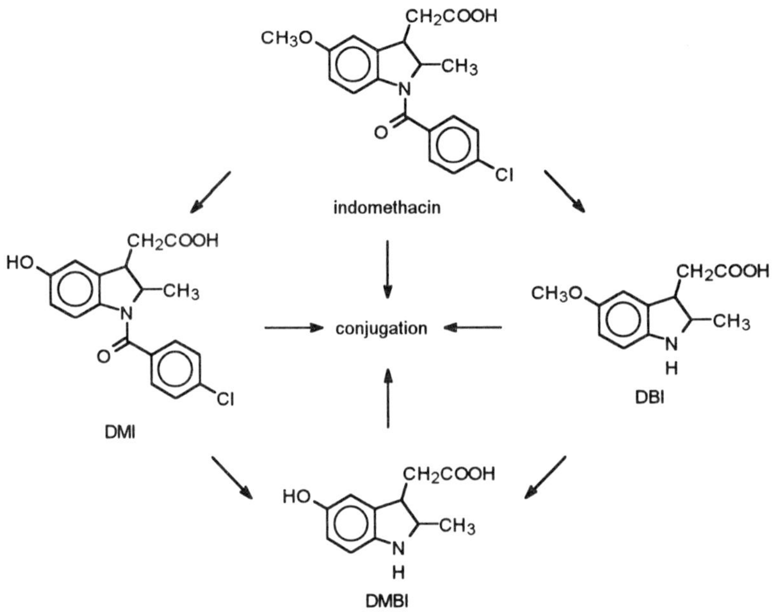

Toxicity. Adverse reactions to indomethacin therapy include gastritis, hypertension, renal toxicity and toxic hepatitis. Symptoms reported in overdose situations include nausea, vomiting, mental confusion, disorientation, paresthesias and convulsions.

A 15 year old girl who ingested 900 mg of indomethacin was given syrup of ipecac to precipitate vomiting and required no other treatment; one hour after ingestion, a plasma indomethacin concentration of 84 mg/L was reported. The same authors also reported the case of a 29 year old woman who ingested 500 mg and whose only outward sign was drowsiness; a plasma indomethacin concentration of 21 mg/L was found about 4–6 hours following ingestion (Sheehan et al., 1986).

Analysis. Indomethacin has been determined in biological fluids by gas chromatography (Evans, 1980) and gas chromatography-mass spectrometry (Dawson et al., 1990). Liquid chromatography has also been employed (Stubbs et al., 1986; Roberts and Smith, 1987; Brown et al., 1988; Avgerinos and Malamataris, 1989; Johnson and Ray, 1992; Vree et al., 1993).

References

A. Avgerinos and S. Malamataris. High-performance liquid chromatographic determination of indomethacin in human plasma and urine. J. Chrom. 495: 309–313, 1989.

B. Bannwarth, P. Netter, F. Lapicque et al. Plasma and cerebrospinal concentrations of indomethacin in humans. Eur. J. Clin. Pharm. 38: 343–346, 1990.

Y.L. Brown, R.J. Kandrotas, J.B. Douglas et al. High-performance liquid chromatographic determination of indomethacin serum concentrations. J. Chrom. 459: 275–279, 1988.

M. Dawson, M.D. Smith and C.M. McGee. Gas chromatography/negative ion chemical ionization/tandem mass spectrometric quantification of indomethacin in plasma and synovial fluid. Biomed. Env. Mass Spec. 19: 453–458, 1990.

D.E. Duggan, A.F. Hogans, K.C. Kwan and F.G. McMahon. The metabolism of indomethacin in man. J. Pharm. Exp. Ther. 181: 563–575, 1972.

M.A. Evans. GLC microdetermination of indomethacin in plasma. J. Pharm. Sci. 69: 219–220, 1980.

A.G. Johnson and J.E. Ray. Improved high-performance liquid chromatographic method for the determination of indomethacin in plasma. Ther. Drug Mon. 14: 61–65, 1992.

I. Roberts and I.M. Smith. A high-performance liquid chromatography method for the analysis of total and free indomethacin in serum. Ann. Clin. Biochem. 24: 167–171, 1987.

V.J.A. Settlage, W. Gielsdorf, M. Nieder et al. Die gaschromatographisch/massenspektometrische Bestimmung der Indometacin-Serumspiegel im Verlauf pharmakokinetischer Untersuchungen an gesunden Freiwilligen. Arz. Forsch. 33: 885–888, 1983.

T.M.T. Sheehan, D.A.R. Boldy and J.A. Vale. Indomethacin poisoning. Clin. Tox. 24: 151–158, 1986.

R.J. Stubbs, M.S. Schwartz, R. Chiou et al. Improved method for the determination of indomethacin in plasma and urine by reversed-phase high-performance liquid chromatography. J. Chrom. 383: 432–437, 1986.

A.J. Taggert, J.C. McElnay, B. Kerr and P. Passmore. The chronopharmacokinetics of indomethacin suppositories in healthy volunteers. Eur. J. Clin. Pharm. 31: 617–619, 1987.

T.B. Vree, M. Vandenbiggelaarmarten and C.P.W.G.M. Vernweyvanwissen. Determination of indomethacin, its metabolites and their glucuronides in human plasma and urine by means of direct gradient high-performance liquid chromatographic analysis. J. Chrom. 616: 271–282, 1993.

Insulin

T½: 3.5–4.3 hr
Vd: 0.37 L/kg
Fb: 0.01–0.10

Occurrence and Usage. Insulin (Iletin, Insular) is an endogenous protein hormone consisting of 2 polypeptide chains with a combined molecular weight of about 6000. Complete synthesis of the compound was achieved in 1966. Commercial preparations of insulin for use in the treatment of diabetes contain purified porcine and bovine insulin in the form of an injectable solution. Most preparations have potencies on the order of 22–30 U.S.P. units/mg, contain 100 µunits/mL of solution and are packaged in 10 mL bottles. A number of forms of the drug are available and are classified as fast-, intermediate- or long-acting on the basis of their promptness and duration of activity. They are intended for subcutaneous administration but certain forms can be given by intravenous injection. Most patients are controlled by daily doses of 5–40 units, whereas resistant patients may require doses of 200 units or more.

Blood Concentrations. Endogenous serum insulin levels for 500 normal fasting subjects were found to average 11 µunits/mL (range, 6–24) (Velasco et al., 1974) and 27 µunits/mL (range, 7–37) for 17 nonfasting subjects. These values were measured by radioimmunoassay and represent immunoreactive insulin. Patients who receive exogenous insulin soon develop antibodies that are capable of binding large amounts of the drug in the serum. Concentrations of free insulin in the serum of 21 insulin-treated diabetic patients ranged from 10–440 µunits/mL (average, 47), whereas total insulin (free plus antibody-bound) concentrations in the same subjects ranged from 67–17,020 µunits/mL (average, 2676). A radioimmunoassay technique performed directly on serum without a preliminary separation step will often yield values that are intermediate between the extremes of free and total insulin (Gennaro and Van Norman, 1975).

Metabolism and Excretion. Intravenously injected insulin has a distribution half-life of about 9 minutes in man; the compound has a volume of distribution that somewhat exceeds the volume of the extracellular fluid, and is only slightly bound to plasma protein. Although insulin is filtered at the glomerulus, it is largely reabsorbed and only minor amounts are excreted unchanged (Chamberlain and Stimmler, 1967), with metabolism by the liver and kidney accounting for the bulk of a dose (Larner and Haynes, 1975). Whereas normal subjects exhibit elimination half-lives for insulin that average 3.8 hours, persons with hepatic or renal insufficiency have half-lives of 9–42 hours. The apparent half-life of lente or crystalline insulin averages 6–8 hours in normal subjects (Van Rooyen et al., 1972).

Toxicity. Insulin overdosage ("insulin shock") causes hypoglycemia, resulting in fatigue, nervousness, nausea, chills, sweating, tachycardia, shallow breathing, hypotension and coma. Treatment usually involves administration of glucose or glucagon.

Insulin is occasionally used as a means of committing suicide or homicide; most of the recently investigated cases have involved the direct measurement of postmortem blood insulin, this being justified on the basis of the relatively large amounts of free insulin present in the specimen after acute overdosage compared to the (presumably) smaller amount bound to insulin antibodies. In the case of a diabetic who self-administered a total of 1080 units of insulin and who died within 26 hours, the level of bound insulin in the postmortem serum (1000–1100 μunits/mL) was exceeded by the level of free drug (1600–1800 μunits/mL) (Stofer, 1970). Undoubtedly, measurement of both free and bound drug would provide a higher index of certitude in interpretation of the results. The measurement of serum C-peptide (normally, 0.7–3.3 ng/mL), an inactive remnant of endogenous proinsulin, is recommended to further substantiate exogenous insulin administration (Haibach et al., 1987). Insulin concentrations of 1830–2010 μunits/mL were measured directly in the antemortem serum, drawn some hours after insulin injection, of an adult who self-administered at least 980 units and who died after 9 days. Postmortem serum contained 43 μunits/mL of insulin and the bile contained 768 μunits/mL. Bile insulin concentrations in 20 control cases ranged from 0–488 μunits/mL (average, 91), the highest level being found in a death due to alcoholism (Sturner and Putnam, 1972). An elderly woman who was intentionally administered an estimated 800 units of insulin and who died about 16 hours after being found comatose had antemortem plasma insulin concentrations of 40, 600, 7500, and 630 μunits/mL at 2.5, 8.5, and 13 hours after discovery (Bauman and Yalow, 1981).

In 3 cases in which death occurred within a short time after injection, left heart blood concentrations of 700, 714 and 1390 μunits/mL have been determined (Baselt and Cravey, 1977; Dickson et al., 1977). Another case in which a subject survived for 3 days following the self-administration of insulin showed a postmortem concentration of 224 μunits/mL (Sturner and Putnam, 1972). In 29 cases of sudden death of nondiabetic adults, insulin concentrations in right heart blood averaged 222 μunits/mL (ranging up to 2400) and in femoral venous blood averaged 23 μunits/mL (range, 5–60); these data suggest that femoral blood specimens are more likely to yield a valid result in cases of suspected insulin poisoning, although no comparison was made to left heart blood specimens (Lindquist and Rammer, 1975).

Generally, postmortem specimens of brain, liver or kidney have not shown significant amounts of insulin in either normal subjects or in victims of overdosage (Dickson et al., 1977), but in several instances tissue from the site of injection has been analyzed and the results used to prove administration of an overdose (Birkinshaw et al., 1958; Stofer, 1970; Phillips et al., 1972; Dickson et al., 1977; Heyndrickx et al., 1979). Postmortem tissue from the calf, abdomen, and buttocks of nondiabetics contains from 10–75 μunits/g (average, 30) of insulin, whereas levels as high as 17,000 μunits/g have been detected at recent injection sites. Old injection sites in diabetic patients may also contain fairly high concentrations of unabsorbed insulin, especially if long-acting forms of the drug were used (Fletcher et al., 1979). The determination of increased intracerebral pH and lowered lactic acid content may also be used to confirm insulin overdosage (Stefan, 1975).

Analysis. Insulin is most frequently assayed in biologic specimens by means of commercial radioimmunoassay systems, of which there are a number available. Body fluids may be analyzed directly, or after differential extraction of free and antibody-bound drug (Gennaro and Van Norman, 1975; Kohno et al., 1987). Tissue from injection sites has usually been subjected to extraction prior to analysis (Phillips et al., 1972; Dickson et al., 1977; Fletcher et al., 1979). The drug is relatively stable in serum for up to 7 days at room or refrigerator temperature, but loses approximately 50% of its activity within 3 days at 37° C. (Haibach et al., 1987).

References

R.C. Baselt and R.H. Cravey. A compendium of therapeutic and toxic concentrations of toxicologically significant drugs in human biofluids. J. Anal. Tox. 1: 81–103, 1977.

W.A. Bauman and R.S. Yalow. Insulin as a lethal weapon. J. For. Sci. 26: 594–598, 1981.

V.J. Birkinshaw, M.R. Gurd, S.S. Randall et al. Investigations in a case of murder by insulin poisoning. Brit. Med. J. 2: 463–468, 1958.

M.J. Chamberlain and L. Stimmler. The renal handling of insulin. J. Clin. Invest. 46: 911–919, 1967.

S.J. Dickson, E.R. Cairns and N.D. Blazey. The isolation and quantitation of insulin in postmortem specimens—a case report. For. Sci. 9: 37–42, 1977.

S.M. Fletcher, L. Richards and A.C. Moffat. The detection of fatal insulin poisoning by tissue analysis. Vet. Hum. Tox. 21 (Suppl.): 197–199, 1979.

W.D. Gennaro and J.D. Van Norman. Quantitation of free, total, and antibody-bound insulin in insulin-treated diabetics. Clin. Chem. 21: 873–879, 1975.

H. Haibach, J.D. Dix and J.H. Shah. Homicide by insulin administration. J. For. Sci. 32: 208–216, 1987.

A. Heyndrickx, C. Van Peteghem, M. Van den Heede et al. Insulin murders: isolation and identification by radio-immunoassay after several months of inhumation. In *Forensic Toxicology* (J.S. Oliver, ed.), Croom Helm, London, 1979, pp. 48–57.

T. Kohno, E. Ishikawa, S. Sugiyama et al. Enzyme immunoassay of total insulin in human serum containing anti-insulin antibodies. Clin. Chim. Acta 163: 105–112, 1987.

J. Larner and R.C. Haynes, Jr. Insulin and oral hypoglycemic drugs; glucagon. In *The Pharmacological Basis of Therapeutics*, 5th ed. (L.S. Goodman and A. Gilman, eds.), MacMillan, New York, 1975, pp. 1507–1533.

O. Lindquist and L. Rammer. Insulin in post-mortem blood. Z. Rechtsmed. 75: 275–277, 1975.

A.P. Phillips, B. Webb and A.S. Curry. The detection of insulin in postmortem tissues. J. For. Sci. 17: 460–463, 1972.

J. Stefan. Beitrag zur postmortalen Diagnose der Insulinvergiftung. Zbl. Allg. Path. 119: 56–59, 1975.

A.R. Stofer. Suicid mit Insulin und Nachweis des Insulins an der Leiche. Arch. Tox. 26: 1–7, 1970.

W.Q. Sturner and R.S. Putman. Suicidal insulin poisoning with nine day survival: recovery in bile at autopsy by radioimmunoassay. J. For. Sci. 17: 514–521, 1972.

R.J. Van Rooyen, E.J.P. De Bruin, E.U. Bieller and J.M.C. Hoog. The half-life of ^{131}I-insulin in different groups of patients compared with normal subjects. S. Afr. Med. J. 46: 1927-1931, 1972.

C.A. Velasco, H.S. Cole and R.A. Camerini-Davalos. Radioimmunoassay of insulin, with use of an immunosorbent. Clin. Chem. 20: 700-702, 1974.

Iron

T½: ?
Vd: ?
Fb: 0.99

Fe

Occurrence and Usage. Iron is the most abundant of the trace metals in the human body and is believed essential for all living cells. The average diet supplies the daily 10–20 mg of iron required by adults. In iron deficiency, ferrous sulfate (or fumarate or gluconate) is usually administered orally to adults in daily doses of 150–900 mg, equivalent to 30–180 mg of iron. Flour and some breakfast cereals and vitamin preparations in the United States contain supplemental iron.

Blood Concentrations. Serum iron concentrations undergo a diurnal variation, with the highest levels found during the afternoon or evening in most subjects. Generally, morning specimens are used for the determination of total serum iron; the 10:00 A.M. values for 26 healthy subjects averaged 1.23 mg/L and ranged from 0.27–2.93 mg/L (Wiltink et al., 1973). Serum iron-binding capacity averaged 2.5 mg/L in 15 subjects, ranging from 1.4–4.1 mg/L (Persijn et al., 1971). About two-thirds of the body's iron is present in erythrocyte hemoglobin, which is 0.347% iron by weight;

whole blood iron concentrations range from 380–560 mg/L in healthy females and from 450–625 mg/L in healthy males.

Metabolism and Excretion. Only 2–10% of dietary iron is absorbed by normal adults, but substantially more may be taken up by children and iron-deficient adults. Of that which is absorbed, about 0.2–0.5 mg is excreted in the daily feces and about 0.2–0.3 mg in urine. About one-third of the body's iron is stored in the liver, spleen and bone marrow as ferritin and hemosiderin (Reinhold, 1975). The following tissue concentrations of iron were determined at autopsy in Japanese citizens (Yukawa et al., 1980):

Iron Concentrations in Human Tissues (mg/kg)

	Brain	Lung	Liver	Spleen	Kidney
Average	48	200	120	290	66
(Range)	(8–96)	(112–280)	(29–240)	(57–590)	(7–160)

Toxicity. Acute iron intoxication is much more common in children than adults and is believed responsible for several hundred pediatric deaths annually. Gastrointestinal distress, metabolic acidosis, shock and coma are frequent clinical features of iron poisoning; deferoxamine is often administered as a chelating agent and can markedly enhance the urinary excretion of iron as a reddish-brown complex. Serum iron concentrations of 2.76–25.5 mg/L were observed initially in 11 children who survived the ingestion of up to 10 g of ferrous sulfate (Jacobs et al., 1965). Concentrations in serum are likely to be highest during the 4 hours following ingestion, and those exceeding 5 mg/L are likely to be associated with severe poisoning (James, 1970). Two adults survived the ingestion of 10 g of ferrous sulfate after developing serum iron concentrations of 6.4–9.2 mg/L (Lavender and Bell, 1970; Peck et al., 1983).

The estimated lethal dose of ferrous iron is 0.3 g/kg of body weight. Autopsy findings in victims of fatal poisoning usually include hemorrhage and necrosis of the gastrointestinal mucosa, degenerative changes in the liver, and hemorrhagic bronchopneumonia (Swift et al., 1952; Curtiss and Kosinski, 1954; Charney, 1961). Children who have died 3–5 days after the ingestion of 6–15 g of ferrous sulfate have exhibited serum iron levels of 18.8–50 mg/L on the first or second day (Barr and Fraser, 1968; deCastro et al., 1977). Normal liver and kidney iron concentrations were reported in one fatal case (Swift et al., 1952), while concentrations of 1504 and 982 mg/kg, respectively, were observed in a child who died with a serum iron of 21 mg/L (Berman, 1980). Three adults who ingested 2–23 g of ferrous iron and died within several hours to 7 days exhibited serum iron concentrations of 3.6–17 mg/L (average, 9.0) (Olenmark et al., 1987).

Analysis. Semiquantitative visual tests for serum iron utilize a chromogenic reagent such as bathophenanthroline, deferoxamine or tripyridyltriazine and are intended for emergency purposes (Fischer, 1967; Hosking, 1969; Cooper et al., 1971). Specific quantitative procedures for serum iron and iron-binding capacity rely on the spectrophotometric measurement of a colored complex formed with one of these same reagents (Persijn et al., 1971; Horak and Sunderman, 1974; Walberg, 1975; Ceriotti and Ceriotti, 1980) or on atomic absorption spectrophotometry (Olson and Hamlin, 1969); the preparation of a protein-free supernatant in these techniques avoids interferences from hemoglobin iron.

References

D.G.D. Barr and D.K.B. Fraser. Acute iron poisoning in children: role of chelating agents. Brit. Med. J. 1: 737–741, 1968.

E. Berman. *Toxic Metals and Their Analysis*, Heyden, London, 1980, pp. 110–116.

F. Ceriotti and G. Ceriotti. Improved direct specific determination of serum iron and total iron-binding capacity. Clin. Chem. 26: 327–331, 1980.

E. Charney. A fatal case of ferrous sulfate poisoning. J. Am. Med. Asso. 178: 326–327, 1961.

H.A. Cooper, M.D. Ekblad and V.F. Fairbanks. Emergency semiquantitative estimation of plasma iron concentration. Am. J. Dis. Child. 122: 19–21, 1971.

C.D. Curtiss and A.A. Kosinski. Fatal case of iron intoxication in a child. J. Am. Med. Asso. 156: 1326–1328, 1954.

F.J. deCastro, R. Jaeger and W.A. Gleason, Jr. Liver damage and hypoglycemia in acute iron poisoning. Clin. Tox. 10: 287–289, 1977.

D.S. Fischer. A method for the rapid detection of acute iron toxicity. Clin. Chem. 13: 6–11, 1967.

E. Horak and F.W. Sunderman, Jr. Direct spectrophotometric method for measurements of serum iron and latent iron-binding capacity. Am. J. Clin. Path. 62: 133–134, 1974.

C.S. Hosking. A simple rapid method of determining the approximate serum iron level in acute iron poisoning. Med. J. Aust. 1: 981–982, 1969.

J. Jacobs, H. Greene and B.R. Gendel. Acute iron intoxication. New Eng. J. Med. 273: 1124–1127, 1965.

J.A. James. Acute iron poisoning: assessment of severity and prognosis. J. Pediat. 77: 117–119, 1970.

S. Lavender and J.A. Bell. Iron intoxication in an adult. Brit. Med. J. 2: 406, 1970.

M. Olenmark, B. Biber, O. Dottori and G. Rybo. Fatal iron intoxication in late pregnancy. Clin. Tox. 25: 347–359, 1987.

A.D. Olson and W.B. Hamlin. A new method for serum iron and total iron-binding capacity by atomic absorption spectrophotometry. Clin. Chem. 15: 438–444, 1969.

M.G. Peck, J.F. Rogers and J.F. Rivenbark. Use of high doses of deferoxamine (Desferal) in an adult patient with acute iron overdosage. Clin. Tox. 19: 865–869, 1983.

J.P. Persijn, W. Van der Slik and A. Riethorst. Determination of serum iron and latent iron-binding capacity (LIBC). Clin. Chim. Acta. 35: 91–98, 1971.

J.G. Reinhold. Trace elements—a selective survey. Clin. Chem. 21: 476–500, 1975.

S.C. Swift, V. Cefalu and E.B. Rubell. Ferrous sulfate poisoning. J. Pediat. 40: 6–10, 1952.

C. Walberg. Iron, type B procedure. In *Methodology for Analytical Toxicology* (I. Sunshine, ed.), CRC Press, Cleveland, 1975, pp. 196–197.

W.F. Wiltink, J. Kruithof, C. Mol et al. Diurnal and nocturnal variations of the serum iron in normal subjects. Clin. Chim. Acta 49: 90–104, 1973.

M. Yukawa, M. Suzuki-Yasumoto, K. Amano and M. Terai. Distribution of trace elements in the human body determined by neutron activation analysis. Arch. Env. Health 35: 36–44, 1980.

Isoflurane

T½: ?
Vd: ?
Fb: ?

$CHF_2-O-CHClCF_3$

Occurrence and Usage. Isoflurane (Forane) is a volatile anesthetic used for the induction and maintenance of general anesthesia. It has a low blood:gas solubility coefficient (1.4) that allows a smaller volume of agent to be used, resulting in more rapid induction and recovery from anesthesia. Isoflurane is supplied in 100 mL amber-colored bottles.

Blood Concentrations. Eighteen patients administered isoflurane for 1 hour at end-tidal air concentrations of 0.3, 0.6 or 1.15% exhibited average steady-state blood isoflurane levels of 20, 40 and 77 mg/L, respectively (Davidkova et al., 1988).

Metabolism and Excretion. More than 99% of an inhaled dose of isoflurane is excreted unchanged in the expired breath. The major metabolites are trifluoroacetic acid and fluoride ion, which occur in the ratio of approximately 2:1 and are excreted in the urine with elimination half-lives of 41 and 36 hours, respectively. Isoflurane is eliminated rapidly after discontinuation of anesthesia and its minimal degree of biotransformation causes no significant post-anesthetic increase in plasma fluoride (Mazze et al., 1974; Davidkova et al., 1988; Smiley et al., 1991).

Toxicity. Adverse reactions to isoflurane include respiratory depression, hypotension, cardiac arrthymias, nausea and vomiting. Two deaths have been reported from isoflurane self-administration, involving either abuse or suicidal intent (Kuhlman et al., 1993):

Isoflurane Concentrations in Fatalities (mg/L or mg/kg)

	Blood	Brain	Lung	Liver	Kidney
Case 1	9.9	107	17	31	22
Case 2	46		35	97	27

Analysis. Analysis of isoflurane in biological specimens is most often accomplished by headspace gas chromatography with flame-ionization detection (Davidkova et al., 1988: Kuhlman et al., 1993).

References

T. Davidkova, H. Kikuchi, K. Fuji et al. Biotransformation of isoflurane: urinary and serum fluoride ion and organic fluorine. Anesthesiology 69: 218–222, 1988.

J.J. Kuhlman, Jr., J. Magluilo, Jr., B. Levine and M.L. Smith. Two deaths involving isoflurane abuse. J. For. Sci. 38: 968–971, 1993.

R.I. Mazze, M.J. Cousins and G.A. Barr. Renal effects and metabolism of isoflurane in man. Anesthesiology 40: 536–542, 1974.

R.M. Smiley, E. Ornstein, E.J. Pantuck et al. Metabolism of desflurane and isoflurane to fluoride ion in surgical patients. Can. J. Anaesth. 38: 965–968, 1991.

Isoniazid

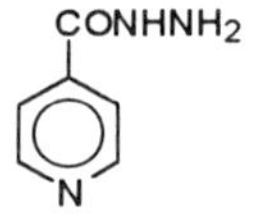

T½: 0.6–6.7 hr (genetically-determined)
Vd: 0.6 L/kg
Fb: 0
pKa: 1.9, 3.5, 10.8

Occurrence and Usage. Isoniazid (isonicotinic acid hydrazide, INH, Nydrazid) is a tuberculostatic agent in clinical use since 1952. It is available as the free base in 100 and 300 mg tablets for oral use or a 100 mg/mL solution for intramuscular injection. Daily doses of 200–500 mg are recommended for prevention or treatment of tuberculosis.

Blood Concentrations. A single 5 mg/kg (350 mg/70 kg) oral dose of isoniazid produced plasma concentrations in 10 subjects that averaged 3.0 mg/L (range, 1.2–4.8) at 1 hour, 1.4 mg/L (range, 0.2–2.7) at 4 hours, and 0.6 mg/L (range, 0.0–1.4) at 8 hours (Peters, 1960). After a 15 mg/kg (1050 mg/70 kg) oral dose, peak plasma isoniazid concentrations occurred at 1 hour and averaged 20 mg/L in 12 slow acetylators and 14 mg/L in 8 rapid acetylators; peak plasma acetylisoniazid concentrations occurred at 5 hours and averaged 4.0 and 10 mg/L, respectively. Isoniazid half-lives range from 0.6–1.8 hours in rapid acetylators and 1.8–6.7 hours in slow acetylators. The drug is completely bioavailable after oral or parenteral administration (Weber and Hein, 1979).

Metabolism and Excretion. Isoniazid is extensively metabolized by N-acetylation, hydrolysis, and hydrazone formation. Acetylhydrazine, liberated by hydrolysis, is believed to be converted to a potent acylating agent and to account for the severe liver injury occasionally encountered with isoniazid use (Mitchell et al., 1976). In rapid and slow acetylators, respectively, 46% and 29% of a single dose is excreted in the 24 hour urine as acetylisoniazid, 1.8% and 2.5% as acetylhydrazine, and 23% and 4.9% as diacetylhydrazine (Timbrell et al., 1977). From 4–20% of a dose is eliminated unchanged in the 24 hour urine (Peters, 1960). Low levels of hydrazine (<0.01 mg/L) are present in the plasma of patients receiving isoniazid (Blair et al., 1985).

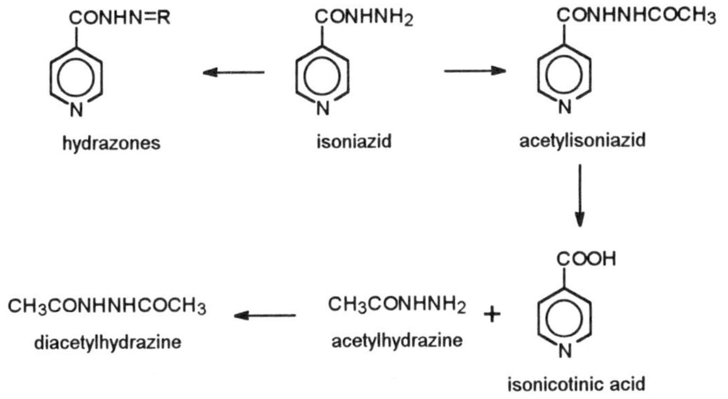

Toxicity. Adverse reactions to isoniazid therapy include peripheral neuropathy, optic neuritis, memory impairment, toxic psychosis, nausea, vomiting, fatigue, hematologic disorders, fever, skin eruptions, systemic lupus erythematosus, convulsions, and severe hepatitis.

Acute overdosage results in nausea, vomiting, blurred vision, slurred speech, hallucinations, respiratory and central nervous system depression, metabolic acidosis, hyperglycemia, seizures, and coma. Treatment is supportive and may involve peritoneal or hemodialysis or hemoperfusion. Pyridoxine is a specific antidote, replacing the endogenous pyridoxine depleted by combination with isoniazid. Pyridoxine depletion results in lowered cerebral gamma-aminobutyric acid levels, causing seizures (Terman and Teitelbaum, 1970; Mottram et al., 1974; Sievers and Herrier, 1975). Twelve persons survived the ingestion of 2–50 g of isoniazid after developing maximal plasma concentrations of 20–143 mg/L and urine concentrations of 412–1440 mg/L; several individuals suffered permanent neurological damage. Hemodialysis reduced the plasma half-life to 20 minutes in one case (Cocco and Pazourek, 1963; Sitprija and Holmes, 1964; Brown, 1972; Konigshausen et al., 1979; Sturner et al., 1985).

Two subjects died following ingestion of 10–15 g of isoniazid after achieving serum concentrations of 72 mg/L (Brown, 1972). Postmortem blood concentrations of 65–168 mg/L were measured in 3 individuals who died within a few hours of ingesting overdoses (McBay, 1968; Mathis and Noguchi, 1981; Sturner et al., 1985). An adult male who died soon after ingesting approximately 8 g of isoniazide exhibited the following tissue distribution of the drug (LoDico et al., 1992):

Isoniazid Concentrations in a Fatal Case (mg/L or mg/kg)

Blood	Liver	Kidney	Urine	Gastric
43	650	110	470	4 mg

Analysis. Isoniazid may be determined in blood or plasma after derivatization by colorimetry (Bjornesjo and Jarnulf, 1967), ultraviolet spectrophotometry (Eidus and Harnanansingh, 1971), or fluorometry (Peters, 1960; Reiss et al., 1967; Boxenbaum and Riegelman, 1974; Miceli et al., 1975; Olson et al., 1977). The drug and its metabolites have been simultaneously assayed by gas chromatography-mass spectrometry (Lauterberg et al., 1981) and liquid chromatography (Saxena et al., 1977; Moulin et al., 1981; Holdiness, 1982; Hutchings et al., 1983; Kohno et al., 1991). A significant loss of isoniazid and acetylisoniazid occurs in plasma during frozen storage, but this can be prevented by initial deproteinization of the specimen (Huffman and Dujovne, 1976).

References

K.B. Bjornesjo and B. Jarnulf. Determination of isonicotinic acid hydrazide in blood serum. Scand. J. Clin. Lab. Invest. 20: 39–40, 1967.

I.A. Blair, R.M. Tinoco, M.J. Brodie et al. Plasma hydrazine concentrations in man after isoniazid and hydralazine administration. Hum. Tox. 4: 195–202, 1985.

H.G. Boxenbaum and S. Riegelman. Determination of isoniazid and metabolites in biological fluids. J. Pharm. Sci. 63: 1191–1197, 1974.

C.V. Brown. Acute isoniazid poisoning. Am. Rev. Resp. Dis. 105: 206–216, 1972.

A.E. Cocco and L.J. Pazourek. Acute isoniazid intoxication—management by peritoneal dialysis. New Eng. J. Med. 269: 852–853, 1963.

L. Eidus and A.M.T. Harnanansingh. A more sensitive spectrophotometric method for determination of isoniazid in serum or plasma. Clin. Chem. 17: 492–494, 1971.

M.R. Holdiness. High pressure liquid chromatographic determination of isoniazid and acetylisoniazid in human plasma. J. Liq. Chrom. 5: 707–714, 1982.

D.H. Huffman and C.A. Dujovne. The instability of isoniazid and acetylisoniazid in frozen plasma. Res. Comm. Chem. Path. Pharm. 15: 203–204, 1976.

A. Hutchings, R.D. Monie, B. Spragg and P.A. Routledge. High-performance liquid chromatographic analysis of isoniazid and acetylisoniazid in biological fluids. J. Chrom. 277: 385–390, 1983.

H. Kohno, H. Kubo, K. Furukawa et al. Fluorometric determination of isoniazid and its metabolites in urine by high-performance liquid chromatography using in-line derivatization. Ther. Drug Mon. 13: 428–432, 1991.

T. Konigshausen, G. Altrogge, D. Hein et al. Hemodialysis of hemoperfusion in the treatment of most severe INH-poisoning. Vet. Hum. Tox. 21: 12–15, 1979.

B.H. Lauterburg, C.V. Smith and J.R. Mitchell. Determination of isoniazid and its hydrazino metabolites acetylisoniazid, acetylhydrazine, and diacetylhydrazine in human plasma by gas chromatography-mass spectrometry. J. Chrom. 224: 431–438, 1981.

C.P. LoDico, B.S. Levine, B.A. Goldberger and Y.H. Caplan. Distribution of isoniazid in an overdose death. J. Anal. Tox. 16: 57–59, 1992.

D.F. Mathis and T.T. Noguchi. Determination of isoniazid in blood using G.C. and T.L.C. Presented at the 33rd annual meeting of the American Academy of Forensic Sciences, Los Angeles, February 19, 1981.

A.J. McBay. Personal communication, 1968.

J.N. Miceli, W.A. Olson and W.W. Weber. An improved micro spectrofluorometric assay for determining isoniazid in serum. Biochem. Med. 12: 348–355, 1975.

J.R. Mitchell, H.J. Zimmerman, K.G. Ishak et al. Isoniazid liver injury: clinical spectrum, pathology, and probable pathogenesis. Ann. Int. Med. 84: 181–192, 1976.

P.E. Mottram, P.B. Johnson and J.E. Hoffman. Isoniazid toxicity. Minn. Med. 57: 81–83, 1974.

M.A. Moulin, F. Albessard, J. Lacotte and R. Camsonne. Hydrophilic ion-pair reversed-phase high-performance liquid chromatography for the simultaneous assay of isoniazid and acetylisoniazid in serum: a microscale procedure. J. Chrom. 226: 250–254, 1981.

W.A. Olson, P.G. Dayton, Z.H. Israili and A.W. Pruitt. Spectrophotofluorometric assay for isoniazid and acetyl isoniazid in plasma adapted to pediatric studies. Clin. Chem. 23: 745–748, 1977.

J.H. Peters. Studies on the metabolism of isoniazid. Am. Rev. Resp. Dis. 81: 485–497, 1960.

O.K. Reiss, W.C. Morse and R.W. Putsch. A chemical determination of isoniazid in serum. Am. Rev. Resp. Dis. 96: 111–114, 1967.

J. Saxena, J.T. Stewart, I.L. Honigberg et al. Liquid chromatography in pharmaceutical analysis VIII: determination of isoniazid and acetyl derivative in plasma and urine samples. J. Pharm. Sci. 66: 813–816, 1977.

M.L. Sievers and R.N. Herrier. Treatment of acute isoniazid toxicity. Am. J. Hosp. Pharm. 32: 202–206, 1975.

V. Sitprija and J.H. Holmes. Isoniazid intoxication. Am. Rev. Resp. Dis. 90: 248–254, 1964.

W.Q. Sturner, N. Haley, H. Martin and P. Ullucci. Suicidal isoniazid intoxication in Cambodian-refugee teenage girls. In *Proceedings of the 21st International Meeting*, International Association of Forensic Toxicologists, Brighton, England, September 13–17, 1985.

D.S. Terman and D.T. Teitelbaum. Isoniazid self-poisoning. Neurology 20: 299–304, 1970.

J.A. Timbrell, J.M. Wright and T.A. Baillie. Monoacetylhydrazine as a metabolite of isoniazid in man. Clin. Pharm. Ther. 22: 602–608, 1977.

W.W. Weber and D.W. Hein. Clinical pharmacokinetics of isoniazid. Clin. Pharmacokin. 4: 401–422, 1979.

Isopropanol

T½: 2.5–3.0 hr
Vd: 0.6 L/kg
Fb: ?

CH₃CHOHCH₃

Occurrence and Usage. Isopropanol (isopropyl alcohol, 2-propanol) is a common industrial and laboratory chemical that is also readily available to the public in a 70% aqueous solution for use as rubbing alcohol. It has about twice the central nervous system depressant potency of ethanol, but is less toxic than methanol. The current threshold limit value in industrial situations is 400 ppm (983 mg/m³) and the estimated anesthetic concentration is 10,000 ppm. Exposure may occur by either inhalation or dermal absorption.

Blood Concentrations. In 3 workers exposed to 470–493 mg/m³ isopropanol in air for 8 hours, blood isopropanol concentrations were below the level of detectability (0.001 g/dL); blood acetone concentrations ranged from 0.004–0.016 g/dL during the exposure (Brugnone et al., 1983). After a sponge bath with isopropanol, one adult subject was noted to have a blood isopropanol level of 0.010 g/dL (Wise, 1969).

Metabolism and Excretion. Isopropanol is slowly metabolized in man, probably by alcohol dehydrogenase, to acetone, which contributes to the depressant effects of the alcohol. Both compounds are eliminated to a small degree in the breath and urine, and acetone is probably further metabolized to acetate, formate and carbon dioxide (Kemal, 1927). Isopropanol exhibits first-order kinetics in man, with an average elimination half-life in 2 subjects of 2.8 hours (Daniel et al., 1981). The acetone that is formed has a half-life on the order of 22 hours (Natowicz et al., 1985). Urine isopropanol and acetone concentrations ranged from 0–2.5 and 0–20 mg/L, respectively, in workers exposed to air isopropanol levels of 1–66 ppm for 8 hours (Kawai et al., 1990).

Toxicity. Exposure to isopropanol at air concentrations of 400–800 ppm produces primarily irritation of the eyes, nose and throat. Higher concentrations may cause nausea, headache, dizziness and coma. Chronic toxicity from isopropanol has not been reported, although muscle weakness, hemolytic anemia, and acute renal failure were observed in a chronic alcoholic believed to have been abusing isopropanol (Juncos and Taguchi, 1968).

An acute lethal dose of isopropanol by ingestion has been estimated at 240 mL for an adult. Several poisoning episodes in children have been reported following excessive use of the alcohol for sponging; blood isopropanol concentrations of 0.040, 0.128 and 0.130 g/dL were noted in 3 comatose children (Garrison, 1953; Senz and Goldfarb, 1958; McFadden and Haddow, 1969). Each of these children survived the intoxication, which probably resulted from inhalation of the alcohol vapors. Hemodialysis has been used successfully in the treatment of 2 comatose adults who each ingested about 1 liter of 70% isopropanol. In the first case, blood concentrations were initially 0.346 and 0.117 g/dL of isopropanol and acetone, respectively, and were 0.060 and 0.150 g/dL, respectively, when the patient awoke. Urine concentrations of isopropanol and acetone over the 2 day period of observation were 7–9% higher an the respective blood concentrations (Freireich et al., 1967). In the second case, the blood concentrations of isopropanol and acetone when hemodialysis was begun were 0.440 and 0.040 g/dL, respectively, and converged to 0.100 g/dL for each substance when the subject revived, after 5 hours of dialysis (King et al., 1970). The apparent elimination half-lives of isopropanol and acetone in 5 poisoned adults ranged from 2.9–16 hours and 7.6–26 hours, respectively (Pappas et al,. 1991).

Adelson (1962) has presented clinical and laboratory data in 5 cases of fatal isopropanol intoxication; the victims, all adults, died within 3.5 hours to 15 days of ingesting an estimated 1 pint of 70% isopropanol in most cases. Two men who died within 6 hours of ingestion were both found to have blood isopropanol concentrations of 0.150 g/dL at autopsy. The tissues of the persons who survived for longer periods were observed to contain only acetone. In a study of 31 deaths attributed to isopropanol poisoning, postmortem blood isopropanol concentrations ranged from 0.01–0.25 g/dL (average, 0.14) and acetone blood concentrations ranged from 0.04–0.30 g/dL (average, 0.17) (Alexander et al., 1982). A woman who died about 3 hours after ingesting isopropanol was found to have the following distribution of the chemical and its metabolite (Cravey, 1978):

Isopropanol and Acetone Concentrations in a Fatal Case (g/dL or g/100 g)

	Blood	Brain	Urine	Gastric
Isopropanol	0.33	0.18	0.20	3.4
Acetone	0.12	0.06	0.07	0.1

Analysis. Isopropanol and its metabolite acetone are frequently determined in body fluids and tissues using the gas chromatographic techniques cited in the section on ethanol.

References

L. Adelson. Fatal intoxication with isopropyl alcohol (rubbing alcohol). Am. J. Clin. Path. 38: 144–151, 1962.

C.B. Alexander, A.J. McBay and R.P. Hudson. Isopropanol and isopropanol deaths—ten years experience. J. For. Sci. 27: 541–548, 1982.

F. Brugnone, L. Perbellini, P. Apostoli et al. Isopropanol exposure: environmental and biological monitoring in a printing works. Brit. J. Ind. Med. 40: 160–168, 1983.

R.H. Cravey. Personal communication, 1978.

D.R. Daniel, B.H. McAnalley and J.C. Garriott. Isopropyl alcohol metabolism after acute intoxication in humans. J. Anal. Tox. 5: 110–112, 1981.

A.W. Freireich, T.J. Cinque, G. Xanthaky and D. Landau. Hemodialysis for isopropanol poisoning. New Eng. J. Med. 277: 699–700, 1967.

R.F. Garrison. Acute poisoning from use of isopropanol alcohol in tepid sponging. J. Am. Med. Asso. 152: 317–318, 1953.

L. Juncos and J.T. Taguchi. Isopropyl alcohol intoxication; report of a case associated with myopathy, renal failure, and hemolytic anemia. J. Am. Med. Asso. 204: 186–188, 1968.

T. Kawai, T. Yasugi, S. Horiguchi et al. Biological monitoring of occupational exposure to isopropyl alcohol vapor by urinalysis for acetone. Int. Arch. Occ. Env. Health 62: 409–413, 1990.

H. Kemal. Beitrag zur Kenntnis der Schicksale des Isopropylalkohols in menschlichen Organismus. Biochem. Z. 187: 461–466, 1927.

L.H. King, Jr., K.P. Bradley and D.L. Shires, Jr. Hemodialysis for isopropyl alcohol poisoning. J. Am. Med. Asso. 211: 1855, 1970.

S.W. McFadden and J.E. Haddow. Coma produced by topical application of isopropanol. Pediatrics 43: 622–623, 1969.

M. Natowicz, J. Donahue, L. Gorman et al. Pharmacokinetic analysis of a case of isopropanol intoxication. Clin. Chem. 31: 326–328, 1985.

A.A. Pappas, B.H. Ackerman, K.M. Olsen and E.H. Taylor. Isopropanol ingestion: a report of six episodes with isopropanol and acetone serum concentration time data. Clin. Tox. 29: 11–21, 1991.

E.H. Senz and D.L. Goldfarb. Coma in a child following use of isopropyl alcohol in sponging. J. Pediat. 53: 322–323, 1958.

J.R. Wise, Jr. Alcohol sponge baths. New Eng. J. Med. 280: 840, 1969.

Isoproterenol

T½: 2.5 hr
Vd: 0.5 L/kg
Fb: 0.65
pKa: 8.6

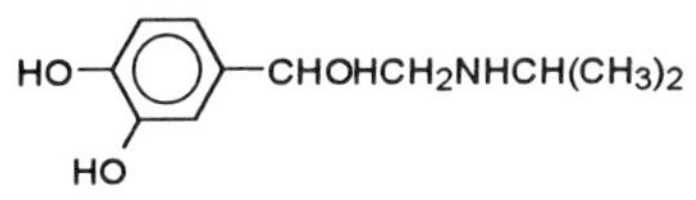

HO—⟨○⟩—CHOHCH$_2$NHCH(CH$_3$)$_2$
HO

Occurrence and Usage. Isoproterenol (isoprenaline, isopropylnoradrenaline, Isuprel, Norisodrine) is a synthetic beta-receptor stimulant that was first investigated in 1940. The drug is frequently administered orally for the treatment of bronchial asthma in daily doses of 30–180 mg, or by inhalation of an aerosol that delivers from 0.25–2.5 mg per usage. Intravenous infusion at the rate of 0.5–30 μg/min may be performed in the therapy of shock, cardiac arrest, ventricular arrhythmia and anesthetic bronchospasm. It is available as the hydrochloride or sulfate of the racemate, although the l-isomer has 50 times the activity of the d-isomer.

Blood Concentrations. An intravenous injection of 0.063 μg/kg (4.4 μg/70 kg) produced an initial maximal plasma concentration of about 0.0004 mg/L; the elimination half-life was estimated at 2.5 hours. The only available data are based on ^{3}H-labeled drug, however, and it has been shown that after 15–30 minutes less than 10% of the plasma radioactivity represents unchanged drug. With intravenous administration, up to 48% of the radioactivity in plasma is represented by 3-0-methylisoproterenol, a metabolite that is said to have weak beta-blocking activity. After an oral dose of 0.2 mg/kg essentially all of the detectable plasma radioactivity is conjugated isoproterenol, with levels approaching 0.5 mg/L at 1.5 hours (Conolly et al., 1972; Kadar et al., 1974).

Metabolism and Excretion. Isoproterenol is rapidly metabolized by 3-0-methylation and by sulfate conjugation of this methylated metabolite and the parent drug. After oral administration, nearly the entire dose is excreted in the 24 hour urine as free (4%) and conjugated (68–94%) isoproterenol and free (0–1%) and conjugated (2–8%) 3-0-methylisoproterenol. The metabolite pattern after aerosol inhalation resembles that of oral administration, since much of an inhaled dose is swallowed. After intravenous administration, up to 93% of a dose is eliminated in the 24 hour urine as unchanged drug (5–14%) and its conjugate (7–16%) and as 3-0-methylisoproterenol (4–9%) and its conjugate (70–82%) (Morgan et al., 1969; Blackwell et al., 1970; Kadar et al., 1974).

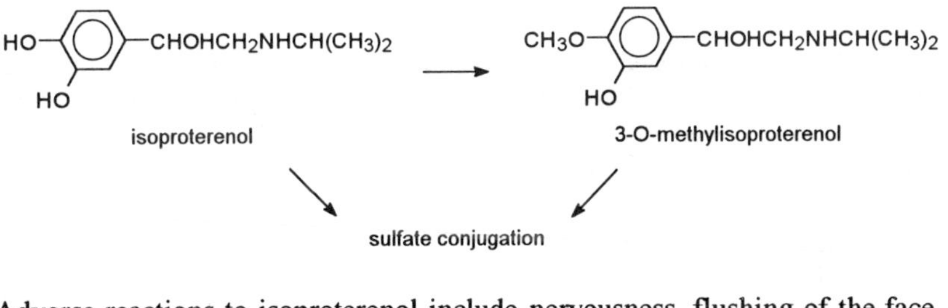

HO—⟨○⟩—CHOHCH$_2$NHCH(CH$_3$)$_2$ $\longrightarrow$ CH$_3$O—⟨○⟩—CHOHCH$_2$NHCH(CH$_3$)$_2$
HO   HO
isoproterenol   3-O-methylisoproterenol

sulfate conjugation

Toxicity. Adverse reactions to isoproterenol include nervousness, flushing of the face, sweating, tremors, headache, nausea, dizziness, weakness, heart palpitation, and pulmonary edema in hypersensitive individuals.

The excessive use of pressurized isoproterenol inhalers has been implicated in the deaths of a number of asthmatic patients (Speizer et al., 1968). It is theorized that either acute tolerance develops to isoproterenol, with cross-tolerance to endogenous sympathomimetics (Conolly et al., 1971), or the fluorocarbon propellants in these units sensitize the myocardium to the adrenergic effects of the drug and of circulating epinephrine, resulting in ventricular fibrillation (Taylor and Harris, 1970; Dollery et al., 1974). One asthmatic patient who died in this manner was found to have a postmortem blood concentration of 0.106 mg/L as unconjugated isoproterenol (Backer et al., 1978).

Analysis. The estimation of isoproterenol in body fluids may be accomplished quantitatively by fluorimetry or semi-quantitatively by thin-layer chromatography (Morgan et al., 1969). Liquid chromatography has also been described (Kishimoto et al., 1982).

References

R.C. Backer, I.M. Sopher and G.A. Johnson. An unusually high isoproterenol blood level in a bronchial asthma death. Presented at the 8th international meeting of the International Association of Forensic Sciences, Wichita, Kansas, May 22–26, 1978.

E.W. Blackwell, M.E. Conolly, D.S. Davies and C.T. Dollery. The fate of isoprenaline administered by pressurized aerosols. Brit. J. Pharm. 39: 194P–195P, 1970.

M.E. Conolly, D.S. Davies, C.T. Dollery and C.F. George. Resistance to α-adrenoceptor stimulants (a possible explanation for the rise in asthma deaths). Brit. J. Pharm. 43: 389–402, 1971.

M.E. Conolly, D.S. Davies, C.T. Dollery et al. Metabolism of isoprenaline in dog and man. Brit. J. Pharm. 46: 458–472, 1972.

C.T. Dollery, F.M. Williams, G.H. Draffan et al. Arterial blood levels of fluorocarbons in asthmatic patients following use of pressurized aerosols. Clin. Pharm. Ther. 15: 59–66, 1974.

D. Kadar, H.Y. Tang and A.W. Conn. Isoproterenol metabolism in children after intravenous administration. Clin. Pharm. Ther. 16: 789–795, 1974.

Y. Kishimoto, S. Ohgitani, A. Yamatodani et al. Method for the simplified analysis of deproteinized plasma and urinary isoproterenol by high-performance liquid chromatography. J. Chrom. 231: 121–127, 1982.

C.D. Morgan, C.R.J. Ruthven and M. Sandler. The quantitative assessment of isoprenaline metabolism in man. Clin. Chim. Acta 26: 381–386, 1969.

F.E. Speizer, R. Doll, P. Heaf and L.B. Strang. Investigation into use of drugs preceding death from asthma. Brit. Med. J. 1: 339–343, 1968.

G.J. Taylor and W.S. Harris. Cardiac toxicity of aerosol propellants. J. Am. Med. Asso. 214: 81–85, 1970.

Isosorbide Dinitrate

T½: 30–50 min
Vd: 6.3–8.9 L/kg
Fb: ?

Occurrence and Usage. Isosorbide dinitrate (Dilatrate, Isordil, Sorbitrate) is an organic nitrate vasodilator that has been in clinical use since 1960. Other such agents include nitroglycerin and pentaerythritol tetranitrate. The drug is available in the form of sublingual tablets (2.5–5 mg), chewable tablets (5–10 mg), or regular (5–40 mg) or sustained-release (40 mg) tablets and capsules. Daily doses of 40–120 mg are recommended.

Blood Concentrations. The oral administration of 5 mg of isosorbide dinitrate to 6 subjects produced an average peak plasma concentration of 3.1 µg/L at 30 minutes, declining to 0.7 µg/L by 2 hours. After sublingual administration of 5 mg, plasma concentrations in the same subjects averaged 8.9 µg/L at 15 minutes and fell to 0.8 µg/L by 2 hours. The elimination half-life averaged 40 minutes (Assinder et al., 1977). In another study, the sublingual administration of 5 mg to 6 subjects resulted in an average peak plasma concentration of 15.9 µg/L at 30 minutes (Mansel-Jones et al., 1978). In a similar study, peak plasma concentrations of isosorbide dinitrate, 2-isosorbide mononitrate, and 5-isosorbide mononitrate averaged 17.9, 9.0, and 38.4 µg/L at 10, 52, and 88 minutes, respectively. The respective average half-lives were 0.48, 1.76, and 7.56 hours (Sporl-Radun et al., 1980). Oral administration of a 40 mg sustained-release formulation produced peak plasma concentrations of these 3 agents of 2.1, 5.8, and 25.8 µg/L at 5, 3.5, and 9 hours, respectively (Gladigau et al., 1981).

Peak plasma concentrations of these 3 agents in 8 patients receiving chronic high dose oral therapy (360–720 mg daily) ranged from 46–224, 179–512, and 912–1975 µg/L, respectively (Shane et al., 1978).

Metabolism and Excretion. A total of 99.8% of a labeled dose of isosorbide dinitrate is excreted in the 5 day urine, primarily as isosorbide glucuronide. 2-Isosorbide mononitrate and 5-isosorbide mononitrate, which accumulate in the plasma and have some pharmacological activity, are minor urinary metabolites (Chasseaud et al., 1975).

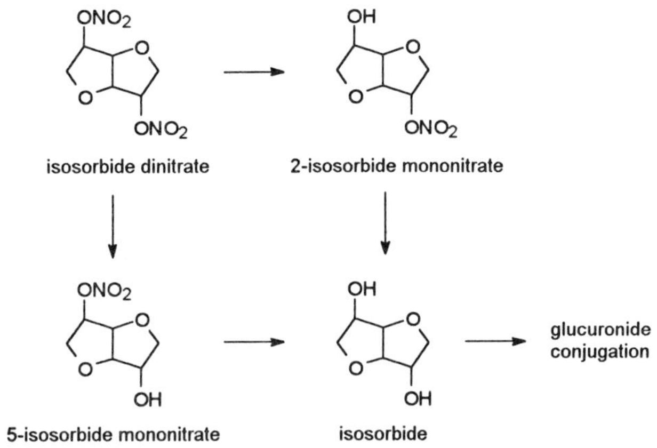

Toxicity. Adverse reactions to isosorbide dinitrate include flushing of the skin, headache, dizziness, weakness, restlessness, postural hypotension, sweating, and collapse. Mild hypotension and tachycardia developed in 15 of 18 volunteers receiving a 5 mg sublingual dose; the other 3 subjects became severely hypotensive even though recumbent (Sporl-Radun et al., 1980). Resistance to these effects seems to develop in patients on high dose therapy (Shane et al., 1978).

Analysis. Isosorbide dinitrate and its mononitrate metabolites are commonly assayed in plasma by electron-capture gas chromatography (Rosseel and Bogaert, 1973; Chin et al., 1977; Malbica et al., 1977; Laufen et al., 1978; Doyle et al., 1980; Sioufi and Pommier, 1982).

References

D.F. Assinder, L.F. Chasseaud and T. Taylor. Plasma isosorbide dinitrate concentrations in human subjects after administration of standard and sustained-release formulations. J. Pharm. Sci. 66: 775–778, 1977.

L.F. Chasseaud, W.H. Down and R.K. Grundy. Concentrations of the vasodilator isosorbide dinitrate and its metabolites in the blood of human subjects. Eur. J. Clin. Pharm. 8: 157–160, 1975.

D.A. Chin, D.G. Prue, J. Michelucci et al. Quantitative determination of isosorbide dinitrate and two metabolites in plasma. J. Pharm. Sci. 66: 1143–1145, 1977.

E. Doyle, L.F. Chasseaud and T. Taylor. Measurement of plasma concentrations of isosorbide dinitrate. Biopharm. Drug Disp. 1: 141–147, 1980.

V. Gladigau, G. Neurath, M. Dunger et al. Plasma levels of isosorbide dinitrate and its main metabolites following oral administration of two sustained release formulations in normal man. Arz. Forsch. 31: 835–840, 1981.

H. Laufen, F. Scharpf and G. Bartsch. Improved method for the rapid determination of isosorbide dinitrate in human plasma and its application in pharmacokinetic studies. J. Chrom. 146: 457–464, 1978.

J.O. Malbica, K. Monson, K. Neilson and R. Sprissler. Electron-capture GLC determination of nanogram to picogram amounts of isosorbide dinitrate. J. Pharm. Sci. 66: 384–386, 1977.

D. Mansel-Jones, T. Taylor, E. Doyle et al. Plasma concentrations of isosorbide dinitrate after cutaneous and sublingual doses to human subjects. J. Clin. Pharm. 18: 544–548, 1978.

M.T. Rosseel and M.G. Bogaert. GLC determination of nitroglycerin and isosorbide dinitrate in human plasma. J. Pharm. Sci. 62: 754–758, 1973.

S.J. Shane, J.J. Iazzetta, A.W. Chisholm et al. Plasma concentrations of isosorbide dinitrate and its metabolites after chronic high oral dosage in man. Brit. J. Clin. Pharm. 6: 37–41, 1978.

A. Sioufi and F. Pommier. Gas chromatographic determination of isosorbide dinitrate in human plasma and urine. J. Chrom. 229: 347–353, 1982.

S. Sporl-Radun, G. Betzien, B. Kaufmann et al. Effects and pharmacokinetics of isosorbide dinitrate in normal man. Eur. J. Clin. Pharm. 18: 237–244, 1980.

Kanamycin

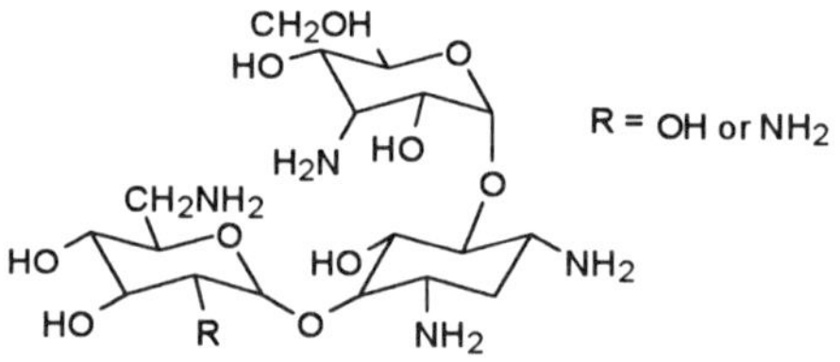

T½: 2–5 hr
Vd: 0.2–0.3 L/kg
Fb: 0.03
pKa: 7.2

Occurrence and Usage. Kanamycin (Kantrex) is an aminoglycoside antibiotic, first described in 1957, used to treat serious gram-negative bacillary infections. The drug is a mixture of kanamycin A (95%) and kanamycin B (5%). It is supplied as the sulfate in 500 mg capsules for oral administration and as a 38–333 mg/mL solution for intravenous or intramuscular injection. In adults, daily oral doses may range from 6–12 g, while injected doses should not exceed 1.5 g daily.

Blood Concentrations. Peak plasma kanamycin concentrations averaged 22 mg/L at 1.0–1.5 hours after a 7.5 mg/kg (525 mg/70 kg) intramuscular dose in 10 normal subjects. When this dose was repeated every 12 hours for 3 days, the average pre-dose plasma concentration was 1.1 mg/L and the peak concentration was essentially unchanged at 23 mg/L. A 2 g intramuscular dose produced an average peak plasma concentration of 92 mg/L at 1 hour. The mean elimination half-life in these subjects was 2.4 hours (Doluisio et al., 1973). The half-life of kanamycin increases with decreasing renal function, and correlates well with serum creatinine. The half-life is approximately 10 hours at a serum creatinine concentration of 3 mg/dL, 18 hours at 6 mg/dL, and 28 hours at 10 mg/dL (Cutler and Orme, 1969). Peak serum kanamycin concentrations should fall in the range of 10–30 mg/L for therapeutic efficacy and trough levels in the range of 5–10 mg/L for safety (Mawer et al., 1972).

Metabolism and Excretion. Kanamycin is believed to be eliminated unchanged in the urine. An average of 81% of a single dose is eliminated in the 12 hour urine, and during chronic therapy essentially the entire dose may be accounted for in the daily urine (Doluisio et al., 1973).

Toxicity. Kanamycin produced ototoxicity, characterized by tinnitus, dizziness, or hearing loss, in 22 of 106 patients who received the drug parenterally. Impairment of renal function may also occur, manifested by oliguria and azotemia, but is usually reversible (Finegold, 1966). Serum concentrations above 30–35 mg/L are considered potentially toxic (Mawer et al., 1972).

Analysis. Microbiological assays for kanamycin and other aminoglycoside antibiotics have largely been supplanted by more sensitive and specific tests involving enzyme immunoassay, radioimmunoassay, and enzymatic radiochemical assay (Maitra et al., 1979). Fluorometry (Csiba, 1979), gas chromatography (Mayhew and Gorbach, 1978), and high-pressure liquid chromatography (Anhalt and Brown, 1978) have also been investigated.

References

J.P. Anhalt and S.D. Brown. High-performance liquid-chromatographic assay of aminoglycoside antibiotics in serum. Clin. Chem. 24: 1940–1947, 1978.

A. Csiba. Spectrofluorimetric method for aminoglycoside antibiotics. J. Pharm. Pharmac. 31: 115–116, 1979.

R.E. Cutler and B.M. Orme. Correlation of serum creatinine concentration and kanamycin half-life. J. Am. Med. Asso. 209: 539–542, 1969.

J.T. Doluisio, L.W. Dittert and J.C. LaPiana. Pharmacokinetics of kanamycin following intramuscular administration. J. Pharmacokin. Biopharm. 1: 253–265, 1973.

S.M. Finegold. Toxicity of kanamycin in adults. Ann. N.Y. Acad. Sci. 132: 942–956, 1966.

S.K. Maitra, T.T. Yoshikawa, L.B. Guze and M.C. Schotz. Determination of aminoglycoside antibiotics in biological fluids: a review. Clin. Chem. 25: 1361–1367, 1979.

G.E. Mawer, B.R. Knowles, S.B. Lucas et al. Computer-assisted prescribing of kanamycin for patients with renal insufficiency. Lancet 1: 12–15, 1972.

J.W. Mayhew and S.L. Gorbach. Gas-liquid chromatographic method for the assay of aminoglycoside antibiotics in serum. J. Chrom. 151: 133–146, 1978.

Kerosene

T½: ?
Vd: ?
Fb: ?

Occurrence and Usage. Kerosene (kerosine) is a petroleum distillate of moderate volatility that consists largely of straight-chain hydrocarbons between 9 and 16 carbons in length. It also contains varying amounts of aromatic, cyclic, and unsaturated straight-chain hydrocarbons. The compound is widely used as a fuel, a vehicle for pesticides, and a cleaning agent and paint thinner.

Blood Concentrations. Kerosene has not been measured in the blood of asymptomatic or occupationally-exposed individuals.

Metabolism and Excretion. In rats, kerosene is slowly absorbed from the gastrointestinal tract, reaching maximal levels in lungs, liver, kidneys, and brain within 8–24 hours after ingestion (Ashkenazi and Berman, 1961).

Toxicity. Ingestion of kerosene typically produces vomiting with aspiration of the liquid into the lungs, resulting in fulminating, hemorrhagic bronchopneumonia. Absorption causes central nervous system depression and mild degenerative changes of the major visceral organs. Death results in about 7% of all cases and may occur within 2–24 hours of the ingestion of several ounces. Authorities differ on the management of acute kerosene poisoning, with some strongly advising gastric lavage to remove unabsorbed chemical (Deichmann et al., 1944; Olstad and Lord, 1952; McNally, 1956) while others feel lavage should be avoided except in the most severe cases to prevent possible aspiration (Lesser et al., 1943; Reed et al., 1950; Foley et al., 1954; Baldachin and Melmed, 1964; Cachia and Fenech, 1964). Brown et al. (1974) found experimentally that corticosteroid therapy may be deleterious in kerosene bronchopneumonia.

Analysis. Kerosene may be quantitatively determined in blood by colorimetry (Gerarde and Skiba, 1960). It has been qualitatively identified in lung tissue by thermal conductivity gas chromatography and infrared spectrophotometry after isolation by steam distillation (Johnston et al., 1965). Gas chromatography-mass spectrometry has also been described (Kimura et al., 1988; Shiono et al., 1989).

References

A.E. Ashkenazi and S.E. Berman. Experimental kerosene poisoning in rats. Pediatrics 28: 642–649, 1961.

B.J. Baldachin and R.N. Melmed. Clinical and therapeutic aspects of kerosene poisoning: a series of 200 cases. Brit. Med. J. 2: 28–30, 1964.

J. Brown, B. Burke and A.S. Dajani. Experimental kerosene pneumonia: evaluation of some therapeutic regimens. J. Pediat. 84: 396–401, 1974.

E.A. Cachia and F.F. Fenech. Kerosene poisoning in children. Arch. Dis. Child. 39: 502–504, 1964.

W.B. Deichmann, K.V. Kitzmiller, S. Witherup and R. Johansmann. Kerosene intoxication. Ann. Int. Med. 21: 803–823, 1944.

J.C. Foley, N.B. Dreyer, A.B. Soule, Jr. and E. Woll. Kerosene poisoning in young children. Radiology 62: 817–829, 1954.

H.W. Gerarde and P. Skiba. Toxicologic studies on hydrocarbons. VI. A colorimetric method for the determination of kerosine in blood. Clin. Chem. 6: 327–331, 1960.

G.W. Johnston, W.S. Hoch and W.C. Butz. Recovery of hydrocarbons from lung tissue in fatal ingestion of furniture polish. Am. J. Clin. Path. 43: 570–574, 1965.

L.I. Lesser, H.S. Weens and J.D. McKey. Pulmonary manifestations following ingestion of kerosene. J. Pediat. 23: 352–364, 1943.

K. Kimura, T. Nagata, K. Hara and M. Kageura. Gasoline and kerosene components in blood—a forensic analysis. Hum. Tox. 7: 299–305, 1988.

W.D. McNally. Kerosene poisoning in children. J. Pediat. 48: 296–299, 1956.

R.B. Olstad and R.M. Lord, Jr. Kerosene intoxication. Am. J. Dis. Child. 83: 446–453, 1952.

E.S. Reed, S. Leikin and H.D. Kerman. Kerosene intoxication. Am. J. Dis. Child. 79: 623–632, 1950.

H. Shiono, K. Matsubara, A. Akane et al. Immolation after drinking kerosene. Am. J. For. Med. Path. 10: 229–231, 1989.

Ketamine

T½: 3–4 hr
Vd: 3–5 L/kg
Fb: 0.30
pKa: 7.5

Occurrence and Usage. Ketamine (Ketaject, Ketalar) is a weakly basic amino compound, available as the hydrochloride salt, that has been used in the United States as an anesthetic induction agent since 1972. It is structurally and pharmacologically related to phencyclidine, a drug that failed clinical trials due to its unpleasant side effects during anesthetic recovery. Phencyclidine is now a popular street drug, and ketamine, which is capable of producing some of the same halucinogenic side effects, has reportedly received attention as a drug of abuse. It is supplied as a 10–100 mg/mL solution for intravenous injection of 1–4.5 mg/kg or intramuscular injection of 6.5–13 mg/kg.

Blood Concentrations. Following intravenous administration of 2.5 mg/kg (175 mg/70 kg) to 5 patients, an average serum concentration of 1.0 mg/L was observed at 12 minutes after injection, declining to 0.5 mg/L by 30 minutes. The serum half-life was estimated at 3.4 hours for the unchanged drug (Wieber et al., 1975). In another study, plasma concentrations as high as 5.8–6.3 mg/L were found 5 minutes after the intravenous injection of 4 mg/kg (280 mg/70 kg) ketamine in 3 patients (Hodshon et al., 1972). The intravenous administration to 31 patients of 2 mg/kg of the drug followed by continuous infusion of 41 µg/kg/min produced an average steady-state plasma ketamine concentration of 2.21 mg/L; peak concentrations of norketamine (1.05 mg/L) and dehydronorketamine (0.71 mg/L) occurred near the end of the 3 hour infusion. After the procedure, patients awoke at an average plasma ketamine concentration of 0.64 mg/L (Idvall et al., 1979).

Metabolism and Excretion. Ketamine is metabolized to at least 2 compounds of pharmacological interest: first, by N-demethylation, to norketamine, which then undergoes dehydrogenation to dehydronorketamine. These 2 metabolites achieve concentrations in serum similar to those of ketamine itself (Wieber et al., 1975). Norketamine has been shown to exhibit depressant effects similar to those of ketamine (Cohen and Trevor, 1974) and it is likely that dehydronorketamine is also active, although the contribution of these 2 metabolites to the overall effects of the drug remains to be elucidated. Over a 72 hour period a single dose of ketamine is eliminated primarily in the urine as unchanged drug (2.3%), norketamine (1.6%), dehydronorketamine (16.2%), and conjugates of hydroxylated derivatives of ketamine (80%) (Wieber et al., 1975; Anonymous, 1970). It has been suggested that dehydronorketamine is an artifact of the analytical procedure rather than a metabolite (Stenberg and Idvall, 1981).

A 46 year old male trauma patient who received 100 mg ketamine intravenously prior to surgery and died from his wounds within 40 minutes had the following postmortem results (Peyton et al., 1988):

Ketamine Concentrations During Therapy (mg/L or mg/kg)

Blood	Brain	Liver	Kidney
3.0	4.0	0.8	0.6

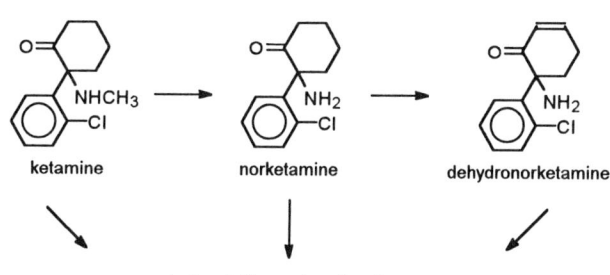

Toxicity. Adverse reactions to ketamine include hallucinations, delerium, irrational behavior, blurred vision, nausea, vomiting, respiratory stimulation or depression, tachycardia or bradycardia, hypertension or hypotension, seizures, and cardiac arrhythmia. The drug has been abused by medical personnel for its hallucinogenic effects (Ahmed and Petchkovsky, 1980).

A 31 year old woman found dead after apparently self-administering as much as 900 mg of ketamine intravenously had the following postmortem findings (Peyton et al., 1988):

Ketamine Concentrations in a Fatality (mg/L or mg/kg)

Blood	Liver	Kidney
7.0	6.3	3.2

Analysis. Analysis of the drug and its demethylated metabolites has been accomplished by flame-ionization (Hodshon et al., 1972; Wieber et al., 1975) or nitrogen-specific (Davisson, 1978; Pitts et al., 1980; Stiller et al., 1982) gas chromatography of the underivatized drugs or by electron-capture detection of their heptafluorobutyryl derivatives (Chang and Glazko, 1972). Liquid chromatography after conversion to p-nitrobenzamide derivatives (Needham and Kochhar, 1975) or of the underivatized forms (Seay et al., 1993) has been reported.

References

S.N. Ahmed and L. Petchkovsky. Abuse of ketamine. Brit. J. Psych. 137: 303, 1980.

Anonymous. Ketamine. Parke-Davis and Company, Morris Plains, New Jersey, 1970.

T. Chang and A.J. Glazko. A gas chromatographic assay for ketamine in human plasma. Anesthesiology 36: 401–404, 1972.

M.L. Cohen and A.J. Trevor. On the cerebral accumulation of ketamine and the relationship between metabolism of the drug and its pharmacological effects. J. Pharm. Exp. Ther. 180: 351–358, 1974.

J.N. Davisson. Rapid gas chromatographic analysis of plasma levels of ketamine and major metabolites employing either nitrogen selective or mass spectroscopic detection. J. Chrom. 146: 344–349, 1978.

B.J. Hodshon, T. Ferrer-Allado, V.L. Brechner and A.K. Cho. A gas chromatographic assay procedure for ketamine in plasma. Anesthesiology 36: 506–508, 1972.

J. Idvall, I. Ahlgren, K.F. Aronsen and P. Stenberg. Ketamine infusions: pharmacokinetics and clinical effects. Brit. J. Anaesth. 51: 1167–1173, 1979.

L.L. Needham and M.M. Kochhar. Determination of ketamine and some in vivo metabolites using high-pressure liquid chromatography. J. Chrom. 114: 220–222, 1975.

S.H. Peyton, A.T. Couch and R.O. Bost. Tissue distribution of ketamine: two case reports. J. Anal. Tox. 12: 268–269, 1988.

F.N. Pitts, Jr., L.S. Yago, O. Aniline and A.F. Pitts. Capillary gas chromatography with a nitrogen detector for measurement of phencyclidine, ketamine and other arylcycloalkylamines in the picogram range. J. Chrom. 193: 157–159, 1980.

S.S. Seay, D.P. Aucoin and K.L. Tyczkowska. Rapid hplc method for the determination of ketamine and its metabolite dehydronorketamine in equine serum. J. Chrom. 620: 281–287, 1993.

P. Stenberg and J. Idvall. Does ketamine metabolite II exist *in vivo*? Brit. J. Anaesth. 53: 778, 1981.

R.L. Stiller, P.G. Dayton, J.M. Perel and C.C. Hug. Gas chromatographic analysis of ketamine and norketamine in plasma and urine: nitrogen-sensitive detection. J. Chrom. 232: 305–314, 1982.

J. Wieber, R. Gugler, J.H. Hengstmann and H.J. Dengler. Pharmacokinetics of ketamine in man. Anaesthesia 24: 260–263 1975.

Ketoprofen

T½: 1.1–4.2 hr
Vd: 0.1–0.5 L/kg
Fb: 0.99
pKa: 4.0

Occurrence and Usage. Ketoprofen (Profenid, Orudis) is a propionic acid derivative, related to fenoprofen, ibuprofen and naproxen, that has been used as an analgesic and antiinflammatory agent in European countries since 1973 and in the United States since 1988. It is available in oral dosage forms of 25–150 mg as the free acid. Daily doses range from 75–900 mg.

Blood Concentrations. The oral administration of 50 mg of ketoprofen to 12 volunteers produced an average peak plasma level of 4.8 mg/L (range, 1.9–8.4) at an average time of 72 minutes; the levels declined with a mean half-life of 1.5 hours (Upton et al., 1981). The oral administration of 100 mg to 9 subjects resulted in peak plasma concentrations averaging 8.6 mg/L (range, 4.1–11.3) and occurring between 40–120 minutes (Brazier et al., 1981). A single 150 mg oral dose given to 10 young adults produced an average maximal plasma concentration of 13 mg/L (range, 5.3–20) at an average time of 1.3 hours (Advenier et al., 1987).

Metabolism and Excretion. Over a 5 day period, 85% of a labeled dose of ketoprofen is eliminated in the urine and from 1–8% in feces. Only about 1% of a dose is eliminated unchanged, the remainder consisting of conjugated ketoprofen or its (unidentified) conjugated metabolites (Delbarre et al., 1976; Kaye et al., 1981).

Toxicity. Ketoprofen is capable of causing nausea, vomiting, abdominal pain, dizziness, confusion, headache, and somnolence with normal or excessive usage. A 12 year old girl who survived a deliberate overdose developed seizures, coma and metabolic acidosis; the serum ketoprofen concentration measured 3–4 hours post-dose was 1128 mg/L (Bond et al., 1989).

Analysis. Ketoprofen has been assayed in plasma by electron-capture gas chromatography after methylation (Stenberg et al., 1979). Several liquid chromatographic methods have been developed for the analysis of plasma and urine (Ballerini et al., 1979; Farinotti and Mahuzier, 1979; Jeffries et al., 1979; Bannier et al., 1980; Upton et al., 1980; Kaye et al., 1981; Oka et al., 1985; Wanwimolruk et al., 1991). The glucuronide of ketoprofen is easily hydrolyzed upon standing in sodium hydroxide solution for 10 minutes (Farinotti and Mahuzier, 1979).

References

C. Advenier, A. Roux, C. Gobert et al. Pharmacokinetics of ketoprofen in the elderly. Brit. J. Clin. Pharm. 16: 65–70, 1983.

R. Ballerini, A. Cambi, P. Del Soldato et al. Determination of ketoprofen by direct injection of deproteinized body fluids into a high-pressure liquid chromatographic system. J. Pharm. Sci. 68: 366–368, 1979.

A. Bannier, J.L. Brazier, R. Ribon and C. Quincy. Determination of ketoprofen in biological fluids by reversed-phase chromatography. J. Pharm. Sci. 69: 763–765, 1980.

G.R. Bond, S.C. Curry, P.A. Arnold-Capell et al. Generalized seizures and metabolic acidosis after ketoprofen overdose. Vet. Hum. Tox. 31: 369, 1989.

J.L. Brazier, J.N. Tamisier, D. Ambert and A. Bannier. Bioavailability of ketoprofen in man with and without concomitant administration of aluminium phosphate. Eur. J. Clin. Pharm. 19: 305–307, 1981.

F. Delbarre, J.C. Roucayrol, B. Amor et al. Pharmacokinetic study of ketoprofen (19.583 R.P.) in man using the tritiated compound. Scand. J. Rheum. (Suppl. 14): 45–52, 1976.

R. Farinotti and G. Mahuzier. High-performance liquid chromatographic determination of ketoprofen in blood and urine. J. Pharm. Sci. 68: 484–485, 1979.

T.M. Jefferies, W.O.A. Thomas and R.T. Parfitt. Determination of ketoprofen in plasma and urine by high-performance liquid chromatography. J. Chrom. 162: 122–124, 1979.

C.M. Kaye, M.G. Sankey and J.E. Holt. A high-pressure liquid chromatographic method for the assay of ketoprofen in plasma and urine, and its application to determining the urinary excretion of free and conjugated ketoprofen following oral administration of Orudis to man. Brit. J. Clin. Pharm. 11: 395–398, 1981.

K. Oka, S. Aoshima and M. Noguchi. Highly sensitive determination of ketoprofen in human serum and urine and its application to pharmacokinetic study. J. Chrom. 345: 419–424, 1985.

P. Stenberg, T.E. Jonsson, B. Nilsson and F. Wollheim. Determination of ketoprofen in plasma by extractive methylation and electron-capture gas chromatography. J. Chrom. 177: 145–148, 1979.

R.A. Upton, J.N. Buskin, T.W. Guentert et al. Convenient and sensitive high-performance liquid chromatography assay for ketoprofen, naproxen and other allied drugs in plasma or urine. J. Chrom. 190: 119–128, 1980.

R.A. Upton, R.L. Williams, T.W. Guentert et al. Ketoprofen pharmacokinetics and bioavailability based on an improved sensitive and specific assay. Eur. J. Clin. Pharm. 20: 127–133, 1981.

S. Wanwimolruk, S.Z. Wanwimolruk and A.R. Zoest. Sensitive hplc assay for ketoprofen in human plasma and its application to pharmacokinetic study. J. Liq. Chrom. 14: 3685–3694, 1991.

Ketorolac

T½: 3.5–9.2 hr
Vd: 0.15–0.33 L/kg
Fb: 0.99
pKa: 3.5

Occurrence and Usage. Ketorolac (Acular, Toradol) is a nonsteroidal anti-inflammatory drug that has been in clinical use in the United States since 1990. The drug is structually related to tolmetin and zomepirac and exhibits analgesic, anti-inflammatory, and antipyretic activity similar to those drugs. Ketorolac appears to be as effective as morphine, but is without potential side-effects such as respiratory depression or constipation. The drug is available as the tromethamine salt in 15–30 mg/mL solutions for intramuscular use, and in 10 mg tablets for oral administration. The recommended oral dose is 10 mg every 4–6 hours, with a daily maximum of 40 mg.

Blood Concentrations. Peak plasma ketorolac concentrations averaged 0.87 mg/L following a single 10 mg oral dose and 3.0 mg/L after a single 30 mg oral dose in young, healthy volunteers (Montoya-Iraheta et al., 1986; Martinez et al., 1987). Peak plasma concentrations in adults following a single intramuscular dose averaged 1.0–1.4 mg/L with 15 mg, 2.2–3.0 mg/L with 30 mg, and 4.0–4.5 mg/L with 60 mg (PDR, 1993).

Metabolism and Excretion. Ketorolac is extensively metabolized by oxidation and conjugation to largely inactive metabolites. The major metabolites are the acyl glucuronide and p-hydroxyketorolac, which represent 77% and 12%, respectively, of an oral dose as urinary excretion products. p-Hydroxyketorolac has about 20% of the anti-inflammatory activity and 1% of the analgesic activity of ketorolac. Other unidentified metabolites in urine account for only 6–7% of the urinary recovery (Mroszczak et al., 1987; Brocks and Jamali, 1992).

Toxicity. Adverse effects following ketorolac administration include nausea, rash, edema, headache and hypertension. Such effects are said to be frequent at plasma ketorolac concentrations above 5 mg/L (PDR, 1993). Anaphylactoid reaction (Goetz et al., 1992) and acute renal failure (Schoch et al., 1992; Quan and Kayser, 1994) have been reported following a single dose.

Analysis. Ketorolac has been determined in biological specimens by liquid chromatography (Wu and Massey, 1990; Chaudhary et al., 1993). Spontaneous hydrolysis of the acyl glucuronide may occur during specimen storage or analysis, liberating free parent drug (Upton et al., 1980).

References

D.R. Brooks and F. Jamali. Clinical pharmacokinetics of ketorolac tromethamine. Clin. Pharmacokin. 23: 415–427, 1992.

R.S. Chaudhary, S.S. Gangwai, K.C. Jindal and S. Khanna. Reversed-phase high-performance liquid chromatography of ketorolac and its application to bioequivalence studies in human serum. J. Chrom. 614: 180, 1993.

C.M. Goetz, J.A. Sterchele and F.P. Harchelroad. Anaphylactoid reaction following ketorolac tromethamine administration. Ann. Pharmacother. 26: 1237–1238, 1992.

J.J. Martinez, D.C. Garg, L.J. Pages et al. Single dose pharmacokinetics of ketorolac in healthy young and renal impaired subjects. J. Clin. Pharm. 27: 722, 1987.

C. Montoya-Iraheta, D.C. Garg, N.S. Jallad et al. Pharmacokinetics of single dose oral and intramuscular ketorolac tromethamine in elderly vs. young healthy subjects. J. Clin. Pharm. 26: 545, 1986.

E.J. Mroszczak, F.W. Lee, D. Combs et al. Ketorolac tromethamine absorption distribution, metabolism, excretion, and pharmacokinetics in animals and humans. Drug Met. Disp. 15: 618–626, 1987.

Physicians' Desk Reference, Medical Economics Co., Montvale, New Jersey, 1993, pp. 2411–2415.

D.J. Quan and S.R. Kayser. Ketorolac induced acute renal failure following a single dose. Clin. Tox. 32: 305–309, 1994.

B.H. Resman-Targoff. Ketorolac: a parenteral nonsteroidal antiiflammatory drug. Drug Int. Clin. Pharm. 24: 1098–1104, 1990.

P.H. Schoch, A. Ranno and D.S. North. Acute renal failure in an elderly woman following intramuscular ketorolac administration. Ann. Pharmacother. 26: 1233–1236, 1992.

R.A. Upton, J.N. Buskin, R.L. Williams et al. Negligible excretion of unchanged ketoprofen, naproxen, and probenecid in urine. J. Pharm. Sci. 69: 1254–1257, 1980.

A.T. Wu and I.J. Massey. Simultaneous determination of ketorolac and its hydroxylated metabolite in plasma by high-performance liquid chromatography. J. Chrom. 534: 241–246, 1990.

Labetalol

T½: 5–8 hr
Vd: 10 L/kg
Fb: 0.50
pKa: 7.4 (acid), 8.7 (base)

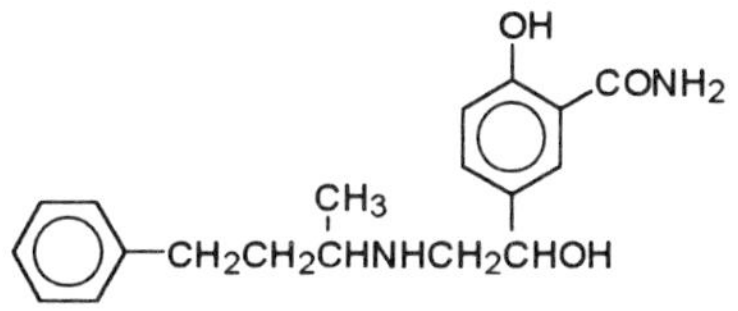

Occurrence and Usage. Labetalol (Normodyne, Trandate) is a competitive alpha- and beta-adrengergic receptor antagonist used in the treatment of hypertension. Tablets of 100, 200 and 300 mg containing the hydrochloride salt are available for oral administration; maintenance doses range from 200–2400 mg/day. It is also available in 20 mL ampules (5 mg/mL) for intravenous administration.

Blood Concentrations. A hypertensive 31 year old male patient given a single dose of 50 mg labetalol intravenously exhibited a plasma concentration of 50 µg/L after one hour and approximately 10 µg/L after 6 hours (Abernethy et al., 1986). After a single oral dose of 100 mg given to 6 subjects, age 21–65 with a mean weight of 76 kg, peak plasma concentrations of 96–250 µg/L (average, 157) were attained in 20–60 minutes. Following a 200 mg single oral dose in the same subjects, peak plasma concentrations of 93–271 µg/L (average, 191) were attained in 40–90 minutes. After chronic administration of 200 mg daily, steady-state plasma concentrations ranged from 36–183 µg/L (average, 91); after 400 mg daily, the steady-state range was 84–205 µg/L (average, 140) (McNeil et al., 1982).

Metabolism and Excretion. In man, labetalol is rapidly absorbed from the gastrointestinal tract and undergoes extensive first-pass metabolism to polar glucuronide metabolites, which are rapidly excreted in the urine. Less than 5% of a single dose is excreted as parent drug and up to 50% is excreted in 24 hours as conjugates (Kanto et al., 1981; Reid et al., 1981; Abernethy et al., 1986).

Toxicity. Labetelol in overdosage produces severe and prolonged hypotension and may cause acute renal failure. A 19 year old woman who survived the acute ingestion of 16 g of labetelol had an admission serum labetelol concentration of 2850 µg/L; her blood pressure was 80/60 mm Hg at the time of initial examination (Smit et al., 1986).

Analysis. Labetalol has been determined in serum and plasma by radioreceptor assay (Kelly et al., 1981), spectrofluorometry (Martin et al., 1976), and liquid chromatography using fluorometric (Dusci and Hackett, 1979; Meredith et al., 1981; Oosterhuis et al., 1981; Wood et al., 1982; Alton et al., 1984; Chung et al., 1986), ultraviolet (Woodman and Johnson, 1981; Hidalgo and Muir, 1984) or electrochemical detection (Abernethy et al., 1986). Liquid chromatography has also been used for the analysis of blood and tissues from fatal cases (Pannell et al., 1982).

References

D.R. Abernethy, E.L. Todd, J.L. Egan and G. Carrum. Labetalol analysis in human plasma using liquid chromatography with electrochemical detection: application to pharmacokinetic studies. J. Liq. Chrom. 9: 2153–2163, 1986.

K.B. Alton, F. Leitz, S. Bariletto et al. High-performance liquid chromatographic assay for labetalol in human plasma using a PRP-1 column and fluorimetric detection. J. Chrom. 311: 319–328, 1984.

M. Chung, F.H. Leitz, G. Maier et al. Rising multiple-dose pharmacokinetics of labetalol in hypertensive patients. J. Clin. Pharm. 26: 248–252, 1986.

T.J. Dusci and L.P. Hackett. Determination of labetalol in human plasma by high-performance liquid chromatography. J. Chrom. 175: 208–210, 1979.

I.J. Hidalgo and K.T. Muir. High-performance liquid chromatographic method for the determination of labetalol in plasma using ultraviolet detection. J. Chrom. 305: 222–227, 1984.

J. Kanto, H. Allonen, T. Kleimola et al. Pharmacokinetics of labetalol in healthy volunteers. Int. J. Clin. Pharm. Ther. Tox. 19: 41–44, 1981.

J.G. Kelly, K. McGarry and K. O'Malley. Radioreceptor assay for labetalol. Brit. J. Clin. Pharm. 8 (Suppl.): 695–710, 1976.

J.J. McNeil, A.E. Anderson, W.J. Louis and D.J. Morgan. Pharmacokinetics and pharmacodynamic studies of labetalol in hypertensive subjects. Brit. J. Clin. Pharm. 8: 157S–161S, 1979.

J.J. McNeil, A.E. Anderson, W.J. Louis and K. Raymond. Labetalol steady-state pharmacokinetics in hypertensive patients. Brit. J. Clin. Pharm. 13 (Suppl. 1): 75S–80S, 1982.

P.A. Meredith, D. McSharry, H.L. Elliott and J.L. Reid. The determination of labetalol in plasma by high-performance liquid chromatography using fluorescent detection. J. Pharm. Meth. 6: 309–314, 1981.

B. Oosterhuis, M. VandenBerg and C.J. Van Boxtel. Sensitive high-performance liquid chromatographic method for the determination of labetalol in human plasma using fluorimetric detection. J. Chrom. 226: 259–265, 1981.

L.K. Pannell, B.M. Thompson and L.F. Wilkinson. Determination of labetalol in a postmortem case using HPLC. J. Anal. Tox. 6: 193–195, 1982.

J.L. Reid, P.A. Meredith and H.L. Elliott. Labetalol and the management of hypertension. J. Cardiovasc. Pharm. 3 (Suppl. 1): 560–568, 1981.

A.J. Smit, P.O.M. Mulder, P.E. de Jong and G.K. van der Hem. Acute renal failure after overdose of labetalol. Brit. Med. J. 293: 1142–1143, 1986.

A.J. Wood, D.G. Ferry and R.R. Bailey. Elimination kinetics of labetalol in severe renal failure. Brit. J. Clin. Pharm. 13 (Suppl. 1): 81S–86S, 1982.

T.F. Woodman and B. Johnson. High pressure liquid chromatography of labetalol in serum or plasma. Ther. Drug Mon. 3: 371–375, 1981.

Lead

T½: 0.4–3.6 yr

Vd: ?

Fb: ?

Pb

Occurrence and Usage. Lead and inorganic lead compounds are found in a variety of commercial products and industrial materials, including paints, plastics, storage batteries, bearing alloys, insecticides and ceramics. Tetraethyllead is a volatile organic liquid that is covered in a separate section. The average urban adult inhales 20–40 µg of inorganic lead daily as atmospheric pollution primarily from automobile exhaust, retaining 30–45%, and ingests about 300 µg in the diet, absorbing only 5–10%. The threshold limit value for inorganic lead fumes and dusts in industrial situations is 0.15 mg/m³.

Blood Concentrations. The average blood lead concentration in 103 members of a remote Himalayan population was 0.03 mg/L (Piomelli et al., 1980). Blood lead concentrations in healthy children gradually increase from a mean of 0.03 mg/L in those less than 1 year old to an average of 0.11

mg/L in 5 year olds (Haas et al., 1972). In healthy suburban adults, a range of 0.07–0.22 mg/L was observed for blood lead, 7–14% of which was derived from atmospheric sources (Manton, 1977). A group of 50 London taxi drivers was found to have a mean blood lead level of 0.29 mg/L, with a range of 0.16–0.49 mg/L (Jones et al., 1972). Children living within a kilometer of a lead smelter had blood lead concentrations that averaged 0.25–0.30 mg/L over a period of 5 years (Roels et al., 1980). Blood lead concentrations ranged from 0.20–1.08 mg/L in 62 workers in a battery plant, where air lead concentrations averaged 0.015–0.187 mg/m^3 in the various departments (Richter et al., 1979). Generally, 0.40 mg/L is considered the normal upper limit for blood lead, 99% of which is contained within erythrocytes. Lead workers exposed at the current TLV may be expected to develop blood lead concentrations averaging 0.60 mg/L (Williams et al., 1969).

Metabolism and Excretion. Humans are in a state of positive lead balance from the day of birth, such that a slow accumulation occurs until a total body burden of 50–350 mg of lead exists by age 60. Over 90% of absorbed lead is deposited in bone, primarily in dense bone, with only minor amounts excreted in hair, nails or urine. Men have higher concentrations in nearly all tissues than women. The following tissue distribution of lead was determined in 60 urban adult males from northwestern England (Barry, 1975):

Lead Concentrations in Normal Subjects (mg/L or mg/kg)

	Brain	Liver	Kidney	Hair	Nails	Urine
Average	0.10	1.0	0.78	6.6	4.7	0.04
(Range)	(0.02–0.78)	(0.18–3.1)	(0.15–1.9)	(1.0–20)	(0.65–15)	(0.01–0.19

Urine lead concentrations in lead workers average 0.12 mg/L during exposure to 0.15 mg/m^3 lead in air, and 0.14 mg/L during exposure to 0.20 mg/m^3 (Williams et al., 1969).

Toxicity. Lead adversely affects many enzyme systems, but most noteworthy in regard to clinical indices of lead poisoning are the effects on heme synthesis. Many diagnostic tests are based on the abnormalities that result, including increases in erythrocyte zinc protoporphyrin, urinary coproporphyrin and urinary delta-aminolevulinic acid (ALA), and inhibition of erythrocyte ALA dehydrase. These parameters, together with blood lead determinations, are most frequently used in the assessment of lead poisoning (Beattie, 1974; Haeger-Aronsen, 1971).

The symptoms of chronic lead poisoning include gastrointestinal disturbances, anemia, insomnia, weight loss, motor weakness, muscle paralysis and nephropathy. Current sources of exposure to toxic quantities of lead include paint and plumbing in older houses, industrial processes, glazed ceramic vessels, and, rarely, the intentional self-administration of organic or inorganic lead compounds. Chelation therapy with BAL, EDTA or penicillamine, or a combination of these, is usually indicated when the blood lead concentration is found to exceed 0.80 mg/L; above this level, encephalopathy can develop with the possiblility of permanent brain damage (Green et al., 1976).

A study of blood lead levels in children of industrially-exposed fathers revealed that 42% were in excess of 0.30 mg/L and 11% exceeded 0.80 mg/L, a result of lead dust carried home on clothing (Baker et al., 1977). Several instructors exposed to lead fumes at an indoor pistol range who complained of abdominal pain were found to have blood lead concentrations of 1.09–1.39 mg/L (Landrigan et al., 1975).

Three persons have been reported poisoned following treatment with Chinese herbal pills, which may contain up to 7.5 mg of lead per dosage unit: a 4 year old child died 7 days after treatment by an herbalist, with lead concentrations of 3 mg/kg in brain and 17 mg/kg in liver (Leung, 1975); a 4 month old child developed a blood lead concentration of 1.37 mg/L and became comatose, but survived with treatment (Chan et al., 1977); and a 59 year old woman with joint pain, insomnia and irritability was found to have a blood lead level of 0.90 mg/L (Kalman, 1977). An aphrodisiac medication from Bangladesh was involved in a similar case, causing a blood lead concentration of 1.20 mg/L in a 24 year old man (Brearly and Forsythe, 1978). A 4 year old child who ingested a hair-darkening agent containing 3% lead acetate developed toxic symptoms and a blood lead concentration of 1.36 mg/L (Waldron, 1979).

Although acute lead poisoning is a rare event, death may occur in 1–2 days after the ingestion of 10–30 g of a lead salt by an adult; one women survived the ingestion of 7 g of lead acetate after achieving a blood lead level of 2.28 mg/L (Karpatkin, 1961).

Three young children who died of lead poisoning had histories of pica and blood lead concentrations of 1.11–3.50 mg/L (Alexander and Delves, 1972). A woman, shot in the leg 5 months before, died of lead poisoning due to the retained bullet; a postmortem blood level concentration of 5.3 mg/L was measured (DiMaio and Garriott, 1980). A 2 year old boy died after drinking for several weeks apple juice stored in a glazed earthenware container; postmortem specimens of brain contained 0.4–2.2 mg/kg of lead, liver contained 13 mg/kg, and kidney, 18 mg/kg (Klein et al., 1970). The following tissue distribution was noted in the death of a child from lead poisoning (Kehoe, 1976):

Lead Concentrations in a Fatal Case (mg/kg)

Brain	Liver	Kidney	Flat Bone	Long Bone
5.8	40	8.8	268	132

Analysis. Analytical procedures for the determination of lead in blood have been reviewed by Delves (1977). Two of the most reliable methods for routine usage are anodic stripping voltammetry (Morrell and Giridhar, 1976; Pinchin and Newham, 1977) and atomic absorption spectrometry. Many variations of the latter method have been developed; flame techniques require preconcentration of lead (Hessel, 1968; Berman et al., 1968) or direct introduction of discrete samples (Delves, 1970), while electrothermal techniques allow direct introduction of measured amounts of both fluids and solid tissues (Evenson and Pendergast, 1974; Fernandez, 1975; Stegavik et al., 1976; Pleban and Pearson, 1979; Shuttler and Delves, 1986; Jacobson et al., 1991). Precautions must be taken when storing specimens for lead analysis and when preparing standards, due to the loss of lead from solutions by adsorption to containers (Unger and Green, 1977). Blood lead is stable for up to 10 weeks when collected in evacuated tubes with heparin or EDTA anticoagulant and refrigerated (Wang and Peter, 1985).

ALA in urine is conveniently measured by colorimetry after column chromatography (Davis and Andelman, 1967).

References

F.W. Alexander and H.T. Delves. Deaths from acute lead poisoning. Arch. Dis. Child. 47: 446–448, 1972.

E.L. Baker, Jr., D.S. Folland, T.A. Taylor et al. Lead poisoning in children of lead workers. New Eng. J. Med. 296: 260–261, 1977.

P.S.I. Barry. A comparison of concentrations of lead in human tissues. Brit. J. Ind. Med. 32: 119–139, 1975.

A.D. Beattie. Clinical and biochemical effects of lead. In *Forensic Toxicology* (B. Ballantyne, ed.), John Wright & Sons, England, 1974, pp. 121–134.

E. Berman, V. Valavanis and A. Dubin. A micromethod for determination of lead in blood. Clin. Chem. 14: 239–242, 1968.

R.L. Brearley and A.M. Forsythe. Lead poisoning from aphrodisiacs: potential hazard in immigrants. Brit. Med. J. 2: 1748–1749, 1978.

H. Chan, Y. Yeh, G.J. Billmeier, Jr. and W.E. Evans. Lead poisoning from ingestion of Chinese herbal medicine. Clin. Tox. 10: 273–281, 1977.

J.R. Davis and S.L. Andelman. Urinary delta-aminolevulinic acid (ALA) levels in lead poisoning. Arch. Env. Health 15: 53–59, 1967.

H.T. Delves. A microsampling method for the rapid determination of lead in blood by atomic-absorption spectrophotometry. Analyst 95: 431–438, 1970.

H.T. Delves. Analytical techniques for blood-lead measurements. J. Anal. Tox. 1: 261–264, 1977.

V.J.M. DiMaio and J. Garriott. A fatal case of lead poisoning due to a retained bullet. Vet. Hum. Tox. 22: 390–391, 1980.

M.A. Evenson and D.D. Pendergast. Rapid ultramicro direct determination of erythrocyte lead concentration by atomic absorption spectrophotometry, with use of a graphite-tube furnace. Clin. Chem. 20: 163–171, 1974.

F.J. Fernandez. Micromethod for lead determination of whole blood by atomic absorption, with use of the graphite furnace. Clin. Chem. 21: 558–561, 1975.

V.A. Green, G.W. Wise and J. Callenbach. Lead poisoning. Clin. Tox. 9: 33–51, 1976.

T. Haas, K. Mache, K.H. Schaller et al. Investigations into ecological lead levels in children. Zbl. Bakt. Hyg. I. Abt. Orig. B. 156: 353–360, 1972.

B. Haeger-Aronsen. An assessment of the laboratory tests used to monitor the exposure of lead workers. Brit. J. Ind. Med. 28: 52–58, 1971.

D.W. Hessel. A simple and rapid quantitative determination of lead in blood. At. Abs. Newsl. 7: 55–56, 1968.

B.E. Jacobson, G. Lockitch and G. Quigley. Improved sample preparation for accurate determination of low concentrations of lead in whole blood by graphite furnace analysis. Clin. Chem. 37: 515–519, 1991.

D.W. Jones, B.T. Commins and A.A. Cernik. Blood lead and carboxyhaemoglobin levels in London taxi drivers. Lancet 2: 302–303, 1972.

S.M. Kalman. The pathophysiology of lead poisoning: a review and a case report. J. Anal. Tox. 1: 277–281, 1977.

S. Karpatkin. Lead poisoning after taking Pb acetate with suicidal intent. Arch. Env. Health 2: 679–684, 1961.

R.A. Kehoe. Pharmacology and toxicology of heavy metals: lead. Pharm. Ther. 1: 161–188, 1976.

M. Klein, R. Namer, E. Harpur and R. Corbin. Earthenware containers as a source of fatal lead poisoning. New Eng. J. Med. 283: 669–672, 1970.

P.J. Landrigan, A.S. McKinney, L.C. Hopkins et al. Chronic lead absorption. J. Am. Med. Asso. 234: 394–397, 1975.

S.C. Leung. Personal communication, 1975.

W.I. Manton. Sources of lead in blood. Arch. Env. Health 32: 149–159, 1977.

G. Morrell and G. Giridhar. Rapid micromethod for blood lead analysis by anodic stripping voltammetry. Clin. Chem. 22: 221–223, 1976.

M.J. Pinchin and J. Newham. The determination of lead, copper and cadmium by anodic stripping voltammetry at a mercury thin-film electrode. Anal. Chim. Acta 90: 91–102, 1977.

S. Piomelli, L. Corash, M.B. Corash et al. Blood lead concentrations in a remote Himalayan population. Science 210: 1135–1136, 1980.

P.A. Pleban and K.H. Pearson. Determination of lead in whole blood and urine using Zeeman effect flameless atomic absorption spectroscopy. Anal. Letters 12: 935–950, 1979.

E.D. Richter, Y. Yaffe and N. Gruener. Air and blood lead levels in a battery factory. Env. Res. 20: 87–98, 1979.

H.A. Roels, J.P. Buchet, R.R. Lauwerys et al. Exposure to lead by the oral and pulmonary routes of children living in the vicinity of a primary lead smelter. Env. Res. 22: 81–94, 1980.

I.L. Shuttler and H.T. Delves. Determination of lead in blood by atomic absorption spectrometry with electro-thermal atomisation. Analyst 111: 651–656, 1986.

K. Stegavik, G. Mikalsen, E.M. Ophus and E.A. Mylius. Determination of lead in human lungs by direct flameless atomic absorption analysis of small tissue samples. Bull. Env. Cont. Tox. 15: 734–738, 1976.

B.C. Unger and V.A. Green. Blood lead analysis—lead loss to storage containers. Clin. Tox. 11: 237–243, 1977.

H.A. Waldron. Lead poisoning from cosmetics. Lancet 2: 1070–1071, 1979.

S.T. Wang and F. Peter. The stability of human blood level in storage. J. Anal. Tox. 9: 85–88, 1985.

M.E. Williams, E. King and J. Walford. An investigation of lead absorption in an electric accumulator factory with the use of personal samplers. Brit. J. Ind. Med. 26: 202–216, 1969.

Levorphanol

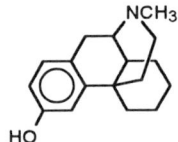

T½: 11 hr
Vd: 10–13 L/kg
Fb: 0.40
pKa: 9.2

Occurrence and Usage. The 1-isomer of 3-hydroxy-N-methylmorphinan is known as levorphanol (Dromoran, Levo-Dromoran), a synthetic compound having 4–5 times the analgesic potency of morphine on a weight basis. The d-isomer, dextrorphan, is essentially devoid of narcotic activity, while the N-allyl derivative, levallorphan, is used as a narcotic antagonist. Levorphanol is administered every 6–8 hours either orally or subcutaneously in amounts of 2–12 mg as the tartrate.

Blood Concentrations. A single 2 mg intravenous dose given to a patient produced plasma levorphanol concentrations that initially exceeded 0.007 mg/L but fell to less than 0.002 mg/L by 4 hours (Dixon et al., 1983). A cancer patient receiving 2 mg of levorphanol by intravenous injection every 4 hours had a peak plasma concentration of 0.008 mg/L after 1 hour, declining to 0.006 mg/L by 3 hours. A patient taking 12 mg orally every 4–6 hours developed plasma concentrations that varied between 0.016–0.021 mg/L in the first 2 hours after each dose (Dixon et al., 1980). The plasma concentrations of conjugated levorphanol may exceed those of the parent by five to ten-fold (Dixon et al., 1983).

Metabolism and Excretion. Very little work has been reported on the fate of the drug in man. Rats excrete about 60% of a labeled dose in urine and 37% in feces over a 4 day period. The urine contains 7% of the dose as unchanged drug, 31% as conjugated levorphanol, 2.5% norlevorphanol, 14% conjugated norlevorphanol, and 6% as an unidentified polar metabolite (Misra et al., 1974).

Toxicity. Two adults died after ingesting overdoses of levorphanol, one within 19 hours of the ingestion of 30 mg; postmortem blood levorphanol concentrations of 0.8 mg/L were observed in both cases (Franc, 1978; Bednarczyk, 1979). One case of suicide by levorphanol ingestion investigated by Turner and Richards (1977) showed the following concentrations of acid-hydrolyzed total drug by gas chromatography:

Levorphanol Concentrations in a Fatal Case (mg/L or mg/kg)

Blood	Brain	Lung	Liver	Bile	Kidney	Urine	Gastric
2.7	1.8	17	5.4	24	3.4	2.3	47 mg

Analysis. Levorphanol has been included in an opiate analysis scheme that involved the formation of silyl derivatives prior to quantitation by flame-ionization gas chromatography (Nakamura and Way, 1975). Methods employing gas chromatography-mass spectrometry (Min et al., 1982) and liquid chromatography (Lucek and Dixon, 1985) have been reported.

References

L.R. Bednarczyk. A death due to levorphanol. J. Anal. Tox. 3: 217–219, 1979.

R. Dixon, T. Crews, E. Mohacsi et al. Levorphanol: radioimmunoassay and plasma concentrations. Res. Comm. Chem. Path. Pharm. 29: 535–547, 1980.

R. Dixon, T. Crews, C. Inturrisi and K. Foley. Levorphanol: pharmacokinetics and steady-state plasma concentrations in patients with pain. Res. Comm. Chem. Path. Pharm. 41: 3–17, 1983.

A.M.L. Franc. Personal communication, 1978.

R. Lucek and R. Dixon. Quantitation of levorphanol in plasma using high-performance liquid chromatography with electrochemical detection. J. Chrom. 341: 239–243, 1985.

B.H. Min, W.A. Garland and J. Pao. Determination of levorphanol (Levo-Dromoran) in human plasma by combined gas chromatography-negative ion chemical ionization mass spectrometry. J. Chrom. 231: 194–199, 1982.

A.L. Misra, N.L. Vadlamani, R. Bloch and S.J. Mule. Differential pharmacokinetic and metabolic profiles of the stereoisomers. Res. Comm. Chem. Path. Pharm. 7: 1–16, 1974.

G.R. Nakamura and E.L. Way. Determination of morphine and codeine in postmortem specimens. Anal. Chem. 47: 775–778, 1975.

J.E. Turner and R.G. Richards. A fatal case involving levorphanol. J. Anal. Tox. 1: 103–104, 1977.

Lidocaine

T½: 0.7–1.8 hr
Vd: 1.3 L/kg
Fb: 0.55–0.79 for lidocaine; 0.14 for MEGX; 0.05 for GX
pKa: 7.9

Occurrence and Usage. Lidocaine (lignocaine, Xylocaine) was first synthesized in 1948 for use as a local anesthetic, and is currently available for topical or injection anesthesia, usually as the hydrochloride salt, in solutions of 0.5–5.0%, with or without epinephrine. More recently, it has achieved popularity as an antiarrhythmic drug, and is administered for this purpose by intravenous injection of 50–100 mg or intramuscular injection of 300 mg.

Blood Concentrations. The subcutaneous administration of 200 mg of lidocaine for infiltration anesthesia produced a mean peak plasma level of 0.42 mg/L at 30 minutes in 8 subjects (Schwartz et al., 1974). An oral dose of 500 mg resulted in peak plasma concentrations of 0.6–1.1 mg/L in 5 subjects after 1–2 hours (Boyes et al., 1971). Following a 1 mg/kg (70 mg/70 kg) intravenous bolus injection, plasma concentrations in 4 healthy subjects averaged 0.96 mg/L at 0.25 hours and 0.40 mg/L at 1.0 hours, declining with an elimination half-life of 44 minutes (Caille et al., 1977). Other authors have reported a half-life of 107 minutes in normal subjects (Rowland et al., 1971).

A 200 mg dose administered by endotracheal spray resulted in an average peak plasma lidocaine concentration of 3.5 mg/L at 20 minutes in 6 subjects (Chu et al., 1975), whereas the same dose given by intramuscular injection produced an average peak plasma level of 2.4 mg/L at 30 minutes (Scott et al., 1968). During a continuous intravenous infusion of 2.5 mg/min of lidocaine in 3 patients, steady-state blood concentrations of 1.9–4.1 mg/L (average, 2.8) for lidocaine and 0.5–1.9 mg/L (average, 1.0) for monoethylglycinexylidide were achieved (Halkin et al., 1975). Glycinexylidide plasma concentrations have ranged from undetectable levels to 2.7 mg/L (Strong et al., 1973). Plasma lidocaine concentrations of 2–5 mg/L are considered desirable for antiarrhythmic control, and this level can be produced in most patients by the constant intravenous infusion of 20–30 μg/kg/min in combination with one or two 50–100 mg loading doses (Melmon et al., 1973; Greenblatt et al., 1976).

Metabolism and Excretion. Lidocaine is metabolized by mono- and di-desethylation to monoethylglycinexylidide (MEGX) and glycinexylidide (GX). Both are active antiarrhythmic agents (83% and 10% as active as lidocaine, respectively) and accumulate to a certain extent in plasma, but only MEGX is thought to contribute significantly to the toxic effects of lidocaine (Blumer et al., 1973). Minor inactive metabolites include 3-hydroxylidocaine, a cyclization product of MEGX, and 2,6-xylidine; the latter compound is probably a precursor in the formation of a major metabolite, 4-hydroxy-2,6-xylidine (Breck and Trager, 1971; Keenaghan and Boyes, 1972). N-hydroxy metabolites have also been suggested as urinary excretion products (Mather and Thomas, 1972).

During conditions of acid urine up to 7% of a dose may be recovered in the 12 hour urine as unchanged lidocaine (Beckett et al., 1966), although under normal conditions only about 3% is excreted unchanged in 24 hours; most of the remainder of a dose has been accounted for in the urine as MEGX (4%), GX (2%), conjugated 3-hydroxylidocaine (1%), 2,6-xylidine (1%) and conjugated 4-hydroxy-2,6-xylidine (73%) (Keenaghan and Boyes, 1972).

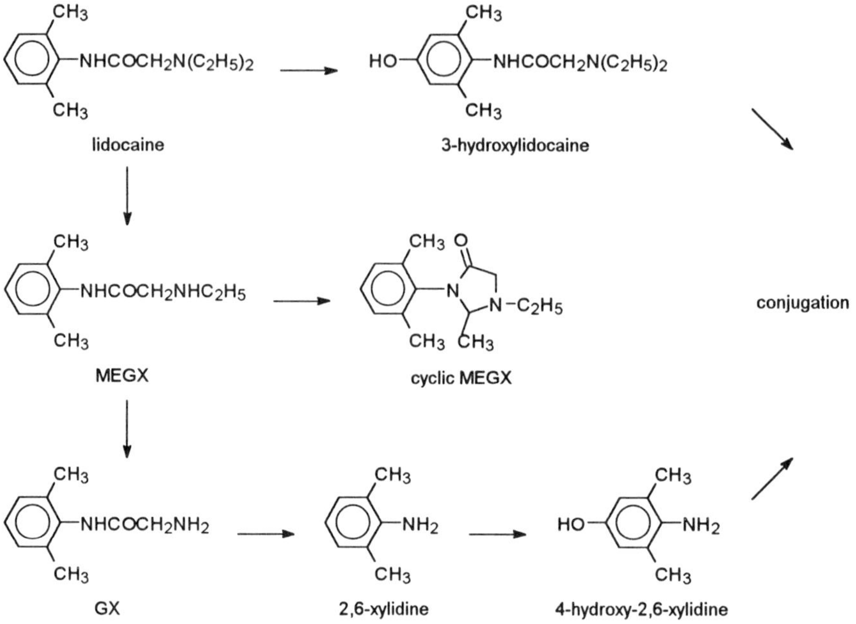

Toxicity. Lidocaine toxicity is manifested by confusion, dizziness, apprehension, delirium, paresthesia, hypotension, central nervous system depression and convulsions; signs of toxicity may appear at plasma concentrations exceeding 8 mg/L. An intravenous infusion of 425–1000 mg given to 4 subjects produced peak blood concentrations of lidocaine that averaged 10.7 mg/L (range, 9.0–14.0) and elicited toxic signs in each subject (Bromage and Robson, 1961). Three individuals who accidentally ingested lidocaine solutions intended for topical anesthesia developed serum concentrations of 7.3–12 mg/L and exhibited agitation, seizures and cardiac abnormalities (Fruncillo et al., 1982; Gorman et al., 1984). A 6 year old child survived the accidental intravenous injection of 1200 mg of lidocaine after achieving a serum level of 19 mg/L and exhibiting asystole and grand mal seizures (Edgren et al., 1986).

Death has resulted within minutes after the accidental intravenous administration of 250–2000 mg of lidocaine to 6 adults, with postmortem blood concentrations of 6–33 mg/L (average, 21) having been determined (Christie, 1976; Alha, 1977; Baselt and Cravey, 1977; Poklis et al., 1984). Two fatalities were reported following paracervical administration of lidocaine (500 mg in one case) in which postmortem blood concentrations of 5 and 9 mg/L were found (Grimes and Cates, 1976). Oral overdosage with up to 25 g of the drug has caused the death of at least 4 persons, in whom blood concentrations of 11–92 mg/L (average, 54) and liver concentrations of 20–96 mg/kg (average, 61) were measured (Borkowski, 1976; Baselt and Cravey, 1977). The following data is representative of tissue concentrations of lidocaine in fatal cases after drug administration by 3 routes (Sunshine and Fike, 1964; Borkowski, 1976; Alha, 1977):

Lidocaine Concentrations in Fatal Cases (mg/L or mg/kg)

Dose	Route	Blood	Brain	Liver	Kidney	Urine
1000	I.V	33	21	23	56	10
2500	S.C.	12	66	96	84	18
25 g	P.O.	44	17	70	66	6

Lidocaine concentrations of greater than 15 mg/kg in brain, lung, heart, liver and kidney are consistent with the presence of toxic and potentially fatal levels of the drug (Peat et al., 1985).

Analysis. Lidocaine has been assayed in biologic media by a methyl orange colorimetric technique (Bromage and Robson, 1961) and by ultraviolet spectrophotometry at 262 nm after extraction from aqueous alkaline solution (Christie, 1976). Gas chromatography is frequently used for the analysis of this drug; flame-ionization (Keenaghan, 1968; Rowland et al., 1971; Benowitz and Rowland, 1973; Caille et al., 1977; Kline and Martin, 1978; Karch and Chmielewski, 1981) and nitrogen-specific detection (Abernethy et al., 1982) have been applied to the measurement of parent drug and electron-capture detection to the measurement of MEGX after derivatization (Halkin et al., 1975). Lidocaine, MEGX, and in some procedures, GX, have been assayed simultaneously in plasma by flame-ionization (DiFazio and Brown, 1971; Nation and Triggs, 1976), or nitrogen-selective gas chromatography (Irgens et al., 1976; Hawkins et al., 1982), by gas chromatography-mass spectrometry (Strong and Atkinson, 1972; Hignite et al., 1978), by direct insertion mass spectrometry (Garland et al., 1974), and by liquid chromatography (Nation et al., 1979; Wisnicki et al., 1979; Lindberg et al., 1983; Angelo et al., 1987). Immunoassay reagents are commercially available for the parent drug.

Contact with the stoppers of Vacutainer blood collection tubes has been shown to lower lidocaine concentrations in plasma or serum by an average of 25% (Stargel et al., 1979). Lidocaine is stable for up to 70 days in blood or serum during storage at either 4° C. or 25° C. (Levine et al., 1983).

References

D.R. Abernethy, D.J. Greenblatt and H.R. Ochs. Lidocaine determination in human plasma with application to single low-dose pharmacokinetic studies. J. Chrom. 232: 180–185, 1982.

A. Alha. Personal communication, 1977.

H.R. Angelo, J. Bonde, J.P. Kampmann and J. Kastrup. A HPLC method for the simultaneous determination of disopyramide, lidocaine and their monodealkylated metabolites. Scand. J. Clin. Lab. Invest. 46: 623–627, 1986.

R.C. Baselt and R.H. Cravey. A compendium of therapeutic and toxic concentrations of toxicologically significant drugs in human biofluids. J. Anal. Tox. 1: 81–103, 1977.

A.H. Beckett, R.N. Boyes and P.J. Appleton. The metabolism and excretion of lignocaine in man. J. Pharm. Pharmac. 18: 76S–81S, 1966.

N. Benowitz and M. Rowland. Determination of lidocaine in blood and tissues. Anesthesiology 39: 639–641, 1973.

J. Blumer, J.M. Strong and A.J. Atkinson, Jr. The convulsant potency of lidocaine and its N-dealkylated metabolites. J. Pharm. Exp. Ther. 186: 31–36, 1973.

T. Borkowski. Personal communication, 1976.

R.N. Boyes, D.B. Scott, P.J. Jebson et al. Pharmacokinetics of lidocaine in man. Clin. Pharm. Ther. 12: 105–116, 1971.

G.D. Breck and W.F. Trager. Oxidative N-dealkylation: a Mannich intermediate in the formation of a new metabolite of lidocaine in man. Science 173: 544–546, 1971.

P.R. Bromage and J.G. Robson. Concentrations of lignocaine in the blood after intravenous, intramuscular, epidural and endotracheal administration. Anaesthesia 16: 461–478, 1961.

G. Caille, J. Lelorier, Y. Latour and J.G. Besner. GLC determination of lidocaine in human plasma. J. Pharm. Sci. 66: 1383–1385, 1977.

J.L. Christie. Fatal consequences of local anesthesia: report of five cases and a review of the literature. J. For. Sci. 21: 671–679, 1976.

S.S. Chu, K.H. Rah, M.D. Brannan and J.L. Cohen. Plasma concentration of lidocaine after endotracheal spray. Anesth. Anal. 54: 438–441, 1975.

C.A. DiFazio and R.E. Brown. The analysis of lidocaine and its postulated metabolites. Anesthesiology 34: 86–88, 1971.

B. Edgren, J. Tilelli and R. Gehrz. Intravenous lidocaine overdosage in a child. Clin. Tox. 24: 51–58, 1986.

R.J. Fruncillo, W. Gibbons and S.M. Bowman. CNS toxicity after ingestion of topical lidocaine. New Eng. J. Med. 306: 426–427, 1982.

W.A. Garland, W.G. Trager and S.D. Nelson. Direct (non-chromatographic) quantification of drugs and their metabolites from human plasma utilizing chemical ionization mass spectrometry and stable isotope labeling: quinidine and lidocaine. Biomed. Mass Spec. 1: 124–129, 1974.

R.L. Gorman, J.C. King and G.M. Oderda. Ingestion of topical lidocaine: it's time to stop the pain. Vet. Hum. Tox. 26: 413, 1984.

D.J. Greenblatt, V. Bolognini, J. Koch-Weser and J.S. Harmatz. Pharmacokinetic approach to the clinical use of lidocaine intravenously. J. Am. Med. Asso. 236: 273–277, 1976.

D.A. Grimes and W. Cates, Jr. Deaths from paracervical anesthesia used for first-trimester abortion, 1972–1975. New Eng. J. Med. 295: 1397–1399, 1976.

H. Halkin, P. Meffin, K.L. Melmon and M. Rowland. Influence of congestive heart failure on blood levels of lidocaine and its active monodeethylated metabolite. Clin. Pharm. Ther. 17: 669–676, 1975.

J.D. Hawkins, R.R. Bridges and T.A. Jennison. A single-step assay for lidocaine and its major metabolite, monoethylglycinexylidide, in plasma by gas-liquid chromatography and nitrogen phosphorus detection. Ther. Drug Mon. 4: 103–106, 1982.

C.E. Hignite, C. Tschanz, J. Steiner et al. Quantitation of lidocaine and its deethylated metabolites in plasma and urine by gas chromatography-mass fragmentography. J. Chrom. 161: 243–249, 1978.

T.R. Irgens, W.M. Henderson and W.H. Shelver. GLC analysis of lidocaine in blood using an alkaline flame-ionization detector. J. Pharm. Sci. 65: 608–610, 1976.

F.E. Karch and K.F. Chmielewski. GLC assay for lidocaine in human plasma. J. Pharm. Sci. 70: 229–230, 1981.

J.B. Keenaghan. The determination of lidocaine and prilocaine in whole blood by gas chromatography. Anesthesiology 29: 110–112, 1968.

J.B. Keenaghan and R.N. Boyes. The tissue distribution, metabolism and excretion of lidocaine in rats, guinea pigs, dogs and man. J. Pharm. Exp. Ther. 180: 454–463, 1972.

B.J. Kline and M.F. Martin. Simplified GLC assay for lidocaine in plasma. J. Pharm. Sci. 67: 887–888, 1978.

B. Levine, R. Blanke and J. Valentour. Lidocaine is stable in serum and blood. Clin. Chem. 29: 1564, 1983.

R. Lindberg, J.S. Salomen and E. Laurikainen. Improved liquid-chromatographic determination of lidocaine and its desethylated metabolites in serum. Clin. Chem. 29: 1572–1573, 1983.

L.E. Mather and J. Thomas. Metabolism of lidocaine in man. Life Sci. 11: 915–919, 1972.

K.L. Melmon, M. Rowland, L. Sheiner and W. Trager. Clinical implications of the disposition of lidocaine in man: a multidisciplinary study. In *Biological Effects of Drugs in Relation to Their Plasma Concentrations* (D.S. Davies and B.N.C. Prichard, eds.), University Park Press, Baltimore, 1973, pp. 107–122.

R.L. Nation and E.J. Triggs. Gas chromatographic method for the quantitative determination of lidocaine and its metabolite monoethylglycinexylidide in plasma. J. Chrom. 116: 188–193, 1976.

R.L. Nation, G.W. Peng and W.L. Chiou. High-performance liquid chromatographic method for the simultaneous determination of lidocaine and its N-dealkylated metabolites in plasma. J. Chrom. 162: 466–473, 1979.

M.A. Peat, M.E. Deyman, D.J. Crouch et al. Concentrations of lidocaine and monoethylglycinexylidide (MEGX) in lidocaine associated deaths. J. For. Sci. 30: 1048–1057, 1985.

A. Poklis, M.A. MacKell and E.F. Tucker. Tissue distribution of lidocaine after fatal accidental injection. J. For. Sci. 29: 1229–1236, 1984.

M. Rowland, P.D. Thomson, A. Guichard and K.L. Melmon. Disposition kinetics of lidocaine in normal subjects. Ann. N.Y. Acad. Sci. 179: 383–398, 1971.

M.L. Schwartz, B.G. Covino, R.M. Narang et al. Blood level of lidocaine following subcutaneous administration prior to cardiac catheterization. Am. Heart J. 88: 721–723, 1974.

D.B. Scott, P.J. Jebson, C.W. Vellani and D.G. Julian. Plasma levels of lignocaine after intramuscular injection. Lancet 2: 1209–1210, 1968.

W.W. Stargel, C.R. Roe, P.A. Routledge and D.G. Shand. Importance of blood-collection tubes in plasma lidocaine determinations. Clin. Chem. 25: 617–619, 1979.

J.M. Strong and A.J. Atkinson, Jr. Simultaneous measurement of plasma concentrations of lidocaine and its desethylated metabolite by mass fragmentography. Anal. Chem. 44: 2287–2290, 1972.

J.M. Strong, M. Parker and A.J. Atkinson, Jr. Identification of glycinexylidide in patients treated with intravenous lidocaine. Clin. Pharm. Ther. 14: 67–72, 1973.

I. Sunshine and W.W. Fike. Value of thin-layer chromatography in two fatal cases of intoxication due to lidocaine and mepivacaine. New Eng. J. Med. 271: 487–490, 1964.

J.L. Wisnicki, W.P. Tong and D.B. Ludlum. Analysis of lidocaine and its dealkylated metabolites by high-pressure liquid chromatography. Clin. Chim. Acta 93: 279–282, 1979.

Lindane

T½: 21 hr
Vd: ?
Fb: ?

Occurrence and Usage. Lindane (Kwell, Gammene), an organochlorine insecticide, is the gamma-isomer of hexachlorocyclohexane (benzene hexachloride, BHC), one of 8 such isomers isolated and the most toxic. Technical BHC contains 12–15% lindane, 65–70% alpha-BHC, 6–8% beta-BHC and 2–5% delta-BHC. The mixture has been extensively used since 1950 for agricultural and domestic purposes (as a fumigant and for the control of body lice) but, as with other organochlorine derivatives, it has recently come under governmental restrictions due to its accumulation in soil, plants and animals. The current threshold limit value for lindane in the industrial atmosphere is 0.5 mg/m³. Exposure may be via inhalation, dermal absorption or ingestion.

Blood Concentrations. Although lindane itself is not found in the blood or plasma of most members of the general population, blood concentrations of beta-BHC in United States residents were found to average 0.0015 and 0.0031 mg/L in 2 separate studies (Dale et al., 1966; Radomski et al., 1971). Blood lindane concentrations in lindane plant workers averaged 0.004 mg/L (range, 0.001–0.009) in those with low exposure and 0.031 mg/L (range, 0.006–0.093) in those with high dermal exposure. The blood concentrations did not appear to increase with continued low-level exposure, but were primarily an index of recent exposure (Milby et al., 1968). Blood lindane concentrations in 8 normal infants, age 5–99 months, who received total body dermal application of 1% lindane lotion reached an average peak level of 0.024 mg/L (range, 0.007–0.064) at 6 hours; the levels declined with an average half-life of 21 hours (Ginsburg et al., 1977).

A group of 57 workers in a lindane factory had average plasma concentrations of 0.070, 0.190, and 0.037 mg/L for alpha, beta, and gamma-BHC, respectively; beta-BHC was the only isomer that was observed to accumulate in serum with chronic exposure (Baumann et al., 1980).

Metabolism and Excretion. Lindane is rapidly metabolized in man by oxidation and dehydrohalogenation to a series of chlorinated phenols that are excreted primarily in urine, in both free and conjugated form (Starr and Clifford, 1972). Lindane concentrations in the urine of unexposed subjects were less than 0.001 mg/L (Cueto and Biros, 1967) and averaged 0.48 mg/kg (range, 0–12.3) in adipose tissue obtained randomly at 994 autopsies (Hoffman et al., 1967). The ratio of fat concentration to serum concentration for beta-BHC, the most lipid-soluble of the common BHC isomers, averaged approximately 220 in a group of lindane factory workers (Baumann et al., 1980).

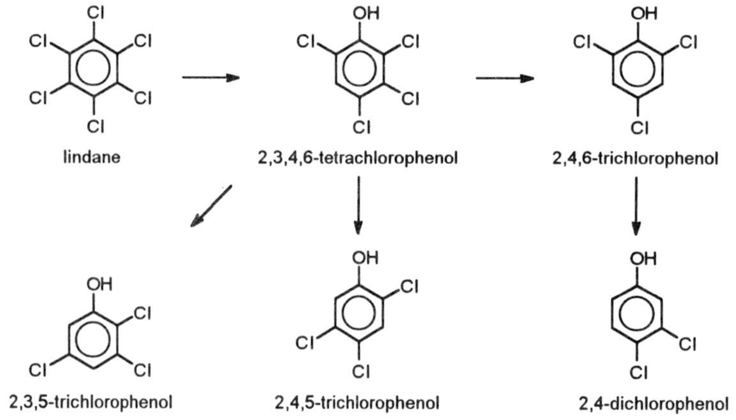

| lindane | 2,3,4,6-tetrachlorophenol | 2,4,6-trichlorophenol |
| 2,3,5-trichlorophenol | 2,4,5-trichlorophenol | 2,4-dichlorophenol |

Toxicity. Blood lindane concentrations exceeding 0.02 mg/L were associated with neurological abnormalities, including EEG changes, muscular jerking and emotional changes, in workers exposed to lindane (Czegledi-Janko and Avar, 1970). Chronic exposure to lindane through the use of home vaporizers has been presumptively implicated in one nonfatal and seven fatal cases of aplastic anemia (Loge, 1965; West, 1967; Morgan et al., 1980). Lindane that was probably absorbed dermally was responsible for a mass poisoning episode, producing weakness, mental confusion, anemia, convulsions and the death of 6 persons (Danopoulos et al., 1953).

A young boy who ingested lindane developed a plasma concentration of 0.29 mg/L after 6 hours, 3 hours after the last convulsion; after 7 days the patient was asymptomatic and the plasma level has declined to 0.02 mg/L (Dale et al., 1966). An 18 month old child developed seizures and a serum lindane concentration of 0.45 mg/L after whole-body application of lindane lotion (Telch and Jarvis, 1982). A young girl who ingested 1.6 g of lindane achieved a serum concentration of 0.84 mg/L after 2 hours, just following grand mal seizures; by 4 hours the concentration decreased to 0.49 mg/L. Concentrations of individual free phenolic metabolites in urine collected 5.5 hours after ingestion ranged from 0.04–0.74 mg/L (Starr and Clifford, 1972). Oral cholestyramine, activated charcoal or liquid paraffin have been recommended as adsorbents in poisoning cases (Jaeger et al., 1984).

The mean fatal dose of technical lindane in adults is believed to be 28 g. A fat concentration of 343 mg/kg was observed in a fatality due to lindane (Hayes and Vaughn, 1977). A woman ingested 8 oz of 20% lindane solution and exhibited seizures, unconsciousness and a serum lindane concentration of 1.3 mg/L; she developed coagulopathy and renal failure and died after 11 days (Rao et al., 1988). An adult male who ingested 2 ounces of 1% lindane lotion developed coma and a blood lindane concentration of 1.3 mg/L on the first day; he was pronounced dead 7 days later and the following postmortem concentrations were found (Kurt et al., 1986):

Lindane Concentrations in a Fatal Case (mg/L or mg/kg)

Blood	Brain	Liver	Kidney	Fat	Gastric
0.02	0.05	0.16	0.05	1.5	1.0 mg

Analysis. Lindane is measureable in body fluids and tissues using general procedures for the electron-capture gas chromatographic determination of organochlorine insecticides (Dale et al., 1966; Cueto and Biros, 1967; Radomski et al., 1971). The phenolic metabolites of lindane may be analyzed in urine by electron-capture gas chromatography after acid hydrolysis and acetylation (Angerer et al., 1981).

References

J. Angerer, R. Heinrich and H. Laudehr. Occupational exposure to hexachlorocyclohexane. V. Gas chromatographic determination of monohydroxychlorobenzenes (chlorophenols) in urine. Int. Arch. Occ. Env. Health 48: 319–324, 1981.

K. Baumann, J. Angerer, R. Heinrich and G. Lehnert. Occupational exposure to hexachlorocyclohexane. I. Body burden of HCH-isomers. Int. Arch. Occ. Env. Health 47: 119–127, 1980.

C. Czegledi-Janko and P. Avar. Occupational exposure to lindane: clinical laboratory findings. Brit. J. Ind. Med. 27: 283–286, 1970.

C. Cueto, Jr. and F.J. Biros. Chlorinated insecticides and related materials in human urine. Tox. Appl. Pharm. 10: 261–269, 1967.

W.E. Dale, A. Curley and C. Cueto, Jr. Hexane extractable chlorinated insecticides in human blood. Life Sci. 5: 47–54, 1966.

E. Danopoulos, K. Mellissinos and G. Katsas. Serious poisoning by hexachlorocyclohexane. Arch. Ind. Hyg. Occ. Med. 8: 582–587, 1953.

C.M. Ginsburg, W. Lowry and J.S. Reisch. Absorption of lindane (gamma benzene hexachloride) in infants and children. J. Pediat. 91: 998–1000, 1977.

W.J. Hayes, Jr and W.K. Vaughn. Mortality from pesticides in the United States in 1973 and 1974. Tox. Appl. Pharm. 42: 235–252, 1977.

W.S. Hoffman, H. Adler, W.I. Fishbein and F.C. Bauer. Relation of pesticide concentration in fat to pathological changes in tissues. Arch. Env. Health 15: 758-765, 1967.

U. Jaeger, A. Podczeck, A. Haubenstock et al. Acute oral poisoning with lindane-solvent mixtures. Vet. Hum. Tox. 26: 11–14, 1984.

T.L. Kurt, R. Bost, M. Gilliland et al. Accidental Kwell (lindane) ingestions. Vet. Hum. Tox. 28: 569–571, 1986.

J.P. Loge. Aplastic anemia following exposure to benzene hexachloride (lindane). J. Am. Med. Asso. 193: 110–114, 1965.

T.H. Milby, A.J. Samuels and F. Ottoboni. Human exposure to lindane: blood lindane levels as a function of exposure. J. Occ. Med. 10: 584–587, 1968.

D.P. Morgan, E.M. Stockdale, R.J. Roberts and A.W. Walter. Anemia associated with exposure to lindane. Arch. Env. Health 35: 307–310, 1980.

J.L. Radomski, W.B. Deichmann, A.A. Rey and T. Merkin. Human pesticide blood levels as a measure of body burden and pesticide exposure. Tox. Appl. Pharm. 20: 175–185, 1971.

C.V.S.R. Rao, R. Shreenivas, V. Singh et al. Disseminated intravascular coagulation in a case of fatal lindane poisoning. Vet. Hum. Tox. 30: 132–134, 1988.

H.G. Starr, Jr. and N.J. Clifford. Acute lindane intoxication. Arch. Env. Health 25: 374–375, 1972.

J. Telch and D.A. Jarvis. Acute intoxication with lindane (gamma benzene hexachloride). Can. Med. Asso. J. 126: 662–663, 1982.

I. West. Lindane and hematologic reactions. Arch. Env. Health 15: 97–101, 1967.

Lithium

T½: 17–58 hr
Vd: 0.4–1.4 L/kg
Fb: 0
pKa: 6.8 (carbonate)

Li

Occurrence and Usage. Lithium (Eskalith, Lithane) has been recognized since 1949 as an effective treatment for certain forms of mania and endogenous depression. Its mood-stabilizing effects are poorly understood but are believed to be centrally-mediated. The metal is administered orally as the carbonate (300 mg tablets and capsules) or citrate (8 mmol/5 mL syrup) in daily doses of 600–2400 mg. The optimum maintenance dosage is often determined by monitoring the serum concentration.

Blood Concentrations. In most persons, the physiological serum lithium concentration ranges from 0.0001–0.0003 mmol/L. In persons living in areas of Chile where drinking water has an unusually high lithium content, plasma lithium averages 0.003–0.012 mmol/L (Zaldivar, 1980).

Following a single oral dosage of 1500 mg of the carbonate to 3 adult subjects, an average peak plasma concentration of 1.66 mmol/L was observed at 1 hour. Plasma concentrations declined rapidly during the first 20 hours, with a half-life of 5.2 hours, and then more slowly over the next 6 days, with an elimination half-life of 17–24 hours (Groth et al., 1974). Optimum serum lithium concentrations for most patients have been found to range from 0.5–1.3 mmol/L in early morning specimens drawn 12 hours after the last dose (Amdisen, 1975). In patients receiving average daily doses of 1500–1700 mg of lithium carbonate, serum concentrations were in the range of 0.7–0.9 mmol/L (Marini and Sheard, 1976). The plasma half-life has been found to average 31 hours in patients just beginning lithium therapy, 40 hours in those receiving the drug for less than 1 year, and 58 hours in those receiving it for over 1 year (Goodnick et al., 1981). The erythrocyte/plasma lithium concentration ratio averages between 0.35 and 0.55 in different groups of patients (Ramsey et al., 1979).

Metabolism and Excretion. In normal subjects lithium is excreted essentially quantitatively in the urine, an average of 97% of a single dose being eliminated within 10 days (Groth et al., 1974). Hyponatremia causes lithium retention and, conversely, the administration of large doses of sodium chloride hastens the renal excretion of the drug. During therapy, brain and cerebrospinal fluid concentrations of lithium average 65% of the serum value (Terhaag et al., 1978).

Toxicity. Lithium toxicity is often manifested at serum concentrations exceeding 2 mmol/L. The symptoms of intoxication include nausea, vomiting, diarrhea, drowsiness, weakness, ataxia, blurred vision, tinnitus, polyuria, confusion, stupor, seizures, and coma. Forced diuresis, alkalinization of urine, and theophylline administration can increase the renal elimination of lithium several fold during poisoning (Thomsen, 1969). Amdisen (1978) recommends that serum lithium levels be measured every 3 hours in intoxicated patients; if a plot of the values reveals that the serum concentration has exceeded 2.5 mmol/L or that it will not fall below 1.0 mmol/L within 30 hours of the onset of symptoms, hemodialysis should be instituted. Clinical manifestations tend to be milder in acute poisoning as opposed to chronic toxicity, and serum lithium levels generally decline more rapidly; a rebound in serum lithium concentrations after hemodialysis may indicate a need for further dialysis (Jacobsen et al., 1987).

A 59 year old man became comatose at a serum lithium concentration of 1.76 mmol/L, which had accumulated during chronic therapy; even with measures to increase renal elimination of lithium, it required 8 days for his serum level to decline by half (Herrero, 1973). A 29 year old pregnant woman who developed chronic toxicity became comatose and exhibited seizure activity about 60 hours after a normal delivery; her lithium elimination half-life was approximately 24 hours, with no special attempts to enhance excretion (Aoki and Ruedy, 1971). Serum half-lives of 30–100 hours were observed in 8 patients who developed lithium toxicity (Schou et al., 1968). One patient survived the ingestion of 22.5 g of lithium carbonate after developing a serum concentration of 8.2 mmol/L; diuresis succeeded in lowering the level to 3.4 mg/L within 22 hours (Horowitz and Fisher, 1969).

In one patient who ingested 60 g of the drug, a peak serum concentration of 14 mmol/L was recorded after 50 hours, at which time the patient was comatose; the level dropped to 5 mmol/L by 64 hours and death occurred at 92 hours (Achong et al., 1975). The following tissue levels were noted in 5 subjects, who developed initial serum lithium concentrations of 2.4–8.0 mmol/L and died within 1–21 days of hospital admission (Chapman and Lewis, 1972; Amdisen et al., 1974; Geldmacher-von Mallinckrodt et al., 1979; Winek et al., 1980; Alha, 1982):

Lithium Concentrations in Fatal Cases (mmol/L or mmol/kg)

	Blood	Brain	Liver	Kidney	Urine
Average	1.9	2.0	2.8	3.6	6.7
(Range)	(0.3–4.6)	(0.9–4.2)	(0.2–6.7)	(0.6–9.6)	(6.7)

Analysis. Lithium is routinely determined in serum or urine by flame emission (van der Helm and Andriesse, 1961) or atomic absorption spectrometry (Hansen, 1968; Scott, 1982). The use of an ion-selective electrode has also been described (Bertholf et al., 1988). Since the lithium ion is not bound to plasma protein, ultrafiltrates of whole blood may be analyzed directly by these procedures with little loss of drug. Some investigators hold that the erythrocyte/plasma lithium ratio is of greater diagnostic value than the serum concentration in toxic situations; this determination may also be performed by emission photometry (Eisenberg and Lantz, 1977) or atomic absorption spectrometry (Hisayasu et al., 1977). Serum stored in clot tubes for 3 days lost 26% of its lithium when refrigerated but only 6% at room temperature; when analysis must be delayed, it is preferable to remove the serum from the clot and store in glass or plastic at 4° C. (Mulyran et al., 1987).

References

M.R. Achong, P.G. Fernandez and P.J. McLeod. Fatal self-poisoning with lithium carbonate. Can. Med. Asso. J. 112: 868–870, 1975.

A. Alha. Personal communication, 1982.

A. Amdisen. Monitoring of lithium treatment through determination of lithium concentration. Dan. Med. Bull. 22: 277–291, 1975.

A. Amdisen, C.G. Gottsfries, L. Jacobsson and B. Winblad. Grave lithium intoxication with fatal outcome. Acta Psych. Scand. Supp. 4: 25–33, 1974.

A. Amdisen. Clinical and serum-level monitoring in lithium therapy and lithium intoxication. J. Anal. Tox. 2: 193–202, 1978.

F.Y. Aoki and J. Ruedy. Severe lithium intoxication: management without dialysis and report of a possible teratogenic effect of lithium. Can. Med. Asso. J. 105: 847–848, 1971.

R.L. Bertholf, M.G. Savory, K.H. Winborne et al. Lithium determined in serum with an ion-selective electrode. Clin. Chem. 34: 1500–1502, 1988.

A.J. Chapman and G. Lewis. Iatrogenic lithium poisoning: a case report with necropsy findings. Okla. State Med. Asso. J. 65: 491–494, 1972.

R. Eisenberg and R. Lantz. Erythrocyte lithium analysis. Clin. Chem. 23: 900, 1977.

M. Geldmacher-von Mallinckrodt, G. Jacob and K.H. Scaller. Lithium distribution in body fluids and organs after treatment with Quilonum Retard (R) (lithium carbonate). Vet. Hum. Tox. 21: 187–190, 1979.

P.J. Goodnick, R.R. Fieve, H.L. Meltzer and D.L. Dunner. Lithium elimination half-life and duration of therapy. Clin. Pharm. Ther. 29: 47–50, 1981.

U. Groth, W. Prellwitz and E. Jahnchen. Estimation of pharmacokinetic parameters of lithium from saliva and urine. Clin. Pharm. Ther. 16: 490–498, 1974.

D. Jacobsen, G. Aasen, P. Fredericksen and B. Eisenga. Lithium intoxication: pharmacokinetics during and after terminated hemodialysis in acute intoxications. Clin. Tox. 25: 81–94, 1987.

J.L. Hansen. The measurement of serum and urine lithium by atomic absorption spectrophotometry. Am. J. Med. Tech. 34: 1–9, 1968.

F.A. Herrero. Lithium carbonate toxicity. J. Am. Med. Asso. 226: 1109–1110, 1973.

G.H. Hisayasu, J.L. Cohen and R.W. Nelson. Determination of plasma and erythrocyte lithium concentrations by atomic absorption spectrophotometry. Clin. Chem. 23: 41–45, 1977.

L.C. Horowitz and G.U. Fisher. Acute lithium toxicity. New Eng. J. Med. 281: 1369, 1969.

J.L. Marini and M.H. Sheard. Sustained-release lithium carbonate in a double-blind study: serum lithium levels, side effects, and placebo response. J. Clin. Pharm. 16: 276–283, 1976.

G. Mulyran, N. Brazil, D. Day-Cody and P. McKeon. Lithium stability in clotted blood: storage guidelines. Clin. Chem. 33: 1944, 1987.

T.A. Ramsey, A. Frazer, J. Mendels and W.L. Dyson. The erythrocyte lithium-plasma lithium ratio in patients with primary affective disorder. Arch. Gen. Psych. 36: 457–461, 1979.

M. Schou, A. Amdisen and J. Trap-Jensen. Lithium poisoning. Am. J. Psych. 125: 520–527, 1968.

I.M.B. Scott. The determination of lithium in blood serum by atomic absorption spectrophotometry. J. For. Sci. Soc. 22: 41–42, 1982.

B. Terhaag, A. Scherber, P. Schaps and H. Winkler. The distribution of lithium into cerebrospinal fluid, brain tissue and bile in man. Int. J. Clin. Pharm. 16: 333–335, 1978.

K. Thomsen. Renal lithium elimination in man and active treatment of lithium poisoning. Acta Psych. Scand. Suppl. 207: 83–84, 1969.

V.J. van der Helm and D. Andriesse. The determination of lithium in serum during therapy with lithium salts. Clin. Chim. Acta 6: 747–748, 1961.

C.L. Winek, J.D. Bricker and F.W. Fochtman. Lithium intoxication. A case study. For. Sci. Int. 15: 227–231, 1980.

R. Zaldivar. High lithium concentrations in drinking water and plasma of exposed subjects. Arch. Tox. 46: 319–320, 1980.

Lorazepam

T½: 9–16 hr
Vd: 0.9–1.3 L/kg
Fb: 0.80
pKa: 1.3, 11.5

Occurrence and Usage. Lorazepam (Ativan) is a 3-hydroxy benzodiazepine, one of a group that includes oxazepam and temazepam. It is available as the free base in 0.5–2 mg tablets or a 2–4 mg/mL solution, and is administered orally or parenterally in daily doses of 1–10 mg as an antianxiety agent.

Blood Concentrations. After a single 2 mg oral dose, lorazepam concentrations in plasma averaged 0.018 mg/L at 2 hours, declining to 0.009 mg/L by 12 hours, with an apparent half-life of 12 hours (Greenblatt et al., 1976). During chronic daily administration of 10 mg, steady-state plasma lorazepam concentrations averaged 0.181 mg/L (range, 0.140–0.240) in 9 subjects (Kyriakopoulos, 1976).

Intramuscular administration of 4 mg to 6 subjects resulted in an average peak plasma concentration of 0.057 mg/L at 1.5 hours (Greenblatt et al., 1977a). Following intravenous injection of 5 mg of the drug, peak plasma concentrations measured in the first few minutes averaged approximately 0.140 mg/L (Greenblatt et al., 1977b).

Lorazepam exhibits linear kinetics, describable by a 1 or 2-compartment model; it is 91–95% bioavailable after oral administration (Greenblatt et al., 1979; Bradshaw et al., 1981).

Metabolism and Excretion. Lorazepam is rapidly conjugated with glucuronic acid, forming an inactive metabolite. Rather than being immediately excreted, however, lorazepam glucuronide accumulates in plasma, achieving concentrations that exceed those of its parent, and has a somewhat longer half-life, about 16 hours. About 75% of a dose is eliminated in urine as lorazepam glucuronide over a 5 day period, with another 14% as conjugates of minor metabolites, which include ring hydroxylation products and quinazoline derivatives. Only negligible amounts of unchanged drug are found in urine (Elliott, 1976; Greenblatt et al., 1976).

Toxicity. Several children who ingested 2.5–25 mg of lorazepam have exhibited symptoms of drowsiness, ataxia, and visual and auditory hallucinations; the patients recovered within 12–30 hours with supportive treatment (Jeffrey and Whitfield, 1974; Vlachos et al., 1978). Three adults intentionally ingested lorazepam (100 and 120 mg in 2 cases) and developed lethargy or light coma; they recovered spontaneously within 24–30 hours. Peak plasma lorazepam concentrations of 0.30–0.60 mg/L were measured in the 3 patients, and the levels declined with half-lives of 9–22 hours (Allen et al., 1980).

Blood lorazepam concentrations of 0.28–1.0 mg/L were measured at autopsy in 3 adult victims of acute drug overdosage, but at least one other depressant drug was involved in each instance (Koves and Yen, 1989). A 6 year old child who accidentally ingested an overdose and died within 6 hours had a postmortem blood lorazepam concentration of 2.8 mg/L (Registry, 1983).

Analysis. Lorazepam is frequently analyzed using electron-capture gas chromatography; it has been chromatographed as the hydrolysis product (Greenblatt et al., 1976), as a trimethylsilyl derivative (deSilva et al., 1976; Higuchi et al., 1979), and as the intact drug (de Groot et al., 1976; Greenblatt et al., 1978). In the latter procedure, however, lorazepam undergoes thermolytic dehydration during analysis to yield a quinazoline-2-carboxyaldehyde, with a deleterious effect on precision. The glucuronide metabolite may be measured in a similar manner after enzyme hydrolysis (Higuchi et al., 1979). Koves and Yen (1989) found that thermal rearrangement of the intact drug was complete and reproducible in their gas chromatographic-mass spectrometric method. A liquid chromatographic procedure has also been described (Egan and Abernethy, 1986).

References

M.D. Allen, D.J. Greenblatt, Y. Lacasse and R.I. Shader. Pharmacokinetic study of lorazepam overdosage. Am. J. Psych. 137: 1414–1415, 1980.

E.G. Bradshaw, A.A. Ali, B.A. Mulley and R.M. Rye. Plasma concentrations and clinical effects of lorazepam after oral administration. Brit. J. Anaesth. 53: 517–522, 1981.

G. de Groot, R.A.A. Maes and H.H.J. Lemmens. Determination of lorazepam in plasma by electron capture GLC. Arch. Tox. 35: 229–234, 1976.

J.A.F. deSilva, I. Bekersky, C.V. Puglisi et al. Determination of 1,4-benzodiazepines and -diazepin-2-ones in blood by electron-capture gas-liquid chromatography. Anal. Chem. 48: 10–19, 1976.

J.M. Egan and D.R. Abernethy. Lorazepam analysis using liquid chromatography: improved sensitivity for single-dose pharmacokinetic studies. J. Chrom. 380: 196–201, 1986.

H.W. Elliott. Metabolism of lorazepam. Brit. J. Anesth. 48: 1017–1023, 1976.

D.J. Greenblatt, R.T. Schillings, A.A. Kyriakopoulos et al. Clinical pharmacokinetics of lorazepam. I. Absorption and disposition of oral ^{14}C-lorazepam. Clin. Pharm. Ther. 20: 329–341, 1976.

D.J. Greenblatt, T.H. Joyce, W.H. Comer et al. Clinical pharmacokinetics of lorazepam II. Intramuscular injection. Clin. Pharm. Ther. 21: 222–230, 1977a.

D.J. Greenblatt, W.H. Comer, H.W. Elliott et al. Clinical pharmacokinetics of lorazepam. III. Intravenous injection. J. Clin. Pharm. 17: 490–494, 1977b.

D.J. Greenblatt, K. Franke and R.I. Shader. Analysis of lorazepam and its glucuronide metabolite by electron-capture gas-liquid chromatography. J. Chrom. 146: 311–320, 1978.

D.J. Greenblatt, R.I. Shader, K. Franke et al. Pharmacokinetics and bioavailability of intravenous, intramuscular, and oral lorazepam in humans. J. Pharm. Sci. 68: 57–63, 1979.

S. Higuchi, H. Urabe and Y. Shiobara. Simplified determination of lorazepam and oxazepam in biological fluids by gas chromatography-mass spectrometry. J. Chrom. 164: 55–61, 1979.

D.J. Jeffrey and M.F. Whitfield. Lorazepam poisoning. Brit. Med. J. 2: 719, 1974.

E.M. Koves and B. Yen. The use of gas chromatography/negative ion chemical ionization mass spectrometry for the determination of lorazepam in whole blood. J. Anal. Tox. 13: 69–72, 1989.

A.A. Kyriakopoulos. Bioavailability of lorazepam in humans. In *Pharmacokinetics of Psychoactive Drugs* (L.A. Gottschalk and S. Merlis, eds.), Spectrum Publications, New York, 1976, pp. 45–60.

Registry of Human Toxicology, American Academy of Forensic Sciences, Colorado Springs, Colorado, 1983.

P. Vlachos, P. Kentarchou, L. Poulos and G. Aloupogiannis. Lorazepam poisoning. Tox. Letters 2: 109–110, 1978.

Loxapine

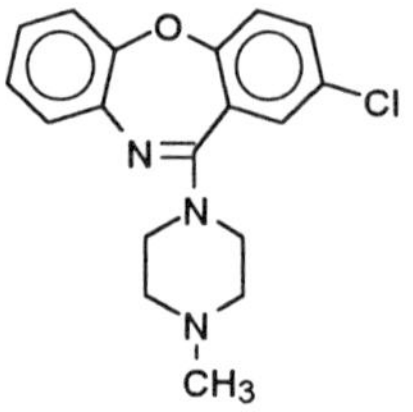

T½: 3–4 hr
Vd: ?
Fb: ?
pKa: 6.6

Occurrence and Usage. Loxapine (Loxitane, Daxoline) is a tricyclic antipsychotic drug that has been in clinical use since 1976. Amoxapine, a related drug, is a metabolite of loxapine. Loxapine is available for oral use as the succinate in 5–50 mg capsules or as the hydrochloride in a 25 mg/mL concentrate; a solution for intramuscular injection contains 50 mg/mL as the hydrochloride. Daily maintenance doses may range from 20–250 mg.

Blood Concentrations. An intramuscular dose averaging 29.5 mg given to 10 subjects produced an average peak plasma loxapine concentration of 0.017 mg/L at 2 hours; concentrations of 2 metabolites, 8-hydroxyloxapine and 8-hydroxyamoxapine, reached peak levels of 0.014 and 0.002 mg/L, respectively, at 24 hours. An average oral dose of 29.5 mg resulted in average peak plasma concentrations of 0.017, 0.030 and 0.005 mg/L at 1, 2 and 6 hours, respectively, for loxapine, 8-hydroxyloxapine, and 8-hydroxyamoxapine (Simpson et al., 1978).

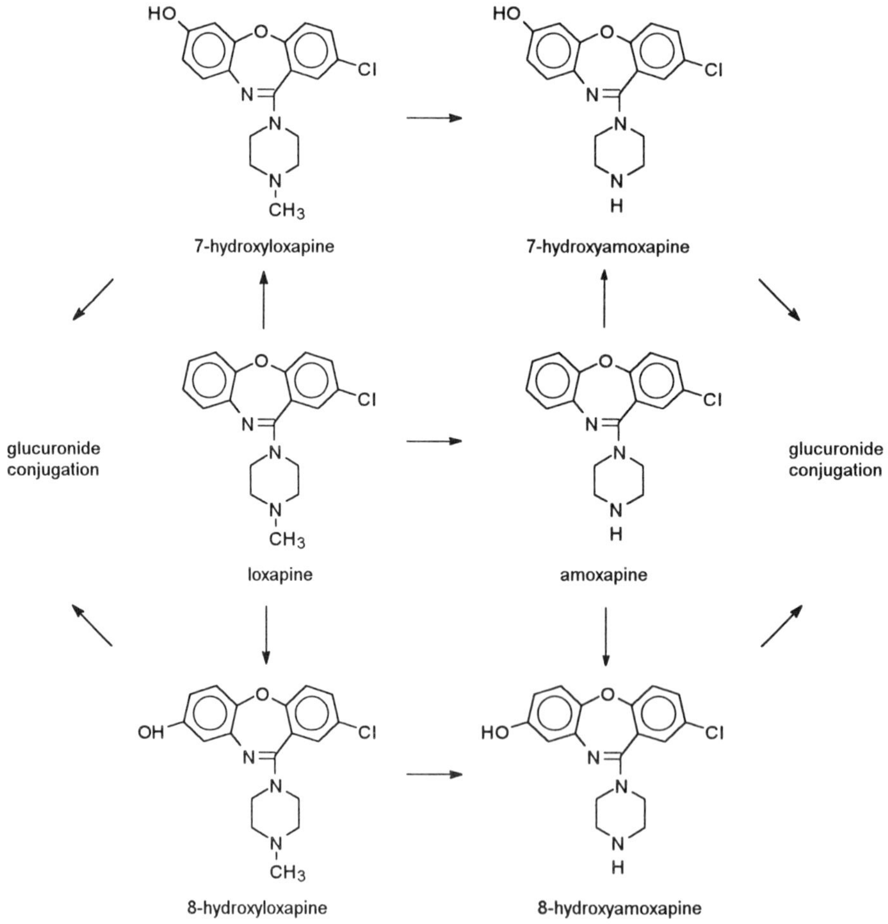

7-hydroxyloxapine   7-hydroxyamoxapine

glucuronide   glucuronide
conjugation   conjugation

loxapine   amoxapine

8-hydroxyloxapine   8-hydroxyamoxapine

Metabolism and Excretion. Loxapine is metabolized by N-demethylation, 7- and 8-hydroxylation, and glucuronide conjugation. N-oxide formation is also believed to take place. The disposition of the drug has not been quantitatively studied, but urinary excretion of glucuronide conjugates probably accounts for a major portion of a dose. Urine concentrations of unchanged loxapine in patients receiving 80 mg daily range from undetectable levels to 0.031 mg/L (Cooper et al., 1979; Cooper et al., 1981).

Toxicity. The manifestations of loxapine toxicity include dizziness, confusion, weakness, extrapyramidal effects, stupor, tachycardia, profound hypotension, respiratory depression, seizures, and coma. Seizures and cardiovascular abnormalities were the most serious complications in 10 adults who survived the acute ingestion of 450–2750 mg of the drug (Peterson, 1981). A 25 year old female was stuporous but easily arousable with a serum loxapine concentration of 0.192 mg/L (Vasiliades et al., 1979). A 20 month old child developed coma and a blood loxapine concentration of 0.72 mg/L, but eventually survived this accidental poisoning (Hepler et al., 1982).

A blood loxapine concentration of 1.9 mg/L was measured upon hospital admission in a young woman who ingested 2500 mg of the drug and died 12 days later. Postmortem blood and liver concentrations of 7.7 mg/L and 150 mg/kg were observed in another woman found dead with 2.9 g of drug remaining unabsorbed in her stomach (Reynolds et al., 1979). The following tissue distribution was observed in a 70 year old woman who died after an acute overdose of loxapine (Registry, 1983):

Loxapine Concentrations in a Fatality (mg/L or mg/kg)

Blood	Brain	Liver	Kidney	Gastric
3.0	40	110	22	710 mg

Analysis. Intact loxapine has been assayed in serum by gas chromatography with nitrogen-specific or mass spectrometric detection (Vasiliades et al., 1979; Lutz et al., 1982). Loxapine and its hydroxylated metabolites may be analyzed by electron-capture gas chromatography after trifluoroacetylation and silylation (Cooper and Kelly, 1979).

References

T.B. Cooper and R.G. Kelly. GLC analysis of loxapine, amoxapine, and their metabolites in serum and urine. J. Pharm. Sci. 68: 216–219, 1979.

S.F. Cooper, R. Dugal and M.J. Bertrand. Determination of loxapine in human plasma and urine and identification of three urinary metabolites. Xenobiotica 9: 405–414, 1979.

T.B. Cooper, R. Bost and I. Sunshine. Postmortem blood and tissue levels of loxapine and its metabolites. J. Anal. Tox. 5: 99–100, 1981.

B.R. Hepler, R. Solano, J.R. Weber et al. Acute loxapine intoxication in a child. J. Anal. Tox. 6: 258–259, 1982.

T. Lutz, S.P. Jindal and T.B. Cooper. GLC/MS assay for loxapine in human biofluids and tissues with deuterium labeled analog as an internal standard. J. Anal. Tox. 6: 301–304, 1982.

C.D. Peterson. Seizures induced by acute loxapine overdose. Am. J. Psych. 138: 1089–1091, 1981.

Registry of Human Toxicology, American Academy of Forensic Sciences, Colorado Springs, Colorado, 1983.

P.C. Reynolds, C.W. Som and P.W. Herrmann. Loxapine fatalities. Clin. Tox. 14: 181–185, 1979.

G.M. Simpson, T.B. Cooper, J.H. Lee and M.A. Young. Clinical and plasma level characteristics of intramuscular and oral loxapine. Psychopharmacology 56: 225–232, 1978.

J. Vasiliades, T.M. Sahawneh and C. Owens. Determination of therapeutic and toxic concentrations of doxepin and loxapine using gas-liquid chromatography with a nitrogen-sensitive detector and gas chromatography-mass spectrometry of loxapine. J. Chrom. 164: 457–470, 1979.

Lysergic Acid Diethylamide

(C$_2$H$_5$)$_2$NCO

N–CH$_3$

N
H

T½: 3–4 hr
Vd: 0.28 L/kg
Fb: ?
pKa: 7.8

Occurrence and Usage. Lysergic acid diethylamide (LSD, lysergamide, Delysid) is an indole de-rivative that was first synthesized in 1938 by A. Hoffman of Sandoz Laboratories. The d-isomer is one of the most potent hallucinogenic agents known (the l-isomer is apparently inactive) and yet has a remarkably low acute toxicity, its therapeutic index being on the order of 1000. LSD is usually administered by drug abusers as the tartrate salt in oral doses of 100–250 µg, being readily synthe-sized from lysergic acid and diethylamine. A closely related but less active compound, lysergic acid amide, occurs naturally in the seeds of the morning glory and the Hawaiian baby wood rose.

Blood Concentrations. Following a single intravenous administration of 2 µg/kg (140 µg/70 kg) of the drug, a maximal plasma concentration of 0.005 mg/L was observed at 1 hour, with a decline to 0.001 mg/L by 8 hours; a plasma half-life of 3.5–4.0 hours was determined using a fluorometric method (Aghajanian and Bing, 1964). Using a similar procedure, plasma concentrations as high as 0.009 mg/L were found within the first 5 hours in subjects who ingested a single 160 µg dose of LSD (Upshall and Wailling, 1972). Wagner et al. (1968) found that LSD behaved according to a 2 compartment open model, with an average elimination half-life of 3 hours.

Metabolism and Excretion. The metabolism of LSD has not been investigated in man. On the basis of animal studies it is known to undergo extensive biotransformation via N-demethylation, N-deethylation, and hydroxylation to inactive metabolites (Axelrod et al., 1956). Monkeys excreted 24% of a labeled oral dose in the urine and none in the feces over a 48 hour period; only a small fraction of the dose was eliminated unchanged (Sullivan et al., 1978).

Urine concentrations of unchanged drug ranged from 0.001–0.055 mg/L in the 24 hours after ingestion of 200–400 µg of the drug by humans (Taunton-Rigby et al., 1973). LSD or its cross-reactive metabolites were detectable for periods of 34–120 hours at concentrations of 0.002–0.028 mg/L in the urine of 7 subjects who received a 300 µg oral dose (Peel and Boynton, 1980).

Toxicity. A common side-effect of LSD usage is the unpredictable recurrence of hallucinations for weeks or months after the last dose (Horowitz, 1969). Hysterical behavior, hyperactivity, and life-threatening hyperthermia were exhibited by a young man who took a large dose of the drug (Friedman and Hirsch, 1971). Two girls took a single dose of LSD and developed delayed psychotic reactions 2 weeks later. Both were hospitalized and received chlorpromazine, a major tranquilizer, for con-trol of their symptoms (Cooper, 1974).

Persons receiving treatment for LSD intoxication, manifested by agitation or unconsciousness, have exhibited plasma and urine levels as high as 0.004 and 0.008 mg/L, respectively (Widdop, 1970; McCarron et al., 1990). A 12 year old child hospitalized with hyperactivity had a serum LSD concentration of 0.002 mg/L (Twitchett et al., 1978).

Eight individuals "snorted" a white powder that they believed to be cocaine. Within 5 minutes they developed restlessness, anxiety, numbness, vomiting and collapse. They were brought to the emergency room of a hospital. Two persons were comatose, 1 was catatonic and 5 were hyperactive, delirious, and hyperpyrexic. Four developed fever, 2 had diarrhea, and all 8 showed evidence of blood coagulation disorders. Only supportive therapy was used, and all patients recovered com-pletely within 12 hours. Admission blood specimens contained LSD in levels ranging from 0.002–0.026 mg/L. Clinically insignificant amounts of ethanol or benzoylecgonine (a cocaine metabolite) were found in 3 of the patients' specimens. The white powder inhaled by the subjects was found to contain 80–90% LSD (Klock et al., 1973).

One case of LSD overdosage was reported in which an uneventful recovery followed the ingestion of 10 mg of the drug (Cohen, 1967). A case in which death was directly attributed to LSD involved a 25 year old male who died 16 hours after hospital admission; antemortem serum and postmortem blood contained 0.014 and 0.005 mg/L LSD, respectively (Fysh et al., 1985).

Analysis. A fluorimetric method for the analysis of LSD in biological materials has been described (Axelrod et al., 1957) and used successfully by several groups of investigators. Paper chromatography (Faed and McLeod, 1973), thin-layer chromatography and high-pressure liquid chromatography methods (Christie et al., 1976) for urine screening with quantitative capabilities have been reported. A number of articles have appeared that deal with the determination of LSD by radioimmunoassay techniques, the reagents for which are now commercially available (Taunton-Rigby et al., 1973; Castro et al., 1973; Loeffler and Pierce, 1973; Ratcliffe et al., 1977). Twitchett et al. (1978) proposed a combination of liquid chromatography with fluorescence detection and radioimmunoassay for analysis of the drug in plasma or urine. Gas chromatography-mass spectrometry has been described for LSD in plasma (Papac and Foltz, 1990) and urine (Francom et al., 1988; Paul et al., 1990). LSD degrades readily in biological specimens unless protected from light and elevated temperature (Peel and Boynton, 1980; Francom et al., 1988); the drug may also bind to glass containers at an acid pH (Paul et al., 1990).

References

G.K. Aghajanian and O.H.L. Bing. Persistence of lysergic acid diethylamide in the plasma of human subjects. Clin. Pharm. Ther. 5: 611–614, 1964.

J. Axelrod, R.O. Brady, B. Witkop and E.V. Evarts. Metabolism of lysergic acid diethylamide. Nature 178: 143–144, 1956.

J. Axelrod, R.O. Brady, B. Witkop and E.V. Evarts. The distribution and metabolism of lysergic acid diethylamide. Ann. N.Y. Acad. Sci. 66: 435–444, 1957.

A. Castro, D.P. Grettie, F. Bartos and D. Bartos. LSD radioimmunoassay. Res. Comm. Chem. Path. Pharm. 6: 879–886, 1973.

J. Christie, M.W. White and J.M. Wiles. A chromatographic method for the detection of LSD in biological liquids. J. Chrom. 120: 496–501, 1976.

S. Cohen. Psychotomimetic agents. Ann. Rev. Pharm. 7: 301–318, 1967.

P. Cooper. *Poisoning by Drugs and Chemicals*, 3rd ed., Year Book Medical Publishing, Chicago, 1974, p. 130.

E.M. Faed and W.R. McLeod. A urine screening test for lysergide (LSD-25). J. Chrom. Sci. 11: 4–6, 1973.

P. Francom, D. Andrenyak, H.K. Lim et al. Determination of LSD in urine by capillary column gas chromatography and electron impact mass spectrometry. J. Anal. Tox. 12: 1–8, 1988.

S.A. Friedman and S.E. Hirsch. Extreme hyperthermia after LSD ingestion. J. Am. Med. Asso. 217: 1549–1550, 1971.

R.R. Fysh, M.C.H. Oon, K.N. Robinson et al. A fatal poisoning with LSD. For. Sci. Int. 28: 109–113, 1985.

M.J. Horowitz. Flashbacks: recurrent intrusive images after the use of LSD. Am. J. Psych. 126: 147–151, 1969.

J.C. Klock, U. Boerner and C.E. Becker. Coma, hyperthermia and bleeding associated with massive LSD overdose. West. J. Med. 120: 183–188, 1973.

L.J. Loeffler and J.V. Pierce. Radioimmunoassay for lysergide (LSD) in illicit drugs and biological fluids. J. Pharm. Sci. 62: 1817–1820, 1973.

M.M. McCarron, C.B. Walberg and R.C. Baselt. Confirmation of LSD intoxication by analysis of serum and urine. J. Anal. Tox. 14: 165–167, 1990.

D.I. Papac and R.L. Foltz. Measurement of lysergic acid diethylamide (LSD) in human plasma by gas chromatography/negative ion chemical ionization mass spectrometry. J. Anal. Tox. 14: 189–190, 1990.

B.D. Paul, J.M. Mitchell, R. Burbage et al. Gas chromatographic-electron impact mass fragmentographiuc determination of lysergic acid diethylamide in urine. J. Chrom. 529: 103–112, 1990.

H.W. Peel and A.L. Boynton. Analysis of LSD in urine using radioimmunoassay—excretion and storage effects. Can. Soc. For. Sci. J. 13: 23–28, 1980.

W.A. Ratcliffe, S.M. Fletcher, A.C. Moffat et al. Radioimmunoassay of lysergic acid diethylamide (LSD) in serum and urine by using antisera of different specificities. Clin. Chem. 23: 169–174, 1977.

A.T. Sullivan, P.J. Twitchett, S.M. Fletcher and A.C. Moffat. The fate of LSD in the body: forensic considerations. J. For. Sci. 18: 89–98, 1978.

A. Taunton-Rigby, S.E. Sher and P.R. Kelley. Lysergic acid diethylamide: radioimmunoassay. Science 181: 165–166, 1973.

P.J. Twitchett, S.M. Fletcher, A.T. Sullivan and A.C. Moffat. Analysis of LSD in human body fluids by high-performance liquid chromatography, fluorescence spectroscopy and radioimmunoassay. J. Chrom. 150: 73–84, 1978.

D.G. Upshall and D.G. Wailling. The determination of LSD in human plasma following oral administration. Clin. Chim. Acta 36: 67–73, 1972.

J.G. Wagner, G.K. Aghajanian and O.H.L. Bing. Correlation of performance test scores with "tissue concentration" of lysergic acid diethylamide in human subjects. Clin. Pharm. Ther. 9: 635–638, 1968.

B. Widdop. Personal communication, 1970.

Magnesium

T½: ?
Vd: 0.2–0.4 L/kg
Fb: 0.34

Mg^{+2}

Occurrence and Usage. Magnesium is an essential trace element whose dietary deficiency may result in irritability, neuromuscular abnormalities, and cardiac and renal damage. Magnesium salts are taken orally as antacids and cathartics and are applied externally to relieve inflammation. Magnesium sulfate is occasionally injected parenterally for the treatment of toxemia of pregnancy. The metal is widely used industrially in various lightweight alloys and in refractory materials. The current threshold limit value for industrial exposure to magnesium oxide fume is 10 mg/m³.

Blood Concentrations. Normal serum magnesium concentrations in several studies have been found to range from 0.5–1.3 mmol/L (1.0–2.6 mEq/L or 1.2–3.2 mg/dL), averaging 0.87–0.93 mmol/L in adults of either sex. An average of 34% of total serum magnesium is bound to protein (Stewart et al., 1963; Hansen and Freier, 1967; Speich et al., 1981).

Patients who received a single oral 30 g dose of magnesium sulfate as a cathartic showed no significant change in serum magnesium level after 1 hour, but those patients who received 3 such doses at 4 hour intervals exhibited an average increase of 51% in serum magnesium at 1 hour after the last dose (Smilkstein et al., 1987).

A single 2 g intravenous dose of magnesium sulfate produced an average peak serum magnesium concentration in 3 pregnant women of 2 mmol/L, but this quickly declined to a level of 1 mmol/L. A 10 g intramuscular dose given to 20 patients resulted in an average peak level of 1.85 mmol/L at 2 hours (Chesley and Tepper, 1957). The combination of a 3 g intravenous dose and 10 g intramuscular dose of magnesium sulfate in 10 patients caused an elevation of serum magnesium to an average peak of 2.3 mmol/L at 1 and 2 hours, declining to about 1.8 mmol/L by 6 hours (Chesley, 1979). Flowers et al. (1962) recommended the maintenance of serum magnesium between 1.2 and 2.5 mmol/L for the treatment of convulsive toxemia of pregnancy. The use of magnesium in this manner is considered controversial (Dinsdale, 1988; Kaplan et al., 1988).

Metabolism and Excretion. Normal urine contains from 1–6 mmol/L of magnesium (Stewart et al., 1963). In dogs, administered magnesium is quickly distributed throughout the body, with the highest concentrations in kidney, liver, and heart. About 22% of a dose is eliminated in urine within 3 hours, and 25% within 24 hours. Only about 1% is excreted in feces. Skeletal muscle and bone account for a large portion of the body burden of magnesium (Brandt et al., 1958). From 38–53% of a 13 g dose of magnesium sulfate is eliminated in the urine of female patients within 4 hours of parenteral administration (Chesley, 1979). Large oral dose of magnesium sulfate may undergo a certain degree of absorption; healthy volunteers receiving a 14 g dose excreted 0.8–8.7% (average, 4.0) of the dose in the 24 hour urine (Morris et al., 1987).

Toxicity. Excessive magnesium administration may cause central nervous system depression, loss of muscle tone, and respiratory and cardiac arrest. Symptoms of toxicity begin to appear at serum magnesium levels of 3.5–5.0 mmol/L, and respiratory arrest may occur at a level of 8.5–13.5 mmol/L. Intravenous calcium gluconate is used as a specific antidote to hypermagnesemia (Chesley, 1979). An adult male who received multiple oral doses of magnesium salts for catharsis developed sedation, bradycardia and respiratory arrest; the serum magnesium level was initially 6.6 mmol/L but fell to 1.4 mmol/L within 24 hours (Fassler et al., 1985). A 25 day old infant given a total of 3112 mg of magnesium hydroxide orally as a laxative over 3 days developed hypotonia and coma; her initial serum magnesium level of 3.8 mmol/L declined quickly with calcium gluconate administration and the child fully recovered (Mofenson and Caraccio, 1991).

An apparent 10-fold error in preparing an intravenous magnesium sulfate solution resulted in cardiorespiratory arrest and eventually death of a pregnant woman after 1.5 hours of infusion; her serum magnesium level 45 minutes post-arrest was 8.7 mmol/L (Baselt, 1990).

Analysis. Serum magnesium may be determined by colorimetry (Simonsen et al., 1947; Heaton, 1960; Wimmer et al., 1986), fluorometry (Schachter, 1959; Ioannou and Konstantianos, 1989), or emission spectrometry (Alcock et al., 1960; Montgomery, 1961). Atomic absorption spectrometry is less subject to interference and may also be applied to urine specimens (Stewart et al., 1963; Hansen and Freier, 1967).

References

N. Alcock, I. MacIntyre and I. Radde. The determination of magnesium in biological fluids and tissues by flame spectrophotometry. J. Clin. Path. 13: 506–510, 1960.

R.C. Baselt. Unpublished results, 1990.

J.L. Brandt, W. Glaser and A. Jones. Soft tissue distribution and plasma disappearance of intravenously administered isotopic magnesium with observations on uptake in bone. Metabolism 7: 355–363, 1958.

L.C. Chesley and I. Tepper. Plasma levels of magnesium attained in magnesium sulfate therapy for preeclampsia and eclampsia. Surg. Clin. No. Am. 37: 353–367, 1957.

L.C. Chesley. Parenteral magnesium sulfate and the distribution, plasma levels, and excretion of magnesium. J. Ob. Gyn. 133: 1–7, 1979.

H.B. Dinsdale. Does magnesium sulfate treat eclamptic seizures? Arch. Neurol. 45: 1360–1361, 1988.

C.A. Fassler, R.M. Rodriguez, D.B. Badesch et al. Magnesium toxicity as a cause of hypotension and hypoventilation. Arch. Int. Med. 145: 1604–1606, 1985.

C.E. Flowers, Jr., W.E. Easterling, Jr., F.D. White et al. Magnesium sulfate in toxemia of pregnancy. J. Ob. Gyn. 19: 315–327, 1962.

J.L. Hansen and E.F. Freier. The measurement of serum magnesium by atomic absorption spectrophotometry. J. Med. Tech. 33: 1–9, 1967.

F.W. Heaton. Determination of magnesium by the Titan yellow and ammonium phosphate methods. J. Clin. Path. 13: 358–360, 1960.

P.C. Ioannou and D.G. Konstantianos. Fluorometric determination of magnesium in serum with 2-hydroxy-1-naphthaldehyde salicyloylhydrazone. Clin. Chem. 35: 1492–1496, 1989.

P.W. Kaplan, R.P. Lesser, R.S. Fisher et al. No, magnesium sulfate should not be used in treating eclamptic seizures. Arch. Neurol. 45: 1361–1364, 1988.

H.C. Mofenson and T.R. Caraccio. Magnesium intoxication in a neonate from oral magnesium hydroxide laxative. Clin. Tox. 29: 215–222, 1991.

R.D. Montgomery. The estimation of magnesium in small biological samples by flame spectrophotometry. J. Clin. Path. 14: 400–402, 1961.

M.E. Morris, S. Leroy and S.C. Sutton. Absorption of magnesium from orally administered magnesium sulfate in man. Clin. Tox. 25: 371–382, 1987.

G.D. Schachter. The fluorometric estimation of magnesium in serum and in urine. J. Lab. Clin. Med. 54: 763–768, 1959.

D.G. Simonsen, L.M. Westover and M. Wertman. The determination of serum magnesium by the molybdivanadate method for phosphate. J. Biol. Chem. 169: 39–47, 1947.

M.J. Smilkstein, D. Steedle, K.W. Kulig et al. Magnesium levels after magnesium-containing cathartics. Vet. Hum. Tox. 29: 458, 1987.

M. Speich, B. Bousquet and G. Nicolas. Reference values for ionized, complexed, and protein-bound plasma magnesium in men and women. Clin. Chem. 27: 246–248, 1981.

W.K. Stewart, F. Hutchinson and L.W. Fleming. The estimation of magnesium in serum and urine by atomic absorption spectrophotometry. J. Lab. Clin. Med. 61: 858–872, 1963.

M.C. Wimmer, J.D. Artiss and B. Zak. A kinetic colorimetric procedure for quantifying magnesium in serum. Clin. Chem. 32: 629–632, 1986.

Malathion

T½: 2.9 hr
Vd: ?
Fb: ?

$$S\ COOC_2H_5$$
$$(CH_3O)_2PSCHCH_2COOC_2H_5$$

Occurrence and Usage. Malathion is one of the least toxic of the commercially available organophosphate insecticides, and therefore one of the safest for domestic usage. It is commonly employed as a dusting powder in concentrations of 1–5% and in solutions of up to 50% strength for spraying. The pure compound is an oily liquid that decomposes when heated or moistened; it is biologically degradable and so does not present an environmental threat. Occupational exposure is commonly by inhalation or dermal absorption. The current threshold limit value is 10 mg/m³.

Blood Concentrations. Persons occupationally exposed to malathion were found to have dimethyldithiophosphate serum concentrations ranging from 0–3.50 mg/L, the level being directly proportional to the degree of exposure (Shafik and Enos, 1969). Subjects who were exposed to controlled amounts of 5% and 20% malathion sprays at atmospheric concentrations of 5–85 mg/m³ for 1 hour periods over 6 consecutive weeks exhibited erythrocyte and plasma cholinesterase values of 90% or greater on all but a few sampling occasions (Golz, 1959). In another study, volunteers ingested 16 mg of malathion daily for 47 days without effect on plasma or erythrocyte cholinesterase activity. Doses of 24 mg, however, when administered for 56 days caused 25% depression of cholinesterase activity, with maximal effects occurring 3 weeks after cessation of administration; no toxic effects were apparent in spite of depression of both plasma and erythrocyte cholinesterase (Moeller and Rider, 1962).

Metabolism and Excretion. In man, malathion is believed to be activated by conversion to malaoxon, an oxygen analogue, with hydrolysis and inactivation of both malathion and malaoxon to dimethyldithiophosphoric acid (DMDTP) and dimethylthiophosphoric acid (DMTP), respectively.

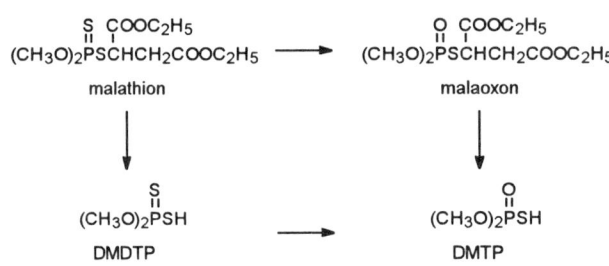

DMDTP and DMTP have been identified in the urine of exposed workers in concentrations of 0.20–1.86 mg/L and 0–0.11 mg/L, respectively, with the levels correlating to the severity of exposure (Shafik and Enos, 1969). Up to 23% of a single oral dose of malathion is excreted in the 16 hour urine as ether-extractable phosphates (Mattson and Sedlak, 1960). In animals and probably in man, the compound is also detoxified by hydrolysis of either or both of its carboxy ester functions (Matsumura, 1975).

Toxicity. Malathion has resulted in fewer episodes of poisoning than most other organophosphate derivatives due to its lower toxicity; the mean fatal dose in man is estimated at 60 g. A number of individuals, both children and adults, have survived the ingestion of up to 50 g of malathion with atropine administration and supportive treatment; 2-PAM was found to be without benefit in several cases. The patients recovered within 2–46 days after admission (Tuthill, 1958; Wenzl and Burke, 1962; Richards, 1964; Crowley and Johns, 1966; Gitelson et al., 1966; Windsor, 1968; Mathewson and Hardy, 1970; Hassan et al., 1981). Cholinesterase activity was reduced to 22% and 10% of normal in the serum and erythrocytes, respectively, of a woman who survived the ingestion of 60 g of malathion due to treatment with atropine and PAM; the levels gradually returned to normal after a period of 31 days for plasma and 130 days for erythrocytes, though clinical recovery occurred the tenth day (Goldin et al., 1964). A 24 year old man was treated and survived a suicidal intravenous injection of 3 mL of 50% malathion (1.8 g); 2 hours post-injection his pseudocholinesterase was undetectable and only began to rise after 24 hours. Serum malathion concentrations ranged from 0.35 mg/L to 0.03 mg/L at 6 and 28 hours post-injection, respectively (Lyon et al., 1987). Chronic domestic use of large amounts of malathion caused weakness, paresthesias, and collapse in a 44 year old male; muscle weakness, fatigue, and loss of appetite were still present a year later (Petty, 1958).

Several hundred fatalities have been reported, usually after ingestion of large amounts of the chemical (Nalin, 1973). One such case involved an adult who died 6 days after ingestion of 60–90 g of malathion; the following cholinesterase levels were determined at autopsy (Namba et al., 1970):

Cholinesterase Activity in a Malathion Fatality (% of normal)

Plasma	Cerebrum	Cerebellum	Muscle	Liver	Kidney
4	32	3	1	19	13

The following malathion concentrations were measured by liquid chromatography in 6 instances of fatal oral suicidal poisoning (Jadhav et al., 1992):

Malathion Concentrations in Fatal Cases (mg/L or mg/kg)

	Blood	Brain	Liver	Kidney	Urine
Average	281	178	274	377	96
(Range)	(175–517)	(84–387)	(198–303)	(280–616)	(33–189)

Analysis. Intact malathion has been estimated in biologic specimens by colorimetry (Farago, 1967) and liquid chromatography (Jadhav et al., 1992) in overdose situations and by electron-capture gas chromatography when only trace amounts were present (Ragab, 1968). Methods for the determination of organic phosphate metabolites of malathion in urine have included colorimetry (Mattson and Sedlak, 1960) and gas chromatography with flame photometric detection (Shafik and Enos, 1969; Shafik et al., 1973; Reid and Watts, 1981). Methods for blood cholinesterase estimation were cited in the section on carbaryl.

References

W.J. Crowley, Jr. and T.R. Johns. Accidental malathion poisoning. Arch. Neurol. 14: 611–616, 1966.

A. Farago. Fatal, suicidal malathion poisonings. Arch. Tox. 23: 11–16, 1967.

S. Gitelson, L. Aladjemoff, S.B. Hador and R. Katznelson. Poisoning by a malathion-xylene mixture. J. Am. Med. Asso. 197: 819–821, 1966.

A.R. Goldin, A.H. Rubenstein, B.A. Bradlow and G.A. Elliott. Malathion poisoning with special reference to the effect of cholinesterase inhibition on erythrocyte survival. New Eng. J. Med. 271: 1289–1293, 1964.

H.H. Golz. Controlled human exposures to malathion aerosols. Arch. Ind. Health 19: 516–523, 1959.

R.M. Hassan, A.J. Pesce, P. Sheng and I.B. Hanenson. Correlation of serum pseudocholinesterase and clinical course in two patients poisoned with organophosphate insecticides. Clin. Tox. 18: 401–406, 1981.

R.K. Jadhav, V.K. Sharma, G.J. Rao et al. Distribution of malathion in body tissues and fluids. For. Sci. Int. 52: 223–229, 1992.

J. Lyon, H. Taylor and B. Ackerman. A case report of intravenous malathion injection with determination of serum half-life. Clin. Tox. 25: 243–249, 1987.

I. Mathewson and E.A. Hardy. Treatment of malathion poisoning. Anaesthesia 25: 265–271, 1970.

F. Matsumura. *Toxicology of Insecticides*, Plenum Press, New York, 1975, pp. 224–226.

A.M. Mattson and V.A. Sedlak. Ether-extractable urinary phosphates in man and rats derived from malathion and similar compounds. J. Agr. Food Chem. 8: 107–110, 1960.

H.C. Moeller and J.A. Rider. Plasma and red blood cell cholinesterase activity as indications of the threshold of incipient toxicity of ethyl-p-nitrophenyl thionobenzenephosphonate (EPN) and malathion in human beings. Tox. Appl. Pharm. 4: 123–130, 1962.

D.R. Nalin. Epidemic of suicide by malathion poisoning in Guyana. Trop. Geog. Med. 25: 8–14, 1973.

T. Namba, M. Greenfield and D. Grob. Malathion poisoning. A fatal case with cardiac manifestation. Arch. Env. Health 21: 533–541, 1970.

C.S. Petty. Organic phosphate insecticide poisoning. Am. J. Med. 23: 467–470, 1958.

M.T.H. Ragab. Gas chromatographic analysis of malathion in water and in fish. Bull. Env. Cont. Tox. 3: 155–163, 1968.

S.J. Reid and R.R. Watts. A method for the determination of dialkyl phosphate residues in urine. J. Anal. Tox. 5: 126–132, 1981.

A.G. Richards. Malathion poisoning successfully treated with large doses of atropine. Can. Med. Asso. J. 91: 82–83, 1964.

M.T. Shafik and H.F. Enos. Determination of metabolic and hydrolytic products of organophosphorus pesticide chemicals in human blood and urine. J. Agr. Food Chem. 17: 1186–1189, 1969.

T. Shafik, D.E. Bradway, H.F. Enos and A.R. Yobs. Human exposure to organophosphorus pesticides. A modified procedure for the gas-liquid chromatographic analysis of alkyl phosphate metabolites in urine. J. Agr. Food Chem. 21: 625–629, 1973.

J.W.G. Tuthill. Toxic hazards. Malathion poisoning. New Eng. J. Med. 258: 1018–1019, 1958.

J.E. Wenzl and E.C. Burke. Poisoning from a malathion-aerosol mixture. J. Am. Med. Asso. 182: 495–497, 1962.

P.W.M. Windsor. Malathion. Practitioner 200: 600, 1968.

Manganese

T½: 12–36 days

Vd: ?

Fb: ?

Mn

Occurrence and Usage. Manganese is widely used industrially in the manufacture of steel, welding rods, batteries, ceramics and refractory materials. It is also an essential trace element and is supplied in daily amounts of 3–7 mg by dietary intake. Occupational exposure usually occurs by inhalation or ingestion of fumes and dusts produced during the refining of manganese ores or the treatment of manganese alloys. The current threshold limit value for manganese fume is 1 mg/m³ and for manganese and its compounds, 5 mg/m³ (both expressed as Mn).

Blood Concentrations. Whole blood manganese, most of which is bound to hemoglobin in the erythrocytes, averages 9 μg/L (range, 3.9–15) in normal adults when measured by atomic absorption spectrometry. Serum manganese in normal adults averages 0.6 μg/L, ranging from 0.2–1.1 μg/L (Neve and Leclercq, 1991). Other authors, using either similar techniques, colorimetry or neutron activation analysis, are in general agreement with this data (Cotzias et al., 1966; Cotzias et al., 1968; Weissman and Pileggi, 1974; Buchet et al., 1976; Pleban and Pearson, 1979; Roels et al., 1992). However, many discrepancies exist in the literature on endogenous manganese concentrations, probably as a result of methodological difficulties and problems with contamination, with some authors claiming normal blood or serum levels 5–40 times higher than those cited above (Nilubol et al., 1968; Mahoney et al., 1969; Jonderko et al., 1971).

Metabolism and Excretion. Most inhaled manganese is mobilized up the trachea and swallowed. The efficiency of gastrointestinal absorption of the element is low, usually less than 10%, but is quite variable and appears to correlate inversely to the amount available for absorption (Mena et al., 1969). The absorbed manganese leaves the blood quickly and is stored in parenchymatous tissues; the half-time for excretion of manganese from the body in normal subjects is about 40 days. Elimination of injected manganese is largely via the feces, which contain from 14–54% of a single dose after 15 days, and to a very minor extent in urine (Mena et al., 1967; Mahoney and Small, 1968).

Urinary manganese concentrations in normal persons have been reported to range from less than 1 to 10 μg/L (Cholak and Hubbard, 1960; Nilubol et al., 1968; Ajemian and Whitman, 1969; Weissman and Pileggi, 1974; Buchet et al., 1976). These concentrations in asymptomatic manganese workers have ranged from 25–124 μg/L (Nilubol et al., 1968), although it has been found that urine concentrations do not usually exceed 8 μg/L when occupational manganese exposure is limited to 5 mg/m³ (Tanaka and Lieben, 1969).

The following average manganese concentrations were present in the tissues of Japanese citizens (Sumino et al., 1975):

Manganese Concentrations in Normal Human Tissues (mg/kg)

Brain	Lung	Liver	Kidney	Bone	Fat
0.25	0.22	1.2	0.56	0.07	0.05

Toxicity. Typical metal fume fever may develop after exposure to manganese oxide fumes, with symptoms of fever, muscle pains, chills and dryness of the mouth and throat. However, chronic overexposure to manganese is more frequently encountered. This may require a year or more of exposure prior to the manifestation of CNS symptoms such as headache, restlessness, irritability, personality change, hallucinations and hearing impairment. Severe toxicity results in muscle weakness and rigidity, tremor and other extrapyramidal symptoms. Administration of levodopa has been successfully employed in the treatment of manganism (Hine and Pasi, 1975).

Manganese concentrations in a patient with chronic poisoning were elevated in blood (75 μg/L) but normal in urine (Rosenstock et al., 1971); another patient demonstrated a blood concentration of 20 μg/L and urine concentrations of 100–150 μg/L (Hine and Pasi, 1975). Blood manganese levels in 4 patients with chronic industrial poisoning ranged from 102–405 μg/L (Huang et al., 1989). Urine manganese concentrations in other manganism patients have ranged from less than 10 to as high as 260 μg/L (Nilubol et al., 1968; Tanaka and Lieben, 1969; Smyth et al., 1973; Chandra et al., 1981).

Analysis. Manganese has been analyzed in urine by a colorimetric procedure that is best suited to toxic levels of the metal (Weissman and Pileggi, 1974). Atomic absorption spectrometry is capable of the determination of endogenous levels of manganese, when precautions are taken to avoid contamination (Ajemian and Whitman, 1969; Buchet et al., 1976; Tsalev et al., 1977; Watanabe et al., 1978; Pleban and Pearson, 1979; Casey et al., 1987; Hams and Fabri, 1988; Neve and Leclercq, 1991). Neutron activation analysis is also recommended (Cotzias et al., 1966; Versieck et al., 1974).

References

R.S. Ajemian and N.E. Whitman. Determination of manganese in urine by atomic absorption spectrometry. Am. Ind. Hyg. Asso. J. 30: 52–56, 1969.

J.P. Buchet, R. Lauwerys and H. Roels. Determination of manganese in blood and urine by flameless atomic absorption spectrophotometry. Clin. Chim. Acta 73: 481–486, 1976.

C.E. Casey, M.A.T. Goodall and K.M. Hambridge. Atomic absorption spectrophotometry of manganese in plasma. Clin. Chem. 33: 1253–1254, 1987.

S.V. Chandra, G.S. Shukla, R.S. Srivastava et al. An exploratory study of manganese exposure to workers. Clin. Tox. 18: 407–416, 1981.

J. Cholak and D.M. Hubbard. Determination of manganese in air and biological material. Am. Ind. Hyg. Asso. J. 21: 356–360, 1960.

G.C. Cotzias, S.T. Miller and J. Edwards. Neutron activation analysis: the stability of manganese concentrations in human blood and serum. J. Lab. Clin. Med. 67: 836–849, 1966.

G.C. Cotzias, P.S. Papavasiliou, E.R. Hughes et al. Slow turnover of manganese in active rheumatoid arthritis accelerated by prednisone. J. Clin. Invest. 47: 992–1001, 1968.

G.A. Hams and J.K. Fabri. An analysis for blood manganese used to assess environmental exposure. Clin. Chem. 34: 1121–1123, 1988.

C.H. Hine and A. Pasi. Manganese intoxication. West. J. Med. 123: 101–107, 1975.

C.C. Huang, N.S. Chu, C.S. Lu et al. Chronic manganese intoxication. Arch. Neurol. 46: 1104–1106, 1989.

G. Jonderko, A. Kujawska and H. Langauer-Lewowicka. Problems of chronic manganese poisoning on the basis of investigations of workers at a manganese alloy foundry. Int. Arch. Arbeitsmed. 28: 250–264, 1971.

J.P. Mahoney and W.J. Small. Studies on manganese. III. The biological half-life of radiomanganese in man and factors which affect this half-life. J. Clin. Invest. 47: 643–653, 1968.

J.P. Mahoney, K. Sargent, M. Greland and W. Small. Studies on manganese. I. Determination in serum by atomic absorption spectrophotometry. Clin. Chem. 15: 312–322, 1969.

I. Mena, O. Marin, S. Fuenzalida and G.C. Cotzias. Chronic manganese poisoning. Clinical picture and manganese turnover. Neurology 17: 128–136, 1967.

I. Mena, K. Horiuchi, K. Burke and G.C. Cotzias. Chronic manganese poisoning. Individual susceptibility and absorption of iron. Neurology 19: 1000–1006, 1969.

J. Neve and N. Leclercq. Factors affecting determinations of manganese in serum by atomic absorption spectrometry. Clin. Chem. 37: 723–728, 1991.

M.L.A. Nilubol, K. Chayawatanangkur and S. Kritalugsana. Manganese toxication in the human body determined by activation analysis. J. Nucl. Med. 9: 178–180, 1968.

P.A. Pleban and K.H. Pearson. Determination of manganese in whole blood and serum. Clin. Chem. 25: 1915–1918, 1979.

H.A. Roels, P. Ghyselen, J.P. Buchet et al. Assessment of the permissible exposure level to manganese in workers exposed to manganese dioxide dust. Brit. J. Int. Med. 49: 25–34, 1992.

H.A. Rosenstock, D.G. Simons and J.S. Meyer. Chronic manganism. Neurologic and laboratory studies during treatment with levodopa. J. Am. Med. Asso. 217: 1354–1358, 1971.

L.T. Smyth, R.C. Ruhf, N.E. Whitman and T. Dugan. Clinical manganism and exposure to manganese in the production and processing of ferromanganese alloy. J. Occ. Med. 15: 101–109, 1973.

K. Sumino, K. Hayakawa, T. Shibata and S. Kitamura. Heavy metals in normal Japanese tissues. Arch. Env. Health 30: 487–494, 1975.

S. Tanaka and J. Lieben. Manganese poisoning and exposure in Pennsylvania. Arch. Env. Health 19: 674–684, 1969.

D.L. Tsalev, F.J. Langmyhr and N. Gunderson. Direct atomic absorption spectrometric determination of manganese in whole blood of unexposed individuals and exposed workers in a Norwegian manganese alloy plant. Bull. Env. Cont. Tox. 17: 660–666, 1977.

J. Versieck, F. Barbier, A. Speecke and J. Hoste. Normal manganese concentrations in human serum. Acta Endocrin. 76: 783–788, 1974.

T. Watanabe, R. Tokunaga, T. Iwahana et al. Determination of urinary manganese by the direct chelation-extraction method and flameless atomic absorption spectrophotometry. Brit. J. Ind. Med. 35: 73–77, 1978.

N. Weissman and W.J. Pileggi. Inorganic ions. In *Clinical Chemistry, Principles and Techniques* (R.J. Henry, D.C. Cannon and J.W. Winkelman, eds.), Harper and Row, New York, 2nd ed., 1974, pp. 707–712.

Maprotiline

T½: 36–105 hr
Vd: 14–22 L/kg
Fb: 0.88
pKa: 10.5

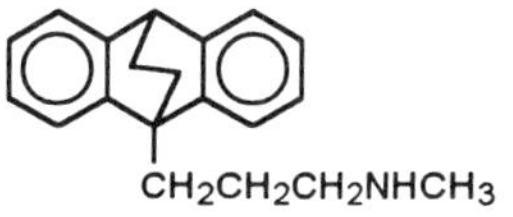

CH2CH2CH2NHCH3

Occurrence and Usage. Maprotiline (Ludiomil) is a tetracyclic antidepressant drug used clinically since 1972. It is available as the hydrochloride in tablets of 25–100 mg for oral use or as a solution for parenteral injection. Daily doses range from 75–300 mg.

Blood Concentrations. Peak blood concentrations in 6 subjects after a single 50 mg oral dose averaged 0.050 mg/L (range, 0.045–0.060) at a mean time of 12 hours (range, 8–24); the concentrations declined with a mean half-life of 58 hours (Alkalay et al., 1980). A 150 mg oral dose given to 9 subjects produced an average peak blood concentration of 0.091 mg/L at 8 hours, with a decline to 0.074 mg/L by 24 hours. The blood/plasma concentration ratio for maprotiline has been reported to average 2.0–2.2 (Maguire et al., 1980).

Steady-state serum maprotiline concentrations in 10 patients receiving 150 mg daily for 14 days ranged from 0.168–0.718 mg/L, averaging 0.346 mg/L (Fischbach, 1979). Normaprotiline concentrations were 23–86% of the steady-state maprotiline value in 5 patients receiving 150 mg daily doses of the drug (Gupta et al., 1977). Plasma maprotiline concentrations as high as 1.558 mg/L (plus normaprotiline, 0.180 mg/L) have been measured in patients on chronic therapy (Jindal et al., 1980).

Metabolism and Excretion. A single intravenous labeled dose of maprotiline is excreted over a 21 day period in the urine (57%) and feces (30%), largely as metabolites. Only about 6% of the dose is eliminated unchanged in urine. The metabolites are chiefly products of N-demethylation, deamination, hydroxylation, and conjugation. About 43% of a dose consists of urinary glucuronide conjugates (Riess et al., 1975). Seven minor urinary ring-hydroxylated metabolites have been structurally elucidated (Breyer-Pfaff et al., 1985).

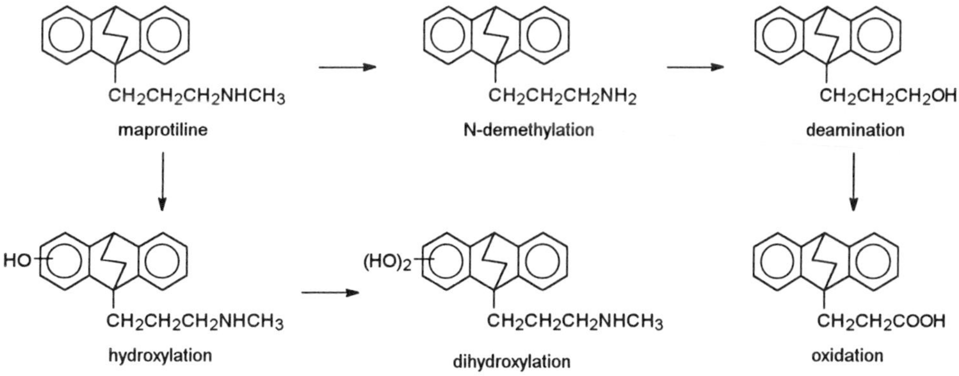

CH2CH2CH2NHCH3
maprotiline

CH2CH2CH2NH2
N-demethylation

CH2CH2CH2OH
deamination

HO—
CH2CH2CH2NHCH3
hydroxylation

(HO)2—
CH2CH2CH2NHCH3
dihydroxylation

CH2CH2COOH
oxidation

Toxicity. Maprotiline taken in excess causes drowsiness, tremor, muscular twitching, ataxia, vertigo, confusion, hallucinations, convulsions, and coma. Several patients receiving therapeutic amounts of maprotiline have developed seizures at serum concentrations of 0.237–0.317 mg/L (Gupta et al., 1977; Marks et al., 1979). Four adults survived overdosage with maprotiline after developing peak plasma concentrations of 0.401–0.800 mg/L; hemoperfusion was used in 2 cases, but was of questionable efficacy due to the very large volume of distribution of this drug (Hofmann et al., 1980; Charette et al., 1981; Rodgers et al., 1982).

The following tissue concentrations were observed in 9 adult victims of fatal poisoning (Meinhart et al., 1974; Clarke, 1976; Robinson et al., 1979; Shaw, 1981; Cravey, 1983; Farr, 1985; Okoye et al., 1985):

Maprotiline Concentrations in Fatal Cases (mg/L or mg/kg)

	Blood	Brain	Liver	Bile	Kidney	Urine	Gastric
Average	5.4	45	223	70	38	15	32 mg
(Range)	(1.3–13)	(13–79)	(34–380)	(15–161)	(21–60)	(4–25)	(3–123)

Additionally, Rejent and Doyle (1982) reported a maprotiline fatality with postmortem levels of 45 mg/L in blood and 605 mg/kg in liver. Maprotiline is subject to postmortem redistribution; heart blood/femoral blood concentration ratios averaged 4.7 (range, 1.4–11) in 3 victims of fatal overdosage (Anderson and Prouty, 1989).

Analysis. Maprotiline and normaprotiline have been assayed in plasma by gas chromatography with flame-ionization (Karkkainen and Seppala, 1980), nitrogen-specific (Gupta et al., 1977; Sioufi and Richard, 1980; Charette et al., 1981; Drebit et al., 1988), electron-capture (Geiger et al., 1975) or mass spectrometric detection (Alkalay et al., 1979; Jindal et al., 1980; Skrinska et al., 1984). Liquid chromatographic methods have also been described (Kuss and Feistenauer, 1981; Wong and Waugh, 1983; Breyer-Pfaff et al., 1984).

References

D. Alkalay, S. Carlsen, L. Khemani and M.F. Bartlett. Selected ion monitoring assay for the antidepressant maprotiline. Biomed. Mass Spec. 6: 435–438, 1979.

D. Alkalay, W.E. Wagner, Jr., S. Carlsen et al. Bioavailability and kinetics of maprotiline. Clin. Pharm. Ther. 27: 697–703, 1980.

W.H. Anderson and R.W. Prouty. Postmortem redistribution of drugs. In *Advances in Analytical Toxicology* (R.C. Baselt, ed.), Vol. 2, YearBook Medical, Chicago, 1987, pp. 70–102.

U. Breyer-Pfaff, R. Wiatr and K. Nill. Measurement of maprotiline and oxaprotiline in plasma by high-performance liquid chromatography of fluorescent derivatives. J. Chrom. 309: 107–114, 1984.

U. Breyer-Pfaff, M. Kroeker, T. Winkler and P. Kriemler. Isolation and identification of hydroxylated maprotiline metabolites. Xenobiotica 15: 57–66, 1985.

C. Charette, I.J. McGilveray and K.K. Midha. Gas-liquid chromatographic procedure with alkali flame ionization detection for the determination of maprotiline in plasma. J. Chrom. 224: 128–132, 1981.

D.G. Clarke. Personal communication, 1976.

R.H. Cravey. Personal communication, 1983.

R. Drebit, G.B. Baker and W.G. Dewhurst. Determination of maprotiline and desmethylmaprotiline in plasma and urine by gas chromatography with nitrogen-phosphorus detection. J. Chrom. 432: 334–339, 1988.

L.M. Farr. Personal communication, 1985.

R. Fischbach. Maprotiline in adult depressed patients. Arz. Forsch. 29: 352–355, 1979.

U.P. Geiger, T.G. Rajagopalan and W. Riess. Quantitative assay of maprotiline in biological fluids by gas-liquid chromatography. J. Chrom. 114: 167–173, 1975.

R.N. Gupta, G. Molnar and M.L. Gupta. Estimation of maprotiline in serum by gas-chromatography, with use of a nitrogen-specific detector. Clin. Chem. 23: 1849–1852, 1977.

V. Hofmann, W. Riess, C. Descoudres and H. Studer. Zur Frage der Haemoperfusion bei Vergiftungen: Unwirksamkeit bei Maprotilin-Intoxikation. Schweiz. Med. Wochenshr. 110: 291–294, 1980.

S.P. Jindal, T. Lutz and P. Vestergaard. GLC-mass spectrometric determination of maprotiline and its major metabolite using stable isotope-labeled analog as internal standard. J. Pharm. Sci. 69: 684–687, 1980.

S. Karkkainen and E. Seppala. Gas chromatographic analysis of therapeutic concentrations of maprotiline in serum, using flame-ionization detection. J. Chrom. 221: 319–326, 1980.

H.J. Kuss and E. Feistenauer. Quantitative high-performance liquid chromatographic assay for the determination of maprotiline and oxaprotiline in human plasma. J. Chrom. 204: 349–353, 1981.

K.P. Maguire, G.D. Burrows, T.R. Norman and B.A. Scoggins. Blood/plasma distribution ratios of psychotropic drugs. Clin. Chem. 26: 1624–1625, 1980.

P. Marks, J. Anderson, R. Vincent et al. Epileptiform seizures with maprotiline hydrochloride. Postgrad. Med. J. 55: 742, 1979.

K. Meinhart, A. Nikiforov and W. Vycudilik. Der Nachweis und die Bestimmung von Maprotilin (Ludiomil) in Leichenmaterial. Arch. Tox. 33: 65–71, 1974.

M.I. Okoye, D.T. Dummer, P.L. Stephens and W.F. Mueller, Jr. A fatal maprotiline intoxication. Am. J. For. Med. Path. 6: 45–47, 1985.

T.A. Rejent and R.E. Doyle. Maprotiline fatality: case report and analytical determinations. J. Anal. Tox. 6: 199–201, 1982.

W. Riess, L. Dubey, E.W. Fuenfgeld et al. The pharmacokinetic properties of maprotiline (Ludiomil) in man. J. Int. Med. Res. 3 (Suppl. 2): 16–41, 1975.

A.E. Robinson, R.D. McDowall, H. Sattar et al. Tricyclic and tetracyclic antidepressant drugs: forensic toxicology of some autopsy cases. J. Anal. Tox. 3: 3–13, 1979.

G.C. Rodgers, C.H. Jarboe and J.T. Ramsey. Pharmacokinetics of maprotiline in overdose, a report of two cases. Vet. Hum. Tox. 24 (Suppl.): 71–72, 1982.

R. Shaw. Presented at the quarterly meeting of the California Association of Toxicologists, San Diego, November 7, 1981.

A. Sioufi and A. Richard. Gas chromatographic determination of maprotiline and its N-desmethyl metabolite in human blood using nitrogen detection. J. Chrom. 221: 393–398, 1980.

V. Skrinska, J. Ohman, C. Wellstead and K. Hahn. Gas chromatography-mass spectrometry of maprotiline in serum. Clin. Chem. 30: 1276–1277, 1984.

S.H.Y. Wong and S.W. Waugh. Determination of the antidepressants maprotiline and amoxapine, and their metabolites, in plasma by liquid chromatography. Clin. Chem. 29: 314–318, 1983.

Medazepam

T½: 1–2 hr
Vd: ?
Fb: >0.90
pKa: 6.2

Occurrence and Usage. Medazepam (Nobrium) is a close analogue of diazepam, lacking only the 2-keto moiety, and is a metabolic precursor of that compound. It is available in Europe for the treatment of anxiety and is administered orally as the hydrochloride in daily doses of 10–50 mg.

Blood Concentrations. Following a single oral dose of 50 mg, the blood medazepam concentration reached a peak of 0.98 mg/L at 1 hour and declined rapidly to 0.12 mg/L at 2 hours; the diazepam concentration reached a maximum of 0.03 mg/L at 1 hour. After administration of 50 mg per day for 4 days, the blood medazepam concentrations reached a maximum of 0.58 mg/L within 1 hour, but again declined rapidly; the levels of diazepam remained fairly constant at 0.05–0.07 mg/L during each 24 hour period; nordiazepam gradually accumulated in the blood and appeared to reach a plateau of 0.45 mg/L; and normedazepam reached a peak concentration of 0.22 mg/L at 1 hour, showing moderate accumulation during the dosing period (deSilva and Puglisi, 1970). During chronic administration of 10–50 mg of the drug daily, plasma concentrations of the nordiazepam metabolite averaged 0.71 mg/L (range, 0.21–1.68) in 20 patients (Bond et al., 1977).

Metabolism and Excretion. Medazepam is metabolized by oxidation at the 2-position to diazepam, which then undergoes its usual route of biotransformation, primarily to nordiazepam and oxazepam. Medazepam is also N-demethylated to normedazepam and this compound may be subsequently oxidized to nordiazepam. The major blood species is nordiazepam, which may account for much of the efficacy of medazepam. As much as 55% of a dose is excreted in urine over an 8 day period, primarily as oxazepam glucuronide. Small amounts of nordiazepam and temazepam are found in urine, but medazepam, normedazepam and diazepam have not been detected in measurable quantities (Schwartz and Carbone, 1970; deSilva and Puglisi, 1970).

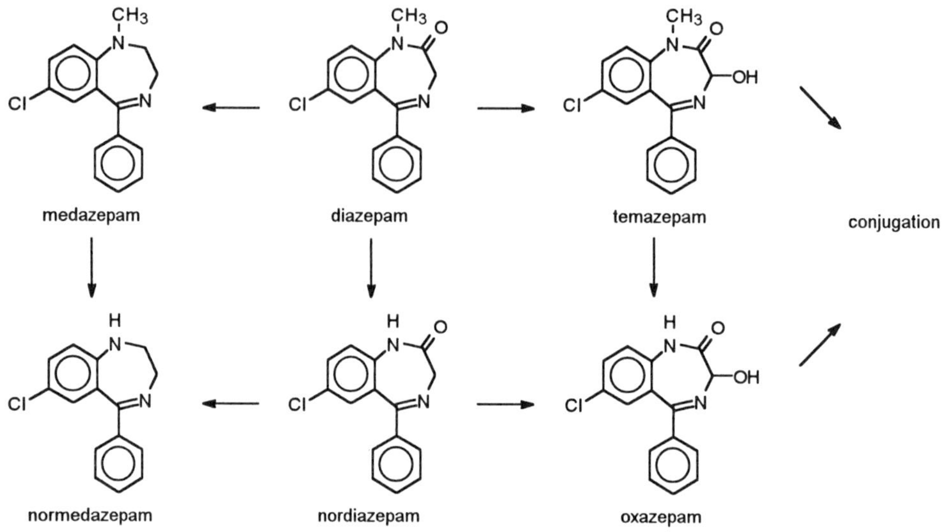

Toxicity. Medazepam produces symptoms of central nervous system depression when taken in overdosage.

Analysis. Methods for the analysis of medazepam and its metabolites have been reported using electron-capture gas chromatography of the intact drugs, with either external standardization (deSilva and Puglisi, 1970) or with prazepam as internal standard (Baird et al., 1973). Techniques employing flame-ionization (Greaves, 1974) and nitrogen-selective detection (Mallach et al., 1973) have also been described.

References

E.S. Baird, D.M. Hailey and S. Malcolm. A gas chromatographic assay for medazepam and its major metabolites in plasma. Clin. Chim. Acta 48: 105–108, 1973.

A.J. Bond, D.M. Hailey and M.H. Lader. Plasma concentrations of benzodiazepines. Brit. J. Clin. Pharm. 4: 51–56, 1977.

J.A.F. deSilva and C.V. Puglisi. Determination of medazepam (Nobrium), diazepam (Valium) and their major biotransformation products in blood and urine by electron capture gas-liquid chromatography. Anal. Chem. 42: 1725–1736, 1970.

M.S. Greaves. Quantitative determination of medazepam, diazepam and nitrazepam in whole blood by flame-ionization gas-liquid chromatography. Clin. Chem. 20: 141–147, 1974.

H.J. Mallach, A. Moosmayer and J.M. Rupp. Zur gaschromatographischen Analytik der Benzodiazepine. Arz. Forsch. 23: 614–616, 1973.

M.A. Schwartz and J.J. Carbone. Metabolism of ^{14}C-medazepam hydrochloride in dog, rat and man. Biochem. Pharm. 19: 343–361, 1970.

Mefenamic Acid

T½: 2–4 hr
Vd: ?
Fb: 0.99
pKa: 4.2

Occurrence and Usage. Mefenamic acid (Ponstel) is an anthranilic acid derivative used as an analgesic and anti-inflammatory agent since 1963. It is supplied as the free acid in 250 mg capsules for oral use. Daily doses range from 1000–1500 mg for a period not to exceed one week.

Blood Concentrations. A single 1000 mg oral dose of mefenamic acid given to 6 subjects resulted in an average peak plasma concentration of 10 mg/L at 2 hours, declining to about 4 mg/L by 4 hours and 1 mg/L by 8 hours. Subjects receiving 4000 mg daily divided into 4 equal doses developed plasma mefenamic acid concentrations of about 20 mg/L by the second day (Glazko, 1968).

Metabolism and Excretion. Mefenamic acid is metabolized by oxidation of the m-methyl group and by glucuronide conjugation. Conjugated parent drug appears in plasma at concentrations exceeding those of the unconjugated drug, together with similar levels of 3'-hydroxymethylmefenamic acid in both free and conjugated form. About 52% of a dose is excreted in the 48 hour urine as conjugated mefenamic acid (6%), conjugated 3'-hydroxymethylmefenamic acid (25%), and free (14%) and conjugated 3'-carboxymefenamic acid (7%). Another 10–20% of a dose appears in feces, mainly as free 3'-carboxymefenamic acid (Glazko, 1968).

mefenamic acid → 3'-hydroxymethylmefenamic accid → 3'-carboxymefenamic acid

glucuronide conjugation

Toxicity. Side-effects of mefenamic acid include nausea, vomiting, diarrhea, blood dyscrasias, drowsiness, blurred vision, headache, and nephrotoxicity. Overdosage has produced drowsiness, muscular twitching and, in about 10% of the patients, grand mal seizures. Five patients with the most severe intoxication had plasma mefenamic acid concentrations of 25–110 mg/L and plasma half-lives of 3–14 hours; all patients recovered without specific treatment (Robson et al., 1979; Balali-Mood et al., 1980).

Analysis. Mefenamic acid has been determined in plasma by fluorometry (Glazko, 1968), flame-ionization or electron-capture gas chromatography after derivatization (Bland et al., 1976; Dusci and Hackett, 1978), and liquid chromatography (Dusci and Hackett, 1979; Sato et al., 1989; Poirier et al., 1992).

References

M. Balali-Mood, J.A.J.H. Critchley and L.F. Prescott. Overdosage with mefenamic acid (Ponstan). Presented at the IX Congress of the European Association of Poison Control Centers, Thessaloniki, Greece, August, 1980.

S.A. Bland, J.W. Blake and R.S. Ray. Mefenamic acid blood and urine levels in the horse determined by derivative gas-liquid chromatography—electron capture. J. Chrom. Sci. 14: 201–203, 1976.

L.J. Dusci and L.P. Hackett. Gas-liquid chromatographic determinations of mefenamic acid in human serum. J. Chrom. 161: 340–342, 1978.

L.J. Dusci and L.P. Hackett. Determination of some anti-inflammatory drugs in serum by high-performance liquid chromatography. J. Chrom. 172: 516–519, 1979.

A.J. Glazko. Pharmacology of fenamates. III. Metabolic disposition. Ann. Phys. Med. (Suppl.) 9: 23–36, 1968.

J.M. Poirier, M. Lebot and G. Cheymol. Rapid and sensitive liquid chromatographic assay of mefenamic acid in plasma. Ther. Drug Mon. 14: 322–326, 1992.

R.H. Robson, M. Balali, J. Critchley et al. Mefenamic acid poisoning and epilepsy. Brit. Med. J. 2: 1438, 1979.

J. Sato, E. Owada, K. Ito et al. Simple, rapid and sensitive reversed-phase high-performance liquid chromatographic method for the determination of mefenamic acid in plasma. J. Chrom. 493: 239–243, 1989.

Meperidine

T½: 2–5 hr
Vd: 3.7–4.2 L/kg
Fb: 0.64
pKa: 8.6

Occurrence and Usage. Meperidine (pethidine, Demerol) is a synthetic narcotic analgesic introduced in 1931. It has approximately one-eighth the potency of morphine on a weight basis, with a somewhat shorter duration of action. It is supplied as the hydrochloride in the form of 50 and 100 mg tablets and a 50 mg/5 mL syrup for oral use, or solutions of 25–100 mg/mL for parenteral injection. Single doses of 50–150 mg and daily doses of 150–1200 mg are given.

Blood Concentrations. Peak plasma meperidine concentrations in 4 subjects administered a single 100 mg oral dose averaged 0.17 mg/L at 1.3 hours and declined with an average half-life of 4.4 hours; the oral bioavailability of the drug was 48–56% due to rapid hepatic metabolism (Mather and Tucker, 1976). A single 100 mg intramuscular injection given to 7 patients produced an average peak plasma concentration of 0.31 mg/L (range, 0.16–0.36) at 1 hour, declining to 0.21 mg/L (range, 0.15–0.2 8) by 3 hours (Mather et al., 1975b). After a 50 mg intravenous injection given to 6 volunteers, serum concentrations averaged 0.52 mg/L at 12 minutes and 0.18 mg/L by 1 hour (Stambaugh et al., 1976). The half-life of meperidine after intravenous administration averages 3.2 hours; the blood/plasma concentration ratio increases from 1.2–1.4 as the whole blood concentration increases from 0.2–2.0 mg/L (Mather et al., 1975a). In patients with liver cirrhosis, the half-life has been found to average 7.0 hours (Klotz et al., 1974). In infants aged 1–5 months, the elimination half-life averaged 15 hours (range, 6–32) and the volume of distribution averaged 9.2 L/kg (range, 4.9–11) (Pokela et al., 1992).

Plasma meperidine concentrations in 7 cancer patients receiving intramuscular meperidine as needed for pain ranged from 0.10–0.55 mg/L at 1 hour after the last dose, while normeperidine concentrations were 0.05–0.28 mg/L. The normeperidine half-life was estimated at 14 and 21 hours in 2 cancer patients, and 34 hours in a patient with renal failure (Szeto et al., 1977).

Metabolism and Excretion. About 7% of a dose of meperidine is eliminated unchanged in the urine together with about 17% as normeperidine; under conditions of acid urine, these values increase to about 27% and 23%, respectively, while during alkaline conditions they decline to 0.6% and 3.6%, respectively. Both of these compounds are de-esterified in man and the 2 hydrolysis products, meperidinic acid and normeperidinic acid, account for approximately 42% and 23% of the dose, respectively, in the urine as conjugates. Normeperidine, a metabolite with about half the analgesic activity of meperidine, is not usually found in plasma after a single administration, but can accumulate with chronic administration and may even exceed its parent in concentration. Normeperidine is 2–3 times as toxic as meperidine, is more active as a convulsant and appears to have a longer half-life.

Urinary concentrations for meperidine and normeperidine of 1–10 mg/L are typical following therapeutic usage, although these values may be considerably higher if the urine is acidic. N-hydroxyl, N-oxide, and hydroxyphenyl metabolites have been identified in relatively minor amounts in urine (Burns et al., 1955; Chan et al., 1975; Lindberg et al., 1975; Stillwell et al., 1976; Lindberg et al., 1980; Chan et al., 1985).

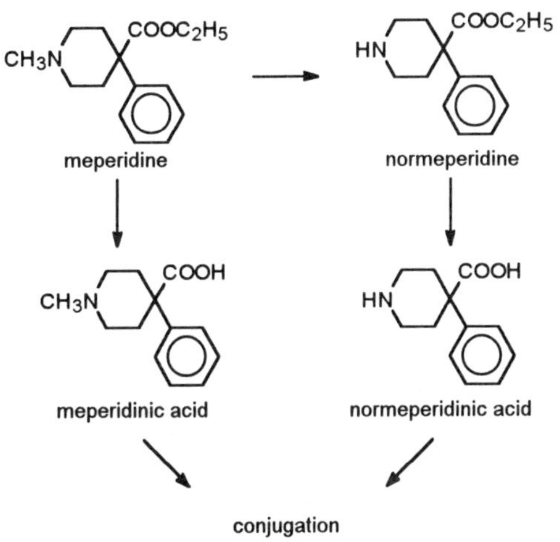

Toxicity. In overdosage, meperidine causes stupor, muscle flaccidity, respiratory depression, hypotension, cold and clammy skin, and coma. Naloxone is considered a specific antagonist. Normeperidine accumulation has been cited as the cause of convulsive seizures or respiratory arrest in 3 adult patients who developed normeperidine blood levels of 1.5–9.9 mg/L after receiving parenteral meperidine for at least 24 hours; the normeperidine elimination half-life was 35 hours in one of these individuals (Armstrong and Bersten, 1986; Geller, 1993).

The following drug concentrations were measured in 6 cases of death due to meperidine overdosage; 3 cases involved oral ingestion and 3 involved intravenous injection (Siek, 1978):

Drug Concentrations in Meperidine Fatalities (mg/L or mg/kg)

Route	Drug	Blood	Liver	Urine
Oral	Meperidine			
	Average	12	7	150
	(Range)	(8–20)	(5–10)	(150)
	Normeperidine			
	Average	19	31	50
	(Range)	(8–30)	(11–66)	(50)
Intravenous	Meperidine			
	Average	4.3	8.3	15
	(Range)	(1–8)	(2–16)	(2–24)
	Normeperidine			
	Average	2.5	7.3	49
	(Range)	(0–7)	(0–12)	(0.1–79)

Meperidine is subject to postmortem redistribution; heart blood/femoral blood concentration ratios of 1.2–3.2 (average, 2.1) were observed in 5 autopsy cases (Anderson and Prouty, 1989).

Analysis. Meperidine has been assayed in biological specimens by colorimetry (Burns et al., 1955), ultraviolet spectrophotometry (Kazyak, 1959), and fluorometry (Dal Cortivo et al., 1970). Gas chromatographic techniques involve flame-ionization (Mather and Tucker, 1974; Shih et al., 1976; Evans and Harbison, 1977), nitrogen-phosphorus (Jacob et al., 1982; Kintz et al., 1989), electron-capture (Hartvig and Fagerlund, 1983) or mass spectrometric detection (Todd et al., 1979; Verbeeck et al., 1980). Many of these procedures require the formation of a normeperidine derivative prior to chromatography. Liquid chromatography has also been employed (Meatherall et al., 1985). The use of chloroform as an extraction solvent may result in the formation of the ethylcarbamate of normeperidine due to reaction with an impurity in the solvent; Siek et al. (1977) recommended the use of dichloromethane in lieu of chloroform.

Meperidinic acid and normeperidinic acid have been measured in urine by gas chromatography after hydrolysis and derivatization (Lindberg et al., 1978; Wainer and Stambaugh, 1978).

References

W.H. Anderson and R.W. Prouty. Postmortem redistribution of drugs. In *Advances in Analytical Toxicology* (R.C. Baselt, ed.), Vol. 2, YearBook Medical, Chicago, 1989, pp. 70–102.

P.J. Armstrong and A. Bersten. Normeperidine toxicity. Anesth. Anal. 65: 536–538, 1986.

J.J. Burns, B.L. Berger, P.A. Lief et al. The physiological disposition and fate of meperidine (Demerol) in man and a method for its estimation in plasma. J. Pharm. Exp. Ther. 114: 289–298, 1955.

K. Chan, M.J. Kendall, W.D.E. Wells et al. Factors influencing the excretion and relative physiological availability of pethidine in man. J. Pharm. Pharmac. 27: 235–241, 1975.

K. Chan, J. Tse, F. Jennings and M.L.E. Orme. Influence of urinary pH on pethidine kinetics in healthy volunteer subjects. Meth. Find. Exp. Clin. Pharm. 7: 245–251, 1985.

L.A. Dal Cortivo, M.M. De Mayo and S.B. Weinberg. Fluorometric determination of microgram amounts of meperidine. Anal. Chem. 42: 941–942, 1970.

M.A. Evans and R.D. Harbison. Micromethod for determination of meperidine in plasma. J. Pharm. Sci. 66: 599–600, 1977.

R.J. Geller. Meperidine in patient-controlled analgesic: a near fatal mishap. Anesth. Anal. 76: 655–657, 1993.

P. Hartvig and C. Fagerlund. A simplified method for the gas chromatographic determination of pethidine and norpethidine after derivatization with trichloroethyl chloroformate. J. Chrom. 274: 355–360, 1983.

P. Jacob, J.F. Rigod, S.M. Pond and N.L. Benowitz. Gas chromatographic analysis of meperidine and normeperidine: determination in blood after a single dose of meperidine. J. Pharm. Sci. 71: 166–168, 1982.

L. Kazyak. Determination of meperidine in biological specimens in conjunction with a case of Demerol intoxication. J. For. Sci. 4: 264–275, 1959.

P. Kintz, B. Godelar, P. Mangin et al. Simultaneous determination of pethidine, phenoperidine, and norpethidine by gas chromatography with selective nitrogen detection. For. Sci. Int. 43: 267–273, 1989.

U. Klotz, T.S. McHorse, G.R. Wilkinson and S. Schenker. The effect of cirrhosis on the disposition and elimination of meperidine in man. Clin. Pharm. Ther. 16: 667–675, 1974.

C. Lindberg, C. Bogentoft, U. Bondesson et al. Mass spectrometric identification of a new metabolite of pethidine. J. Pharm. Pharmac. 27: 975–976, 1975.

C. Lindberg, U. Bondesson and P. Hartvig. Investigation of the urinary excretion of pethidine and five of its metabolites in man using selected ion monitoring. Biomed. Mass Spec. 7: 88–92, 1980.

L.E. Mather and G.T. Tucker. Meperidine and other basic drugs: general method for their determination in plasma. J. Pharm. Sci. 63: 306–307, 1974.

L.E. Mather, G.T. Tucker, A.E. Pflug et al. Meperidine kinetics in man. Clin. Pharm. Ther. 17: 21–30, 1975a.

L.E. Mather, M.J. Lindop, G.T. Tucker and A.E. Pflug. Pethidine revisited: plasma concentrations and effects after intramuscular injection. Brit. J. Anaesth. 47: 1269–1275, 1975b.

L.E. Mather and G.T. Tucker. Systemic availability of orally administered meperidine. Clin. Pharm. Ther. 20: 535–540, 1976.

R.C. Meatherall, D.R.P. Guay and J.L. Chalmers. Analysis of meperidine and norpeperidine in serum and urine by high-performance liquid chromatography. J. Chrom. 338: 141–149, 1985.

M.L. Pokela, K.T. Olkkola, M. Koivisto and P. Ryhanen. Pharmacokinetics and pharmacodynamics of intravenous meperidine in neonates and infants. Clin. Pharm. Ther. 52: 342–349, 1992.

A.P.L. Shih, K. Robinson and W.Y.W. Au. Determination of therapeutic serum concentrations of oral and parenteral meperidine by gas liquid chromatography. Eur. J. Clin. Pharm. 9: 451–456, 1976.

T.J. Siek, L.S. Eichmeier, M.E. Caplis and F.E. Esposito. The reaction of normeperidine with an impurity in chloroform. J. Anal. Tox. 1: 211–214, 1977.

T.J. Siek. The analysis of meperidine and normeperidine in biological specimens. J. For. Sci. 23: 6–13, 1978.

J.E. Stambaugh, I.W. Wainer, J.K. Sanstead et al. The clinical pharmacology of meperidine—comparison of routes of administration. J. Clin. Pharm. 16: 245–256, 1976.

W.G. Stillwell, C.S. Myram and J.T. Stewart. Meperidine metabolites: identification of N-hydroxynormeperidine and hydroxy-methoxy derivative of meperidine in biological fluids. Res. Comm. Chem. Path. Pharm. 14: 605–619, 1976.

H.H. Szeto, C.E. Inturrisi, R. Houde et al. Accumulation of normeperidine, an active metabolite of meperidine, in patients with renal failure or cancer. Ann. Int. Med. 86: 738–741, 1977.

E.L. Todd, D.T. Stafford and J.C. Morrison. Determination of meperidine and normeperidine in serum by gas chromatography/mass spectrometry. J. Anal. Tox. 3: 256–259, 1979.

R.K. Verbeeck, R.C. James, D.F. Taber et al. The determination of meperidine, noremeperidine and deuterated analogs in blood and plasma by gas chromatography mass spectrometry selected ion monitoring. Biomed. Mass Spec. 7: 58–60, 1980.

I.W. Wainer and J.E. Stambaugh. GLC determination of meperidinic and normeperidinic acids in urine. J. Pharm. Sci. 67: 116–118, 1978.

Mephenytoin

T½: 12–32 hr
Vd: ?
Fb: 0.20–0.50
pKa: ?

Occurrence and Usage. Mephenytoin (3-methyl-5-ethyl-5-phenylhydantoin, Mesantoin) is a hydantoin derivative that has been available since 1945 for the treatment of convulsive disorders. It is the N-methyl derivative of 5-ethyl-5-phenylhydantoin (Nirvanol), a drug introduced in 1916 that fell into disuse by 1930 as a result of its excessive toxicity. Mephenytoin is administered as the racemic mixture of the free acid in daily oral doses of 100–600 mg, and is used primarily in patients who fail to respond to less toxic agents.

Blood Concentrations. It was found after daily administration for 14 days of 300 mg of mephenytoin to a volunteer that the metabolite, normephenytoin or Nirvanol, reached a peak concentration of 26 mg/L, and it was suggested that the parent drug concentration was much lower. The metabolite concentration in the plasma was still climbing steadily when the drug was withdrawn (Butler and Waddell, 1958). The plasma half-life of mephenytoin ranges from 12–32 hours and for normephenytoin, from 74–144 hours. Autoinduction of metabolism may occur with continued usage. The suggested therapeutic range for combined plasma mephenytoin and normephenytoin concentrations during chronic therapy is 25–40 mg/L; the mephenytoin concentration averages 8% of the combined level in epileptic patients receiving the drug (Troupin et al., 1976).

Metabolism and Excretion. Mephenytoin is metabolized initially by N-demethylation to normephenytoin, which is considerably more active as an anticonvulsant, has a longer half-life and is more toxic than its parent. It is believed on the basis of animal experiments that most of the anticonvulsant activity of mephenytoin is due to this metabolite (Kupferberg and Yonekawa, 1975). Both mephenytoin and normephenytoin undergo p-hydroxylation and glucuronide conjugation. An average of 61% of a labeled dose is excreted in the 72 hour urine; conjugated p-hydroxymephenytoin accounts for 46% (91% of which is formed from S-mephenytoin), normephenytoin for 3%, and mephenytoin for less than 0.5%. Minor amounts of conjugated o-hydroxy-, m-hydroxy-, and 5-hydroxyethylmephenytoin and p-hydroxynormephenytoin have also been reported (Butler; 1956; Lynn et al., 1979; Kupfer et al., 1980; Kupfer et al., 1981). During chronic therapy, normephenytoin accounts for at least 22% of the daily dose in the 24 hour urine (Butler, 1952). Certain subjects exhibit a hydroxylation deficiency for mephenytoin that results in plasma normephenytoin concentrations approximately twice those of normal individuals (Kupfer et al., 1984).

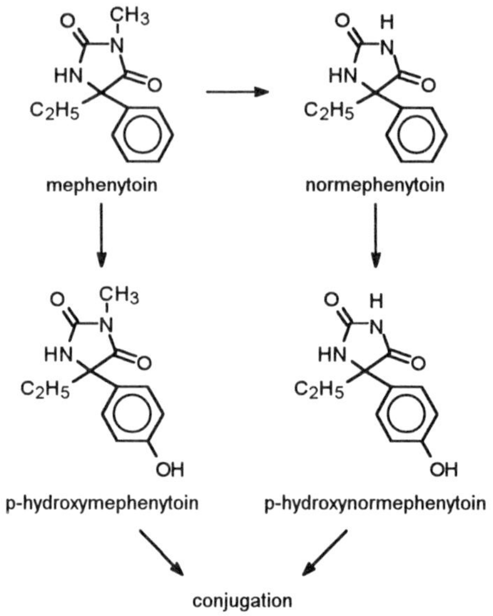

mephenytoin   normephenytoin

p-hydroxymephenytoin   p-hydroxynormephenytoin

conjugation

Toxicity. The side-effects of mephenytoin administration include drowsiness, ataxia, confusion, tremor, dermatitis, blood dyscrasias, and hepatitis. A number of cases involving severe hematologic disorders have been reported with several deaths (Bercel et al., 1950; Hofstatter, 1951; Witkind and Waid, 1951). A 10 year old girl developed a skin rash less than 2 weeks after being placed on mephenytoin; it progressed to fulminating dermatitis with secondary leukocytosis, and the patient died suddenly 12 days after discontinuation of the drug (Ruskin, 1948). Mephenytoin is considered safe for the majority of patients if a periodic blood count is performed routinely (Abbott and Schwab, 1954).

Analysis. Mephenytoin and normephenytoin may be analyzed in plasma by gas chromatography with flame-ionization (Kupferberg and Yonekawa, 1975; Raisys et al., 1979) or mass spectrometric detection (Yonekawa and Kupferberg, 1979). Liquid chromatographic procedures have also been described (Kabra et al., 1978; Kupfer et al., 1982).

References

J.A. Abbott and R.S. Schwab. Mesantoin in the treatment of epilepsy. New Eng. Med. J. 250: 197–199, 1954.

N.A. Bercel, B. Finesilver, P. Solomon et al. Mesantoin in epilepsy. J. Am. Med. Asso. 143: 1460–1462, 1950.

T.C. Butler. Metabolic demethylation of 3-methyl-5-ethyl-5-phenylhydantoin (Mesantoin). J. Pharm. Exp. Ther. 104: 299–308, 1952.

T.C. Butler. The metabolic conversion of 3-methyl-5-ethyl-5-phenylhydantoin (Mesantoin) and of 5-ethyl-5-phenylhydantoin (Nirvanol) to 5-ethyl-5-(p-hydroxyphenyl)hydantoin. J. Pharm. Exp. Ther. 117: 160–165, 1956.

T.C. Butler and W.J. Waddell. N-mythelated derivatives of barbituric acid, hydantoin and oxazolidinedione used in the treatment of epilepsy. Neurology 8: 106–112, 1958.

L. Hofstatter. Mesantoin in the management of the hospitalized psychotic epileptic. South. Med. J. 44: 827–832, 1951.

P.M. Kabra, D.M. McDonald and L.J. Marton. A simultaneous high-performance liquid chromatographic analysis of the most common anticonvulsants and their metabolites in the serum. J. Anal. Tox. 2: 127–133, 1978.

A. Kupfer, G.M. Brilis, J.T. Watson and T.M. Harris. A major pathway of mephenytoin metabolism in man. Drug Met. Disp. 8: 1–4, 1980.

A. Kupfer, R.K. Roberts, S. Schenker and R.A. Branch. Stereoselective metabolism of mephenytoin in man. J. Pharm. Exp. Ther. 218: 193–199, 1981.

A. Kupfer, J.K. Carr and R. Branch. Analysis of hydroxylated and demethylated metabolites of mephenytoin in man and laboratory animals using gas-liquid chromatography and high-performance liquid chromatography. J. Chrom. 232: 93–100, 1982.

A. Kupfer, P. Desmond, R. Patwardhan et al. Mephenytoin hydroxylation deficiency: kinetics after repeated doses. Clin. Pharm. Ther. 35: 33–39, 1984.

H.J. Kupferberg and W. Yonekawa. The metabolism of 3-methyl-5-ethyl-5-phenylhydantoin (mephenytoin) to 5-ethyl-5-phenylhydantoin (Nirvanol) in mice in relation to anticonvulsant activity. Drug Met. Disp. 3: 26–29, 1975.

R.K. Lynn, J.E. Bauer, W.P. Gordon et al. Characterization of mephenytoin metabolites in human urine by gas chromatography and mass spectrometry. Drug Met. Disp. 7: 138–144, 1979.

V.A. Raisys, A.M. Zebelman and S.F. MacMillan. Gas-chromatographic determination of mephenytoin and desmethylmephenytoin, after off-column alkylation. Clin. Chem. 25: 172–175, 1979.

D.B. Ruskin. Fulminating dermatitis bullosa medicamentosa due to "Mesantoin". J. Am. Med. Asso. 137: 1031–1035, 1948.

A.S. Troupin, L.M. Ojemann and C.B. Dodrill. Mephenytoin: a reappraisal. Epilepsia 17: 403–414, 1976.

E. Witkind and M.E. Waid. Aplasia of the bone marrow during Mesantoin therapy. J. Am. Med. Asso. 147: 757–759, 1951.

W. Yonekawa and H.J. Kupferberg. Measurement of mephenytoin (3-methyl-5-ethyl-5-phenylhydantoin) and its demethylated metabolite by selective ion monitoring. J. Chrom. 163: 161–167, 1979.

Mephobarbital

T½: 48–52 hr
Vd: 2.6 L/kg
Fb: 0.40–0.60
pKa: 7.8

Occurrence and Usage. Mephobarbital (N-methylphenobarbital, Mebaral), is a methylated barbiturate that has been employed since the 1930s for the treatment of epilepsy. It is administered as the free acid in daily oral maintenance doses of 200–600 mg, somewhat higher than for phenobarbital itself, since mephobarbital is presumably less well absorbed. It is not commonly used today since it offers no advantages over phenobarbital.

Blood Concentrations. A single 800 mg oral dose given to 2 volunteers produced peak mephobarbital plasma concentrations of 2.5–3.5 mg/L after 2–8 hours; phenobarbital concentrations reached 1.5–3.0 mg/L by the sixth day after ingestion. The mephobarbital half-life averaged 50 hours while that for phenobarbital averaged 121 hours; the bioavailability of the parent drug was 71–75% by the oral route (Hooper et al., 1981a). Two subjects who received 200–240 mg daily oral doses for 3 weeks reached plateau plasma levels of 2.0–2.5 mg/L for mephobarbital and 9–17 mg/L for phenobarbital (Hooper et al., 1981b). In 6 epileptic patients receiving 100–400 mg daily oral doses, plasma mephobarbital concentrations ranged from 0.5–1.7 mg/L and phenobarbital, from 11–32 mg/L; on average, mephobarbital represented only 5% of the total plasma drug level (Kupferberg and Longacre-Shaw, 1979).

Metabolism and Excretion. Mephobarbital is rapidly metabolized by N-demethylation to phenobarbital, its active metabolite, which probably accounts for most of its pharmacologic activity. Both mephobarbital and phenobarbital undergo p-hydroxylation and conjugation. Less than 1% of a dose of mephobarbital is excreted unchanged in the urine, while as much as 15% is present as phenobarbital. About 35% is eliminated as conjugated p-hydroxymephobarbital and about 1% as conjugated p-hydroxyphenobarbital (Butler, 1952; Svendsen and Brochmann-Hanssen, 1962; Hooper et al., 1981b).

Toxicity. Adverse reactions to mephobarbital include sedation, dizziness, confusion, nausea, allergic dermatitis, blood dyscrasias, and hepatic damage. Overdosage may result in hypotension, respiratory depression, and coma. A 38 year old woman ingested 13 g of drug and developed coma that persisted for 6 days; blood concentrations of both mephobarbital and phenobarbital were relatively constant at 40–60 mg/L for the first 5 days and only began to decline after hemoperfusion was instituted (Pond et al., 1982).

Analysis. Gas chromatographic procedures have been described for the simultaneous measurement of underivatized mephobarbital and phenobarbital in biological specimens (Svendsen and Brochmann-Hanssen, 1962; Cremers and Verheesen, 1973; Ritz and Warren, 1975). Others have involved the preparation of butyl (Hooper et al., 1975) or propyl derivatives (Kupferberg and Longacre-Shaw, 1979; Hooper et al., 1981c). Procedures that require the formation of methyl derivatives of the anticonvulsants will result in the conversion of phenobarbital to mephobarbital and so are not applicable to the differential measurement of these two drugs. For most purposes, however, the measurement of total drug (mephobarbital plus phenobarbital) will suffice.

Liquid chromatography can be used for the simultaneous assay of these drugs in plasma (Kabra et al., 1978) as well as their metabolites in urine (Kunze et al., 1981).

References

T.C. Butler. Quantitative studies of the metabolic fate of mephobarbital (N-methylphenobarbital). J. Pharm. Exp. Ther. 106: 235–245, 1952.

H.M.H.G. Cremers and P.E. Verheesen. A rapid method for the estimation of anti-epileptic drugs in blood serum by gas-liquid chromatography. Clin. Chim. Acta 48: 413–420, 1973.

W.D. Hooper, D.K. Dubetz, M.J. Eadie and J.H. Tyrer. Simultaneous assay of methylphenobarbitone and phenobarbitone using gas-liquid chromatography with on-column butylation. J. Chrom. 110: 206–209, 1975.

W.D. Hooper, H.E. Kunze and M.J. Eadie. Pharmacokinetics and bioavailability of methylphenobarbital in man. Ther. Drug Mon. 3: 39–44, 1981a.

W.D. Hooper, H.E. Kunze and M.J. Eadie. Qualitative and quantitative studies of methylphenobarbital metabolism in man. Drug Met. Disp. 9: 381–385, 1981b.

W.D. Hooper, H.E. Kunze and M.J. Eadie. Simultaneous assay of methylphenobarbital and phenobarbital in plasma using gas chromatography-mass spectrometry with selected ion monitoring. J. Chrom. 223: 426–431, 1981c.

P.M. Kabra, D.M. McDonald and L.J. Marton. A simultaneous high-performance liquid chromatographic analysis of the most common anticonvulsants and their metabolites in the serum. J. Anal. Tox. 2: 127–133, 1978.

H.E. Kunze, W.D. Hooper and M.J. Eadie. High performance liquid chromatographic assay of methylphenobarbital metabolites in urine. Ther. Drug Mon. 3: 45–49, 1981.

H.J. Kupferberg and J. Longacre-Shaw. Mephobarbital and phenobarbital plasma concentrations in epileptic patients treated with mephobarbital. Ther. Drug Mon. 1: 117–122, 1979.

S. Pond, P. Jacob, M. Humphreys et al. Impaired metabolism of methylphenobarbital after a combined drug overdose: treatment by resin hemoperfusion. Clin. Tox. 19: 187–196, 1982.

D.P. Ritz and C.G. Warren. Single extraction GLC analysis of six commonly prescribed antiepileptic drugs. Clin. Tox. 8: 311–324, 1975.

A.B. Svendsen and E. Brochmann-Hanssen. Gas chromatography of barbiturates II. Application to the study of their metabolites and excretion in humans. J. Pharm. Sci. 51: 494–495, 1962.

Mepivacaine

T½: 1.9 hr
Vd: 1.2 L/kg
Fb: 0.77
pKa: 7.6

Occurrence and Usage. Mepivacaine (Carbocaine), an anilide local anesthetic related to bupivacaine, was synthesized in 1957. It is often used for paracervical, caudal, epidural and infiltration anesthesia as the hydrochloride of the racemate, in single doses of up to 400 mg and in daily doses of up to 1000 mg.

Blood Concentrations. The local administration of 36–51 mg of mepivacaine to 3 subjects produced maximal blood concentrations of 0.28–0.53 mg/L at 30–60 minutes, which declined to 0.10–0.21 mg/L by 4 hours; concentrations were up to 40% higher in 1 subject when the drug was administered without a vasoconstrictor, compared to the same dose with a vasoconstrictor (Pratt et al., 1967). After paracervical administration of 200 mg to 13 patients, arterial blood concentrations reached a mean peak of 2.3 mg/L at 6 minutes, decreasing to 1.6 mg/L at 30 minutes and 1.3 mg/L at 60 minutes (Shnider et al., 1968). During lumbar peridural obstetric anesthesia (initial 140 mg dose with reinforcing doses of 100 mg/hour) in 19 patients, plasma mepivacaine concentrations averaged 1.7 mg/L (Hook et al., 1971). In a similar situation after doses of 250–580 mg to 8 patients, plasma concentrations averaged 4.7 mg/L (range, 3.7–5.5) for mepivacaine and 0.23 mg/L for normepivacaine, a metabolite (Meffin et al., 1973). In a third such study with doses of 200–300 mg initially and 200 mg every hour thereafter, blood mepivacaine concentrations reached an average peak of 7.7 mg/L at 5 hours, with levels in several patients exceeding 10 mg/L (Takasaki et al., 1987).

Metabolism and Excretion. Mepivacaine is biotransformed in man by hydroxylation of the aromatic ring, with subsequent conjugation of the phenolic metabolites, and to a slight extent by N-demethylation. Normepivacaine is found in low levels in plasma and is less toxic than its parent. With intravenous administration, only 36% of a dose has been accounted for in the 30 hour urine as unchanged drug (4.0%), normepivacaine (2.4%), conjugated 3'-hydroxymepivacaine (17%) and conjugated 4'-hydroxymepivacaine (12%) (Hansson et al., 1965; Thomas and Meffin, 1972; Meffin et al., 1973).

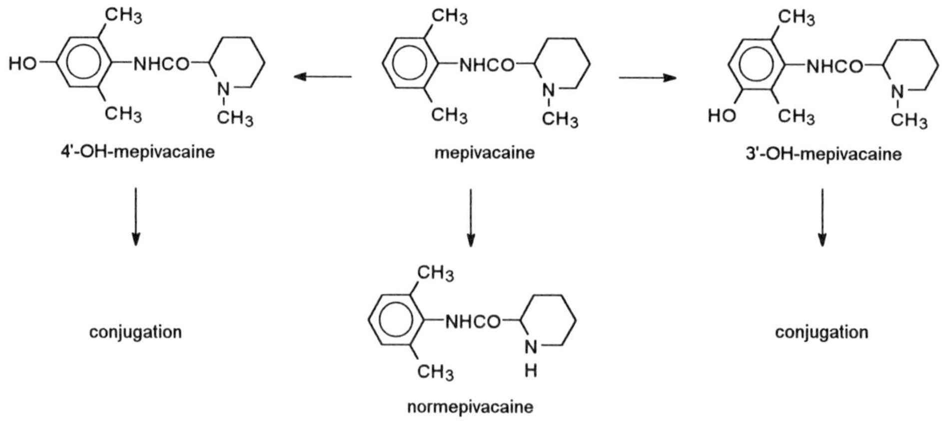

Toxicity. Adverse reactions to mepivacaine administration include headache, drowsiness or excitation, hypotension, bradycardia, respiratory depression, coma, and convulsions. Five female patients who developed apprehension, confusion, muscular twitching, nausea, and vomiting during the perinatal use of mepivacaine had plasma mepivacaine concentrations of 4.4–8.6 mg/L, averaging 6.3 mg/L (Morishima et al., 1966). Accidental administration of mepivacaine to fetuses has resulted in a number of intoxications. Bradycardia was noted in 4 neonates whose scalp blood mepivacaine levels averaged 4.0 mg/L, compared to a mean level of 1.0 mg/L in normal infants following paracervical administration of the drug to the mothers (Shnider et al., 1968). Two neonates with blood levels of 31 and 75 mg/L required respiratory support and exchange transfusions; the signs of toxicity disappeared after some hours when the blood levels had fallen to about 8 mg/L (Finster et al., 1965).

The deaths of 3 neonates have been reported in which postmortem mepivacaine concentrations ranged from 9.8–52 mg/L in blood, 47–84 mg/kg in brain and 88–133 mg/kg in liver (Sinclair et al., 1965; Dodson et al., 1975). One adult has died from intolerance to or inadvertent intravenous administration of 200 mg of the drug for paracervical block, with resulting hypotension and convulsions (Grimes and Cates, 1976). The following tissue distribution was observed in the death of an adult after infiltration of up to 3 g of mepivacaine for breast surgery (Sunshine and Fike, 1964):

Mepivacaine Concentrations in a Fatal Case (mg/L or mg/kg)

Blood	Brain	Liver	Bile	Kidney	Urine
50	51	75	50	51	100

Analysis. Flame-ionization gas chromatography has been used to determine mepivacaine in biological samples (Pratt et al., 1967; Asling et al., 1969); normepivacaine has been similarly measured as an acetyl derivative (Thomas and Meffin, 1972). Gas chromatography with nitrogen-selective detection has also been employed (Bjork et al., 1990).

References

J.H. Asling, S.M. Shnider, G.R. Wilkinson and E.L. Way. Gas chromatographic determination of mepivacaine in capillary blood. Anesthesiology 31: 458–461, 1969.

M. Bjork, K.J. Pettersson and G. Osterlop. Capillary gas chromatographic method for the simultaneous determination of local anaesthetics in plasma samples. J. Chrom. 533: 229–234, 1990.

W.E. Dodson, R.E. Hillman and L.S. Hillman. Brain tissue levels in a fatal case of neonatal mepivacaine (Carbocaine) poisoning. J. Pediat. 86: 624–627, 1975.

M. Finster, P.J. Poppers, J.C. Sinclair et al. Accidental intoxication of the fetus with local anesthetic drug during caudal anesthesia. Am. J. Obs. Gyn. 92: 922–924, 1965.

D.A. Grimes and W. Cates, Jr. Deaths from paracervical anesthesia used for first-trimester abortion, 1972–1975. New Eng. J. Med. 295: 1397–1399, 1976.

E. Hansson, P. Hoffmann and L. Kristerson. Fate of mepivacaine in the body: II. Excretion and biotransformation. Acta Pharm. Tox. 22: 213–223, 1965.

R. Hook, R.A. Greenberg and F.W. Hehre. Continuous lumbar peridural anesthesia in obstetrics. Anesth. Anal. 50: 693–698, 1971.

P. Meffin, G.J. Long and J. Thomas. Clearance and metabolism of mepivacaine in the human neonate. Clin. Pharm. Ther. 14: 218–225, 1973.

H.O. Morishima, S.S. Daniel, M. Finster et al. Transmission of mepivacaine hydrochloride (Carbocaine) across the human placenta. Anesthesiology 27: 147–154, 1966.

E.L. Pratt, H.P. Warrington and J. Grego. The gas chromatographic determination of mepivacaine in blood with a note on other local anesthetics. Anesthesiology 28: 432–437, 1967.

S.M. Shnider, J.H. Asling, A.J. Margolis et al. High fetal blood levels of mepivacaine and fetal bradycardia. New Eng. J. Med. 279: 947–948, 1968.

J.C. Sinclair, H.A. Fox, J.F. Lentz et al. Intoxication of the fetus by a local anesthetic. New Eng. J. Med. 273: 1173–1177, 1965.

I. Sunshine and W.W. Fike. Value of thin-layer chromatography in two fatal cases of intoxication due to lidocaine and mepivacaine. New Eng. J. Med. 271: 487–490, 1964.

M. Takasaki, T. Oh-Oka, K. Doi and Y. Kosaka. Blood levels of mepivacaine during continuous epidural anesthesia. Anesth. Anal. 66: 337–340, 1987.

J. Thomas and P. Meffin. Aromatic hydroxylation of lidocaine and mepivacaine in rats and humans. J. Med. Chem. 15: 1046–1049, 1972.

Meprobamate

T½: 6–17 hr
Vd: 0.7 L/kg
Fb: 0.20

$$NH_2OCOCH_2\underset{\underset{C_3H_7}{|}}{\overset{\overset{CH_3}{|}}{C}}CH_2OCONH_2$$

Occurrence and Usage. Meprobamate (Equanil, Miltown) is the prototype of the medicinal carbamates, having been synthesized in 1950 and introduced in 1955 for clinical usage. It is frequently employed as a sedative, antianxiety agent, and muscle relaxant and is available for oral administration in doses of 200–400 mg, alone or in combination with other drugs. As much as 2400 mg may be consumed in a single day.

Blood Concentrations. A single 400 mg oral dose given to 6 subjects produced average plasma meprobamate concentrations of 7.7 mg/L at 2 hours, 4.4 mg/L at 8 hours, and 1.6 mg/L at 24 hours (Meyer et al., 1978). Peak plasma concentrations of 12–19 mg/L (average, 16) were achieved by 6 volunteers 2 hours after the ingestion of 800 mg of meprobamate (Hoffman and Ludwig, 1959). An average plasma half-life of 11 hours (range, 6.4–17) has been determined in 12 subjects (Hollister and Levy, 1964). An average blood concentration of 24 mg/L (range, 8.6–27) was observed at 2 hours after the ingestion of 1600 mg by 5 volunteers over a 1.5 hour period; this level declined to 20 mg/L by 6 hours and 7.7 mg/L by 19.5 hours (Parker et al., 1970).

Metabolism and Excretion. Meprobamate is metabolized by oxidation of the propyl side-chain to hydroxymeprobamate, an inactive metabolite, and by N-glucuronidation of the parent drug (Ludwig et al., 1961). There is some evidence that chronic administration of meprobamate causes induction of the microsomal enzyme system, enhancing the production of hydroxymeprobamate (Douglas et al., 1963). Meprobamate concentrations in urine after a 1600 mg oral dose ranged from 24–176 mg/L during the 18 hour post-ingestion period in 5 subjects; this represented an average excretion of 5.3% of the dose in unchanged form (Parker et al., 1970). Up to 11% of a single dose is excreted in the urine in 24 hours (Maddock and Bloomer, 1967). A comparable portion of a dose is excreted as hydroxymeprobamate (Douglas et al., 1963), and as much as 65% may be eliminated in the 48 hour urine as the N-glucuronide (Ludwig et al., 1961).

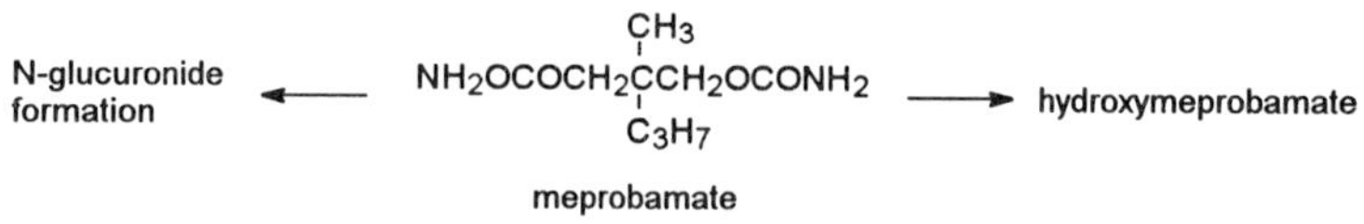

$$\text{N-glucuronide formation} \longleftarrow NH_2OCOCH_2\underset{\underset{C_3H_7}{|}}{\overset{\overset{CH_3}{|}}{C}}CH_2OCONH_2 \longrightarrow \text{hydroxymeprobamate}$$

meprobamate

Toxicity. Side-effects of meprobamate usage include drowsiness, headache, dizziness, nausea, and paradoxical excitement. Several cases of severe hypotension and one case of fatal aplastic anemia have also been reported (Scott et al., 1957; Meyer et al., 1957).

Numerous instances of both nonfatal and fatal intoxication following overdosage with meprobamate have been described. While death has occurred after the ingestion of 12 g of the drug, survival has been reported after a dose of 40 g (Powell et al., 1958). Blood concentrations as high as 90 and 96 mg/L of meprobamate were found in 2 persons who were arrested while driving motor vehicles (Graves, 1974). Plasma concentrations of 60–120 mg/L were determined in 6 intoxicated patients who were in light coma, and concentrations of 100–240 mg/L for 9 persons in deep coma (Maddock and Bloomer, 1967). Large amounts of unabsorbed meprobamate may remain in the stomach of intoxicated patients (Schwartz, 1976). Hemoperfusion has permitted a more than 3-fold reduction in the plasma half-life of the drug in poisoned patients (Jacobsen et al., 1987).

Felby (1970) reported 12 fatal cases that involved the ingestion of 16–40 g of meprobamate and in which blood concentrations averaged 226 mg/L (range, 142–346) and liver concentrations, 238 mg/kg (range, 147–412). Another 16 deaths were investigated and attributed solely to overdosage with meprobamate; postmortem blood levels averaged 95 mg/L (range, 35–240) and liver levels averaged 148 mg/kg (range, 58–360) (Baselt and Cravey, 1977). The following tissue distribution of the drug was observed in 2 cases of intentional oral overdosage by adults with 36–38 g of meprobamate (Jenis et al., 1969; Kintz et al., 1988a):

Meprobamate Concentrations in Fatalities (mg/L or mg/kg)

	Blood	Brain	Liver	Kidney	Urine	Fat	Gastric
Case 1	180	140	300	500		600	25 g
Case 2	205	118	255	286	237		1.1 g

Analysis. A popular procedure for the determination of meprobamate in biological fluids has been the colorimetric assay of Hoffman and Ludwig (1959), which apparently does not measure metabolites of the drug but which will react with other carbamates. Meprobamate is amenable to gas chromatographic analysis, and this more specific technique has been approached by flame-ionization detection of the underivatized drug (Finkle, 1967; Douglas et al., 1967; Kintz et al., 1988b; Trenque et al., 1993) and of a derivative of the hydrolyzed drug (Martis and Levy, 1974; Gupta and Eng, 1980). Gas chromatography-mass spectrometry (Kintz and Mangin, 1993) and liquid chromatography (Gupta and Eng, 1980) have also been described.

References

R.C. Baselt and R.H. Cravey. A compendium of therapeutic and toxic concentrations of toxicologically significant drugs in human biofluids. J. Anal. Tox. 1: 81–103, 1977.

J.F. Douglas, B.J. Ludwig and N. Smith. Studies on the metabolism of meprobamate. Proc. Soc. Exp. Biol. Med. 112: 436–438, 1963.

J.F. Douglas, T.F. Kelley, N.B. Smith and J.A. Stockage. Gas chromatographic determination of meprobamate, 2-methyl-2-propyl-1,3-propanediol dicarbamate, in plasma and urine. Anal. Chem. 39: 956–958, 1967.

S. Felby. Concentrations of meprobamate in blood and liver following fatal meprobamate poisoning. Acta Pharm. Tox. 28: 334–337, 1970.

B.S. Finkle. The identification, quantitative determination and distribution of meprobamate and glutethimide in biological material. J. For. Sci. 12: 509–528, 1967.

M.H. Graves. Personal communication, 1974.

R.N. Gupta and F. Eng. GC and HPLC determination of meprobamate in plasma. J. High Res. Chrom. Chrom. Comm. 3: 419–420, 1980.

A.J. Hoffman and B.J. Ludwig. An improved colorimetric method for the determination of meprobamate in biological fluids. J. Am. Pharm. Asso. 48: 740–742, 1959.

L.E. Hollister and G. Levy. Kinetics of meprobamate elimination in humans. Chemotherapia 9: 20–24, 1964.

D. Jacobsen, E. Wiik-Larsen, E. Saltvedt and J.E. Bredesen. Evaluation of hemoperfusion in severe meprobamate intoxications. Vet. Hum. Tox. 29: 484, 1987.

E.H. Jenis, R.J. Payne and L.R. Goldbaum. Acute meprobamate poisoning. J. Am. Med. Asso. 207: 361–362, 1969.

P. Kintz. A. Tracqui, P. Mangin and A.A.J. Lugnier. Fatal meprobamate self-poisoning. Am. J. For. Med. Path. 9: 139–140, 1988a.

P. Kintz, P. Mangin, A.A.J. Lugnier and A.J. Chaumont. A rapid and sensitive gas chromatographic analysis of meprobamate or carisoprodol in urine and plasma. J. Anal. Tox. 12: 73–74, 1988b.

P. Kintz and P. Mangin. Determination of meprobamate in human plasma, urine and hair by gas chromatography and electron impact mass spectrometry. J. Anal. Tox. 71: 408–410, 1993.

B.J. Ludwig, J.F. Douglas, L.S. Powell et al. Structures of the major metabolites of meprobamate. J. Med. Pharm. Chem. 3: 53–64, 1961.

R.K. Maddock and H.A. Bloomer. Meprobamate overdosage. J. Am. Med. Asso. 201: 999–1003, 1967.

L. Martis and R.H. Levy. GLC determination of meprobamate in water, plasma and urine. J. Pharm. Sci. 63: 834–837, 1974.

L.M. Meyer, W.L. Heeve and R.W. Bertscher. Aplastic anemia after meprobamate (2-methyl-2-n-propyl-1,3-propanediol dicarbamate) therapy. New Eng. J. Med. 256: 1232–1233, 1957.

M.C. Meyer, A.P. Melikian and A.B. Straughn. Relative bioavailability of meprobamate tablets in humans. J. Pharm. Sci. 67: 1290–1293, 1978.

K.D. Parker, H.W. Elliott, J.A. Wright et al. Blood and urine concentrations of subjects receiving barbiturates, meprobamate, glutethimide, or diphenylhydantoin. Clin. Tox. 3: 131–145, 1970.

L.W. Powell, Jr., G.T. Mann and S. Kaye. Acute meprobamate poisoning. New Eng. J. Med. 259: 716–718, 1958.

H.S. Schwartz. Acute meprobamate poisoning with gastrotomy and removal of a drug-containing mass. New Eng. J. Med. 295: 1177–1178, 1976.

P.A.L. Scott, L. Grimshaw and H.M.P. Molony. Severe hypotensive crisis following treatment with meprobamate. Arch. Int. Med. 100: 484–486, 1957.

T. Trenque, D. Lamiable, H. Millart et al. Gas chromatographic determination of meprobamate in human plasma. J. Chrom. 615: 343–346, 1993.

Mercury

T½: 24 days (inorganic mercury)

52 days (methylmercury)

Hg

Vd: ?

Fb: ?

Occurrence and Usage. Mercury is a nonessential trace element, the presence of which in human tissues represents uptake from both natural and man-made sources. Inorganic mercury released by industries into waterways can b̶ ˙ ʋerted to methylmercury by microflora; this lipid-soluble organic form of the element is efficiently concentrated by fish and other aquatic organisms. In the United States, a total mercury limit of 0.5 mg/kg has been established for commercial fish; mercury levels in marine fish have ranged from undetectable to 5.0 mg/kg, averaging 0.2–0.5 mg/kg in some species, while freshwater fish in contaminated areas have accumulated concentrations of up to 40 mg/kg (80–90% of which is methylmercury). Organic mercury compounds are used as preservatives in paints and for agricultural purposes, and as diuretics in clinical medicine. Mercury is widely used industrially, especially in electrical components, and also in dentistry. The daily dietary intake of mercury ranges from 1–30 µg for most persons. The current threshold limit value for mercury and its inorganic compounds is 0.05 mg/m^3, while for alkyl mercury compounds it is 0.01 mg/m^3 (as Hg). Industrial exposure is usually by inhalation or dermal absorption.

Blood Concentrations. Total blood mercury ranges up to 0.006 mg/L in persons having low fish consumption, up to 0.050 mg/L in dieters eating moderate quantities of tunafish and up to 0.200 mg/L or higher in those consuming large amounts of predatory marine fish. About 95% of the mercury in whole blood is contained in red cells, largely as methylmercury (Clarkson, 1977). A group of 205 dentists had significantly higher total blood mercury concentrations (average, 0.006 mg/L) than control subjects (average, 0.004 mg/L) (Chang et al., 1987). A concentration of 0.020 mg/L is considered an acceptable level of mercury in whole human blood (Panel on Mercury, 1978). Following a 3 day occupational exposure to metallic mercury vapor, blood mercury values exhibited a biphasic decline with elimination half-lives averaging 3 and 18 days (Barregard et al., 1992).

Metabolism and Excretion. Methylmercury is well-absorbed from dietary sources and has a whole body half-life of about 70 days in man. It is slowly converted in man, possibly by the intestinal flora, to inorganic divalent mercury at the rate of about 1% of the body burden daily. Individuals in mercury equilibrium have a body burden of approximately 100 times the daily intake, and about 1% of the daily intake is found in 1 liter of blood. About 50% of an oral dose of methylmercury localizes initially in the liver. Over a period of 10 days, 13–14% of the dose is excreted in the feces and 0.2– 0.3% in urine; over 49 days, the corresponding figures are 33–35% and 3.3% (Aberg et al., 1969). Hair concentrations correlate well with blood concentrations during exposure to methylmercury, but urine concentrations are not considered a good index to the body burden of methylmercury (Lundgren et al., 1967; Clarkson, 1977).

Metallic mercury vapor is approximately 74% absorbed by the lung during inhalation. It is very rapidly oxidized to divalent mercury. Over a 7 day period, 9% of the absorbed dose is excreted in feces and 2% in urine (Cherian et al., 1978). Urine concentrations are the best guide to blood levels following exposure to inorganic or metallic mercury (Clarkson, 1977).

Urine mercury concentrations in normal persons are nearly always less than 0.010 mg/L. A weak positive correlation exists between urine mercury concentration and the number of dental amalgams in an individual (Langworth et al., 1991). In Japanese workers, urine mercury concentrations averaged 0.119 mg/L in an unexposed group and 0.403 mg/L in an asymptomatic group exposed to mercury vapor (Nakayama et al., 1977). Following a 3 day occupational exposure to metallic mercury vapor, urine mercury concentrations reached peak values 19 days later and then began a biphasic decline with elimination half-lives averaging 28 and 141 days (Barregard et al., 1992). Urine mercury levels in exposed workers may remain elevated for some years following cessation of the exposure (Goldwater and Nicolau, 1966).

The following total mercury concentrations were determined in normal Japanese autopsy specimens; the methylmercury content of most tissues averages 10–20% of the total mercury value, except in kidney and hair, where it is 2% and 63%, respectively (Sumino et al., 1975):

Total Mercury Concentrations in Normal Tissues (mg/L or mg/kg)

	Blood	Brain	Lung	Liver	Kidney	Hair
Average	0.06	0.10	0.08	0.47	1.1	4.1
(Range)	(0.02–0.11)	(0.04–0.23)	(0.02–0.30)	(0.16–1.3)	(0.2–2.6)	(1.4–15)

Toxicity. The average lethal dose of mercury is about 100 mg for organic mercury and 1 g for inorganic mercuric salts. The organic mercury compounds can produce severe and often irreversible central nervous system toxicity in overdosage, while inorganic compounds result in primarily peripheral effects, including gastroenteritis and tubular nephritis leading to renal failure. Elemental mercury by inhalation produces central effects initially, progressing to renal toxicity after its oxidation to mercuric ion.

Several mass poisonings, involving over 8000 people, have been caused by accidental ingestion of organic mercury in contaminated seafood (Minimata disease) or of mercury-treated seed grain. A daily intake of methylmercury exceeding 0.3 mg will produce chronic mercury poisoning in the average 70 kg adult; this level of intake is associated with steady-state concentrations of 0.200 mg/L in blood, 60 mg/kg in hair and a body burden of 20–30 mg of mercury (Panel on Mercury, 1978). Hair concentrations of methylmercury have ranged from 200–800 mg/kg during moderate intoxication (Gerstner and Huff, 1977) and up to 2436 mg/kg in severe intoxication (Pierce et al., 1972). Liver concentrations in 51 Iraqi victims of methylmercury poisoning ranged from 1.4–76 mg/kg, while liver concentrations in the Minimata cases ranged from 22–71 mg/kg (Magos et al., 1976). The following tissue levels were established in 8 victims of accidental methylmercury poisoning and are expressed as total mercury (Al-Saleem, 1976):

Concentrations in Fatal Methylmercury Poisoning (mg/L or mg/kg)

	Blood	Brain	Liver	Kidney	Urine
Average	2.6	27	30	22	0.8
(Range)	(0.6–6.0)	(18–35)	(4.2–78)	(2.4–41)	(0.8)

Deaths have occurred in both children and adults following extensive dermal application of solutions of mercurochrome, a mercury-containing fluorescein derivative (Yeh et al., 1978; Battista et al., 1979).

Poisoning from inorganic mercury has been described after both ingestion and external application of soluble mercuric salts. Urine mercury concentrations of 0.09–0.25 mg/L were reported in nephrotic patients who had developed chronic intoxication through the use of a skin-lightening cream (Gerstner and Huff, 1977). A number of poisonings have occurred following chronic oral ingestion of Chinese herbal medicines, which may contain mercuric sulfide or mercurous chloride; urine levels of up to 2.8 mg/L were mesured in several victims (Kang-Yum and Oransky, 1992). Postmortem blood mercury concentrations of 1.7 and 2.1 mg/L were observed in 2 adults who received peritoneal lavage with mercuric chloride during surgery and who absorbed lethal amounts of the metal (Cross et al., 1979). The following tissue concentrations were observed in 2 adults who died 2 hours or 8 days after the ingestion of large amounts of mercuric chloride (Klenshoj and Rejent, 1966; Steentoft, 1968):

Concentrations in Fatal Inorganic Mercury Poisoning (mg/L or mg/kg)

Period of Survival	Blood	Brain	Liver	Kidney
2 hours	22	3	56	136
8 days	0.8	1.1	33	47

Mercury concentrations in 3 patients, 2 of whom died, suffering from acute mercury vapor poisoning, were 0.4–0.9 mg/L in blood and 0.5–1.6 mg/L in urine (Jaeger et al., 1979). In 5 victims of chronic mercury vapor poisoning who suffered symptoms of nervousness, lassitude, tremor, burning eyes and bleeding gums, blood mercury concentrations ranged from 0.18–0.62 mg/L and urine concentrations, from 2.4–8.3 mg/L (Sexton et al., 1978). Exposure to metallic mercury vapor has produced elevated body burdens in many dental personnel and toxicity in some (Joselow et al., 1968; Cook and Yates, 1969; Buchwald, 1972; Gutenmann et al., 1973; Battistone et al., 1977;

Kelman, 1978). The following mercury concentrations were measured in the tissues of a 3 year old girl who died, 8–9 weeks after playing with elemental mercury, of acrodynia and neutropenia (Johnson et al., 1978):

Concentrations in Fatal Elemental Mercury Poisoning (mg/L or mg/kg)

Brain	Lung	Liver	Kidney	Antemortem Urine
1.3	3.7	3.9	14–30	0.16–0.86

Intoxication by mercury in all its various chemical forms is usually treated by chelation therapy employing BAL, N-acetylpenicillamine or penicillamine; a latent period of days to months before development of symptoms is often noted, especially after exposure to organomercurials (Gerstner and Huff, 1977).

Analysis. Extensive losses of mercury from solutions during several days' storage have been noted, and it was suggested that acidification with nitric acid and prompt analysis be performed to reduce mercury loss (Rosain and Wai, 1973). Numerous procedures for the determination of mercury in biologic specimens have been published, many of which are described in a recent review (Van Ormer, 1975). The somewhat insensitive dithizone colorimetric procedure was once frequently employed (Simonsen, 1953). Atomic absorption spectrometry with the cold vapor technique is highly sensitive and is now used routinely for the determination of total mercury in urine (Richardson, 1976; Gaffin and Hornung, 1977; Sharma and Davis, 1979; Margel and Hirsh, 1984; Ngim et al., 1988) and for the differential analysis of inorganic and organic mercury in various body fluids and tissues (Clarkson et al., 1977; Greenwood et al., 1977; Farant et al., 1981; Chang et al., 1987). Gas chromatographic methods have been developed for inorganic mercury (Luckow and Russel, 1978), methylmercury (Longbottom et al., 1973; Von Burg et al., 1974; Cappon and Smith, 1978; Goolvard and Smith, 1980; Brunmark et al., 1992) and the differential measurement of both the inorganic and organic forms (Cappon and Smith, 1977); these techniques require electron-capture detection and the conversion of inorganic mercury to organic derivatives.

References

B. Aberg, L. Ekman, R. Falk et al. Metabolism of methyl mercury (^{203}Hg) compounds in man. Arch. Env. Health 19: 478–484, 1969.

T. Al-Saleem. Levels of mercury and pathological changes in patients with organomercury poisoning. Bull. W.H.O. 53 (Suppl): 99–104, 1976.

L. Barregard, G. Sallsten, A. Schutz et al. Kinetics of mercury in blood and urine after brief occupational exposure. Arch. Env. Health 47: 176–184, 1992.

H.J. Battista, R. Henn, J. Wilske et al. Mercury intoxications during application of pharmaceutical preparations. In *Forensic Toxicology* (J.S. Oliver, ed.), Croom Helm, London, 1979, pp. 268–271.

G.C. Battistone, J.J. Hefferren, R.A. Miller and D.E. Cutright. Mercury as an occupational hazard in the practice of dentistry. In *Clinical Chemistry and Chemical Toxicology of Metals* (S.S. Brown, ed.), Elsevier/North Holland, New York, 1977, pp. 205–208.

P. Brunmark, G. Skarping and A. Schutz. Determination of methylmercury in human blood using capillary gas chromatography and selected-ion monitoring. J. Chrom. 573: 35–41, 1992.

H. Buchwald. Exposure of dental workers to mercury. Am. Ind. Hyg. Asso. J. 33: 492–502, 1972.

C.J. Cappon and J.C. Smith. Gas-chromatographic determination of inorganic mercury and organomercurials in biological materials. Anal. Chem. 49: 365–369, 1977.

C.J. Cappon and J.C. Smith. A simple and rapid procedure for the gas-chromatographic determination of methylmercury in biological specimens. Bull. Env. Cont. Tox. 19: 600–607, 1978.

S.B. Chang, C. Siew and S.E. Gruninger. Examination of blood levels of mercurials in practicing dentists using cold-vapor atomic absorption spectrometry. J. Anal. Tox. 11: 149–153, 1987.

M.G. Cherian, J.B. Hursh, T.W. Clarkson and J. Allen. Radioactive mercury distribution in biological fluids and excretion in human subjects after inhalation of mercury vapor. Arch. Env. Health 33: 109–114, 1978.

T.W. Clarkson. Mercury poisoning. In *Clinical Chemistry and Chemical Toxicology of Metals* (S.S. Brown, ed.), Elsevier/North Holland, New York, 1977, pp. 189–200.

T.W. Clarkson, M.R. Greenwood and L. Magos. Atomic absorption determination of total, inorganic, and organic mercury in biological fluids. In *Clinical Chemistry and Chemical Toxicology of Metals* (S.S. Brown, ed.), Elsevier/North Holland, New York, 1977, pp. 201–208.

T.A. Cook and P.O. Yates. Fatal mercury intoxication in a dental surgery assistant. Brit. Dent. J. 127: 553–555, 1969.

J.D. Cross, I.M. Dale, H.L. Elliott and H. Smith. Postoperative mercury poisoning. Med. Sci. Law 19: 202–204, 1979.

J.P. Farant, D. Brissette, L. Moncion et al. Improved cold-vapor atomic absorption technique for the microdetermination of total and inorganic mercury in biological samples. J. Anal. Tox. 5: 47–51, 1981.

S.L. Gaffin and H. Hornung. Rapid determination of mercury in urine by flameless atomic absorption spectrometry. Clin. Tox. 10: 345–351, 1977.

H.G. Gerstner and J.E. Huff. Selected case histories and epidemiologic examples of human mercury poisoning. Clin. Tox. 11: 131–150, 1977.

L.J. Goldwater and A. Nicolau. Absorption and excretion of mercury in man. Arch. Env. Health 12: 196–198, 1966.

L. Goolvard and H. Smith. Determination of methylmercury in human blood. Analyst 105: 726–729, 1980.

M.R. Greenwood, P. Dhahir, T.W. Clarkson et al. Epidemiological experience with the Magos' reagents in the determination of different forms of mercury in biological samples by flameless atomic absorption. J. Anal. Tox. 1: 265–269, 1977.

W.H. Gutenmann, J.J. Silvin and D.J. Lisk. Elevated concentrations of mercury in dentists' hair. Bull. Env. Cont. Tox. 9: 318–320, 1973.

A. Jaeger, J.D. Tempe, J.M. Haegy et al. Accidental acute mercury vapor poisoning. Vet. Hum. Tox. 21: 62–63, 1979.

K.G. Johnson, A. Evanger and W. Van Meter. Elemental mercury poisoning manifest by acrodynia and neutropenia. Vet. Hum. Tox. 20: 404–409, 1978.

M.M. Joselow, L.J. Goldwater, A. Alvarez and J. Herndon. Absorption and excretion of mercury in man. XV. Occupational exposure among dentists. Arch. Env. Health 17: 39–43, 1968.

E. Kang-Yum and S.H. Oransky. Chinese patent medicine as a potential source of mercury poisoning. Vet. Hum. Tox. 34: 235–238, 1992.

G.R. Kelman. Urinary mercury excretion in dental personnel. Brit. J. Ind. Med. 35: 262–265, 1978.

N.C. Klendshoj and T.A Rejent. Tissue levels of some poisoning agents less frequently encountered. J. For. Sci. 11: 75–80, 1966.

S. Langworth, C.G. Elinder, C.J. Gothe and O. Vesterberg. Biological monitoring of environmental and occupational exposure to mercury. Int. Arch. Occ. Env. Health 63: 161–167, 1991.

J.E. Longbottom, R.C. Dressman and J.J. Lichtenberg. Gas chromatographic determination of methyl mercury in fish, sediment, and water. J. Asso. Off. Anal. Chem. 56: 1297–1303, 1973.

V. Luckow and H.A. Russel. Gas chromatographic determination of trace amounts of inorganic mercury. J. Chrom. 150: 187–194, 1978.

K.D. Lundgren, A. Swensson and U. Ulfvarson. Studies in humans on the distribution of mercury in the blood and the excretion in urine after exposure to different mercury compounds. Scand. J. Clin. Lab. Invest. 20: 164–166, 1967.

L. Magos, F. Bakir, T.W. Clarkson et al. Tissue levels of mercury in autopsy specimens of liver and kidney. Bull. W.H.O. 53 (Suppl.): 93–97, 1976.

S. Margel and J. Hirsh. Reduction of organic mercury in water, urine, and blood by sodium borohydride for direct determination of total mercury content. Clin. Chem. 30: 243–245, 1984.

E. Nakayama, H. Momotani and S. Ishizu. A pattern of urinary mercury excretion in workers exposed to mercury vapor of relatively low and constant concentration. In *Clinical Chemistry and Chemical Toxicology of Metals* (S.S. Brown, ed.), Elsevier/North Holland, New York, 1977, pp. 209–212.

C.H. Ngim, S.C. Foo and W.O. Phoon. Atomic absorption spectrophotometric microdetermination of total mercury in undigested biological samples. J. Anal. Tox. 12: 132–135, 1988.

Panel on Mercury. *An Assessment of Mercury in the Environment*, National Academy of Sciences, Washington, D.C., 1978.

P.E. Pierce, J.F. Thompson, W.H. Likosky et al. Alkyl mercury poisoning in humans. J. Am. Med. Asso. 220: 1439–1442, 1972.

R.A. Richardson. Automated method for determination of mercury in urine. Clin. Chem. 22: 1604–1607, 1976.

R.M. Rosain and C.M. Wai. The rate of loss of mercury from aqueous solution when stored in various containers. Anal. Chim. Acta 65: 279–284, 1973.

D.J. Sexton, K.E. Powell, J. Liddle et al. A nonoccupational outbreak of inorganic mercury vapor poisoning. Arch. Env. Health 33: 186–191, 1978.

D.C. Sharma and P.S. Davis. Direct determination of mercury in blood by use of sodium borohydride reduction and atomic absorption spectrophotometry. Clin. Chem. 25: 769–772, 1979.

D.G. Simonsen. Determination of mercury in biologic materials. Am. J. Clin. Path. 23: 789–797, 1953.

D.A. Steentoft. Personal communication, 1968.

K. Sumino, K. Hayakawa, T. Shibata and S. Kitamura. Heavy metals in normal Japanese tissues. Arch. Env. Health 30: 487–494, 1975.

D.G. Van Ormer. Atomic absorption analysis of some trace metals of toxicological interest. J. For. Sci. 20: 595–623, 1975.

R. Von Burg, F. Farris and J.C. Smith. Determination of methylmercury in blood by gas chromatography. J. Chrom. 97: 65–70, 1974.

T.F. Yeh, R.S. Pildes, H.V. Firor and P.B. Szanto. Mercury poisoning from mercurochrome therapy of infected omphalocele. Lancet 1: 210,1978.

Mescaline

T½: 6 hr
Vd: ?
Fb: ?
pKa: ?

Occurrence and Usage. Mescaline (3,4,5-trimethoxyphenethylamine) is a hallucinogenic alkaloid first isolated in 1896 from the peyote cactus *(Lophophora williamsii)* of northern Mexico. It is related to the more potent synthetic amphetamine derivatives, methylenedioxyamphetamine and p-methoxyamphetamine, used as street drugs. Mescaline is employed by certain Indian tribes to produce psychedelic experiences during religious rituals, usually in the form of a tea brewed from the cactus button. Gelatin capsules containing powdered cactus buttons, which contain about 6% mescaline and lesser amounts of numerous related alkaloids such as N-acetylmescaline, are infrequently encountered in illicit drug traffic. An oral hallucinogenic dose of mescaline is estimated at 200–500 mg as the hydrochloride or sulfate salt; the effects of a single administration persist for approximately 12 hours.

Blood Concentrations. Blood concentrations of total radioactivity in 12 subjects given a 500 mg labeled dose of mescaline hydrochloride averaged approximately 3.8 mg/L at 2 hours and 1.5 mg/L at 7 hours after ingestion; the half-life was estimated at 6 hours (Charalampous et al., 1966). A 5 mg/kg (350 mg/70 kg) intravenous dose of mescaline sulfate given to 11 subjects produced an average peak blood concentration of 14.8 mg/L at 15 minutes, declining to 4.9 mg/L by 1 hour and 2.1 mg/L by 2 hours; maximal psychological effects occurred at 2 hours and recovery was 80% complete by 9 hours (Mokrasch and Stevenson, 1959).

Metabolism and Excretion. An average of 87% of a labeled oral dose of mescaline is excreted in the 24 hour urine. The urinary excretion products consist of mescaline (55–60%), 3,4,5-trimethoxyphenylacetic acid (27–30%), 3,4,5-trimethoxybenzoic acid (not quantitated), N-acetylmescaline (0.1%), and N-acetyl-3,4-dimethoxy-5-hydroxyphenethylamine (5%). All of the metabolites are believed to be pharmacologically inactive (Charalampous et al., 1964; Charalampous et al., 1966; Demisch et al., 1978).

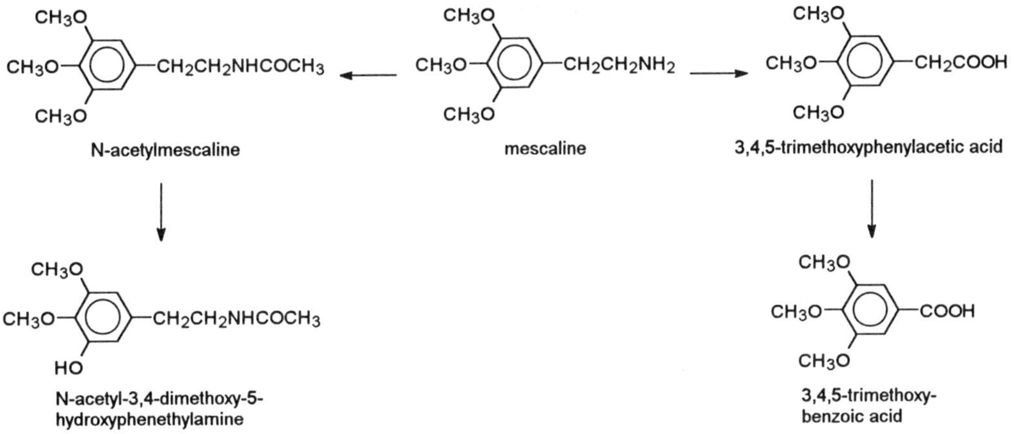

Toxicity. Adverse effects associated with mescaline administration include nausea, vomiting, abdominal cramps, diarrhea, sweating, tremor, anxiety, visual and perceptual distortions, and disturbing hallucinations. The gastrointestinal effects may persist for several days and have been mistaken for acute gastroenteritis (Teitelbaum and Wingeleth, 1977). An adult male who died of head injuries after jumping from a height of 600 feet while under the influence of mescaline was found to have postmortem concentrations of 9.7 mg/L in blood, 71 mg/kg in liver, and 1163 mg/L in urine (Reynolds and Jindrich, 1985).

Analysis. Mescaline in urine has been qualitatively determined by thin-layer chromatography and flame-ionization gas chromatography (Teitelbaum and Wingeleth, 1977). Quantitative analysis of plasma and urine may be accomplished by fluorometry (Cohen and Vogel, 1970) or by gas chromatography/mass spectrometry after trifluoroacetylation (Van Peteghem et al., 1980).

References

K.D. Charalampous, A. Orengo, K.E. Walker and J.K. Wright. Metabolic fate of β–(3,4,5-trimethoxyphenyl)-ethylamine (mescaline) in humans: isolation and identification of 3,4,5-trimethoxyphenylacetic acid. J. Pharm. Exp. Ther. 145: 242–246, 1964.

K.D. Charalampous, K.E. Walker and J. Kinross-Wright. Metabolic fate of mescaline in man. Psychopharmacologia 9: 48–63, 1966.

I. Cohen and W.H. Vogel. An assay procedure for mescaline and its determination in rat brain, liver and plasma. Experientia 26: 1231–1232, 1970.

L. Demisch, P. Kaczmarczyk and N. Seiler. 3,4,5-Trimethoxybenzoic acid, a new mescaline metabolite in humans. Drug Met. Disp. 6: 507–509, 1978.

L.C. Mokrasch and I. Stevenson. The metabolism of mescaline with a note on correlations between metabolism and psychological effects. J. Nerv. Ment. Dis. 129: 177–183, 1959.

P.C. Reynolds and E.J. Jindrich. A mescaline associated fatality. J. Anal. Tox. 9: 183–184, 1985.

D.T. Teitelbaum and D.C. Wingeleth. Diagnosis and management of recreational mescaline self poisoning. J. Anal. Tox. 1: 36–37, 1977.

C. Van Peteghem, A. Heyndrickx and W. Van Zele. GLC-mass spectral determination of mescaline in plasma of rabbits after intravenous injection. J. Pharm. Sci. 69: 118–120, 1980.

Mesoridazine

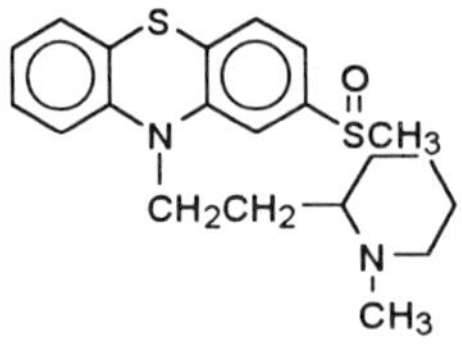

T½: 2–9 hr
Vd: 3–6 L/kg
Fb: ?
pKa: ?

Occurrence and Usage. Mesoridazine (Lidanil, Serentil) is the side-chain sulfoxide of thioridazine and is an active antipsychotic drug in its own right. It was first synthesized in 1963 and has been in clinical use since 1965. The drug is administered either orally or by intramuscular injection as the besylate salt in doses of 50–400 mg per day. It is somewhat more potent than thioridazine and has significant antiemetic activity.

Blood Concentrations. Following a single intramuscular injection of 2 mg/kg (140 mg/70 kg) to normal subjects, plasma concentrations of mesoridazine reached an average peak level of 0.51 mg/L (range, 0.10–1.05) at 4 hours, while the major metabolite, sulforidazine, reached a peak level of 0.31 mg/L (range, 0.10–0.59) at the same time. These concentrations were determined by gas chromatography, and it was found that simultaneous spectrofluorometric analysis yielded apparent mesoridazine concentrations 2–3 times those obtained with the former method (Gottschalk et al., 1976).

Metabolism and Excretion. The metabolism and excretion of mesoridazine have not been more than briefly investigated. The compound is itself a major metabolite of thioridazine, and it may have a number of metabolic products in common with that drug. A major active metabolite of mesoridazine, sulforidazine (mesoridazine side-chain sulfone), is also found after thioridazine administration (Gruenke et al., 1975). Other possible metabolites are the ring sulfoxides of both mesoridazine and sulforidazine and products of N-demethylation. Judging from the disparity between simultaneous gas chromatographic and fluorometric measurements of mesoridazine, metabolites other than sulforidazine accumulate in plasma.

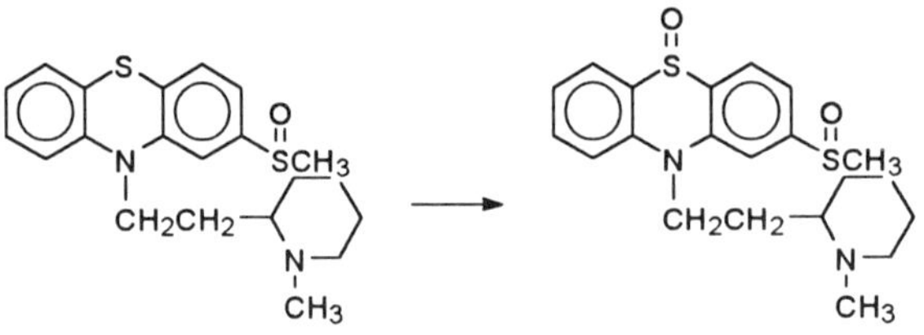

mesoridazine   sulforidazine

Toxicity. An adult ingested 5–10 g of drug and became comatose about 4 hours later with a blood mesoridazine level of 16 mg/L; she died about 6 hours post-ingestion after developing hypotension, a seizure and ventricular fibrillation (Vertrees and Siebel, 1987). As with other phenothiazines, blood or plasma concentrations of mesoridazine in fatal cases may not differ greatly from those observed during high-dose chronic therapy. In 2 cases of death due to ingestion of 2.5 and 8.0 g of the drug, postmortem blood concentrations were 3 and 4 mg/L, respectively; in the first case, a liver concentration of 114 mg/kg and kidney concentration of 17 mg/kg were also determined (Donlon and Tupin, 1977).

Analysis. A popular procedure for the determination of this drug in plasma is the fluorometric technique (Pacha, 1969), although it has the disadvantage of nonspecificity. Methods allowing for the simultaneous analysis of mesoridazine and its major metabolites have employed gas chromatography (Dinovo et al., 1976; Shvartsburd et al., 1984) and liquid chromatography (McKay et al., 1985; Chakraborty et al., 1987).

References

B.S. Chakraborty, E.M. Hawes and K.K. Midha. Development of a radioimmunoassay procedure for mesoridazine and its comparison with a high-performance liquid chromatographic method. Ther. Drug Mon. 9: 464–471, 1987.

E.C. Dinovo, L.A. Gottschalk, B.R. Nandi and P.G. Geddes. GLC analysis of thioridazine, mesoridazine, and their metabolites. J. Pharm. Sci. 65: 667–669, 1976.

P.T. Donlon and J.P. Tupin. Successful suicides with thioridazine and mesoridazine. Arch. Gen. Psych. 34: 955–957, 1977.

L.A. Gottschalk, E. Dinovo, R. Biener et al. Plasma levels of mesoridazine and its metabolites and clinical response in acute schizophrenia after a single intramuscular drug dose. In *Pharmacokinetics of Psychoactive Drugs* (L.A. Gottschalk and S.

Merlis, eds.), Spectrum Publications, New York, 1976, pp. 171–189.

L.D. Gruenke, J.C. Craig, E.C. Dinovo et al. Identification of a metabolite of thioridazine and mesoridazine from human plasma. Res. Comm. Chem. Path. Pharm. 10: 221–225, 1975.

G. McKay, J.K. Cooper, T. Gurnsey and K.K. Midha. A simple, sensitive and simultaneous assay of thioridazine, sulforidazine and mesoridazine in plasma by HPLC. Liq. Chrom. 3: 256–258, 1985.

W.L. Pacha. A method for the fluorimetric determination of thioridazine (Mellaril) or mesoridazine (Lidanil) in plasma. Experientia 25: 103–104, 1969.

A. Shvartsburd, B. Nwokeafor and R.C. Smith. Red blood cell and plasma levels of thioridazine and mesoridazine in schizophrenic patients. Psychopharmacology 82: 55–61, 1984.

J.E. Vertrees and G. Siebel. Rapid death resulting from mesoridazine overdose. Vet. Hum. Tox. 29: 65–67, 1987.

Metaldehyde

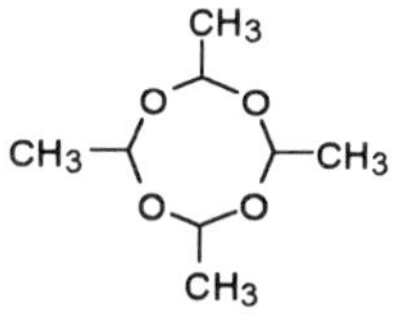

T½: 27 hr
Vd: ?
Fb: ?

Occurrence and Usage. Metaldehyde, a cyclic tetramer of acetaldehyde, is the active ingredient of many of the snail and slug baits used in the United States and Europe. It has also been used as a portable solid fuel. The concentration of metaldehyde is molluscicides in the United States has been limited to less than 4%, but in Europe the concentration may be considerably higher.

Blood Concentrations. Blood concentrations have not been measured in persons occupationally exposed to metaldehyde.

Metabolism and Excretion. The metabolism of metaldehyde in man has not been studied. It is apparently hydrolyzed to acetaldehyde by gastric acidity, but acetaldehyde has not been detected in blood or urine in instances of human poisoning (Dreisbach, 1977; Keller et al., 1991; Moody and Inglis, 1992).

Toxicity. From 1966–1970, the U.S. Environmental Protection Agency's Pesticide Incident Monitoring System recorded 52 case reports of metaldehyde poisoning, 70% of which were in children 5 years old or younger. Toxic symptoms include nausea, vomiting, respiratory distress, decreased blood pressure, rapid pulse, dilated pupils, confusion, convulsions and memory loss. In the case of a 32 year old woman who swallowed 16 ounces of slug bait (18.9 g metaldehyde) in a suicide attempt, coma persisted for 7 days and mental status improved very slowly; she was discharged from hospital after 51 days with memory still impaired (Longstreth and Pierson, 1982). An adult male presented in coma after ingesting 7–10 g of metaldehyde, but recovered with treatment; his serum metaldehyde concentration peaked 11 hours post-admission at 125 mg/L and declined with a half-life of 27 hours (Moody and Inglis, 1992). Another adult male ingested approximately 19 g of metaldehyde and presented with coma and seizures 10 hours later; at 16 hours post-ingestion, serum and urine metaldehyde levels were 10 and 30 mg/L, respectively (Keller et al., 1991).

A 2.5 year old boy ingested a solid fuel tablet containing metaldehyde and died 33 hours later after exhibiting convulsive seizures, vomiting, hyperpyrexia, tachycardia and coma (Lewis et al., 1939).

Analysis. Gas chromatography with flame-ionization detection has been used to measure metaldehyde both before (Booze and Oehme, 1985) and after conversion to acetaldehyde (Griffiths, 1984).

References

T.F. Booze and F.W. Oehme. Gas chromatographic analysis of metaldehyde in urine and plasma. J. Anal. Tox. 9: 172–173, 1985.

R.H. Dreisbach. *Handbook of Poisoning*, 9th ed. Lange Medical Publications, Los Altos, California, 1977, pp. 173–177.

C.J. Griffiths. The determination of metaldehyde in biological material by head-space chromatography. J. Chrom. 295: 240–247, 1984.

K.H. Keller, G. Shimizu, F.G. Walter and K.R. Olson. Acetaldehyde analysis in severe metaldehyde poisoning. Vet. Hum. Tox. 33: 374, 1991.

D.R. Lewis, G.A. Madel and J. Drury. Fatal poisoning by "meta fuel" tablets. Brit. Med. J. 1: 1283–1284, 1939.

W.T. Longstreth and D.J. Pierson. Metaldehyde poisoning from slug bait ingestion. West. J. Med. 137: 134–137, 1982.

J.P. Moody and F.G. Inglis. Persistence of metaldehyde during acute molluscicide poisoning. Hum. Exp. Tox. 11: 361–362, 1992.

D.P. Stubbings, A.B. Edginton, D.G. Lyon et al. Three cases of metaldehyde poisoning in cattle. Vet. Rec. 98: 356–357, 1976.

Metformin

T½: 4–8 hr
Vd: 3.7 L/kg
Fb: 0
pKa: 11.5

$$(CH_3)_2NCNHCNH_2$$
$$\overset{NH}{\|} \quad \overset{NH}{\|}$$

Occurrence and Usage. Metformin (1,1-dimethylbiguanide, Glucophage) is an oral hypoglycemic agent that has been in clinical use in Europe since 1970 in the treatment of maturity-onset diabetes. It is chemically related to buformin and phenformin, the latter drug having been removed from the United States market in 1977 due to its propensity for causing severe lactic acidosis. Daily oral doses of metformin, as the hydrochloride, range from 500–2500 mg.

Blood Concentrations. Five subjects administered a single oral 500 mg dose of metformin achieved peak plasma concentrations of 1.0–2.3 mg/L (average, 1.6) at 1–3 hours (Pentikainen et al., 1979). An average peak plasma concentration of 3.1 mg/L (range, 1.8–4.0) was achieved at 1.5 hours by 4 subjects given a 1500 mg oral dose; the elimination half-life averaged 6.0 hours and the drug was 50–60% bioavailable. The peak drug concentrations did not increase in persons taking the drug chronically, but there was a slow rise in trough levels indicative of drug accumulation in tissues (Tucker et al., 1981).

Metabolism and Excretion. Metformin is not believed to be metabolized in man. An average of 50% of a single oral dose is eliminated in the 5 day urine, with 27% appearing in the feces as unabsorbed drug. Urine metformin concentrations in patients on therapy range up to 1600 mg/L (Charles et al., 1981; Tucker et al., 1981).

Toxicity. Plasma metformin concentrations in 3 patients who developed lactic acidosis due to drug accumulation, secondary to renal failure, while on chronic therapy ranged from 45–70 mg/L. Treatment involved reversal of acidosis, forced diuresis, and hemodialysis.

An adult ingested 24 g of metformin in a suicide attempt and developed coma, metabolic acidosis, and a plasma metformin level of 110 mg/L; he died approximately 40 hours after ingestion (Assan et al., 1977). A similar situation involved the ingestion of 25.5 g of drug; the patient achieved plasma and urine concentrations of 85 and 389 mg/L, respectively, 12 hours after ingestion, and died 2 weeks later (Larcan et al., 1979).

Analysis. Metformin may be assayed in plasma at toxic levels using the colorimetric method cited in the section on phenformin. More sensitive and specific techniques have been developed using gas chromatography with nitrogen-phosphorus (Brohon and Noel, 1978) or electron-capture detection (Lennard et al., 1978) and high-pressure liquid chromatography (Ross, 1977; Charles et al., 1981; Keal and Somogyi, 1986; Huupponen et al., 1992).

References

A. Assan, C. Heuelin, D. Ganeval et al. Metformin-induced lactic acidosis in the presence of acute renal failure. Diabetologia 13: 211–217, 1977.

J. Brohon and M. Noel. Determination of metformin in plasma at therapeutic levels by gas-liquid chromatography using a nitrogen detector. J. Chrom. 146: 148–151, 1978.

B.G. Charles, N.W. Jacobsen and P.J. Ravenscroft. Rapid liquid-chromatographic determination of metformin in plasma and urine. Clin. Chem. 27: 434–436, 1981.

R. Huupponen, P. Ojala-Karlsson, J. Rouru and M. Koulu. Determination of metformin in plasma by high-performance liquid chromatography. J. Chrom. 583: 270–273, 1992.

J. Keal and A. Somogyi. Rapid and sensitive high-performance liquid chromatographic assay for metformin in plasma and urine using ion-pair extraction techniques. J. Chrom. 378: 503–508, 1986.

A. Larcan, H. Lambert and F. Ginsbourger. Acute intoxication by phenformine hyperlactatemia reversible with extra-renal purification. Vet. Hum. Tox. 21 (Suppl.): 19–22, 1979.

M.S. Lennard, C. Casey, G.T. Tucker and H.F. Woods. Determination of metformin in biological samples. Brit. J. Clin. Pharm. 6: 183–185, 1978.

P.J. Pentikainen, P.J. Neuvonen and A. Penttila. Pharmacokinetics of metformin after intravenous and oral administration to man. Eur. J. Clin. Pharm. 16: 195–202, 1979.

M.S.F. Ross. Determination of metformin in biological fluids by derivatization followed by high-performance liquid chromatography. J. Chrom. 133: 408–411, 1977.

G.T. Tucker, C. Casey, P.J. Phillips et al. Metformin kinetics in healthy subjects and in patients with diabetes mellitus. Brit. J. Clin. Pharm. 12: 235–246, 1981.

Methadone

T½: 15–55 hr
Vd: 4–5 L/kg
Fb: 0.87
pKa: 8.6

$$C_2H_5COCCH_2CHN(CH_3)_2$$

with CH$_3$ group

Occurrence and Usage. Methadone (Dolophine) was first synthesized as a morphine substitute in Germany during World War II and was made clinically available in the United States in 1947. It possesses many of the pharmacologic properties of morphine and is approximately equipotent as an analgesic when administered parenterally. Unlike morphine, however, methadone produces marked sedative effects with repeated administration as a result of drug accumulation. This undesirable property restricted clinical usage of the drug until 1965 when Dole and Nyswander began narcotic maintenance treatment of former heroin addicts using large daily oral doses of dl-methadone. Whereas maintenance patients may receive as much as 180 mg of the drug daily, doses of 50 mg or less have been known to prove fatal to nontolerant adults. The drug is available commercially as a hydrochloride salt of the racemic mixture, in tablets of 5–10 mg or diskets of 40 mg for oral usage and a 10 mg/mL solution for parenteral injection. The pharmacologic activity is due almost entirely to the l-isomer. The d-methadone isomer does have analgesic properties in large doses and this may be due to its conversion to minor amounts of alpha-l-methadone and alpha-l-normethadol, both of which are potent analgesics (Sullivan et al., 1972b).

Blood Concentrations. Plasma methadone concentrations reached an average peak of 0.034 mg/L at 50 minutes after a 10 mg intramuscular injection into the gluteal region, and an average peak of 0.096 mg/L at 34 minutes after injection of the same dose into the deltoid region (Grabinski et al., 1983). Following a single 15 mg oral dose, plasma concentrations of methadone reached a peak at 4 hours of 0.075 mg/L and declined slowly (plasma half-life of 15 hours) until 24 hours after administration when the concentration was still 0.030 mg/L; pupillary constriction coincided closely with the plasma concentration of methadone (Inturrisi and Verebely, 1972c). A single 10 mg intravenous dose produced plasma concentrations that were initially as high as 0.50 mg/L, but declined rapidly to 0.04–0.05 mg/L after 1–2 hours (Inturrisi et al., 1987).

With chronic administration of 100–200 mg daily oral doses of the drug to tolerant subjects, the plasma concentration again peaked at 4 hours, with an average value of 0.83 mg/L (range, 0.57–1.06), and declined to 0.46 mg/L (range, 0.28–0.79) 24 hours after the last dose (average plasma half-life of 25 hours) (Inturrisi and Verebely, 1972b). The plasma half-life averaged 20 hours in 5 subjects during conditions of acid urine, and 42 hours in the same subjects when the urine was maintained alkaline (Nilsson et al., 1982). Plasma methadone concentrations in maintenance patients increased by an average of 0.263 mg/L for every 1 mg/kg increase in oral dosage (Wolff et al., 1991). Omission of a single daily dose during chronic maintenance therapy with methadone has been found to cause a 50% reduction in the average preomission plasma concentration (Verebely and Kutt, 1975). It has been estimated that trough plasma methadone levels should be at least 0.05–0.10 mg/L to prevent withdrawal symptoms in narcotic maintenance patients (Bell et al., 1988; Wolff et al., 1992). The average blood/plasma ratio for methadone is 0.75 (Inturrisi et al., 1987).

Metabolism and Excretion. Methadone is metabolized largely by mono- and di-N-demethylation, with spontaneous cyclization of the resulting unstable metabolites to form 2-ethylidene-1,5-dimethyl-3,3-diphenylpyrrolidine (EDDP) and 2-ethyl-5-methyl-3,3-diphenylpyrroline (EMDP) (Pohland et al., 1971). All 3 compounds are hydroxylated to a minor extent in the para-position of one of the phenyl rings, with subsequent glucuronide conjugation (Sullivan et al., 1972a; Baselt and Bickel, 1973). Aside from the small amounts of methadol and normethadol that are produced, none of the metabolites of methadone has any apparent pharmacologic activity and none is found to any significant extent in plasma during therapeutic usage. The major urinary excretion products are methadone, EDDP and EMDP. The importance of the hydroxylated and conjugated derivatives in urine has not been quantitatively established in man.

Following a 5 mg oral dose, methadone and EDDP each accounted for 5% of the dose in the 24 hour urine, with less than 1% as EMDP. Acidification of the urine resulted in excretion of 22% of the dose as unchanged methadone and only 2% as EDDP. In maintenance subjects, 24 hour urinary methadone may account for 5–50% of the dose and EDDP for 3–25%, with large individual variations due to urine pH, urine volume, dose and rate of metabolism. Urinary concentrations of methadone and EDDP in these subjects ranging from 1–50 mg/L are commonly encountered (Baselt and Casarett, 1972; Bellward et al., 1977).

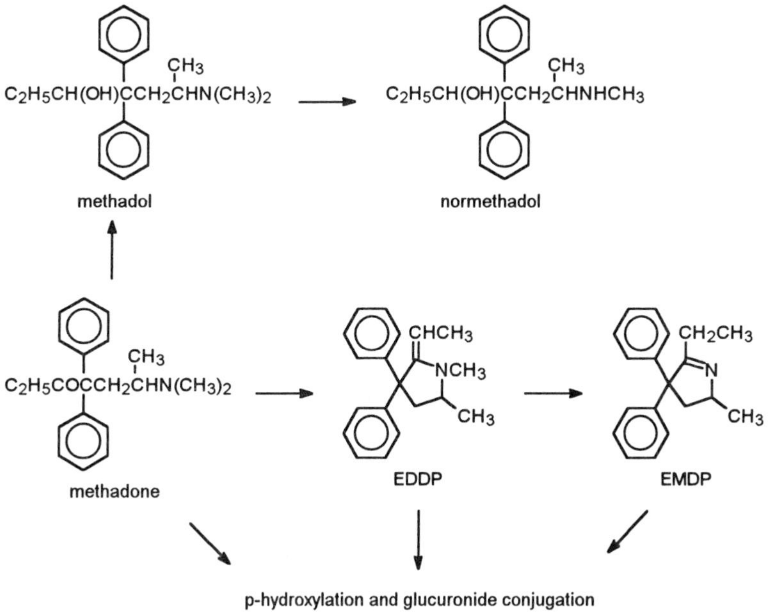

p-hydroxylation and glucuronide conjugation

Toxicity. Methadone maintenance patients receiving 60–100 mg of the drug daily did not exhibit impairment in the performance of complex tasks (Moskowitz and Robinson, 1985). Overdosage with methadone is characterized by stupor, muscle flaccidity, respiratory depression, cold and clammy skin, pupillary constriction, hypotension, coma, and circulatory collapse. Naloxone is considered a specific antidote. The deaths of 4 children were reported following accidental ingestion of methadone; postmortem blood methadone concentrations ranged from 0.06–1.1 mg/L (Smialek et al., 1977).

Fatalities in adults from methadone overdosage have increased significantly in many urban areas as a result of widespread availability of the drug, both from licit and illicit sources (Segal and Catherman, 1974). In one study, most of the deaths were found to have occurred following oral administration of the drug, and lack of opiate tolerance was considered to play a major role (Greene et al., 1974). In a series of 10 fatal cases attributed to methadone, it was found that liver was the tissue with the highest concentration of those studied and that blood and brain were usually comparable in methadone content (Manning et al., 1976):

Methadone Concentrations in Fatalities (mg/L or mg/kg)

	Blood	Brain	Liver	Bile	Kidney
Average	1.0	1.0	3.8	7.5	2.9
(Range)	(0.4–1.8)	(0.5–1.4)	(1.8–7.5)	(2.9–18.0)	(1.1–6.0)

The span of blood concentrations of victims of methadone overdosage overlaps that of methadone maintenance subjects and it is difficult, if not impossible, to distinguish between the two on this basis alone. In some cases it may be useful to quantitate EDDP concentrations, as the presence of the metabolite in substantial amounts may indicate prior usage of the drug and therefore tolerance to its effects, although the relative amounts of methadone and EDDP in the organs would of course depend as well on survival time after administration (Robinson and Williams, 1971; Garriott et al., 1973). Blood methadone concentrations averaged 0.28 mg/L (range, 0.06–3.1) in 59 victims of fatal methadone overdosage; in comparison, blood levels averaged 0.11 mg/L (range, 0.03–0.56) in 62 methadone maintenance subjects included as controls (Worm et al., 1993).

Analysis. Gas chromatography with flame-ionization detection is the most popular means for the determination of methadone in biological samples; EDDP and EMDP can be included in most schemes without derivatization, and SKF-525A is often used as internal standard (Inturrisi and Verebely, 1972a; Sullivan and Blake, 1972; Lynn et al., 1977; Thompson and Caplan, 1977; Greizerstein and McLaughlin, 1983). Electron-capture detection following oxidation of the drug to benzophenone has also been utilized (Hartvig and Naslund, 1975), and several methods involving gas chromatography/mass spectrometry have appeared (Sullivan et al., 1975; Hachey et al., 1977; Kang and Abbott, 1982; Baugh et al., 1991). Liquid chromatographic methods have also been reported (Rio et al., 1987; Wolff et al., 1991). Urine screening procedures based on enzyme immunoassay or radioimmunoassay are commercially available; diphenhydramine and doxylamine have been found to cause false positive results with enzyme immunoassay for methadone (Hausmann et al., 1983; Kelner, 1984).

References

R.C. Baselt and M.H. Bickel. Biliary excretion of methadone by the rat: identification of a para-hydroxylated major metabolite. Biochem. Pharm. 22: 3117–3120, 1973.

R.C. Baselt and L.J. Casarett. Urinary excretion of methadone in man. Clin. Pharm. Ther. 13: 64–70, 1972.

E.D. Baugh, R.H. Liu and A.S. Walia. Simultaneous gas chromatography-mass spectrometry assay of methadone and 2-ethyl-1,5-dimethyl-3,3-diphenylpyrrolidine (EDDP) in urine. J. For. Sci. 36: 548–555, 1991.

J. Bell, V. Seres, P. Bowdron et al. The use of serum methadone levels in patients receiving methadone maintenance. Clin. Pharm. Ther. 43: 623–629, 1988.

G.D. Bellward, P.M. Warren, W. Howald and J.E. Axelson. Methadone maintenance: effect of urinary pH on renal clearance in chronic high and low doses. Clin. Pharm. Ther. 22: 92–99, 1977.

J.C. Garriott, W.Q. Sturner and M.F. Mason. Toxicologic findings in six fatalities involving methadone. Clin. Tox. 6: 163–173, 1973.

P.Y. Grabinski, R.F. Kaiko, A.G. Rogers and R.W. Houde. Plasma levels and analgesia following deltoid and gluteal injections of methadone and morphine. J. Clin. Pharm. 23: 48–55, 1983.

M.H. Greene, J.L. Luke and R.L. DuPont. Opiate overdose deaths in the District of Columbia. Part II. Methadone-related fatalities. J. For. Sci. 19: 575–584, 1974.

H.B. Greizerstein and I.G. McLaughlin. Sensitive method for the determination of methadone in small blood samples. J. Chrom. 264: 312–315, 1983.

D.L. Hachey, M.J. Kreek and D.H. Mattson. Quantitative analysis of methadone in biological fluids using deuterium-labeled methadone and GLC-chemical-ionization mass spectrometry. J. Pharm. Sci. 66: 1579–1582, 1977.

P. Hartvig and B. Naslund. Electron-capture gas chromatography of methadone after oxidation to benzophenone. J. Chrom. 111: 347–354, 1975.

H.A. Hausmann, V. Kohl, H. von Boehmer and H.H. Wellhoner. False-positive EMIT indication of opiates and methadone in a doxylamine intoxication. J. Clin. Chem. Clin. Biochem. 21: 599–600, 1983.

C. Inturrisi and K. Verebely. A gas-liquid chromatographic method for the quantitative determination of methadone in human plasma and urine. J. Chrom. 65: 361–369, 1972a.

C.E. Inturrisi and K. Verebely. The levels of methadone in the plasma in methadone maintenance. Clin. Pharm. Ther. 13: 633–637, 1972b.

C.E. Inturrisi and K. Verebely. Disposition of methadone in man after a single oral dose. Clin. Pharm. Ther. 13: 923–930, 1972c.

C.E. Inturrisi, W.A. Colburn, R.F. Kaiko et al. Pharmacokinetics and pharmacodynamics of methadone in patients with chronic pain. Clin. Pharm. Ther. 41: 392–401, 1987.

G.I. Kang and F.S. Abbott. Analysis of methadone and metabolites in biological fluids with gas chromatography-mass spectrometry. J. Chrom. 231: 311–319, 1982.

M.J. Kelner. Positive diphenhydramine interference in the EMIT-d.a.u. assay. Clin. Chem. 30: 1430, 1984.

R.K. Lynn, R.M. Leger, W.P. Gordon et al. New gas chromatographic assay for the quantitation of methadone. Application in human and animal studies. J. Chrom. 131: 329–340, 1977.

T. Manning, J.H. Bidanset, S. Cohen et al. Evaluation of the Abuscreen for methadone. J. For. Sci. 21: 112–120, 1976.

H. Moskowitz and C.D. Robinson. Methadone maintenance and tracking performance. In *Alcohol, Drugs and Traffic Safety* (S. Kaye and G.W. Meier, eds.), University of Puerto Rico, 1985, pp. 995–1004.

M.I. Nilsson, E. Widerlov, U. Meresaar and E. Anggard. Effect of urinary pH on the disposition of methadone in man. Eur. J. Clin. Pharm. 22: 337–342, 1982.

A. Pohland, H.E. Boaz and H.R. Sullivan. Synthesis and identification of metabolites resulting from the biotransformation of dl-methadone in man and the rat. J. Med. Chem. 14: 194–197, 1971.

J. Rio, N. Hodnett and J.H. Bidanset. The determination of propoxyphene, norpropoxyphene and methadone in post-mortem blood and tissues by high-performance liquid chromatography. J. Anal. Tox. 11: 222–224, 1987.

A.E. Robinson and F.M. Williams. The distribution of methadone in man. J. Pharm. Pharmac. 23: 353–358, 1971.

R.J. Segal and R.L. Catherman. Methadone—a cause of death. J. For. Sci. 19: 64–71, 1974.

J.E. Smialek, J.R. Monforte, R. Aronow and W.U. Spitz. Methadone deaths in children. J. Am. Med. Asso. 238: 2516–2517. 1977.

H.R. Sullivan, S.L. Due and R.E. McMahon. The identification of three new metabolites of methadone in man and in the rat. J. Am. Chem. Soc. 94: 4050–4051, 1972a.

H.R. Sullivan, S.E. Smits, S.L. Due et al. Metabolism of d-methadone: isolation and identification of analgesically active metabolites. Life. Sci. 11: 1093–1104, 1972b.

H.R. Sullivan and D.A. Blake. Quantitative determination of methadone concentrations in human blood, plasma and urine by gas chromatography. Res. Comm. Chem. Path. Pharm. 3: 467–478, 1972.

H.R. Sullivan, F.J. Marshall, R.E. McMahon et al. Mass fragmentographic determination of unlabeled and deuterium labeled methadone in human plasma. Possibilities for measurement of steady state pharmacokinetics. Biomed. Mass Spec. 2: 179–200, 1975.

B.C. Thompson and Y.H. Caplan. A gas chromatographic method for the determination of methadone and its metabolites in biological fluids and tissues. J. Anal. Tox. 1: 66–69, 1977.

K. Verebely and H. Kutt. Methadone plasma levels in maintenance patients: the effect of dose omission. Res. Comm. Chem. Path. Pharm. 11: 373–386, 1975.

K. Wolff, M. Sanderson, A.W.M. Hay and D. Raistrick. Methadone concentrations in plasma and their relationship to drug dosage. Clin. Chem. 37: 205–209, 1991.

K. Wolff, A.W.M. Hay and D. Raistrick. Plasma methadone measurements and their role in methadone detoxification programs. Clin. Chem. 38: 420–425, 1992.

K. Worm, A. Steentoft and B. Kringsholm. Methadone and drug addicts. Int. J. Leg. Med. 106: 119–123, 1993.

d-Methamphetamine

T½: 6–15 hr (urine pH-dependent)
Vd: 3.0–7.0 L/kg
Fb: 0.10–0.20
pKa: 9.9

$$\text{C}_6\text{H}_5-\text{CH}_2\text{CHNHCH}_3 \quad (\text{CH}_3)$$

Occurrence and Usage. d-Methamphetamine (d-desoxyephedrine, Desoxyn, Methedrine), the N-methyl derivative of amphetamine, was first prepared in 1919. As the hydrochloride salt, it is utilized in the treatment of obesity in single oral doses of 2.5–15 mg. The l-isomer, covered in a separate section, is used in certain non-prescription inhalers as a decongestant. d-Methamphetamine has received a great deal of attention as a drug of abuse in past years and at one time was available by prescription as an injectable solution in ampule form. It is now available as conventional tablets of 2.5–5 mg and prolonged-release tablets of 5–15 mg for oral use. Illicit methamphetamine is readily synthesized from phenylacetone and N-methylformamide (dl-mixture), or from ephedrine using red phosphorus/hydriodic acid reduction (d-isomer). d-Methamphetamine is also formed as a metabolite of benzphetamine and famprofazone.

Blood Concentrations. A single oral methamphetamine dose of 0.125 mg/kg (8.75 mg/70 kg) given to 6 adults produced an average peak plasma concentration of 0.020 mg/L at 3.6 hours. The plasma elimination half-life averaged 10 hours (range, 6–15) for 24 subjects (Cook et al., 1992). A maximal blood concentration of 0.03 mg/L was observed at 1 hour after a single oral dose of 10 mg of methamphetamine in a volunteer (Lebish et al., 1970). A 12.5 mg oral dose given to 10 subjects resulted in an average peak blood level of 0.020 mg/L at 2.5 hours, declining to 0.016 mg/L by 6 hours and 0.010 mg/L by 24 hours (Driscoll et al., 1971). A blood/plasma concentration ratio of 0.65 was noted in an overdose case (Katsumata et al., 1993).

Metabolism and Excretion. Methamphetamine undergoes some N-demethylation to amphetamine, its major active metabolite. During normal conditions up to 43% of a dose is eliminated unchanged in the 24 hour urine, with about 4–7% as amphetamine. In acid urine, up to 76% is found as unchanged drug and 7% as amphetamine in 24 hours, whereas in alkaline urine the corresponding values are 2% and less than 0.1% (Beckett and Rowland, 1965). About 15% is excreted as p-hydroxymethamphetamine and the remainder of the dose is accounted for as minor amounts of the same metabolites found after amphetamine administration (Caldwell et al., 1972). Methamphetamine urine concentrations of 0.5–4.0 mg/L are commonly observed during the first 24 hours after ingestion of 10 mg. Methamphetamine concentrations of 24–333 mg/L (average, 142) and amphetamine concentrations of 1–90 mg/L (average, 18) were observed in the urine of methamphetamine abusers (Lebish et al., 1970). Concentrations of total (free plus conjugated) p-hydroxymethamphetamine and p-hydroxyamphetamine in the urine of another group of abusers were less than 10 mg/L and less than 0.5 mg/L, respectively (Shimosato et al., 1986).

deamination, p-hydroxylation and conjugation

Toxicity. Methamphetamine in overdosage causes restlessness, confusion, anxiety, hallucinations, cardiac arrhythmias, hypertension, hyperthermia, circulatory collapse, convulsions, and coma. Chronic abusers may develop paranoid psychosis. Concentrations of 0.15–0.56 mg/L were detected in the blood of 7 methamphetamine abusers who exhibited violent and irrational behavior; amphetamine, if present, was below the 0.01 mg/L limit of detectability (Lebish et al., 1970). Two women found by police asleep in a car had blood methamphetamine concentrations of 1.7 and 2.1 mg/L, as well as substantial levels of diazepam (Weingarten, 1984). Methamphetamine blood concentrations of 1.4–13 mg/L (average, 5.1) were found postmortem in 9 drug abusers who died of traumatic injury by violent means (Reynolds and Weingarten, 1983).

Methamphetamine has been implicated in fatal poisonings following both intravenous and oral administration. In 4 cases of death after intravenous injection of the drug, blood methamphetamine concentrations ranged as high as 0.8 mg/L (Cravey and Reed, 1970; Kojima et al., 1983). A case of oral administration of 140 mg was reported in which a blood concentration of 1.33 mg/L was apparent 48 hours after ingestion, with a decline to 0.98 mg/L by 96 hours and death at 120 hours

(Zalis and Parmley, 1963). Methamphetamine concentrations of 4.3 and 5.6 mg/L in blood and 28 and 320 mg/L in urine were measured postmortem in 2 cases of death by oral ingestion of the drug (Patterson and Peat, 1976; Kojima et al., 1984). Concentrations of 40 mg/L in blood and 206 mg/kg in liver were observed in a youth who developed hyperpyrexia and died 5.5 hours after ingestion of a large amount of methamphetamine (Cravey and Baselt, 1968). The following concentrations were measured in a woman who died after nasal insufflation of methamphetamine (Baselt, 1986):

Drug Concentrations in a Methamphetamine Fatality (mg/L or mg/kg)

Drug	Blood	Liver	Urine	Gastric
Methamphetamine	2.0	4.8	28	1.5 mg
Amphetamine	0.3	0.7	2.7	0.1 mg

Analysis. Commercial immunoassays for the amphetamines exhibit variable cross-reactivity with methamphetamine, but those designed especially for methamphetamine are relatively specific for d-methamphetamine. The gas chromatographic techniques cited for amphetamine are applicable for the most part to the simultaneous assay of methamphetamine and amphetamine. Methods capable of differentiating the isomeric forms of methamphetamine are described in the section on l-methamphetamine. Certain gas chromatographic-mass spectrometric schemes for methamphetamine employing derivatization may yield false positive results when high concentrations of ephedrine or pseudoephedrine are present in the specimen (Wu et al., 1992; Hornbeck et al., 1993).

References

R.C. Baselt. Unpublished results, 1986.

A.H. Beckett and M. Rowland. Urinary excretion kinetics of methylamphetamine in man. J. Pharm. Pharmac. 17: 109S–114S, 1965.

J. Caldwell, L.G. Dring and R.T. Williams. Metabolism of (^{14}C) methamphetamine in man, the guinea pig and the rat. Biochem. J. 129: 11–22, 1972.

C.E. Cook, A.R. Jeffcoat, B.M. Sadler et al. Pharmacokinetics of oral methamphetamine and effects of repeated daily dosing in humans. Drug Met. Disp. 20: 856–862, 1992.

R.H. Cravey and R.C. Baselt. Methamphetamine poisoning. J. For. Sci. Soc. 8: 118–120, 1968.

R.H. Cravey and D. Reed. Intravenous amphetamine poisoning: report of three cases. J. For. Sci. Soc. 10: 109–112, 1970.

R.C. Driscoll, F.S. Barr, B.J. Gragg and G.W. Moore. Determination of therapeutic blood levels of methamphetamine and pentobarbital by GC. J. Pharm. Sci. 60: 1492–1495, 1971.

C.L. Hornbeck, J.E. Carrig and R.J. Czarny. Detection of GC/MS artifact peak as methamphetamine. J. Anal. Tox. 17: 257–263, 1993.

S. Katsumata, K. Sato, H. Kashiwade et al. Sudden death due presumably to internal use of methamphetamine. For. Sci. Int. 62: 209–215, 1993.

T. Kojima, I. Une and M. Yashiki. CI-Mass fragmentographic analysis of methamphetamine and amphetamine in human autopsy tissues after acute methamphetamine poisoning. For. Sci. Int. 21: 253–258, 1983.

T. Kojima, I. Une, M. Yashiki, J. Noda et al. A fatal methamphetamine poisoning associated with hyperpyrexia. For. Sci. Int. 24: 87–93, 1984.

P. Lebish, B.S. Finkle and J.W. Brackett, Jr. Determination of amphetamine, methamphetamine, and related amines in blood and urine by gas chromatography with hydrogen-flame ionization detector. Clin. Chem. 16: 195–200, 1970.

S. Patterson and M.A. Peat. Personal communication, 1976.

P.C. Reynolds and H. Weingarten. Presented at the quarterly meeting of the California Association of Toxicologists, Yosemite National Park, California, November 5, 1983.

K. Shimosato, M. Tomita and I. Ijiri. Urinary examination of p-hydroxylated methamphetamine metabolites in man. Arch. Tox. 59: 135–140, 1986.

H. Weingarten. Presented at the quarterly meeting of the California Association of Toxicologists, San Francisco, August 4, 1984.

A.H.B. Wu, S.S. Wong, K.G. Johnson et al. The conversion of ephedrine to methamphetamine and metham-
    phetamine-like compounds during and prior to gas chromatographic/mass spectrometric analysis of CB and
    HFB derivatives. Biol. Mass Spec. 21: 278–284, 1992.
E.G. Zalis and L.F. Parmley, Jr. Fatal amphetamine poisoning. Arch. Int. Med. 112: 822–826, 1963.

l-Methamphetamine

T½: ?
Vd: ?
Fb: ?
pKa: 9.9

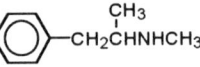

Occurrence and Usage. l-Methamphetamine (l-desoxyephedrine, ingredient of Vicks Inhaler), reported to have weaker central stimulant action and greater peripheral sympathomimetic activity than the d-isomer, has been employed for many years as a nasal decongestant in certain nonprescription inhalers. Currently, such inhalers contain 50 mg of the free base within a plastic cylinder; the user is directed to inhale twice through each nostril every 2 hours as needed for up to 7 days. Abusers of the drug have been known to remove the contents of the inhaler in preparation for oral or intravenous administration. l-Methamphetamine is also formed as a metabolite of selegiline.

Blood Concentrations. l-Methamphetamine concentrations in blood or plasma following therapeutic administration have not been reported.

Metabolism and Excretion. l-Methamphetamine is believed to follow generally the same biotransformation pathways as the d-isomer, but at a slower rate. Following a 13.7 mg oral dose, the 24 hour urine contained an average of 34% and 1.7% of the dose as l-methamphetamine and l-amphetamine, respectively, whereas corresponding figures for the d-isomer were 20% and 4.9% (Beckett and Rowland, 1965). l-Amphetamine is also metabolized at a slower rate than its corresponding d-isomer, having an average elimination half-life of 19 hours versus 13 hours for d-amphetamine (Wan et al., 1978).

    Three subjects who used Vicks Inhalers every 20 minutes for 6 hours developed peak urinary l-methamphetamine and l-amphetamine concentrations of 1.5–6.0 mg/L and 0.25–0.46 mg/L, respectively, within 24 hours of beginning the use (Fitzgerald et al., 1988).

Toxicity. A 13.7 mg oral dose of l-methamphetamine given to 3 male volunteers did not produce any observable central nervous system effects (Beckett and Rowland, 1965), yet a 30 mg dose was reported to have caused agitation, muscle fasciculations, irregular pulse and respiration, delerium, hallucinations and periods of unconsciousness in a patient (Haley, 1947).

    The intraperitoneal LD50 for l-methamphetamine in mice is 82 mg/kg, only slightly higher than the 70 mg/kg value for the d-isomer (Christensen, 1974). A 41 year old male observed shoplifting a quantity of nasal inhalers was chased and apprehended by witnesses, but he suffered a cardiorespiratory arrest during the struggle; he was pronounced dead shortly thereafter, and postmortem blood and urine specimens contained 0.50 and 13 mg/L l-methamphetamine, respectively (Leis, 1991).

Analysis. Most immunoassays for amphetamine or methamphetamine show some cross-reactivity with l-methamphetamine (Fitzgerald et al., 1988; Poklis et al., 1993). Methods capable of distinguishing the optical isomers have included gas chromatography-mass spectrometry (Czarny and Hornbeck, 1989; Hughes et al., 1991; Cody, 1992; Cooke, 1994) and liquid chromatography (Nagai and Kamiyama, 1991; Cody, 1992). Urine testing results showing only the presence of l-methamphetamine are consistent with use of Vicks Inhaler, while those showing only d-methamphetamine would indicate either prescription methamphetamine use or abuse of illicit drug prepared by reduction of l-ephedrine or d-pseudoephedrine; the presence of the racemate in urine would be consistent with abuse of illicit drug synthesized from phenyl-2-propanone (Fitzgerald et al., 1988; Cody and Schwarzhoff, 1993; Hornbeck and Czarny, 1993).

References

A.H. Beckett and M. Rowland. Urinary excretion kinetics of methylamphetamine in man. J. Pharm. Pharmac. 17 (Suppl.): 109–114, 1965.

H.E. Christensen (ed). *The Toxic Substances List*, National Institute for Occupational Safety and Health, Rockville, Maryland, 1974, p. 573.

J.T. Cody. Determination of methamphetamine enantiomer ratios in urine by gas chromatography-mass spectrometry. J. Chrom. 580: 77–95, 1992.

J.T. Cody and R. Schwarzhoff. Interpretation of methamphetamine and amphetamine enantiomer data. J. Anal. Tox. 17: 321–326, 1993.

B.J.A. Cooke. Chirality of methamphetamine and amphetamine from workplace urine samples. J. Anal. Tox. 18: 49–51, 1994.

R.J. Czarny and C.L. Hornbeck. Quantitation of methamphetamine and amphetamine in urine by capillary GC/MS. J. Anal. Tox. 13: 257–262, 1989.

R.L. Fitzgerald, J.M. Ramos, S.C. Bogema and A. Poklis. Resolution of methamphetamine stereoisomers in urine drug testing. J. Anal. Tox. 12: 255–259, 1988.

T.J. Haley. Desoxyephedrine—a review of the literature. J. Am. Pharm. Asso. 36: 161–169, 1947.

C.L. Hornbeck and R.J. Czarny. Retrospective analysis of some l-methamphetamine/l-amphetamine urine data. J. Anal. Tox. 17: 23–25, 1993.

R.O. Hughes, W.E. Bronner and M.L. Smith. Detection of amphetamine and methamphetamine in urine by gas chromatography/mass spectrometry following derivatization with (-)-menthyl chloroformate. J. Anal. Tox. 15: 256–259, 1991.

E. Leis. Personal communication, 1991.

T. Nagai and S. Kamiyama. Simultaneous HPLC analysis of optical isomers of methamphetamine and its metabolites. J. Anal. Tox. 15: 299–304, 1991.

A. Poklis, S.A. Jortani, C.S. Brown and C.R. Crooks. Response of the EMIT II amphetamine/methamphetamine assay to specimens collected following use of Vicks Inhalers. J. Anal. Tox. 17: 284–286, 1993.

S.H. Wan, S.B. Matin and D.L. Azarnoff. Kinetics, salivary excretion of amphetamine isomers, and effect of urinary pH. Clin. Pharm. Ther. 23: 585–590, 1978.

Methanol

T½: 2–24 hr (zero-order)
Vd: 0.6 L/kg CH_3OH
Fb: 0

Occurrence and Usage. Methanol finds widespread commercial use as a solvent, especially in paints and varnishes. It is also a constituent of some antifreeze solutions, is used to denature ethanol and is being considered as an alternative energy source. The current threshold limit value for methanol in industry is 200 ppm (262 mg/m³). The methanol content of 20 commercial wines was found to range from 50–325 mg/L (Lee et al., 1975) and of 24 distilled liquors, from 13–106 mg/L (Carroll, 1970). Occupational exposure may be via inhalation, dermal absorption or ingestion.

Blood Concentrations. Normal blood methanol concentrations, derived from endogenous production and dietary sources, are on the order of 1.5 mg/L or less (Eriksen and Kulkarni, 1963). Blood methanol levels in volunteers increased from an average baseline of 1.8 mg/L to an average of 7.0 mg/L following a 6 hour exposure to 200 ppm of methanol in air (Lee et al., 1992). During a 10–15 day period of chronic bourbon consumption by volunteers, blood methanol concentrations rose steadily to an average peak of 27 mg/L, and did not decline until blood ethanol concentrations fell to less than 200–700 mg/L. This accumulation was believed due to the inhibition of metabolism of endogenous and exogenous methanol by ethanol (Majchrowicz and Mendelson, 1971). A peak blood concentration of 117 mg/L was attained at 1 hour after the ingestion of 7 mL of methanol by a 78.5 kg adult male volunteer (Leaf and Zatman, 1952).

Blood formic acid concentrations in normal subjects average about 5 mg/L. In workers exposed to 85–134 ppm of methanol vapor, blood formic acid increased from an average of 3.2 mg/L in pre-exposed specimens to 7.9 mg/L by the late afternoon (Baumann and Angerer, 1979). In another study, background blood formate levels (average, 9.1 mg/L) were undistinguishable from those present after 6 hours exposure to 200 ppm of air methanol (average, 8.7 mg/L) (Lee et al., 1992).

Metabolism and Excretion. Methanol exhibits zero-order elimination kinetics in man with a half-life of 2–24 hours, being oxidized by liver alcohol dehydrogenase at about one-tenth the rate of ethanol (Kane et al., 1968; Mani et al., 1970). The highly toxic formaldehyde that is formed has not been found to accumulate, but is oxidized to formic acid, which is 6 times more toxic than methanol and which probably accounts for the insidious toxicity of its parent. Formic acid is further oxidized to carbon dioxide by a folate-dependent pathway in the rat (Palese and Tephly, 1975). From 10–20% of a dose of methanol is eliminated unchanged through the lungs and about 3% by the kidneys; up to 60% is oxidized and, although formaldehyde is not found in urine, urinary formic acid may account for 2–5% over a 4–10 day period (Lund, 1948; Keeney and Mellinkoff, 1951). The average urine/blood concentration ratio for methanol in man is 1.30, identical to that for ethanol (Leaf and Zatman, 1952).

Methanol breath concentrations in workers exposed to 85–134 ppm of methanol vapor averaged 0.8 ppm before work and 2.5 ppm by late afternoon (Baumann and Angerer, 1979). Urinary methanol concentrations averaged 1.9 mg/L in nonexposed subjects and 42 mg/L in workers exposed to 200 ppm methanol in air for 8 hours (Kawai et al., 1991).

Urine formic acid concentrations average from 12–17 mg/L in unexposed subjects as a result of normal metabolism (Triebig et al., 1978; Baumann and Angerer, 1979). After oral ingestion of 4 mL of methanol by volunteers, urinary formic acid levels reached a maximum of about 56 mg/L within 2 hours and declined rapidly thereafter (Kendal and Ramanathan, 1953). In workers exposed to methanol at vapor concentrations of 85–134 ppm, urine formic acid concentrations increased from an average of 13 mg/L in the morning to 20 mg/L by late afternoon (Baumann and Angerer, 1979). On the fifth day of worker exposure to methanol air concentrations of 40–160 ppm, urine formic acid levels ranged from 26–98 mg/g creatinine (Liesivuori and Savolainen, 1987). Yasugi et al. (1992) found that the high background urinary formic acid levels in workers (average, 29 mg/L) made interpretation of post-shift levels (average of 38 mg/L after 200 ppm exposure) very difficult.

Toxicity. The accumulation of formic acid has been held primarily responsible for the severe metabolic acidosis and ocular toxicity of methanol (Makar and Tephly, 1977). The initial narcotic effects of methanol are much milder than those of ethanol, and the characteristic toxic syndrome may not appear until 6–30 hours after ingestion; treatment may include administration of ethanol to inhibit methanol metabolism, administration of folate to induce formic acid detoxification and hemodialysis for the removal of methanol and formic acid (Gosselin et al., 1976; Manoguerra et al., 1977). Hemodialysis is especially important if the blood methanol concentration exceeds 500–1000 mg/L; additional ethanol must be administered to replace that lost during dialysis, maintaining the blood ethanol concentration at approximately 1000 mg/L (McCoy et al., 1979; Swartz et al., 1981).

Chronic exposure to air concentrations of 3000 ppm or greater is believed to cause accumulation of methanol in the body, with resulting toxicity (Leaf and Zatman, 1952). However, exposure for long periods of time to levels of only 800–1000 ppm may be sufficient to produce serious eye damage in some persons (ACGIH, 1971).

The acute ingestion of as little as 10 mL of methanol has caused permanent blindness and 100–200 mL is fatal to most adults. Of 725 cases of methanol poisoning by ingestion that occurred prior to 1939, 54% resulted in death, 12% in total blindness and 12% in visual impairment (Keeney and

Mellinkoff, 1951). Blood methanol concentrations are not necessarily a good prognostic index. Bennett et al. (1953) reported blood concentrations ranging from 0–3900 mg/L (average, 1300) in 11 patients who survived, and concentrations of 0–4000 mg/L (average, 1600) in 7 who died during treatment. In 9 hospitalized patients, Lund (1948) found blood methanol concentrations of 0–1200 mg/L (average, 600) and blood formic acid levels of 8–134 mg/L (average, 56).

A blood methanol concentration of 400 mg/L is believed to be a minimum lethal level in individuals receiving no medical treatment. Blood methanol concentrations in 20 fatal cases averaged 1900 mg/L with a range of 200–6300 mg/L (Kane et al., 1968; Tonkabony, 1975). A comatose adult admitted to the hospital with a serum methanol concentration of 2400 mg/L and serum formic acid level of 450 mg/L was eventually declared brain dead after 10 days (Shahangian and Ash, 1986). The body distribution of methanol in man has been found to be very similar to that of ethanol (Harger et al., 1938; Wu Chen et al., 1985). Postmortem blood formic acid concentrations of 230 and 320 mg/L were measured in 2 adult victims of accidental methanol poisoning (Tanaka et al., 1991).

Analysis. The gas chromatographic techniques cited previously for ethanol are applicable as well to the determination of methanol. Methods for formic acid analysis were discussed in the section on formaldehyde.

References

ACGIH. *Documentation of the Threshold Limit Values*, American Conference of Governmental Industrial Hygienists, Cincinnati, Ohio, 1971, pp. 155–156.

K. Baumann and J. Angerer. Occupational chronic exposure to organic solvents. Int. Arch. Occ. Env. Health 42: 241–249, 1979.

I.L. Bennett, Jr., F.H. Cary, G.L. Mitchell, Jr. and M.N. Cooper. Acute methyl alcohol poisoning: a review based on experiences in an outbreak of 323 cases. Medicine 32: 431–463, 1953.

R.B. Carroll. Analysis of alcoholic beverages by gas-liquid chromatography. Quart. J. Stud. Alc. Suppl. 5: 6–19, 1970.

S.P. Eriksen and A.B. Kulkarni. Methanol in normal human breath. Science 141: 639–640, 1963.

R.E. Gosselin, H.C. Hodge, R.P. Smith and M.N. Gleason. *Clinical Toxicology of Commercial Products*, 4th ed., Williams and Wilkins, Baltimore, 1976, pp. 229–233 (Section III).

R.N. Harger, S.L. Johnson and E.G. Bridwell. Detection and estimation of methanol, with results in human cases of methanol poisoning. J. Biol. Chem. (Suppl.) 23: 50–51, 1938.

R.L. Kane, W. Talbert, J. Harlan et al. A methanol poisoning outbreak in Kentucky. Arch. Env. Health 17: 119–129, 1968.

T. Kawai, T. Yasugi, K. Mizunuma et al. Methanol in urine as a biological indicator of occupational exposure to methanol vapor. Int. Arch. Occ. Env. Health 63: 311–318, 1991.

A.H. Keeney and S.M. Mellinkoff. Methyl alcohol poisoning. Ann. Int. Med. 34: 331–338, 1951.

L.P. Kendal and A.N. Ramanathan. Excretion of formate after methanol ingestion in man. Biochem. J. 54: 424–426, 1953.

G. Leaf and L.J. Zatman. A study of the conditions under which methanol may exert a toxic hazard in industry. Brit. J. Ind. Med. 9: 19–31, 1952.

C.Y. Lee, T.E. Acree and R.M. Butts. Determination of methyl alcohol in wine by gas chromatography. Anal. Chem. 47: 747–748, 1975.

E.W. Lee, T.S. Terzo, J.B. D'Arcy et al. Lack of blood formate accumulation in humans following exposure to methanol vapor. Am. Ind. Hyg. Asso. J. 53: 99–104, 1992.

J. Liesivuori and H. Savolainen. Urinary formic acid as an indicator of occupational exposure to formic acid and methanol. Am. Ind. Hyg. Asso. J. 48: 32–34, 1987.

A. Lund. Excretion of methanol and formic acid in man after methanol consumption. Acta Pharm. Tox. 4: 205–212, 1948.

E. Majchrowicz and J.H. Mendelson. Blood methanol concentrations during experimentally induced ethanol intoxication in alcoholics. J. Pharm. Exp. Ther. 179: 293–300, 1971.

A.B. Makar and T.R. Tephly. Methanol poisoning VI: role of folic acid in the production of methanol poisoning in the rat. J. Tox. Env. Health 2: 1201–1209, 1977.

J.C. Mani, R. Pietruszko and H. Theorell. Methanol activity of alcohol dehydrogenases from human liver, horse liver, and yeast. Arch. Biochem. Biophys. 140: 52–59, 1970.

A.S. Manoguerra, R.J. Cipolle, D.E. Zaske and S.M. Ehlers. Serum concentration studies during hemodialysis in a patient with severe methanol intoxication. In *Management of the Poisoned Patient* (B.H. Rumack and A.R. Temple, eds.), Science Press, Princeton, 1977, pp. 103–114.

H.G. McCoy, R.J. Cipolle, S.M. Ehlers et al. Severe methanol poisoning. Am. J. Med. 67: 804–807, 1979.

M. Palese and T.R. Tephly. Metabolism of formate in the rat. J. Tox. Env. Health 1: 13–24, 1975.

S. Shahangian and K.O. Ash. Formic and lactic acidosis in a fatal case of methanol intoxication. Clin. Chem. 32: 395–397, 1986.

R.D. Swartz, R.P. Millman, J.E. Billi et al. Epidemic methanol poisoning: clinical and biochemical analysis of a recent episode. Medicine 60: 373–382, 1981.

E. Tanaka, K. Honda, H. Horiguchi and S. Misawa. Postmortem determination of the biological distribution of formic acid in methanol intoxication. J. For. Sci. 36: 936–938, 1991.

S.E.H. Tonkabony. Post-mortem blood concentration of methanol in 17 cases of fatal poisoning from contraband vodka. For. Sci. 6: 1–3, 1975.

G. Triebig, K.H. Schaller and K. Gossler. Eineinfache und zuverlaessige gas-chromatographische Bestimmung von Ameisensaeure im Urin. Z. Anal. Chem. 290: 114, 1978.

N.B. Wu Chen, E.R. Donoghue and M.I. Schaffer. Methanol intoxication: distribution in postmortem tissues and fluids including vitreous humor. J. For. Sci. 30: 213–216, 1985.

T. Yasugi, T. Kawai, K. Mizunuma et al. Formic acid excretion in comparison with methanol excretion in urine of workers occupationally exposed to methanol. Int. Arch. Occ. Env. Health 64: 329–337, 1992.

Methapyrilene

T½: 1.1–2.1 hr
Vd: 2.1–6.6 L/kg
Fb: ?
pKa: 3.7, 8.9

Occurrence and Usage. Methapyrilene (Thenylene, Histadyl) is an ethylenediamine derivative that was synthesized in 1947. As an antihistamine, it has been available in various oral formulations as the hydrochloride or fumarate salt in doses of 5–81 mg. It has also received widespread attention due to its sedative properties, and until 1980 was used as a component of numerous nonprescription soporific preparations in doses of 15–50 mg, frequently in combination with other agents.

Blood Concentrations. Peak plasma methapyrilene concentrations in 8 subjects averaged 0.014 mg/L (range, 0.003–0.032) after a 25 mg oral dose and 0.024 mg/L (range, 0.006–0.050) after a 50 mg oral dose; the peak levels occurred approximately 1.5 hours after ingestion. Sedation was not apparent in the volunteers (Calandre et al., 1981).

Metabolism and Excretion. From 0.04–1.3% of a dose of methapyrilene is excreted unchanged in the 24 hour urine. The bioavailabililty after oral administration is highly variable, ranging from 4–46%. A polar urinary metabolite, possibly a hydroxylated compound, has been observed on thin-layer chromatograms (Schirmer and Pierson, 1973; Baselt and Franch, 1980; Calandre et al., 1981).

Toxicity. Methapyrilene was recently removed from the United States over-the-counter market due to its carcinogenicity in rats (Lijinsky et al., 1980). In acute overdosage the drug causes nausea, vomiting, stupor, respiratory depression, hyperthermia, convulsions, coma, and tachycardia (Rives et al., 1949; Snyderman, 1949).

Methapyrilene has been implicated in a fair number of instances of drug intoxication in which toxicological analysis was performed. Urine concentrations of 8–228 mg/L were found for 5 intoxicated individuals who later recovered (Ainsworth and Biggs, 1977). One person survived the ingestion of 2.5 g of the drug (Winek et al., 1977), while 2 fatalities were known to have resulted from overdosage with 7.4–8.2 g (Cravey et al., 1977).

Blood concentrations of methapyrilene in 10 fatal cases ranged from 4.4–30 mg/L (average, 18), with liver concentrations of 25–160 mg/kg (average, 86) (O'Dea and Liss, 1953; Fatteh and Dudley, 1972; Ainsworth and Biggs, 1977; Baselt and Cravey, 1977; Cravey et al., 1977; Winek et al., 1977). One of these cases showed the following tissue distribution of the drug (Ainsworth and Biggs, 1977):

Methapyrilene Concentrations in a Fatal Case (mg/L or mg/kg)

Blood	Lung	Liver	Kidney	Urine
9	119	82	52	200

Analysis. The determination of toxic levels of methapyrilene in human body fluids and tissues has been performed by ultraviolet spectrophotometry and by gas chromatography with flame-ionization detection (Winek et al., 1977). Therapeutic plasma concentrations may be measured by gas chromatography with nitrogen-phosphorus detection (Baselt and Franch, 1980; Calandre et al., 1981).

References

C.A. Ainsworth and J.D. Biggs. A fatality involving methapyrilene. Clin. Tox. 11: 281–286, 1977.

R.C. Baselt and R.H. Cravey. A compendium of therapeutic and toxic concentrations of toxicologically significant drugs in human biofluids. J. Anal. Tox. 1: 81–103, 1977.

R.C. Baselt and S. Franch. Plasma and urine concentrations of methapyrilene by nitrogen-phosphorus gas-liquid chromatography. J. Chrom. 183: 234–238, 1980.

E.P. Calandre, N. Alferez, K. Hassanein and D.L. Azarnoff. Methapyrilene kinetics and dynamics. Clin. Pharm. Ther. 29: 527–532, 1981.

R.H. Cravey, D. Reed, P.R. Sedgwick and J.E. Turner. Toxicologic data from documented drug-induced or drug-related fatal cases. Clin. Tox. 10: 327–339, 1977.

A. Fatteh and J.B. Dudley. Fatal poisoning involving methapyrilene. J. Am. Med. Asso. 219: 756–757, 1972.

W. Lijinsky, M.D. Reuber and B.N. Blackwell. Liver tumors induced in rats by oral administration of the antihistaminic methapyrilene hydrochloride. Science 209: 817–819, 1980.

A.E. O'Dea and M. Liss. Suicidal poisoning by methapyrilene hydrochloride with documentation by paper chromatography. New Eng. J. Med. 249: 566–567, 1953.

H.F. Rives, B.B. Ward and M.L. Hicks. A fatal reaction to methapyrilene (Thenylene). J. Am. Med. Asso. 140: 1022–1024, 1949.

R.E. Schirmer and R.J. Pierson. GLC analysis of methapyrilene in plasma and urine using a sulfur-specific flame-photometric detector. J. Pharm. Sci. 62: 2052–2054, 1973.

H.S. Snyderman. Accidental Thenylene hydrochloride poisoning. J. Pediat. 35: 376–377, 1949.

C.L. Winek, F.W. Fochtman, W.J. Trogus et al. Methapyrilene toxicity. Clin. Tox. 11: 287–294, 1977.

Methaqualone

T½: 20–60 hr
Vd: 6 L/kg
Fb: 0.80
pKa: 2.4

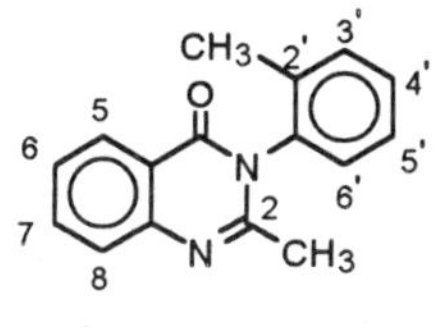

Occurrence and Usage. Methaqualone (Quaalude, Sopor) is a quinazoline derivative that was synthesized in 1951 and found clinically effective as a sedative and hypnotic in 1956. The compound acts primarily like a weak base but is also soluble in dilute alkaline solutions. It is supplied for oral use in amounts of 75–300 mg as the free base and 200–400 mg as the hydrochloride. Methaqualone has received a great deal of attention as a drug of abuse, being self-administered in oral doses of up to 3 g daily; chronic usage can result in tolerance and physical dependence. The drug was removed from the U.S. market in 1984 due to its extensive misuse. It is still occasionally encountered in illicit form, and is also available in European countries in combination with diphenhydramine (Mandrax).

Blood Concentrations. A 250 mg oral dose of methaqualone base given to 7 subjects produced a mean peak plasma level of 2.2 mg/L (range, 1.0–4.0) at 2 hours, declining to 1.1 mg/L by 5 hours; an equivalent dose of the hydrochloride given to 8 subjects resulted in a peak concentration of 3.7 mg/L (range, 2.0–4.9) at 1 hour, also declining to 1.1 mg/L at 5 hours. The free base caused little subjective effect throughout the course of the experiment, whereas the hydrochloride caused a marked sedative effect during the first hour after ingestion (Brown, 1976). A 600 mg oral dose of the free base produced an average maximum serum concentration of 7.0 mg/L at 1 hour in 3 subjects (Smyth et al., 1973). Estimates of the plasma half-life of methaqualone have ranged from 2.6–41.5 hours; however, the low figure is representative of the distributive phase and not of the terminal elimination phase, the half-life for which averages 33–38 hours (Morris et al., 1972; Alvan et al., 1973; Alvan et al., 1974).

With chronic administration of the drug, plasma concentrations show initial accumulation but eventually return to the levels seen with single doses; this is due to a moderate decline in the elimination phase half-life during chronic dosing (Alvan et al., 74; Nayak et al., 1974). Cerebrospinal fluid concentrations of the drug average 18% of the serum concentrations (Christensen and Holfort, 1975).

Metabolism and Excretion. Methaqualone is extensively metabolized *in vivo* principally by hydroxylation at virtually every possible position on the molecule. At least 12 hydroxylated metabolites have been identified in urine, including a dihydroxy derivative, and most are excreted as glucuronide conjugates. N-oxidation and ring cleavage, with production of 2-nitrobenzo-o-toluidide, also occur to a certain extent. None of the metabolites has been found to exhibit significant pharmacologic activity (Brown and Goenechea, 1973). From 40–50% of a labeled dose is excreted in the 72 hour urine and only 1–4% in the feces; only traces of unchanged drug are present in urine after normal doses (Smyth et al., 1973). Following a single oral dose to healthy young adults, the following amounts (as a percentage of the dose) were excreted in the 24 hour urine: 0.2% as methaqualone, 6.6% as methaqualone-N-oxide, 10.3% conjugated 4'-hydroxymethaqualone, 4.7% conjugated 2'-hydroxymethylmethaqualone, 3.5% conjugated 3'-hydroxymethaqualone, 2.8% conjugated 2-hydroxymethylmethaqualone, and 2.8% conjugated 6-hydroxymethaqualone (Reynolds et al., 1978).

Methaqualone urine concentrations after a 250 mg oral dose usually do not exceed 0.2 mg/L, whereas total (free plus conjugated) 6-hydroxymethaqualone concentrations range up to 4 mg/L (McReynolds et al., 1975). Total urine concentrations of the 3'- and 4'-hydroxy and 2'- and 2-hydroxymethyl metabolites range from 0.8–32 mg/L in the first 24 hours after a similar dose (Permisohn et al., 1976). There is considerable variation in the relative amounts of the different metabolites formed by individuals (Kazyak et al., 1977). The urinary excretion of 6-hydroxymethaqualone has been followed for up to 29 days in a subject who ingested a single 300 mg methaqualone tablet; the detectability limit of the assay used was approximately 0.001 mg/L (Heck, 1978).

Toxicity. Numerous instances of intoxication with methaqualone have been recorded and there is substantial analytical data regarding blood or plasma concentrations of the drug in these cases. Blood concentrations of the drug in 14 persons arrested for erratic driving have ranged from 2–12 mg/L (average, 6) (Graves, 1973). Twenty chronic drug users who were titrated to the point of mild toxicity (ataxia, slurred speech, drowsiness and nystagmus) with 600 mg of methaqualone per hour achieved blood levels of 2–16 mg/L after total doses of 300–4900 mg of the drug (Comstock, 1974).

Concentrations in the plasma of overdose victims have ranged from 2–230 mg/L, with concentrations greater than 8 mg/L being associated with unconsciousness (Proudfoot et al., 1968; Bailey and Jatlow, 1973). Twenty-five hospitalized subjects in grade I coma exhibited serum methaqualone concentrations of 6–17 mg/L, averaging 11 mg/L (Lundberg, 1973). Blood concentrations of unconjugated 2'-hydroxymethylmethaqualone exceeded the concentrations of parent drug by up to 50% in a comatose patient; since this metabolite has twice the acute lethal potency of methaqualone, it may contribute to morbidity following overdosage with the drug (Kazyak et al., 1979).

In 6 fatal cases, postmortem blood concentrations of 5–42 mg/L (average, 22) and liver concentrations of 26–89 mg/kg (average, 55) were observed (Baselt and Cravey, 1977). The following data were obtained from a fatal case that involved the ingestion of methaqualone and ethchlorvynol, and illustrates the tissue distribution of this drug (Cravey, 1977):

Tissue Distribution of Methaqualone (mg/L or mg/kg)

Blood	Liver	Kidney	Urine	Gastric
6.4	58	69	17	264 mg

Analysis. Methaqualone has been assayed in biologic fluids and tissues by fluorometry (Brown and Smart, 1969; Smyth et al., 1973) and by ultraviolet spectrophotometry (Bailey and Jatlow, 1973). More specific procedures involving gas chromatography of the parent drug in plasma (Berry, 1969; Mitchard and Williams, 1972; Evenson and Lensmeyer, 1974; Peat and Finkle, 1980) and of its metabolites (as trimethylsilyl derivatives after hydrolysis) in urine (Bonnichsen et al., 1972; Kazyak et al., 1977) have been described. Commercial immunoassays are available that exhibit cross-reactivity with many of the metabolites of the drug (Berman et al., 1975; Bost et al., 1976; Sutheimer et al., 1983). Hydrolysis of conjugated urinary metabolites is more efficiently performed using beta-glucuronidase or sodium metaperiodate than with hydrochloric acid, which partially destroys the compounds (Bonnichsen et al., 1974; Sleeman et al., 1975).

References

G. Alvan, J.E. Lindgren, C. Bogentoft and O. Ericsson. Plasma kinetics of methaqualone in man after single oral doses. Eur. J. Clin. Pharm. 6: 187–190, 1973.

G. Alvan, O. Ericsson, S. Levander and J.E. Lindgren. Plasma concentrations and effects of methaqualone after single and multiple oral doses in man. Eur. J. Clin. Pharm. 7: 449–454, 1974.

D.N. Bailey and P.I. Jatlow. Methaqualone overdose: analytical methodology, and the significance of serum drug concentrations. Clin. Chem. 19: 615–620, 1973.

R.C. Baselt and R.H. Cravey. A compendium of therapeutic and toxic concentrations of toxicologically significant drugs in human biofluids. J. Anal. Tox. 1: 81–103, 1977.

A.R. Berman, J.P. McGrath, R.C. Permisohn and J.A. Cella. Radioimmunoassay of methaqualone and its monohydroxy metabolites in urine. Clin. Chem. 21: 1878–1881, 1975.

D.J. Berry. Gas chromatographic determination of methaqualone, 2-methyl-3-o-tolyl-4(^{3}H)-quinazolinone, at therapeutic levels in human plasma. J. Chrom. 42: 39–44, 1969.

R. Bonnichsen, C.G. Fri, C. Negoita and R. Ryhage. Identification of methaqualone metabolites from urine extract by gas chromatography-mass spectrometry. Clin. Chim. Acta 40: 309–318, 1972.

R. Bonnichsen, Y. Marde and R. Ryhage. Identification of free and conjugated metabolites of methaqualone by gas chromatography-mass spectrometry. Clin. Chem. 20: 230–235, 1974.

R.O. Bost, C.A. Sutheimer and I. Sunshine. Methaqualone assay by radioimmunoassay and gas chromatography. Clin. Chem. 22: 689–690, 1976.

S.S. Brown and G.A. Smart. Fluorimetric assay of methaqualone in plasma by reduction to 1,2,3,4-tetrahydro-2-methyl-4-oxo-3-o-tolyl-quinazoline. J. Pharm. Pharmac. 21: 466–468, 1969.

S.S. Brown and S. Goenechea. Methaqualone: metabolic, kinetic and clinical pharmacologic observations. Clin. Pharm. Ther. 14: 314–324, 1973.

S.S. Brown. Assay of methaqualone in blood. In *Assay of Drugs and Other Trace Compounds in Biological Fluids* (E. Reid, ed.), North-Holland, New York, 1976, pp. 179–194.

J.M. Christensen and S. Holfort. Methaqualone in human serum and cerebrospinal fluid after oral intake. J. Pharm. Pharmac. 27: 538–539, 1975.

E.G. Comstock. Personal communication, 1974.

R.H. Cravey. Personal communication, 1977.

M.A. Evenson and G.L. Lensmeyer. Qualitative and quantitative determination of methaqualone in serum by gas chromatography. Clin. Chem. 20: 249–254, 1974.

M. Graves. Personal communication, 1973.

H.d'A. Heck, K. Maloney and M. Anbar. Long-term urinary excretion of methaqualone in a human subject. J. Pharmacokin. Biopharm. 6: 111–121, 1978.

L. Kazyak, J.A. Kelly, J.A. Cella et al. Methaqualone metabolites in human urine after therapeutic doses. Clin. Chem. 23: 2001–2006, 1977.

L. Kazyak, R.M. Anthony and I. Sunshine. Methaqualone metabolites and their significance in acute intoxication. J. Anal. Tox. 3: 67–71, 1979.

G. Lundberg. Personal communication, 1973.

J.H. McReynolds, H.d'A. Heck and M. Anbar. Determination of picomole quantities of methaqualone and 6-hydroxymethaqualone in urine. Biomed. Mass Spec. 2: 299–303, 1975.

M. Mitchard and M.E. Williams. An improved quantitative gas-liquid chromatographic assay for the estimation of methaqualone in biological fluids. J. Chrom. 72: 29–34, 1972.

R.N. Morris, G.A. Gunderson, S.W. Babcock and J.F. Zaroslinski. Plasma levels and absorption of methaqualone after oral administration to man. Clin. Pharm. Ther. 13: 719–723, 1972.

R.K. Nayak, R.D. Smyth, J.H. Chamberlain et al. Methaqualone pharmacokinetics after single- and multiple-dose administration in man. J. Pharm. Biopharm. 2: 107–121, 1974.

M.A. Peat and B.S. Finkle. Determination of methaqualone and its major metabolite in plasma and saliva after single oral doses. J. Anal. Tox. 4: 114–118, 1980.

R.C. Permisohn, L.R. Hilpert and L. Kazyak. Determination of methaqualone in urine by metabolite detection via gas chromatography. J. For. Sci. 21: 98–107, 1976.

A.T. Proudfoot, J. Noble, J. Nimmo et al. Peritoneal dialysis and haemodialysis in methaqualone (Mandrax) poisoning. Scot. Med. J. 13: 232–236, 1968.

C.N. Reynolds, K. Wilson and D. Burnett. Metabolism of methaqualone in geriatric patients. Eur. J. Clin. Pharm. 13: 285–289, 1978.

H.K. Sleeman, J.A. Cella, J.L. Harvey and D.J. Beach. Thin-layer chromatographic detection and identification of methaqualone metabolites in urine. Clin. Chem. 21: 76–80, 1975.

R.D. Smyth, J.K. Lee, A. Polk et al. Bioavailability of methaqualone. J. Clin. Pharm. 13: 391–400, 1973.

C.A. Sutheimer, B.R. Hepler and I. Sunshine. EMIT-st screening for drugs of abuse: methaqualone. J. Anal. Tox. 7: 83–85, 1983.

Metharbital

T½: ?
Vd: ?
Fb: ?
pKa: 8.5

Occurrence and Usage. Metharbital (N-methylbarbital, Gemonil) is a methylated barbiturate derivative that was first synthesized in 1903, but was not applied to the therapy of epilepsy until about 1950. It probably offers no advantages over other drugs such as phenobarbital nor even over its major metabolite, barbital. The compound is available in 100 mg tablets and is administered in daily oral doses of 100–600 mg as the free acid.

Blood Concentrations. Only one study has been reported in which plasma concentrations of the drug were measured. Following the daily administration of 300 mg of metharbital for 14 days to a single adult male, the peak plasma barbital concentration was 26 mg/L and still climbing, while the metharbital concentration, which had reached 5 mg/L initially, declined to undetectable levels (Butler and Waddell, 1958).

Metabolism and Excretion. Metharbital is metabolized extensively by N-demethylation to barbital, an active metabolite that probably accounts for most or all of the activity of the parent, especially with chronic usage. The rate of demethylation is considerably slower than for mephobarbital, a related drug (Butler, 1953). Slightly over 1% of a dose of metharbital is excreted unchanged in the 48 hour urine, and about 9% is excreted as barbital. It is believed that much of the remainder of the dose is excreted as barbital over a 2 or 3 week period following a single administration (Butler, 1953; Svendsen and Brochmann-Hanssen, 1962).

metharbital   barbital

Toxicity. Adverse reactions to metharbital include gastric distress, drowsiness, irritability, and dizziness.

Analysis. A gas-liquid chromatographic procedure using flame-ionization detection has been described for the analysis of underivatized metharbital and barbital (Svendsen and Brochmann-Hanssen, 1962). Any assay that involves methylation of the drugs would of course prevent the differentiation of metharbital and its metabolite.

References

T.C. Butler. Quantitative studies of the demethylation of N-methyl barbital (metharbital, Gemonil). J. Pharm. Exp. Ther. 108: 474–480, 1953.

T.C. Butler and W.J. Waddell. N-methylated derivatives of barbituric acid, hydantoin and oxazolidinedione used in the treatment of epilepsy. Neurology 8: 106–112, 1958.

A.B. Svendsen and E. Brochmann-Hanssen. Gas chromatography of barbiturates II. Application to the study of their metabolism and excretion in humans. J. Pharm. Sci. 551: 494–495, 1962.

Methocarbamol

T½: 1.2–2.2 hr
Vd: ?
Fb: ?

Occurrence and Usage. Methocarbamol (Robaxin) is a carbamate derivative that was synthesized in 1956 and that is used occasionally as a sedative or muscle relaxant. It may be administered by intravenous or intramuscular injection in single doses of 1–3 g, or orally in single doses of 500–1500 mg and daily doses of 4–8 g. One oral formulation contains 400 mg of methocarbamol and 325 mg of aspirin.

Blood Concentrations. Serum concentrations of methocarbamol peaked at 25.8 mg/L in a subject at 1 hour after the ingestion of 2000 mg; this level diminished to 14.5 mg/L by 4 hours and 2.2

mg/L by 8 hours. Estimates of the half-life of the drug have ranged from 1.2–2.2 hours (Forist and Judy, 1971; Bruce et al., 1971). After a single oral 4000 mg dose given to 10 subjects, an average peak plasma concentration of about 41 mg/L was attained at 2 hours (Huf et al., 1959).

Metabolism and Excretion. The biotransformation of methocarbamol is known to proceed primarily via O-demethylation and hydroxylation of the phenyl ring; the parent drug and the 2 major metabolites are excreted largely in conjugated form. Up to 99% of a single oral dose is eliminated in the urine over a 3 day period, with less than 1% present as free methocarbamol. The following amounts of total metabolites (free plus conjugated) were found in the 72 hour urine of 2 volunteers 9–15% methocarbamol, 21–28% O-desmethylmethocarbamol, and 24–28% 4-hydroxy-methocarbamol. Unidentified metabolites constitute the remainder of the dose (Campbell et al., 1961; Bruce et al., 1971).

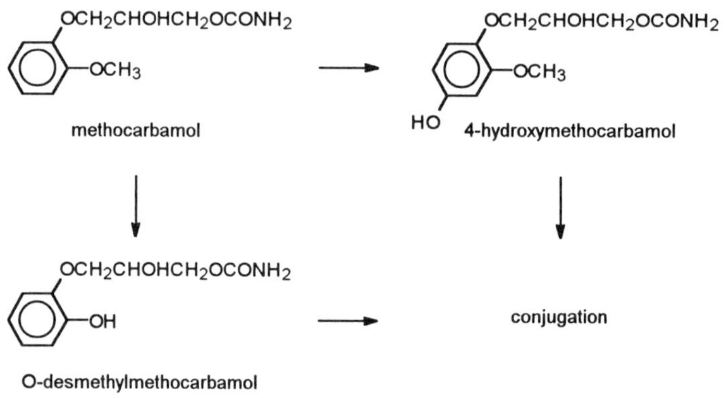

Toxicity. Overdosage with methocarbamol results in nausea, drowsiness, blurred vision, fever, hypotension, convulsions, and coma. In 3 acute fatalities involving the drug, the following concentrations were measured (Cravey, 1974; Kemal et al., 1982; Ferslew et al., 1990):

Methocarbamol Concentrations in Fatal Cases* (mg/L or mg/kg)

	Blood	Brain	Liver	Urine	Gastric
Average	367	133	378	415	3.6 g
(Range)	(257–525)	(133)	(296–459)	(255–575)	(3.4–3.7)

* Each case also involved significant levels of either ethanol or secobarbital.

Analysis. Colorimetric assays for the determination of methocarbamol in biological fluids have been described and require either diazotization (Titus et al., 1948) or reaction with chromotropic acid (Forist and Judy, 1971). Specific gas and liquid chromatographic procedures have been reported more recently (Kemal et al., 1982).

References

R.B. Bruce, L.B. Turnbull and J.H. Newman. Metabolism of methocarbamol in the rat, dog, and human. J. Pharm. Sci. 60: 104–106, 1971.

A.D. Campbell, F.K. Coles, L.L. Eubank and E.G. Huf. Distribution and metabolism of methocarbamol. J. Pharm. Exp. Ther. 131: 18–25, 1961.

R.H. Cravey. Personal communication, 1974.

K.E. Ferslew, A.N. Hagardorn and W.F. McCormick. A fatal interaction of methocarbamol and ethanol in an accidental poisoning. J. For. Sci. 35: 477–482, 1990.

A.A. Forist and R.W. Judy. Comparative pharmacokinetics of chlorphenesin carbamate and methocarbamol in man. J. Pharm. Sci. 60: 1686–1688, 1971.

E.G. Huf, F.K. Coles and L.L. Eubank. Comparative plasma levels of mephenesin carbamate and methocarbamol. Proc. Soc. Exp. Biol. Med. 102: 276–277, 1959.

M. Kemal, R.H. Imami and A. Poklis. A fatal methocarbamol intoxication. J. For. Sci. 27: 217–222, 1982.

E. Titus, S. Ulick and A.P. Richardson. The determination of 3-(orthotoloxyl)-1,2-propanediol (Myanesin) in body fluids and tissues, and its disappearance from the blood following intravenous injections in the dog. J. Pharm. Exp. Ther. 93: 129–134, 1948.

Methohexital

T½: 1.2–2.1 hr
Vd: 1.1–2.6 L/kg
Fb: 0.73
pKa: 7.9

Occurrence and Usage. Methohexital (methohexitone, Brevital) was first introduced as an intravenous anesthetic in the United States in 1957. The compound is an N-methylated ultrashort-acting barbiturate that is available commercially in the alpha-dl isomeric form. It is often used as the sole agent in ambulatory anesthesia, but also as an induction agent with subsequent administration of a gaseous or volatile anesthetic. It is considered to be of shorter duration than thiopental and several times as potent on a weight basis. The drug is supplied in vials containing 500–5000 mg of the sodium salt for reconstitution into a 10 mg/mL solution. Intravenous induction doses often range from 50–120 mg.

Blood Concentrations. Following a bolus injection of 1.5–2.0 mg/kg of methohexital to 6 patients, maximal venous blood concentrations of 3.9–8.6 mg/L were observed within the first 3 minutes with a rapid decline (Sunshine et al., 1966). During a 60 minute intravenous infusion of 3.0 mg/kg (210 mg/70 kg) of the drug, a peak plasma concentration of 3.0 mg/L was achieved, with reduction to 0.4 mg/L 2 hours after the end of infusion (Breimer, 1976). Plasma methohexital concentrations of 3.4–10.7 mg/L are believed to produce the necessary range of responses in anesthetized individuals, from sleep induction to suppression of EEG activity (Lauven et al., 1987). After a 40 minute intravenous infusion of the exceptionally large dose of 2340 mg of methohexital, plasma concentrations as high as 39.6 mg/L were reached (Brand et al., 1963).

Metabolism and Excretion. Although the fate of methohexital in man has not been fully investigated, it is believed that rapid metabolism rather than tissue uptake accounts for its very short duration of action. Less than 1% of a dose is excreted unchanged in the 24 hour urine and bile (Sunshine et al., 1966), and it is likely that the remainder will be accounted for as products of side-chain hydroxylation, as is the case in experimental animals (Welles et al., 1963). 4'-Hydroxy-methohexital has been reported present in human plasma (Heusler et al., 1981).

Toxicity. Adverse reactions to methohexital administration include hypotension, respiratory depression, laryngospasm, cardiorespiratory arrest, convulsions, coma and death.

A fatal case involving the intravenous self-administration of methohexital was reported in which the following concentrations were observed: blood, 103 mg/L; liver, 41 mg/kg; and kidney, 45 mg/kg (Clarke, 1969). In a similar case, blood and liver concentrations of 98 mg/L and 82 mg/kg were observed (Kirkwood and Yip, 1978).

Analysis. Methohexital is suitable for analysis by ultraviolet spectrophotometry (Brand et al., 1963). Gas chromatography with flame-ionization (Sunshine et al., 1966; Giovanniello and Peeci, 1977), nitrogen-selective (Breimer, 1976), electron-capture (Bjorkman et al., 1983) and mass spectrometric detection (Kestin and Fennessey, 1988) has been reported. Liquid chromatography has also been described (Bjorkmann and Iduall, 1984).

References

S. Bjorkman, J. Idvall and P. Stenberg. Gas-liquid chromatographic determination of methohexital in plasma or whole blood with electron-capture detection of the pentafluorobenzyl derivative. J. Chrom. 278: 424–428, 1983.

S. Bjorkman and J. Idvall. A high-performance liquid chromatographic method for methohexital and thiopental in plasma or whole blood. J. Chrom. 307: 481–487, 1984.

L. Brand, L.D. Mark, M.M. Snell et al. Physiologic disposition of methohexital in man. Anesthesiology 24: 331–335, 1963.

D.D. Breimer. Pharmacokinetics of methohexitone following intravenous infusion in humans. Brit. J. Anaesth. 48: 643–649, 1976.

E.G.C. Clarke (ed.). *Isolation and Identification of Drugs*, Pharmaceutical Press, London, 1969, p. 415.

T.J. Giovanniello and J. Pecci. Isothermal gas-chromatographic separation of barbiturates with use of on-column hexylation and heptylation. Clin. Chem. 23: 2154–2155, 1977.

H. Heusler, J. Epping, S. Heusler et al. Simultaneous determination of blood concentrations of methohexital and its hydroxy metabolite by gas chromatography and identification of 4'-hydroxy-methohexital by combined gas-liquid chromatography-mass spectrometry. J. Chrom. 226: 403–412, 1981.

K.J. Kestin and P.V. Fennessey. Microtechnique for quantitation of plasma methohexital using gas chromatography and mass spectrometry. Anesth. Anal. 67: 466–468, 1988.

C.M. Kirkwood and M.W. Yip. Methohexital poisoning—a case report. Can. Soc. For. Sci. J. 11: 283, 1978.

P.M. Lauven, H. Schwilden and H. Stoeckel. Threshold hypnotic concentration of methohexitone. Eur. J. Clin. Pharm. 33: 261–265, 1987.

I. Sunshine, J.G. Whitman, W.W. Fike et al. Distribution and excretion of methohexitone in man. Brit. J. Anaesth. 38: 23–28, 1966.

J.S. Welles, R.E. McMahon and W.J. Doran. The metabolism and excretion of methohexital in the rat and dog. J. Pharm. Exp. Ther. 139: 166–171, 1963.

Methotrexate

T½: 5–9 hr
Vd: 2.6 L/kg
Fb: 0.50
pKa: 4.3, 5.5

$$HOOCCH_2CH_2CHNHCO-\bigcirc-NCH_2$$

with COOH and CH_3 substituents, linked to a pteridine ring system bearing N, N, NH_2 groups.

Occurrence and Usage. Methotrexate (Mexate) is a folic acid antagonist used as an antineoplastic agent since the 1950s. The compound competitively inhibits folic acid reductase, an enzyme necessary for cellular replication. The drug is available as the free acid in 2.5 mg tablets for oral administration, and as the sodium salt in 20–100 mg vials or in 2.5–25 mg/mL solutions for parenteral injection. Dosage schedules vary, but often involve daily oral administration of 2.5–25 mg for up to 8 days or once weekly administration of 10–50 mg by any route. High-dose methotrexate therapy, currently used against certain cancers, consists of rapid (4–6 hours) or slow (20–42 hours) intravenous infusion of up to 15 g/m² of the drug. This is followed by the frequent administration of leucovorin (citrovorum factor, 5-formyltetrahydrofolinic acid), an antidote that acts by restoring the body pools of reduced folate, to prevent damage to normal cells.

Blood Concentrations. Patients receiving high-dose methotrexate therapy (1–15 g/m²) by either rapid or slow intravenous infusion achieved initial serum concentrations of 10–1000 μmol/L. An average half-life of 6 hours (range, 5–9) has been demonstrated for patients not developing toxicity

(Tattersall et al., 1975). Therapeutic monitoring is generally performed to insure that plasma methotrexate concentrations are below 1 μmol/L at 48 hours after an infusion, or below 0.1 μmol/L at 72 hours (Sadee, 1980).

Metabolism and Excretion. An average of 81% of a labeled dose of methotrexate is eliminated in urine and only 1% in feces in the 4 days after an intravenous dose. Approximately 16% of a dose is eliminated in the urine as 7-hydroxymethotrexate; this metabolite accumulates in plasma, but is relatively inactive (Huffman et al., 1973; Chan et al., 1980; Sadee, 1980).

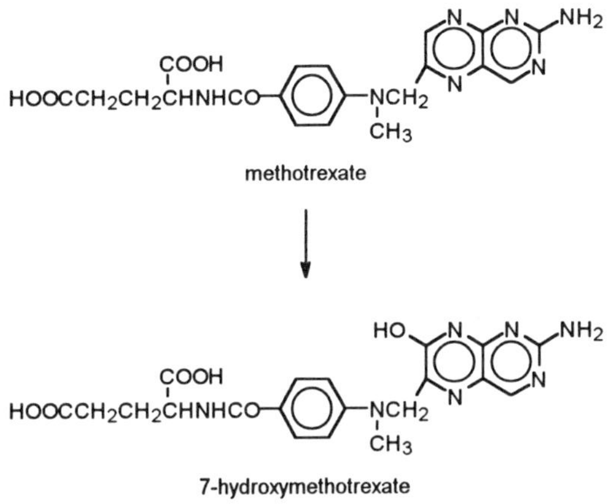

methotrexate

7-hydroxymethotrexate

Toxicity. Adverse reactions to methotrexate include nausea, vomiting, diarrhea, fatigue, dizziness, ulcerative stomatitis, hepatic toxicity, renal damage, and blood dyscrasias. Patients who develop serious toxicity, usually expressed as myelosuppression, after high-dose therapy generally exhibit drug half-lives greater than 10 hours and plasma methotrexate concentrations in excess of 0.9 μmol/L at 48 hours after infusion (Tattersall et al., 1975; Stoller et al., 1977).

Analysis. Methotrexate has been frequently measured in serum by competitive protein binding (Myers et al., 1975) and enzymatic inhibition (Falk et al., 1976; Finley and Williams, 1977; Persijn, 1979). The antibiotic drug trimethoprim is known to interfere with each of these techniques (Bock and Pierce, 1980; Hande et al., 1980). Recently, liquid chromatography has been applied to the simultaneous determination of methotrexate and its 7-hydroxy metabolite (Watson et al., 1978; Canfell and Sadee, 1980; Cohen et al., 1980; Lawson et al., 1981; Buice and Sidhu, 1982; So et al., 1985; Najjar et al., 1992). Reagents for radioimmunoassay and enzyme immunoassay are commercially available and exhibit less than 4% cross-reactivity with 7-hydroxymethotrexate (Buice et al., 1980). Alcoholic solutions of methotrexate exhibit considerable loss of the drug through binding to glassware (Chen and Chiou, 1982).

References

J.L. Bock and R. Pierce. Trimethoprim interference in methotrexate assays. Clin. Chem. 26: 1510–1511, 1980.

R.G. Buice, W.E. Evans, J. Karas et al. Evaluation of enzyme immunoassay, radioassay, and radioimmunoassay of serum methotrexate, as compared with liquid chromatography. Clin. Chem. 26: 1902–1904, 1980.

R.G. Buice and P. Sidhu. Reversed-phase high-pressure liquid chromatographic determination of serum methotrexate and 7-hydroxymethotrexate. J. Pharm. Sci. 71: 74–77, 1982.

C. Canfell and W. Sadee. Methotrexate and 7-hydroxymethotrexate: serum level monitoring by high-performance liquid chromatography. Cancer Treat. Rep. 64: 165–169, 1980.

K.K. Chan, M.S.B. Nayar, J.L. Cohen et al. Metabolism of methotrexate in man after high and conventional doses. Res. Comm. Chem. Path. Pharm. 28: 551–561, 1980.

M.L. Chen and W.L. Chiou. Adsorption of methotrexate onto glassware and syringes. J. Pharm. Sci. 71: 129–131, 1982.

J.L. Cohen, G.H. Hisayasu, A.R. Barrientos et al. Reversed-phase high-performance liquid chromatographic analysis of methotrexate and 7-hydroxymethotrexate in serum. J. Chrom. 181: 478–483, 1980.

L.C. Falk, D.R. Clark, S.M. Kalman and T.F. Long. Enzymatic assay for methotrexate in serum and cerebrospinal fluid. Clin. Chem. 22: 785–788, 1976.

P.R. Finley and R.J. Williams. Methotrexate assay by enzymatic inhibition, with use of the centrifugal analyzer. Clin. Chem. 23: 2139–2141, 1977.

K. Hande, J. Gober and R. Fletcher. Trimethoprim interferes with serum methotrexate assay by the competitive protein binding technique. Clin. Chem. 26: 1617–1619, 1980.

D.H. Huffman, S.H. Wan, D.L. Azarnoff and B. Hoogstraten. Pharmacokinetics of methotrexate. Clin. Pharm. Ther. 14: 572–579, 1973.

G.J. Lawson, P.F. Dixon and G.W. Aherne. Rapid and simple method for the measurement of methotrexate and 7-hydroxymethotrexate in serum by high-performance liquid chromatography. J. Chrom. 223: 225–231, 1981.

C.E. Myers, M.E. Lippman, H.M. Eliot and B.A. Chabner. Competitive protein binding assay for methotrexate. Proc. Nat. Acad. Sci. 72: 3683–3686, 1975.

T.A.O. Najjar, K.M. Matar and J.M. Alfawaz. Comparison of a new high-performance liquid chromatography method with fluorescence polarization immunoassay for analysis of methotrexate. Ther. Drug Mon. 14: 142–146, 1992.

J.P. Persijn. A rapid enzymatic assay for methotrexate in serum. J. Clin. Chem. Clin. Biochem. 17: 235–239, 1979.

W. Sadee. Antineoplastic agents: high-dose methotrexate and citrovorum factor rescue. Ther. Drug Mon. 2: 177–185, 1980.

N. So, D.P. Chandra, I.S. Alexander et al. Determination of serum methotrexate and 7-hydroxymethotrexate concentrations. J. Chrom. 337: 81–90, 1985.

R.G. Stoller, K.R. Hande, S.A. Jacobs et al. Use of plasma pharmacokinetics to predict and prevent methotrexate toxicity. New Eng. J. Med. 297: 630–634, 1977.

M.H.N. Tattersall, L.M. Parker, S.W. Pitman and E. Frie. Clinical pharmacology of high-dose methotrexate (NSC-740). Cancer Chemother. Rep. 6 (Part 3): 25–29, 1975.

E. Watson, J.L. Cohen and K.K. Chan. High-pressure liquid chromatographic determination of methotrexate and its major metabolite, 7-hydroxymethotrexate, in human plasma. Cancer Treat. Rep. 62: 381–387, 1978.

Methotrimeprazine

T½: 17–78 hr
Vd: 23–42 L/kg
Fb: ?
pKa: 9.2

$CH_2CHCH_2N(CH_3)_2$
CH_3

Occurrence and Usage. Methotrimeprazine (levomepromazine, Levoprome) is a phenothiazine derivative that has been in clinical use since 1958. In Europe it has found widespread acceptance as an antipsychotic drug with pronounced sedative effect, and is administered as the hydrochloride in chronic oral doses of 100–400 mg daily. The compound also has analgesic activity comparable to that of morphine; in the United States it is used only for this purpose, and is administered by intramuscular injection in single doses of 5–40 mg.

Blood Concentrations. Following a single intramuscular 25 mg dose to 4 patients, an average peak plasma concentration of 0.022 mg/L was observed at 1.5 hours; the sulfoxide metabolite was not detected in these specimens (Dahl, 1976). During chronic daily oral administration of 300–400 mg of the drug, plasma methotrimeprazine concentrations averaged 0.082 mg/L (range, 0.051–0.141) 3 hours after the last dose, while methotrimeprazine sulfoxide concentrations averaged 0.271 mg/L (range, 0.208–0.389) (Dahl and Garle, 1977). Estimates of the plasma half-life of the drug have ranged from 17–78 hours (Dahl et al., 1977).

Metabolism and Excretion. Methotrimeprazine may rival chlorpromazine in the complexity of its biologic disposition. The sulfoxide is a major metabolite, and is known to have *in vitro* pharmacologic (cardiac) activity (Dahl and Refsum, 1976); mono- and di-N-demethylation and O-demethylation are known to occur, hydroxylation and conjugation products have been tentatively identified, and N-oxidation has been postulated (Allgen et al., 1963; Afifi and Way, 1968; Dahl and Garle, 1977; Johnsen and Dahl, 1982). Combinations of many of the above biotransformation pathways are of course possible.

Less than 1% of a dose of methotrimeprazine is eliminated unchanged in the 24 hour urine (Afifi and Way, 1968). Methotrimeprazine sulfoxide accounts for about 10% of a dose and has been found at concentrations of 4–11 mg/L in the urine of patients, while the concentrations of unchanged drug, the mono-N-desmethyl metabolite and its sulfoxide, and the di-N-desmethyl metabolite were less than 1 mg/L (Dahl and Garle, 1977).

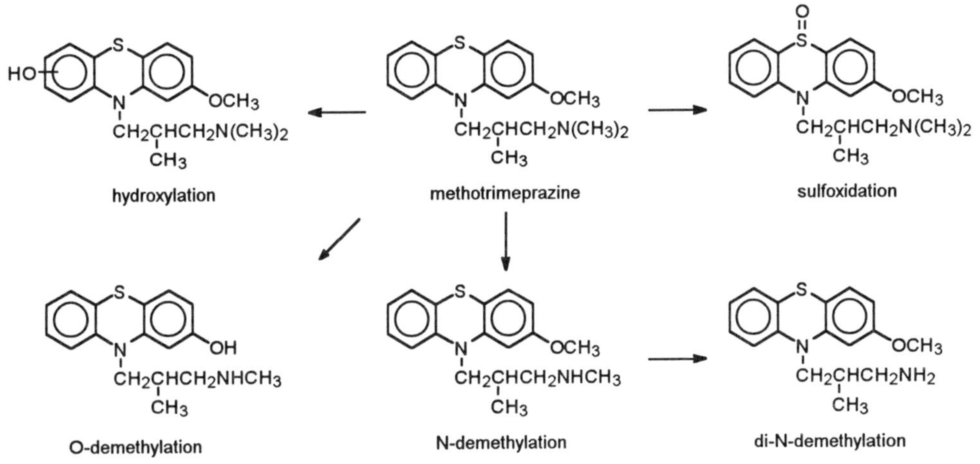

Toxicity. Adverse reactions to methotrimeprazine include sedation, dizziness, weakness, orthostatic hypotension, hepatotoxicity, agranulocytosis, and extrapyramidal symptoms. Overdosage usually results in nausea, vomiting, coma, convulsions, hyperpyrexia and tachycardia.

In a single fatal case, a blood concentration of 8 mg/L and a liver concentration of 160 mg/kg were observed (Bonnichsen et al., 1970).

Analysis. Methotrimeprazine and its major metabolites have been analyzed by a specific gas chromatographic procedure (Dahl and Jacobsen, 1976; Dahl et al., 1982); gas chromatography-mass spectrometry has been applied to the detection of the drug and several of its non-hydroxylated metabolites in plasma and urine (Dahl and Garle, 1977). Liquid chromatography has also been reported (Holt et al., 1981; Loennechen et al., 1990).

References

A.M. Afifi and E.L. Way. Studies on the biologic disposition of methotrimeprazine. J. Pharm. Exp. Ther. 160: 397–406, 1968.

E.G. Allgen, L. Hellstrom and C.J. Sant Orp. On the metabolism and elimination of psychotropic phenothiazine drug levomepromazine (Nozinan) in man. Acta Psych. Scand. Supp. 169: 366–381, 1963.

R. Bonnichsen, P. Geertinger and A.C. Maehley. Toxicological data on phenothiazine drugs in autopsy cases. Z. Rechtsmed. 67: 158–169, 1970.

S.G. Dahl. Pharmacokinetics of methotrimeprazine after single and multiple doses. Clin. Pharm. Ther. 19: 435–442, 1976.

S.G. Dahl and S. Jacobsen. GLC determination of methotrimeprazine and its sulfoxide in plasma. J. Pharm. Sci. 65: 1329–1333, 1976.

S.G. Dahl and H. Refsum. Effects of levomepromazine, chlorpromazine and their sulfoxides on isolated rat atria. Eur. J. Pharm. 37: 241–248, 1976.

S.G. Dahl and M. Garle. Identification of nonpolar methotrimeprazine metabolites in plasma and urine by GLC-mass spectrometry. J. Pharm. Sci. 66: 190–193, 1977.

S.G. Dahl, R.E. Strandjor and S. Sigfusson. Pharmacokinetics and related bioavailability of levomepromazine after repeated administration of tablets and syrup. Eur. J. Clin. Pharm. 11: 305–310, 1977.

S.G. Dahl, T. Bratlid and O. Lingjaerde. Plasma and erythrocyte levels of methotrimeprazine and two of its nonpolar metabolites in psychiatric patients. Ther. Drug Mon. 4: 81–87, 1982.

H. Johnsen and S.G. Dahl. Identification of O-demethylated and ring-hydroxylated metabolites of methotrimeprazine (levomepromazine) in man. Drug Met. Disp. 10: 63–67, 1982.

J.E. Holt, C.M. Kaye and M.G. Sankey. Sensitive high-performance liquid chromatographic assay methods for monitoring methotrimeprazine and dimethothiazine levels in plasma. Brit. J. Clin. Pharm. 12: 282P, 1981.

T. Loennechen, A. Anderson, P.A. Hals and S.G. Dahl. High-performance liquid chromatographic determination of levomepromazine (methotrimeprazine) and its main metabolites in serum and urine. Ther. Drug Mon. 12: 574–581, 1990.

p-Methoxyamphetamine

T½: ?
Vd: ?
Fb: ?
pKa: ?

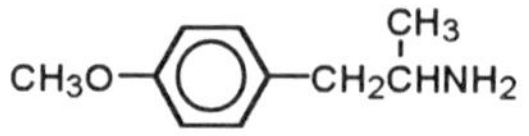

Occurrence and Usage. Para-methoxyamphetamine (PMA) is one of a group of methoxylated phenethylamine derivatives with hallucinogenic properties. This group includes a naturally-occurring compound, mescaline, and synthetic compounds such as methylenedioxyamphetamine (MDA), 2,5-dimethoxy-4-methylamphetamine (STP, DOM), and 2,4,5-trimethoxyamphetamine (TMA). PMA has about 5 times the potency of mescaline, and has been used as an illicit drug both orally and intravenously in doses of 50–100 mg.

Blood Concentrations. Concentrations of PMA in blood or plasma after hallucinogenic doses have not been determined, but by analogy to amphetamine they probably do not exceed 0.2 mg/L.

Metabolism and Excretion. From 49–83% of a labeled dose of PMA is excreted in the 24 hour urine. An average of 15% is eliminated as unchanged drug, 18% as free p-hydroxyamphetamine, 21% as conjugated p-hydroxyamphetamine, 7% as conjugated N-hydroxy-PMA, and 4% as p-hydroxynorephedrine (Kitchen et al., 1979). The N-hydroxy metabolite is unstable and is converted to an oxime during extraction and analysis (Beckett and Midha, 1974).

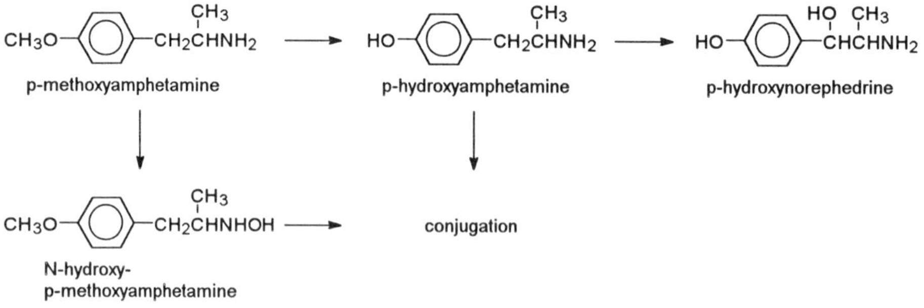

Toxicity. At least 15 fatalities resulting from the oral or intravenous use of PMA have been reported. Hyperpyrexia, tachycardia, agitation, shallow labored breathing, and hypertension are common manifestations of overdosage. Nine cases were described by Cimbura (1974) in which the following ranges of concentrations were determined in the postmortem specimens: blood, 0.3–1.9 mg/L; liver, 0.5–10 mg/kg; and urine, 6–175 mg/L. Additionally, the following data is representative of the distribution of the drug after oral (Tucker, 1973) and intravenous (Wright, 1974) administration:

PMA Concentrations in Fatalities (mg/L or mg/kg)

Route	Blood	Brain	Liver	Bile	Kidney	Urine
Oral	0.4	6.6	6.8	10	24	123 mg
I.V.	1.8	2.8	18	5.5	151	0

Analysis. The analytical methods described for amphetamine are applicable as well to PMA. Both ultraviolet spectrophotometry and flame-ionization gas chromatography of the N-acetyl derivative (Schweitzer and Friedhoff, 1970) have been used successfully.

References

A.H. Beckett and K.K. Midha. The identification of four metabolic products after incubation of p-methoxy-amphetamine with liver preparations of various species. Xenobiotica 4: 297–311, 1974.

G. Cimbura. PMA deaths in Ontario. Can. Med. Asso. J. 110: 1263–1264, 1974.

I. Kitchen, J. Tremblay, J. Andre et al. Interindividual and interspecies variation in the metabolism of the hallucinogen 4-methoxyamphetamine. Xenobiotica 9: 397–404, 1979.

J.W. Schweitzer and A.J. Friedhoff. Amphetamines in human urine: rapid estimation by gas-liquid chromatography. Clin. Chem. 16: 786–788, 1970.

R. Tucker. Personal communication, 1973.

J. Wright. Personal communication, 1974.

Methoxyflurane

T½: ?
Vd: ?
Fb: ?

$CH_3OCF_2CHCl_2$

Occurrence and Usage. Methoxyflurane (Penthrane) is a potent halogenated anesthetic agent that was first used clinically in 1959. It is highly soluble in blood and fat, requiring long periods for induction and recovery, and produces profound respiratory depression at maintenance concentrations of 0.2–0.8% in the inspired air. Methoxyflurane has been implicated in high-output renal failure resembling fluoride intoxication, possibly a result of its extensive biotransformation.

Blood Concentrations. Following conscious obstetric analgesic administration of 0.2–0.5% methoxyflurane in oxygen, maternal arterial blood concentrations of the drug averaged 21 mg/L at delivery, while fetal umbilical venous blood averaged 15 mg/L (Young et al., 1976). During surgical anesthesia lasting 92–280 minutes with administration of 0.24% methoxyflurane, arterial blood concentrations ranged from 126–200 mg/L, with total uptake of 8.4–31 g of the agent (Yoshimura et al., 1976).

Metabolism and Excretion. Only 19% of a dose of methoxyflurane was eliminated unchanged in the expired air during 10 post-operative days. Blood fluoride concentrations usually reached a maximum on the second day, ranging from about 25–132 μmol/L, and renal clearance of blood fluoride was depressed in most patients. The urinary excretion of organic fluorine, inorganic fluoride and oxalic acid accounted for 29%, 8% and 7%, respectively, of the administered dose of the drug over the 10 day period studied. Approximately 37% of the dose was unaccounted for (Yoshimura et al., 1976). Other biotransformation products of methoxyflurane in man are carbon dioxide, dichloroacetic acid and methoxydifluoroacetic acid (Holaday et al., 1970).

The following tissue distribution has been determined for methoxyflurane at body temperature (Wollman and Smith, 1975):

Partition Coefficients for Methoxyflurane

Blood:Gas	Brain:Blood	Liver:Blood	Kidney:Blood	Fat:Blood
11	1.8–2.7	2.3	1.8	61

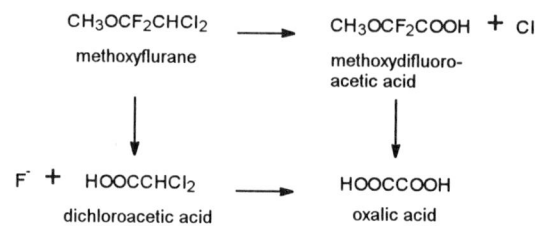

Toxicity. Sixteen of 94 patients administered methoxyflurane developed a toxic nephropathy characterized by diuresis; renal impairment lasted only 10–20 days in most cases, but 3 patients had elevated blood urea nitrogen values for up to 29 months (Crandell et al., 1966). One patient who became nephrotoxic had a serum inorganic fluoride level of 275 μmol/L 8 days after anesthesia, about 10 times the values observed in 2 nontoxic patients; his renal fluoride excretion was also decreased to about 10% of normal (Taves et al., 1970). Two patients developed polyuria and progressive azotemia after methoxyflurane anesthesia, and died 16–84 days later of renal failure; crystals resembling calcium oxalate were found in the renal tubules of both patients at autopsy (Panner et al., 1970). Jaundice and hepatocellular necrosis have been rarely reported following methoxyflurane administration (Klein and Jeffries, 1966).

Analysis. Gas chromatographic procedures for the determination of methoxyflurane in blood or plasma have included a direct injection technique (Cole et al., 1975) and solvent extraction (Yoshimura et al., 1976; Young et al., 1976). Methods for inorganic fluoride in plasma or urine are cited in the section on fluoride.

References

W.J. Cole, R.F. Salamonsen and K.J. Fish. A method for the gas chromatographic analysis of inhalation anaesthetics in whole blood by direct injection into a simple precolumn device. Brit. J. Anaesth. 47: 1043–1047, 1975.

W.B. Crandell, S.G. Pappas and A. MacDonald. Nephrotoxicity associated with methoxyflurane anesthesia. Anesthesiology 27: 591–607, 1966.

D.A. Holaday, S. Rudofsky and P.S. Treuhaft. The metabolic degradation of methoxyflurane in man. Anesthesiology 33: 579–593, 1970.

N.C. Klein and G.H. Jeffries. Hepatotoxicity after methoxyflurane administration. J. Am. Med. Asso. 197: 1037–1039, 1966.

B.J. Panner, R.B. Freeman, L.A. Roth-Moyo and W. Markowitch, Jr. Toxicity following methoxyflurane anesthesia. I. Clinical and pathological observations in two fatal cases. J. Am. Med. Asso. 214: 86–90, 1970.

D.R. Taves, B.W. Fry, R.B. Freeman and A.J. Gillies. Toxicity following methoxyflurane anesthesia. II. Fluoride concentrations in nephrotoxicity. J. Am. Med. Asso. 214: 91–95, 1970.

H. Wollman and T.C. Smith. Uptake, distribution, elimination, and administration of inhalation anesthetics. In *The Pharmacological Basis of Therapeutics*, 5th ed. (L.S. Goodman and A. Gilman, eds.), MacMillan, New York, 1975, pp. 71–80.

N. Yoshimura, D.A. Holaday and V. Fiserova-Bergerova. Metabolism of methoxyflurane in man. Anesthesiology 44: 372–378, 1976.

S.R. Young, R.K. Stoelting, V.K. Bond and C. Peterson. Methoxyflurane biotransformation and renal function following methoxyflurane administration for vaginal delivery or Caesarean section. Anesth. Anal. 55: 415–419, 1976.

Methsuximide

T½: 0.7–2.6 hr (methsuximide)
 28–57 hr (normethsuximide)

Vd: ?

Fb: 0

pKa: ?

Occurrence and Usage. Methsuximide (Celontin) is a substituted succinimide first made available in 1951 and now widely used for the treatment of petit mal and psychomotor epilepsy. The compound is administered in doses of up to 1200 mg daily.

Blood Concentrations. Following a single oral administration of 1200 mg of methsuximide, plasma concentrations averaged 6.8 mg/L after 1 hour and declined to 0.4 mg/L by 12 hours (Glazko and Dill, 1972). Patients receiving 600–1200 mg of methsuximide daily and exhibiting good to excellent seizure control had almost negligible plasma concentrations of unchanged drug (average, 0.036 mg/L; range, 0.010–0.113) compared to those of the active metabolite, normethsuximide, which averaged 25 mg/L (range, 16–37). On the basis of these and other patients, it was concluded that effective plasma concentrations during methsuximide therapy lie between 10 and 40 mg/L, expressed as the metabolite (Strong et al., 1974). The plasma half-lives of methsuximide and normethsuximide in patients on therapy averaged 1.4 and 38 hours, respectively (Porter et al., 1979).

3-hydroxymethsuximide   methsuximide   normethsuximide

2-hydroxymethyl-methsuximide   m-, p-, and di-hydroxy-phenylmethsuximide   conjugation

Metabolism and Excretion. Methsuximide is extensively metabolized, primarily by N-demethylation to normethsuximide, which possesses significant anticonvulsant activity, has a longer half-life, and probably accounts for most of the effectiveness of the parent drug (Zimmerman, 1953; Nicholls and Orton, 1972). There is good evidence that methsuximide induces the rate of its own metabolism, since the 2.6 hour half-life found with the initial dose was only one-fourth as long after the fourth dose (Glazko and Dill, 1972). Methsuximide also undergoes oxidation of the phenyl ring, yielding both p- and m-hydroxymethsuximide in significant amounts. Less than 1% of an administered dose is excreted as unchanged methsuximide in the urine. Normethsuximide has been identified in urine qualitatively but not quantitatively, and it seems likely that it would undergo further metabolism. The major urinary metabolites are the conjugated p-hydroxyphenyl compounds, while minor metabolites include the 3-hydroxy, 2-hydroxymethyl and 2-dihydrodihydroxyphenyl derivatives (Glazko and Dill, 1972; Nicholls and Orton, 1972; Horning et al., 1973).

Toxicity. Adverse reactions to methsuximide administration include nausea, vomiting, diarrhea, drowsiness, ataxia, blurred vision, and blood dyscrasias. A case of nonfatal suicidal overdosage with methsuximide was described in which a teenager ingested approximately 10 g of the drug. Blood concentrations of methsuximide and normethsuximide 14 hours after ingestion were 18 and 44 mg/L, respectively. Coma lasted about 80 hours and correlated with the continued presence of the metabolite (Karch, 1973).

Analysis. A gas chromatographic method for the determination of underivatized succinimide anticonvulsants, including methsuximide and its major metabolite, has been reported (Bonitati, 1976). Liquid chromatography is also suitable to the simultaneous analysis of both compounds (Kabra et al., 1978). Procedures that include formation of methyl derivatives of antiepileptic drugs would be unsuitable for the simultaneous differential measurement of methsuximide and normethsuximide.

References

J. Bonitati. Gas chromatographic analysis for succinimide anticonvulsants in serum: macro- and micro-scale methods. Clin. Chem. 22: 341–345, 1976.

A.J. Glazko and W.A. Dill. Other succinimides. Methsuximide and phensuximide. In *Antiepileptic Drugs* (D.M. Woodbury, J.K. Penry and R.P. Schmidt eds.), Raven Press, New York, 1972, pp. 455–464.

M.G. Horning, C. Butler, D.J. Harvey et al. Metabolism of N,2-dimethyl-2-phenylsuccinimide (methsuximide) by the epoxide-diol pathway in rat, guinea pig and human. Res. Comm. Chem. Path. Pharm. 6: 565–577, 1973.

P.M. Kabra, D.M. McDonald and L.J. Marton. A simultaneous high-performance liquid chromatographic analysis of the most common anticonvulsants and their metabolites in the serum. J. Anal. Tox. 2: 127–133, 1978.

S.B. Karch. Methsuximide overdose. J. Am. Med. Asso. 223: 1463–1465, 1973.

P.J. Nicholls and T.C. Orton. The physiological disposition of ^{14}C-methsuximide in the rat. Brit. J. Pharm. 45: 48–59, 1972.

R.J. Porter, J.K. Penry, J.R. Lacy et al. Plasma concentrations of phensuximide, methsuximide, and their metabolites in relation to clinical efficacy. Neurology 29: 1509–1513, 1979.

J.M. Strong, T. Abe, E.L. Gibbs and A.J. Atkinson, Jr. Plasma levels of methsuximide and N-desmethyl-methsuximide during methsuximide therapy. Neurology 24: 250–255, 1974.

R.T. Zimmerman. New drugs in the treatment of petit mal epilepsy. Am. J. Psych. 109: 767–773, 1953.

Methyl Bromide

T½: ?
Vd: ?
Fb: ?

CH_3Br

Occurrence and Usage. Methyl bromide is a gaseous chemical (b.p. 5° C..) that is frequently employed as a fumigant for large enclosed residential, industrial and agricultural areas. It has also been used as a refrigerant and fire extinguishant. The threshold limit value for industrial usage is 5 ppm (19 mg/m³) in the atmosphere; at this level the compound has practically no detectable odor, but at higher concentrations the odor resembles that of chloroform. Exposure may be by inhalation or dermal absorption.

Blood Concentrations. Blood concentrations of intact methyl bromide after low-level occupational exposure have not been established. However, inorganic bromide blood concentrations have been measured in 12 asymptomatic methyl bromide workers and found to average 15 mg/L, with a range of 4–36 mg/L (Rathus and Landy, 1961). In another study, a range of 0–114 mg/L (average, 55) was found in workers (Drawneek et al., 1964). By contrast, patients receiving sodium bromide as an anticonvulsant or sedative often develop serum bromide concentrations of at least 75–100 mg/L (Maynert, 1965). Baseline blood bromide concentrations in normal subjects average 3 mg/L, with a range of 1–5 mg/L (Cross and Smith, 1978). The half-life of bromide in blood is about 12 days (Soremark, 1960).

Metabolism and Excretion. Methyl bromide is known to be partially converted in man to inorganic bromide. The contribution of this metabolite to the toxicity of the parent is not clear, but since inorganic bromide blood concentrations after methyl bromide poisoning are generally much lower than during intoxication by bromide salts, it is felt that methyl bromide itself is the primary toxic agent. Its ability to methylate sulfhydryl groups and thus inactivate enzymes has been postulated to play an important role in methyl bromide poisoning (Gosselin et al., 1976). There is a suggestion that a fraction of a dose (2–3%) may be eliminated in the urine as a mercapturic acid conjugate (Drawneek et al., 1964). Undoubtedly, much of the compound is rapidly exhaled unchanged, whereas the inorganic bromide that is formed as a metabolite has a serum half-life of about 15 days and is slowly excreted in the urine (Maynert, 1965).

Urinary bromide levels in non-exposed controls averaged 6.3 mg/L and, in workers exposed to an average methyl bromide air concentration of 3.8 ppm, averaged 9.0 mg/L; urine bromide levels correlated positively (r=0.60) with air concentrations of the chemical (Tanaka et al., 1991).

Toxicity. Methyl bromide toxicity following exposure often develops after a latent period of several hours, and is manifested by confusion, abdominal pain, weakness, nausea, convulsions, coma and occasionally pulmonary edema. Exposure to atmospheric concentrations of 600 ppm for a period of several hours may prove fatal. Persons who survive often require a long period of convalescence and may experience permanent disability due to continued weakness, vertigo and mental and motor impairment (Hine, 1969).

The serum inorganic bromide level in poisoned patients can often be correlated with severity of symptoms and has ranged from 24 mg/L in a person experiencing dizziness to 550 mg/L in a subject who suffered convulsions, with an overall average of 164 mg/L for 25 survivors (Clarke et al., 1945; Benatt and Courtney, 1948; Longley and Jones, 1965; Hine, 1969; Hustinx et al., 1993).

In 11 fatal cases of methyl bromide intoxication, blood bromide concentrations of 40–656 mg/L (average, 237) were noted (Clarke et al., 1945; Hine, 1969; Marraccini et al., 1983; Behrens and Dukes, 1986; Dempsey et al., 1992; Fuortes, 1992). These concentrations of inorganic bromide are only one-eighth those observed in fatalities due to carbromal, a brominated monoureide used as a sedative, and one-tenth those measured in nonfatal intoxications with inorganic bromide salts (Wenk et al., 1976). The following bromide concentrations were determined in an adult who died at least 6 hours after occupational exposure to methyl bromide (Alha, 1974):

Bromide Concentrations in a Methyl Bromide Fatality (mg/L or mg/kg)

Blood	Liver	Spleen	Kidney	Urine
144	84	114	90	200

Analysis. Intact methyl bromide has not been isolated from human tissues following exposure. Procedures for the analysis of inorganic bromide are cited in the section on bromide.

References

A. Alha. Personal communication, 1974.

R.H. Behrens and D.C.D. Duke. Fatal methyl bromide poisoning. Brit. J. Ind. Med. 43: 561–562, 1986.

A.J. Benatt and T.R.B. Courtney. Uraemia in methyl bromide poisoning: a case report. Brit. J. Ind. Med. 5: 21–25, 1948.

C.A. Clarke, C.G. Roworth and H.E. Holling. Methyl bromide poisoning. Brit. J. Ind. Med. 2: 17–23, 1945.

J.D. Cross and H. Smith. Bromine in human tissue. For. Sci. 11: 147–153, 1978.

D.A. Dempsey, C.E. Becker and F.C. Mihm. Death after entering an apartment building fumigated with methyl bromide and cleared for habitation. Vet. Hum. Tox. 34: 356, 1992.

W. Drawneek, M.J. O'Brien, H.J. Goldsmith, and R.E. Bourdillion. Industrial methyl-bromide poisoning in fumigators. Lancet 2: 855–856, 1964.

L.A. Fuortes. A case of fatal methyl bromide poisoning. Vet. Hum. Tox. 34: 240–241, 1992.

R.E. Gosselin, H.C. Hodge, R.P. Smith and M.N. Gleason. *Clinical Toxicology of Commercial Products*, 4th ed., Williams and Wilkins, Baltimore, 1976, pp. 233–237 (Section III).

C.H. Hine. Methyl bromide poisoning. A review of ten cases. J. Occ. Med. 11: 1–10, 1969.

W.N.M. Hustinx, R.T.H. van de Laar, A.C. van Huffelen et al. Systemic effects of inhalational methyl bromide poisoning. Brit. J. Ind. Health 50: 155–159, 1993.

E.O. Longley and A.T. Jones. Methyl bromide poisoning in man. Ind. Med. Surg. 34: 499–502, 1965.

J.V. Marraccini, G.E. Thomas, J.P. Ongley et al. Death and injury caused by methyl bromide, an insecticide fumigant. J. For. Sci. 28: 601–607, 1983.

E.W. Maynert. Sedatives and hypnotics I: nonbarbiturates. In *Drill's Pharmacology in Medicine* (J.R. DiPalma, ed.), 3rd ed., McGraw-Hill, New York, 1965, p. 184.

E.M. Rathus and P.J. Landy. Methyl bromide poisoning. Brit. J. Ind. Med. 18: 53–57, 1961.

R. Soremark. The biological half-life of bromide ions in human blood. Acta Physiol. Scand. 50: 119–123, 1960.

S. Tanaka, S. Abuku, Y. Seki and S. Imamiya. Evaluation of methyl bromide exposure on the plant quarantine fumigators by environmental and biological monitoring. Ind. Health 29: 11–21, 1991.

R.E. Wenk, J.A. Lustgarten, N.J. Pappas et al. Serum chloride analysis, bromide detection and the diagnosis of bromism. Am. J. Clin. Path. 64: 49–57, 1976.

Methyl n-Butyl Ketone

T½: ?
Vd: ?
Fb: 0 $CH_3COC_4H_9$

Occurrence and Usage. Methyl n-butyl ketone (2-hexanone) has been widely used as a solvent for plastic resins, inks and various cleaning agents. Its use has been limited recently due to concern over its potential to cause peripheral neuropathy. The current threshold limit value is 5 ppm (20 mg/m³).

Blood Concentrations. Serum concentrations of methyl n-butyl ketone reached an average peak level of 1.2 mg/L in 3 volunteers exposed to 100 ppm of the vapor for 1.5 hours; concentrations of the metabolite, 2,5-hexanedione, achieved an average peak of 0.9 mg/L at 0.5 hour after the exposure ended (DiVincenzo et al., 1978).

Metabolism and Excretion. In experimental animals, methyl-n-butyl ketone is metabolized to 2-hexanol, 5-hydroxy-2-hexanone, 2,5-hexanedione, and carbon dioxide (DiVincenzo et al., 1976; Abdel-Rahman et al., 1976). Humans given a labeled oral dose excreted 40% as carbon dioxide in breath and 26% as metabolites in urine over an 8 day period (DiVincenzo et al., 1978). 2,5-Hexanedione is also a metabolite of hexane (Krasavage et al., 1980).

Between 75–92% of inhaled methyl n-butyl ketone is absorbed by the human lung. Alveolar breath concentrations of the chemical reached average peak levels of 1.8, 10.8 and 24.7 ppm during a 7.5 hour exposure to air concentrations of 10, 50 or 100 ppm, respectively; these levels fell to 0.1, 0.3 and 0.6 ppm by 0.5 hour after the exposure ended (DiVincenzo et al., 1978).

Toxicity. Exposure of workers to methyl n-butyl ketone at moderate concentrations for periods of 6 months or more has caused peripheral neuropathy, characterized by loss of sensation and weakness of the extremities. Most individuals have shown improvement after removal from exposure (Billmaier et al., 1974; Allen et al., 1975). A metabolite, 2,5-hexanedione, is believed to be responsible for this syndrome (Raleigh et al., 1975). Air concentrations of 1000 ppm for more than several minutes cause eye and nose irritation.

Analysis. Methyl n-butyl ketone may be analyzed in breath or blood using a gas chromatographic technique (DiVincenzo et al., 1977).

References

M.S. Abdel-Rahman, L.B. Hetland and D. Couri. Toxicity and metabolism of methyl n-butyl ketone. Am. Ind. Hyg. Asso. J. 37: 95–102, 1976.

M. Allen, J.R. Mendell, D.J. Billmaier et al. Toxic polyneuropathy due to methyl n-butyl ketone. Arch. Neurol. 32: 209–218, 1975.

D. Billmaier, H.T. Yee, N. Allen et al. Peripheral neuropathy in a coated fabrics plant. J. Occ. Med. 16: 665–671, 1974.

G.D. DiVincenzo, C.J. Kaplan and J. Dedinas. Characterization of the metabolites of methyl n-butyl ketone, methyl iso-butyl ketone, and methyl ethyl ketone in guinea pig serum and their clearance. Tox. Appl. Pharm. 36: 511–522, 1976.

G.D. DiVincenzo, M.L. Hamilton, C.J. Kaplan and J. Dedinas. Metabolic fate and disposition of ^{14}C-labeled methyl n-butyl ketone in the rat. Tox. Appl. Pharm. 41: 547–560, 1977.

G.D. DiVincenzo, M.L. Hamilton, C.J. Kaplan et al. Studies on the respiratory uptake and excretion and the skin absorption of methyl n-butyl ketone in humans and dogs. Tox. Appl. Pharm. 44: 593–604, 1978.

W.J. Krasavage, J.L. O'Donoghue, G.D. DiVincenzo and C.J. Terhaar. The relative neurotoxicity of methyl-n-butyl ketone, n-hexane and their metabolites. Tox. Appl. Pharm. 52: 433–441, 1980.

R.L. Raleigh, P.S. Spencer and H.H. Schaumburg. Methyl n-butyl ketone. J. Occ. Med. 17: 286, 1975.

Methyl Chloride

T½: 50–90 min

Vd: ?

Fb: 0

CH_3Cl

Occurrence and Usage. Methyl chloride (chloromethane) is a colorless, odorless gas at room temperature that has been used as a refrigerant, blowing agent for plastic foams, and chemical intermediate. The current threshold limit value for industrial exposure is 50 ppm (105 mg/m³).

Blood Concentrations. Human volunteers exposed to methyl chloride for 6 hours have been shown to fall into 1 of 2 distinct subgroups; those exposed to an air concentration of 10 ppm developed approximate average blood methyl chloride concentrations of either 7 or 30 µg/L, while those exposed to 50 ppm developed blood levels of either 35 or 100 µg/L. Upon termination of exposure, those with the lower levels exhibited excretion half-lives averaging 50 minutes, while those with the higher levels exhibited half-lives averaging 90 minutes. Only 20–40% of the population is estimated to be in the latter group (Nolan et al., 1985).

Metabolism and Excretion. Methyl chloride is believed to be metabolized to formaldehyde and carbon dioxide; N-acetyl-S-methyl cysteine is purportedly a urinary excretion product (Torkelson and Rowe, 1981). Breath methyl chloride concentrations in volunteers averaged 10–15 µg/L or 50–80 µg/L during a 6 hour exposure to air concentrations of 10 or 50 ppm, respectively, and declined rapidly after the exposure ended (Nolan et al., 1985).

Toxicity. Methyl chloride is toxic to the nervous system, liver, kidneys and bone marrow. Toxicity may be expressed as drowsiness, dizziness, headache, slurred speech, confusion, staggering gait, nausea, vomiting, blurred vision, weakness, personality changes, cyanosis, convulsions, coma and death. These effects may occur following exposure to concentrations exceeding 200 ppm for several days or weeks; recovery may be complete but usually requires several months after removal from exposure. This syndrome was more common when methyl chloride was used as a refrigerant, but is still encountered occasionally in people who work with polystyrene foam, from which the chemical may offgas (McNally, 1946; Smith and von Oettingen, 1947; Hansen et al., 1953; Mackie, 1961; MacDonald, 1964; Scharnweber et al., 1974; Spevak et al., 1976; Lanham, 1982; Pasternak and Becker, 1986).

Analysis. Methyl chloride may be analyzed in blood or breath using an electron-capture gas chromatographic method (Landry et al., 1983).

References

H. Hansen, N.K. Weaver and F.S. Venable. Methyl chloride intoxication. AMA Arch. Ind. Hyg. Occ. Med. 8: 328–334, 1953.

T.D. Landry, T.S. Gushow, P.W. Langvardt et al. Pharmacokinetics and metabolism of inhaled methyl chloride in the rat and dog. Tox. Appl. Pharm. 68: 473–486, 1983.

J.M. Lanham. Methyl chloride: an unusual incident of intoxication. Can. Med. Asso. J. 126: 593, 1982.

J.D.C. MacDonald. Methyl chloride intoxication. J. Occ. Med. 6: 81–84, 1964.

I.J. Mackie. Methyl chloride intoxication. Med. J. Aust. 1: 203–205, 1961.

W.D. McNally. Eight cases of methyl chloride poisoning with three deaths. J. Ind. Hyg. Tox. 28: 94–97, 1946.

R.J. Nolan, D.L. Rick, T.D. Landry et al. Pharmacokinetics of inhaled methyl chloride (CH₃C1) in male volunteers. Fund. Appl. Tox. 5: 361–369, 1985.

G.A. Pasternak and C.E. Becker. Methyl chloride neurotoxicity—case report of cerebellar degeneration. Vet. Hum. Tox. 28: 473, 1986.

H.C. Scharnweber, G.N. Spears and S.R. Cowles. Chronic methyl chloride intoxication in six industrial workers. J. Occ. Med. 16: 112–113, 1974.

W.W. Smith and W.F. von Oettingen. The acute and chronic toxicity of methyl chloride. J. Ind. Hyg. Tox. 29: 47–52, 1947.

L. Spevak, V. Nadj and D. Felle. Methyl chloride poisoning in four members of a family. Brit. J. Ind. Med. 33; 272–278, 1976.

T.R. Torkelson and V.K. Rowe. Halogenated aliphatic hydrocarbons. In *Patty's Industrial Hygiene and Toxicology*, 3rd ed., Vol. IIB (G.D. Clayton and F.E. Clayton, eds.), John Wiley & Sons, New York, 1981, pp. 3436–3442.

Methyldopa

T½: 4–14 hours
Vd: 0.3 L/kg
Fb: less than 0.20
pKa: 2.2, 9.2, 10.6, 12.0

Occurrence and Usage. Methyldopa (alpha-methyl-3,4-dihydroxyphenylalanine, Aldomet) was synthesized as early as 1954 and was found to be an effective antihypertensive agent in 1960. The drug is known to inhibit dopa decarboxylase in peripheral adrenergic neurons, but recent evidence indicates that its effects are mediated primarily via a central mechanism. Methyldopa is available for oral use as the hydrochloride of the l-isomer in tablets of 125–250 mg, sometimes in combination with a diuretic, and is administered in daily doses of 500–2000 mg. The compound is also available as the hydrochloride of the ethyl ester (methyldopate) for intravenous infusion in doses of 250–1000 mg.

Blood Concentrations. Plasma concentrations of free methydopa, after the oral administration of 750 mg to 12 subjects, peaked at an average of 2.6 mg/L at 3 hours and declined to 1.8 mg/L by 5 hours; after a 90-minute intravenous infusion of 250 mg, an average maximal plasma level of 7.5 mg/L occurred at 1.5 hours (at the end of the infusion) and declined to 2.1 mg/L by 3.5 hours (Kwan et al., 1976). By contrast, the intravenous injection of 250 mg of methyldopa ethyl ester in a 5 minute period produced plasma concentrations of free and esterified drug that averaged 1.7 mg/L at 1 hour and 1.0 mg/L by 4 hours (Saavedra et al., 1975). The terminal half-life of the free drug has been found to range from 4–14 hours (Stenbaek et al., 1977). Plasma concentrations averaged 2.2 mg/L (range, 0.8–4.5) in 5 persons on chronic therapy with 500–1000 mg of the drug daily, 4 hours after the morning dose (Myhre et al., 1972a).

Metabolism and Excretion. Methyldopa is metabolized primarily by conjugation with sulfate at the p-hydroxy position. The sulfate conjugate accumulates in plasma, especially in patients with renal disease, and may reach concentrations as high as 67 mg/L during chronic oral therapy; there is some indication that it may contribute to the hypotensive effects of the drug (Myhre et al., 1972a). Methyldopa may also undergo p-O-methylation, and both this metabolite and the parent may be decarboxylated to yield the corresponding dopamine derivatives.

Normal subjects excrete within 2 days about 40% of an oral dose in the urine and 60% in the feces; the fecal product is entirely unchanged drug and represents unabsorbed methyldopa. Urinary constituents include unchanged drug (10–18%), methyldopa-O-sulfate (9–20%), free and conjugated 3-0-methyl-alpha-methyldopa (4%), alpha-methyldopamine (2–4%), 3,4-dihydroxyphenylacetone (3–5%) and 3-O-methyl-alpha-methyldopamine (0.3%) (Buhs et al., 1964; Au et al., 1972; Kwan et al., 1976). After intravenous injection, 100% of the dose is recovered in the 48 hour urine as unchanged drug (45–64%) and methyldopa-O-sulfate (1–2%), with the remainder as unquantitated amounts of the previously discussed metabolites (Myhre et al., 1972b; Kwan et al., 1976; Stenbaek et al., 1977).

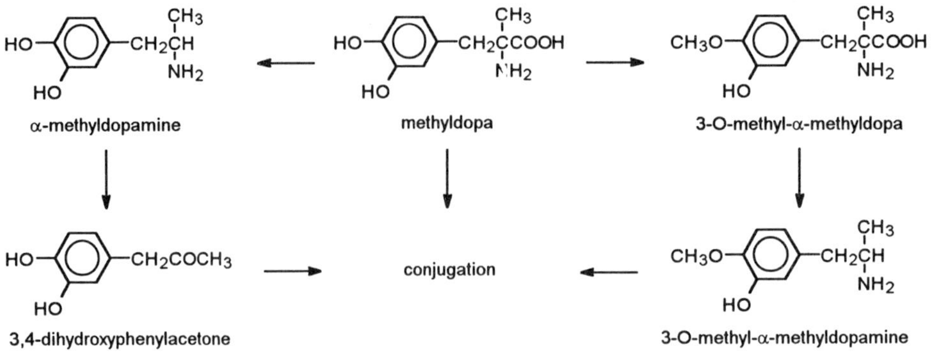

α-methyldopamine   methyldopa   3-O-methyl-α-methyldopa

3,4-dihydroxyphenylacetone   conjugation   3-O-methyl-α-methyldopamine

Toxicity. Adverse reactions to methyldopa administration include sedation, headache, weakness, nausea, vomiting, diarrhea, parasthesias, psychic disturbances, involuntary movements, orthostatic hypotension, blood dyscrasias, and liver damage. An elderly woman died of drug-induced hepatitis while on methyldopa therapy (Bezahler, 1982). Two cases of suspected drug overdosage were described in which methyldopa concentrations of 7.2 and 9.4 mg/L in serum and 126 and 129 mg/L in urine were determined (Clarke, 1969). A young man who survived the ingestion of 2.5 g of methyldopa had a serum concentration of 19 mg/L about 10 hours later, at which time he was comatose (Shnaps et al., 1982).

An adult who died within 1 day of overdosage with methyldopa was found to have postmortem concentrations of 9 mg/L in blood and 1400 mg/L in urine (Tamminen, 1970).

Analysis. Methyldopa may be assayed in biological fluids by ultraviolet spectrophotometry of the intact drug. A fluorometric technique has been widely used for the measurement of the drug and its conjugate (after acid hydrolysis), and involves oxidation to a highly fluorescent trihydroxyindole derivative (Sjoerdsma et al., 1963; Myhre et al., 1972c; Kim and Koda, 1977). Liquid chromatography has been applied to the determination of methyldopa in serum (Cooper et al., 1979; Kochak and Mason, 1980; Ong et al., 1982) and urine (Mell and Gustafson, 1978; Kochak and Mason, 1981).

References

W.Y.W. Au, L.G. Dring, D.G. Grahame-Smith et al. The metabolism of ^{14}C-labelled α-methyldopa in normal and hypertensive human subjects. Biochem. J. 129: 1–10 1972.

G.H. Bezahler. Fatal methyldopa-associated granulomatous hepatitis and myocarditis. Am. J. Med. Sci. 283: 41–45, 1982.

R.P. Buhs, J.L. Beck, O.C. Speth et al. The metabolism of methyldopa in hypertensive human subjects. J. Pharm. Exp. Ther. 143: 205–214, 1964.

E.G.C. Clarke (ed.). *Isolation and Identification of Drugs*, Pharmaceutical Press, London, 1969, pp. 422–423.

M.J. Cooper, R.F. O'Dea and B.L. Mirkin. Determination of methyldopa and metabolites in human serum by high-performance liquid chromatography with electrochemical detection. J. Chrom. 162: 601–604, 1979.

B.K. Kim and R.T. Koda. Fluorometric determination of methyldopa in biological fluids. J. Pharm. Sci. 66: 1632–1634, 1977.

G.M. Kochak and W.D. Mason. Determination of free methyldopa in plasma by high-pressure liquid chromatography and electrochemical detection. J. Pharm. Sci. 69: 897–900, 1980.

G.M. Kochak and W.D. Mason. A simplified method of determining free methyldopa in urine. Anal. Letters 14: 439–449, 1981.

K.C. Kwan, E.L. Foltz, G.O. Breault et al. Pharmacokinetics of methyldopa in man. J. Pharm. Exp. Ther. 198: 264–277, 1976.

L.D. Mell and A.B. Gustafson. Urinary free methyldopa determined by reversed-phase high-performance liquid chromatography. Clin. Chem. 24: 23–26, 1978.

E. Myhre, O. Stenbaek, E.K. Brodwall and T. Hansen. Conjugation of methyldopa in renal failure. Scand. J. Clin. Lab. Invest. 29: 195–199, 1972a.

E. Myhre, E.K. Brodwall, O. Stenbaek and T. Hanson. The renal excretion of methyldopa. Scand. J. Clin. Lab. Invest. 29: 201–204, 1972b.

E. Myhre, E.K. Brodwall, O. Stenbaek and T. Hansen. Plasma turnover of methyldopa in advanced renal failure. Acta Med. Scand. 191: 343–347, 1972c.

H. Ong, S. Sued and N. Beaudoin. Assay and stability of α-methyldopa in man using high-performance liquid chromatography with electrochemical detection. J. Chrom. 229: 433–438, 1982.

J.A. Saavedra, J.L. Reid, W. Jordan et al. Plasma concentration of α-methyldopa and sulphate conjugate after oral administration of methyldopa and intravenous administration of methyldopa and methyldopa hydro-chloride ethyl ester. Eur. J. Clin. Pharm. 8: 381–386, 1975.

Y. Shnaps, S. Almog, H. Halkin and M. Tirosh. Methyldopa poisoning. Clin. Tox. 19: 501–502, 1982.

S. Sjoerdsma, V. Vendsalu and K. Engelman. Studies on the metabolism and mechanism of action of methyldopa. Circulation 28: 492–502, 1963.

O. Stenbaek, E. Myhre, H.E. Rugstad et al. Pharmacokinetics of methyldopa in healthy man. Eur. J. Clin. Pharm. 12: 117–123, 1977.

V. Tamminen. Personal communication, 1970.

4,4'-Methylenebis(2-chloroaniline)

T½: ?
Vd: ?
Fb: ?
pKa: ?

Occurrence and Usage. 4,4'-Methylenebis(2-chloroaniline), or MOCA, is used as a curing agent for epoxy resins and isocyanate polymers. The substance is a solid at room temperature and may be absorbed following inhalation or dermal contact. The currently assigned threshold limit value is 0.02 ppm (0.22 mg/m^3), with a warning of suspected carcinogenic potential for man.

Blood Concentrations. Blood concentrations of MOCA in man have not been reported.

Metabolism and Excretion. Rats given 50 mg of MOCA orally excreted less than 0.1% of the dose unchanged in the 96 hour urine (Ducos et al., 1985). Mono- and di-N-acetyl-MOCA have been identified in human urine (Ducos et al., 1985), and the presence of an N-glucuronide conjugate has been demonstrated (Gristwood et al., 1984; Cocker et al., 1990).

Workers exposed to MOCA at air concentrations that generally averaged less than 0.01 mg/m^3 exhibited urine MOCA concentrations by gas chromatography that averaged 0.16–1.26 mg/L over a 12 month period, with individual maximum levels as high as 6.7 mg/L (Linch et al., 1971). In a French factory, workers' urine MOCA concentrations were lowered from an initial average of 0.600 mg/L to 0.062 mg/L through improved manufacturing procedures (Ducos et al., 1985).

Toxicity. MOCA is known to be a mild skin irritant. It causes lung and liver cancer in rats and urinary tumors in dogs. Due to its structural similarity to benzidine, it is suspected of being a human carcinogen, but workers exposed for up to 16 years showed no unusual signs compared to controls (Linch et al., 1971). A worker who was accidentally sprayed with MOCA suffered only eye irritation and nausea; his urine contained 3.6 mg/L MOCA on the day of exposure, but only 0.03 mg/L the day after (Hosein and Van Roosmalen, 1978).

Analysis. Total urinary diazotizable amines, including MOCA and its metabolites, may be measured by colorimetry (Linch et al., 1971). More sensitive and specific electron-capture gas chromatographic (Gristwood et al., 1984; Thomas and Wilson, 1984) and liquid chromatographic procedures (Okayama et al., 1988; Ichikawa et al., 1990) have also been described. Urine specimens that are allowed to stand for 24 hours at room temperature show a 2–5 fold increase in apparent MOCA concentration due to the lability of the N-glucuronide conjugate (Cocker and Wilson, 1989).

References

J. Cocker and H.K. Wilson. Determination of 4,4'-methylenebis(2-chloroaniline) in urine. Clin. Chem. 35: 506, 1989.

J. Cocker, A.R. Boobis, H.K. Wilson and D. Gompertz. Evidence that a β-N-glucuronide of 4,4'-methylenebis(2-chloroaniline) (MbOCA) is a major urinary metabolite in man. Brit. J. Ind. Med. 47: 154–161, 1990.

P. Ducos, C. Maine and R. Gaudin. Assessment of occupational exposure to 4,4'-methylene-bis-(2-chloroaniline) "MOCA" by a new sensitive method for biological monitoring. Int. Arch. Occ. Env. Health 55: 159–167, 1985.

W. Gristwood, S.M. Robertson and H.K. Wilson. The determination of 4,4'-methylenebis (2-chloroaniline) in urine by electron-capture gas chromatography. J. Anal. Tox. 8: 101–105, 1984.

H.R. Hosein and P.B. Van Roosmalen. Acute exposure to methylene-bis-ortho chloroaniline (MOCA). Am. Ind. Hyg. Asso. J. 39: 496–497, 1978.

Y. Ichikawa, M. Yoshida, A. Okayama et al. Biological monitoring for workers exposed to 4,4'-methylenebis(2-chloroaniline). Am. Ind. Hyg. Asso. J. 51: 5–7, 1990.

A.L. Linch, G.B. O'Connor, J.R. Barnes et al. Methylene-bis-ortho-chloroaniline (MOCA): evaluation of hazards and exposure control. Am. Ind. Hyg. Asso. J. 32: 802–819, 1971.

A. Okayama, Y. Ichikawa, M. Yoshida et al. Determination of 4,4'-methylenebis(chloroaniline) in urine by liquid chromatography with ion-paired solid-phase extraction and electrochemical detection. Clin. Chem. 34: 2122–2125, 1988.

J.D. Thomas and H.K. Wilson. Biological monitoring of workers exposed to 4,4'-methylenebis(2-chloraniline) (MBOCA). Brit. J. Ind. Med. 41: 547–551, 1984.

Methylenedioxyamphetamine

T½: ?
Vd: ?
Fb: ?
pKa: ?

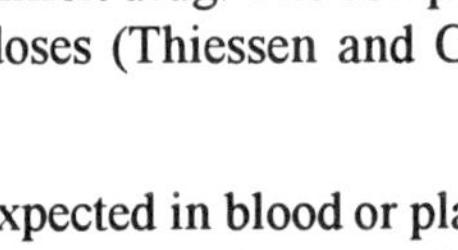

Occurrence and Usage. 3,4-Methylenedioxyamphetamine (MDA) is a psychotropic amphetamine derivative first synthesized in 1910. It is similar in potency to p-methoxyamphetamine, and is administered both orally and intravenously in doses of 50–250 mg as an illicit drug. The compound is primarily a central stimulant and may be hallucinogenic in large doses (Thiessen and Cook, 1973).

Blood Concentrations. No information is available on concentrations expected in blood or plasma after usual doses of MDA, although an analogy with amphetamine suggests that these would not exceed 0.4 mg/L.

Metabolism and Excretion. The human metabolism of this compound has not been studied; urine concentrations in fatal cases of up to 160 mg/L have been recorded and are indicative of excretion of substantial portions of unchanged drug (Cimbura, 1972). In animals, MDA is metabolized by O-dealkylation, deamination, and conjugation (Midha et al., 1978).

Toxicity. Overdosage with MDA causes agitation, tremor, tachycardia, rapid breathing, pupillary dilation, hyperthermia, muscular rigidity, convulsions and coma. These effects were produced in 3 subjects by the ingestion of 500 mg; they were discharged 12–24 hours after admission (Richards and Borgstedt, 1971). A 1 year old child who survived an MDA overdose developed unconsciousness, muscle rigidity and seizures; an admission urine specimen contained 131 mg/L MDA (Vidal, 1992).

The following distribution has been noted in 12 fatalities that followed ingestion of as little as 1000 mg of MDA by young adults (Cimbura, 1972; Kier, 1972, Reed et al., 1972; Fiorese, 1974, 1975; Lukaszewski, 1979; Poklis et al., 1979; Gottschalk and Cravey, 1980):

MDA Concentrations in Fatal Cases (mg/L or mg/kg)

	Blood	Liver	Bile	Kidney	Urine	Gastric
Average	9.3	12	7	18	108	6 mg
(Range)	(1.8–26)	(8–17)	(5–9)	(18)	(2–175)	(0.2–22)

Analysis. MDA may be determined in biologic media using most methods that are relevant to amphetamine analysis. Quantitative procedures include colorimetry (DeMayo et al., 1972), ultraviolet spectrophotometry (Cimbura, 1972) and gas chromatography (Midha et al., 1976).

References

G. Cimbura. 3,4-Methylenedioxyamphetamine (MDA): analytical and forensic aspects of fatal poisoning. J. For. Sci. 17: 329–333, 1972.

M.M. DeMayo, E.J. Briglia, Jr. and L.A. Dal Cortivo. Colorimetric determination of 3,4-methylenedioxyamphetamine (MDA). J. For. Sci. 17: 444–446, 1972.

F. Fiorese. Personal communication, 1974.

F. Fiorese. Personal communication, 1975.

L.A. Gottschalk and R.H. Cravey. *Toxicological and Pathological Studies on Psychoactive Drug-Involved Deaths*, Biomedical Publications, Davis, California, 1980, pp. 255–256.

L. Kier. Personal communication, 1972.

T. Lukaszewski. 3,4-Methylenedioxyamphetamine overdose. Clin. Tox. 15: 405–409, 1979.

K.K. Midha, I.J. McGilveray, S.P. Bhatnager and J.K. Cooper. GLC identification and determination of 3,4-methylenedioxyamphetamine in vivo in dog and monkey. Drug Met. Disp. 6: 623–630, 1978.

K.K. Midha, J.W. Hubbard, K. Bailey and J.K. Cooper. α-Methyldopamine, a key intermediate in the metabolic disposition of 3,4-methylenedioxyamphetamine in vivo in dog and monkey. Drug Met. Disp. 6: 623–630, 1978.

A. Poklis, M.A. Mackell and W.K. Drake. Fatal intoxication from 3,4-methylenedioxyamphetamine. J. For. Sci. 24: 70–75, 1979.

D. Reed, R.H. Cravey and P.R. Sedgwick. A fatal case involving methylenedioxyamphetamine. Clin. Tox. 5: 3–6, 1972.

K.C. Richards and H.H. Borgstedt. Near fatal reaction to ingestion of the hallucinogenic drug MDA. J. Am. Med. Asso. 218: 1826–1827, 1971.

P.M. Thiessen and D.A. Cook. The properties of 3,4-methylenedioxyamphetamine (MDA). Clin. Tox. 6: 45–52, 1973.

D.L. Vidal. Personal communication, 1992.

Methylenedioxymethamphetamine

T½: 7.6 hours
Vd: ?
Fb: ?
pKa: ?

Occurrence and Usage. 3,4-Methylenedioxymethamphetamine (MDMA, Ecstasy, XTC) is a ring-substituted derivative of methamphetamine that has been evaluated as an adjunct to psychotherapy. In recent years, its widespread use as a recreational drug caused the U.S. Drug Enforcement Administration to place the compound in Schedule I. The drug is usually taken in oral doses of 100–150 mg as the hydrochloride.

Blood Concentrations. A peak plasma MDMA level of 0.106 mg/L was measured 2 hours after oral ingestion of 50 mg by a 74 kg male adult; the peak level of the metabolite, methylenedioxyamphetamine, was 0.028 mg/L and occurred at 4 hours (Verebey et al., 1988). An oral 1.5 mg/kg (105 mg/70 kg) dose given to adult patients produced an average maximum plasma MDMA concentration of 0.300 mg/L at 2.3 hours (Helmlin et al., 1993).

Metabolism and Excretion. MDMA is known to be metabolized by N-demethylation to methylenedioxyamphetamine (MDA); urinary excretion accounts for 65% of the dose as parent drug and 7% as MDA within 3 days (Verebey et al., 1988). Urinary MDMA concentrations following a 1.5 mg/kg (105 mg/70 kg) oral dose may exceed 17 mg/L. Other urinary metabolites include mono- and di-hydroxy derivatives of MDMA and MDA, resulting from fission of the methylene bridge, which are eliminated as conjugates (Helmlin et al., 1993).

Toxicity. Symptoms of MDMA toxicity occurring in a 32 year old woman after ingestion of about 200 mg included visual hallucinations, confusion, agitation, coma and hypotension; a serum MDMA concentration of 7 mg/L was reported (Brown et al., 1986). Several abusers of the drug have experienced long-lasting neurobehavioral disturbances following cessation of use (McCann and Ricaurte, 1991; McGuire and Fahy, 1991).

Following the ingestion of approximately 150 mg of MDMA, a healthy 18 year old woman collapsed and died in ventricular fibrillation; postmortem toxicology revealed 1.0 mg/L MDMA and 0.04 g/dL ethanol in the blood (Dowling et al., 1987). Five other adults who succumbed to MDMA overdosage had postmortem blood concentrations of 0.6–2.8 mg/L (average, 1.8) (Reynolds, 1987; Suarez and Riemersma, 1988; Rohrig and Prouty, 1992; Forrest et al., 1994).

Analysis. MDMA can be determined in biological specimens using most methods that are applicable to amphetamine analysis. A specific gas chromatographic-mass spectrometric technique has been described (Gan et al., 1991).

References

C.R. Brown, H. McKinney, J.D. Osterloh et al. Severe adverse reaction to 3,4-methylenedioxymethamphetamine (MDMA). Vet. Hum. Tox. 28: 490, 1986.

G.P. Dowling, E.T. McDonough and R.O. Bost. 'Eve' and 'Ecstasy', a report of five deaths associated with the use of MDEA and MDMA. J. Am. Med. Asso. 257: 1615–1617, 1987.

A.R.W. Forrest, J.H. Halloway, I.D. Marsh et al. A fatal overdose with 3,4-methylenedioxyamphetamine derivatives. For. Sci. Int. 64: 57–59, 1994.

B.K. Gan, D. Baugh, R.H. Liu and A.S. Walia. Simultaneous analysis of amphetamine, methamphetamine, and 3,4-methylenedioxymethamphetamine (MDMA) in urine samples. J. For. Sci. 36: 1331–1341, 1991.

H.J. Helmlin, K. Bracher, S.J. Salamone and R. Brenneisen. Analysis of 3,4-methylenedioxymethamphetamine (MDMA) and its metabolites in human plasma and urine. Presented at the annual meeting of the Society of Forensic Toxicologists, Phoenix, Arizona, October 15, 1993.

U.D. McCann and G.A. Ricaurte. Lasting neuropsychiatric sequelae of (+) methylenedioxymethamphetamine ('Ecstasy') in recreational users. J. Clin. Psychopharm. 11: 302–305, 1991.

P. McGuire and T. Fahy. Chronic paranoid psychosis after misuse of MDMA ("ecstasy"). Brit. Med. J. 302: 697, 1991.

P. Reynolds. Personal communication, 1987.

T.P. Rohrig and R.W. Prouty. Tissue distribution of methylenedioxymethamphetamine. J. Anal. Tox. 16: 52–53, 1992.

R.V. Suarez and R. Riemersma. "Ecstasy" and sudden cardiac death. Am. J. For. Med. Path. 9: 339–341, 1988.

K. Verebey, J. Alrazi and J.H. Jaffe. The complications of 'Ecstasy' (MDMA). J. Am. Med. Asso. 259: 1649–1650, 1988.

Methyl Ethyl Ketone

T½: 1.3 hours
Vd: ? $CH_3COC_2H_5$
Fb: 0

Occurrence and Usage. Methyl ethyl ketone (2-butanone, MEK) is commonly employed as a solvent in paints, varnishes, paint removers and thinners, cleaning agents and adhesives. The odor threshold is approximately 25 ppm, while the current threshold limit value for occupational exposure is 200 ppm (590 mg/m^3).

Blood Concentrations. Workers exposed to MEK at air concentrations of 10–175 mg/m^3 (3–60 ppm) developed blood MEK levels of 0.8–9.6 mg/L, averaging 2.6 mg/L. The blood/breath ratio averaged 116 and the blood/environmental air ratio averaged 35 (Perbellini et al., 1984). Exposure of volunteers to average MEK air concentrations of 100 or 200 ppm for 4 hours resulted in average peak blood MEK levels of 1.9 and 3.5 mg/L, respectively, at the end of the exposure; the levels had declined to 0.5 and 1.0 mg/L, respectively, by 1.5 hours after the end of the exposure (Dick et al., 1988).

Metabolism and Excretion. In experimental animals, MEK is known to be metabolized to 2-butanol, 3-hydroxy-2-butanone and 2,3-butanediol (DiVincenzo et al., 1976). Humans excrete about 0.1% of an absorbed dose unchanged in the urine, with a similar amount present as 3-hydroxy-2-butanone. MEK and this metabolite were present at concentrations averaging 0.5 and 0.6 mg/L, respectively, in workers exposed to air levels of MEK averaging 101 mg/m^3 (34 ppm). Alveolar breath concentrations average 30% of the environmental air concentration of MEK in exposed workers (Miyasaka et al., 1982; Perbellini et al., 1984). Ong et al. (1991) reported a good correlation between urinary MEK levels and the atmospheric concentration of the chemical; urine levels in workers averaged 3.6 mg/L at the TLV of 200 ppm.

Toxicity. MEK causes nose and throat irritation at concentrations of 100 ppm, eye irritation at 200 ppm, headache at 300 ppm, and weakness and paresthesias at levels of 300–600 ppm. Higher levels lead to greater degrees of control nervous system depression, including confusion, loss of coordination, and drowsiness. MEK by itself has not been shown to cause peripheral neuropathy in animals or man, but it does markedly potentiate the ability of n-hexane to cause that condition, even in small amounts (Altenkirch et al., 1978). An adult male who intentionally ingested 240 mL of a solution containing MEK and methanol was successfully treated with ethanol infusion and hemodialysis; his admission blood contained 1240 mg/L MEK and 240 mg/L 2-butanol, as well as 2020 mg/L methanol (Price et al., 1944).

Analysis. MEK may be determined in blood, breath or urine using flame-ionization gas chromatography (DiVincenzo et al., 1976; Miyasaka et al., 1982; Kezic and Monster, 1988). Liquid chromatography has also been reported (van Doorn et al., 1989).

References

H. Altenkirch, G. Stoltenburg and H.M. Wagner. Experimental studies on hydrocarbon neuropathies induced by methyl-ethyl-ketone (MEK). J. Neurol. 219: 159–170, 1978.

R.B. Dick, W.D. Brown, J.V. Setzer et al. Effects of short duration exposures to acetone and methyl ethyl ketone. Tox. Letters 43: 31–49, 1988.

G.D. DiVincenzo, C.J. Kaplan and J. Dedinas. Characterization of the metabolites of methyl n-butyl ketone, methyl iso-butyl ketone, and methyl ethyl ketone in guinea pig serum and their clearance. Tox. Appl. Pharm. 36: 511–522, 1976.

S. Kezic and A.C. Monster. Determination of methyl ethyl ketone and its metabolites in urine using capillary gas chromatography. J. Chrom. 428: 275–280, 1988.

M. Miyasaka, M. Kumar, A. Koizumi et al. Biological monitoring of occupational exposure to methyl ethyl ketone by means of urinalysis for methyl ethyl ketone itself. Int. Arch. Occ. Env. Health 50: 131–137, 1982.

C.N. Ong, G.L. Sia, H.Y. Ong et al. Biological monitoring of occupational exposure to methyl ethyl ketone. Int. Arch. Occ. Env. Health 63: 319–324, 1991.

L. Perbellini, F. Brugnone, P. Mozzo et al. Methyl ethyl ketone exposure in industrial workers. Int. Arch. Occ. Env. Health 54: 73–81, 1984.

E.A. Price, A. D'Alessandro, T. Kearney et al. Osmolar gap with minimal acidosis in combined methanol and methyl ethyl ketone ingestion. Clin. Tox. 32: 79–84, 1994.

J.E. van Doorn, J. de Cock, S. Kezic and A.C. Monster. Determination of methyl ethyl ketone in human urine after derivatization with o-nitrophenylhydrazine, using solid-phase extraction and reversed-phase high-performance liquid chromatography and ultraviolet detection. J. Chrom. 489: 411–418, 1989.

Methylfentanyl

T½: ?
Vd: ?
Fb: ?
pKa: ?

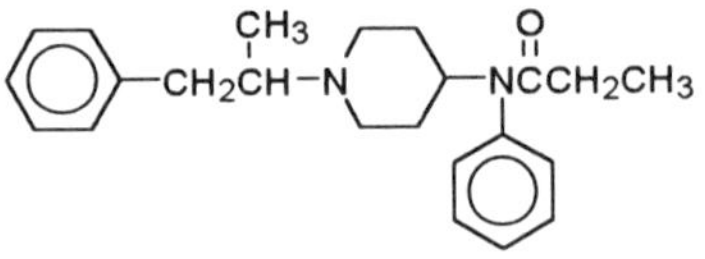

Occurrence and Usage. Methylfentanyl (alpha-methylfentanyl, "China white") is a narcotic analgesic closely related to and approximately equipotent with fentanyl. It was first detected as a street drug in California in late 1979. The drug is administered by intravenous injection or by insufflation; 5–10 µg is believed to constitute a typical dose. Street samples of the drug have been found to contain 0.4–0.9 µg/mg methylfentanyl. Recently, 3-methylfentanyl, believed to be more than 10 times as potent as fentanyl, has been detected as a street drug.

Blood Concentrations. Blood concentrations of methylfentanyl have not been measured in man following recreational usage. By analogy to fentanyl, concentrations are probably in the 1–5 µg/L range during the first hour after intravenous injection.

Metabolism and Excretion. The biotransformation of methylfentanyl has not been studied, but the drug is probably extensively metabolized. Despropionylmethylfentanyl has been identified in human tissues as a potential metabolite (Gillespie et al., 1982).

Toxicity. Methylfentanyl is capable of causing coma and severe respiratory depression. The following concentrations of the drug were found in postmortem specimens from 8 adults who died after intravenous overdosage (Reed, 1981; Gillespie et al., 1982):

Methylfentanyl Concentrations in Fatal Cases (µg/L or µg/kg)

	Blood	Liver	Bile	Urine
Average	7	78	47	47
(Range)	(2–11)	(78)	(6–75)	(5–151)

Analysis. Methylfentanyl may be assayed in biological specimens using the methods cited in the section on fentanyl. A nitrogen-phosphorus gas chromatographic procedure was developed specifically for the drug (Gillespie et al., 1982).

References

T.J. Gillespie, A.J. Gandolfi, T.P. Davis and R.A. Morano. Identification and quantification of alpha-methylfentanyl in post mortem specimens. J. Anal. Tox. 6: 139–142, 1982.

D. Reed. Presented at the quarterly meeting of the California Association of Toxicologists, San Jose, August 1, 1981.

Methylphenidate

T½: 2.4–4.2 hr
Vd: 11–33 L/kg
Fb: 0.15
pKa: 8.8

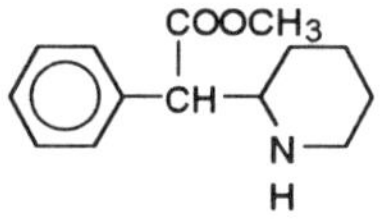

Occurrence and Usage. Methylphenidate (Ritalin) is a phenethylamine derivative used in the treatment of depression, narcolepsy and childhood hyperkinesis. The compound was first synthesized in 1944 and is currently marketed as the hydrochloride of the threo racemate. It is administered orally in single doses of 5–20 mg and daily doses of 20–60 mg. Methylphenidate has achieved popularity as a drug of abuse, being administered by intravenous injection of the dissolved tablets.

Blood Concentrations. Plasma methylphenidate concentrations in 2 women averaged 0.019 and 0.036 mg/L at 1 and 3 hours after a single oral dose of 20 mg; plasma ritalinic acid concentrations averaged 0.151 and 0.120 mg/L at the same times (Milberg et al., 1975). Plasma concentrations in 4 children given a 10–15 mg oral dose ranged from 0.004–0.025 mg/L for methylphenidate and 0.080–0.250 mg/L for ritalinic acid, 3–6 hours after ingestion (Hungund et al., 1978). The plasma half-life of the drug averaged 2.6 hours in 4 children (Hungund et al., 1979). In adults, plasma half-lives averaged 2.1 hours for methylphenidate and 4.0 hours for ritalinic acid (Wargin et al., 1983). The blood/plasma concentration ratio of methylphenidate in one subject was 0.7–0.8 (Redalieu et al., 1982).

Metabolism and Excretion. Methylphenidate is rapidly biotransformed by hydrolysis of the ester linkage to ritalinic acid (alpha-phenyl-2-piperidineacetic acid), an inactive metabolite. This hydrolysis step also occurs in aqueous alkaline solutions during storage, and during incubation with blood or plasma; it may be retarded by acidification or addition of EDTA (Schubert, 1970; Perel and Black, 1970). About 80% of a dose of methylphenidate is eliminated in the urine in a 24 hour period (Dayton et al., 1970), primarily as ritalinic acid (60–81%) and 6-oxo-alpha-phenyl-2-piperidineacetic acid (5–12%) (Bartlett and Egger, 1972). Normally less than 1% of a dose is excreted unchanged in the urine, although this may be enhanced by acidification of the urine. Minor urinary metabolites include p-hydroxymethylphenidate and p-hydroxyritalinic acid (Faraj et al., 1974).

Wells et al. (1974) found methylphenidate and ritalinic acid concentrations as high as 3.3 and 64 mg/L, respectively, in the 6 hour urine of children treated with a 10 mg dose. Urine methylphenidate concentrations ranged from 0.107–0.940 mg/L in the 8 hours following a 25 mg oral dose to 5 adults (Dugal et al., 1978).

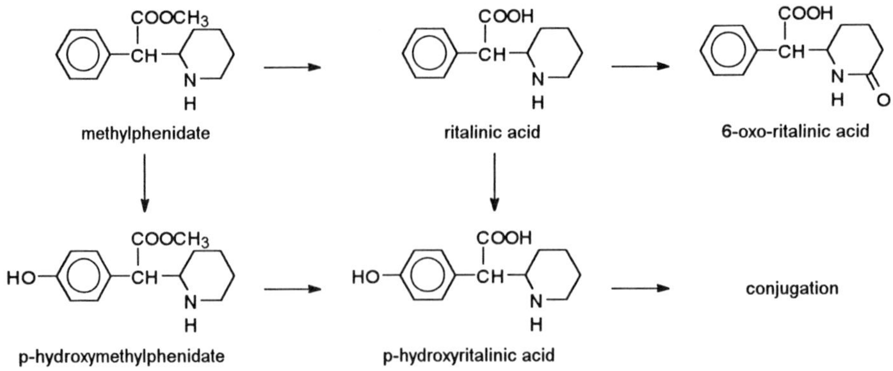

methylphenidate → ritalinic acid → 6-oxo-ritalinic acid

p-hydroxymethylphenidate → p-hydroxyritalinic acid → conjugation

Toxicity. Overdosage with methylphenidate may cause nausea, vomiting, agitation, tremors, twitching, delerium, hallucinations, sweating, flushing of the skin, headache, tachycardia, hyperpyrexia, cardiac arrhythmias, hypertension, convulsions, and coma. Relatively few instances of serious toxicity due to overdosage with this drug have been recorded. A related hazard of intravenous methylphenidate abuse is the development of talc granulomatosis, which has proven fatal (Lewman, 1972). Schubert (1970) found methylphenidate concentrations ranging from 0.8–40 mg/L (average, 16) in the urine of 6 arrested drivers who exhibited symptoms of hyperactivity or drowsiness. One of these persons demonstrated a blood concentration of 0.5 mg/L 12 hours after the ingestion of an unknown quantity of the drug.

Postmortem concentrations of 2.8 mg/L in blood and 2.1 mg/kg in liver were found in an adult woman who became hypertensive and died in cardiac arrest about 1 hour after intravenously injecting 40 mg of methylphenidate (Levine et al., 1986).

Analysis. Screening of urine specimens for ritalinic acid may be performed by thin-layer chromatography (van Boven and Daenens, 1979; Manno et al., 1986). Quantitative assays of this drug in biological fluids have involved the differential extraction of methylphenidate and ritalinic acid, with conversion of the latter to methylphenidate by reaction with diazomethane. Determination of both is accomplished by gas chromatography with flame-ionization (Schubert, 1970; Wells et al., 1974), nitrogen-phosphorus (Dugal et al., 1978; Hungund et al., 1978), or mass spectrometric detection (Milberg et al., 1975; Iden and Hungund, 1979). Gas chromatographic techniques for methylphenidate alone have employed nitrogen-phosphorus (Potts et al., 1984), electron-capture (Huffman et al., 1974) and mass spectrometric detection (Chan et al., 1980; Patrick and Jarvi, 1990). Liquid chromatography has also been applied to the measurement of the drug (Soldin et al., 1979b; Lalande et al., 1987) and its major metabolite (Soldin et al., 1979a) in serum.

References

M.F. Bartlett and H.P. Egger. Disposition and metabolism of methylphenidate in dog and man. Fed. Proc. 31: 537, 1972.

Y.M. Chan, S.J. Soldin, J.M. Swanson et al. Gas chromatographic/mass spectrometric analysis of methylphenidate (Ritalin) in serum. Clin. Biochem. 13: 266–272, 1980.

P.E. Dayton, J.M. Read and V. Ong. Physiological disposition of methylphenidate C-14 in man. Fed. Proc. 29: 345, 1970.

R. Dugal, M.A. Rouleau and M.J. Bertrand. The nitrogen-phosphorus detector in the gas chromatographic assay of unmetabolized methylphenidate. J. Anal. Tox. 2: 101–106, 1978.

B.A. Faraj, Z.H. Israili, J.M. Perel et al. Metabolism and disposition of methylphenidate-^{14}C: studies in man and animals. J. Pharm. Exp. Ther. 191: 535–547, 1974.

R. Huffman, J.W. Blake, R. Ray et al. Methylphenidate blood plasma levels in the horse determined by derivative gas-liquid chromatography-electron capture. J. Chrom. Sci. 12: 383–384, 1974.

B.L. Hungund, M. Hanna and B.G. Winsberg. A sensitive gas chromatographic method for the determination of methylphenidate (Ritalin) and its major metabolite α-phenyl-2-piperidine acetic acid (ritalinic acid) in human plasma using nitrogen-phosphorus detector. Comm. Psychopharm. 2: 203–208, 1978.

B.L. Hungund, J.M. Perel, M.J. Hurwic et al. Pharmacokinetics of methylphenidate in hyperkinetic children. Brit. J. Clin. Pharm. 8: 571–576, 1979.

C.R. Iden and B.L. Hungund. A chemical ionization selected ion monitoring assay for methylphenidate and ritalinic acid. Biomed. Mass Spec. 6: 422–426, 1979.

M. Lalande, D.L. Wilson and I.J. McGilveray. HPLC determination of methylphenidate in human plasma. J. Liq. Chrom. 10: 2257–2264, 1987.

B. Levine, Y.H. Caplan and G. Kauffman. Fatality resulting from methylphenidate overdose. J. Anal. Tox. 10: 209–210, 1986.

L.V. Lewman. Fatal pulmonary hypertension from intravenous injection of methylphenidate (Ritalin) tablets. Hum. Path. 3: 67–70, 1972.

B.R. Manno, J.E. Manno and C.A. Dempsey. A thin layer chromatographic method for high volume screening of urine for methylphenidate abuse. J. Anal. Tox. 10: 116–119, 1986.

R. Milberg, K.L. Rinehart, Jr., R.L. Sprague and E.K. Sleator. A reproducible gas chromatographic mass spectrometric assay for low levels of methylphenidate and ritalinic acid in blood and urine. Biomed. Mass Spec. 2: 2–8, 1975.

K.S. Patrick and E.J. Jarvi. Capillary gas chromatographic-mass spectrometric analysis of plasma methylphenidate. J. Chrom. 528: 214–220, 1990.

J.M. Perel and N. Black. In vitro metabolism studies with methylphenidate. Fed. Proc. 29: 345, 1970.

B.D. Potts, C.A. Martin and M. Vore. Gas-chromatographic quantification of methylphenidate in plasma with use of solid-phase extraction and nitrogen-sensitive detection. Clin. Chem. 30: 1374–1377, 1984.

E. Redalieu, M.F. Bartlett, L.M. Waldes et al. A study of methylphenidate in man with respect to its major metabolite. Drug Met. Disp. 10: 708–709, 1982.

B. Schubert. Detection and identification of methylphenidate in human urine and blood samples. Acta Chem. Scand. 24: 433–438, 1970.

S.J. Soldin, B.M. Hill, Y.P.M. Chan et al. A liquid-chromatographic analysis for ritalinic acid [α-phenyl-α-(2-piperidyl)acetic acid] in serum. Clin. Chem. 25: 51–54, 1979a.

S.J. Soldin, Y.P.M. Chan, B.M. Hill and J.M. Swanson. Liquid-chromatographic analysis for methylphenidate (Ritalin) in serum. Clin. Chem. 25: 401–404, 1979b.

M. van Boven and P. Daenens. Determination at the nanogram range of ritalinic acid in urine after ion-pair extraction. J. For. Sci. 24: 55–60, 1979.

R. Wells, K.B. Hammond and D.O. Rodgerson. Gas-liquid chromatographic procedure for measurement of methylphenidate hydrochloride and its metabolite, ritalinic acid, in urine. Clin. Chem. 20: 440–443, 1974.

W. Wargin, K. Patrick, C. Kilts et al. Pharmacokinetics of methylphenidate in man, rat and monkey. J. Pharm. Exp. Ther. 226: 382–386, 1983.

Methyl Salicylate

T½: ?
Vd: ?
Fb: ?

Occurrence and Usage. Methyl salicylate (oil of wintergreen) is found in the leaves of *Gaultheria procumbens* or the bark of *Betula lenta*. Commercial methyl salicylate is synthesized by esterification of salicylic acid with methanol. The compound is used medicinally as a counter-irritant and an analgesic. Due to its irritating effect on the gastric mucosa, medicinal use has been restricted to external application. It is available for topical use in solutions, liniments, creams and ointments in concentrations of 10% and higher.

Blood Concentrations. Blood methyl salicylate concentrations following therapeutic administration of the drug have not been reported.

Metabolism and Excretion. Although the disposition of methyl salicylate has been little studied in man, rat studies have shown that the conversion of methyl salicylate to salicylate occurs predominately in the liver. In human studies, it was noted that very little hydrolysis occurred in blood, either in the plasma or red blood cells (Davison et al., 1960).

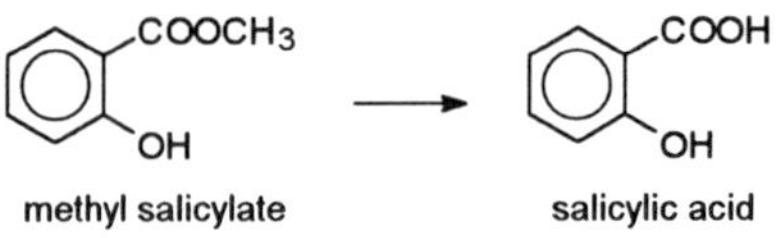

methyl salicylate   salicylic acid

Toxicity. Allergy to methyl salicylate, with the production of urticaria and angioedema, has been described (Speer, 1979). A 35 year old woman who survived ingestion of 60 mL of oil of wintergreen had a blood salicylate concentration of 1200 mg/L 45 hours after ingestion (Tabor et al., 1981). A 22 month old child was hospitalized after ingestion of an unknown quantity of oil of wintergreen; a blood salicylate concentration of 980 mg/L was reported from a sample taken 6 hours post-ingestion (Lester, 1984).

A 60 year old senile, alcoholic woman wandering the streets holding an empty bottle of oil of wintergreen was hospitalized, but died the following day of metabolic acidosis; a serum salicylate concentration of 1050 mg/L was reported on admission, while postmortem blood contained 650 mg/L (Levine and Caplan, 1984). A 59 year old woman who died 8.5 hours after ingestion of oil of wintergreen had salicylate concentrations of 615 mg/L in the postmortem blood and 455 mg/kg in the liver (Ryall, 1974). A 2.5 year old girl who was hospitalized following persistent application of oil of wintergreen on her knees for relief of pain died 3 days after admission; blood taken at autopsy contained 100 mg/L salicylate (Lawson and Kaiser, 1937).

Analysis. The methods cited for acetylsalicylic acid are applicable to the analysis of salicylate following methyl salicylate ingestion or exposure. Liquid chromatography has been employed for the determination of both methyl salicylate and salicylate in biological samples (Levine and Caplan, 1984).

References

C. Davison, E.F. Zimmerman and P.K. Smith. On the metabolism and toxicity of methyl salicylate. J. Pharm. Exp. Ther. 132: 207–211, 1960.

R.B. Lawson and A.D. Kaiser. Methyl salicylate poisoning. Arch. Pediat. 54: 509–515, 1937.

H. Lester. Oil of wintergreen. Vet. Hum. Tox. 26: 308, 1984.

B. Levine and Y.H. Caplan. Liquid chromatographic determination of salicylate and methyl salicylate in blood and application to a postmortem case. J. Anal. Tox. 8: 239–241, 1984.

J. Ryall. Personal communication, 1974.

F. Speer. Allergy to methyl salicylate. Ann. Allergy 43: 36–37, 1979.

K.J. Tabor, J.D. Hull, D.P. Hays and S. Kumar. Methyl salicylate poisoning—a case report and literature review. Vet. Hum. Tox. 23: 350, 1981.

Methyprylon

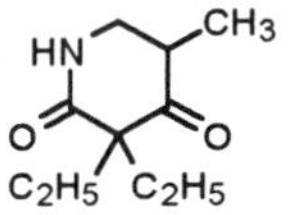

T½: 7–11 hr
Vd: 0.6–1.5 L/kg
Fb: ?
pKa: 12.0

Occurrence and Usage. Methyprylon (Noludar), like glutethimide, is a piperidinedione derivative, and bears a structural resemblance to barbital. It has been in clinical use since 1955 as a
sedative and hypnotic, and is currently available for oral use as the free acid in doses of 50–300 mg.

Blood Concentrations. A single 300 mg oral dose given to 10 adults produced peak plasma levels
of 3.5–8.4 mg/L (average, 5.6) at times ranging from 1.0–2.2 hours (Gwilt et al., 1985). A single
oral dose of 650 mg of methyprylon administered to 6 subjects resulted in an average peak plasma
concentration of 10.2 mg/L at 2 hours, which fell to 7.9 mg/L by 4 hours (Randall et al., 1956).

Metabolism and Excretion. Methyprylon is metabolized by dehydrogenation and oxidation to a
series of more polar compounds. At least one of these, 5-methylpyrithyldione (methylpersedon), is
an active hypnotic (Pribilla, 1959) and it is likely that 6-oxomethyprylon also exhibits activity.
Concentrations of the 4 metabolites in urine have only been assessed in overdose cases, where they
usually exceed that of the parent drug (Boesche, 1969; Dickson, 1974). Probably 5-hydroxy-
methylpyrithyldione and 5-carboxypyrithyldione are excreted largely as conjugates (Bernhard et
al., 1957). About 3% of a dose is excreted in the 24 hour urine as unchanged drug and an equal
amount as 5-methylpyrithyldione (Randall et al., 1956).

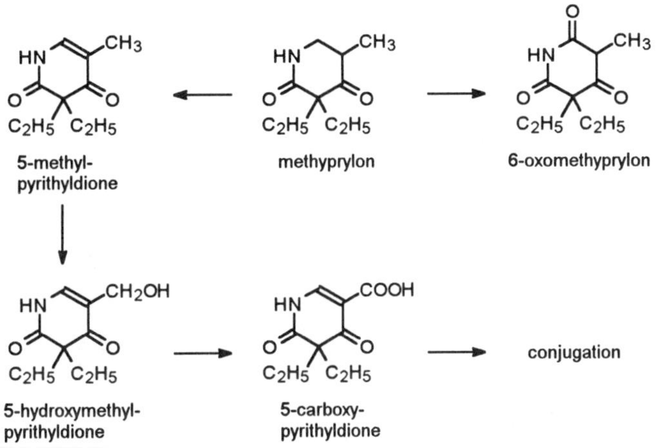

Toxicity. Numerous cases of nonfatal overdosage with methyprylon have been reported, in which
the total amount of ingested drug ranged from 0.8–27 g and initial methyprylon serum concentrations from 5–209 mg/L (Pellegrino and Henderson, 1957; Xanthaky et al., 1966; Yudis et al., 1968;
de Silva and D'Arconte, 1969; Mandelbaum and Simon, 1971; Bailey and Shaw, 1983). Serum
concentrations in excess of 30 mg/L are generally consistent with unconsciousness in the acutely
poisoned patient (Bailey and Jatlow, 1973). A comatose patient achieved maximal methyprylon and
5-methylpyrithyldione concentrations of 168 and 143 mg/L in blood and 250 and 1930 mg/L in
urine; the plasma half-life of the parent drug prior to hemodialysis was 50 hours (Bridges and Peat,
1979).

A fatality has occurred after ingestion of as little as 6 g of the drug (Reidt, 1956). Blood concentrations of methyprylon in fatal cases have ranged up to 1140 mg/L (Clarke, 1969). In one individual, postmortem tissue concentrations of 5-methylpyrithyldione were 23–44% of the parent drug value; the urine metabolite concentration, however, was twice that of methyprylon (van Boven, 1979). Liquid chromatographic methods have also been described (Pankaskie and Brooks, 1983; Gwilt et al., 1985). The following concentrations were observed in 4 fatal cases and are indicative of the nearly uniform tissue distribution of this essentially neutral drug (Cravey, 1972; Baselt, 1977):

Methyprylon Concentrations in Fatal Cases (mg/L or mg/kg)

	Blood	Liver	Kidney	Urine	Gastric
Average	59	118	62	86	96 mg
(Range)	(53–66)	(62–260)	(10–108)	(17–166)	(1–272)

Analysis. Methyprylon has been assayed in biologic specimens by visible spectrophotometry of a colored complex formed with Folin-Ciocalteau reagent (Randall et al., 1956; Xanthaky et al., 1966; Kivela, 1975a). The various metabolites of the drug undoubtedly interfere to some extent, and specific gas chromatographic procedures may be preferred under some circumstances (Dickson, 1974; Kivela, 1975b; Anweiler et al., 1976; Bridges and Peat, 1979; van Boven, 1979). Liquid chromatographic methods have also been described (Pankaskie and Brooks, 1983; Gwilt et al., 1985). The major metabolite of methyprylon has been found to interfere in the determination of barbiturates by ultraviolet spectrophotometry (Wells et al., 1981).

References

J. Anweiler, G. Bender and M. Hobel. Simultaneous determination of glutethimide, methyprylon, and methaqualone in serum by gas liquid chromatography. Arch. Tox. 35: 187–193, 1976.

D.N. Bailey and P.I. Jatlow. Methyprylon overdose: interpretation of serum drug concentrations. Clin. Tox. 6: 563–569, 1973.

D.N. Bailey and R.F. Shaw. Interpretation of blood glutethimide, meprobamate, and methyprylon concentrations in nonfatal and fatal intoxications involving a single drug. Clin. Tox. 20: 133–145, 1983.

R. Baselt. Unpublished results, 1977.

K. Bernhard, M. Just, A.H. Lutz and J.P. Vuilleumier. Ueber das Verhalten in 5-Stellung methylierter Dioxodiaethyl-hydropyridine im Stoffwechsel. Helv. Chim. Acta 40: 436–444, 1957.

J. Boesche. Konzentrationen von Methylprylon und dessen Metaboliten im Harn bei Vergiftsfaellen. Arz. Forsch. 19: 123–125, 1969.

R.R. Bridges and M.A. Peat. Gas-liquid chromatographic analysis of methyprylon and its major metabolite (2,4-dioxo-3,3-diethyl-5-methyl-1,2,3,4-tetrahydropyridine) in an overdose case. J. Anal. Tox. 3: 21–25, 1979.

E.G.C. Clarke (ed.). *Isolation and Identification of Drugs*, Pharmaceutical Press, London, 1969, pp. 426–427.

R.H. Cravey. Personal communication, 1972.

J.A.F. de Silva and L. D'Arconte. The use of spectrophotofluorometry in the analysis of drugs in biological materials. J. For. Sci. 14: 184–204, 1969.

S.J. Dickson. The determination of methyprylon and its metabolites in biological fluids by gas chromatography. For. Sci. 4: 177–182, 1974.

P.R. Gwilt, M.C. Pankaskie, J.E. Thornburg et al. Pharmacokinetics of methyprylon following a single oral dose. J. Pharm. Sci. 74: 1001–1003, 1985.

E.W. Kivela. Methyprylon. Type B procedure. In *Methodology for Analytical Toxicology* (I. Sunshine, ed.), CRC Press, Cleveland, 1975a, pp. 260–262.

E.W. Kivela. *ibid*, 1975b, pp. 262–264.

J.M. Mandelbaum and N.M. Simon. Severe methyprylon intoxication treated by hemodialysis. J. Am. Med. Asso. 216: 139–140, 1971.

M.C. Pankaskie and M.A. Brooks. Determination of methyprylon and its dehydro metabolite, 5-methylpyrithyldione, in plasma by high-performance liquid chromatography. J. Chrom. 278: 458–463, 1983.

E.D. Pellegrino and R.R. Henderson. Clinical toxicity of methyprylon (Noludar). J. Med. Soc. N. J. 54: 515–518, 1957.

O. Pribilla. Studien zur Toxikologie der Schlafmittel aus der Tetrahydro-pyridin- und Piperidine-Reihe. Arch. Tox. 18: 1–86, 1959.

L.O. Randall, V. Iliev and O. Brandman. Metabolism of methyprylon. Arch. Int. Pharm. Ther. 106: 388–394, 1956.

W.U. Reidt. Fatal poisoning with methyprylon (Noludar), a nonbarbiturate sedative. New Eng. J. Med. 255: 231–232, 1956.

M. van Boven. Capillary gas chromatography for drug analysis. J. Anal. Tox. 3: 174–176, 1979.

J. Wells, I. Moftah, G. Cimbura and K. Koves. The identification of a methyprylon metabolite which interferes with the UV differential spectra of barbiturates. Can. Soc. For. Sci. J. 14: 47–53, 1981.

G. Xanthaky, A.W. Freireich, W. Matusiak and L. Lukash. Hemodialysis in methyprylon poisoning. J. Am. Med. Asso. 198: 190–191, 1966.

M. Yudis, C. Swartz, G. Onesti et al. Hemodialysis for methyprylon (Noludar) poisoning. Ann. Int. Med. 68: 1301–1304, 1968.

Metoprolol

T½: 2.5–7.5 hr
Vd: 2.5–5.6 L/kg
Fb: 0.11
pKa: 9.7

$$OCH_2CHCH_2NHCH(CH_3)_2$$
(with OH on the central carbon)

$$CH_2CH_2OCH_3$$

Occurrence and Usage. Metoprolol (Lopressor, Toprol) is a beta-adrenergic blocking agent chemically related to practolol and, less closely, to oxprenolol. It has been used as an antihypertensive drug since 1975. Tablets of 50 and 100 mg containing the tartrate salt are available for oral administration; daily doses range from 100–450 mg. The tartrate salt is also available in a 5 mg/5 mL ampule for intravenous injection, and the succinate salt is available as extended-release tablets of 50–200 mg.

Blood Concentrations. A single 50 mg oral dose given to 8 patients produced peak plasma levels that averaged 0.072 mg/L (range, 0.035–0.125) at 0.8–2.5 hours, declining with a mean half-life of 3.8 hours (Bengtsson et al., 1975). Maximal plasma levels averaged 0.135 mg/L (range, 0.046–0.270) at 0.7–2.7 hours after a 100 mg oral dose in 6 volunteers (Regardh et al., 1975). Steady-state plasma concentrations averaging 0.116 mg/L (range, 0.020–0.341) were measured in 16 patients receiving 300 mg of the drug daily in 3 divided doses (von Bahr et al., 1976). Concentrations of the active metabolite III are approximately one-third those of the parent drug in young adults on chronic oral therapy, but are approximately equal to those of the parent in the elderly (Quarterman et al., 1981). The blood/plasma concentration ratio for metoprolol averages 1.1 (Regardh et al., 1974).

Metabolism and Excretion. Metoprolol is well-absorbed from the gastrointestinal tract, but is only 40–50% bioavailable due to rapid metabolism. An average of 99.6% of a single labeled oral dose is eliminated in the 72 hour urine, with only 3% present as unchanged drug (Regardh et al., 1975). The major urinary metabolites are products of O-demethylation and oxidation (metabolite I), oxidative deamination (II), and aliphatic hydroxylation (III); these substances account for 65%, 10%, and 10% of a single oral dose, respectively. Metabolite III has about one-tenth the beta-blocking activity of metoprolol, and the others are essentially inactive (Borg et al., 1975).

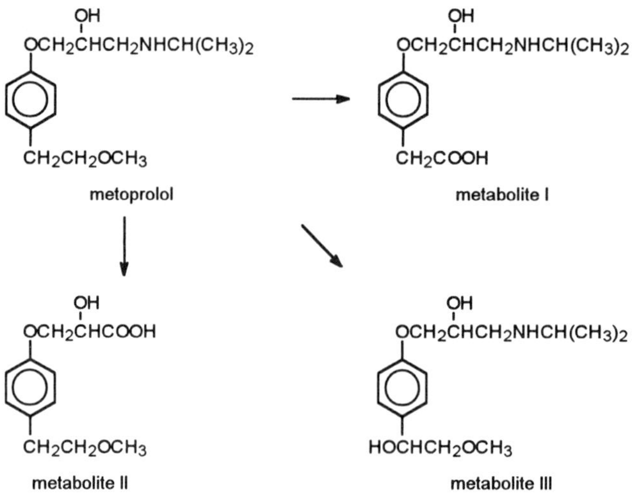

metoprolol → metabolite I

metabolite II   metabolite III

Toxicity. Adverse reactions to metoprolol have included dizziness, fatigue, shortness of breath, bradycardia, diarrhea, bronchospasm, and depression. A young adult who ingested 10 g of the drug developed cyanosis and severe hypotension; he achieved a plasma metoprolol concentration of 12.2 mg/L, but recovered completely in 12 hours with supportive therapy (Moller, 1976). A man who survived the ingestion of 50 g exhibited coma, hypotension, bradycardia, seizures and metabolic acidosis; a plasma metoprolol level of 18 mg/L was measured 2.5 hours after ingestion (Wallin and Hulting, 1983).

The following concentrations were observed in 5 fatalities arising from acute overdosage with metoprolol (Holzbecher et al., 1982; Reynolds, 1984; Stajic et al., 1984; Riker et al., 1987; Rohring et al., 1987):

Metoprolol Concentrations in Fatalities (mg/L or mg/kg)

	Blood	Liver	Urine	Gastric
Average	60	173	66	75 mg
(Range)	(4.7–142)	(6.3–296)	(1.0–194)	(35–95)

Metoprolol may exhibit postmortem redistribution; in a case of fatal overdosage, the heart blood/ femoral blood concentration ratio was 3.8 (Prouty and Anderson, 1990).

Analysis. Metoprolol has been assayed in plasma by electron-capture gas chromatography after formation of a halogenated derivative (Zak et al., 1980; Kinney, 1981; Sioufi et al., 1983; Ervik et al., 1986). A method for metoprolol and its active metabolites in plasma and urine utilizes gas chromatography/mass spectrometry (Ervik et al., 1981). Liquid chromatographic schemes have also been described (Lennard and Silas, 1983; Lecaillon et al., 1984; Balmer et al., 1987; Rutledge and Garrick, 1989).

References

K. Balmer, Y. Zhang, P.O. Lagerstrom and B.A. Persson. Determination of metoprolol and two major metablites in plasma and urine by column liquid chromatography and fluorometric detection. J. Chrom. 417: 357–365, 1987.

C. Bengtsson, G. Johnsson and C.G. Regardh. Plasma levels and effects of metoprolol on blood pressure and heart rate in hypertensive patients after an acute dose and between two doses during long-term treatment. Clin. Pharm. Ther. 17: 400–408, 1975.

K.O. Borg, E. Carlsson, K.J. Hoffmann et al. Metabolism of metoprolol-(^{3}H) in man, the dog and the rat. Acta Pharm. Tox. 36: 125–135, 1975.

M. Ervik, K.J. Hoffmann and K. Kylberg-Hanssen. Selected ion monitoring of metoprolol and two metabolites in plasma and urine using deuterated internal standards. Biomed. Mass Spec. 8: 322–326, 1981.

M. Ervik, K. Kylberg-Hanssen and L. Johansson. Determination of metoprolol in plasma and urine using high-resolution gas chromatography and electron-capture detection. J. Chrom. 381: 168–174, 1986.

M. Holzbecher, R.A. Perry and H.A. Ellenberger. Report of a metoprolol-associated death. J. For. Sci. 27: 715–717, 1982.

C.D. Kinney. Determination of metoprolol in plasma and urine by gas-liquid chromatography with electron-capture detection. J. Chrom. 225: 213–218, 1981.

J.B. Lecaillon, J. Godbillon, F. Abadie and G. Gossett. Determination of metoprolol and its α-hydroxylated metabolite in human plasma by high-performance liquid chromatography. J. Chrom. 305: 411–417, 1984.

M.A. Lefebvre, J. Girault and J.B. Fourtillan. β-Blocking agents: determination of biological levels using high performance liquid chromatography. J. Liq. Chrom. 4: 483–500, 1981.

M.S. Lennard and J.H. Silas. Rapid determination of metoprolol and α-hydroxymetoprolol in human plasma and urine by high-performance liquid chromatography. J. Chrom. 272: 205–209, 1983.

B.H.J. Moller. Massive intoxication with metoprolol. Brit. Med. J. 24: 222, 1976.

R.W. Prouty and W.H. Anderson. The forensic science implications of site and temporal influences on post-mortem blood-drug concentrations. J. For. Sci. 35: 243–270, 1990.

C.P. Quarterman, M.J. Kendall and D.B. Jack. The effect of age on the pharmacokinetics of metoprolol and its metabolites. Brit. J. Clin. Pharm. 11: 287–294, 1981.

C.G. Regardh, K.O. Borg, R. Johansson et al. Pharmacokinetic studies on the selective β$_1$-receptor antagonist metoprolol in man. J. Pharmacokin. Biopharm. 2: 347–354, 1974.

C.G. Regardh, G. Johnsson, L. Jordo and L. Solvell. Comparative bioavailability and effect studies on metoprolol administration as ordinary and slow-release tablets in single and multiple doses. Acta Pharm. Tox. 36: 45–58, 1975.

P. Reynolds. Presented at the quarterly meeting of the California Association of Forensic Toxicologists, San Francisco, August 4, 1984.

C.D. Riker, R.K. Wright, W. Matusiak and B.E. de Tuscan. Massive metoprolol ingestion associated with a fatality—a case report. J. For. Sci. 32: 1447–1452, 1987.

T.P. Rohrig, D.A. Rundle and W.N. Leifer. Fatality resulting from metoprolol overdose. J. Anal. Tox. 11: 231–232, 1987.

D.R. Rutledge and C. Garrick. Determination of metoprolol and its α-hydroxide metabolite in serum by reversed-phase high-performance liquid chromatogrphy. J. Chrom. Sci. 27: 561–565, 1989.

A. Sioufi, F. Leroux and N. Sandrenan. Gas chromatographic determination of metoprolol in human plasma. J. Chrom. 272: 103–110, 1983.

M. Stajic, R.H. Granger and J.C. Beyer. Fatal metoprolol overdose. J. Anal. Tox. 8: 228–230, 1984.

C. von Bahr, P. Collste, M. Frisk-Holmberg et al. Plasma levels and effects of metoprolol on blood pressure, adrenergic beta receptor blockade, and plasma renin activity in essential hypertension. Clin. Pharm. Ther. 20: 130–137, 1976.

C.J. Wallin and J. Hulting. Massive metoprolol poisoning treated with prenalterol. Acta Med. Scand. 214: 253–255, 1983.

S. Zak, F. Honc and T.G. Gilleran. A sensitive gas chromatographic method for the determination of metoprolol in human plasma. Anal. Letters 13: 1359–1371, 1980.

Mexiletine

T½: 8–17 hr (urine pH-dependent)
Vd: 6–12 L/kg
Fb: 0.70
pKa: 8.4

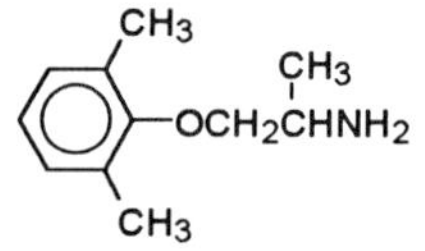

Occurrence and Usage. Mexiletine (Mexitil) is an antiarrhythmic agent used since 1972 in the treatment of ventricular arrhythmia. It is available as the hydrochloride salt for oral, intramuscular, or intravenous administration in single doses of 50–400 mg and daily doses of up to 1500 mg.

Blood Concentrations. A 300 mg oral dose of mexiletine to one patient produced a peak plasma level of 0.4 mg/L at 4 hours (Frydman et al., 1978). In 5 volunteers who received a single oral 400 mg dose, peak plasma concentrations of 0.9–1.6 mg/L were achieved at 2–4 hours after ingestion, and an average elimination half-life of 9.3 hours was measured (Prescott et al., 1977). Peak plasma concentrations following a 200 mg intravenous dose averaged about 2.5 mg/L at 10 minutes and fell below 0.5 mg/L by 65 minutes; the elimination half-life in the 10 patients averaged 13 hours.

Patients receiving 750 mg of the drug daily, in divided oral doses of 250 mg every 8 hours, achieved steady-state trough mexiletine concentrations averaging 0.9–1.4 mg/L over a 14 day period. Plasma concentrations of 0.75–1.00 mg/L were found to be effective in 77% of the patients tested, and concentrations of 0.75–2.00 mg/L were effective in 79% (Campbell et al., 1978). The blood/plasma concentration ratio for mexiletine averages 1.1 (Turgeon et al., 1987).

Metabolism and Excretion. The bioavailability of mexiletine is 80–90% by the oral route and is 100% by intramuscular injection. From 30–55% of a dose is eliminated unchanged in 24 hours by the kidney when the urine is maintained acidic, only 10–23% during normal urine pH conditions, and only 0.4% during alkaline urine conditions. The major urinary metabolites are p-hydroxy-mexiletine (5–13%) and hydroxymethylmexiletine (5–15%), both of which may be further metabolized by N-deamination to alcohols. Minor metabolites include N-oxides, deaminated mexiletine, m-hydroxymexiletine and N-methylmexiletine (Kiddie et al., 1974; Beckett and Chidomere, 1977; Grech-Belanger et al., 1991).

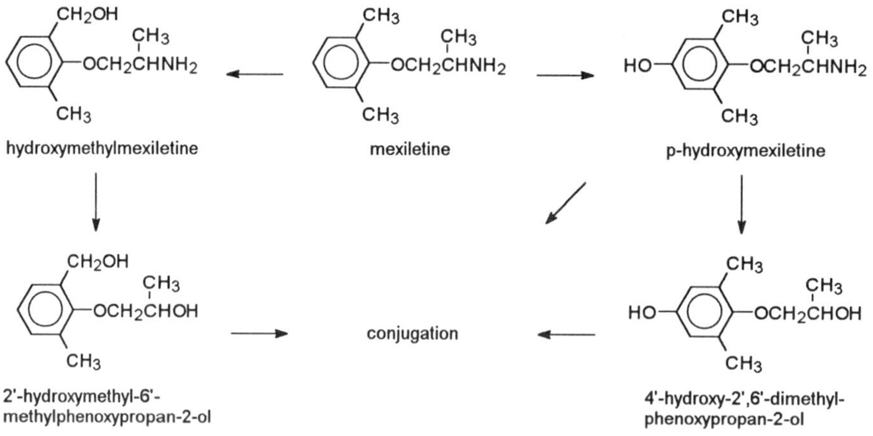

hydroxymethylmexiletine   mexiletine   p-hydroxymexiletine

2'-hydroxymethyl-6'-
methylphenoxypropan-2-ol   conjugation   4'-hydroxy-2',6'-dimethyl-
phenoxypropan-2-ol

Toxicity. Plasma mexiletine concentrations exceeding 2 mg/L are associated with a high incidence of side-effects, including hypotension, bradycardia, vomiting, dizziness, blurred vision, tremor, and confusion (Talbot et al., 1976; Campbell et al., 1978). A 62 year old male cardiac patient became agitated, confused, and tremulous when his plasma mexiletine concentration inadvertently exceeded 4 mg/L (Bradbrook et al., 1977).

Four deaths have been reported in adults who acutely ingested 4–8 g of mexiletine; blood concentrations of 21–37 mg/L and liver concentrations of 55–433 mg/kg were determined in postmortem specimens (Jequir et al., 1976; Hruby et al., 1980; Oliver and Harland, 1980; Blackmore, 1982).

Mexiletine may exhibit postmortem redistribution; in a fatal overdosage, the heart blood/subclavian blood concentration ratio was 2.7 (Kempton et al., 1993).

Analysis. Mexiletine may be assayed in plasma or urine by fluorometry (Kelly et al., 1973). Gas chromatographic procedures have utilized flame-ionization (Kelly, 1977; Holt et al., 1979; Grech-Belanger, 1984; Ji et al., 1993), nitrogen-phosphorus (Kelly et al., 1973; Bradbrook et al., 1977; Smith and Meffin, 1980; Vasiliades et al., 1984), and electron-capture detection (Willox and Singh, 1976; Frydman et al., 1978). Liquid chromatography has also been employed (Farid and White, 1983; Mastropaolo et al., 1984; Gupta and Lew, 1985; Kramer et al., 1989; Packowski et al., 1992).

References

A.H. Beckett and E.C. Chidomere. The distribution, metabolism and excretion of mexiletine in man. Postgrad. Med. J. 53: 60–66, 1977.

R.C. Blackmore. Personal communication, 1982.

I.D. Bradbrook, C. James and H.J. Rogers. A rapid method for the determination of plasma mexiletine levels by gas chromatography. Brit. J. Clin. Pharm. 4: 380–382, 1977.

N.P.S. Campbell, J.G. Kelly, A.A.J. Adgey and R.G. Shanks. The clinical pharmacology of mexiletine. Brit. J. Clin. Pharm. 6: 103–108, 1978.

N.A. Farid and S.M. White. Determination of mexiletine and its metabolites in serum by liquid chromatography with fluorescence detection. J. Chrom. 275: 458–462, 1983.

A. Frydman, J.P. Lafarge, F. Vial et al. New electron-capture gas-liquid chromatographic method for the determination of mexiletine plasma levels in man. J. Chrom. 145: 401–411, 1978.

O. Grech-Belanger. Gas chromatographic method for the routine serum monitoring of mexiletine. J. Chrom. 309: 165–169, 1984.

O. Grech-Belanger, J. Turgeon, M. Lalande and P.M. Belanger. Meta-hydroxymexiletine, a new metabolite of mexiletine. Drug Met. Disp. 19: 458–461, 1991.

R.N. Gupta and M. Lew. Liquid chromatographic determination of mexiletine and tocainide in human plasma with fluorescence detection after reaction with a modified o-phthalaldehyde reagent. J. Chrom. 344: 221–230, 1985.

D.W. Holt, R.J. Flanagan, A.M. Hayler and M. Loizou. Simple gas-liquid chromatographic method for the measurement of mexiletine and lignocaine in blood-plasma or serum. J. Chrom. 169: 295–301, 1979.

K. Hruby, J. Missliwetz and K. Lenz. Poisoning with oral antiarrhythmic drugs. In *Toxicological Aspects* (A. Kovatsis, ed.), Thessaloniki, Greece, 1980, pp. 485–492.

P. Jequir, R. Jones and A. MacKintosh. Fatal mexiletine overdose. Lancet 1: 492, 1976.

S.G. Ji, Q.H. Kong, X.L. Li and P. Li. Gas chromatographic determination of mexiletine in human plasma with flame ionization detection after reaction with carbon disulphide. Biomed. Chrom. 7: 196–199, 1993.

J.G. Kelly, J. Nimmo, R. Rae et al. Spectrophotofluorometric and gas-liquid chromatographic methods for the estimation of mexiletine (Ko 1173) in plasma and urine. J. Pharm. Pharmac. 25: 550–553, 1973.

J.G. Kelly. Measurement of plasma mexiletine concentrations. Postgrad. Med. J. 53: 48–49, 1977.

J. Kempton, B. Levine, A. Manoukian and J.E. Smialek. A mexiletine intoxication. Presented at the annual meeting of the Society of Forensic Toxicologists, Phoenix, Arizona, October 15, 1993.

M.A. Kiddie, C.M. Kaye, P. Turner and T.R.D. Shaw. The influence of urinary pH on the elimination of mexiletine. Brit. J. Clin. Pharm. 1: 229–232, 1974.

B.K. Kramer, K.M. Ress, F. Mayer et al. Rapid high-performance liquid chromatographic method for the quantitation of mexiletine and its metabolies in serum. J. Chrom. 493: 414–420, 1989.

W. Mastropaola, D.R. Holmes, M.J. Osborn et al. Improved liquid-chromatographic determination of mexiletine, an antiarrhythmic drug, in plasma. Clin. Chem. 30: 319–322, 1984.

J.S. Oliver and W.A. Harland. Mexiletine ('Mexitil') poisoning. In *Toxicological Aspects* (A. Kovatsis, ed.), Thessaloniki, Greece, 1980, pp. 345–350.

D. Paczkowski, M. Filipek, Z. Mielniczuk et al. Simultaneous determination of mexiletine and four hydroxylated metabolites in human serum by high-performance liquid chromatography. J. Chrom. 573: 235–246, 1992.

L.F. Prescott, A. Pottage and J.A. Clements. Absorption, distribution and elimination of mexiletine. Postgrad. Med. J. 53: 50–55, 1977.

K.J. Smith and P.J. Meffin. Mexiletine analysis in blood and plasma using gas chromatography and nitrogen-selective detection. J. Chrom. 181: 469–472, 1980.

R.G. Talbot, D.G. Julian and L.F. Prescott. Long-term treatment of ventricular arrhythmias with oral mexiletine. Am. Heart J. 91: 58–65, 1976.

J. Turgeon, O. Grech-Belanger and M. Gilbert. Erythrocyte and serum distribution of mexiletine in man. Biopharm. Drug Disp. 8: 571–576, 1987.

J. Vasiliades, J. Kellett and R.S. Cox. Gas-chromatographic determination of mexiletine with a nitrogen-selective detector. Am. J. Clin. Path. 81: 776–779, 1984.

S. Willox and B.N. Singh. Sensitive gas chromatographic method for the estimation of a new antiarrhythmic compound, mexiletine (Ko1173), in biological fluids. J. Chrom. 128: 196–198, 1976.

Mianserin

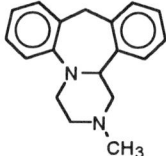

T½: 6–39 hr
Vd: 10–29 L/kg
Fb: 0.90
pKa: 7.1

Occurrence and Usage. Mianserin (ORG GB-94, Bolvidon, Norval) is a tetracyclic antidepressant used clinically since 1975. It is available as the hydrochloride in tablets of 10–20 mg for oral use; daily doses range from 20–90 mg.

Blood Concentrations. A single 20 mg oral dose given to 4 male adults resulted in an average peak plasma concentration of 0.026 mg/L (range, 0.023–0.030) at a mean time of 1.7 hours. The average elimination half-life was 17 hours. Steady-state plasma concentrations in patients receiving 60 mg of the drug daily averaged 0.037 mg/L (range, 0.012–0.081); in patients receiving 90 mg daily, concentrations averaged 0.062 mg/L (range, 0.017–0.158) (Coppen and Kopera, 1978). Montgomery et al. (1978) observed the best clinical response in patients with steady-state plasma mianserin levels of 0.015 to 0.070 mg/L. The blood/plasma concentration ratio for the drug averages 0.66 (Maguire et al., 1982). The elimination half-life is increased by age, averaging 9.6 hours in young adults and 27 hours in elderly patients (Shami et al., 1983).

Metabolism and Excretion. Mianserin is known to be metabolized by N-demethylation, N-oxidation, and 8-hydroxylation. From 64–74% of a labeled dose is eliminated in the urine over a period of several days, largely as conjugated metabolites; only 5% is excreted unchanged in urine (van Riezen et al., 1981). The oral bioavailability of the drug is 30% (Coppen and Kopera, 1978).

Toxicity. Mianserin apparently does not cause the cardiac toxicity characteristic of the tricyclic antidepressants, although 2 women did exhibit first-degree heart block for up to 14 hours after ingesting 580–900 mg of the drug and achieving plasma levels, 3.5–5.0 hours following ingestion, of 0.439–0.700 mg/L (Green and Kendall-Taylor, 1977; Hla and Boyd, 1987). Five adults who acutely ingested 250–800 mg of mianserin and developed plasma concentrations of 0.070–0.500 mg/L (average, 0.209) exhibited only drowsiness and hypertension (Newman and Crome, 1979). A 53 year old woman ingested at least 600 mg of the drug and became unconscious; her peak plasma drug level was 0.780 mg/L 5 hours after ingestion, and she awoke 12 hours later. Hemodialysis was without effect on the elimination kinetics of the drug, which were consistent with those observed after therapeutic administration (Coppen and Kopera, 1978).

An elderly woman ingested 600 mg of mianserin and an unknown amount of lorazepam, became comatose, and died the next day; plasma concentrations on admission were 0.110 mg/L for mianserin and 0.500 mg/L for lorazepam (Crome and Newman, 1977). The following concentrations were determined in the tissues of an elderly man who died after ingesting large amounts of digoxin and mianserin (Geyer, 1983):

Mianserin Concentrations in a Digoxin/Mianserin Fatality (mg/L or mg/kg)

Blood	Brain	Liver	Urine	Gastric
2.3	4.3	8.1	19	28 mg

Analysis. Mianserin may be determined in plasma by gas chromatography utilizing nitrogen-phosphorus (Vink and van Hal, 1980; Lewis and Cairncross, 1981) or mass spectrometric detection (de Ridder et al., 1977; Vink et al., 1980; Jindal et al., 1982). Liquid chromatography has also been employed (Suckow et al., 1982; Wong et al., 1984).

References

A. Coppen and H. Kopera. Workshop on the clinical pharmacology and efficacy of mianserin. Brit. J. Clin. Pharm. 5: 91S–99S, 1978.

P. Crome and B. Newman. Poisoning with maprotiline and mianserin. Brit. Med. J. 2: 260, 1977.

J.J. de Ridder, P.C.J.M. Koppens and H.J.M. van Hal. Mass fragmentographic assay of nanogram amounts of the antidepressant drug mianserin hydrochloride (Org GB94) in human plasma. J. Chrom. 143: 289–297, 1977.

R. Geyer. Personal communication, 1983.

S.D.R. Green and P. Kendall-Taylor. Heart block in mianserin hydrochloride overdose. Brit. Med. J. 2: 1190, 1977.

K.K. Hla and O. Boyd. Mianserin and complete heart block. Hum. Tox. 6: 401–402, 1987.

S.P. Jindal, T. Lutz and P. Vestergaard. Selected ion monitoring assay for the antidepressant mianserin in human plasma with stable isotope labeled analog as internal standard. J. Anal. Tox. 6: 34–37, 1982.

J. Lewis and K.D. Cairncross. A simplified method for the estimation of mianserin in plasma. Brit. J. Clin. Pharm. 12: 583–585, 1981.

K.P. Maguire, T.R. Norman, G.D. Burrows and B.A. Scoggins. A pharmacokinetic study of mianserin. Eur. J. Clin. Pharm. 21: 517–520, 1982.

S. Montgomery, R. McAuley and D.B. Montgomery. Relationship between mianserin plasma levels and anti-depressant effect in a double-blind trial comparing a single night-time and divided daily dose regimens. Brit. J. Clin. Pharm. 5: 71S–76S, 1978.

B. Newman and P. Crome. The clinical toxicology of mianserin hydrochloride. Vet. Hum. Tox. 21: 60–62, 1979.

M. Shami, H.L. Elliott, A.W. Kelman and B. Whiting. The pharmacokinetics of mianserin. Brit. J. Clin. Pharm. 15: 313S–322S, 1983.

R.F. Suckow, T.B. Cooper, F.M. Quitkin and J.W. Stewart. Determination of mianserin and metabolites in plasma by liquid chromatography with electrochemical detection. J. Pharm. Sci. 71: 889–892, 1982.

H. van Riezen, R.M. Pinder, V.J. Nickolson et al. Mianserin. In *Pharmacological and Biochemical Properties of Drug Substances*, Vol. 3 (M.E. Goldberg, ed.), American Pharmaceutical Association, Washington, D.C., 1981, pp. 56–93.

J. Vink and H.J.M. van Hal. Simplified method for determination of the tetracyclic antidepressant mianserin in human plasma using gas chromatography with nitrogen detection. J. Chrom. 181: 25–31, 1980.

J. Vink, H.J.M. van Hal and B. Delver. Comparative statistical study of assay methods using mass fragmentography and gas chromatography with nitrogen detection for determination of the tetracyclic anti-depressant mianserin in human plasma. J. Chrom. 181: 115–119, 1980.

S.H.Y. Wong, S.W. Waugh, M. Draz and N. Jain. Liquid-chromatographic determination of two antidepressants, trazodone and mianserin, in plasma. Clin. Chem. 30: 230–233, 1984.

Midazolam

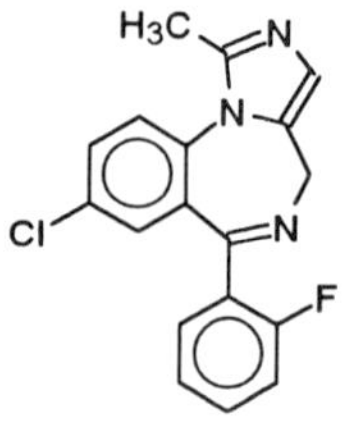

T½: 1–4 hr
Vd: 1.0–2.5 L/kg
Fb: 0.96
pKa: 6.2

Occurrence and Usage: Midazolam (Versed), an imidazobenzodiazepine derivative, was first synthesized in 1976. The drug is utilized as a preoperative medication, sedative-hypnotic and anesthetic induction agent. When the drug is used alone for intravenous sedation during diagnostic procedures, a total dose of 0.10–0.15 mg/kg is used. For intramuscular preoperative sedation, 0.07–0.08 mg/kg (4.9–5.6 mg/70 kg) is administered 1 hour before surgery. For induction of anesthesia, an initial dose of 0.30–0.35 mg/kg (21–25 mg/70 kg) is usually given to patients less than 55 years of age and not receiving premedication. The drug is currently available in the United States as the hydrochloride salt in a 1–5 mg/mL injectable solution, and in many European countries as the maleate salt in forms intended for oral administration.

Blood Concentrations. A peak plasma concentration of 50 µg/L was observed 30 minutes following oral ingestion of 10 mg of midazolam by a male adult. Another subject was given a single dose of 5.5 mg intramuscularly and a peak plasma concentration of 103 µg/L was reached within 20 minutes (Dixon et al., 1982). Following a 10 mg oral dose in 20 normal subjects aged 24–37 years, the time of peak plasma concentration was about 1 hour; the average peak plasma concentration for the 10 males was 69 µg/L and for the 10 females, 53 µg/L. In the same study, 20 individuals aged 60–79 were given an oral dose of 10 mg; the average peak plasma concentration for the men was 85 µg/L and for the women, 96 µg/L (Greenblatt et al., 1984). As a preoperative medication in doses of 0.13 mg/kg (9.1 mg/70 kg) intramuscularly, average peak plasma concentrations of 68 µg/L were found (Mattila et al., 1983).

The elimination half-life of the drug is prolonged in cardiac surgery patients to an average of 10.4 hours. The midazolam plasma concentration required to obtain a sedative effect in post-surgical patients is about 100 µg/L; this concentration can be maintained in most patients by continuous infusion of 1–3 mg/hour (Maitre et al., 1989). Surgical patients receiving 3 intravenous doses of 0.3 mg/kg every 45 minutes for anesthetic induction and maintenance had peak plasma midazolam concentrations averaging 1103 µg/L at 5 minutes after the last injection; the average plasma level upon arousal 2–4 hours later was 131 µg/L (Crevat-Pisano et al., 1986).

Metabolism and Excretion. The major metabolite of midazolam in man is 1-hydroxymidazolam. Smaller amounts of 4-hydroxymidazolam are formed together with yet smaller amounts of 1,4-dihydroxymidazolam (Reves et al., 1985; Heizmann and Ziegler, 1981). 1-Hydroxymidazolam is pharmacologically less active than the parent drug, has a 30% shorter half-life, and is present at much lower concentrations in plasma (Heizmann et al., 1983; Mandema et al., 1992). These metabolites are eliminated in the urine in the form of glucuronide conjugates; very little unchanged drug is found in the urine.

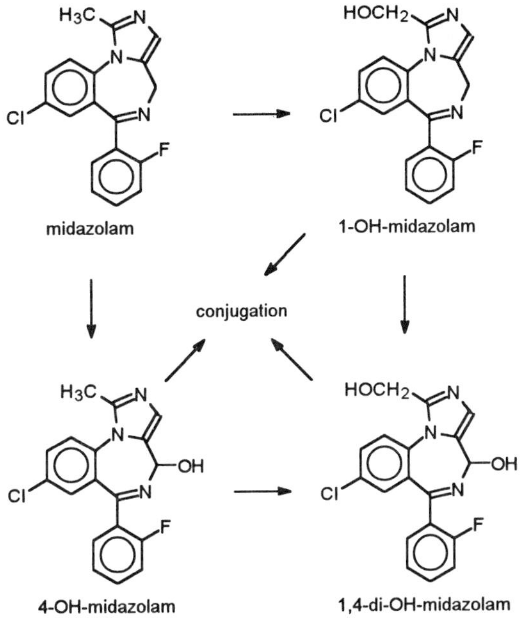

midazolam

1-OH-midazolam

conjugation

4-OH-midazolam

1,4-di-OH-midazolam

Toxicity. Midazolam can cause respiratory depression, apnea and hypotension. Anterograde amnesia may last as long as 2 hours after injection.

Midazolam concentrations of 50 µg/L in blood, 930 µg/kg in liver and 300 µg/L in urine were found postmortem in an individual who intravenously self-administered 10 mg midazolam and 100 µg sufentanil (Ferslew et al., 1989).

Analysis. Assays for the quantitation of midazolam and its major metabolite include gas chromatography with electron-capture (Puglisi et al, 1978; Greenblatt et al., 1981; Smith et al., 1981; Arendt et al., 1984; Sunzel, 1989), nitrogen-selective (Vasiliades and Owens, 1980; Vasiliades and Sahawneh, 1982) and mass spectrometric detection (Rubio et al., 1982). Liquid chromatography (Vasiliades and Sahawneh, 1981, 1982; Puglisi et al., 1985; Sautou et al., 1991) and radioimmunoassay (Dixon et al., 1982) have also been reported.

References

R.M. Arendt, D.J. Greenblatt and W.A. Garland. Quantitation by gas chromatography of the 1- and 4-hydroxy metabolites of midazolam in human plasma. Pharmacology 29: 158–164, 1984.

P. Crevat-Pisano, S. Dragna, C. Granthil et al. Plasma concentrations and pharmacokinetics of midazolam during anaesthesia. J. Pharm. Pharmac. 38: 578–582, 1986.

R. Dixon, R. Lucek, D. Todd and A. Walser. Midazolam: radioimmunoassay for pharmacokinetic studies in man. Res. Comm. Chem. Path. Pharm. 37: 11–20, 1982.

K.E. Ferslew, A.N. Hagardorn and W.F. McCormick. Postmortem determination of the biological distribution of sufentanil and midazolam after an acute intoxication. J. For. Sci. 34: 249–257, 1989.

D.J. Greenblatt, D.R. Abernethy, A. Locniskar et al. Effect of age, gender, and obesity on midazolam kinetics. Anesthesiology 61: 27–35, 1984.

D.J. Greenblatt, A. Locniskar, H.R. Ochs and P.M. Lauven. Automated gas chromatography for studies of midazolam pharmacokinetics. Anesthesiology 55: 176–179, 1981.

P. Heizmann and W.H. Ziegler. Excretion and metabolism of ^{14}C-midazolam in humans following oral dosing. Arz. Forsch. 31: 2220–2223, 1981.

P. Heizmann, M. Eckert and W.H. Ziegler. Pharmacokinetics and bioavailability of midazolam in man. Brit. J. Clin. Pharm. 16: 43S–49S, 1983.

P.O. Maitre, B. Funk, C. Crevoisier and H.R. Ha. Pharmacokinetics of midazolam in patients recovering from cardiac surgery. Eur. J. Clin. Pharm. 37: 161–166, 1989.

J.W. Mandema, B. Tuk, A.L. van Steveninck et al. Pharmacokinetic-pharmacodynamic modeling of the central nervous system effects of midazolam. Clin. Pharm. Ther. 51: 715–728, 1992.

M.A.K. Mattila, S. Suurinkeroinen, K. Saila and J.J. Himgerg. Midazolam and fat-emulsion diazepam as intramuscular premedication. A double blind clinical trial. Acta Anaesth. Scand. 27: 345–348, 1983.

C.V. Puglisi, J.C. Meyer, L. D'Arconte et al. Determination of water soluble imidazo-1,4-benzodiazepines in blood by electron-capture gas-liquid chromatography and in urine by differential pulse polargraphy. J. Chrom. 145: 81–96, 1978.

C.V. Puglisi, J. Pao, F.J. Ferrara and J.A.F. de Silva. Determination of midazolam (Versed) and its metabolites in plasma by high-performance liquid chromatography. J. Chrom. 344: 199–209, 1985.

J.G. Reves, R.J. Fragen, H.R. Vinik and D.J. Greenblatt. Midazolam: pharmacology and uses. Anesthesiology 62: 310–324, 1985.

F. Rubio, B.J. Miwa and W.A. Garland. Determination of midazolam and two metabolites of midazolam in human plasma by gas chromatography-negative chemical-ionization mass spectrometry. J. Chrom. 233: 157–165, 1982.

V. Sautou, J. Chopineau, M.P. Terrisse and P. Bastide. Solid-phase extraction of midazolam and two of its metabolites from plasma for high performance liquid chromatographic analysis. J. Chrom. 571: 298–304, 1991.

M.T. Smith, M.J. Eadie and T.O. Brophy. The pharmacokinetics of midazolam in man. Eur. J. Clin. Pharm. 19: 271–278, 1981.

M. Sunzel. Determination of midazolam and the α-hydroxy metabolite by gas chromatography in small plasma volumes. J. Chrom. 491: 455–460, 1989.

J. Vasiliades and C. Owens. Determination of midazolam in serum by gas chromatography with a nitrogen selective detector. J. Chrom. 182: 439–444, 1980.

J. Vasiliades and T.H. Sahawneh. Determination of midazolam by high-performance liquid chromatography. J. Chrom. 225: 266–271, 1981.

J. Vasiliades and T. Sahawneh. Midazolam determination by gas chromatography, liquid chromatography and gas chromatography-mass spectrometry. J. Chrom. 228: 195–203, 1982.

Molindone

T½: 2.0 hr
Vd: ?
Fb: ?
pKa: 6.9

Occurrence and Usage. Molindone (Moban) is a dihydroindolone compound used for the management of psychotic disorders. It is available in tablets of 5–100 mg as the hydrochloride salt. The usual adult dose is 5–25 mg 3 or 4 times a day.

Blood Concentrations. A single 50 mg oral dose given to 3 subjects produced an average plasma molindone level of 5.0 µg/L at 0.5 hours, declining to 2.8 µg/L by 7 hours. Nine psychiatric inpatients given 100 mg/day of molindone for a period of 2 weeks exhibited average molindone plasma concentrations of 44 µg/L at 6 hours after the last dose and 9 µg/L at 12 hours (Wolf et al., 1985). Eight patients receiving daily doses of 200–400 mg exhibited serum molindone levels averaging 137 µg/L (range, 44–374) (Narasimhachari et al., 1988).

Metabolism and Excretion. Molindone is extensively metabolized after oral administration. There are 36 recognized metabolites, with less than 2–3% unchanged drug excreted in urine and feces.

Toxicity. Adverse reactions to molindone include drowsiness, depression, muscle rigidity, tremors, tardive dyskinesia, blood dyscrasias and alterations in liver function. The following tissue distribution was observed in a suicide attributed to molindone (Reynolds, 1982):

Molindone Concentrations in a Fatal Case (mg/L or mg/kg)

Blood	Liver	Urine	Gastric
9.3	69	247	23 mg

Analysis. Molindone has been determined in plasma by radioreceptor assay (Tune et al., 1980) and liquid chromatography (Wolf et al., 1985; Narasimhachari et al., 1988).

References

N. Narasimhachari, A.K. Pandurangi and B. Landa. A simple hplc method for the quantitation of molindone in human plasma or serum. J. Liq. Chrom. 11: 983–989, 1988.

P.C. Reynolds. Personal communication, 1982.

L.E. Tune, I. Creese, J.R. Depaulo et al. Clinical state and serum levels measured by radioreceptor assay in schizophrenics. Am. J. Psych. 137: 187–190, 1980.

M.E. Wolf, A.D. Mosnaim, R. Owen et al. Molindone pharmacokinetics in psychiatric patients. Res. Comm. Psych. Behavior 10: 215–220, 1985.

Moricizine

T½: 1.5–3.5 hr
Vd: 11 L/kg
Fb: 0.95
pKa: 6.4

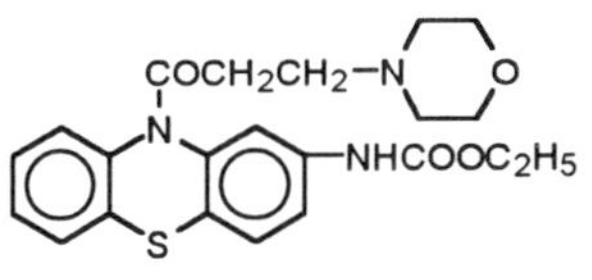

Occurrence and Usage. Moricizine (Ethmozine) is a class I antiarrhythmic drug with potent local anesthetic activity and myocardial membrane-stabilizing effects. It is available as the hydrochloride salt for oral administration in tablets containing 200–300 mg. Dosage must be individualized, but typically is 600–900 mg/day in divided doses.

Blood Concentrations. The oral administration of a single 250 mg dose of moricizine to 24 fasting healthy males produced a maximum plasma concentration ranging from 0.26–1.91 mg/L (average, 0.72); when this dose was repeated following a normal breakfast, the peak plasma concentration ranged from 0.12–1.27 mg/L (average, 0.55) (Pieniaszek et al., 1991). Following the administration of a single 500 mg oral dose to 3 fasting males weighing 50–75 kg, peak plasma concentrations ranging from 0.48–1.54 mg/L occurred between 1 and 3 hours (Whitney et al., 1981).

Peak steady-state plasma concentrations ranged from 0.50–0.55 mg/L following 7 days of treatment in 12 healthy, young males given oral doses of moricizine ranging from 150–300 mg every 8 hours (Benedek et al., 1991).

Metabolism and Excretion. Moricizine is extensively metabolized in man, with less than 1% of a dose excreted in urine as unchanged drug. It is metabolized primarily by sulfoxidation, hydroxylation, N-dealkylation, and glucuronide or sulfate conjugation. The drug has at least 26 metabolites, of which 9 have been identified and 2 have some degree of antiarrhythmic activity. The 2 pharmacologically active metabolites are moricizine sulfoxide and phenothiazine-2-carbamic acid ethyl ester sulfoxide. They represent less than 1% of the administered dose and have plasma half-lives of about 3 hours. Approximately 56% of an oral radioactive dose is excreted in the feces and 39% in the urine (Howrie et al., 1987; Mann, 1990).

Toxicity. Adverse reactions to moricizine include syncope, hypotension, emesis, lethargy, coma and respiratory failure. Two deaths in adults have been attributed to overdoses of 2250 mg and 10,000 mg (Mann, 1990).

Analysis. Moricizine has been determined in biological fluids by liquid chromatography (Whitney et al., 1981; Piotrovski and Metelitsa, 1982: Martin-Light et al., 1984; Poirier, 1985; Yang et al., 1989).

References

I.H. Benedek, D.M. Garner and H.J. Pieniaszek. Dose proportionality of moricizine after escalating multiple doses in healthy volunteers. J. Clin. Pharm. 31: 229–232, 1991.

D.L. Howrie, H.J. Pieniaszek, Jr., R.N. Fogoros et al. Disposition of moricizine (Ethmozine) in healthy subjects after oral administration of radiolabelled drug. Eur. J. Clin. Pharm. 32: 607–610, 1987.

H.J. Mann. Moricizine: a new class I antiarrhythmic. Clin. Pharm. 9: 842–852, 1990.

G. Martin-Light, W.L. Gee, R. Williams et al. High-pressure liquid chromatographic determination of Ethmozine (moricizine HCl) in human plasma. Acad. Pharm. Sci. 14: 94, 1984.

H.J. Pieniaszek, Jr., D.C. Rakeshaw, W.L. Schary and R.L. Williams. Influence of food on the oral absorption and bioavailability of moricizine. J. Clin. Pharm. 31: 792–795, 1991.

V.K. Piotrovski and V.I. Metelitsa. Ion-exchange high-performance liquid chromatography in drug assay in biological fluids. I. Ethmozin. J. Chrom. 231: 205–209, 1982.

J.M. Poirier. Sensitive high performance liquid chromatographic analysis of Ethmozin in plasma. Ther. Drug Mon. 7: 439–441, 1985.

C.C. Whitney, S.H. Weinstein and J.C. Gaylord. High-performance liquid chromatographic determination of Ethmozin in plasma. J. Pharm. Sci. 70: 462–463, 1981.

J.M. Yang, K. Chan and W.D. Jiang. Improved column liquid chromatographic method for the determination of moricizine in plasma or serum. J. Chrom. 490: 458–463, 1989.

Morphine

T½: 1.3–6.7 hr
Vd: 2–5 L/kg
Fb: 0.35
pKa: 8.1

Occurrence and Usage. Morphine is prototypical of the narcotic analgesics, having been available for thousands of years as the primary constituent of crude opium and finally isolated as a pure alkaloid in 1803. It remains a popular drug for treatment of moderate to severe pain, usually by subcutaneous or intramuscular injection of the sulfate salt at an initial dose of 10 mg/70 kg. Morphine is available for oral administration, but as its effects are considerably diminished and somewhat unpredictable with this route, it is not commonly used. Poppy seed, a common food ingredient, may contain morphine at concentrations of 4–200 mg/kg, leading to oral morphine doses as high as 5–10 mg per helping of poppy seed food.

Blood Concentrations. Using an assay specific for unconjugated morphine, it was found that a single 0.125 mg/kg (8.75 mg/70 kg) intravenous dose of morphine to adults produced an average serum concentration of 0.44 mg/L at 0.5 minutes, with a rapid early decline to 0.02 mg/L by 2 hours (Aitkenhead et al., 1984). Intramuscular injection of the same dose results in similar concentrations, an average peak level of 0.07 mg/L being observed 10–20 minutes after administration with a decline to 0.02 mg/L in serum by 4 hours post-dosing; in this study it was noted that morphine-3-glucuronide, a metabolite devoid of pharmacologic activity, appeared in serum within 20 minutes after administration and exceeded the free morphine concentration after 2 hours (Berkowitz et al.,

1975). The epidural administration of 0.1 mg/kg (7 mg/70 kg) of the drug to 9 adult surgical patients produced an average maximal serum concentration of 0.08 mg/L at 10 minutes, declining to less than 0.01 mg/L by 4 hours (Drost et al., 1986). The plasma half-life of morphine in surgical patients averages 1.8 hours for women and 2.9 hours for men (Rigg et al., 1978). The half-life is not significantly increased in renal failure patients (Aitkenhead et al., 1984), but is approximately doubled in cirrhotic subjects (Mazoit et al., 1987). In neonates, it averages 6.8 hours (Lynn and Slattery, 1987). A longer terminal elimination phase (18–60 hours) observed in some studies using radioimmunoassay may be a result of cross-reactivity of morphine antibodies with morphine-3-glucuronide (Stanski et al., 1978).

Plasma morphine concentrations of 0.046–0.083 mg/L (average, 0.065) were found necessary to produce surgical analgesia in pediatric patients (Dahlstrom et al., 1979). Large doses (55–65 mg) of morphine given by intravenous infusion to surgical patients produced peak plasma concentrations of 0.8–2.6 mg/L with concentrations of 0.3–0.5 mg/L still detected after 1.5 hours; this amount of drug produced profound respiratory depression in all patients and assisted ventilation was required (Stanski et al., 1976). The oral bioavailability of morphine ranges from 15–64% and averages 38%; a 20–30 mg oral dose in adult terminal cancer patients was sufficient to maintain serum morphine levels above 0.020 mg/L (considered to be analgesic) for 4–6 hours in most patients (Sawe et al., 1981). In cancer patients receiving 15 mg oral doses every 6 hours for 5 days, steady-state plasma concentrations averaged 0.014 mg/L morphine, 0.515 mg/L morphine-3-glucuronide and 0.077 mg/L morphine-6-glucuronide (an active metabolite). The elimination half-life of morphine-6-glucuronide is similar to that of morphine in patients with normal renal function, but may be prolonged in renal disease (Peterson et al., 1990; Hasselstrom et al., 1991). The blood/plasma concentration ratio for morphine averages 1.02 (Hand et al., 1988).

Metabolism and Excretion. Approximately 5% of a dose of morphine is N-demethylated to normorphine, which is less active than morphine as an analgesic and which probably does not contribute significantly to overall pharmacologic effects; normorphine is found as a urinary metabolite in both the free (1%) and conjugated (4%) forms.

With its free phenolic hydroxyl group, morphine is an excellent substrate for glucuronide formation; indeed, the majority of administered morphine is converted to morphine-3-glucuronide. Most of this highly water-soluble metabolite is excreted in the bile and a portion is eventually eliminated in the feces. However, there is substantial enterohepatic circulation of conjugated and intestinally-deconjugated morphine, with the result that up to 87% of a morphine dose is eliminated in the 72 hour urine, with 75% present as morphine-3-glucuronide. Enterohepatic circulation, as well as hepatocyte secretion into blood, of the glucuronide may account for its presence in plasma and serum. Free morphine in the urine accounts for about 10% of the dose, while very small amounts of morphine-6-glucuronide, morphine-3-ethereal sulfate, and morphine-3,6-diglucuronide are also present (Boerner et al., 1975; Yeh, 1975; Hahn et al., 1977; Yeh et al., 1977). There is evidence that morphine-6-glucuronide is an active metabolite and speculation that it is a significant contributor to analgesia during chronic morphine treatment (Hanks et al., 1987; Osborne et al., 1990).

Certain investigators have suggested that codeine is a minor metabolite of morphine in man, but others have shown that codeine arises as an impurity in commercial morphine to the extent of 0.04%, and that this is the source of urinary codeine following morphine administration (Boerner and Abbott, 1973; Boerner et al., 1974; Yeh, 1974).

The following morphine concentrations were found in a subject who received multiple administrations of intravenous morphine during a 48 hour period of hospitalization and who died of traumatic causes (Cravey and Reed, 1977):

Morphine Concentrations in a Trauma Patient (mg/L or mg/kg)

Blood	Brain	Lung	Liver	Bile
0.67	0.04	0.21	0.11	0.44

As expected from animal studies on the blood-brain barrier penetration by morphine (Oldendorf et al., 1972), the brain concentration is very low. Since the radioimmunoassay procedure used in the above body distribution study is 80% cross-reactive with morphine-3-glucuronide, it is likely that this metabolite accounts for a portion of the above concentrations. This contribution may be especially important in the case of the blood concentration, since the data of Spiehler and Brown (1987) show that unconjugated morphine averages just 42% (range, 0–100%) of the total blood morphine level in forensic cases.

Eating of poppy seed foods has resulted in morphine and codeine concentrations as high as 0.100 and 0.007 mg/L, respectively, in serum and 4.5 and 0.2 mg/L, respectively, in urine (Bjerver et al., 1982; Fritschi et al., 1985; Hayes et al., 1987; Pettitt et al., 1987; Streumpler, 1987; Zebelman et al., 1987).

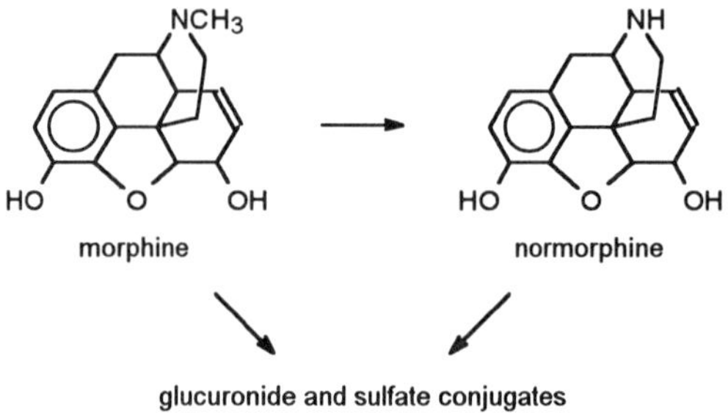

Toxicity. Adverse or toxic effects of morphine usage include pupillary constriction, constipation, urinary retention, nausea, vomiting, hypothermia, drowsiness, dizziness, apathy, confusion, respiratory depression, hypotension, cold and clammy skin, coma, and pulmonary edema. Impairment of cognition and motor control is demonstrable in healthy volunteers at plasma morphine concentrations equal to or greater than 0.040 mg/L (Kerr et al., 1991). Doses greater than 30 mg parenterally and 100 mg orally are toxic to the nontolerant adult, and death may occur following doses of 120 mg or more. Three renal failure patients exhibited prolonged respiratory failure after morphine administration, at a time when plasma morphine concentrations were less than 0.004 mg/L but morphine-6-glucuronide levels were 0.130–1.171 mg/L (Osborne et al., 1986). Two neonates receiving intravenous morphine infusions experienced seizures at serum morphine concentrations of 0.061 and 0.090 mg/L (Koren et al., 1985).

Morphine *per se* is rarely used by addicts in the United States and there is little information on tissue concentrations to be expected following fatal overdosage. However, the drug is apparently used more commonly in Europe, and one report of 10 fatalities involving the intravenous administration of morphine, with no other drugs found, presented the following information (Felby et al., 1974):

Total Morphine Concentrations in Fatalities (mg/L or mg/kg)

	Blood	Muscle	Liver	Urine
Average	0.7	0.8	3.0	52
(Range)	(0.2–2.3)	(0.1–2.0)	(0.4–18)	(14–81)

* By gas chromatography after acid hydrolysis and silylation

Chan et al. (1986) presented 2 additional fatalities, involving oral and intravenous morphine administration, with findings of 0.07–0.35 mg/L unconjugated morphine in blood and 2.9–7.0 mg/kg total drug in liver.

Analysis. The assay of morphine is discussed in the section on heroin.

References

A.R. Aitkenhead, M. Vater, K. Achola et al. Pharmacokinetics of single-dose i.v. morphine in normal volunteers and patients with end-stage renal failure. Brit. J. Anaesth. 56: 813–818, 1984.

B.A. Berkowitz, S.H. Ngai, J.C. Yang et al. The disposition of morphine in surgical patients. Clin. Pharm. Ther. 17: 629–635, 1975.

K. Bjerver, J. Jonsson, A. Nilsson et al. Morphine intake from poppy seed food. J. Pharm. Pharmac. 34: 798–801, 1982.

U. Boerner and S. Abbott. New observations in the metabolism of morphine. The formation of codeine from morphine in man. Experientia 29: 180–181, 1973.

U. Boerner, R.L. Roe and C.E. Becker. Detection, isolation and characterization of normorphine and norcodeine as morphine metabolites in man. J. Pharm. Pharmac. 26: 393–398, 1974.

U. Boerner, S. Abbott and R.L. Roe. The metabolism of morphine and heroin in man. Drug Met. Rev. 4: 39–73, 1975.

S.C. Chan, E.M. Chan and H.A. Kaliciak. Distribution of morphine in body fluids and tissues in fatal overdose. J. For. Sci. 31: 1487–1491, 1986.

R.H. Cravey and D. Reed. The distribution of morphine in man following chronic intravenous administration. J. Anal. Tox. 1: 166–167, 1977.

B. Dahlstrom, P. Bolme, H. Feychting et al. Morphine kinetics in children. Clin. Pharm. Ther. 26: 354–365, 1979.

R.H. Drost, T.I. Ionescu, J.M. van Rossum and R.A.A. Maes. Pharmacokinetics of morphine after epidural administration in man. Arz. Forsch. 36: 1096–1100, 1986.

S. Felby, H. Christensen and A. Lund. Morphine concentrations in blood and organs in cases of fatal poisoning. For. Sci. 3: 77–81, 1974.

G. Fritschi and W.R. Prescott. Morphine levels in urine subsequent to poppy seed consumption. For. Sci. Int. 27: 111–117, 1985.

E.F. Hahn, H. Roffwarg and J. Fishman. Morphine metabolism in opiate dependent and normal men by double isotope techniques. Res. Comm. Chem. Path. Pharm. 18: 401–414, 1977.

C.W. Hand, R.A. Moore and J.W. Sear. Comparison of whole blood and plasma morphine. J. Anal. Tox. 12: 234–235, 1988.

G.W. Hanks, P.J. Hoskin, G.W. Aherne et al. Explanation for potency of repeated oral doses of morphine? Lancet 2: 723–725, 1987.

J. Hasselstrom, N. Alexander, C. Bringel et al. Single-dose and steady-state kinetics of morphine and its metabolites in cancer patients. Eur. J. Cln. Pharm. 40: 585–591, 1991.

L.W. Hayes, W.G. Krasselt and P.A. Mueggler. Concentrations of morphine and codeine in serum and urine after ingestion of poppy seeds. Clin. Chem. 33: 806–808, 1987.

B. Kerr, H. Hill, B. Coda et al. Concentration-related effects of morphine on cognition and motor control in human subjects. Neuropsychopharmacology 5: 157–166, 1991.

G. Koren, W. Butt, K. Pape and H. Chinyanga. Morphine-induced seizures in newborn infants. Vet. Hum. Tox. 27: 519–520, 1985.

A.M. Lynn and J.T. Slattery. Morphine pharmacokinetics in early infancy. Anesthesiology 66: 136–139, 1987.

J.X. Mazoit, P. Sandouk, P. Zetlauoi and J.M. Scherrmann. Pharmacokinetics of unchanged morphine in normal and cirrhotic subjects. Anesth. Anal. 66: 293–298, 1987.

W.H. Oldendorf, S. Hyman, L. Braun and S.Z. Oldendorf. Blood-brain barrier: penetration of morphine, codeine, heroin, and methadone after carotid injection. Science 178: 984–986, 1972.

R.J. Osborne, S.P. Joel and M.L. Slevin. Morphine intoxication in renal failure: the role of morphine-6-glucuronide. Brit. Med. J. 292: 1548–1549, 1986.

R. Osborne, S. Joel, D. Trew and M. Slevin. Morphine and metabolite behaviour after different routes of morphine administration. Clin. Pharm. Ther. 47: 12–19, 1990.

G.M. Peterson, C.T.C. Randall and J. Paterson. Plasma levels of morphine and morphine glucuronides in the treatment of cancer pain. Eur. J. Clin. Pharm. 38: 121–124, 1990.

B.C. Pettitt, S.M. Dyszel and L.V.S. Hood. Opiates in poppy seed: effect on urinalysis results after consumption of poppy seed cake-filling. Clin. Chem. 33: 1251–1252, 1987.

J.R.A. Rigg, R.A. Browne, C. Davis et al. Variation in the disposition of morphine after I.M. administration in surgical patients. Brit. J. Anaesth. 50: 1125–1130, 1978.

J. Sawe, B. Dahlstrom, L. Paalzow and A. Rane. Morphine kinetics in cancer patients. Clin. Pharm. Ther. 30: 629–635, 1981.

V. Spiehler and R. Brown. Unconjugated morphine in blood by radioimmunoassay and gas chromatography-mass spectrometry. J. For. Sci. 32: 906–916, 1987.

D.R. Stanski, D.J. Greenblatt, D.G. Lappas et al. Kinetics of high-dose intravenous morphine in cardiac surgery patients. Clin. Pharm. Ther. 19: 752–756, 1976.

D.R. Stanski, D.J. Greenblatt and E. Lowenstein. Kinetics of intravenous and intramuscular morphine. Clin. Pharm. Ther. 24: 52–59, 1978.

R.E. Streumpler. Excretion of codeine and morphine following ingestion of poppy seed. J. Anal. Tox. 11: 97–99, 1987.

S.Y. Yeh. Absence of evidence of biotransformation of morphine to codeine in man. Experientia 30: 264–266, 1974.

S.Y. Yeh. Urinary excretion of morphine and its metabolites in morphine-dependent subjects. J. Pharm. Exp. Ther. 192: 201–210, 1975.

S.Y. Yeh, S.W. Gorodetzky and H.A. Krebs. Isolation and identification of morphine 3- and 6-glucuronides, morphine 3,6-diglucuronide, morphine 3-ethereal sulfate, normorphine, and normorphine 6-glucuronide as morphine metabolites in humans. J. Pharm. Sci. 66: 1288–1293, 1977.

A.M. Zebelman, B.L. Troyer, G.L. Randall and J.D. Batjer. Detection of morphine and codeine following consumption of poppy seeds. J. Anal. Tox. 11: 131–132, 1987.

Nadolol

T½: 11–18 hr
Vd: 1.5–3.6 L/kg
Fb: 0.20
pKa: 9.7

Occurrence and Usage. Nadolol (Corgard) is a beta-adrenergic blocking agent used for the treatment of hypertension and angina. It is available for oral administration in tablets containing 40, 80, 120 or 160 mg of the free base. For the treatment of angina pectoris, doses of up to 240 mg daily are sometimes used. For hypertension, doses of up to 320 mg daily may be needed.

Blood Concentrations. After a single 80 mg oral dose of nadolol in 4 subjects, maximum plasma concentrations ranging from 0.04–0.21 mg/L (average, 0.14) were attained in 1–4 hours. In those same patients following a multiple-dosage regimen (80 mg daily for 11 days and 40 mg daily for 3 days), maximum plasma concentrations ranging from 0.11–0.34 mg/L (average, 0.22) were observed in 2–4 hours. A study with 8 mildly hypertensive patients who were given 80 mg of nadolol once daily showed that steady-state concentrations were attained in 6 days; the average plasma concentration of nadolol 24 hours after the fifth daily dose was 0.045 mg/L (Dreyfuss et al., 1979).

Metabolism and Excretion. Absorption of nadolol after oral dosing is variable, averaging about 30%. Unlike other beta-blockers, the drug is not metabolized to any great extent, being excreted largely unchanged (Gupta et al., 1983). An average of 15–21% of a dose is excreted unchanged in the urine and an average of 68–85% eliminated in the feces within a 4 day period (Dreyfuss et al., 1979).

Toxicity. Since nadolol is water-soluble and does not readily cross the blood-brain barrier, central nervous system effects occur less frequently than with lipophilic beta-blockers. However, dizziness, fatigue, sedation and behavioral changes have been reported. Other adverse effects include bradycardia, cardiac failure, hypotension, blood dyscrasias, disorientation and hallucinations.

Analysis. Fluorometry has been effectively utilized for quantitation of nadolol in serum (Ivashkiv, 1977). Gas chromatographic methods with nitrogen-selective (Yamaguchi et al., 1982) and mass spectrometric detection (Funke et al., 1978; Cohen et al., 1984; Ribick et al., 1986) have been described. Liquid chromatography using electrochemical (Surmann, 1980) and fluorescence detection (Gupta et al., 1983; Moncrieff, 1985; Noguchi et al., 1992) has been employed.

References

A.I. Cohen, R.G. Devlin, E. Ivashkiv et al. Determination of orally coadministered nadolol and its deuterated analogue in human serum and urine by gas chromatography with selected ion monitoring mass spectrometry. J. Pharm. Sci. 73: 1571–1575, 1984.

J. Dreyfuss, D.L. Griffith, S.M. Singhvi et al. Pharmacokinetics of nadolol, a beta-receptor antagonist: administration of therapeutic single and multiple-dosage regimens to hypertensive patients. J. Clin. Pharm. 19: 712–720, 1979.

P.T. Funke, M.F. Malley, E. Ivashkiv and A.I. Cohen. Determination of serum nadolol levels by GLC-selected ion monitoring mass spectrometry: comparison with a spectrofluorometric method. J. Pharm. Sci. 67: 653–656, 1978.

R.N. Gupta, R.B. Haynes, A.G. Logan et al. Liquid-chromatographic determination of nadolol in plasma. Clin. Chem. 29: 1085–1087, 1983.

E. Ivashkiv. Fluorometric determination of nadolol in human serum and urine. J. Pharm. Sci. 66: 1168–1171, 1977.

J. Moncrieff. Assay of nadolol in serum by reversed-phase high-performance liquid chromatography with fluorometric detection. J. Chrom. 342: 206–211, 1985.

H. Noguchi, K. Yoshida, M. Murano and S. Naruto. Determination of nadolol in serum by high-performance liquid chromatography with fluorimetric detection. J. Chrom. 573: 336–338, 1992.

M. Ribick, E. Ivashkiv, M. Jemal and A.I. Cohen. Use of an inexpensive mass-selective detector for the high-sensitivity gas chromatographic determination of nadolol in plasma. J. Chrom. 381: 419–423, 1986.

P. Surmann. Determination of nadolol in serum. Arch. Pharm. 313: 1052–1054, 1980.

T. Yamaguchi, Y. Morimoto, Y. Sekine and M. Hashimoto. Determination of beta-adrenergic blocking drugs as cyclic boronates by gas chromatography with nitrogen-selective detection. J. Chrom. 239: 609–615, 1982.

Nalbuphine

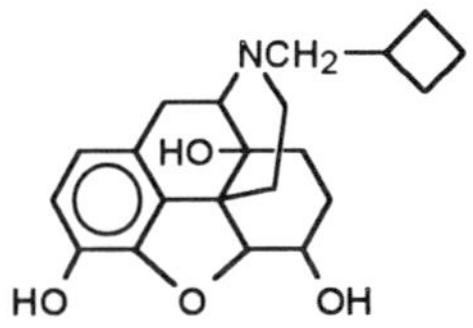

T½: 1.9–7.7 hr
Vd: 2.4–7.3 L/kg
Fb: ?
pKa: ?

Occurrence and Usage. Nalbuphine (Nubain) is a synthetic narcotic agonist/antagonist of the phenanthrene series that is chemically related to both naloxone and oxymorphone. It is equipotent to morphine on a weight basis. The usual dose is 10 mg every 3–6 hours as needed. Nalbuphine is available in ampules containing 10–20 mg/mL as the hydrochloride for intramuscular, intravenous or subcutaneous administration.

Blood Concentrations. An average peak plasma nalbuphine concentration of about 0.015 mg/L was attained in 1 hour following a single oral dose of 30 mg to three subjects. Peak plasma nalbuphine concentrations ranging from 0.038–0.059 mg/L (average, 0.052) were reached within 15–30 minutes following a single intramuscular dose of 10 mg to 6 subjects (Bullingham, 1984). The plasma half-life averaged 2.2–2.6 hours after intravenous, intramuscular or subcutaneous administration (Lo et al., 1987). In another study of 10 healthy subjects with intravenous administration of 20 mg, plasma nalbuphine concentrations averaged 0.559 mg/L at 1 minute and 0.069 mg/L at 15 minutes; elimination half-lives averaged 3.7 hous (range, 1.9–7.7) (Aitkenhead et al., 1988).

Metabolism and Excretion. Nalbuphine is metabolized by N-dealkylation and conjugation. Urinary excretion accounts for about 71% of a dose as free and conjugated nalbuphine and nornalbuphine. The remaining drug is thought to be eliminated in the feces as a result of biliary excretion (Lake et al., 1982).

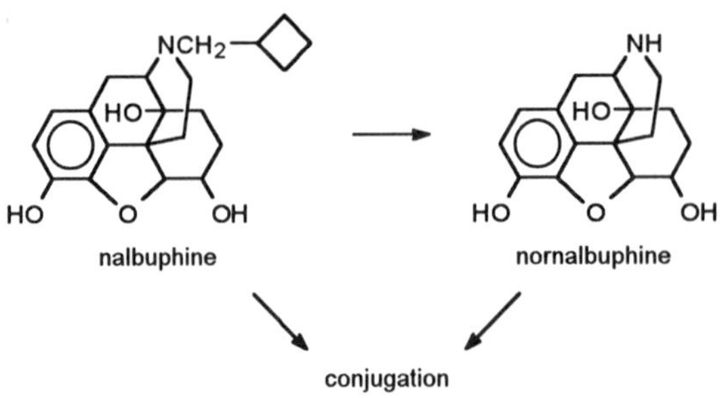

Toxicity. Nalbuphine is capable of producing sedation, central nervous system depression, hostility, confusion, delusions, hallucinations, bradycardia, tachycardia, respiratory depression, coma and cardiac arrest.

Analysis. Nalbuphine has been determined in plasma by gas chromatography with electron-capture detection (Weinstein et al., 1978) and by liquid chromatography (Lake et al., 1982; Keegan and Kay, 1984; Lo et al., 1984; Dube et al., 1988).

References

A.R. Aitkenhead, E.S. Lin and K.J. Achola. The pharmacokinetics of oral and intravenous nalbuphine in healthy volunteers. Brit. J. Clin. Pharm. 25: 264–268, 1988.

R.E.S. Bullingham. Pharmacokinetics of nalbuphine. In *Opioid Agonist/Antagonist Drugs in Clinical Practice* (W.S. Nimmo and G. Smith, eds.), Excerpta Medica, Oxford, 1984, pp. 115–122.

L.M. Dube, N. Beaudoin, M. LaLande and I.J. McGilveray. Determination of nalbuphine by high-performance liquid chromatography with electrochemical detection. J. Chrom. 427: 113–120, 1988.

M. Keegan and B. Kay. Detection of nalbuphine in plasma: an improved high-performance liquid chromatography assay. J. Chrom. 311: 223–226, 1984.

C.L. Lake, C.A. DiFazio, E.N. Duckworth et al. High-performance liquid chromatographic analysis of plasma levels of nalbuphine in cardiac surgical patients. J. Chrom. 233: 410–416, 1982.

M.W. Lo, G.P. Juergens and C.C. Whitney, Jr. Determination of nalbuphine in human plasma by automated high-performance liquid chromatography with electrochemical detection. Res. Comm. Chem. Path. Pharm. 43: 159–168, 1984.

M.W. Lo, F.H. Lee, W.L. Schary and C.C. Whitney, Jr. The pharmacokinetics of intravenous, intramuscular, and subcutaneous nalbuphine in healthy subjects. Eur. J. Clin. Pharm. 33: 297–301, 1987.

S.H. Weinstein, M. Alteras and J. Gaylord. Quantitative determination of nalbuphine in plasma using electron-capture detection. J. Pharm. Sci. 67: 547–548, 1978.

Naloxone

T½: 30–80 min
Vd: 2.6–2.8 L/kg
Fb: ?
pKa: 7.9

Occurrence and Usage. Naloxone (N-allylnoroxymorphone, Narcan) is a synthetic narcotic antagonist that has been used clinically since 1962. The drug is the allyl analogue of oxymorphone, a potent narcotic analgesic, but is without agonist activity of its own. It is available for parenteral injection as a 0.4 mg/mL solution of the hydrochloride; the usual adult dose is 0.4 mg, repeated at frequent intervals as needed.

Blood Concentrations. The intravenous injection of 0.4 mg in 9 subjects produced plasma naloxone concentrations that averaged 0.010 mg/L at 2 minutes and 0.004 mg/L at 5 minutes; the levels declined with an average half-life of 64 minutes (Ngai et al., 1976). Steady-state plasma naloxone levels of 0.069–0.084 mg/L were produced in 2 adult volunteers by the intravenous administration of a 20 mg bolus injection followed by a 0.24 mg/min constant infusion (Reid et al., 1993).

Metabolism and Excretion. From 60–68% of a labeled intravenous dose of naloxone is excreted in the 72 hour urine, with about half of that appearing in the first 6 hours; all of the excreted material was in conjugated form (Fishman et al., 1973). Naloxone is known to be metabolized by N-dealkylation, reduction of the 6-keto group, and O-glucuronidation. Human urinary metabolites include, largely in conjugated form, naloxone, nornaloxone (noroxymorphone), and naloxol (Weinstein et al., 1971, 1974).

Toxicity. Up to 10 mg of naloxone has been given intravenously to patients without apparent effect. The drug is routinely administered to all comatose patients in many emergency facilities, in the event that a narcotic analgesic is the cause of the intoxication.

Analysis. Naloxone has been quantitatively determined in plasma by radioimmunoassay (Berkowitz et al., 1975) and by electron-capture gas chromatography after formation of a halogenated derivative (Sams and Malspeis, 1976; Meffin and Smith, 1980). Liquid chromatographic methods have also been described (Asali et al., 1983; Terry et al., 1984; Albeck et al., 1989; Reid et al., 1993).

References

H. Albeck, S. Woodfield and M.J. Kreek. Quantitative and pharmacokinetic analysis of naloxone in plasma using high-performance liquid chromatography with electrochemical detection and solid-phase extraction. J. Chrom. 488: 435–445, 1989.

L.A. Asali, R.L. Nation and K.F. Brown. Determination of naloxone in blood by high-performance liquid chromatography. J. Chrom. 278: 329–335, 1983.

B.A. Berkowitz, S.H. Ngai, J. Hempstead and S. Spector. Disposition of naloxone: use of a new radioimmunoassay. J. Pharm. Exp. Ther. 195: 499–504, 1975.

J. Fishman, H. Roffwarg and L. Hellman. Disposition of naloxone-7,8-^{3}H in normal and narcotic-dependent men. J. Pharm. Exp. Ther. 187: 575–580, 1973.

P.J. Meffin and K.J. Smith. Gas chromatographic analysis of naloxone in biological fluids. J. Chrom. 183: 352–356, 1980.

S.H. Ngai, B.A. Berkowitz, J.C. Yang et al. Pharmacokinetics of naloxone in rats and in man: basis for its potency and short duration of action. Anesthesiology 44: 398–401, 1976.

R.W. Reid, A. Deakin and D.J. Loehey. Measurement of naloxone in plasma using hplc with electrochemical detection. J. Chrom. 614: 117–122, 1993.

R.A. Sams and L. Malspeis. Determination of naloxone and naltrexone as perfluoroalkyl ester derivatives by electron-capture gas-liquid chromatography. J. Chrom. 125: 409–420, 1976.

M.D. Terry, G.H. Hisayasu, J.W. Kern and J.L. Cohen. High-performance liquid chromatographic analysis of naloxone in human serum. J. Chrom. 311: 213–217, 1984.

S.H. Weinstein, M. Pfeffer, J.M. Schor et al. Metabolites of naloxone in human urine. J. Pharm. Sci. 60: 1567–1568, 1971.

S.H. Weinstein, M. Pfeffer and J.M. Schor. Metabolism and pharmacokinetics of naloxone. Adv. Biochem. Psychopharm. 8: 525–535, 1974.

Naltrexone

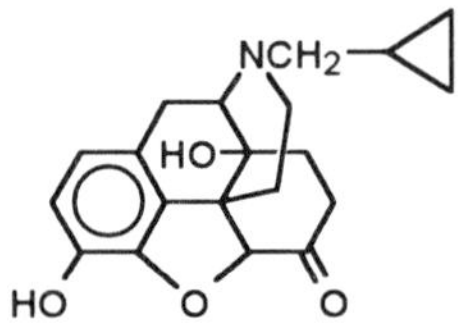

T½: 1–2 hr
Vd: 3 L/kg
Fb: 0.21
pKa: 7.9

Occurrence and Usage. Naltrexone (Trexan) is a potent narcotic antagonist first synthesized in 1965. It is a synthetic congener of oxymorphone and naloxone. The drug markedly attenuates or reversibly blocks the subjective effects of heroin and other opiates for up to 24 hours. The usual oral dose is 25 mg with an additional 25 mg an hour later if no withdrawal symptoms occur. The usual adult maintenance dose is 50 mg every 24 hours. Naltrexone is available as the hydrochloride in tablets containing 50 mg.

Blood Concentrations. Following the oral administration of 100 mg of naltrexone to 4 subjects, peak plasma concentrations averaged 44 µg/L at 1 hour for naltrexone and 87 µg/L at 2 hours for the major metabolite, 6β-naltrexol (Verebey et al., 1976a). The average plasma naltrexone concentration in 6 schizophrenic patients following 100 mg daily oral doses was 1.9 µg/L, while the concentration of 6β-naltrexol averaged 40 µg/L (Verebey and Mule, 1979).

Metabolism and Excretion. Naltrexone undergoes extensive first-pass metabolism with approximately 95% of the absorbed drug being converted to several metabolites. The major metabolites observed in plasma, urine and feces are conjugated naltrexone and free and conjugated 6β-naltrexol, with the latter being the major urinary metabolite in man (Cone et al., 1974; Verebey et al., 1975; Verebey et al., 1976a). 2-Hydroxy-3-0-methyl-6β-naltrexol is found in urine in minor quantities (Wall et al., 1981). Up to 70% of an oral labeled dose has been recovered in urine within 24 hours, with less than 0.5% in the feces (Verebey et al., 1976b).

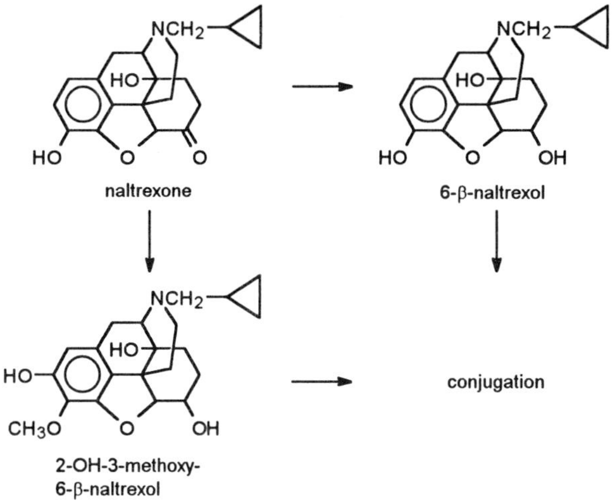

naltrexone

6-β-naltrexol

2-OH-3-methoxy-
6-β-naltrexol

conjugation

Toxicity. Adverse reactions to naltrexone administration include sedation, lightheadedness and weakness. In one study, patients who received 800 mg daily for 1 week showed no signs of toxicity (Verebey and Mule, 1979). In acute toxicity studies in laboratory animals, the cause of death was clonic-tonic convulsions and/or respiratory failure.

Analysis. Naltrexone and its metabolites have been analyzed in biological samples employing gas chromatography (Verebely et al., 1975; Verebey et al., 1976b; Verebey et al., 1980), liquid chromatography (Ventura et al., 1988; Zuccaro et al., 1991), and gas chromatography-mass spectrometry (Cone et al., 1978; Monti et al., 1991).

References

E.J. Cone, C.W. Gorodetzky and S.Y. Yeh. The urinary excretion profile of naltrexone and metabolites in man. Drug Met. Disp. 2: 506–512, 1974.

E.J. Cone, C.W. Gorodetzky, W.D. Darwin et al. The identification and measurement of two new metabolites of naltrexone in human urine. Res. Comm. Chem. Path. Pharm. 20: 413–433, 1978.

K.M. Monti, R.L. Foltz and D.M. Chinn. Analysis of naltrexone and 6β-naltrexol in plasma and urine by gas chromatography/negative ion chemical ionization mass spectrometry. J. Anal. Tox. 15: 136–140, 1991.

R. Ventura, R. de la Torre and J. Segura. Analysis of naltrexone urinary metabolites. J. Pharm. Biomed. Anal. 6: 887–893, 1988.

K. Verebely, S.J. Mule and D. Jukofsky. A gas-liquid chromatographic method for the determination of naltrexone and beta-naltrexol in human urine. J. Chrom. 111: 141–148, 1975.

K. Verebey, M.A. Chedekel, S.J. Mule and D. Rosenthal. Isolation and identification of a new metabolite of naltrexone in human blood and urine. Res. Comm. Chem. Path. Pharm. 12: 67–84, 1975.

K. Verebey, J. Volavka, S.J. Mule et al. Naltrexone: disposition, metabolism, and effects after acute and chronic dosing. Clin. Pharm. Ther. 20: 315–328, 1976a.

K. Verebey, M.J. Kogan, A. de Pace and S.J. Mule. Quantitative determination of naltrexone and beta-naltrexol in human plasma using electron capture detection. J. Chrom. 118: 331–335, 1976b.

K. Verebey and S.J. Mule. Naltrexone and β-naltrexol plasma levels in schizophrenic patients after large oral doses of naltrexone. Res. Comm. Psych. Psychiat. Behav. 4: 311–317, 1979.

K. Verebey, A. De Pace, D. Jukofsky et al. Quantitative determination of 2-hydroxy-3-methoxy-6β-naltrexol (HMN), naltrexone, and 6β-naltrexol in human plasma, red blood cells, saliva and urine by gas liquid chromatography. J. Anal. Tox. 4: 33–37, 1980.

M.E. Wall, D.R. Brine and M. Perez-Reyes. Metabolism and disposition of naltrexone in man after oral and intravenous administration. Drug Met. Disp. 9: 369–375, 1981.

P. Zuccaro, I. Altieri, P. Betto et al. Determination of naltrexone and 6-β-naltrexol in plasma by high-performance liquid chromatography with coulometric detection. J. Chrom. 567: 485–490, 1991.

Naproxen

T½: 9–22 hr
Vd: 0.09 L/kg
Fb: 0.99
pKa: 5.0

Occurrence and Usage. Naproxen (Aleve, Anaprox, Naprosyn) is a propionic acid derivative used clinically since 1972 as an antiinflammatory, analgesic and antipyretic agent. It is chemically related to fenoprofen, ibuprofen and ketoprofen. The drug is available for oral administration as the free acid in tablets of 250 or 375 mg, and as the sodium salt in tablets of 275 mg. Daily doses range from 250–1250 mg.

Blood Concentrations. A single 250 mg oral dose of naproxen given to 11 volunteers resulted in an average peak serum concentration of 31 mg/L at 3.1 hours, which declined with an average half-life of 16 hours (Weber et al., 1981). A single 500 mg oral dose produced peak levels of 49–69 mg/L in 3 subjects after 2 hours; the concentration of O-desmethylnaproxen was less than 1% of the parent drug (Tomson et al., 1981). Trough serum levels in volunteers receiving 250 mg twice daily for 7 days averaged 31 mg/L, and peak levels averaged 46 mg/L (Weber et al., 1981). A single 750 mg oral dose in 12 healthy subjects produced peak plasma naproxen levels of 60–102 mg/L (average, 89) at 1–4 hours post-dose (Strocchi et al., 1991). Peak levels exceeding 120 mg/L were observed in subjects receiving 1500 mg of the drug daily for 5 days (Weber et al., 1981).

Naproxen exhibits nonlinear kinetics at daily doses exceeding 1000 mg, probably due to saturation of plasma protein binding sites leading to accelerated renal clearance (Runkel et al., 1974, 1976). Plasma naproxen concentrations were only 36% of normal in patients with hypoproteinemia (Calvo et al., 1981). Plasma concentrations were lowered to 71% or 61% of normal in patients with moderate or severe renal failure, respectively, and the renal clearance of the drug was increased proportionally in these patients, due to decreased binding to plasma protein (Anttila et al., 1980).

Metabolism and Excretion. An average of 87% of a single labeled oral dose is excreted in the 96 hour urine, with 2.3% in feces (Runkel et al., 1974). Approximately 10% of a daily dose is reported to be excreted as unchanged drug in urine; 60% appears as conjugated naproxen, 5% as O-desmethyl-naproxen, and 23% as conjugated O-desmethylnaproxen (Segre, 1975). Upton et al. (1980a) found that only 0.6% of a dose is eliminated unchanged, and that higher values are due to the facile hydrolysis of naproxen conjugates in stored specimens (especially if alkaline).

Toxicity. The toxic reactions most commonly associated with naproxen include nausea, abdominal pain, constipation, headache, dizziness, drowsiness, tinnitus, and skin eruptions. One patient acutely ingested 25 g of the drug and achieved a serum concentration of 414 mg/L, but experienced only nausea and indigestion (Fredell and Strand, 1977).

Analysis. Naproxen has been assayed in plasma by ultraviolet spectrophotometry (Holzbecher et al., 1979), fluorometry (Antilla, 1977; Mortensen et al., 1979) and flame-ionization gas chromatography of a methyl derivative (Weber et al., 1981). Gas chromatography has been applied to the determination of the urinary metabolites of naproxen (Wan and Matin, 1979), and liquid chromatographic procedures are available for both plasma and urine (Slattery and Levy, 1979; Upton et al., 1980b; Broquaire et al., 1981; van Loenhout et al., 1982; Satterwhite and Boudinot, 1988; Wanwimolruk, 1990).

References

M. Anttila. Fluorometric determination of naproxen in serum. J. Pharm. Sci. 66: 433–434, 1977.

M. Anttila, M. Haataja and A. Kasanen. Pharmacokinetics of naproxen in subjects with normal and impaired renal function. Eur. J. Clin. Pharm. 18: 263–268, 1980.

M. Broquaire, V. Rovei and R. Braithwaite. Quantitative determination of naproxen in plasma by a simple high-performance liquid chromatographic method. J. Chrom. 224: 43–49, 1981.

M.V. Calvo, A. Dominguez-Gil and C. Muriel. Pharmacokinetics of naproxen in patients with hypoproteinemia. Int. J. Clin. Pharm. Ther. Tox. 19: 326–330, 1981.

E.W. Fredell and L.J. Strand. Naproxen overdose. J. Am. Med. Asso. 238: 938, 1977.

M. Holzbecher, H.A. Ellenberger, J.M. Marsh and S. Boudreau. An ultraviolet spectrophotometric procedure for the routine determination of naproxen. Clin. Biochem. 12: 66–67, 1979.

A. Mortensen, E.B. Jensen, P.B. Petersen et al. The determination of proxen by spectrofluorometry and its binding to serum proteins. Acta Pharm. Tox. 44: 277–283, 1979.

R. Runkel, E. Forchielli, H. Sevelius et al. Nonlinear plasma level response to high doses of naproxen. Clin. Pharm. Ther. 15: 261–266, 1974.

R. Runkel, M.D. Chaplin, H. Sevelius et al. Pharmacokinetics of naproxen overdose. Clin. Pharm. Ther. 20: 269–277, 1976.

J.H. Satterwhite and F.D. Boudinot. High performance liquid chromatographic determination of ketoprofen and naproxen in rat plasma. J. Chrom. 431: 444–449, 1988.

E.J. Segre. Naproxen metabolism in man. J. Clin. Pharm. 15: 316–323, 1975.

J.T. Slattery and G. Levy. Determination of naproxen and its desmethyl metabolite in human plasma or serum by high performance liquid chromatography. Clin. Biochem. 12: 100–103, 1979.

E. Strocchi, E. Ambrosioni, E. Palazzini and G. Galli. Pharmacokinetics of a controlled release preparation of naproxen. Int. J. Clin. Pharm. Ther. Tox. 29: 253–256, 1991.

G. Tomson, N.O. Lunell, E. Oliw and A. Rane. Relation of naproxen kinetics to effect on platelet prostaglandin release in men and dysmenorrheic women. Clin. Pharm. Ther. 29: 168–173, 1981.

R.A. Upton, J.N. Buskin, R.L. Williams et al. Negligible excretion of unchanged ketoprofen, naproxen, and probenecid in urine. J. Pharm. Sci. 69: 1254–1257, 1980a.

R.A. Upton, J.N. Buskin, T.W. Guentert et al. Convenient and sensitive high-performance liquid chromatography assay for ketoprofen, naproxen and other allied drugs in plasma or urine. J. Chrom. 190: 119–128, 1980b.

J.W.A. van Loenhout, C.A.M. van Ginneken, H.C.J. Ketelaars et al. A high-performance liquid chromatographic method for the quantitative determination of naproxen and des-methyl-naproxen in biological samples. J. Liq. Chrom. 5: 549–561, 1982.

S.H. Wan and S.B. Matin. Quantitative gas-liquid chromatographic analysis of naproxen, 6-O-desmethyl-naproxen and their conjugates in urine. J. Chrom. 170: 473–478, 1979.

S. Wanwimolruk. A simple isocratic high-performance liquid chromatographic (HPLC) determination of naproxen in human plasma using a microbore column technique. J. Liq. Chrom. 13: 1611–1626, 1990.

S.S. Weber, A.D. Bankhurst, E. Mroszczak and T.L. Ding. Effect of Mylanta on naproxen bioavailability. Ther. Drug Mon. 3: 75–83, 1981.

Nickel

T½: 11 hr   **Ni**
Vd: ?
Fb: 0.59

Occurrence and Usage. Nickel is a component of many alloys, being present in amounts of up to 15% in stainless steel. It is used to plate other metals and is widely used in electrical devices. Nickel is an essential trace element and is supplied at the rate of 0.3–0.6 mg per day by the diet. The metal or its compounds are absorbed following inhalation or ingestion. The threshold limit values for nickel in the industrial atmosphere range from 0.1 mg/m^3 for soluble compounds of nickel to 1 mg/m^3 for the metal itself. Nickel carbonyl is dealt with in the subsequent section.

Blood Concentrations. Nickel in the plasma of healthy subjects averages 2.1 µg/L (range, 1.4–3.4). In 6 asymptomatic nickel-exposed workers, plasma concentrations ranged from 3.2–11.1 µg/L (Andersen et al., 1978). Patients who have experienced myocardial infarction exhibit serum nickel concentrations averaging 5.2–6.0 µg/L in the 9 days following the episode (Howard, 1980). Serum nickel concentrations following the oral ingestion of 25 mg of nickel sulfate (5.6 mg Ni) by 8 volunteers reached an average peak concentration of 34 µg/L at 2.5 hours, and declined with a half-life of 11 hours (Christensen and Lagesson, 1980). Plasma concentrations as high as 100 µg/L have been observed in nickel refinery workers (Hogetveit et al., 1978). Whole blood concentrations are approximately twice those of plasma or serum (Sunderman, 1977).

Metabolism and Excretion. Of the nickel that is ingested, over 90% is excreted unabsorbed in the feces (Sunderman, 1977). Absorbed nickel tends to localize in the connective tissue, kidney and lungs (Oskarsson and Tjalve, 1977). Nickel concentrations in parenchymal tissues are generally quite low, usually less than 25 µg/kg in lung and less than 10 µg/kg in liver, and do not appear to increase with age in healthy non-occupationally exposed subjects (Panel on Nickel, 1975). Most of the absorbed nickel is believed to be excreted in urine, with an average of 4.5 µg/L (range, 1.9–9.6) found in the urine of unexposed persons (Andersen et al., 1978). Urine nickel concentrations in healthy electroplating shop employees have ranged from 4–65 µg/L in one study (Bernacki et al., 1978) and 10–120 µg/L in another (Tola et al., 1979). Urine levels as high as 1200 µg/L have been observed in nickel refinery workers (Hogetveit and Barton, 1976).

Insoluble nickel compounds that are inhaled tend to accumulate in the nasal mucosa and lungs, and nickel levels in these tissues may remain elevated for years after cessation of exposure (Torjussen and Andersen, 1979). The following tissue concentrations were found in adults at autopsy (Sunderman, 1980):

Nickel Concentrations in Normal Tissues (µg/kg)

	Heart	Lung	Liver	Kidney	Bone
Average	6.4	85	8.2	10.5	333
(Range)	(4.3–9.3)	(8–221)	(5.2–13.2)	(6.9–18.2)	(190–640)

Toxicity. Nickel is well-known for producing contact dermatitis in sensitized persons that can become quite severe. Chelation therapy with dithiocarb or disulfiram has been found useful in treating such individuals (Menne et al., 1980; Sunderman, 1981). Nickel-induced asthma has also been reported (Block and Yeung, 1982; Novey et al., 1983).

Nickel intoxication occurred in 23 dialysis patients due to leaching of the metal from a plated stainless steel water heater in the dialysis unit; symptoms of nausea, vomiting, weakness and headache occurred with plasma nickel concentrations on the order of 3 mg/L (Webster et al., 1980). The acute oral ingestion of approximately 10 g of nickel sulfate by an adult male resulted in postmortem levels of 7.5 mg/L in blood, 27 mg/kg in liver and 47 mg/L in urine (Szathmary and Daldrup, 1982).

Acute exposure to nickel fume has occasionally produced typical metal fume fever. Few industrial problems have arisen in regard to acute toxicity from exposure to soluble or insoluble nickel compounds, with the exception of nickel carbonyl (see next section) and the rare instance of accidental ingestion of a soluble salt. Nickel carcinogenicity, especially with exposure to insoluble compounds, is a more serious cause for concern, having been demonstrated experimentally and in a number of epidemiologic studies involving refinery workers (Panel on Nickel, 1975).

Analysis. Analytical techniques for the determination of nickel in biological specimens were recently reviewed (Sunderman, 1980). Currently, the most frequently used technique is electrothermal atomic absorption spectrometry, with or without prior sample digestion (Mikac-Devic et al., 1977; Andersen et al., 1978; Adams, 1980; Dornemann and Kleist, 1980; Brown et al., 1981; Long-zhu and Zhe-ming, 1985; Ong et al., 1990).

References

D.B. Adams. The routine determination of nickel and creatinine in urine. In *Nickel Toxicology* (S.S. Brown and F.W. Sunderman, Jr., eds.), Academic Press, London, 1980, pp. 99–102.

I. Andersen, W. Torjussen and H. Zachariasen. Analysis for nickel in plasma and urine by electrothermal atomic absorption spectrometry, with sample preparation by protein precipitation. Clin. Chem. 24: 1198–1202, 1978.

E.J. Bernacki, G.E. Parsons, B.R. Roy et al. Urine nickel concentrations in nickel-exposed workers. Ann. Clin. Lab. Sci. 8: 184–189, 1978.

G.T. Block and M. Yeung. Asthma induced by nickel. J. Am. Med. Asso. 247: 1600–1602, 1982.

S.S. Brown, S. Nomoto, M. Stoeppler and F.W. Sunderman, Jr. IUPAC reference method for analysis of nickel in serum and urine by electrothermal atomic absorption spectrometry. Pure Appl. Chem. 53: 773–781, 1981.

O.B. Christensen and V. Lagesson. Concentrations of nickel in blood and urine after oral administration. In *Nickel Toxicology* (S.S. Brown and F.W. Sunderman, Jr., eds.), Academic Press, London, 1980, pp. 95–98.

A. Dornemann and H. Kleist. Determination of nanogram amounts of nickel in liver and kidney samples. In *Nickel Toxicology* (S.S. Brown and F.W. Sunderman, eds.), Academic Press, London, 1980, pp. 175–178.

A.C. Hogetveit and R.T. Barton. Preventive health program for nickel workers. J. Occ. Med. 18: 805–808, 1976.

A.C. Hogetveit, R.T. Barton and C.O. Kostol. Plasma nickel as a primary index of exposure in nickel refining. Ann. Occ. Hyg. 21: 113–120, 1978.

J.M.H. Howard. Serum nickel in myocardial infarction. Clin. Chem. 26: 1515, 1980.

J. Long-zhu and N. Zhe-ming. Determination of nickel in urine and other biological samples by graphite furnace atomic absorption spectrometry. Fres. Z. Anal. Chem. 321: 72–76, 1985.

T. Menne, K. Kaaber and J.C. Tjell. Treatment of nickel dermatitis. Ann. Clin. Lab. Sci. 10: 160–164, 1980.

D. Mikac-Devic, F.W. Sunderman, Jr. and S. Nomoto. Furildioxime method for nickel analysis in serum and urine by electrothermal atomic absorption spectrometry. Clin. Chem. 23: 948–956, 1977.

H.S. Novey, M. Habib and I.D. Wells. Asthma and IgE antibodies induced by chromium and nickel salts. J. Allerg. Clin. Imm. 72: 407–412, 1983.

C.N. Ong, L.H. Chua, B.L. Lee et al. Electrothermal atomic absorption spectrometric determination of cadmium and nickel in urine. J. Anal. Tox. 14: 29–33, 1990.

A. Oskarsson and H. Tjalve. Autoradiography of nickel chloride and nickel carbonyl in mice. Acta Pharm. Tox. 41: 158–159, 1977.

Panel on Nickel. *Nickel*, National Academy of Sciences, Washington, DC, 1975.

F.W. Sunderman, Jr. A review of the metabolism and toxicology of nickel. Ann. Clin. Lab. Sci. 7: 377–398, 1977.

F.W. Sunderman, Jr. Analytical biochemistry of nickel. Pure Appl. Chem. 52: 527–544, 1980.

F.W. Sunderman, Sr. Chelation therapy in nickel poisoning. Ann. Clin. Lab. Sci. 11: 1–8, 1981.

S.C. Szathmary and T. Daldrup. Zum Nachweis von Nickel in biologischen Materialien mittels GC, GC-MS und AAS nach einer todlichen Vergiftung. Zeitschr. Anal. Chem. 313: 48, 1982.

S. Tola, J. Kilpio and M. Virtamo. Urinary and plasma concentrations of nickel as indicators of exposure to nickel in an electroplating shop. J. Occ. Med. 21: 184–188, 1979.

W. Torjussen and I. Andersen. Nickel concentrations in nasal mucosa, plasma, and urine in active and retired nickel workers. Ann. Clin. Lab. Sci. 9: 289–298, 1979.

J.D. Webster, T.F. Parker, A.C. Alfrey et al. Acute nickel intoxication by dialysis. Ann. Int. Med. 92: 631–633, 1980.

Nickel Carbonyl

T½: ?

Vd: ?

Fb: ?

$Ni(CO)_4$

Occurrence and Usage. Nickel carbonyl is an especially toxic form of nickel produced as an intermediate in the purification of nickel ore and used in organic synthesis and in electroplating operations. It may be formed inadvertently whenever carbon monoxide comes into contact with active nickel; tobacco smoke has been found to contain an average of approximately 3.5 ppm of nickel carbonyl. The substance is generally encountered in industry as a vapor (b.p. of the liquid is 43° C.), which is rapidly absorbed after inhalation. The current threshold limit value is 0.05 ppm (0.12 mg/m³); it had been set as low as 0.001 ppm in earlier years due to concern over the carcinogenic potential of the compound.

Blood Concentrations. Due to its rapid metabolism and elimination, intact nickel carbonyl has not been measured in the blood of exposed subjects. Ionic nickel, a metabolite of nickel carbonyl, has been found at concentrations of 4.3–4.8 µg/L in the serum of 2 asymptomatic workers exposed to nickel carbonyl; by comparison, serum nickel concentrations average 2.6 µg/L (range, 1.1–4.6) in healthy exposed subjects (Nomoto and Sunderman, 1970).

Metabolism and Excretion. Inhaled nickel carbonyl is rapidly absorbed into the blood and distributed primarily to the lungs, brain, adrenal glands, and kidney. Oxidation to divalent nickel takes place intracellularly within minutes (Oskarsson, 1979). Slightly more than one-third of a dose is exhaled unchanged by rats over a period of 6 hours (Kasprzak and Sunderman, 1969). The divalent nickel that is formed is nearly totally excreted in the urine within 6 days (Tedeschi and Sunderman, 1957).

Urine nickel concentrations in asymptomatic nickel carbonyl workers have been observed to range from 10–50 µg/L (Kincaid et al., 1956), compared to a range of 2–10 µg/L in normal unexposed persons (Andersen et al., 1978). Two workers who were exposed to excessive amounts of nickel carbonyl but did not develop symptoms of toxicity were found to have nickel levels of 110 and 180 µg/L in urine collected during the 8 hours following exposure (Sunderman and Kincaid, 1954).

Toxicity. The immediate effects of nickel carbonyl exposure include headache, chest pain and dizziness. These may disappear after a few hours, to be followed within 12 hours to 5 days by the delayed effects. In severe cases, nausea, cough, dyspnea, cyanosis and weakness have been observed. Death usually occurs within 3–7 days and is the result of diffuse interstitial pneumonitis and cerebral edema (Sunderman, 1977). In those who survive, recovery of pulmonary function and muscular strength are generally complete within 3–6 months (Vuopala et al., 1970).

Several hundred instances of acute nickel carbonyl poisoning have occurred, with between 20 and 30 reported deaths (Panel on Nickel, 1975; Sunderman, 1979; Shi, 1986). In these cases, urine specimens taken on the first day of exposure have contained nickel at concentrations of 100–2470 µg/L, the concentrations being reasonably well-correlated with the severity of the symptoms. Sunderman and Sunderman (1958) have suggested that if an initial 8 hour urine specimen contains less than 100 µg/L nickel, the exposure should be classified as mild; if it contains 100–500 µg/L, as moderately severe; and if more than 500 µg/L, as severe. Oral administration of sodium diethyldithiocarbamate (dithiocarb) is often prescribed for chelation treatment of serious cases of nickel carbonyl poisoning.

One individual who died 3 days after industrial exposure to nickel carbonyl had a urine nickel concentration of 535 µg/L in a specimen collected 24 hours after exposure; at autopsy, lung and liver specimens contained 173 and 53 µg/kg, respectively, of nickel (Jones, 1973; Sunderman, 1979). Normal tissue nickel concentrations are cited in the section on nickel.

Analysis. Procedures for the analysis of nickel in biological specimens are cited in the section on nickel.

References

I. Andersen, W. Torjussen and H. Zachariasen. Analysis for nickel in plasma and urine by electrothermal atomic absorption spectrometry, with sample preparation by protein precipitation. Clin. Chem. 24: 1198–1202, 1978.

C.C. Jones. Nickel carbonyl poisoning. Arch. Env. Health 26: 245–248, 1973.

K.S. Kasprzak and F.W. Sunderman, Jr. The metabolism of nickel carbonyl-¹⁴C. Tox. Appl. Pharm. 15: 295–303, 1969.

J.F. Kincaid, E.L. Stanley, C.H. Beckworth and F.W. Sunderman. Nickel poisoning. Am. J. Clin. Path. 26: 107–119, 1956.

S. Nomoto and F.W. Sunderman. Atomic absorption spectrometry of nickel in serum, urine, and other biological materials. Clin. Chem. 16: 477–485, 1970.

A. Oskarsson. Tissue localization of some nickel compounds. Abstract of Doctoral Dissertation, University of Uppsala, Sweden, 1979.

Panel on Nickel. *Nickel*, National Academy of Sciences, Washington, D.C., 1975.

Z. Shi. Acute nickel carbonyl poisoning: a report of 179 cases. Brit. J. Ind. Med. 43: 422–424, 1986.

F.W. Sunderman and J.F. Kincaid. Nickel poisoning. II. Studies on patients suffering from acute exposure to vapors of nickel carbonyl. J. Am. Med. Asso. 155: 889–894, 1954.

F.W. Sunderman and F.W. Sunderman, Jr. Nickel poisoning. VIII. Dithiocarb: a new therapeutic agent for persons exposed to nickel carbonyl. Am. J. Med. Sci. 236: 26–31, 1958.

F.W. Sunderman, Jr. A review of the metabolism and toxicology of nickel. Ann. Clin. Lab. Sci. 7: 377–398, 1977.

F.W. Sunderman, Sr. Efficacy of sodium diethyldithiocarbamate (dithiocarb) in acute nickel carbonyl poisoning. Ann. Clin. Lab. Sci. 9: 1–10, 1979.

R.E. Tedeshi and F.W. Sunderman. Nickel poisoning. V. The metabolism of nickel under normal conditions and after exposure to nickel carbonyl. Arch. Ind. Health 16: 486–488, 1957.

U. Vuopala, E. Huhti, J. Takkunen and M. Huikko. Nickel carbonyl poisoning. Ann. Clin. Res. 2: 214–222, 1970.

Nicotine

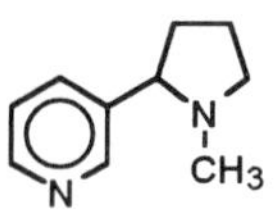

T½: 24–84 min (urine pH-dependent)
Vd: 1.0 L/kg
Fb: 0.05
pKa: 7.8, 3.0

Occurrence and Usage. Nicotine is a highly toxic alkaloid that causes stimulation of autonomic ganglia and the central nervous system. In its free state it is a liquid (b.p., 247° C.) that slowly darkens on exposure to air. The compound was first isolated in 1828 from tobacco, in which it is present in amounts of 0.5–8.0% by weight; certain varieties of tobacco also contain nornicotine to the extent of 10–20% of the nicotine content. The average cigarette in the United States contains 1.5% nicotine; of the amount that survives the combustion process and is presented to the respiratory tract (0.2–2.4 mg), 10–50% is absorbed during mouth puffing and 80–100% during deep lung inhalation. Nicotine is a drug to which virtually every member of a tobacco-smoking society is exposed. The concentrations of nicotine in the air of public places range from 1–10 μg/m³ (Hinds and First, 1975), and nicotine can be found in the urine of most nonsmokers. The drug is now available as replacement therapy for smokers in the form of chewing gum containing 2–4 mg (Nicorette) or transdermal patches containing 8–114 mg and capable of delivering 5–22 mg over 24 hours (Habitrol, Nicoderm, Nicotrol, Prostep). Nicotine is also used as a horticultural pesticide and is commercially available in a crude 40% solution of the sulfate, which is applied as a spray. The threshold limit value for industrial exposure is 0.5 mg/m³. The compound is absorbed following inhalation, ingestion or dermal contact.

Blood Concentrations. Of a group of 39 urban nonsmokers, about half had measurable amounts of nicotine in their plasma, with a concentration range of 0–0.006 mg/L (Russell and Feyerabend, 1975). Six nonsmoking flight attendants had an average blood nicotine concentration of 0.0016 mg/L prior to working and 0.0032 mg/L 1 hour after completion of a Tokyo to San Francisco flight (Foliart et al., 1983). Plasma nicotine concentrations were found to range from 0.012–0.044 mg/L 30 minutes after a 6.5 hour *ad libitum* smoking period, during which the total abstracted nicotine dose ranged from 7.8–33 mg (Isaac and Rand, 1972). In a study performed with multiple sampling of plasma during the smoking of 7 cigarettes at the rate of 1 per hour, it was found that the plasma nicotine concentrations peaked rapidly after each cigarette (peak level range, 0.035–0.054 mg/L) and declined rapidly, with only moderate accumulation of nicotine over the 7 hour period (Russell et al., 1976). The plasma half-life of nicotine in smokers has been found to range from 24–84 minutes, with an average of 40 minutes (Armitage et al., 1975). Plasma nicotine averaged only 0.004 mg/L in pipe smokers (McCusker et al., 1982), while persons chewing nicotine gum of 2 or 4 mg size developed average steady-state plasma levels of 0.012 or 0.023 mg/L, respectively (McNabb et al., 1982). Subjects wearing transdermal patches intended to deliver 22 mg nicotine per day developed serum nicotine levels of 0.004–0.444 mg/L and serum cotinine levels of 0.035–0.249 mg/L (Hurt et al., 1993).

Plasma concentrations of cotinine, a metabolite, averaged 0.001 mg/L in children from non-smoking homes versus 0.004 mg/L for children from homes in which smokers were present (Pattishall et al., 1985).

Metabolism and Excretion. The fate of nicotine in man has not been thoroughly elucidated, but it is known to be extensively transformed to largely inactive metabolites. The first step in its biotransformation appears to be oxidation to cotinine, which is further degraded by oxidation to hydroxycotinine and a ring cleavage product. Nicotine-1'-N-oxide, nornicotine, cotinine-N-oxide and norcotinine have also been identified as metabolites. A number of these compounds may undergo glucuronide conjugation. Only about 5% of a dose of nicotine is excreted unchanged in the 24 hour urine, with 10% as cotinine, 35% as hydroxycotinine and about 4% as nicotine-1'-N-oxide; the quantities of the other known metabolites are generally less than 5% of the dose (Bowman et al., 1959; Bowman and McKennis, 1962; Beckett et al., 1971; Armitage et al., 1975; Neurath et al., 1987; Kyerematen et al., 1990; Byrd et al., 1992). The excretion of nicotine is enhanced by acidification of the urine (Matsukura et al., 1979a), whereas cotinine excretion is less affected by pH changes (Matsukura et al., 1979b). In urban nonsmokers the average urinary nicotine concentration was 0.010 mg/L (range, 0–0.064), although after spending 78 minutes in a smoky room this average increased to 0.080 mg/L (range, 0.013–0.208). By contrast, the urine nicotine concentrations in a group of 18 smokers (8–70 cigarettes/day) averaged 1.236 mg/L (range, 0.104–2.743) (Russell and Feyerabend, 1975).

Early morning urine contained average cotinine levels of 0.7 mg/g creatinine in nonsmokers and 8.6 mg/g creatinine in smokers (Matsukura et al., 1984).

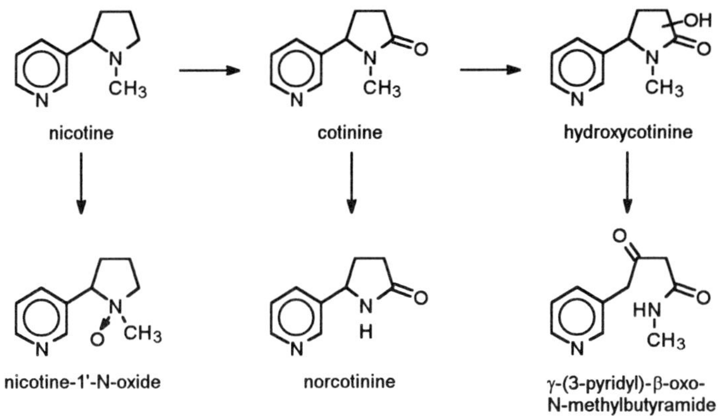

nicotine — cotinine — hydroxycotinine

nicotine-1'-N-oxide — norcotinine — γ-(3-pyridyl)-β-oxo-N-methylbutyramide

Toxicity. Small doses of nicotine produce nausea, vomiting, dizziness, pinpoint pupils, tachycardia, hypertension, sweating and salivation. The estimated minimal lethal dose of nicotine in an adult is 40–60 mg, an amount that will cause prostration, convulsions, respiratory paralysis and death within a few minutes to 1 hour after ingestion. Nonfatal poisoning has occurred in children following ingestion of cigarettes or used transdermal patches (McGee et al., 1991,; Yuen et al., 1993). A common means of exposure is by accidental or intentional ingestion of a solution that is commercially available for insecticidal purposes. Toxicity has been observed in tobacco harvesters, probably as a result of dermal absorption of nicotine (Gehlbach et al., 1975). Dermal exposure to concentrated nicotine solutions has caused nonfatal poisoning in several adults (Faulkner, 1933; Lockhart, 1933; Benowitz et al., 1986). One person survived the accidental intramuscular injection of 240 mg of nicotine from an animal tranquilizing dart; atropine was administered as an antidote (Brady et al., 1979).

Postmortem blood concentrations of 11–63 mg/L (average, 29) were observed in 5 adult subjects who swallowed 20–25 g of nicotine sulfate solution and who died within 1 hour (Baselt and Cravey, 1977). In other fatal cases, blood concentrations of 5–600 mg/L and urine concentrations of 17–58 mg/L have been reported (Clarke, 1969). Nicotine was the second most frequently encountered toxin in suicidal poisonings in Hungary in 1967; blood nicotine concentrations of 16–5800 mg/L (average, 472) and liver concentrations of 4–2270 mg/kg (average, 493) were reported for 24 such cases (Grusz-Harday, 1967).

Analysis. Spectrophotometry is used routinely in the assay of nicotine for toxicological purposes (Kivela, 1975). Nicotine and cotinine have been determined by gas chromatography using a flame-ionization technique for urine (Beckett and Triggs, 1966) and nitrogen-selective (Isaac and Rand, 1972; Feyerabend et al., 1975; Hengen and Hengen, 1978; Jacob et al., 1981; Kogan et al., 1981; Verebey et al., 1982) or electron-capture detection (Neelakantan and Kostenbauder, 1974; Hartvig et al., 1979) for blood and plasma. The latter method requires formation of halogenated derivatives. Liquid chromatographic analysis has also been reported (Watson, 1977; Maskarinec et al., 1978; Kyerematen et al., 1982; Barlow et al., 1987; Parviainen and Barlow, 1988; Hariharan and Van Noord, 1991). The analysis of very low concentrations of nicotine in biological specimens requires careful precautions to prevent interference from extraneous nicotine (Feyerabend and Russell, 1980).

References

A.K. Armitage, C.T. Dollery, C.F. George et al. Absorption and metabolism of nicotine from cigarettes. Brit. Med. J. 4: 313–316, 1975.

R.D. Barlow, P.A. Thompson and R.B. Stone. Simultaneous determination of nicotine, cotinine and five additional nicotine metabolites in the urine of smokers using pre-column derivatisation and high-performance liquid chromatography. J. Chrom. 419: 375–380, 1987.

R.C. Baselt and R.H. Cravey. A compendium of therapeutic and toxic concentrations of toxicologically signifi-cant drugs in human biofluids. J. Anal. Tox. 1: 81–103, 1977.

A.H. Beckett and E.J. Triggs. Determination of nicotine and its metabolite, cotinine, in urine by gas chroma-tography. Nature 211: 1415–1417, 1966.

A.H. Beckett, J.W. Gorrod and P. Jenner. The analysis of nicotine-1'-N-oxide in urine, in the presence of nicotine and cotinine, and its application to the study of in vivo nicotine metabolism in man. J. Pharm. Pharmac. 23: 55S–61S, 1971.

N.L. Benowitz, T. Lake, K.H. Keller and B.L. Lee. Prolonged absorption and toxicity following cutaneous exposure to nicotine. Vet. Hum. Tox. 28: 490, 1986.

E.R. Bowman, L.B. Turnbull and H. McKennis, Jr. Metabolism of nicotine in the human and excretion of pyridine compounds by smokers. J. Pharm. Exp. Ther. 127: 92–95, 1959.

E.R. Bowman and H. McKennis, Jr. Studies on the metabolism of (-)-cotinine in the human. J. Pharm. Exp. Ther. 135: 306–311, 1962.

M.E. Brady, W.A. Ritschel, D.A. Saelinger et al. Animal model and pharmacokinetic interpretation of nicotine poisoning in man. Int. J. Clin. Pharm. Biopharm. 17: 12–17, 1979.

G.D. Byrd, K.M. Chang, J.M. Greene and J.D. deBethizy. Evidence for urinary excretion of glucuronide conjugates of nicotine, cotinine, and trans-3'-hydroxycotinine in smokers. Drug Met. Disp. 20: 192–197, 1992.

E.G.C. Clarke (ed.). *Isolation and Identification of Drugs,* Pharmaceutical Press, London, 1969, pp. 440–441.

J.M. Faulkner. Nicotine poisoning by absorption through the skin. J. Am. Med. Asso. 100: 1664–1665, 1933.

C. Feyerabend, T. Levitt and M.A.H. Russell. A rapid gas-liquid chromatographic estimation of nicotine in biological fluids. J. Pharm. Pharmac. 27: 434–436, 1975.

C. Feyerabend and M.A.H. Russell. Assay of nicotine in biological materials: sources of contamination and their elimination. J. Pharm. Pharmac. 32: 178–181, 1980.

D. Foliart, N.L. Benowitz and C.E. Becker. Passive absorption of nicotine in airline flight attendants. New. Eng. J. Med. 308: 1105, 1983.

S.H. Gehlbach, W.A. Williams, L.D. Perry and J.I. Freeman. Nicotine absorption by workers harvesting green tobacco. Lancet 1: 478–480, 1975.

E. Grusz-Harday. Toedliche Nicotinvergiftungen. Arch. Tox. 23: 35–41, 1967.

M. Hariharan and T. Van Noord. Liquid-chromatographic determination of nicotine and cotinine in urine from passive smokers. Clin. Chem. 37: 1276–1280, 1991.

P. Hartvig, N.O. Ahnfelt, M. Hammarlund and J. Vessman. Analysis of nicotine as a trichloroethyl carbamate by gas chromatography with electron-capture detection. J. Chrom. 173: 127–138, 1979.

N. Hengen and M. Hengen. Gas-liquid chromatographic determination of nicotine and cotinine in plasma. Clin. Chem. 24: 50–53, 1978.

W.C. Hinds and M.W. First. Concentrations of nicotine and tobacco smoke in public places. New Eng. J. Med. 292: 844–845, 1975.

R.D. Hurt, L.C. Dale, K.P. Offord et al. Serum nicotine and cotinine levels during nicotine-patch therapy. Clin. Pharm. Ther. 54: 98–106, 1993.

P.F. Isaac and M.J. Rand. Cigarette smoking and plasma levels of nicotine. Nature 236: 308–310, 1972.

P. Jacob, M. Wilson and N.L. Benowitz. Improved gas chromatographic method for the determination of nicotine and cotinine in biologic fluids. J. Chrom. 222: 61–70, 1981.

E.W. Kivela. Nicotine. Type B Procedure. In *Methodology for Analytical Toxicology* (I. Sunshine, ed.), CRC Press, Cleveland, 1975, pp. 280–281.

M.J. Kogan, K. Verebey, J.H. Jaffee and S.J. Mule. Simultaneous determination of nicotine and cotinine in human plasma by nitrogen detection gas-liquid chromatography. J. For. Sci. 26: 6–11, 1981.

G.A. Kyerematen, M.D. Damiano, B.H. Dvorchik and E.S. Vesell. Smoking-induced changes in nicotine disposition: application of a new HPLC assay for nicotine and its metabolites. Clin. Pharm. Ther. 32: 769–780, 1982.

G.A. Kyerematen, M.L. Morgan, B. Chattopadhyay et al. Disposition of nicotine and eight metabolites in smokers and nonsmokers. Clin. Pharm. Ther. 48: 641–651, 1990.

L.P. Lockhart. Nicotine poisoning. Brit. Med. J. 1: 246–247, 1933.

M.P. Maskarinec, R.W. Harvey and J.E. Caton. A novel method for the isolation and quantitative analysis of nicotine and cotinine in biological fluids. J. Anal. Tox. 2: 124–126, 1978.

S. Matsukura, N. Sakamoto, K. Takahashi et al. Effect of pH and urine flow on urinary nicotine excretion after smoking cigarettes. Clin. Pharm. Ther. 25: 549–554, 1979a.

S. Matsukura, N. Sakamoto, Y. Seino et al. Cotinine excretion and daily cigarette smoking in habituated smokers. Clin. Pharm. Ther. 25: 555–561, 1979b.

S. Matsukura, T. Taminato, N. Kitano et al. Effects of environmental tobacco smoke on urinary cotinine excretion in nonsmokers. New Eng. J. Med. 311: 828–832, 1984.

K. McCusker, E. McNabb and R. Bone. Plasma nicotine levels in pipe smokers. J. Am. Med. Asso. 248: 577–578, 1982.

D. McGee, M. Picciotti and T. Spevack. Two year review of tobacco ingestions. Vet. Hum. Tox. 33: 370, 1991.

M.E. McNabb, R.V. Ebert and K. McCusker. Plasma nicotine levels produced by chewing nicotine gum. J. Am. Med. Asso. 248: 865–868, 1982.

L. Neelakantan and H.B. Kostenbauder. Electron capture derivative for determination of nicotine in sub-picomole quantities. Anal. Chem. 46: 452–454, 1974.

G.B. Neurath, M. Dunger, D. Orth and F.G. Pein. Trans-3'-hydroxycotinine as a main metabolite in urine of smokers. Int. Arch. Occ. Env. Health 59: 199–201, 1987.

M.T. Parviainen and R.D. Barlow. Assessment of exposure to environmental tobacco smoke using a hplc method for the simultaneous determination of nicotine and two of its metabolites in urine. J. Chrom. 431: 216–221, 1988.

E.N. Pattishall, G.L. Strope, R.A. Etzel et al. Serum cotinine as a measure of tobacco smoke exposure in children. Am. J. Dis. Child. 139: 1101–1104, 1985.

M.A.H. Russell and C. Feyerabend. Blood and urinary nicotine in nonsmokers. Lancet 1: 179–181, 1975.

M.A.H. Russell, C. Feyerabend and P.V. Cole. Plasma nicotine levels after cigarette smoking and chewing nicotine gum. Brit. Med. J. 1: 1043–1046, 1976.

K.G. Verebey, A. DePace, S.J. Mule et al. A rapid, quantitative GLC method for the simultaneous determination of nicotine and cotinine. J. Anal. Tox. 6: 294–296, 1982.

I.D. Watson. Rapid analysis of nicotine and cotinine in the urine of smokers by isocratic high-performance liquid chromatography. J. Chrom. 143: 203–206, 1977.

J.A. Yuen, J.F. Ashbourne and D.R. Croteau. Review of transdermal nicotine exposures. Vet. Hum. Tox. 35: 349, 1993.

Nifedipine

T½: 3–4 hr
Vd: 1.2 L/kg
Fb: 0.98
pKa: ?

Occurrence and Usage. Nifedipine (Adalat, Procardia) is a calcium antagonist that is widely used for the management of angina pectoris, cardiac arrhythmias, and hypertension. The drug is supplied in 10 and 20 mg capsules as the free base. The initial oral dose is 10 mg given 3 times daily, and the effective daily dosage range is 30–120 mg. The total daily dose should not exceed 180 mg.

Blood Concentrations. Peak nifedipine serum concentrations in 6 young adults following sublingual administration ranged from 15–89 µg/L (average, 42), while the range following oral administration was 38–162 µg/L (average, 99); the time to peak serum concentration was longer following sublingual administration (1.2 hours) than with the oral dose (0.7 hour) (Brown et al., 1986). Steady-state serum concentrations were determined in 12 patients aged 53–73 following repeated daily oral doses of 30–120 mg; the mean serum concentration was 115 µg/L and the time necessary to reach this level was 0.7 hour (Gutierrez et al., 1986).

Metabolism and Excretion. Up to 15% of a single oral nifedipine dose is eliminated in the feces as metabolites in 4 days and about 70% of the dose is excreted in urine as inactive metabolites. When the drug is given acutely, the major metabolites found in serum and urine are dehydronifedipinic acid and hydroxydehydronifedipinic acid, which is in equilibrium with dehydronifedipinolactone. When patients are maintained on chronic nifedipine therapy, dehydronifedipinic acid is found to be the major serum metabolite and urinary excretion product (Raemsch and Sommer, 1983; Snedden and Fernandez, 1985; Snedden et al., 1986a; Snedden et al., 1986b).

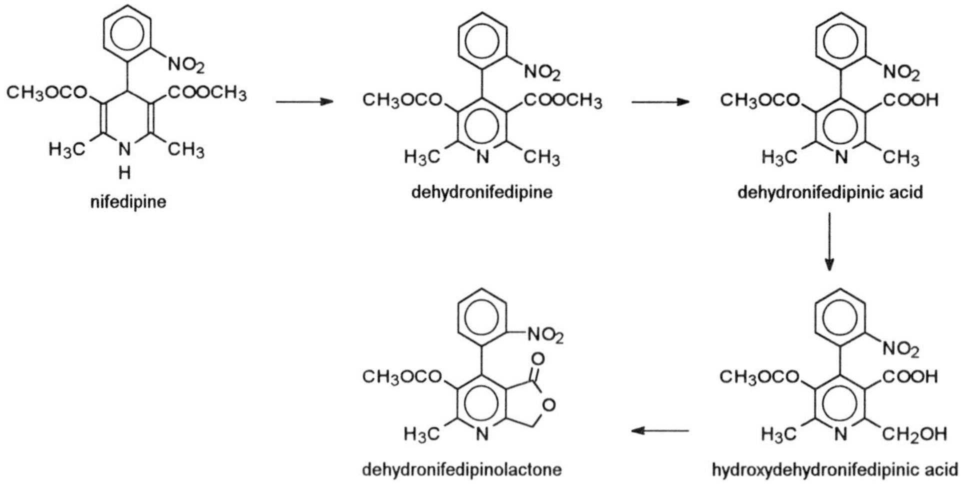

Toxicity. Overdosage with nifedipine results in excessive peripheral vasodilation with subsequent marked and prolonged systemic hypotension. Four hours after ingestion of 280 mg of nifedipine in an unsuccessful suicide attempt, a 23 year old woman experienced throbbing headaches, facial flushing, weakness, vertigo and muscle cramps; plasma nifedipine concentrations were 127 µg/L at 9 hours, 87 µg/L at 12 hours, and 10 µg/L at 45 hours after overdosage (Schiffl et al., 1984).

A 14 month old child exhibited lethargy and bradycardia after ingesting a 10 mg nifedipine capsule; death occurred within 4 hours, and a postmortem blood level of 270 µg/L was measured (Pearigen, 1993). Two young adults each intravenously self-administered 60 mg of nifedipine and died within minutes; postmortem blood levels of 155 and 172 µg/L were determined (Purdue et al., 1991).

Analysis. Nifedipine may be analyzed in plasma or serum by gas chromatography with electron-capture (Jacobsen et al., 1979; Hamann and McAllister, 1983; Lesko et al., 1983; Tanner et al., 1986) or mass spectrometric detection (Patrick et al., 1989). Nifedipine and its major metabolite have been determined in plasma by liquid chromatography (Kleinbloesem et al., 1984; Snedden et al., 1986; Fu and Mason, 1989; Soons et al., 1991). Exposure of biological fluids containing nifedipine to room light for 4 hours caused 62% loss of the drug in plasma but only 11% loss in whole blood (Tucker et al., 1985).

References

G.R. Brown, D.G. Fraser, J.A. Castile et al. Nifedipine serum concentrations following sublingual and oral doses. Int. J. Clin. Pharm. Ther. Tox. 24: 283–286, 1986.

C.J. Fu and W.D. Mason. A simplified method for determination of nifedipine in human plasma by high performance liquid chromatography. Anal. Letters 22: 2985–3002, 1989.

L.M. Gutierrez, L.J. Lesko, R. Whipps et al. Pharmacokinetics and pharmacodynamics of nifedipine in patients at steady state. J. Clin. Pharm. 26: 587–592, 1986.

S.R. Hamann and R.G. McAllister. Measurement of nifedipine in plasma by gas-liquid chromatography and electron-capture detection. Clin. Chem. 29: 158–160, 1983.

P. Jakobsen, O.L. Pedersen and E. Mikkelsen. Gas chromatographic determination of nifedipine and one of its metabolites using electron-capture detection. J. Chrom. 162: 81–87, 1979.

C.H. Kleinbloesem, J. van Harten, P. van Brummelen et al. Liquid chromatographic determination of nifedipine in plasma and of its main metabolite in urine. J. Chrom. 308: 209–216, 1984.

L. Lesko, A. Miller, R.L. Yeager and D.C. Chatterji. Rapid GC method for quantitation of nifedipine in serum using electron capture detection. J. Chrom. Sci. 21: 415–419, 1983.

K.S. Patrick, E.J. Jarvi, A.B. Straughn and M.C. Meyer. Gas chromatographic-mass spectrometric analysis of plasma nifedipine. J. Chrom. 495: 123–130, 1989.

P.D. Pearigen. Death from accidental nifedipine ingestion in a toddler. Vet. Hum. Tox. 35: 345, 1993.

B.N. Purdue, G.C.A. Fernando and A. Busuttil. Two deaths from intravenous nifedipine abuse. Int. J. Leg. Med. 104: 289–291, 1991.

K. Raemsch and J. Sommer. Pharmacokinetics and metabolism of nifedipine. Hypertension 5 (Suppl. 2): 18–24, 1983.

H. Schiffl, J. Ziupa and P. Schollmeyer. Clinical features and management of nifedipine overdosage in a patient with renal insufficiency. Clin. Tox. 22: 387–395, 1984.

W. Snedden and P.G. Fernandez. Metabolism of nifedipine in hypertensives. Clin. Pharm. Ther. 37: 230–234, 1985.

W. Snedden, P.G. Fernandez and C. Nath. HPLC analysis of nifedipine and some of its metabolites in hypertensive patients. Can. J. Physiol. Pharm. 64: 290–296, 1986.

W. Snedden, P.G. Fernandez and C. Nath. The metabolism of nifedipine during long term therapy. Clin. Invest. Med. 9: 244–249, 1986.

P.A. Soons, J.H.M. Schellens, M.C.M. Roosemalen and D.D. Breimer. Analysis of nifedipine and its pyridine metabolite dehydronifedipine in blood and plasma. J. Pharm. Biomed. Anal. 9: 475–484, 1991.

R. Tanner, A. Romagnoli and W.G. Kramer. Simplified method for determination of plasma nifedipine by gas chromatography. J. Anal. Tox. 10: 250–251, 1986.

F.A. Tucker, P.S.B. Minty and G.A. MacGregor. Study of nifedipine photodecomposition in plasma and whole blood using capillary gas-liquid chromatography. J. Chrom. 342: 193–198, 1985.

Nitrazepam

T½: 17–48 hr
Vd: 2–5 L/kg
Fb: 0.87
pKa: 3.2, 10.8

Occurrence and Usage. Nitrazepam (Mogadon) is a 7-nitro benzodiazepine, as are clonazepam and flunitrazepam. It is used in many European countries as a hypnotic agent, in oral doses of 5–10 mg as the free base.

Blood Concentrations. After a single oral dose of 5 mg of nitrazepam, peak serum concentrations averaged 0.035 mg/L at 2 hours in 15 subjects, and declined thereafter with an average half-life of 25–28 hours (Jensen, 1975). Following a single oral dose of 10 mg, peak plasma concentrations averaged 0.084 mg/L in 6 subjects; chronic administration of 5 mg daily resulted in steady-state levels that averaged 0.039 mg/L (Rieder and Wendt, 1973).

Metabolism and Excretion. Nitrazepam is largely converted to inactive metabolites that are subsequently excreted in the urine. Metabolism proceeds via reduction of the 7-nitro group, with acetylation of the resulting 7-amino metabolite. These 2 compounds accumulate to some extent in plasma. Nitrazepam also undergoes ring cleavage to 2-amino-5-nitrobenzophenone (ANB), which is hydroxylated in the 3-position to form hydroxy-ANB (HANB). Only traces of unchanged drug are found in the 24 hour urine; conjugated HANB (5.3%) and free 7-acetamidonitrazepam (4.8%) are the major excretory products, with lesser amounts of 7-aminonitrazepam and ANB present (Sawada and Shinohara, 1971; Rieder and Wendt, 1973). In the 7 day urine, 1% of the dose is found as parent drug, with 31% as free and conjugated 7-aminonitrazepam and 21% as free and conjugated 7-acetamidonitrazepam (Kangas, 1979a).

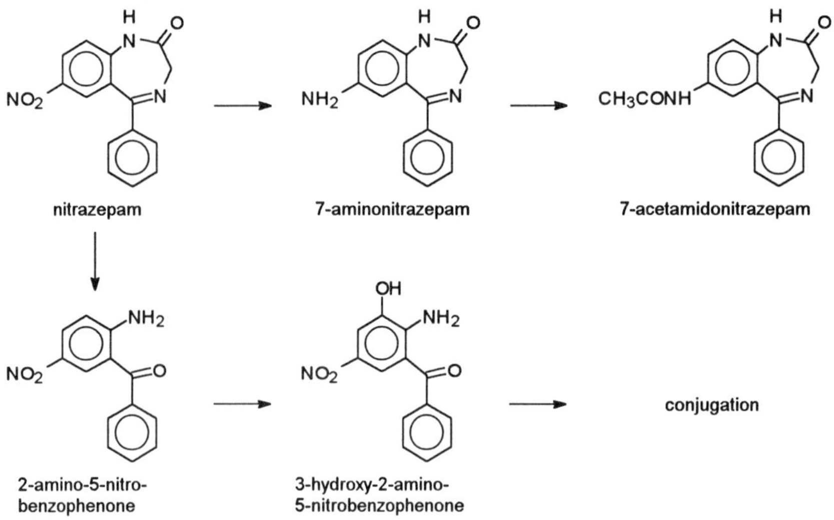

nitrazepam   7-aminonitrazepam   7-acetamidonitrazepam

2-amino-5-nitro-   3-hydroxy-2-amino-   conjugation
benzophenone   5-nitrobenzophenone

Toxicity. Six cases of fatal overdosage with nitrazepam have been reported, one of which involved the ingestion of 250 mg of the drug; blood concentrations of 1.2–9.0 mg/L, liver concentrations of 0.7–4.0 mg/kg, and urine concentrations of 1–10 mg/L were observed in the victims (Loveland, 1974; Oliver and Smith, 1974; Torry, 1976; Giusti and Chiarotti, 1979).

Analysis. Nitrazepam is stable for several weeks in biological specimens that are stored at 4° C. in the dark, but degrades rapidly when exposed to heat or light (Kelly et al., 1982). The methods described for the analysis of nitrazepam in biological specimens, with the necessary sensitivity and specificity to measure the very low concentrations attained after normal usage, have included fluorimetry (Rieder, 1973) and electron-capture gas chromatography (Jensen, 1975) of the hydrolysis products. The latter procedure has also been applied to the determination of the intact drug, although peak tailing is reported to be a disadvantage (Kangas, 1977; Kangas, 1979b; Locniskar et al., 1985). Liquid chromatographic techniques have been developed for the assay of nitrazepam and its metabolites in plasma and urine (Kelly et al., 1982; Kozu, 1984; Tada et al., 1987).

References

G.V. Giusti and M. Chiarotti. Lethal nitrazepam intoxications. Z. Rechtsmed. 84: 75–78, 1979.

K.M. Jensen. Determination of nitrazepam in serum by gas-liquid chromatography. J. Chrom. 111: 389–396, 1975.

L. Kangas. Comparison of two gas-liquid chromatographic methods for the determination of nitrazepam in plasma. J. Chrom. 136: 259–270, 1977.

L. Kangas. Urinary elimination of nitrazepam and its main metabolites. Acta Pharm. Tox. 45: 16–19, 1979a.

L. Kangas. Determination of nitrazepam and its main metabolites in urine by gas-liquid chromatography: use of electron capture and nitrogen-selective detectors. J. Chrom. 172: 273–278, 1979b.

H. Kelly, A. Huggett and S. Dawling. Liquid-chromatographic measurement of nitrazepam in plasma. Clin. Chem. 28: 1478–1481, 1982.

T. Kozu. High-performance liquid chromatographic determination of nitrazepam and its metabolites in human urine. J. Chrom. 310: 213–218, 1984.

A. Locniskar, D.J. Greenblatt and H.R. Ochs. Simplified gas chromatographic assay of underivatized nitrazepam in plasma. J. Chrom. 337: 131–135, 1985.

M.R. Loveland. Personal communication, 1974.

J.S. Oliver and H. Smith. Determination of nitrazepam in poisoning cases. For. Sci. 4: 183–186, 1974.

J. Rieder. A fluorometric method for determining nitrazepam and the sum of its main metabolites in plasma and urine. Arz. Forsch. 23: 207–211, 1973.

J. Rieder and Wendt. Pharmacokinetics and metabolism of the hypnotic nitrazepam. In *The Benzodiazepines* (S. Garattini, E. Mussini and L.O. Randall, eds.), Raven Press, New York, 1973, pp. 99–127.

H. Sawada and K. Shinohara. On the urinary excretion of nitrazepam and its metabolites. Arch. Tox. 28: 214–221, 1971.

K. Tada, A. Miyahira and T. Moroji. Liquid chromatographic assay of nitrazepam and its main metabolites in serum, and its application to pharmacokinetic study in the elderly. J. Liq. Chrom. 10: 465–476, 1987.

J.M. Torry. A case of suicide with nitrazepam and alcohol. Practitioner 217: 648–649, 1976.

Nitrite

T½: ?
Vd: ?
Fb: ?

NO_2^-

Occurrence and Usage. Both sodium nitrite and the organic nitrates (isosorbide dinitrate, nitroglycerin, pentaerythritol tetranitrate), which may release nitrite ion in the body, are commonly used as vasodilators in man. Another effect of inorganic nitrite is methemoglobin formation, and sodium nitrite is employed for this purpose in the treatment of cyanide poisoning. The widespread use of nitrates as fertilizers can lead to accumulation of this ion in food plants and water supplies, presenting a hazard to infants in whom intestinal bacteria cause reduction of nitrate to nitrite. Both nitrates and nitrites are also used as curing agents in processed meats and may legally be present in these products in amounts up to 500 and 200 ppm, respectively.

Blood Concentrations. Sodium nitrite is administered orally in doses of 30–60 mg as a vasodilator for the treatment of angina pectoris. It may also be injected intravenously in amounts of 300–500 mg as an antidote for cyanide poisoning; plasma nitrite levels have not been determined during therapy, although the compound may be monitored indirectly by measuring methemoglobin concentrations. Methemoglobinemia to the extent of 30–40% can protect against several lethal doses of cyanide without severely affecting respiration.

Metabolism and Excretion. While nitrite ion disappears rapidly from the circulation, little is known of its fate (Rath and Krantz, 1942). Only one-third of a dose is excreted unchanged in the urine.

Toxicity. Numerous cases of infant methemoglobinemia have resulted from the consumption of rural well water high in nitrate; death may occur when methemoglobin levels exceed 70% (Ridder and Oehme, 1974). Several persons have experienced weakness, nausea, numbness, shortness of breath, tachycardia, and cyanosis after accidentally ingesting sodium nitrite; methemoglobin levels of 34% and 54% were noted in 2 cases (Thwaites, 1956; Aquanno et al., 1981). Three men developed methemoglobinemia of 42–65% after dermal exposure to sodium and potassium nitrate in an industrial accident that also caused severe burns; the individual with the highest methemoglobin level died within 30 minutes of hospital admission (Harris et al., 1979). Two adults who accidentally ingested sodium nitrite (1 g in one case) became cyanotic and had serum nitrite levels of 0.5 and 0.6 mg/L; both recovered with treatment (Sevier and Barbatis, 1976). Both oxygen and methylene blue, to reduce methemoglobin, are used as antidotes.

A child died after the intravenous administration of 450 mg of sodium nitrite, a dose sufficient to produce 92% methemoglobinemia (Berlin, 1970). In many situations in which death has followed accidental or intentional ingestion of sodium or potassium nitrite, the chemical has been identified in gastric contents but not in other body fluids or tissues (McQuiston, 1936; Padberg and Martin, 1939; Manley, 1945; Barton, 1954; Blunt, 1976). In one case, however, a urine nitrite concentration of 340 mg/L was determined (Naidu and Rao, 1936), and in another, a blood concentration of 0.6 mg/L was reported (Standefer et al., 1979). The following distribution of the substance was observed in an adult who intentionally ingested sodium nitrite and whose postmortem methemoglobin level was 49% (de Beer et al., 1975):

Nitrite Concentrations in a Fatal Case (mg/L or mg/kg)

Blood	Liver	Kidney	Urine	Gastric
0.5	0	0.3	8.7	3.9

Analysis. Nitrite may be determined in biological fluids by a sulfanilic acid-alphanaphthylamine colorimetric diazotization technique, directly (Baselt, 1980) or following isolation of the ion by dialysis, protein precipitation, or steam distillation (Naidu and Rao, 1936; Shechter et al., 1972; de Beer et al., 1975; Blunt, 1976; Standefer et al., 1979; Gutman and Hollywood, 1992). The use of an ion-selective electrode has also been reported (Choi and Fung, 1980), as well as liquid chromatography (Thayer and Huffaker, 1980; Osterloh and Goldfield, 1984). Methods for the analysis of blood methemoglobin were cited in the section on aniline.

References

J.J. Aquanno, K.M. Chan and D.N. Dietzler. Accidental poisoning of two laboratory technologists with sodium nitrite. Clin. Chem. 27: 1145–1146, 1981.

G.M.G. Barton. A fatal case of sodium nitrite poisoning. Lancet 1: 190–191, 1954.

R.C. Baselt. *Analytical Procedures for Therapeutic Drug Monitoring and Emergency Toxicology*, Biomedical Publications, Davis, California, 1980, pp. 182–183.

C.M. Berlin, Jr. The treatment of cyanide poisoning in children. Pediatrics 46: 793–796, 1970.

S.R. Blunt. Rapid death of a child following sodium nitrite ingestion. Bull. Int. Asso. For. Tox. 12 (3):15–17, 1976.

K.K. Choi and F.W. Fung. Determination of nitrate and nitrite in meat products by using a nitrate ion-selective electrode. Analyst 105: 241–245, 1980.

J. de Beer, A. Heyndrickx and J. Timperman. Suidical poisoning by nitrite. Eur. J. Tox. 8: 247–251, 1975.

S.I. Gutman and C.A. Hollywood. Simple, rapid method for determining nitrates and nitrites in biological fluids. Clin. Chem. 38: 2152, 1992.

J.C. Harris, B.H. Rumack, R.G. Peterson and B.M. McGuire. Methemoglobinemia resulting from absorption of nitrates. J. Am. Med. Asso. 242: 2869–2871, 1979.

C.H. Manley. A fatal case of sodium nitrite poisoning. Analyst 70: 50, 1945.

T.A.C. McQuiston. Fatal poisoning by sodium nitrite. Lancet 2: 1153–1154, 1936.

S.R. Naidu and P.V. Rao. Case of nitrite poisoning. Brit. Med. J. 1: 1300, 1936.

J. Osterloh and D. Goldfield. Determination of nitrate and nitrite ions in human plasma by ion exchange-high performance liquid chromatography. J. Liq. Chrom. 7: 753–763, 1984.

L.R. Padberg and T. Martin. Three fatal cases of sodium nitrite poisoning. J. Am. Med. Asso. 113: 1733, 1939.

M.M. Rath and J.C. Krantz, Jr. Nitrites. IX. A further study of the mechanism of the action of organic nitrates. J. Pharm. Exp. Ther. 76: 33–38, 1942.

W.E. Ridder and F.W. Oehme. Nitrates as an environmental, animal, and human hazard. Clin. Tox. 7: 145–159, 1974.

J.N. Sevier and C.G. Berbatis. Accidental sodium nitrite ingestion. Med. J. Aust. 1: 847, 1976.

H. Shechter, N. Gruener and H.I. Shuval. A micromethod for the determination of nitrite in blood. Anal. Chim. Acta 60: 93–99, 1972.

J.C. Standefer, A.M. Jones, E. Street and R. Inserra. Death associated with nitrite ingestion: report of a case. J. For. Sci. 24: 768–771, 1979.

J.R. Thayer and R.C. Huffaker. Determination of nitrate and nitrite by high-pressure liquid chromatography: comparison with other methods for nitrite determination. Anal. Biochem. 102: 110–119, 1980.

C. Thwaites. A case of methaemoglobinaemia due to sodium nitrite poisoning. Med. J. Aust. 2: 185–186, 1956.

Nitrobenzene

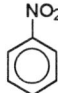

T½: ?
Vd: ?
Fb: ?

Occurrence and Usage. Nitrobenzene is a chemical intermediate frequently employed in commercial organic syntheses. The substance is a liquid at room temperature, and is well-absorbed after inhalation of the vapor or ingestion of or dermal contact with the liquid. The current threshold limit value for nitrobenzene in the industrial atmosphere is 1 ppm (5 mg/m³).

Blood Concentrations. Nitrobenzene or its metabolites have not been measured in the blood of exposed persons at normally encountered levels. Methemoglobinemia, which is produced by exposure to nitrobenzene, does not exceed 2% in healthy non-smokers. Workers exposed daily for 8 hours to nitrobenzene at an average air concentration of 19 mg/m³ were found to develop blood methemoglobin levels averaging 4.3% (Pacseri et al., 1958).

Metabolism and Excretion. Nitrobenzene is metabolized in man by oxidation to p-nitrophenol and by reduction to aniline, which is further oxidized to p-aminophenol. Nitrosobenzene and phenylhydroxylamine, highly toxic compounds, are believed to be produced as intermediates in the reduction of nitrobenzene to aniline. Only about 13–16% of a dose is excreted in the urine as p-nitrophenol, with probably less than 10% as p-aminophenol. Both of these substances are eliminated in the form of sulfate or glucuronide conjugates (Piotrowski, 1977).

In a subject exposed to 6 ppm of nitrobenzene for 6 hours, urine p-nitrophenol concentrations reached a maximum of about 5.2 mg/L at 2 hours after the end of the exposure and declined with a half-life of about 60 hours (Salmowa et al., 1963). With daily exposure to 1–6 ppm of nitrobenzene, urine p-nitrophenol concentrations reached a plateau after 3 days that was equivalent to 2.5 times the peak concentration achieved on the first day. p-Aminophenol was not found in urine in these studies, utilizing a colorimetric procedure with a sensitivity of 10 mg/L (Piotrowski, 1967).

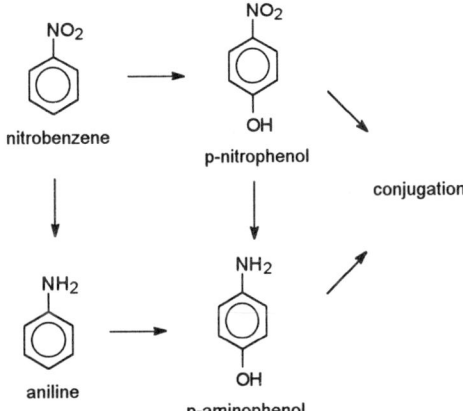

Toxicity. Exposure to 3–6 ppm of nitrobenzene for several hours may cause headache and elevation of blood methemoglobin concentration. Chronic exposure has produced severe headache, cyanosis, anemia, dizziness, loss of appetite, nausea, loss of feeling in the extremities, and severe weakness in a worker; methemoglobinemia at a level of 33% was observed initially, with peak urinary p-nitrophenol and p-aminophenol concentrations of 147 and 45 mg/L, respectively (Ikeda and Kita, 1964).

Numerous instances of acute nonfatal and fatal poisoning due to ingestion or dermal absorption of nitrobenzene have been reported in the older literature, at a time when the chemical was a common constituent of soaps, shoe dyes, inks, and other household products. Methylene blue is recommended for reversal of the often severe methemoglobinemia that results (Nabarro, 1948).

One person has survived the acute ingestion of 50 mL of nitrobenzene; a methemoglobin level of 82% was attained on the first day, accompanied by severe cyanosis and unconsciousness, and peak urinary p-nitrophenol and p-aminophenol excretion rates of 512 mg/24 hours and 198 mg/24 hours were observed on the third and second days, respectively. The half-life for metabolite excretion was estimated at 84 hours and measurable excretion continued for 22 days (Myslak et al., 1971).

Analysis. Procedures for blood methemoglobin and urine p-aminophenol are cited in the section on aniline. Methods for urinary p-nitrophenol are discussed in the section on parathion; an additional colorimetric technique was described by Piotrowski (1967).

References

M. Ikeda and A. Kita. Excretion of p-nitrophenol and p-aminophenol in the urine of a patient exposed to nitrobenzene. Brit. J. Ind. Med. 21: 210–213, 1964.

Z. Myslak, J.K. Piotrowski and E. Musialowicz. Acute nitrobenzene poisoning. Arch. Tox. 28: 208–213, 1971.

J.D.N. Nabarro. A case of acute mononitrobenzene poisoning. Brit. Med. J. 1: 929–931, 1948.

I. Pacseri, L. Magos and L.A. Batskor. Threshold and toxic limits of some amino and nitro compounds. Arch. Ind. Health 18: 1–8, 1958.

J. Piotrowski. Further investigations on the evaluation of exposure to nitrobenzene. Brit. J. Ind. Med. 24: 60–65, 1967.

J.K. Piotrowski. *Exposure Tests for Organic Compounds in Industrial Toxicology*, U.S. Government Printing Office, Washington, D.C., 1977, pp. 76–80.

J. Salmowa, J. Piotrowski and U. Neuhorn. Evaluation of exposure to nitrobenzene. Brit. J. Ind. Med. 20: 41–46, 1963.

Nitroglycerin

T½: 7.5 min
Vd: 2.6 L/kg
Fb: ?

$$\underset{\underset{ONO_2}{|}}{CH_2}\underset{\underset{}{}}{CH}\underset{\underset{ONO_2}{|}}{CH_2}$$
ONO₂ ONO₂

Occurrence and Usage. Nitroglycerin (glyceryl trinitrate, trinitroglycerin, Nitro-Bid, Nitro-Dur, Nitrogard, Nitrospan, Nitrostat) has been used as a coronary vasodilator for over 100 years. Other organic nitrates used for this purpose include isosorbide dinitrate and pentaerythritol tetranitrate. Nitroglycerin is a viscous liquid at room temperature and is almost insoluble in water. The drug is available in the form of sublingual tablets (0.15–0.60 mg), which may be taken every 5 minutes for an acute attack, and in 2.5–9.0 sustained-release capsules, to be swallowed 2–3 times daily. A 2% ointment is available for dermal application in amounts of approximately 30–60 mg every 4–8 hours, and dermal patches have recently been developed to deliver 10 mg of the drug over a 24 hour period.

Blood Concentrations. A peak plasma concentration of 0.25 µg/L was achieved by one volunteer at 40 minutes after the oral administration of a 6.5 mg capsule of nitroglycerin (Blumenthal et al., 1977). Plasma nitroglycerin concentrations in 6 volunteers reached an average peak level of 1.6 µg/L at 5 minutes after the sublingual administration of 0.60 mg, declining to 0.5 µg/L by 30 minutes. An average plasma concentration of 2.3 µg/L was observed 1 hour after dermal application of 45 mg of nitroglycerin as an ointment to 3 patients (Wei and Reid, 1979). Peak plasma levels of 6–13 µg/L were measured in 3 volunteers within 4 minutes of the sublingual administration of 1.2 mg of the drug (Bogaert and Rosseel, 1972). Three different dermal patch preparations intended to deliver 10 mg of nitroglycerin over 24 hours produced steady-state plasma levels that ranged from 0.1–0.2 µg/L during the 24 hour period (McAllister et al., 1986). The plasma half-life of nitroglycerin has been estimated at 7.5 minutes (Armstrong et al., 1979).

Metabolism and Excretion. The metabolism of nitroglycerin has not been thoroughly studied in man. In rats, the drug is degraded to 1,3-glyceryl dinitrate, 1,2-glyceryl dinitrate, 1- and 2-glyceryl mononitrate, glycerol, and inorganic nitrite. Each of the metabolites is more water-soluble and less active as a vasodilator than nitroglycerin. The major urinary metabolites include glyceryl mononitrate (33% of a dose), glycerol (8%), 1,2-glyceryl dinitrate (6%), and 1,3-glyceryl dinitrate (2%) (Needleman, 1976). 1-Glyceryl mononitrate has been studied as a possible vasodilator drug in man and was found to exhibit a plasma half-life of 1.8-3.2 hours (Laufen and Leitold, 1987). Plasma concentrations of the 4 nitro-metabolites generally exceed those of the parent in persons receiving the drug (Han et al., 1994).

Toxicity. Adverse reactions to nitroglycerin include headache, hypotension, tachycardia, dizziness, flushing of the skin, faintness, and nausea. Certain patients with hypertension are intolerant to the drug, exhibiting nausea, vomiting, syncope and collapse with doses as low as 0.24 mg (Lueth and Hanks, 1938). The acute lethal dose has been estimated at 200 mg, with death occurring in 2–6 hours; methemoglobinemia is usually present in severe poisoning, but not to the same extent as with amyl nitrite (Rabinowitch, 1944).

Analysis. Nitroglycerin has been assayed in plasma by electron-capture gas chromatography (Rosseel and Bogaert, 1973; Yap et al., 1978; Armstrong et al., 1979; Wei and Reid, 1979; Taylor et al., 1981; Sioufi and Pommier, 1985; Lee et al., 1988; Han et al., 1992). Liquid chromatography has been used to measure the drug and its nitro-metabolites in the blood of dogs (Spanggord and Keck, 1980). The *in vitro* half-life of nitroglycerin in plasma is about 1 hour; this reaction is inhibited by the addition of iodoacetamide or silver nitrate (Taylor et al., 1981). The *in vitro* degradation of nitroglycerin in whole blood has a half-life of about 20 minutes and results in the production of the 4 major *in vivo* nitro-metabolites (Han et al., 1992).

References

P.W. Armstrong, J.A. Armstrong and G.S. Marks. Blood levels after sublingual nitroglycerin. Circulation 59: 585–588, 1979.

H.P. Blumenthal, H.L. Fung, E.F. McNiff and S.K. Yap. Plasma nitroglycerin levels after sublingual, oral and topical administration. Brit. J. Clin. Pharm. 4: 241–242, 1977.

M.G. Bogaert and M.T. Rosseel. Plasma levels in man of nitroglycerin after buccal administration. J. Pharm. Pharmac. 24: 737–738, 1972.

C.Han, P. Jung, S.W. Sanders et al. Pharmacokinetics of nitroglycerin and its four metabolites during nitroglycerin transdermal application. Biopharm. Drug Disp. 15: 179–183, 1994.

C. Han, M. Gumbleton, D.T.W. Lau and L.Z. Benet. Improved gas chromatographic assay for the simultaneous determination of nitroglycerin and its mono- and dinitrate metabolites. J. Chrom. 579: 237–245, 1992.

H. Laufen and M. Leitold. Glyceryl-1-nitrate pharmacokinetics in healthy volunteers. Brit. J. Clin. Pharm. 23: 287–293, 1987.

F.W. Lee, N. Watari, J. Rigod and L.Z. Benet. Simultaneous determination of nitroglycerin and its dinitrate metabolite by capillary gas chromatography with electron-capture detection. J. Chrom. 426: 259–266, 1988.

H.C. Lueth and T.G. Hanks. Unusual reactions of patients with hypertension to glyceryl trinitrate. Arch. Int. Med. 62: 97–108, 1938.

A. McAllister, H. Mosberg, J.A. Settlage and J.A. Steiner. Plasma levels of nitroglycerin generated by three nitroglycerin patch preparations, Nitradisc, Transiderm-Nitro and Nitro-Dur and one ointment formulation, Nitrobid. Brit. J. Clin. Pharm. 21: 365–369, 1986.

P. Needleman. Organic nitrate metabolism. Ann. Rev. Pharm. Tox. 16: 81–93, 1976.

I.M. Rabinowitch. Acute nitroglycerine poisoning. Can. Med. Asso. J. 50: 199–202, 1944.

M.T. Rosseel and M.G. Bogaert. GLC determination of nitroglycerin and isosorbide dinitrate in human plasma. J. Pharm. Sci. 62: 754–758, 1973.

A. Sioufi and F. Pommier. Quantitative determination of nitroglycerin in human plasma by capillary gas chromatography with electron-caputre detection. J. Chrom. 339: 117–126, 1985.

R.J. Spanggord and R.G. Keck. Application of high-pressure liquid chromatography and thermal energy analyzer to analysis of trinitroglycerin and its metabolites in blood. J. Pharm. Sci. 69: 444–446, 1980.

I.W. Taylor, C. Ioannides, J.C. Turner et al. Micro determination of glyceryl trinitrate in biological fluids; effect of deuteration of glyceryl trinitrate on its pharmacokinetic properties. J. Pharm. Pharmac. 33: 244–246, 1981.

J.Y. Wei and P.R. Reid. Quantitative determination of trinitroglycerin in human plasma. Circulation 59: 588–592, 1979.

P.S.K. Yap, E.F. McNiff and H.L. Fung. Improved GLC determination of plasma nitroglycerin concentrations. J. Pharm. Sci. 67: 582–584, 1978.

Nitroprusside

T½: 11 min
Vd: ?
Fb: ?

$$Na_2Fe(NO)(CN)_5 \cdot 2H_2O$$

Occurrence and Usage. Nitroprusside (nitrosylpentacyanoferrate, Nipride) as the sodium salt is a rapid-acting hypotensive agent. Its effects were recognized as early as 1928, but it has only recently achieved popularity in the treatment of hypertensive crises and to produce controlled hypotension during anesthesia. The drug is administered by intravenous infusion in doses of 0.5–8.0 μg/kg/min and is available in 50 mg ampules.

Blood Concentrations. Nitroprusside plasma concentrations have not been measured in man, but are known to be significant only during continued infusion of the drug (Rodkey and Collison, 1977). Plasma thiocyanate concentrations averaged 5.5 mg/L in 17 subjects prior to infusion with 1.1–10.6 μg/kg/min (average, 5.1) of nitroprusside for 20–90 minutes (average, 58) and after infusion, averaged 5.9 mg/L. The average respective plasma cyanide concentrations were 0.004 mg/L and 0.017 mg/L. After prolonged infusion (several days) of nitroprusside in 2 patients, plasma thiocyanate concentrations were 17.4 and 29.0 mg/L and plasma cyanide concentrations, 0.038 and 0.055 mg/L; in the first patient, the corresponding erythrocyte cyanide concentration was 0.832 mg/L (Vesey et al., 1974). In 50 surgical patients, whole blood cyanide concentrations averaged 0.023 mg/L (range, 0–0.113) before the infusion for 15–120 min of 3–8 μg/kg/min nitroprusside, and averaged 0.333 mg/L (range, 0.021–1.800) just after the infusion (Bogusz et al., 1979). To avoid cyanide accumulation, it has been recommended that the nitroprusside infusion rate not exceed 4 μg/kg/min (5.8 mg/kg/day) (Vesey and Cole, 1985).

Metabolism and Excretion. Nitroprusside is believed to undergo nonenzymatic transformation by reaction with erythrocyte hemoglobin, during which methemoglobin is formed and one of the 5 cyanide equivalents that are released is trapped as cyanmethemoglobin (Smith and Kruszyna, 1974). The cyanide that is formed is subsequently metabolized by conversion to thiocyanate via the liver enzyme rhodanase (Goldstein and Rieders, 1951) and, although most of the thiocyanate is slowly excreted unchanged by the kidney, some is reconverted to cyanide by erythrocytes (Goldstein and Reiders, 1953). Thiocyanate does not accumulate in plasma following nitroprusside except after prolonged administration (Vesey et al., 1974). Free cyanide will be present in plasma only when the blood concentration exceeds the cyanide-binding capacity of the erythrocyte methemoglobin (about 10 mg in adults) (Rodkey and Collison, 1977). The cyanide that accumulates during nitroprusside infusion appears to be responsible for toxicity, although the cardiovascular effects of the drug are believed to be due to the parent structure and, to a lesser degree, thiocyanate (Smith and Kruszyna, 1974).

Toxicity. The toxic effects of nitroprusside may be due to the parent drug or its metabolic products. Nitroprusside itself can cause severe hypotension; during its metabolism by hemoglobin, methemoglobin is formed, leading eventually to cyanosis; the metabolite cyanide causes cellular hypoxia and metabolic acidosis; and a further metabolite, thiocyanate, can produce tinnitus, blurred vision, delerium, hypotension, and hypothyroidism. A 4 day infusion involving a total of 321 mg of nitroprusside produced cyanosis and a blood methemoglobin level of 16% in a 58 year old man (Bower and Peterson, 1975). A 6 day infusion involving approximately 1000 mg nitroprusside resulted in blood cyanide and thiocyanate levels of 5 and 24 mg/L, respectively, in a woman who gradually became unresponsive; she survived with antidotal treatment (Marbury et al., 1982). Metabolic acidosis developed in patients whose erythrocyte cyanide levels exceeded 0.750 mg/L (Cottrell et al., 1978) and in those whose blood cyanide levels exceeded 0.900 mg/L (Aitken et al., 1977).

Nitroprusside-induced cyanide intoxication has been successfully treated by the antidotal administration of hydroxocobalamin (Posner et al., 1976) or thiosulfate (Perschau et al., 1977). Thiocyanate and cyanide blood concentrations are not dependable indicators of nitroprusside toxicity during administration of the drug; it has been suggested that limiting the total dose to 3–3.5 mg/kg and monitoring for biochemical evidence of anerobic metabolism will aid in the prevention of poisoning (Tinker and Michenfelder, 1976).

Several fatalities associated with nitroprusside have been described that involved the administration of a total of 750 mg of the drug (Jack, 1974; Merrifield and Blundell, 1974). A blood cyanide concentration of 5 mg/L and urine concentration of 3 mg/L were observed in a teenager who died following the infusion of 10 mg/kg (total dose, 400 mg) of sodium nitroprusside over an 80 minute period (Davies et al., 1975).

Analysis. Nitroprusside is measurable in blood or plasma by incubation with cysteine and colorimetric determination of the liberated cyanide; a correction for free cyanide must be made by analysis of a separate specimen using a gas transfer or diffusion technique (Rodkey and Collison, 1977). Procedures for analysis of cyanide and thiocyanate are discussed in the section on cyanide. It has been suggested that the cyanide found in blood after nitroprusside administration is largely an artifact of the colorimetric methods commonly used, and that measurement with a cyanide-specific electrode is preferred (Bisset et al., 1981).

References

D. Aitken, D. West, F. Smith et al. Cyanide toxicity following nitroprusside induced hypotension. Can. Anaesth. Soc. J. 24: 651–660, 1977.

W.I.K. Bisset, A.R. Butler, C. Glidewell and J. Reglinski. Sodium nitroprusside and cyanide release: reasons for re-appraisal. Brit. J. Anaesth. 53: 1015–1018, 1981.

M. Bogusz, J. Moroz, J. Karski et al. Blood cyanide and thiocyanate concentrations after administration of sodium nitroprusside as hypotensive agent in neurosurgery. Clin. Chem. 25: 60–63, 1979.

P.J. Bower and J.N. Peterson. Methemoglobin after sodium nitroprusside therapy. New Eng. J. Med. 293: 865, 1975.

J.E. Cottrell, P. Casthely, J.D. Brodie et al. Prevention of nitroprusside-induced cyanide toxicity with hydroxocobalamin. New Eng. J. Med. 298: 809–811, 1978.

D.W. Davies, D. Kadar, D.J. Steward and I.R. Munro. A sudden death associated with the use of sodium nitroprusside for induction of hypotension during anaesthesia. Can. Anaesth. Soc. J. 22: 547–552, 1975.

F. Goldstein and F. Rieders. Formation of cyanide in dog and man following administration of thiocyanate. Am. J. Physiol. 167: 47–51, 1951.

F. Goldstein and F. Rieders. Conversion of thiocyanate to cyanide by an erythrocytic enzyme. Am. J. Physiol. 173: 287–290, 1953.

R.D. Jack. Toxicity of sodium nitroprusside. Brit. J. Anaesth. 46: 952, 1974.

T.C. Marbury, J.E. Sheppard, K. Gibbons and C.S.C. Lee. Combined antidotal and hemodialysis treatments for nitroprusside-induced cyanide toxicity. Clin. Tox. 19: 475–482, 1982.

A.J. Merrifield and M.D. Blundell. Toxicity of sodium nitroprusside. Brit. J. Anaesth. 46: 324, 1974.

R.A. Perschau, J.H. Modell, R.W. Bright and P.D. Shirley. Suspected sodium nitroprusside-induced cyanide intoxication. Anesth. Anal. 56: 533–537, 1977.

M.A. Posner, F.L. Rodkey and R.E. Tobey. Nitroprusside-induced cyanide poisoning: antidotal effect of hydroxocobalamin. Anesthesiology 44: 330–335, 1976.

F.L. Rodkey and H.A. Collison. Determination of cyanide and nitroprusside in blood and plasma. Clin. Chem. 23: 1969–1975, 1977.

R.P. Smith and H. Kruszyna. Nitroprusside produces cyanide poisoning via a reaction with hemoglobin. J. Pharm. Exp. Ther. 191: 557–563, 1974.

J.H. Tinker and J.D. Michenfelder. Sodium nitroprusside: pharmacology, toxicology and therapeutics. Anesthesiology 45: 340–354, 1976.

C.J. Vesey, P.V. Cole, J.C. Linnell and J. Wilson. Some metabolic effects of sodium nitroprusside in man. Brit. Med. J. 2: 140–142, 1974.

C.J. Vesey and P.V. Cole. Blood cyanide and thiocyanate concentrations produced by long-term therapy with sodium nitroprusside. Brit. J. Anaesth. 57: 148–155, 1985.

Nitrous Oxide

T½: ?
Vd: ?
Fb: ?

N_2O

Occurrence and Usage. Nitrous oxide was discovered by Priestly in 1776 and, although its potential as an anesthetic was recognized by Davy in 1799, it did not come into general usage until after 1860. The nonflammable, nearly odorless gas is a good analgesic but will not produce complete anesthesia at safe concentrations (65% in oxygen), and so is used primarily as an analgesic or as an adjunct to other more potent anesthetic agents.

Blood Concentrations. Arterial blood concentrations of nitrous oxide range from 170–220 mL/L during surgical anesthesia (Raginsky and Bourne, 1934).

Metabolism and Excretion. Nitrous oxide is relatively insoluble in tissues and thus induction and recovery are usually quite rapid. The gas is eliminated very rapidly by pulmonary diffusion following exposure, and there is no evidence that any significant biotransformation occurs. The following distribution is seen at body temperature (Wollman and Smith, 1975):

Partition Coefficients for Nitrous Oxide

Blood:Gas	Brain:Blood	Liver:Blood	Kidney:Blood	Fat:Blood
0.47	1.1	0.9	0.9	2.3

Toxicity. Nitrous oxide is often inhaled for its euphoric effects, being easily obtained from whipped cream cans or from medical supplies (Rosenberg et al., 1979). Inhalation of 40% nitrous oxide in air causes confusion and sedation, while a level of 80% causes unconsciousness in most persons (Dohrn et al., 1992; Wagner et al., 1992). Myeloneuropathy has been reported in dentists after chronic exposure to the gas (Layzer, 1978), and bone marrow depression is known to occur in patients receiving the drug for long periods (Amess et al., 1978). Nitrous oxide was held responsible for cardiovascular collapse in a pediatric surgical patient (Davidson and Chinyanga, 1982).

The gas is a central nervous system depressant and can cause asphyxiation by oxygen displacement. In 6 deaths due to abuse of nitrous oxide, postmortem blood concentrations of 46–180 mL/L (average, 100) were observed (Baselt, 1976; DiMaio and Garriott, 1978; Wagner et al., 1992). The following distribution of the gas was determined in a similar case (Shaw, 1980):

Nitrous Oxide Concentrations in a Fatality (mL/L or mL/kg)

Blood	Brain	Lung
88	34	11–16

Analysis. Nitrous oxide has been determined in biological specimens by infrared spectroscopy (Feldstein, 1965), mass spectrometry (Urich et al., 1977), or more commonly by gas chromatography using thermal conductivity detection and a molecular sieve (Yokota et al., 1967; DiMaio and Garriott, 1978) or Porapak Q column (Molloy et al., 1973; Saloojee and Cole, 1978).

References

J.A.L. Amess, J.F. Burman, G.M. Rees et al. Megaloblastic haemopoiesis in patients receiving nitrous oxide. Lancet 2: 339–344, 1978.

R.C. Baselt. Unpublished results, 1976.

J.R. Davidson and H.M. Chinyanga. Cardiovascular collapse associated with nitrous oxide anaesthetic: a case report. Can. Anaesth. Soc. J. 29: 484–488, 1982.

V.J.M. DiMaio and J.C. Garriott. Four deaths resulting from abuse of nitrous oxide. J. For. Sci. 23: 169–172, 1978.

C.S. Dohrn. J.L. Lichtor, R.S. Finn et al. Subjective and psychomotor effects of nitrous oxide in healthy volunteers. Behav. Pharm. 3: 19–30, 1992.

M. Feldstein. Analysis of toxic gases in blood by infrared spectroscopy. J. For. Sci. 10: 207–216, 1965.

R.B. Layzer. Myeloneuropathy after prolonged exposure to nitrous oxide concentrations in whole blood. Brit. J. Anaesth. 45: 556–562, 1973.

M.J. Molloy, I.P. Latto and M. Rosen. Analysis of nitrous oxide concentrations in whole blood. Brit. J. Anaesth. 45: 556–562, 1973.

B.B. Raginsky and W. Bourne. Cyanosis in nitrous oxide oxygen anaesthesia in man. Can. Med. Asso. J. 30: 518–522, 1934.

H. Rosenberg, F.K. Orkin and J. Springstead. Abuse of nitrous oxide. Anesth. Anal. 58: 104–106, 1979.

Y. Saloojee and P. Cole. Estimation of nitrous oxide in blood. Anaesthesia 33: 779–783, 1978.

R. Shaw. Presented at the quarterly meeting of the California Association of Toxicologists, San Francisco, February 2, 1980.

R.W. Urich, D.L. Bowerman, P.H. Wittenberg et al. Head space mass spectrometric analysis for volatiles in biological specimens. J. Anal. Tox. 1: 195–199, 1977.

S.A. Wagner, D.L. Wesche, M.A. Clark et al. Asphyxial deaths from the recreational use of nitrous oxide. J. For. Sci. 37: 1008–1015, 1992.

H. Wollman and T.C. Smith. Uptake, distribution, elimination, and administration of inhalational anesthetics. In *The Pharmacological Basis of Therapeutics*, 5th ed. (L.S. Goodman and A. Gilman, eds.), MacMillan, New York, 1975, pp. 71–80.

T. Yokota, Y. Hitomi, K. Ohta and F. Kosaka. Direct injection method for gas chromatographic measurement of inhalation anesthetics in whole blood and tissues. Anesthesiology 28: 1064–1073, 1967.

Nomifensine

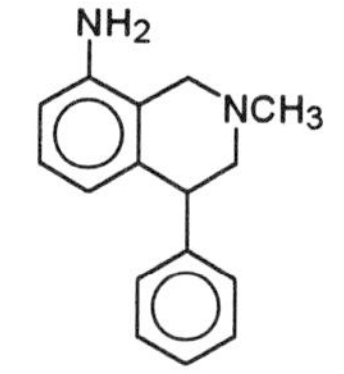

T½: 3–5 hr
Vd: 5.4–8.4 L/kg
Fb: 0.60–0.75
pKa: ?

Occurrence and Usage. Nomifensine (Merital) is an isoquinoline derivative used as an antidepressant agent since 1973. In contrast to the tricyclic antidepressants, the drug has a definite central nervous system stimulant effect due apparently to its ability to inhibit dopamine reuptake by neurons. It is available as the maleate salt in 25 or 50 mg tablets or capsules. Daily oral maintenance doses range from 75–150 mg.

Blood Concentrations. The oral administration of 50 mg of nomifensine to 3 volunteers resulted in an average peak plasma level of 0.122 mg/L (range, 0.055–0.170) at 1.5 hours, declining to 0.068 mg/L by 4 hours and 0.016 mg/L by 8 hours (Vereczkey et al., 1976). A single 150 mg oral dose in 5 patients produced an average peak plasma level of 0.324 mg/L at 1.4 hours that declined to 0.044 mg/L by 8 hours; plasma concentrations of an inactive metabolite, nomifensine-N-glucuronide, reached an average peak level of 3.982 mg/L at 1.7 hours and declined to 0.380 mg/L by 8 hours (Dawling et al., 1980). The plasma half-life of the drug has been found to average 3.9 hours in healthy volunteers (Vereczkey et al., 1975) and ranges from 8–46 hours in patients with impaired renal function (Ringoir et al., 1977). The blood/plasma concentration ratio for nomifensine averages 1.2 (Maguire et al., 1980).

In 9 subjects who received 75 mg daily (in 3 divided doses) for 6 days, plasma nomifensine concentrations averaged 0.011 mg/L (range, 0.005–0.017) at 6 hours after the last dose (Bailey et al., 1977).

Metabolism and Excretion. Nomifensine is known to be metabolized by phenyl hydroxylation and conjugation, and to a minor extent by N-demethylation. An acid-labile conjugate, nomifensine-N-glucuronide, is the major species found in plasma and urine. Urine collected for 12 hours after a

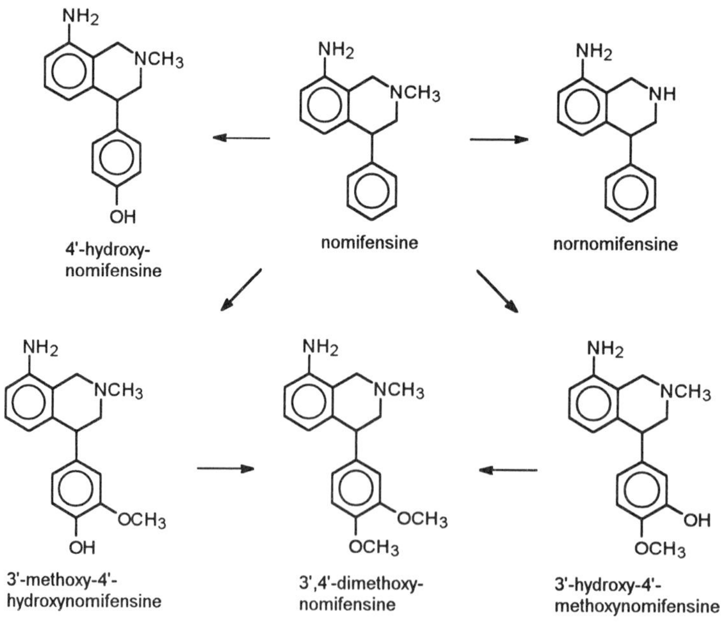

4'-hydroxy-
nomifensine

nomifensine

nornomifensine

3'-methoxy-4'-
hydroxynomifensine

3',4'-dimethoxy-
nomifensine

3'-hydroxy-4'-
methoxynomifensine

single dose contained 57% of the dose as conjugated nomifensine, 7% as 4'-hydroxynomifensine, 7% as 3'-methoxy-4'-hydroxynomifensine, and 7% as 3'-hydroxy-4'-methoxynomifensine. Another 12% was in the form of conjugated metabolites, while nornomifensine and 3',4'-dimethoxy-nomifensine accounted for less than 1%. The parent drug is not believed to be excreted unchanged in urine, although the rapid hydrolysis of the N-glucuronide conjugate under acidic conditions may give the appearance of free drug excretion (Heptner et al., 1978; Lindberg and Syvalahti, 1986).

Toxicity. Overdosage with nomifensine may result in drowsiness or excitation, tachycardia, tremor, hypertension, and coma. Acute hemolysis and renal failure have also been reported (Prescott et al., 1980). The drug is not known to produce convulsions or cardiotoxicity, and is believed to be less toxic than the tricylic antidepressants (Crome and Chand, 1980). A 28 year old woman who ingested 1.5 g of the drug and developed only tachycardia achieved a maximal plasma nomifensine concentration of 2.8 mg/L (Montgomery et al., 1978). A 43 year old woman ingested 3.5 g and exhibited slurred speech as the only manifestation of poisoning; her plasma level 17 hours after ingestion was 3.7 mg/L and it declined with an apparent half-life of 5 hours (Vohra et al., 1978). A 60 year old man became comatose and developed renal failure after overdosage; a plasma nomifensine level of 16 mg/L was measured about 28 hours after drug ingestion, but he recovered within a week (Skinner and Ferner, 1986).

A 23 year old woman who died following the suicidal ingestion of alcohol and nomifensine was found to have a postmortem blood alcohol concentration of 0.50 g/dL and the following levels of nomifensine: blood, 17 mg/L; liver, 32 mg/kg; kidney, 141 mg/kg; and urine, 400 mg/L (Reyfer et al., 1979).

Analysis. Nomifensine has been determined in biological fluids by radioimmunoassay (Heptner et al., 1977) and by gas chromatography using nitrogen-specific (Bailey et al., 1977; Chamberlain and Hill, 1977; Dawling et al., 1980; McIntyre et al., 1981), electron-capture (Vereczkey et al., 1976) or mass spectrometric detection (Bagchi et al., 1985). Liquid chromatography has also been reported (Lindberg et al., 1983). Since the N-glucuronide conjugate of nomifensine decomposes rapidly in specimens at room temperature, releasing free nomifensine, it is important to refrigerate or freeze those specimens that are not to be analyzed immediately (Dawling et al., 1980).

References

S.P. Bagchi, T. Lutz and S.P. Jindal. Gas chromatographic-mass spectrometric determination of nomifensine using a stable isotope-labeled analogue as an internal standard. J. Chrom. 344: 362–366, 1985.

E. Bailey, M. Fenoughty and L. Richardson. Automated high-resolution gas chromatographic analysis of psychotropic drugs in biological fluids using open-tubular glass capillary columns. J. Chrom. 131: 347–355, 1977.

J. Chamberlain and H.M. Hill. A simple gas chromatographic method for the determination of nomifensine in plasma and a comparison of the method with other available techniques. Brit J. Clin. Pharm. 4: 117S–121S, 1977.

P. Crome and S. Chand. The clinical toxicology of nomifensine: comparison with tricyclic antidepressants. Roy. Soc. Med. Int. Cong. Symp. Ser. 25: 55–58, 1980.

S. Dawling, R. Braithwaite and S.A. Montgomery. Analytical measurement and pharmacokinetics of nomifensine. Roy. Soc. Med. Int. Cong. Symp. Ser. 25: 39–45, 1980.

W. Heptner, M.J. Badian, S. Baudner et al. Determination of nomifensine by a sensitive radioimmunoassay. Brit. J. Clin. Pharm. 4: 123S–127S, 1977.

W. Heptner, I. Hornke, F. Cavagna et al. Metabolism of nomifensine in man and animal species. Arz. Forsch. 28: 58–64, 1978.

R.L.P. Lindberg, J.S. Salomen and E.I. Iisalo. Determination of nomifensine in human serum. J. Chrom. 276: 85–92, 1983.

R.L.P. Lindberg and E.K.G. Syvalahti. Metabolism of nomifensine after oral and intravenous administration. Clin. Pharm. Ther. 39: 378–383, 1986.

K.P. Maguire, G.D. Burrows, T.R. Norman and B.A. Scoggins. Blood/plasma distribution ratios of psychotropic drugs. Clin. Chem. 26: 1624–1625, 1980.

I.M. McIntyre, T.R. Norman, G.D. Burrows and K.P. Maguire. Determination of nomifensine plasma concentrations: a comparison of radioimmunoassay and gas chromatography. Brit. J. Clin. Pharm. 12: 691–694, 1981.

S. Montgomery, P. Crome and R. Braithwaite. Nomifensine overdose. Lancet 1: 828–829, 1978.

A.F. Reyfer, O. Frye, T. Krompecher and A.L. Zwahlen. Selbstmord durch Vergiftung mit einem Medikament, dessen aktive Substanz Nomifensin ist. Beit. Gericht. Med. 37: 313–318, 1979.

S. Ringoir, N. Lamiere, M. Munche et al. Pharmacokinetics of nomifensine in impaired renal function. Brit. J. Clin. Pharm. 4: 129S–134S, 1977.

R. Skinner and R.E. Ferner. Acute renal failure without acute intravascular haemolysis after nomifensine overdosage. Hum. Tox. 5: 279–280, 1986.

L. Vereczkey, G. Bianchetti, S. Garattini and P.L. Morselli. Pharmacokinetics of nomifensine in man. Psychopharmacologia 45: 225–227, 1975.

L. Vereczkey, G. Bianchetti, V. Rovei and A. Frigerio. Gas chromatographic method for the determination of nomifensine in human plasma. J. Chrom. 116: 451–456, 1976.

J.K. Vohra, G.D. Burrows, I. McIntyre and B. Davies. Cardiovascular effects of nomifensine. Lancet 2: 902–903, 1978.

Nortriptyline

T½: 15–90 hr
Vd: 20–57 L/kg
Fb: 0.95
pKa: 9.7

$CHCH_2CH_2NHCH_3$

Occurrence and Usage. Nortriptyline (Aventyl, Pamelor) is the mono-N-desmethyl metabolite of amitriptyline and is itself an active antidepressant agent. The compound was first synthesized in 1962 and its efficacy in humans demonstrated in 1963. It is available as the hydrochloride salt in 10–75 mg capsules or as a 10 mg/5 mL syrup; oral doses of 75–150 mg daily are typical.

Blood Concentrations. Following a single oral 1 mg/kg (70 mg/70 kg) dose of nortriptyline, plasma concentrations reached an average peak level of 0.042 mg/L (range, 0.030–0.061) at 5.3 hours, with a plasma half-life of 27 hours (Alexanderson, 1972). During chronic therapy with 75 mg daily, steady-state plasma levels in 15 patients have ranged from 0.010–0.275 mg/L, with an average of 0.055 mg/L (Hammer and Sjoqvist, 1967). In patients on chronic dose regimens of 150 and 250 mg daily, steady-state plasma concentrations averaged 0.171 and 0.375 mg/L, respectively (Burrows et al., 1974). The plasma 10-hydroxynortriptyline/nortriptyline concentration ratio averages 1.2 in young adults and 2.5 in elderly patients on chronic therapy (Young et al., 1984). The blood/plasma concentration ratio for nortriptyline averages 1.5–1.7 (Maguire et al., 1980).

Metabolism and Excretion. Nortriptyline is metabolized by both N-demethylation and 10-hydroxylation, with glucuronide conjugation of the two hydroxy-derivatives (Alexanderson et al., 1971). None of the metabolites seems to accumulate to any significant degree in plasma (Hammer et al., 1971). The 24 hour urinary excretion of unchanged drug does not normally exceed 3% of the dose, but may increase slightly with acid urine conditions; urine nortriptyline concentrations in patients on chronic therapy were found to range from 0.2–7.0 mg/L (Sjoqvist et al., 1969). Nearly an entire dose of nortriptyline can be accounted for as urinary metabolites over a 6 day period, with about equal amounts of free and conjugated 10-hydroxynortriptyline representing 50–70%; an additional 5–20% is present as unidentified polar metabolites (Gram and Overo, 1975). Less than 1% is excreted as free dinortriptyline and about 10% as free and conjugated 10-hydroxydinortriptyline (Alexanderson and Borga, 1973).

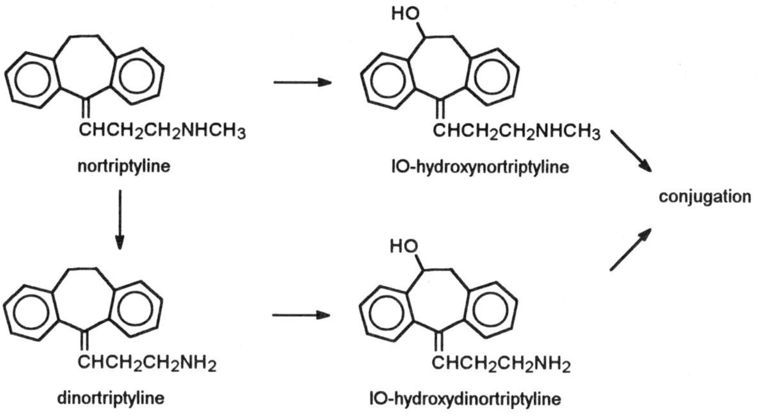

HO

CHCH₂CH₂NHCH₃
nortriptyline

10-hydroxynortriptyline
CHCH₂CH₂NHCH₃

conjugation

CHCH₂CH₂NH₂
dinortriptyline

HO

CHCH₂CH₂NH₂
10-hydroxydinortriptyline

Toxicity. Relatively few episodes of serious intoxication, fatal or otherwise, have been attributed to nortriptyline in comparison to the tertiary amine tricyclic antidepressants. Undesirable side effects, such as hypotension or hypertension, tachycardia, cardiac arrhythmias, confusion, anxiety, blurred vision, dry mouth, and nausea, generally occur at plasma concentrations exceeding 0.200 mg/L (Asberg, 1974). A change in drug formulation in a man who had been stabilized at 175 mg/day of nortriptyline caused a rise in steady-state plasma level from 0.125 mg/L to 0.680 mg/L and the onset of headache, lethargy and confusion (Dubovsky, 1987). Survival has been reported following ingestion of 2500 mg of the drug, after which plasma concentrations of 0.5–0.9 mg/L were observed (Sjoqvist et al., 1969). Another case was described in which a pregnant woman ingested at least 1500 mg of nortriptyline and attained a maximum plasma level of 1.2 mg/L after 17 hours, at which time she was unconscious; consciousness was regained some time after successful delivery of the child, when the plasma level dropped to 0.5 mg/L, 36 hours after ingestion (Sjoqvist et al., 1972).

A 30 year old woman ingested approximately 2000 mg of nortriptyline and was brought to a hospital 12 hours later, awake but disoriented, with a plasma drug level of 0.886 mg/L. She developed ventricular tachycardia and became comatose; pharmacological countermeasures were instituted, but she had a convulsion with cardiovascular collapse, and died 5 hours after admission (Rudorfer and Robins, 1981). The following distribution was observed in 9 fatal cases by means of an ultraviolet spectrophotometric technique (Bonnichsen et al., 1970):

Nortriptyline Concentrations in Fatalities (mg/L or mg/kg)

	Blood	Liver	Kidney	Urine
Average	11	90	43	79
(Range)	(0–26)	(8–220)	(7–94)	(25–120)

Nortriptyline may exhibit postmortem redistribution; the average heart blood/femoral blood concentration ratio in a series of 28 cases was 2.3 (range, 0.5–8.4) (Anderson and Prouty, 1989). A heart blood/femoral blood concentration ratio of 12 was observed in the death of an adult male who acutely ingested as much as 3.75 g of nortriptyline; heart blood, brain and liver concentrations of the drug were 86 mg/L, 97 mg/kg and 253 mg/kg, respectively (Rohrig and Prouty, 1989).

Analysis. The analytical procedures described for amitriptyline are suitable as well for nortriptyline. In addition, nortriptyline alone has been determined by radioacetylation and thin-layer chromatography (Zuleski et al., 1977). Electron-capture gas chromatography (Borga and Garle, 1972; Anliker et al., 1992) and gas chromatography-mass spectrometry (Hammer et al., 1971) have been applied to the detection of the drug and its major metabolties. In this latter technique, it was found that trifluoroacetylation of 10-hydroxynortriptyline resulted in spontaneous conversion of the metabolite to 10,11-dehydronortriptyline-trifluoroacetamide. Liquid chromatography has also been employed (Gupta, 1993).

References

B. Alexanderson, L. Bertilsson, O. Borga and F. Sjoqvist. Studies on the metabolism and pharmacokinetics of nortriptyline and desmethylimipramine in man. Chem. Biol. Int. 3: 235–236, 1971.

B. Alexanderson. Pharmacokinetics of desmethylimipramine and nortriptyline in man after single and multiple oral doses—a cross-over study. Eur. J. Clin. Pharm. 5: 1–10, 1972.

B. Alexanderson and O. Borga. Urinary excretion of nortriptyline and five of its metabolites in man after single and multiple oral doses. Eur. J. Clin. Pharm. 5: 174–180, 1973.

W.H. Anderson and R.W. Prouty. Postmortem redistribution of drugs. In *Advances in Analytical Toxicology* (R.C. Baselt, ed.), Vol. 2, YearBook Medical, Chicago, 1989, pp. 70–102.

S.L. Anliker, M. Hamilton, R.J. Bopp and M.J. Goldberg. Sensitive method for the quantitation of nortriptyline and 10-hydroxynortriptyline in human plasma by capillary gas chromatography with electron-capture detection. J. Chrom. 573: 141–145, 1992.

M. Asberg. Individualization of treatment of tricyclic compounds. Med. Clin. N. Am. 58: 1083–1091, 1974.

R. Bonnichsen, A.C. Maehly and G. Skold. A report on autopsy cases involving amitriptyline and nortriptyline. Z. Rechtsmed. 57: 190–200, 1970.

O. Borga and M. Garle. A gas chromatographic method for the quantitative determination of nortriptyline and some of its metabolites in human plasma and urine. J. Chrom. 68: 77–88, 1972.

G. Burrows, B.A. Scoggins, L.R. Turecek and B. Davies. Plasma nortriptyline and clinical response. Clin. Pharm. Ther. 16: 639–644, 1974.

S.L. Dubovsky. Severe nortriptyline intoxication due to change from a generic to a trade preparation. J. Nerv. Ment. Dis. 175: 115–117, 1987.

L.F. Gram and K.F. Overo. First-pass metabolism of nortriptyline in man. Clin. Pharm. Ther. 18: 305–314, 1975.

R.N. Gupta. An improved solid phase extraction procedure for the determination of antidepressants in serum by column liquid chromatography. J. Liq. Chrom. 16: 2751–2765.

C. Hammar, B. Alexanderson, B. Holmstedt and F. Sjoqvist. Gas chromatography-mass spectrometry of nortriptyline in body fluids of man. Clin. Pharm. Ther. 12: 496–505, 1971.

W. Hammer and F. Sjoqvist. Plasma levels of monomethylated tricyclic antidepressants during treatment with imipramine-like compounds. Life Sci. 6: 1895–1903, 1967.

K.P. Maguire, G.D. Burrows, T.R. Norman and B.A. Scoggins. Blood/plasma distribution ratios of pyschotropic drugs. Clin. Chem. 26: 1624–1625, 1980.

T.P. Rohrig and R.W. Prouty. A nortriptyline death with unusually high tissue concentrations. J. Anal. Tox. 13: 303–304, 1989.

M.V. Rudorfer and E. Robins. Fatal nortriptyline overdose, plasma levels and *in vivo* methylation of tricyclic antidepressants. Am. J. Psych. 138: 982–983, 1981.

F. Sjoqvist, F. Berglund, O. Borga et al. The pH-dependent excretion of monomethylated tricyclic antidepressants. Clin. Pharm. Ther. 10: 826–833, 1969.

F. Sjoqvist, P.G. Bergfors, M. Lind et al. Plasma disappearance of nortriptyline in a newborn infant following placental transfer from an intoxicated mother: evidence for drug metabolism. J. Pediat. 80: 496–500, 1972.

R.C. Young, G.S. Alexopoulos, C.A. Shamoian et al. Plasma 10-hydroxynortriptyline in elderly depressed patients. Clin. Pharm. Ther. 35: 540–544, 1984.

F.R. Zuleski, A. Loh and F.J. DiCarlo. Assay of human plasma for nortriptyline by radioacetylation and thin-layer chromatography. J. Chrom. 132: 45–49, 1977.

Orphenadrine

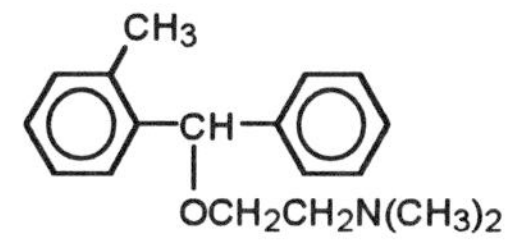

T½: 13–20 hr
Vd: 4.3–7.8 L/kg
Fb: 0.20
pKa: 8.4

Occurrence and Usage. Orphenadrine (Disipal, Norflex, Norgesic) is a diphenhydramine analogue whose synthesis was first described in 1951. It has both sedative and anticholinergic effects
and is used primarily as an antiparkinsonism agent and to control the extrapyramidal side effects of
phenothiazine therapy. The compound is administered orally as a tablet in single doses of 25–100
mg and daily doses of up to 300 mg as the hydrochloride or citrate salt. A 60 mg/2 mL solution is
available for intramuscular or intravenous injection.

Blood Concentrations. Following a single oral 100 mg dose in a volunteer, plasma orphenadrine
concentrations reached a peak of about 0.150 mg/L at 3 hours, declining with a half-life of 16
hours. Nororphenadrine (tofenacine) reached a peak level of about 0.045 mg/L at 6 hours, and had
a slightly longer apparent half-life (Labout et al., 1977). During chronic oral administration of 100
mg of orphenadrine every 8 hours (300 mg daily), plasma concentrations in 12 patients were found
to range from undetectable levels to 0.845 mg/L, with many of the specimens in the 0.100–0.200
mg/L range (Loga et al., 1975). Seven subjects receiving chronic daily doses exhibited average
steady-state plasma orphenadrine levels of 0.229 mg/L at a dose of 150 mg/day, 0.352 mg/L at 225
mg/day and 0.426 mg/L at 300 mg/day (Labout et al., 1982).

Metabolism and Excretion. An average of 60% of a labeled dose of orphenadrine is excreted in the
72 hour urine. The major urinary products include unchanged drug (8%), nororphenadrine (8%),
dinororphenadrine (4%), orphenadrine-N-oxide (5%), conjugated o-methylbenzhydryloxyacetic acid
(13%), and conjugated o-methylbenzhydrol (8%). Up to 30% of a dose may be eliminated unchanged if the urine is maintained at an acidic pH (Beckett and Khan, 1971; Ellison et al., 1971).
Nororphenadrine has been shown to have both muscle relaxant and anticataleptic activity (den
Besten et al., 1970).

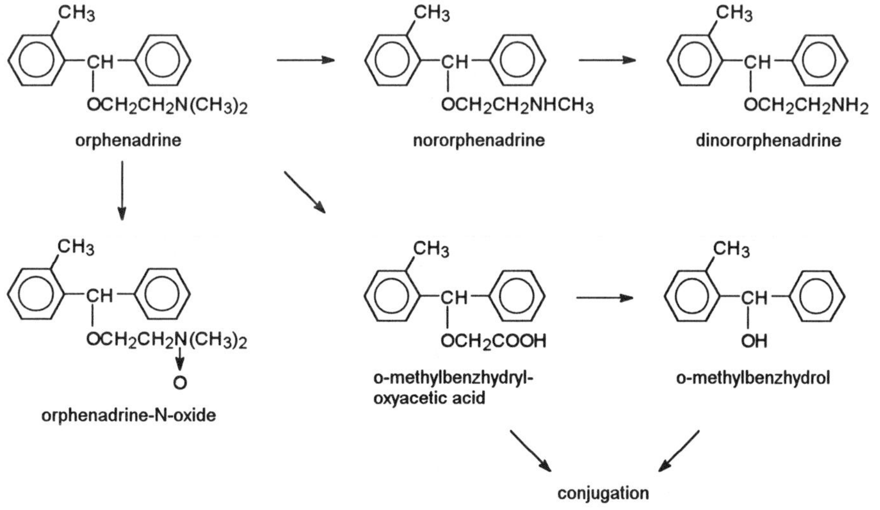

Toxicity. Adverse reactions to orphenadrine include dryness of the mouth, pupillary dilation, blurred
vision, tachycardia, weakness, nausea, vomiting, headache, dizziness, and drowsiness. Coma, convulsions, and cardiac arrest occur frequently in acute poisoning. A male adult survived the inges-

tion of 5 g of drug with supportive treatment; his peak serum orphenadrine level of 3.1 mg/L occurred 16 hours post-ingestion (Furlanut et al., 1985). An 18 month old child accidentally ingested the drug and became comatose; 30 hours later he had orphenadrine concentrations of 4 mg/L in blood and 100 mg/L in urine. The child died 36 hours after ingestion (Bozza-Marrubini et al., 1977). One person has recovered after the ingestion of 7500 mg of the drug, whereas another adult expired following a dose of 1000 mg (Heinonen et al., 1968).

Robinson et al. (1977) reported on a large series of orphenadrine-related fatalities in which blood concentrations in the acute cases ranged from 5.5–37 mg/L and urine concentrations from 3–324 mg/L. Another 8 cases have shown the following postmortem concentrations (Koumides, 1968; Clarke, 1969; Blomquist et al., 1971; Som, 1974; De Mercurio et al., 1979; Wilkinson et al., 1983):

Orphenadrine Concentrations in Fatal Cases (mg/L or mg/kg)

	Blood	Liver	Urine	Gastric
Average	20	144	41	694 mg
(Range)	(4–75)	(8–410)	(7–91)	(40–1452)

Analysis. Orphenadrine may be assayed in biologic media by ultraviolet spectrophotometry, making use of the absorption maximum at 264 nm. A more sensitive and specific method is gas chromatography, with either flame-ionization (Robinson et al., 1977) or nitrogen-selective detection (Bilzer and Gundert-Remy, 1973; Labout et al., 1977; Wilkinson et al., 1983). The deaminated metabolite of orphenadrine has been analyzed in serum by flame-ionization gas chromatography (Huisman et al., 1979).

References

A.H. Beckett and F. Khan. Metabolism, distribution and excretion of orphenadrine in man. J. Pharm. Pharmac. 23 (Suppl.): 222, 1971.

W. Bilzer and U. Gundert-Remy. Determination of nanogram quantities of diphenhydramine and orphenadrine in human plasma using gas-liquid chromatography. Eur. J. Clin. Pharm. 6: 268–270, 1973.

M. Blomquist, R. Bonnichsen and B. Schubert. Lethal orphenadrine intoxication. Z. Rechtsmed. 68: 111–114, 1971.

M. Bozza-Marrubini, A. Frigerio, R. Ghezzi et al. Two cases of severe orphenadrine poisoning with atypical features. Acta Pharm. Tox. 41: (Suppl. 2): 137–152, 1977.

E.G.C. Clarke. *Isolation and Identification of Drugs*, Pharmaceutical Press, London, 1969, p. 456.

D. De Mercurio, M. Chiarotti and G.V. Giusti. Lethal orphenadrine intoxication: report of a case. Z. Rechtsmed. 82: 349–353, 1979.

W. den Besten, D. Mulder, A.B.H. Funcke and W.T. Nauta. The effect of alkyl substitution in drugs. Arz. Forsch. 20: 538–542, 1970.

T. Ellison, A. Snyder, J. Bolger and R. Okun. Metabolism of orphenadrine citrate in man. J. Pharm. Exp. Ther. 176: 284–295 1971.

M. Furlanut, D. Bettio, I. Bertin et al. Orphenadrine serum levels in a poisoned patient. Hum. Tox. 4: 331–333, 1985.

J. Heinonen, J. Heikkila, M.J. Mattila and S. Takki. Orphenadrine poisoning. Arch. Tox. 23: 264–272, 1968.

J. Huisman, L.L. Liebregt and J.H.H. Thyssen. Gas chromatographic determination of (o-methyl-α-phenylbenzyloxy)acetic acid levels in human serum following therapeutic doses of orphenadrin (Disipal). J. Chrom. 164: 510–514, 1979.

O. Koumides. Personal communication, 1968.

J.J.M. Labout, C.T. Thijssen and W. Hespe. Sensitive and specific gas chromatographic and extraction method for the determination of orphenadrine in human body fluids. J. Chrom. 144: 201–208, 1977.

J.J.M. Labout, C.T. Thijssen, G.G.J. Keijser and W. Hespe. Difference between single and multiple dose pharmacokinetics of orphenadrine hydrochloride in man. Eur. J. Clin. Pharm. 21: 343–350, 1982.

S. Loga, S. Curry and M. Lader. Interactions of orphenadrine and phenobarbitone with chlorpromazine: plasma concentrations and effects in man. Brit. J. Clin. Pharm. 2: 197–208, 1975.

A.E. Robinson, A.T. Holder, R.D. McDowell et al. Forensic toxicology of some orphenadrine-related deaths. For. Sci. 9: 53–62, 1977.

S. Som. Personal communication, 1974.

L.F. Wilkinson, B.M. Thomson and L.K. Pannell. A report on the analysis of orphenadrine in post mortem specimens. J. Anal. Tox. 7: 72–74, 1983.

Oxalate

T½: ?
Vd: ?
Fb: 0
pKa: 1.2, 4.2

⁻OOCCOO⁻

Occurrence and Usage. Oxalic acid and oxalate salts may be encountered in industry and at home as cleaning and bleaching agents. Oxalate is also present in relatively high concentrations in certain dietary plants, including spinach, rhubarb and tea. Ingestion of the compound produces local corrosive and irritant effects as well as hypocalcemia, due to the precipitation of calcium. Use is made of this latter property when oxalate is added to blood specimens as an anticoagulant. Oxalate is produced *in vivo* following the ingestion of ethylene glycol. The current threshold limit value for oxalic acid in the industrial atmosphere is 1 mg/m³.

Blood Concentrations. Serum oxalate concentrations in 20 normal subjects were found to average 1.4 mg/L using a specific gas chromatographic procedure; a value of 2.4 mg/L was considered the upper limit for normal serum oxalate (Nuret and Offner, 1978). There is little or no binding of oxalic acid by plasma proteins at physiologic pH, and whole blood oxalate concentrations are only slightly higher (average, 1.7 mg/L) than plasma concentrations. Oxalate concentrations have not been measured in the blood of exposed workers.

Metabolism and Excretion. There is no evidence that oxalate is utilized or further metabolized by human tissues; up to 99% of an intravenously injected radiolabeled dose is excreted in the urine after 36 hours. Only 2–5% of ingested oxalic acid is absorbed in normal adults. Urinary oxalic acid, which usually ranges from 8–40 mg/day, is derived largely from dietary ascorbic acid (35–44%), from the metabolism of glycine (40%), and the remainder from minor metabolic sources and from dietary oxalic acid. Calcium oxalate is a major constituent of urinary calculi and also often occurs as crystals in freshly voided urine (Hodgkinson and Zarembski, 1968). Patients with hyperoxaluria due to increased gastrointestinal absorption of dietary oxalate excrete from 95–380 mg/day in the urine (Stauffer, 1960). Normal tissue concentrations, determined on single specimens, are 0.6 mg/kg in brain, 2.3 mg/kg in liver and 4.0 mg/kg in kidney (Hodgkinson and Zarembski, 1968).

Toxicity. External contact with oxalic acid may cause eye and skin irritation. Systemic oxalate poisoning is characterized by local corrosive effects, renal damage and a marked fall in plasma calcium levels, with resulting shock, collapse and convulsions. By oral ingestion, the mean adult lethal dose is probably 15–30 g, although the intravenous injection of only 1.2 g of sodium oxalate caused the death of a 16 year old girl (Dvorackova, 1966). A number of childhood poisonings have occurred following the ingestion of rhubarb leaves (rather than the stalks), which contain up to 1% oxalic acid; at least 2 deaths resulted (Tallqvist and Vaananen, 1960; Kalliala and Kauste, 1964). One case of poisoning due to chronic occupational exposure to oxalic acid fumes was reported in which the predominant symptoms were severe headache, vomiting, lower back pain, loss of weight, anemia and extreme exhaustion (Howard, 1932).

Following the ingestion of potassium hydrogen oxalate by 4 women, the plasma oxalate concentration at 6 hours in the one survivor was 3.7 mg/L, while those of the 3 who died ranged from 18–

110 mg/L (average, 68). Analysis of postmortem specimens from one of these victims showed the following distribution (Zarembski and Hodgkinson, 1967):

Oxalate Concentrations in a Fatal Case (mg/L or mg/kg)

Plasma	Brain	Liver	Gastric
110	21	382	2250

Analysis. Oxalic acid may be determined in biological fluids by enzyme analysis (Hatch et al., 1977; Yriberri and Posen, 1980; Buttery et al., 1983), complexometric titration (Giterson et al., 1970), colorimetry (Hodgkinson and Williams, 1972; Eswara Dutt and Mottola, 1974; Husdan et al., 1976; Sample et al., 1980), fluorimetry (Zarembski and Hodgkinson, 1965), indirect atomic absorption spectrometry (Fraser and Campbell, 1972), gas chromatography of ester derivatives (Mee and Stanley, 1973; Nuret and Offner, 1978; Farrington and Chalmers, 1979; Park and Gregory, 1980; Moye et al., 1981; DeCorcia et al., 1982), and liquid chromatography (Mayer et al., 1979; Libert, 1981). Procedures for the isolation of oxalate from solid tissues have been described (Rieders and Frere, 1963; Zarembski and Hodgkinson, 1967).

References

J.E. Buttery, N. Ludvigsen, E.A. Braiotta and P.R. Pannall. Determination of urinary oxalate with commercially available oxalate oxidase. Clin. Chem. 29: 700–702, 1983.

A. DiCorcin, R. Samperi, G. Vinci and G. D'Ascenzo. Simple, reliable chromatographic measurement of oxalate in urine. Clin. Chem. 28: 1457–1460, 1982.

I. Dvorackova. Toedliche Vergiftung nach intravenoeser Verabreichung von Natriumoxalat. Arch. Tox. 22: 63–67, 1966.

V.V.S. Eswara Dutt and H.A. Mottola. Detection and initial rate determination of oxalic acid at the microgram level. Biochem. Med. 9: 148–157, 1974.

C.J. Farrington and A.H. Chalmers. Gas-chromatographic estimation of urinary oxalate and its comparison with a colorimetric method. Clin. Chem. 25: 1993–1996, 1979.

J. Fraser and D.J. Campbell. Indirect measure of oxalic acid in urine by atomic absorption spectrophotometry. Clin. Biochem. 5: 99–103, 1972.

A.L. Giterson, P.A.M. Slooff and H. Schouten. Oxalate in urine. Clin. Chim. Acta 29: 342–343, 1970.

M. Hatch, E. Bourke and J. Costello. New enzymic method for serum oxalate determination. Clin. Chem. 23: 76–78, 1977.

A. Hodgkinson and P.M. Zarembski. Oxalic acid metabolism in man: a review. Calc. Tiss. Res. 2: 115–132, 1968.

A. Hodgkinson and A. Williams. An improved colorimetric procedure for urine oxalate. Clin. Chim. Acta 36: 127–132, 1972.

C.D. Howard. Chronic poisoning by oxalic acid: with report of a case and results of a study concerning the volatilization of oxalic acid from aqueous solution. J. Ind. Hyg. 14: 283–290, 1932.

H. Husdan, M. Leung, D. Oreopoulos and A. Rapport. Modified method for urinary oxalate. Clin. Chem. 22: 1538, 1976.

H. Kalliala and O. Kauste. Ingestion of rhubarb leaves as cause of oxalic acid poisoning. Ann. Paed. Fenn. 10: 228–231, 1964.

B. Libert. Rapid determination of oxalic acid by reversed-phase high-performance liquid chromatography. J. Chrom. 210: 540–543, 1981.

W.J. Mayer, J.P. McCarthy and M.S. Greenberg. The determination of oxalic acid in urine by high performance liquid chromatography with electrochemical detection. J. Chrom. Sci. 17: 656–660, 1979.

J.M.L. Mee and R.W. Stanley. A rapid gas-liquid chromatographic method for determining oxalic acid in biological materials. J. Chrom. 76: 242–243, 1973.

H.A. Moye, M.H. Malagodi, D.H. Clarke and C.J. Miles. A rapid gas chromatographic procedure for the analysis of oxalate ion in urine. Clin. Chim. Acta 114: 173–185, 1981.

P. Nuret and M. Offner. A new method for determination of oxalate in blood serum by gas chromatography. Clin. Chim. Acta 82: 9–12, 1978.

K.Y. Park and J. Gregory. Gas-chromatographic determination of urinary oxalate. Clin. Chem. 26: 1170–1172, 1980.

F. Rieders and F.J. Frere. Detection and estimation of toxicologically significant amounts of borate, chlorate and oxalate in biologic material. J. For. Sci. 8: 46–53, 1963.

R.H.B. Sample, M.E. Farber and M.R. Glick. Urinary oxalate indirectly determined by continuous-flow analysis for calcium. Clin. Chem. 26: 1105, 1980.

M. Stauffer. Oxalosis. New Eng. J. Med. 263: 386–390, 1960.

H. Tallqvist and I. Vaananen. Death of a child from oxalic acid poisoning due to eating rhubarb leaves. Ann. Paed. Fenn. 6: 144–147, 1960.

J. Yriberri and S. Posen. A semi-automatic enzymic method for estimating urinary oxalate. Clin. Chem. 26: 881–884, 1980.

P.M. Zarembski and A. Hodgkinson. The fluorimetric determination of oxalic acid in blood and other biological materials. Biochem. J. 96: 717–721, 1965.

P.M. Zarembski and A. Hodgkinson. Plasma oxalic acid and calcium levels in oxalate poisoning. J. Clin. Path. 20: 283–285, 1967.

Oxazepam

T½: 4–11 hr
Vd: 0.7–1.6 L/kg
Fb: 0.87–0.94
pKa: 1.7, 11.6

Occurrence and Usage. Oxazepam (Serax) is the 3-hydroxy metabolite of nordiazepam, and has been used in the United States as an antianxiety agent since 1965. It is available as tablets or capsules containing 10–30 mg of the free base and is administered orally in doses of 30–60 mg, being somewhat less potent than diazepam and nordiazepam.

Blood Concentrations. An average maximal serum concentration of 0.31 mg/L was reached 1.5 hours after a single 15 mg oral dose of oxazepam (Wretlind et al., 1977). Following a single oral dose of 45 mg, an average peak serum concentration of 1.06 mg/L (range, 0.88–1.44) was observed at 2 hours, with a decline to 0.37 mg/L (range, 0.18–0.60) by 8 hours; no accumulation of oxazepam in serum was evident during chronic dosing (Knowles and Ruelius, 1982). The plasma half-life was found to average 5–6 hours regardless of age or liver disease. The blood/plasma concentration ratio of oxazepam is 1.0 (Shull et al., 1976).

Metabolism and Excretion. Oxazepam is rapidly conjugated with glucuronic acid and excreted in the urine. Oxazepam glucuronide, an inactive metabolite, is found to a limited extent in serum, and accounts for 61% of an oral dose in the 48 hour urine. Only trace amounts of free oxazepam are found in urine, and other products of hydroxylation account for less than 5% of a dose (Knowles and Ruelius, 1972).

Toxicity. Fourteen individuals arrested for impaired driving ability had blood oxazepam concentrations of 0.2–8.0 mg/L (average, 2.4) as the only drug-related finding (McLinden, 1987). One case of oxazepam overdosage has been described in which a 2 year old girl ingested 90 mg of the drug; 18 hours after ingestion the serum oxazepam concentration was 0.5 mg/L, at which time the patient was lethargic. The urine concentrations of oxazepam and its glucuronide were 1.3 and 19.5 mg/L, respectively; recovery was slow, but uneventful (Shimkin and Shaivitz, 1966). An adult ingested a large amount of oxazepam and became deeply comatose for several days, but survived with supportive treatment (Zileli et al., 1971).

Analysis. Oxazepam has been analyzed using colorimetry after acid hydrolysis (Walkenstein et al., 1964). Acid hydrolysis has also been employed in the electron-capture gas chromatographic determination of the drug (Knowles and Ruelius, 1972); analysis of the intact drug in the same manner results in thermal dehydration of oxazepam, with some loss of reproducibility and sensitivity (deSilva et al., 1976; Giles et al., 1978). To prevent this, a dimethyl derivative has been prepared for gas chromatography (Vessman et al., 1977; Langner et al., 1991) or, alternatively, liquid chromatography may be employed (Kabra et al., 1978; Moore and Oliver, 1988).

References

J.A.F. deSilva, I. Bekersky, C.V. Puglisi et al. Determination of 1,4-benzodiazepines and -diazepin-2-ones in blood by elecron-capture gas-liquid chromatography. Anal. Chem. 48: 10–19, 1976.

H.G. Giles, T. Fan, C.A. Naranjo and E.M. Sellers. A simple electron-capture gas-chromatographic analysis of oxazepam in plasma by determination of its thermal degradation product. Can. J. Pharm. Sci. 13: 64–65, 1978.

P.M. Kabra, G.L. Stevens and L.J. Marton. High-pressure liquid chromatographic analysis of diazepam, oxazepam and N-desmethyldiazepam in human blood. J. Chrom. 150: 355–360, 1978.

J.A. Knowles and H.W. Ruelius. Absorption and excretion of 7-chloro-1,3-dihydro-3-hydroxy-5-phenyl-^{2}H-1,4-benzodiazepin-2-one(oxazepam) in humans. Arz. Forsch. 22: 687–692, 1972.

J.G. Langner, B.K. Gan, R.H. Liu et al. Enzymatic digestion, solid-phase extraction, and gas chromatography/mass spectrometry of derivatized intact oxazepam in urine. Clin. Chem. 37: 1595–1601, 1991.

V.J. McLinden. Experiences in relation to drugs/driving offences. J. For. Sci. Soc. 27: 73–80, 1987.

C.M. Moore and J.S. Oliver. Rapid extraction of oxazepam from greyhound urine for hplc analysis. For. Sci. Int. 38: 237–241, 1988.

P.M. Shimkin and S.A. Shaivitz. Oxazepam poisoning in a child. J. Am. Med. Asso. 196: 662–663, 1966.

H.J. Shull, Jr., G.R. Wilkinson, R. Johnson and S. Schenker. Normal disposition of oxazepam in acute viral hepatitis and cirrhosis. Ann. Int. Med. 84: 420–425, 1976.

J. Vessman, M. Johansson, P. Magnusson and S. Stromberg. Determination of intact oxazepam by electron capture gas chromatography after an extractive alkylation reaction. Anal. Chem. 49: 1545–1549, 1977.

S.S. Walkenstein, R. Wiser and C.H. Gudmundsen. Absorption, metabolism and excretion of oxazepam and its succinate half-ester. J. Pharm. Sci. 53: 1181–1186, 1964.

M. Wretlind, A. Pilbrandt, A. Sundwall and J. Vessman. Disposition of three benzodiazepines after single oral administration in man. Acta Pharm. Tox. 40: 28–39, 1977.

M.S. Zileli, F. Teletar, S. Deniz et al. Oxazepam intoxication simulating non-keto-acidotic diabetic coma. J. Am. Med. Asso. 215: 1986, 1971.

Oxprenolol

T½: 2–3 hr
Vd: 1.5 L/kg
Fb: 0.78
pKa: 9.5

$OCH_2CH=CH_2$
$OCH_2CHOHCH_2NHCH(CH_3)_2$

Occurrence and Usage. Oxprenolol (Trasicor) is a beta-adrenergic blocking agent synthesized in 1966 and now used as an antihypertensive and antiarrhythmic drug in many countries other than the United States. It is administered orally as the hydrochloride in doses of 80–160 mg daily, or by intravenous injection of 10–20 mg.

Blood Concentrations. Plasma concentrations of the drug after oral administration of 20 mg to 5 subjects reached an average peak of 0.173 mg/L at 0.5 hours and declined to 0.071 mg/L by 2 hours; after an oral dose of 160 mg, plasma concentrations peaked at 0.708 mg/L at 1 hour and declined to 0.063 mg/L after 8 hours. The intravenous infusion of 10 and 20 mg of oxprenolol over a 10 minute period produced average maximal plasma levels of 0.268 and 0.528 mg/L, respectively at the end of infusion; concentrations diminished thereafter with an average elimination half-life of 2.3 hours (Mason and Winer, 1976).

Metabolism and Excretion. Oxprenolol is readily conjugated with glucuronic acid at the side-chain hydroxyl, and the level of this conjugate greatly surpasses the concentration of the parent drug in plasma after oral administration. From 70–95% of a dose is eliminated in the 24 hour urine largely as the glucuronide (Riess et al., 1970). Products of N- and O-dealkylation and ring hydroxylation have been identified as metabolites in animals, but have not yet been detected in man (Garteiz, 1971).

Toxicity. Adverse reactions to the drug include nausea, vomiting, weakness, hypotension, bradycardia, congestive heart failure and bronchospasm. Thrombocytopenia has been associated with the therapeutic usage of oxprenolol.

A fatal case of oxprenolol poisoning in an adult was reported in which a liver concentration of 58 mg/kg was determined (Oliver and Watson, 1977). Postmortem concentrations of 6 mg/L in blood and 27 mg/kg in liver were found in an overdose case that also involved digoxin (Ryall, 1978). The following concentrations were observed in the death of a woman who ingested 4.5 g of the drug and died in coma within 2 hours (Khan and Muscat-Baron, 1977):

Oxprenolol Concentrations in a Fatal Case (mg/L or mg/kg)

Blood	Brain	Liver	Gastric
10	71	230	1050 mg

Analysis. Oxprenolol has been determined in biological specimens by ultraviolet spectrophotometry (Oliver and Watson, 1977) and by electron-capture gas chromatography of a halogenated derivative (Walle, 1974; Degen and Riess, 1976; Sioufi et al., 1983). Direct fluorometry of thin-layer chromatograms has also been used (Schaefer and Mutschler, 1979), and liquid chromatographic methods have been described (Tsuei et al., 1980; Godbillon et al., 1985).

References

P.H. Degen and W. Riess. Simplified method for the determination of oxprenolol and other β–receptor blocking agents in biological fluids by gas-liquid chromatography. J. Chrom. 121: 72–75, 1976.

D.A. Garteiz. Metabolism of a *beta* blocking drug, oxprenolol. J. Pharm. Exp. Ther. 179: 354–358, 1971.

J. Godbillon, M. Duval and G. Gosset. Determination of oxprenolol in human plasma by high-performance liquid chromatography, in comparison with gas chromatography and gas chromatography-mass spectrometry. J. Chrom. 345: 365-371, 1985.

D.L. Hare and B.H. Hicks. Thrombocytopemia due to oxprenolol. Med. J. Aust. 2: 259, 1979.

A. Khan and J.M. Muscat-Baron. Fatal oxprenolol poisoning. Brit. Med. J. 1: 552, 1977.

W.D. Mason and N. Winer. Pharmacokinetics of oxprenolol in normal subjects. Clin. Pharm. Ther. 20: 401–412, 1976.

J.S. Oliver and A.A. Watson. Oxprenolol (Trasicor) poisoning. Med. Sci. Law 17: 279–281, 1977.

W. Reiss, T.G. Rajagopalan, P. Imhof et al. Metabolic studies on oxprenolol in animals and man by means of radio-tracer techniques and GLC-analysis. Postgrad. Med. J. 46 (Nov. Suppl.): 32–39, 1970.

J.E. Ryall. Personal communication, 1978.

M. Schaefer and E. Mutschler. Fluorimetric determination of oxprenolol in plasma by direct evaluation of thin-layer chromatograms. J. Chrom. 164: 247–252, 1979.

A. Sioufi, D. Colussi and P. Mangoni. Gas chromatographic determination of oxprenolol in human plasma. J. Chrom. 278: 185–188, 1983.

S.E. Tsuei, J. Thomas and R.G. Moore. Quantification of oxprenolol in biological fluids using high-performance liquid chromatography. J. Chrom. 181: 135–140, 1980.

T. Walle. GLC determination of propranolol, other β–blocking drugs, and metabolites in biological fluids and tissues. J. Pharm. Sci. 63: 1885–1891, 1974.

Oxycodone

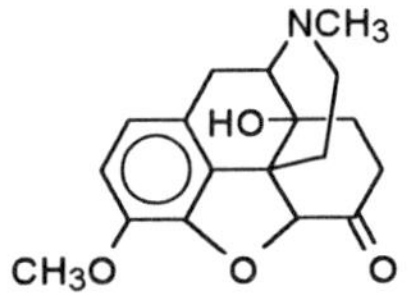

T½: 4–6 hr
Vd: 1.8–3.7 L/kg
Fb: ?
pKa: 8.5

Occurrence and Usage. Oxycodone (ingredient of Percodan, Percocet, Roxicet and Tylox) is a semisynthetic narcotic analgesic, derived from thebaine, that is available in oral formulations often in combination with other drugs such as acetaminophen, aspirin, phenacetin and caffeine. The usual adult dose is 2.5–5 mg as the hydrochloride or terephthalate salt every 6 hours. Given subcutaneously, the drug is approximately equipotent with morphine, but it has a higher oral/parenteral efficacy ratio.

Blood Concentrations. Plasma oxycodone concentrations in 6 subjects following the oral administration of 4.5 mg of the hydrochloride plus 0.38 mg of the terephthalate averaged 0.018 mg/L (range, 0.009–0.037) at 1 hour, 0.016 mg/L at 2 hours, 0.009 mg/L at 4 hours, and 0.005 mg/L at 8 hours (Renzi and Tam, 1979). Peak plasma concentrations in 12 patients receiving a 10 mg oral dose averaged 0.030 mg/L (range, 0.013–0.046) at 0.8–2.5 hours post-dose (Leow et al., 1992). Peak plasma concentrations in 9 volunteers receiving an unusually large 0.28 mg/kg (20 mg/70 kg) oral dose averaged 0.038 mg/L at an average time of 1.0 hours; the elimination half-life averaged 5.1 hours in these subjects (Poyhia et al., 1992).

Metabolism and Excretion. Oxycodone is known to be metabolized by N- and O-demethylation. One of the metabolites, oxymorphone, is a potent narcotic analgesic, while the other, noroxycodone, is relatively inactive. From 33–61% of a single dose of oxycodone is excreted in the 24 hour urine as free (13–19%) and conjugated oxycodone (7–29%), conjugated oxymorphone (13–14%), and an unknown amount of noroxycodone.

Free oxycodone concentrations in urine after a single 5 mg oral dose generally do not exceed 1 mg/L. Urine concentrations of free oxycodone and noroxycodone in a patient taking 700 mg (!) of oxycodone daily were 13 and 18 mg/L, respectively (Baselt and Stewart, 1978; Weinstein and Gaylord, 1979).

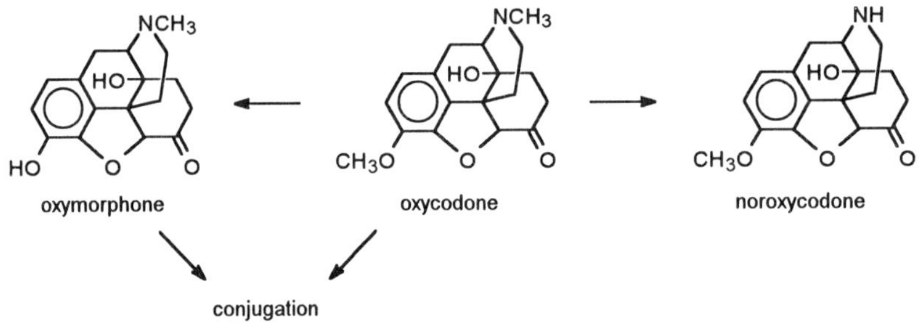

oxymorphone   oxycodone   noroxycodone

conjugation

Toxicity. Oxycodone is capable of producing stupor, coma, muscle flaccidity, severe respiratory depression, hypotension, and cardiac arrest in overdosage. Naloxone is a specific antidote.

Three deaths have been reported involving acute ingestion of oxycodone overdoses by adults who exhibited postmortem blood concentrations of 0.4–0.7 mg/L, but each of these cases involved at least 1 other depressant drug (Baselt, 1993; Drummer, 1993). Two adult suicides by oxycodone overdosage were investigated in which postmortem drug concentrations of 4.3 and 14 mg/L in blood and 22 and 63 mg/kg in liver were observed (Cravey, 1985). The following tissue distribution of oxycodone was reported by Sedgwick (1973) in the case of a man who died while scuba-diving and who presumably had taken a large amount of the drug as a suicidal gesture:

Distribution of Oxycodone in a Fatal Case (mg/L or mg/kg)

Blood	Brain	Liver	Bile	Gastric
5	28	12	28	1.4 mg

Analysis. The reported procedures for determination of oxycodone and its metabolites in plasma or urine have utilized gas chromatography with electron-capture detection of heptafluorobutyryl derivatives (Baselt and Stewart, 1978; Weinstein and Gaylord, 1979) or nitrogen-phosphorus detection (Renzi and Tam, 1979; Kapil et al., 1992). Liquid chromatography has also been described (Schneider et al., 1984; Smith et al., 1991). Other methods applicable to narcotic analgesics in general are cited in the section on heroin.

References

R.C. Baselt and C.B. Stewart. Determination of oxycodone and a major metabolite in urine by electron-capture GLC. J. Anal. Tox. 2: 107–109, 1978.

R.C. Baselt. Unpublished results, 1985.

R.H. Cravey. Unpublished results, 1985.

O.H. Drummer. Unpublished results, 1993.

R.P. Kapil, P.K. Padovani, S.Y.P. King and G.N. Lam. Nanogram level quantitation of oxycodone in human plasma by capillary gas chromatography using nitrogen-phosphorus selective detection. J. Chrom. 577: 283–288, 1992.

K.P. Leow, M.T. Smith, J.A. Watt et al. Comparative oxycodone pharmacokinetics in humans after intravenous, oral and rectal administration. Ther. Drug Mon. 14: 479–484, 1992.

R. Poyhia, T. Seppala, K.T. Olkkola and E. Kalso. The pharmacokinetics and metabolism of oxycodone after intramuscular and oral administration to healthy subjects. Brit. J. Clin. Pharm. 33: 617–621, 1992.

N.L. Renzi, Jr. and J.N. Tam. Quantitative GLC determination of oxycodone in human plasma. J. Pharm. Sci. 68: 43–45, 1979.

J.J. Schneider, E.J. Triggs, D.A. Bourne et al. Determination of oxycodone in human plasma by high-performance liquid chromatography with electrochemical detection. J. Chrom. 308: 359–362, 1984.

P. Sedgwick. Personal communication, 1973.

M.T. Smith, J.A. Watt, G.P. Mapp and T. Cramond. Quantitation of oxycodone in human plasma using high-performance liquid chromatography with electrochemical detection. Ther. Drug Mon. 13: 126–130, 1991.

S.H. Weinstein and J.C. Gaylord. Determination of oxycodone in plasma and identification of a major metabolite. J. Pharm. Sci. 68: 527–528, 1979.

Oxymorphone

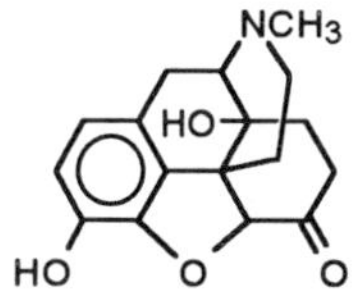

T½: ?
Vd: ?
Fb: ?
pKa: 8.5, 9.3

Occurrence and Usage. Oxymorphone (Numorphan) is a semisynthetic narcotic analgesic derived from thebaine. It is used for the relief of moderate to severe pain and for pre-operative medication. The drug is available in ampules containing 1.0 or 1.5 mg/mL as the hydrochloride for subcutaneous or intramuscular administration and in suppositories containing 5 mg. Oxymorphone is also a metabolite of oxycodone.

Blood Concentrations. Blood concentrations have not been reported in man following therapeutic administration of oxymorphone.

Metabolism and Excretion. Oxymorphone is extensively metabolized, principally by reduction and conjugation. Approximately 49% of an oral dose is eliminated in the 120 hour urine as parent drug (1.9%), conjugated oxymorphone (44%), free and conjugated 6β–oxymorphol (2.9%), and conjugated 6α–oxymorphol (0.1%) (Cone et al., 1983).

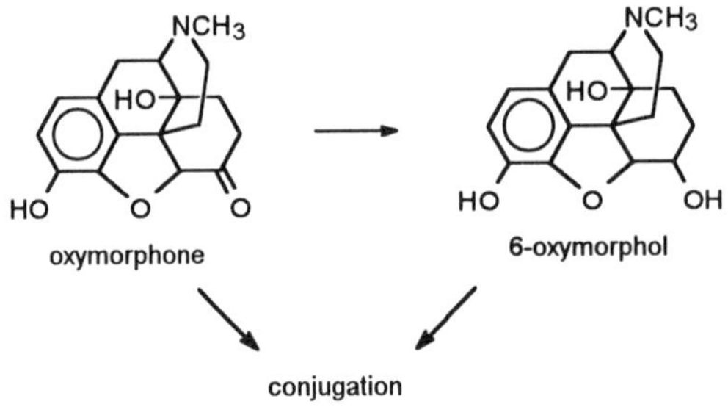

oxymorphone   6-oxymorphol

conjugation

Toxicity. In overdosage, oxymorphone causes hypotension, bradycardia, apnea, coma, circulatory collapse, and cardiac arrest.

Analysis. Oxymorphone has been determined in biological specimens by gas chromatography with electron-capture detection (Baselt and Stewart, 1978), gas chromatography-mass spectrometry (Cone et al., 1983) and liquid chromatography with electrochemical detection (Lam et al., 1987).

References

R.C. Baselt and C.B. Stewart. Determination of oxycodone and a major metabolite in urine by electron-capture GLC. J. Anal. Tox. 2: 107–109, 1978.

E.J. Cone, W.D. Darwin, W.F. Buchwald et al. Oxymorphone metabolism and urinary excretion in human, rat, guinea pig, rabbit, and dog. Drug Met. Disp. 11; 446–450, 1983.

G. Lam, R.M. Williams and C.C. Whitney. Electrochemical determination of oxymorphone in rat plasma by ion-pair reversed-phase high-performance liquid chromatography. J. Chrom. 413: 309–314, 1987.

Oxyphenbutazone

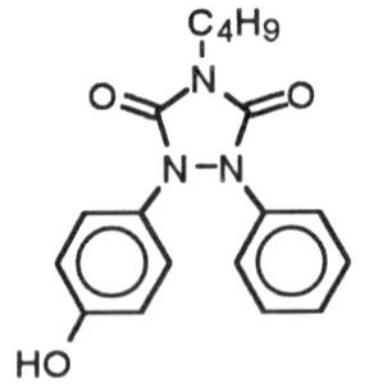

T½: 48–72 hr
Vd: 0.14 L/kg
Fb: 0.99
pKa: 4.7

Occurrence and Usage. Oxyphenbutazone (p-hydroxyphenylbutazone, Oxalid, Tandearil) was recognized as a pharmacologically active metabolite of phenylbutazone in 1955 and has since been used as an anti-inflammatory agent in man. It is available in 100 mg tablets as the free acid and is administered orally in daily doses of 100–600 mg.

Blood Concentrations. Ten normal volunteers administered a single oral 200 mg dose achieved peak plasma concentrations ranging from 11–44 mg/L at 2–12 hours after ingestion. At 4 hours, concentrations averaged about 18 mg/L, declining thereafter to about 11 mg/L by 72 hours (Bertrand et al., 1979). Plasma concentrations of the drug after intravenous administration of 600 mg were initially as high as 70 mg/L and declined to about 25 mg/L after 4 days; at these concentrations oxyphenbutazone exhibits 99% binding to plasma proteins (Perel et al., 1964). Plasma concentrations of persons on chronic oral therapy with 300–400 mg daily, when measured prior to the morning dose, ranged from 27–118 mg/L (Weiner et al., 1967). The plasma half-life of this compound has been estimated at 48–72 hours (Burns et al., 1955; Gutman et al, 1960).

Metabolism and Excretion. Oxyphenbutazone is known to be metabolized by glucuronide conjugation. Less than 2% of a dose is excreted unchanged in the 24 hour urine (Gutman et al., 1960), and 1–5% as the glucuronide. Up to 25% of a dose may eventually be eliminated in the conjugated form. The drug may also undergo hydroxylation of the n-butyl side chain in a manner analogous to that of phenylbutazone (Perel et al., 1964).

Toxicity. Oxyphenbutazone has been linked to serious toxic reactions that include gastrointestinal ulceration, dermatitis, blood dyscrasias, hepatitis and renal failure.

Analysis. Oxyphenbutazone may be determined in biologic fluids by ultraviolet spectrophotometric measurement of the absorption maximum at 225 nm, after ethylene dichloride extraction from aqueous acid solution (Burns et al., 1955). A flame-ionization gas chromatographic procedure involving formation on a methyl derivative has been described (Midha et al., 1974), as well as one utilizing nitrogen-selective detection of a trifluoroacetyl derivative (Bertrand et al., 1979). Liquid chromatography has also been employed (Sioufi et al., 1983).

References

M. Bertrand, C. Dupuis, M.A. Gagnon and R. Dugal. Quantitative determination of plasma oxyphenbutazone by gas-liquid chromatography with selective nitrogen detection. J. Chrom. 171: 377–383, 1979.

J.J. Burns, R.K. Rose, S. Goodwin et al. The metabolic fate of phenylbutazone (Butazolidin) in man. J. Pharm. Exp. Ther. 113: 481–489, 1955.

A.B. Gutman, P.G. Dayton, T.F. Yu et al. A study of the inverse relationship between pKa and rate of renal excretion of phenylbutazone analogs in man and dog. Am. J. Med. 29: 1017–1033, 1960.

K.K. Midha, I.J. McGilveray and C. Charette. GLC determination of plasma concentration of phenylbutazone and its metabolite oxyphenbutazone. J. Pharm. Sci. 63: 1234–1239, 1974.

J.M. Perel, M.M. Snell, W. Chen and P.G. Dayton. A study of structure activity relationships in regard to species difference in the phenylbutazone series. Biochem. Pharm. 13: 1305–1317, 1964.

A. Sioufi, D. Colussi and P. Mangoni. Determination of oxyphenbutazone in human plasma by hplc. J. Chrom. 275: 201–205, 1983.

M. Weiner, A.A. Siddiqui, R.T. Shahani and P.G. Dayton. Effect of steroids on disposition of oxyphenbutazone in man. Proc. Soc. Exp. Biol. Med. 124: 1170–1173, 1967.

Pancuronium

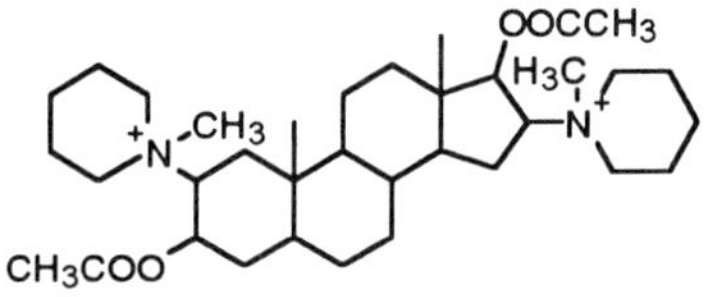

T½: 1.9–2.2 hr
Vd: 0.28 L/kg
Fb: 0.87

Occurrence and Usage. Pancuronium (Pavulon) is a quaternary ammonium derivative that was synthesized in 1964 as a neuromuscular blocking agent. It is a non-depolarizing agent used as an alternative to d-tubocurarine. The compound is supplied in ampules as the dibromide, for intravenous administration in doses of 0.04–0.10 mg/kg (2.8–7.0 mg/70 kg).

Blood Concentrations. Following the intravenous injection of 6 mg, plasma pancuronium concentrations are initially between 1 and 2 mg/L, but decline rapidly with a distribution half-life of 12.5 minutes and an elimination half-life of 2 hours. Recovery (99% paralysis) was first evident when the mean plasma level was 0.218 mg/L, 30–60 minutes after injection. An 80% paralysis was noted at a mean concentration of 0.169 mg/L at about 1 hour (Somogyi et al., 1976), and 50% block was present at an average level of 0.09 mg/L after about 2 hours (Agoston et al., 1977). Both the half-life and volume of distribution of pancuronium are, on average, doubled in patients with renal failure or liver cirrhosis, due possibly to inhibition of plasma protein binding of the drug (Somogyi et al., 1977a; Duvaldestin et al., 1978).

Metabolism and Excretion. Pancuronium is metabolized by deacetylation at the 3-position to a 3-hydroxy derivative, which is 2–6 times less active than the parent (Agoston et al., 1977). Within 30 hours of a single administration, about 40% of the dose is eliminated in urine as unchanged drug (25%) and the metabolite (15%). An additional 11% of a dose is excreted in bile during this period (Agoston et al., 1973). About 5% of a dose is represented by 2 relatively inactive urinary metabolites, 17-hydroxypancuronium and 3,17-dihydroxypancuronium (Buzello, 1975; Somogyi et al., 1977b; Miller et al., 1978).

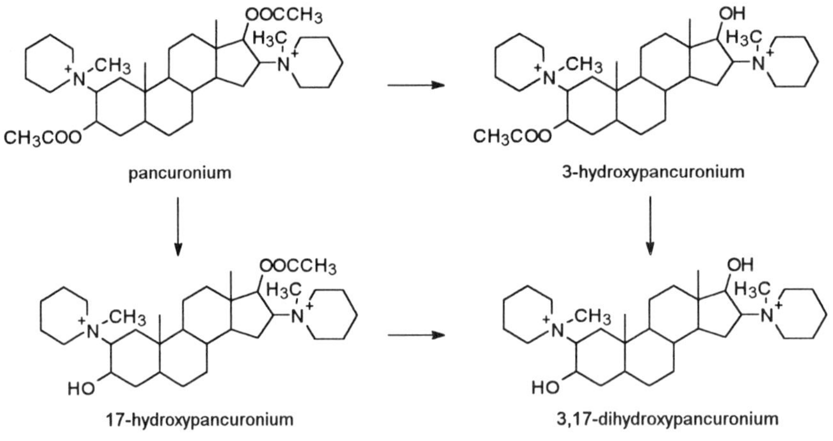

pancuronium

3-hydroxypancuronium

17-hydroxypancuronium

3,17-dihydroxypancuronium

Toxicity. Pancuronium toxicity is often treated by the administration of neostigmine, to reverse the neuromuscular blockade, and atropine, to minimize the cholinergic side effects that neostigmine causes.

A medical resident who committed suicide by intravenous injection of 10 mg of pancuronium exhibited postmortem blood and urine concentrations of 1.6 and 1.5 mg/L, respectively (Poklis and Melanson, 1980).

Analysis. A fluorescence dye technique has been used successfully to measure pancuronium and its hydroxy-metabolite in biologic fluids and tissues, with qualitative confirmation by thin-layer chromatography (Kersten et al., 1973). This procedure has been modified to enhance stability of the fluorescent product; the investigators also found up to 43% loss of pancuronium from serum specimens stored frozen for 1 week (Wingard et al., 1979). Gas chromatography (Furuta et al., 1988) and direct-insertion mass spectrometry (Castagnoli et al., 1988; Nisikawa et al., 1991) have also been employed.

References

S. Agoston, G.A. Vermeer, U.W. Kersten and D.K.F. Meijer. The fate of pancuronium bromide in man. Acta Anaesth. Scand. 17: 267–275, 1973.

S. Agoston, J.F. Crul, U.W. Kersten and A.H.J. Scaf. Relationship of the serum concentration of pancuronium to its neuromuscular activity in man. Anesthesiology 47: 509–512, 1977.

W. Buzello. Der Stoffwechsel von Pancuronium beim Menschen. Anaesthesist 24: 13–18, 1975.

K.P. Castagnoli, Y. Shinohara, T. Furuta et al. Quantitative estimation of quaternary ammonium neuromuscular blocking agents in serum by direct insertion probe chemical ionization mass spectrometry. Biomed. Env. Mass Spec. 13: 327–332, 1986.

P. Duvaldestin, S. Agoston, D. Henzel et al. Pancuronium pharmacokinetics in patients with liver cirrhosis. Brit. J. Anaesth. 50: 1131–1136, 1978.

T. Furuta, P.C. Canfell, K.P. Castagnoli et al. Quantitation of pancuronium, vecuronium, 3-desacetylvecuronium, pipecuronium and 3-desacetylpipecuronium in biological fluids by capillary gas chromatography using nitrogen-sensitive detection. J. Chrom. 427: 41–54, 1988.

U.W. Kersten, D.K.F. Meijer and S. Agoston. Fluorimetric and chromatographic determination of pancuronium bromide and its metabolites in biological materials. Clin. Chim. Acta 44: 59–66, 1973.

R.D. Miller, S. Agoston, L.H.D.J. Booij et al. The comparative potency and pharmacokinetics of pancuronium and its metabolites in anesthetized man. J. Pharm. Exp. Ther. 207: 539–543, 1978.

M. Nisikawa, M. Tatsuno, S. Suzuki and H. Tsuchihashi. The analysis of quaternary ammonium compounds in human urine by direct inlet electron impact ionization mass spectrometry. For. Sci. Int. 51: 131–138, 1991.

A. Poklis and E.G. Melanson. A suicide by pancuronium bromide injection: evaluation of the fluorometric determination of pancuronium in postmortem blood, serum and urine. J. Anal. Tox. 4: 275–280, 1980.

A.A. Somogyi, C.A. Shanks and E.J. Triggs. Clinical pharmacokinetics of pancuronium bromide. Eur. J. Clin. Pharm. 10: 367–372, 1976.

A.A. Somogyi, C.A. Shanks and E.J. Triggs. The effect of renal failure on the disposition and neuromuscular blocking action of pancuronium bromide. Eur. J. Clin. Pharm. 12: 23–29, 1977a.

A.A. Somogyi, C.A. Shanks and E.J. Triggs. Disposition kinetics of pancuronium bromide in patients with total biliary obstruction. Brit. J. Anaesth. 49: 1103–1108, 1977b.

L.B. Wingard, Jr., E. Abouleish, D.C. West and T.J. Goehl. Modified fluorometric quantitation of pancuronium bromide and metabolites in human maternal and umbilical serums. J. Pharm. Sci. 68: 914–916, 1979.

Papaverine

T½: 0.8–1.5 hr
Vd: 0.5–0.6 L/kg
Fb: 0.91
pKa: 6.4

Occurrence and Usage. Papaverine (Cerebid, Pavabid) is an isoquinoline alkaloid that is present in opium to the extent of about 1% by weight. It is a smooth muscle relaxant and is used clinically as a vasodilator and antispasmodic. This drug is administered as the hydrochloride, by intramuscular or intravenous injection of 30–120 mg or orally in daily doses of 300–600 mg.

Blood Concentrations. The oral administration of 150 mg of papaverine as an elixir produced plasma concentrations in 12 subjects that averaged 0.245 mg/L at 0.5 hours and 0.118 mg/L at 1.5 hours (Arnold et al., 1977). Plasma concentrations after ingestion of a 150 mg gelatin capsule by 15 subjects reached an average peak of 0.521 mg/L at 2 hours, compared to 0.256 mg/L for a sustained-release preparation of the same potency (Lee et al., 1978). Concentrations as high as 4 mg/L have been observed 2 hours after the ingestion of 300 mg of the drug (Guttman et al., 1974). Estimates of the plasma half-life of papaverine have ranged from 0.8–1.5 hours (Arnold et al., 1977; Ritschel and Hammer, 1977).

Metabolism and Excretion. The major route of biotransformation of papaverine is O-demethylation to phenolic metabolites, which are excreted as glucuronide conjugates in urine. About 60% of an oral dose is eliminated in 24 hours, with less than 1% as unchanged drug. Conjugated metabolites include 3'-hydroxypapaverine (2.3%), 4'-hydroxypapaverine (8.5%), 6-hydroxypapaverine (36%), 7-hydroxypapaverine (2.2%), and a trace amount of 4',6-dihydroxypapaverine (Axelrod et al., 1958; Belpaire et al., 1978; Wilen and Ylitalo, 1982).

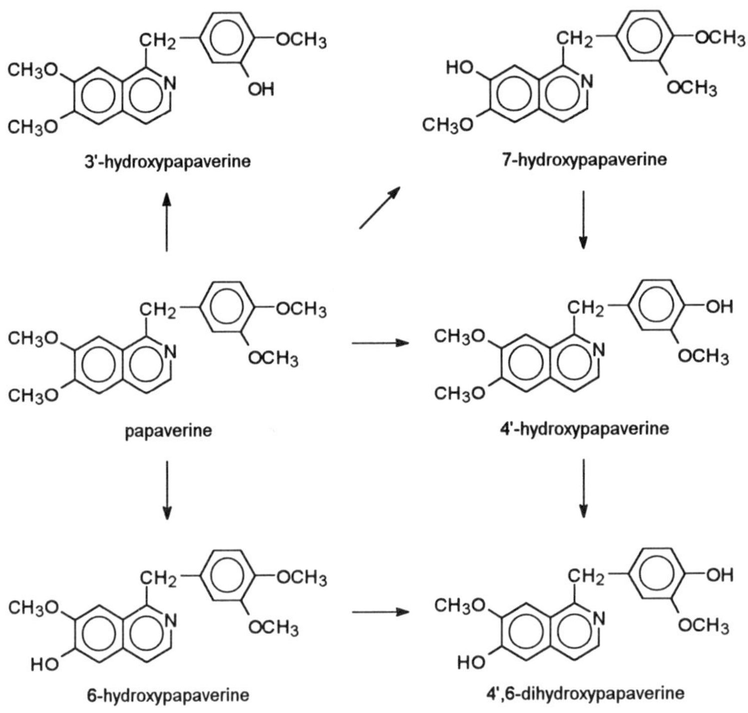

Toxicity. Adverse reaction to papaverine have included headache, dizziness, nausea, sweating, constipation or diarrhea, and jaundice. A woman who ingested 15 g of the drug exhibited reduced consciousness and marked hyperpnea. Severe lactic acidosis, accompanied by intense respiratory alkalosis, persisted for several days (Vaziri et al., 1981).

Analysis. The determination of papaverine in biological specimens has been accomplished by ultraviolet spectrophotometry (Axelrod et al., 1958), flame-ionization or nitrogen-selective gas chromatography (Guttman et al., 1974; Arnold et al., 1977; Bellia et al., 1978), and liquid chromatography (Pierson et al., 1979; Gautam et al., 1980; Hoogewijs et al., 1981).

References

J.D. Arnold, J. Baldridge, B. Riley and G. Brody. Papaverine hydrochloride: the evaluation of two new dosage forms. Int. J. Clin. Pharm. 15: 230–233, 1977.

J. Axelrod, R. Shofer, J.K. Inscoe et al. The fate of papaverine in man and other mammals. J. Pharm. Exp. Ther. 124: 9–15, 1958.

V. Bellia, J. Jacob and H.T. Smith. Determination of papaverine in blood samples by gas chromatography using a flame-ionization and a nitrogen-phosphorus detector. J. Chrom. 161: 231–235, 1978.

F.M. Belpaire, M.T. Rosseel and M.G. Bogaert. Metabolism of papaverine. IV. Urinary elimination of papaverine metabolites in man. Xenobiotica 8: 297–300, 1978.

S.R. Gautam, A. Nahum, J. Baechler and D.W.A. Bourne. Determination of papaverine in plasma and urine by high-performance liquid chromatography. J. Chrom. 182: 482–486, 1980.

D.E. Guttman, H.B. Kostenbauder, G.R. Wilkinson and P.H. Dube. GLC determination of papaverine in biological fluids. J. Pharm. Sci. 63: 1625–1626, 1974.

G. Hoogewijs, Y. Michotte, J. Lambrecht and D.L. Massart. High-performance liquid chromatographic determination of papaverine in whole blood. J. Chrom. 226: 423–430, 1981.

B.Y. Lee, H. Sakamoto, F. Trainor et al. Comparison of soft gelatin capsule vs. sustained release formulation of papaverine HCl: vasodilation and plasma levels. Int. J. Clin. Pharm. 16: 32–39, 1978.

S.L. Pierson, J.J. Hanigan, R.E. Taylor and J.E. McClurg. Simple and rapid high-pressure liquid chromatographic determination of papaverine in plasma. J. Pharm. Sci. 68: 1550–1551, 1979.

W.A. Ritschel and G.V. Hammer. Pharmacokinetics of papaverine in man. Int. J. Clin. Pharm. 15: 227–229, 1977.

N.D. Vaziri, J. Stokes and T.R. Treadwell. Lactic acidosis, a complication of papaverine overdose. Clin. Tox. 18: 417–423, 1981.

G. Wilen and P. Ylitalo. Metabolism of [^{14}C] papaverine in man. J. Pharm. Pharmac. 34: 264–266, 1982.

Paraldehyde

T½: 3–10 hr
Vd: 0.9 L/kg
Fb: ?

Occurrence and Usage. Paraldehyde (Paral) is a cyclic acetaldehyde trimer that was first synthesized in 1872 and first used therapeutically in 1882. At room temperature, it is an aromatic liquid (b.p. 124° C.) that slowly decomposes to acetic acid upon exposure to air. For use as a sedative or hypnotic it is administered in doses of 5–10 mL orally or occasionally by intramuscular or intravenous injection.

Blood Concentrations. A single 10 mL intramuscular dose given to a single subject produced plasma concentrations of 77 mg/L at 1.2 hours, 62 mg/L at 2.3 hours and 15 mg/L at 3.8 hours as determined by gas chromatography (Maes et al., 1969). Ten obstetric patients who received 30 mL of the drug orally developed maximal blood concentrations of 110–332 mg/L (average, 220) within 0.5–4.0 hours after ingestion, which declined to an average of 75 mg/L by 16 hours; patients who received the same dose rectally exhibited maximal concentrations that were only 70–75% of those seen with oral administration. All patients whose blood concentrations exceeded 200 mg/L experienced a period of complete amnesia (Gardner et al., 1940). Cerebrospinal fluid concentrations of paraldehyde were found to average 75% of serum levels at 1 hour after intramuscular injection of the drug; the biological half-life averaged 7.4 hours in 5 children (Thurston et al., 1968).

Metabolism and Excretion. The fate of paraldehyde in man has not been investigated but, on the basis on animal studies, it is believed that paraldehyde is depolymerized in the liver to acetaldehyde, which is then oxidized to acetic acid. Up to 80% of a dose may be transformed in this manner, with less than 3% excreted unchanged in the urine and up to 28% eliminated by the pulmonary route (Levine et al., 1940; Hitchcock and Nelson, 1943). Acetaldehyde itself has not been found in the serum of subjects administered paraldehyde (Thurston et al., 1968).

Toxicity. Paraldehyde has produced hypotension, tachycardia, cyanosis, rapid and shallow breathing, coughing, coma and death in a number of individuals following therapeutic administration; one infant survived a serum paraldehyde level of 1744 mg/L produced by intravenous infusion (Shoor, 1941; Sinal and Crowe, 1976; Bostrom, 1982). Chronic usage may result in addiction, with symptoms resembling those of alcoholism (Williams and Bowie, 1963).

While one subject has survived a dose of 125 mL of paraldehyde, another died following the ingestion of 25 mL. A subject who ingested 120 mL developed a blood concentration of 1300 mg/L and became comatose, but eventually recovered (Kaye and Haag, 1964). Blood concentrations of the drug in 4 fatal cases averaged 936 mg/L (range, 543–1480) (Figot et al., 1952), while in another 17 fatalities the concentrations ranged from 490–1600 mg/L (Hayward and Boshell, 1957; DiMaio and Garriott, 1974; Caplan, 1975). The tissue distribution of this neutral agent is demonstrated by the concentrations found in 3 fatal cases, 2 of which also involved alcohol (Rehling, 1967).

Tissue Distribution of Paraldehyde (mg/L or mg/kg)

	Blood	Brain	Liver	Kidney	Urine
Average	245	273	337	167	130
(Range)	(115–480)	(150–370)	(200–600)	(50–260)	(130)

Analysis. Most methods for the analysis of paraldehyde in biological specimens rely on the facile conversion of the drug to acetaldehyde in dilute acid with heating. The acetaldehyde thus formed may be estimated by oxidimetric titration (Levine and Bodansky, 1940), colorimetrically (Westerfield, 1945), by ultraviolet spectrophotometry (Figot et al., 1952), enzymatically (Thurston et al., 1968) or by gas chromatography (Hancock et al., 1977). Gas chromatography has also been used for the determination of the intact drug after isolation by steam distillation (Maes et al., 1969), headspace sampling (Anthony et al., 1978), or membrane ultrafiltration (Hessel, 1988).

References

R.M. Anthony, R.O. Bost, W.L. Thompson and I. Sunshine. Paraldehyde, toluene, and methylene chloride analysis by headspace gas chromatography. J. Anal. Tox. 2: 262–264, 1978.

B. Bostrom. Paraldehyde toxicity during treatment of status epilepticus. Am. J. Dis. Child. 136: 414–415, 1982.

Y.H. Caplan. Personal communication, 1975.

V.J.M. DiMaio and J.C. Garriott. A fatal overdose of paraldehyde during treatment of a case of delirium tremens. J. For. Sci. 19: 755–758, 1974.

P.P. Figot, C.H. Hine and E.L. Way. Estimation and significance of paraldehyde levels in blood and brain. Acta Pharm. Tox. 8: 290–304, 1952.

H.L. Gardner, H. Levine and M. Bodansky. Concentration of paraldehyde in the blood following its administration during labor. Am. J. Obs. Gyn. 40: 435–439, 1940.

J.P. Hancock, J.C. Harrill and E.T. Solomons. Head space gas chromatographic analysis of paraldehyde in toxicologic specimens. J. Anal. Tox. 1: 161–163, 1977.

J.N. Hayward and B.R. Boshell. Paraldehyde intoxication with metabolic acidosis. Am. J. Med. 23: 965–976, 1957.

D.W. Hessel. The analysis of blood serum for paraldehyde by ultrafiltration and gas chromatography with a wide-bore capillary column. J. Anal. Tox. 12: 350–353, 1988.

P. Hitchcock and E.E. Nelson. The metabolism of paraldehyde. J. Pharm. Exp. Ther. 79: 286–294, 1943.

S. Kaye and H.B. Haag. Study of death due to combined action of alcohol and paraldehyde in man. Tox. Appl. Pharm. 6: 316–320, 1964.

H. Levine and M. Bodansky. Determination of paraldehyde in biological fluids. J. Biol. Chem. 133: 193–198, 1940.

H. Levine, A.J. Gilbert and M. Bodansky. The pulmonary and urinary excretion of paraldehyde in normal dogs and in dogs with liver damage. J. Pharm. Exp. Ther. 69: 316–323, 1940.

R. Maes, N. Hodnett, H. Landesman et al. The gas chromatographic determination of selected sedatives (ethchlorvynol, paraldehyde, meprobamate and carisoprodol) in biological material. J. For. Sci. 14: 235–254, 1969.

C.J. Rehling. Poison residues in human tissues. In *Progress in Chemical Toxicology*, Vol. 3 (A. Stolman, ed.), Academic Press, New York, 1967, pp. 363–386.

M. Shoor. Paraldehyde poisoning. J. Am. Med. Asso. 117: 1534–1535, 1941.

S.H. Sinal and J.E. Crowe. Cyanosis, cough, and hypotension following intravenous administration of paraldehyde. Pediatrics 57: 158–159, 1976.

J.H. Thurston, H.S. Liang, J.S. Smith and E.J. Valentini. New enzymatic method for measurement of paraldehyde: correlation of effects with serum and CSF levels. J. Lab. Clin. Med. 72: 699–704, 1968.

W.W. Westerfield. A colorimetric determination of paraldehyde. J. Lab. Clin. Med. 30: 1076–1077, 1945.

E.Y. Williams and Z. Bowie. Paraldehyde intoxication. J. Nat. Med. Asso. 55: 154–156, 1963.

Paraquat

T½: 12–120 hr
Vd: 1.2–1.6 L/kg
Fb: ?

Occurrence and Usage. Paraquat (Gramoxone W, Weedol) is a bis-quaternary ammonium compound that has seen widespread use since 1962 as a domestic and commercial herbicide. The compound was first synthesized in 1932 and, under the name methyl viologen, was used for many years as an oxidation-reduction indicator dye. The dichloride salt is supplied as a 5% powder for domestic use or a 10–30% aqueous concentrate for agricultural purposes; combinations of paraquat and diquat, an ortho-bipyridyl analogue, are also commercially available. The current threshold limit value for occupational exposure is 0.1 mg/m³. The compound is known to be absorbed after dermal contact, inhalation and ingestion.

Blood Concentrations. Paraquat has not been measured in the blood of asymptomatic exposed persons. It is estimated that less than 5% of an oral dose is absorbed (Conning et al., 1969).

Metabolism and Excretion. Paraquat is not believed to be significantly biotransformed in man. An oral dose given to rats is eliminated in 3 days largely in feces (93–96%) and to a slight extent in urine (6%), whereas a subcutaneous dose appears to a much larger extent in urine (73–96%), indicating poor absorption from the gut. Unabsorbed paraquat appears to undergo substantial microbial degradation in the intestine (Daniel and Gage, 1966). The lung was the organ of highest paraquat concentration in rats given an intravenous LD50 dose, from 4 hours until about 9 days after injection; plasma levels declined with a half-life of 56 hours (Sharp et al., 1972). An unidentified paraquat metabolite has been detected in rat lung (Molnar and Hayes, 1971).

Concentrations of paraquat in the urine of 6 asymptomatic spray operators ranged from undetectable to 0.32 mg/L and averaged 0.04 mg/L during the daily agricultural application of large volumes of 0.25% paraquat solution over a 12 week period (Swan, 1969).

Toxicity. Occupational exposure to paraquat generally produces only skin rash, fingernail damage and epistaxis, although severe eye damage has occurred upon direct contact and several individuals died after extensive dermal contact (Wohlfahrt, 1982). There has been no report of long-term effects with routine exposures of up to several years' duration (Swan, 1969; Howard, 1979).

Several hundred deaths have occurred after the ingestion of paraquat, and it is believed that an oral dose of only 1–2 g is fatal to most adults. Victims of poisoning experience epigastric pain, vomiting, dyspnea, dysuria and jaundice; death usually follows, often after a period of many days, as a result of severe and extensive fibrotic lung changes and renal failure. Some subjects become comatose and die within a few hours, prior to the development of significant organ pathology.

Plasma paraquat concentrations exceeding 0.2 mg/L or a urinary excretion rate greater than 1 mg/hour on the first day of poisoning are usually associated with an unfavorable prognosis (Davies et al., 1977; Wright et al., 1978; Proudfoot et al., 1979). Poisoning has been treated aggressively with forced diuresis (Kerr et al., 1968), hemodialysis (van Dijk et al., 1975) and hemoperfusion (Winchester et al., 1983), but the efficacy of these measures has been questioned (Mascie-Taylor et al., 1983; Bismuth et al., 1987). In several episodes of nonfatal poisoning, maximal serum concentrations of 0.6–3.2 mg/L and urine concentrations of 0.9–64 mg/L have been noted (Tompsett, 1970; van Dijk et al., 1975; Houze et al., 1990). Paraquat has been detected in urine in concentrations exceeding 0.07 mg/L for up to 26 days after acute ingestion, even during forced diuresis (Beebeejaun et al., 1971).

In cases that eventually proved fatal, antemortem paraquat concentrations were initially as high as 19 mg/L in blood and 1766 mg/L in urine (van Dijk et al., 1975); often these are much lower, however, and when death is postponed for a period exceeding 18 days, autopsy specimens may yield negative results for paraquat by some analytical procedures (Tompsett, 1970; Carson and Carson, 1976). The following series of 32 fatalities due to ingestion of paraquat has been subdivided according to survival time in order to illustrate the manner in which tissue concentrations of the chemical decline with time (Tompsett, 1970; Maes, 1973; Leung, 1975; Piper, 1975; Carson and Carson, 1976; Cravey, 1979):

Paraquat Concentrations in Fatal Cases (mg/L or mg/kg)*

Survival	Cases	Blood	Brain	Lung	Liver	Kidney	Urine
0–1 days	9	15 (0–63)	7.0 (1.5–18)	58 (2.6–185)	73 (8.8–386)	100 (12–311)	462 (20–1210)
1–7 days	13	0.8 (0–4.4)		5.2 (0–21)	6.8 (0.2–58)	14 (1.0–74)	4.5 (0–16)
8–21 days	8	0.5 (0–4.0)		1.8 (0–4.7)	1.7 (0–4.4)	1.6 (0.6–3.5)	0.6 (0–2.2)
22 days	1	0.10	0.09	0.02	0.05	0.08	
23 days	1	0		0	0	0	

*All results obtained using the dithionite colorimetric method

Analysis. Paraquat has been frequently analyzed in biologic specimens using a visible spectrophotometric method based on sodium dithionite reduction of the ion under alkaline conditions; the analysis is performed after preliminary isolation by cation-exchange chromatography (Daniel and Gage, 1966; Lott et al., 1978; Kuo, 1987), protein precipitation (Knepil, 1977), ion-pair extraction (Jarvie and Stewart, 1979), or by direct addition of the test reagents to urine (Berry and Grove, 1971; Widdop, 1976). The latter technique has a sensitivity of approximately 1 mg/L and is useful for emergency diagnosis of poisoning. Very sensitive gas chromatographic procedures have been devised for paraquat analysis that are based on borohydride reduction to a tertiary amine (Draffan et al., 1977; van Dijk et al., 1977) or on injection-port pyrolysis (Martens et al., 1977); both flame-ionization and nitrogen-specific detection were utilized, with ethyl viologen as internal standard. Liquid chromatographic techniques have been described (Pryde and Darby, 1975; Miller et al., 1979; Gill et al., 1983; Queree et al., 1985; Croes et al., 1993).

References

A.R. Beebeejaun, G. Beevers and W.N. Rogers. Paraquat poisoning—prolonged excretion. Clin. Tox. 4: 397–407, 1971.

D.J. Berry and J. Grove. The determination of paraquat (1,1'-dimethyl-4,4'-bipyridylium cation) in urine. Clin. Chim. Acta 34: 5–11, 1971.

C. Bismuth, J.M. Scherrmann, R. Garnier et al. Elimination of paraquat. Hum. Tox. 6: 63–67, 1987.

D.J.L. Carson and E.D. Carson. The increasing use of paraquat as a suicidal agent. For. Sci. 7: 151–160, 1976.

D.M. Conning, K. Fletcher and A.A.B. Swan. Paraquat and related bipyridyls. Brit. Med. Bull. 25: 245–249, 1969.

R.H. Cravey. Poisoning by paraquat. Clin. Tox. 14: 195–198, 1979.

K. Croes, F. Martens and K. Desmet. Quantitation of paraquat in serum by HPLC. J. Anal. Tox. 17: 310–312, 1993.

J.W. Daniel and J.C. Gage. Absorption and excretion of diquat and paraquat in rats. Brit. J. Ind. Med. 23: 133–136, 1966.

D.S. Davies, G.M. Hawksworth and P.N. Bennett. Paraquat poisoning. Proc. Eur. Soc. Tox. 18: 21–26, 1977.

G.H. Draffan, R.A. Clare, D.L. Davies et al. Quantitative determination of the herbicide paraquat in human plasma by gas chromatographic and mass spectrometric methods. J. Chrom. 139: 311–320, 1977.

R. Gill, S.C. Qua and A.C. Moffat. High-performance liquid chromatography of paraquat and diquat in urine with rapid sample preparation involving ion-pair extraction on disposable cartridges of octadecyl-silica. J. Chrom. 255: 483–490, 1983.

P. Houze, F.J. Baud, R. Mouy et al. Toxicokinetics of paraquat in humans. Hum. Exp. Tox. 9: 5–12, 1990.

J.K. Howard. A clinical survey of paraquat formulation workers. Brit. J. Ind. Med. 36: 220–223, 1979.

D.R. Jarvie and M.J. Stewart. The rapid extraction of paraquat from plasma using an ion-pairing technique. Clin. Chim. Acta 94: 241–251, 1979.

F. Kerr, A.R. Patel, P.D.R. Scott and S.L. Tompsett. Paraquat poisoning treated by forced diuresis. Brit. Med. J. 3: 290–291, 1968.

J. Knepil. A short, simple method for the determination of paraquat in plasma. Clin. Chim. Acta 79: 387–390, 1977.

T.L. Kuo. Determination of paraquat in tissue using ion-pair chromatography in conjunction with spectrophotometry. For. Sci. Int. 33: 177–185, 1987.

S.C. Leung. Personal communication, 1975.

P.F. Lott, J.W. Lott and D.J. Doms. The determination of paraquat. J. Chrom. Sci. 16: 390–395, 1978.

R.A.A. Maes. Personal communication, 1973.

M. Martens, F. Martens and H. Heyndrickx. The determination of paraquat in 1-mL blood samples by means of pyrolysis-NFID-GLC. Proc. Eur. Soc. Tox. 18: 183–184, 1977.

B.H. Mascie-Taylor, J. Thompson and A.M. Davison. Haemoperfusion ineffective for paraquat removal in life-threatening poisoning. Lancet 1: 1376–1377, 1983.

J.J. Miller, E. Sanders and D. Webb. Measurement of paraquat in serum by high-performance liquid chromatography. J. Anal. Tox. 3: 1–3, 1979.

I.G. Molnar and W.J. Hayes, Jr. Distribution and metabolism of paraquat in the rat. Tox. Appl. Pharm. 19: 405, 1971.

N.H. Piper. Personal communication, 1975.

A.T. Proudfoot, M.S. Stewart, T. Levitt and B. Widdop. Paraquat poisoning: significance of plasma-paraquat concentrations. Lancet 2: 330–332, 1979.

A. Pryde and F.J. Darby. The analysis of paraquat in urine by high-speed liquid chromatography. J. Chrom. 115: 107–116, 1975.

E.A. Queree, S.J. Dickson and S.M. Shaw. Extraction and quantification of paraquat in liver and hemolyzed blood. J. Anal. Tox. 9: 10–14, 1985.

C.W. Sharp, A. Ottolenghi and H.S. Posner. Correlation of paraquat toxicity with tissue concentrations and weight loss of the rat. Tox. Appl. Pharm. 22: 241–251, 1972.

A.A.B. Swan. Exposure of spray operators to paraquat. Brit. J. Ind. Med. 26: 322–329, 1969.

S.L. Tompsett. Paraquat poisoning. Acta Pharm. Tox. 28: 346–358, 1970.

A. van Dijk, R.A.A. Maes, R.H. Drost et al. Paraquat poisoning in man. Arch. Tox. 34: 129–136, 1975.

A. van Dijk, R. Ebberink, G. de Groot et al. A rapid and sensitive assay for the determination of paraquat in plasma by gas-liquid chromatography. J. Anal. Tox. 1: 151–154, 1977.

B. Widdop. Detection of paraquat in urine. Brit. Med. J. 2: 1135, 1976.

J.F. Winchester, M.C. Gelfand and G.E. Schreiner. Haemoperfusion for paraquat poisoning. Lancet 2: 277, 1983.

D.J. Wohlfahrt. Fatal paraquat poisoning after skin absorption. Med. J. Aust. 1: 512–513, 1982.

N. Wright, W.B. Yeoman and K.A. Hale. Assessment of severity of paraquat poisoning. Brit. Med. J. 2: 396, 1978.

Parathion

T½: ?
Vd: ?
Fb: ?

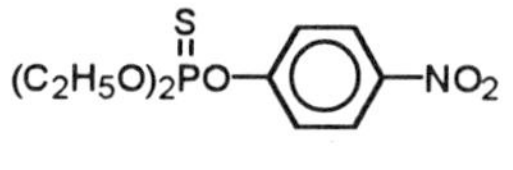

$(C_2H_5O)_2\overset{\overset{S}{\|}}{P}O-\!\!\!\!\bigcirc\!\!\!\!-NO_2$

Occurrence and Usage. Parathion (nitrostigmine, DNTP) is a highly toxic organophosphate in-secticide that has been used frequently and in large quantities since 1949. Parathion and its dim-ethyl analogue, methylparathion, are yellow oily liquids in pure form that are supplied as dusts, wettable powders and aerosols in concentrations of up to 50% for agricultural purposes. The cur-rent threshold limit value for parathion is 0.1 mg/m³. The compound is well-absorbed after inhala-tion, dermal contact or ingestion.

Blood Concentrations. Dosages of 0.05 mg/kg (3.5 mg/70 kg) of parathion have been orally ad-ministered to humans daily for at least 3 weeks with no apparent effect on blood cholinesterase levels (Williams et al., 1958). An oral dose of 7.2 mg, when given daily to volunteers for 6 weeks, caused reduction of cholinesterase activity to levels of 84% of normal in erythrocytes and 63% in plasma; 28 days after the end of the experiment these values were only partially restored to pre-experiment control values (Edson, 1964). Parathion serum concentrations in 23 occupationally exposed asymptomatic workers ranged from 0.004–0.200 mg/L, with no correlation to erythrocyte or plasma cholinesterase activity. Paraoxon has occasionally been detected in the serum of persons exposed to parathion (Roan et al., 1969).

Metabolism and Excretion. Parathion must be activated by conversion via liver microsomal en-zymes to paraoxon, a potent cholinesterase inhibitor; both compounds are rapidly hydrolyzed by plasma and tissue esterases, with production of diethylthiophosphoric acid (DETP), diethylphosphoric acid (DEP) and p-nitrophenol. These products are largely excreted in urine and represent the ma-jority of a dose of parathion. Urinary DETP and DEP are known to be unstable in stored specimens (Comer et al., 1976) and thus p-nitrophenol, which is rapidly excreted in the urine as a conjugate within 48 hours of an exposure, has been used as a sensitive index of exposure to parathion.

Urine p-nitrophenol concentrations ranged from 0.4–13.2 mg/L in 23 asymptomatic occupation-ally exposed workers and correlated well with serum parathion levels, but not with cholinesterase activity in blood (Roan et al., 1969). Due to slow absorption of parathion via the dermal route, p-nitrophenol excretion may be very prolonged after this type of exposure (Durham et al., 1972). Urine p-nitrophenol concentrations were found to average 0.11 mg/L (range, 0.06–0.31) in resi-dents living near orchards where parathion was used, 0.28 mg/L (range, 0.10–0.72) in orchard workers, 2.0 mg/L (range, 0.14–11.3) in parathion mixing-plant personnel and 4.7 mg/L (range, 3.2–6.3) in parathion applicators (Arterberry et al., 1961).

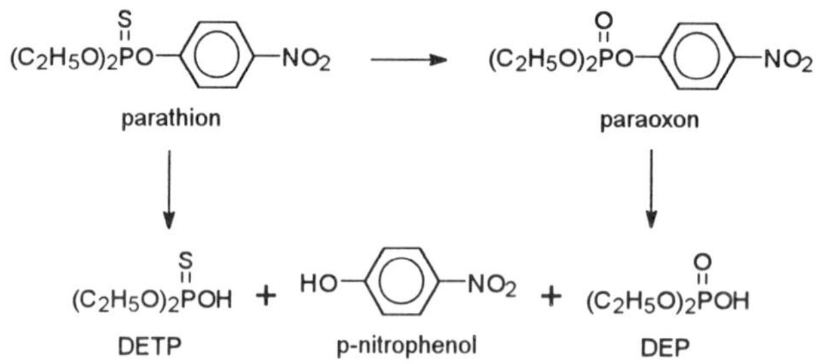

Toxicity. Symptoms of exposure to parathion are similar to those produced by other cholinesterase inhibitors and include respiratory difficulty, excessive salivation, miosis, nausea, vomiting, muscle weakness and paralysis. Atropine and 2-PAM (pralidoxime) are administered as specific antidotes (Hayes, 1965).

Food contamination by parathion has caused several epidemics of poisoning in which numerous deaths have occurred (Askew, 1968; Diggory et al., 1977). Several hundred deaths in Denmark over a 5 year period were attributed to the suicidal use of parathion (Frost and Poulsen, 1964). The estimated fatal dose of parathion for an adult by ingestion or inhalation is 10–300 mg. In a nonfatal poisoning of a worker following dermal exposure to parathion, diethylphosphate (DEP) concentrations in blood were as high as 0.28 mg/L; concentrations of monoethylphosphate reached 0.55 mg/L in blood and 7.0 mg/L in urine (Reichert et al., 1978). Urinary DETP and DEP concentrations in another nonfatal poisoning were initially 3.9 and 0.5 mg/L, respectively (Comer et al., 1976). Urinary p-nitrophenol concentrations in severe poisoning cases have ranged from 1.6–11.6 mg/L (Arterberry et al., 1961), lying within the range of concentrations observed in asymptomatic workers (Roan et al., 1969).

A series of 19 fatalities due to parathion poisoning was investigated quantitatively by means of a bioassay based on cholinesterase inhibition, and provided the following data (Heyndrickx and De Clerc, 1977):

Parathion Concentrations in Fatal Cases (mg/L or mg/kg)

	Blood	Brain	Liver	Kidney	Urine
Average	9.0	4.9	11	3.3	10
(Range)	(0.5–34)	(0.9–13)	(0.1–120)	(0.2–12)	(0.4–78)

In another fatality that occurred about 10 hours after the onset of cholinergic symptoms, parathion was detected in brain, liver and kidney in concentrations of 1.39–1.69 mg/kg; cholinesterase determinations in this case (performed 4 days after death) showed the following results (Grob et al., 1949):

Cholinesterase Activity in a Fatal Parathion Case (% of Normal)

Plasma	Erythrocytes	Cerebrum	Cerebellum	Liver	Kidney
5	12	12	47	43	41

Analysis. Gas chromatographic techniques for the determination of intact parathion in biologic specimens have utilized electron-capture (Kadoum, 1968), phosphorus-specific (Gabica et al., 1971) or mass spectrometric detection (Nielson, 1985). The phosphate metabolites of parathion may be assayed in blood and urine by procedures cited in the section on diazinon. Urinary p-nitrophenol may be measured by colorimetry (Elliot et al., 1960), electron-capture gas chromatography of an ethyl (Bradway and Shafik, 1973) or trimethylsilyl derivative (Cranmer, 1970), or liquid chromatography (Diamond and Quebbemann, 1979; Ott, 1979). Liquid chromatography has also been used to measure tissue levels of paraoxon (deNeef et al., 1981). Postmortem specimens for cholinesterase assay must be kept in cold storage and analyzed as soon as possible to minimize the effects of spontaneous reactivation of the enzyme (Geldmacher-v. Mallinckrodt et al., 1974). Procedures for cholinesterase determination are cited in the section on carbaryl.

References

J.D. Arterberry, W.F. Durham, J.W. Elliott and H.R. Wolfe. Exposure to parathion. Arch. Env. Health 3: 476–485, 1961.

A.B. Askew. History of assistance to Tijuana: acute parathion food poisoning. Clin. Tox. 1: 251–253, 1968.

D.E. Bradway and T.M. Shafik. Parathion exposure studies. A gas chromatographic method for the determination of low levels of p-nitrophenol in human and animal urine. Bull. Env. Cont. Tox. 9: 134–139, 1973.

S.W. Comer, H.E. Ruark and A.L. Robbins. Stability of parathion metabolites in urine samples collected from poisoned individuals. Bull. Env. Cont. Tox. 16: 618–625, 1976.

M. Cranmer. Determination of p-nitrophenol in human urine. Bull. Env. Cont. Tox. 5: 329–332, 1970.

J.H. de Neef, A.J. Porsius and H.H. van Rooy. Quantitative analysis of the cholinesterase inhibitor paraoxon in brain tissue using high-performance liquid chromatography. J. Chrom. 224: 133–138, 1981.

G. Diamond and A.J. Quebbemann. Rapid separation of p-nitrophenol and its glucuronide and sulfate conjugates by reversed-phase high-performance liquid chromatography. J. Chrom. 177: 368–371, 1979.

H.J.P. Diggory, P.J. Landrigan, K.P. Latimer et al. Fatal parathion poisoning caused by contamination of flour in international commerce. Am. J. Epidemiol. 106: 145–153, 1977.

W.F. Durham, H.R. Wolfe and J.W. Elliott. Absorption and excretion of parathion by spraymen. Arch. Env. Health 24: 381–387, 1972.

E.F. Edson. No-effect levels of three organophosphates in the rat, pig and man. Food Cosmet. Tox. 2: 311–316, 1964.

J.W. Elliott, K.C. Walker, A.E. Penick and W.F. Durham. A sensitive procedure for urinary p-nitrophenol determination as a measure of exposure to parathion. J. Agr. Food Chem. 8: 111–113, 1960.

J. Frost and E. Poulsen. Poisoning due to parathion and other organophosphorus insecticides in Denmark. Dan. Med. Bull. 11: 169–177, 1964.

J. Gabica, J. Wyllie, M. Watson and W.W. Benson. Example of flame photometric analysis for methyl parathion in rat whole blood and brain tissue. Anal. Chem. 43: 1102–1105, 1971.

M. Geldmacher-v. Mallinckrodt, H.H. Lindorf, M. Petenyi et al. Zur Bewertung der Serum-Cholinesteraseaktivitaet in Leichenblut bei Verdacht auf eine E 605-Vergiftung. Z. Rechtsmed. 75: 191–199, 1974.

D. Grob, W.L. Garlick, G.G. Merrill and H.C. Freimuth. Death due to parathion, an anticholinesterase insecticide. Ann. Int. Med. 31: 899–904, 1949.

W.J. Hayes, Jr. Parathion poisoning and its treatment. J. Am. Med. Asso. 192: 136–139, 1965.

A. Heyndrickx and F. De Clerc. Toxicological results and criteria of death. J. Pharm. Belg. 32: 149–161, 1977.

A.M. Kadoum. Cleanup procedure for water, soil, animal and plant extracts for the use of electron-capture detector in the gas chromatographic analysis of organophosphorus insecticide residues. Bull. Env. Cont. Tox. 3: 247–253, 1968.

P.G. Nielson. Quantitative analysis of parathion and parathion-methyl by combined capillary column gas chromatography negative ion chemical ionization mass spectrometry. Biomed. Mass Spec. 12: 695–698, 1985.

D.E. Ott. Mechanized system for liquid chromatographic determination of 4-nitrophenol and some other phenolic pesticide metabolites in urine. J. Asso. Off. Anal. Chem. 62: 93–99, 1979.

E.R. Reichert, H.W. Klemmer and T.J. Haley. A note on dermal poisoning from mevinphos and parathion. Clin. Tox. 12: 33–35, 1978.

C.C. Roan, D.P. Morgan, N. Cook and E.H. Paschal. Blood cholinesterases, serum parathion concentrations and urine p-nitrophenol concentrations in exposed individuals. Bull. Env. Cont. Tox. 4: 362–369, 1969.

M.W. Williams, J.W. Cook, J.R. Blake et al. The effect of parathion on human red blood cell and plasma cholinesterase. Arch. Ind. Health 18: 441–445, 1958.

Paroxetine

T½: 7–37 hr
Vd: 3–28 kg
Fb: 0.95
pKa: ?

Occurrence and Usage. Paroxetine (Paxil) is a serotonin reuptake inhibitor used as an antidepressant agent and belonging to a class of drugs that includes fluoxetine and sertraline. It is available as the hydrochloride for oral administration in tablets of 20 and 30 mg; daily oral doses are generally 20–50 mg.

Blood Concentrations. A single 20 mg oral dose produced an average peak plasma level of 11 µg/L (range, 0.8–33) in 29 healthy subjects at times of 3.0–8.0 hours (Kaye et al., 1989). In a study of 15 healthy adult males who received a single 30 mg oral dose daily for 30 days, peak steady-state plasma paroxetine concentrations averaged 62 µg/L at 5.2 hours. The trough concentrations averaged 31 µg/L and the elimination half-life averaged 21 hours in these subjects (PDR, 1994). No correlation has been observed between plasma paroxetine concentrations and either efficicy or the frequency of side-effects (Tasker et al., 1989). The elimination half-life averaged 41 hours in a group of poor metabolizers (about 7% of the population), compared to 16 hours for extensive metabolizers (Sindrup et al.,1992).

Metabolism and Excretion. Paroxetine is extensively biotransformed by oxidation, methylation and conjugation to largely inactive metabolites. Over a 10 day period following a single oral dose, approximately 64% is eliminated in urine and 36% in feces. Less than 2% of a dose is found in the urine as parent drug (Haddock et al., 1989; Kaye et al., 1989).

Following a single oral dose, the 24 hour urine of extensive metabolizers contained 17% as metabolite I sulfate, 8% as metabolite I glucuronide, 3.1% as metabolite II glucuronide, 0.4% as parent drug and only trace amounts of other metabolites (Sindrup et al., 1992).

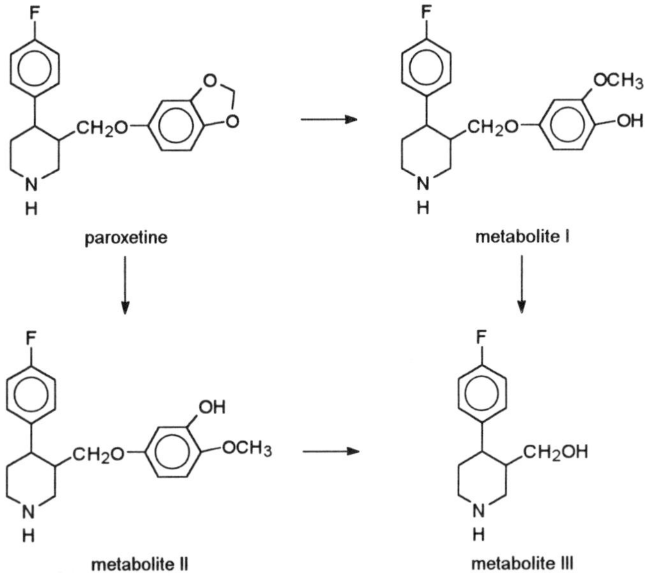

paroxetine

metabolite I

metabolite II

metabolite III

Toxicity. Adverse reactions to paroxetine include somnolence, agitation, tremor, insomnia, nausea and muscular weakness. Concurrent administration of a monoamine oxidase inhibitor may cause extreme agitation, muscle rigidity, hyperthermia, hypertension, delerium and coma. Vertigo, nausea and vomiting have been reported in patients following discontinuation of paroxetine therapy (Barr et al., 1994). Overdosage has produced nausea, vomiting, drowsiness and tachycardia. An adult male who ingested 400 mg of the drug manifested only anxiety during a 10 hour post-dose observation period (Gorman et al., 1993).

A woman who intentionally ingested a drug overdose had postmortem blood and liver paroxetine levels of 0.24 mg/L and 3.5 mg/kg, respectively; the other drug involved in the case was amitriptyline, which was present at corresponding levels of 0.43 mg/L and 6.8 mg/kg (Win, 1994).

Analysis. Paroxetine may be determined in biological specimens using liquid chromatography (Brett et al., 1987).

References

L.C. Barr, W.K. Goodman and L.H. Price. Physical symptoms associated with paroxetine discontinuation. Am. J. Psych. 151: 289, 1994.

M.A. Brett, H.D. Dierdorf, B.D. Zussman and P.E. Coates. Determination of paroxetine in human plasma, using high-performance liquid chromatography with fluorescence detection. J. Chrom. 419: 438–444, 1987.

S.E. Gorman, T. Rice and H.F. Simmons. Paroxetine overdose. Am. J. Emer. Med. 11: 682, 1993.

R.E. Haddock, A.M. Johnson, P.F. Langley et al. Metabolic pathway of paroxetine in animals and man and the comparative pharmacological properties of its metabolites. Acta Psych. Scand. 80 (Suppl. 350): 24–26, 1989.

Physicians' Desk Reference, Medical Economics Company, Montvale, New Jersey, 1994, pp. 2267–2270.

C.M. Kaye, E.E. Haddock, P.F. Langley et al. A review of the metabolism and pharmacokinetics of paroxetine in man. Acta Psych. Scand. 80 (Suppl. 350): 60–75, 1989.

T.C.G. Tasker, C.M. Kaye, B.D. Zussman and C.G.G. Link. Paroxetine plasma levels: lack of correlation with efficacy or adverse events. Acta Psych. Scand. 80 (Suppl. 350): 152–155, 1989.

B. Win. Personal communication, 1994.

Pemoline

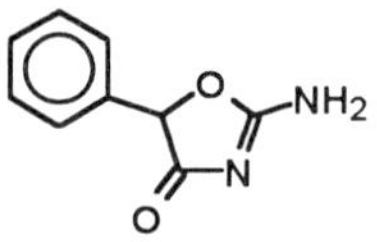

T½: 11 hr
Vd: 0.22–0.59 L/kg
Fb: 0.30
pKa: 10.5

Occurrence and Usage. Pemoline (Cylert) was synthesized in 1913 and introduced into medical practice in the 1950's as a central nervous system stimulant. The drug is used in the treatment of childhood hyperactivity, mildly depressed patients, to counteract drowsiness due to antihistamines, and as an inhibitor of the growth of Ehrlich tumor cells. For the treatment of hyperactivity in children of 5–12 years, the recommended starting dose is 37.5 mg/day; the daily dose is gradually increased at 1 week intervals until the desired clinical response is obtained. Pemoline is available in tablets containing 18.75, 37.5 and 75 mg as the free acid.

Blood Concentrations. Following a single oral dose of 37.5 or 50 mg given to 4 fasting volunteers ranging in age from 25–28 years and weighing 68–87 kg, a maximum plasma concentration ranging from 0.77–1.22 mg/L (average, 0.98) was attained after 2.1–3.5 hours (average, 2.7) (Vermeulen et al., 1979). A single dose of 2 mg/kg of pemoline was given to 10 children, 5–12 years of age and weighing 23–60 kg, following an 18 hour fast; maximum serum pemoline concentrations ranged from 3.2–6.2 mg/L (average, 4.3) after 1.0–5.5 hours (average, 2.8) (Sallee et al., 1985).

Fifteen boys and girls, 6.5–11 years of age, on pemoline therapy, 1.63–4.86 mg/kg, for 6 months attained mean serum pemoline concentrations ranging from 0.88–5.0 mg/L (average, 2.2) between 2 and 8 hours after the morning dose (Collier et al., 1985).

Metabolism and Excretion. After 48 hours, approximately 92% of a dose can be recovered from the urine and feces in man. The urine contains approximately 40% of a dose as unchanged drug, 20% in conjugated form, 35% as unidentified polar metabolites and 4% as 5-phenyl-2,4-oxazolidinedione. Less than 1% of the dose is recovered in the feces (Vermeulen et al., 1979; Tomkins et al., 1980).

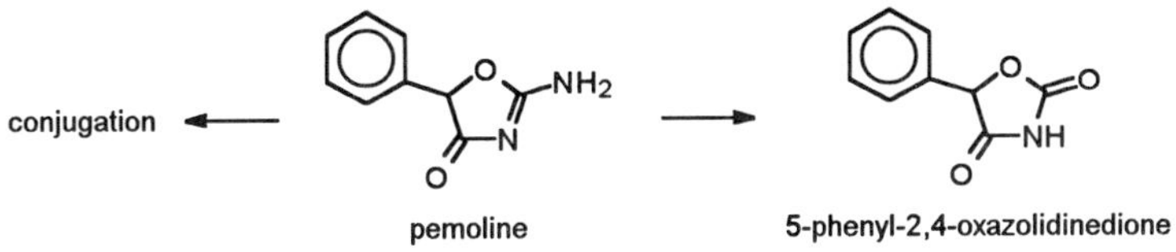

conjugation ← pemoline → 5-phenyl-2,4-oxazolidinedione

Toxicity. Pemoline in overdosage causes restlessness, confusion, anxiety, hallucinations, hyperthermia, convulsions and coma. Chronic abusers may develop mania, psychosis and dependency (Sternbach, 1981; Polchert and Morse, 1985). A fatal case attributed to pemoline and methadone involved a blood pemoline concentration of 5 mg/L in a 27 year old male drug abuser (Forrest, 1985).

Analysis. Pemoline has been determined in biological specimens by ultraviolet spectrophotometry after conversion to benzaldehyde (Cummins and Perry, 1969). More specific gas chromatographic methods employing electron-capture (Chu and Sennello, 1977; Libeer and Schepens, 1978), nitrogen-specific (Veremulen et al., 1978; Hoffman, 1979) and mass spectrometric detection (Van Boven and Daenens, 1977) have been reported. Pemoline and its metabolites have also been determined by liquid chromatography (Cartoni and Natalizia, 1976; Tomkins et al., 1980; Aoyama et al., 1988).

References

T. Aoyama, H. Kotaki, Y. Saitoh and F. Nakagawa. Determination of pemoline in plasma, urine and tissues by reversed phase high-performance liquid chromatography. J. Chrom. 430: 351–360, 1988.

G.P. Cartoni and F. Natalizia. Determination of pemoline by high-pressure liquid chromatography. J. Chrom. 123: 474–478, 1976.

S.Y. Chu and L.T. Sennello. Gas chromatographic determination of pemoline in biological fluids using electron capture detection. J. Chrom. 137: 343–350, 1977.

C.P. Collier, S.J. Soldin, J.M. Swanson et al. Pemoline pharmacokinetics and long term therapy in children with attention deficit disorder and hyperactivity. Clin. Pharm. 10: 269–278, 1985.

L.M. Cummins annd J.E. Perry. Spectrophotometric determination of pemoline and mandelic acid in biological fluids. J. Pharm. Sci. 58: 762–763, 1969.

A.R.W. Forrest. Personal communication, 1985.

D.J. Hoffman. Sensitive GLC assay for pemoline in biological fluids using nitrogen-specific detection. J. Pharm. Sci. 68: 445–447, 1979.

J.C. Libeer and P. Schepens. GLC determination of pemoline in biological fluids. J. Pharm. Sci. 67: 419–421, 1978.

S.E. Polchert and R.M. Morse. Pemoline abuse. J. Am. Med. Asso. 254: 946–947, 1985.

F. Sallee, R. Stiller, J. Perel et al. Oral pemoline kinetics in hyperactive children. Clin. Pharm. Ther. 37: 606–609, 1985.

H. Sternbach. Pemoline-induced mania. Biol. Psych. 16: 987–989, 1981.

C.P. Tomkins, S.J. Soldin, S.M. MacLeod et al. Analysis of pemoline in serum by high performance liquid chromatography: clinical application to optimize treatment of hyperactive children. Ther. Drug Mon. 2: 255–260, 1980.

M. Van Boven and P. Daenens. Combined gas-liquid chromatographic-mass spectrometric analysis of pemoline in biological samples. J. Chrom. 134: 415–421, 1977.

N.P.E. Vermeulen, M.W.E. Teunissen and D.D. Breimer. Assay of pemoline in human plasma, saliva and urine by capillary gas chromatography with nitrogen-selective detection. J. Chrom. 157: 133–140, 1978.

N.P.E. Vermeulen, M.W.E. Teunissen and D.D. Breimer. Pharmacokinetics of pemoline in plasma, saliva and urine following oral administration. Brit. J. Clin. Pharm. 8: 459–463, 1979.

Pentachlorophenol

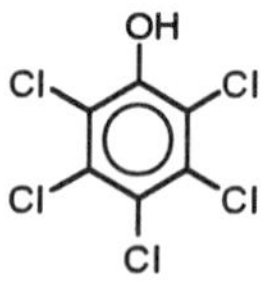

T½: 13–19 days
Vd: 0.35 L/kg
Fb: 0.99
pKa: 5.0

Occurrence and Usage. Pentachlorophenol and its sodium salt (PCP, Penta, Dowicide-G) are frequently employed industrially and in the home as wood preservatives, contact herbicides, disinfectants, and mildew retardants. The compound is often dissolved in hydrocarbon solvents for application by spraying, brushing, or pressure treatment, and is known to be well-absorbed after oral, pulmonary, or dermal exposure. Vaporization from treated wood is a source of chronic inhalation exposure in areas where pentachlorophenol is used extensively for termite control. The average daily dietary intake for U.S. citizens is estimated at 19 µg. The current threshold limit value for industrial exposure is 0.5 mg/m^3.

Blood Concentrations. Serum pentachlorophenol concentrations in unexposed persons in Europe or the U.S. have been found to range from 0.002–0.200 mg/L in various studies (Bomhard et al., 1984; Uhl et al., 1986; Gomez-Catalan et al., 1987; Cline et al., 1989). Plasma concentrations of pentachlorophenol in members of the general population of Hawaii, where use of the chemical is high, ranged from 0.05–1.0 mg/L; plasma concentrations in healthy occupationally-exposed workers in a wood treatment plant were largely in the range of 1.0–10.0 mg/L, with several subjects attaining concentrations a high as 20 mg/L. Plasma contains 99% of the whole blood content of pentachlorophenol (Bevenue et al., 1968; Casarett et al., 1969). Following a single oral dose of 0.1 mg/kg (7 mg/70 kg) given to 4 men, plasma concentrations reached an average peak of 0.2 mg/L at 4 hours (Braun et al., 1979).

Metabolism and Excretion. The metabolism of pentachlorophenol has only been briefly studied in man. The chemical is known to be oxidized to tetrachlorohydroquinone, and this metabolite and its parent are excreted largely in urine in both free and conjugated form (Ahlborg et al., 1974). An average of 74% of a single oral dose is eliminated as free and 12% as conjugated pentachlorophenol over a 7 day period, with an additional 4% found in feces. No other metabolites were found in this single dose study (Braun et al., 1979). The excretion of the chemical is enhanced by alkalinization of the urine (Uhl et al., 1986). During chronic exposure, the urinary levels of conjugated pentachlorophenol exceed those of the free chemical by several-fold (Drummond et al., 1982).

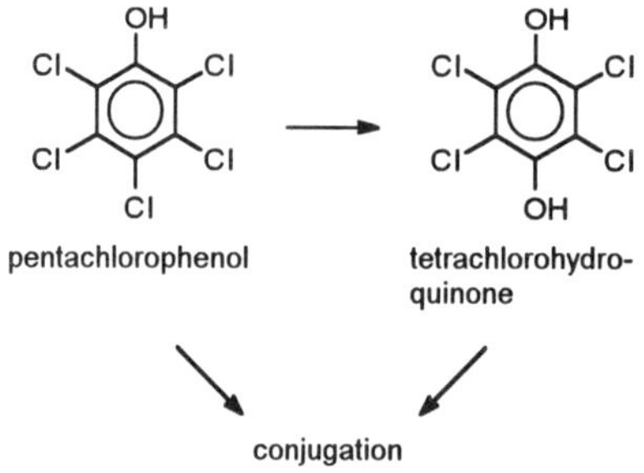

pentachlorophenol → tetrachlorohydroquinone → conjugation

Free pentachlorophenol concentrations in members of the general population averaged 0.025 mg/kg (range, 0.005–0.052) in fat (Shafik, 1973) and 0.044 mg/L (range, 0.003–0.570) in urine. Persons with occupational exposure exhibited urine levels of 0.003–38.6 mg/L, averaging 0.465 mg/L (Bevenue et al., 1967). Morning urine specimens from workers with substantial dermal and respiratory exposure to pentachlorophenol averaged as high as 5.6 mg/L over one 10 day period; a direct correlation was observed between blood and urine concentrations of pentachlorophenol (Casarett et al., 1969). Pentachlorophenol concentrations in adipose tissue from members of the general population in Japan average 0.14 mg/kg, with a range of 0–0.57 mg/kg (Ohe, 1979).

Toxicity. Pentachlorophenol is a highly toxic substance that can result in chloracne and disturbances in lipid metabolism with chronic exposure (Baxter, 1984). Acute overdosage produces delirium, weakness, flushing, hyperpyrexia, tachycardia, tachypnea, coma, and death within several hours of the absorption of approximately 2 g by an adult. Profound rigor mortis is often observed immediately after death, in both man and animals.

Four men who developed excessive sweating, facial flushing, fever, and weight loss during occupational exposure to pentachlorophenol had urine concentrations of the chemical that ranged from 3.8–17.5 mg/L (Bergner et al., 1965). A young child exhibited symptoms of pentachlorophenol poisoning and a urine concentration of 60 mg/L following dermal exposure to contaminated bath water (Chapman and Robson, 1965). Contamination of nursery linens by pentachlorophenol was responsible for an epidemic of poisoning in a hospital; an inital serum pentachlorophenol concentration of 118 mg/L was noted in one infant, successfully treated by exchange transfusion, while concentrations of 28 mg/kg in kidney and 34 mg/kg in fat were determined in another child who died. Serum concentrations of 11.3–25.6 mg/L (average, 18.7) and urine concentrations of 0.02–0.70 mg/L (average, 0.34) were found in 6 healthy infants in the same nursery (Armstrong et al., 1969). The intentional ingestion of pentachlorophenol by an adult was sucessfully treated by forced diuresis; blood concentrations as high as 115 mg/L were observed and were noted to decline with half-lives of 116 and 42 hours before and after diuresis was instituted, respectively (Young and Haley, 1978).

A blood concentration of 39 mg/L was measured in the case of an adult who ingested 11 g of the chemical and died within 4 hours (Burger, 1966). The following concentrations were compiled from 7 fatalities resulting from pulmonary, oral, or dermal exposure to pentachlorophenol (Gordon, 1956; Blair, 1961; Mason et al., 1965; Clarke, 1969; Cretney, 1976; Gray et al., 1985):

Pentachlorophenol Concentrations in Fatal Cases (mg/L or mg/kg)

	Blood	Brain	Liver	Kidney	Urine
Average	107	22	98	164	153
(Range)	(46–173)	(14–35)	(52–225)	(41–639)	(28–520)

Analysis. Pentachlorophenol is generally determined in biological specimens by electron-capture gas chromatography of a methyl or ethyl derivative (Bevenue et al., 1966; Bevenue et al., 1968; Cranmer and Freal, 1970; Rivers, 1972; Shafik, 1973; Bomhard et al., 1984) or an acetyl derivative (Woiwode et al., 1980; Siqueira and Fernicola, 1981), although flame-ionization detection is certainly suitable for measurement of toxic levels of the compound. Formation of the ethyl derivative of pentachlorophenol allows its separation from tetrachlorohydroquinone, which is present as a metabolite in urine specimens (Hoben et al., 1976). Gas chromatography-mass spectrometry (Wagner et al., 1991) and liquid chromatographic methods (Drummond et al., 1982; Chou and Bailey, 1986) have also been reported. Prior hydrolysis of urine specimens is not necessary for most routine monitoring purposes, but has been found to yield pentachlorophenol levels up to 17 times as high as methods not incorporating this step (Edgerton and Moseman, 1979). Tetrachlorohydroquinone was found to be a potent inhibitor of beta-glucuronidase, and urinary conjugates must therefore by hydrolyzed by boiling with strong acid prior to solvent extraction (Ahlborg et al., 1974).

References

U.G. Ahlborg, J.E. Lindgren and M. Mercier. Metabolism of petnachlorophenol. Arch. Tox. 32: 271–281, 1974.

R.W. Armstrong, E.R. Eichner, D.E. Klein et al. Pentachlorophenol poisoning in a nursery for newborn infants. J. Pediat. 75: 317–325, 1969.

R.A. Baxter. Biochemical study of pentachlorophenol workers. Ann. Occ. Hyg. 28: 429–438, 1984.

H. Bergner, P. Constantinidis and J.H. Martin. Industrial pentachlorophenol poisoning in Winnipeg. Can. Med. Asso. J. 92: 448–451, 1965.

A. Bevenue, J.R. Wilson, E.F. Potter et al. A method for the determination of pentachlorophenol in human urine in picogram quantities. Bull. Env. Cont. Tox. 1: 257–266, 1966.

A. Bevenue, J. Wilson, L.J. Casarett and H.W. Klemmer. A survey of pentachlorophenol content in human urine. Bull. Env. Cont. Tox. 2: 319–332, 1967.

A. Bevenue, M.L. Emerson, L.J. Casarett and W.L. Yauger, Jr. A sensitive gas chromatographic method for the determination of pentachlorophenol in human blood. J. Chrom. 38: 467–472, 1968.

D.M. Blair. Dangers in using and handling sodium pentachlorophenate as a molluscicide. Bull. World Health Org. 25: 597–601, 1961.

A. Bomhard, K.H. Schaller and G. Triebig. Capillar-Gas-Chromatographie mit ECD-und MS-Detektion zur quantitaven Bestimmung von Pentachlorphenol im menschlichen Plasma und Harn. Fres. Z. Anal. Chem. 319: 516–519, 1984.

W.H. Braun, G.E. Blau and M.B. Chenoweth. The metabolism/pharmacokinetics of pentachlorophenol in man, and a comparison with the rat and monkey. In *Toxicological and Occupational Medicine* (W.B. Deichmann, ed.), Elsevier, New York, 1979, pp. 289–296.

E. Burger. Akute toediche Vergiftung mit Pentachlorphenolnatrium. Deut. Z. Gericht. Med. 58: 240–247, 1966.

L.J. Casarett, A. Bevenue, W.L. Yauger, Jr. and S.A. Whalen. Observations on pentachlorophenol in human blood and urine. Am. Ind. Hyg. Asso. J. 30: 360–366, 1969.

J.B. Chapman and P. Robson. Pentachlorophenol poisoning from bathwater. Lancet 1: 1266–1267, 1965.

P.P. Chou and J.L. Bailey. Liquid-chromatographic determination of urinary pentachlorophenol. Clin. Chem. 32: 1026–1028, 1986.

E.G.C. Clarke (ed.). *Isolation and Identification of Drugs*, Pharmaceutical Press, London, 1969, pp. 471–472.

R.E. Cline, R.H. Hill, D.L. Phillips and L.L. Needham. Pentachlorophenol measurements in body fluids of people in log homes and workplaces. Arch. Env. Cont. Tox. 18: 475–481, 1989.

M. Cranmer and J. Freal. Gas chromatographic analysis of pentachlorophenol in human urine by formation of alkyl ethers. Life Sci. 9: 121–128, 1970.

M.J. Cretney. Personal communication, 1976.

I. Drummond, P.B. van Roosmalen and M. Kornicki. Determination of total pentachlorophenol in the urine of workers. Int. Arch. Occ. Env. Health 50: 321–327, 1982.

T.R. Edgerton and R.F. Moseman. Determination of pentachlorophenol in urine: the importance of hydrolysis. J. Agr. Food Chem. 27: 197–199, 1979.

J. Gomez-Catalan, J. To-Figueras, J. Planas et al. Pentachlorophenol and hexachlorobenzene in serum and urine of the population of Barcelona. Hum. Tox. 6: 397–400, 1987.

D. Gordon. How dangerous is pentachlorophenol? Med. J. Aust. 2: 485–488, 1956.

R.E. Gray, R.D. Gilliland, E.E. Smith et al. Pentachlorophenol intoxication: report of a fatal case, with comments on the clinical course and pathologic anatomy. Arch. Env. Health 40: 161–164, 1985.

H.J. Hoben, S.A. Ching, L.J. Casarett and R.A. Young. A study of the inhalation of pentachlorphenol by rats. Part I. A method for the determination of pehtachlorophenol in rat plasma, urine and tissue and in aerosol samples. Bull. Env. Cont. Tox. 15: 78–85, 1976.

M.F. Mason, S.M. Wallace, E. Foerster and W. Drummond. Pentachlorophenol poisoning: report of two cases. J. For. Sci. 10: 136–147, 1965.

T. Ohe. Pentachlorophenol residues in human adipose tissue. Bull. Env. Cont. Tox. 22: 287–292, 1979.

J.B. Rivers. Gas chromatographic determination of pentachlorophenol in human blood and urine. Bull. Env. Cont. Tox. 8: 294–296, 1972.

T.M. Shafik. The determination of pentachlorophenol and hexachlorophene in human adipose tissue. Bull. Env. Cont. Tox. 10: 57–63, 1973.

M.E.P.B. Siqueira and N.A.G.G. Fernicola. Determination of pentachlorophenol in urine Bull. Env. Cont. Tox. 27: 380–385, 1981.

S. Uhl, P. Schmid and C. Schlatter. Pharmacokinetics of pentachlorophenol in man. Arch. Tox. 58: 182–186, 1986.

S.L. Wagner, L.R. Durand, R.D. Inman et al. Residues of pentachlorophenol and other chlorinated contaminants in human tissues. Arch. Env. Cont. Tox. 21: 596–606, 1991.

W. Woiwode, R. Wodarz, K. Drysch and H. Weichardt. Bestimmung von freiem Pentachlorophenol in der Luft und im Blut durch leistungsfaehige Routineverfahren. Int. Arch. Occ. Env. Health 45: 153–161, 1980.

J.F. Young and T.J. Haley. A pharmacokinetic study of pentachlorophenol poisoning and the effect of forced diuresis. Clin. Tox. 12: 41–48, 1978.

Pentazocine

T½: 2.1–3.5 hr
Vd: 4.4–7.8 L/kg
Fb: 0.61
pKa: 9.0

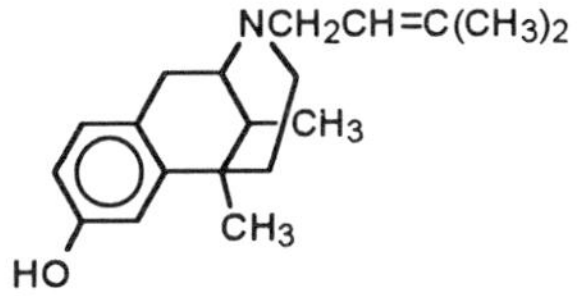

Occurrence and Usage. Pentazocine (Talwin) is a synthetic benzomorphan derivative that, as the racemic form, is one-third to one-sixth as potent an analgesic as morphine and is a weak narcotic antagonist as well. Pentazocine is administered parenterally (usually intramuscularly) as the lactate at an initial dose of 30 mg, and orally as the hydrochloride in doses of 50–100 mg. One oral form of the drug combines 12.5 mg of the hydrochloride and 325 mg of aspirin.

Blood Concentrations. Following intramuscular administration of 45 mg to 8 subjects, peak pentazocine plasma concentrations occurred between 15 and 60 minutes and averaged 0.14 mg/L, declining with a half-life of 2.1 hours; after oral administration of 75 mg, peak concentrations averaged 0.16 mg/L between 2 and 3 hours (Berkowitz et al., 1969). Plasma concentrations ranging from 0.2–1.0 mg/L have been noted in surgical patients 5 or 10 minutes after the intravenous administration of 30 mg of the drug (Agurell et al., 1974). The whole blood/plasma concentration ratio is 1.06 (Ehrnebo et al., 1974).

Metabolism and Excretion. Pentazocine is extensively metabolized both by oxidation of either of the methyl groups on the dimethylallyl side chain and by glucuronide conjugation of the parent drug and the oxidized metabolites. Animal studies indicate that most of the free and conjugated metabolites are present in blood, that penetration of the blood-brain barrier is limited to the unchanged drug and that brain pentazocine concentrations always exceed those of plasma (Pittman, 1973). The oral bioavailability is only 11–32% due to first-pass hepatic metabolism (Ehrnebo et al., 1977).

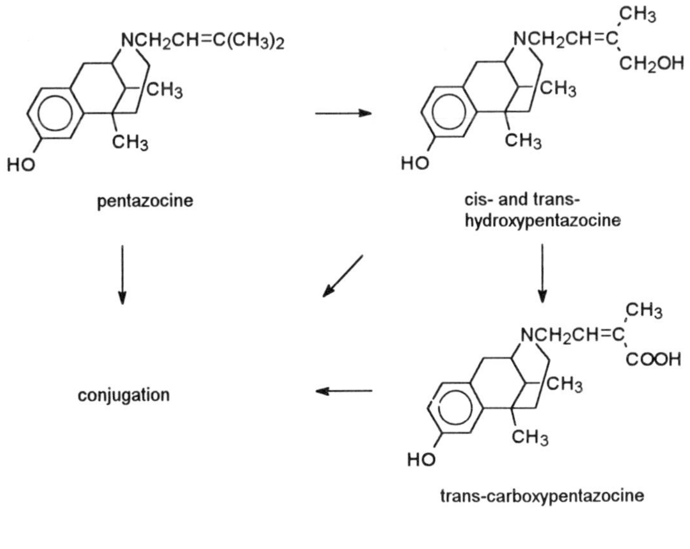

pentazocine

cis- and trans-
hydroxypentazocine

conjugation

trans-carboxypentazocine

The 24 hour urine of 4 male volunteers after ingestion of 56.5 mg of pentazocine contained the following amounts of total metabolites (free plus conjugated), expressed as a percentage of the dose: 9.5% pentazocine, 11.6% cis-hydroxypentazocine and 38.9% trans-carboxypentazocine. No evidence for the presence of trans-hydroxypentazocine in the urine was found (Pittman, 1970). After oral administration of 100 mg, the amount of free pentazocine in the urine of 4 subjects was seen to range from 3–15% of the dose, during conditions of acid urine (Beckett et al., 1970). Although no studies of the analgesic properties of the metabolites of pentazocine have been reported, their apparent inability to cross the blood-brain barrier may make this a moot point.

Toxicity. Adverse effects of pentazocine use include headache, dizziness, nausea, sweating, dry mouth, hypotension, tachycardia, respiratory depression, agitation, hallucinations and tremor. Neither nalorphine nor levallorphan is effective in reversing the respiratory depression produced by pentazocine, although naloxone is. The drug has been reported to have a relatively low potential for abuse and dependence, but cases have been reported involving chronic self-administration of up to 1200 mg daily; withdrawal symptoms were noted in most instances (Neuschatz, 1969; Sandoval and Wang, 1969; Schoolar et al., 1969; Inciardi and Chambers, 1971).

Blood concentrations of pentazocine in fatalities are generally in the 1–5 mg/L range, comparable to those for codeine. Brain concentrations often exceed the blood levels and, except in cases of intravenous administration, the excretory organs contain substantial amounts of the unchanged drug (Finkle, 1974; Baselt, 1976; Cravey, 1977; Poklis and Mackell, 1982):

Pentazocine Concentrations in Fatalities (mg/L or mg/kg)*

Route	n	Blood	Brain	Liver	Kidney	Urine	Gastric
Oral	5	4.7	7.0	42	9.0	3.8	201 mg
		(3.0–9.2)	(7.0)	(23–87)	(9.0)	(3.0–4.5)	(1–590)
I.V.	2	1.0	3.6	1.6	5.9	32	trace
		(1.0–1.0)	(1.1–6.0)	(1.2–2.0)	(2.8–9.0)	(32)	(trace)

* By gas chromatography without prior hydrolysis

Blood pentazocine concentrations of 0.4–11 mg/L (average, 3.7) were measured in 14 victims of accidental intravenous overdosage with a pentazocine-tripelennamine combination (Monforte et al., 1983).

Analysis. Pentazocine is reasonably well-suited to analysis by fluorimetry as shown by Berkowitz et al. (1969) and others (Borg and Mikaelsson, 1970). However, the question of specificity arises when the drug metabolites are present in a sample, and for this reason gas chromatography is the preferred technique. This has been used successfully by analysis of the underivatized drug (Beckett et al., 1970) as well as of a silyl derivative (Pittman, 1970). Many of the flame-ionization and electron-capture techniques for morphine are adaptable to the assay of pentazocine. Gas chromatography-mass spectrometry of underivatized pentazocine has also been reported (Agurell et al., 1974), as has liquid chromatography (Anderson et al., 1982; Shibanoki et al., 1987; Moeller et al., 1990).

It should be noted that acid hydrolysis for the purpose of hydrolyzing conjugated pentazocine will result in partial conversion of the drug to a hydroxy derivative, formed by hydrolysis of the double bond in the side chain; thus, enzymatic hydrolysis of pentazocine conjugates is indicated (Vaughn and Beckett, 1973). This conversion has been used as a confirmation step in the thin-layer chromatographic screening procedure for pentazocine in urine (Reid and Gerbeck, 1981).

References

S. Agurell, L.O. Boreus, E. Gordon et al. Plasma and cerebrospinal fluid concentrations of pentazocine in patients: assay by mass fragmentography. J. Pharm. Pharmac. 26: 1–8, 1974.

R.D. Anderson, K.F. Ilett, L.J. Dusci and L.P. Hackett. High-performance liquid chromatographic analysis of pentazocine in blood and plasma. J. Chrom. 227: 239–243, 1982.

R. Baselt. Unpublished observations, 1976.

A.H. Beckett, J.F. Taylor and P. Kourounakis. The absorption, distribution and excretion of pentazocine in man after oral and intravenous administration. J. Pharm. Pharmac. 22: 123–128, 1970.

B.A. Berkowitz, J.H. Asling, E.L. Way et al. Relationship of pentazocine plasma levels to pharmacological activity in man. Clin. Pharm. Ther. 10: 320–328, 1969.

K.O. Borg and A. Mikaelsson. Fluorimetric determination of pentazocine in biological samples by partition chromatography as ion pair in micro-columns. Acta Pharmac. Suecica 7: 673–680, 1970.

R.H. Cravey. Personal communication, 1977.

M. Ehrnebo, S. Agurell, L.O. Boreus et al. Pentazocine binding to blood cells and plasma proteins. Clin. Pharm. Ther. 16: 424–429, 1974.

M. Ehrnebo, L.O. Boreus and U. Lonroth. Bioavailability and first-pass metabolism of oral pentazocine in man. Clin. Pharm. Ther. 22: 888–892, 1977.

B.S. Finkle. Personal communication, 1974.

J.A. Inciardi and C.D. Chambers. Patterns of pentazocine abuse and addiction. N.Y. State J. Med. 71: 1727–1733, 1971.

N. Moeller, K. Dietzel, B. Nuernberg et al. High-performance liquid chromatographic determination of pentazocine in plasma. J. Chrom. 530: 200–205, 1990.

J.R. Monforte, R. Gault, J. Smialek and T. Goodin. Toxicological and pathological findings in fatalities involving pentazocine and tripelennamine. J. For. Sci. 28; 90–101, 1983.

J. Neuschatz. Pentazocine: massive dosage without side effects. J. Am. Med. Asso. 209: 112–113, 1969.

K.A. Pittman. Human metabolism of orally administered pentazocine. Biochem. Pharm. 19: 1833–1836, 1970.

K.A. Pittman. Pentazocine in rhesus monkey plasma and brain after parenteral and oral administration. Life Sci. 12: 131–143, 1973.

A. Poklis and M.A. Mackell. Toxicological findings in deaths due to ingestion of pentazocine: a report of two cases. For. Sci. Int. 20: 89–95, 1982.

R.W. Reid and C.M. Gerbeck. Detection of pentazocine and tripelennamine in urine. Clin. Chem. 27: 10–13, 1981.

R.G. Sandoval and R.I.H. Wang. Tolerance and dependence on pentazocine. New. Eng. J. Med. 280: 1391–1392, 1969.

J.C. Schoolar, P. Idanpaan-Heikkila and A.S. Keats. Pentazocine addiction? Lancet 1: 1263, 1969.

S. Shibanoki, Y. Imamura, T. Itoh et al. Application of high-performance liquid chromatography with electrochemical detection for monitoring the concentration of pentazocine in human blood. J. Chrom. 421: 425–429, 1987.

D.P. Vaughn and A.H. Beckett. A note on the chemical change of pentazocine in aqueous acidic media. J. Pharm. Pharmac. 25: 993–995, 1973.

Pentobarbital

T½: 20–30 hr
Vd: 0.5–1.0 L/kg
Fb: 0.65
pKa: 7.9

Occurrence and Usage. Pentobarbital (pentobarbitone, Nembutal) is a short-acting barbiturate derivative first prepared in 1930. The drug is available alone and in combination with other agents in amounts of 15–200 mg for oral, intramuscular or rectal administration. It is supplied as the racemic mixture in the form of both the free acid and the sodium salt, the latter being strongly alkaline in aqueous solution.

Blood Concentrations. After a 5 minute intravenous infusion of 50 mg, plasma concentrations in 5 subjects averaged 1.18 mg/L (range, 1.05–1.33) at 0.08 hours, declining to 0.54 mg/L by 1 hour and 0.27 mg/L by 24 hours (Smith et al., 1973). Plasma concentrations averaged 3 mg/L at 6 minutes after intravenous injection of 100 mg of pentobarbital to 7 volunteers and fell to 1.6 mg/L by 1 hour, when they began to decline with a half-life of 22 hours (Ehrnebo, 1974). A single oral dose of 100 mg produced peak serum pentobarbital concentrations of 1.2–3.1 mg/L at 0.5–2.0 hours after administration; these levels diminished slowly, and after 48 hours an average serum concentration of 0.3 mg/L was found (Sun and Chun, 1977). Estimates of the plasma half-life of pentobarbital have ranged from 15–48 hours, with the average between 20 and 30 hours (Breimer, 1977). The oral administration of 600 mg of the drug over a 3 hour period produced a maximal average blood concentration of 3.0 mg/L (range, 1.8–4.7) in 5 subjects by 0.5 hours after the last dose; this level remained unchanged by 4.5 hours and declined to 1.5 mg/L (range, 1.2–1.7) after 18 hours (Parker et al., 1970).

Repeated intravenous doses of pentobarbital, usually 100–200 mg every 30–60 minutes, have been used to reduce intracranial pressure and lower cerebral oxygen demand in patients with severe head trauma, Reye's syndrome, or anoxic brain damage. The doses are adjusted to maintain the plasma drug level at 25–40 mg/L, and therapy may continue for up to several weeks (Marshall et al., 1978, 1979). The plasma 3'-hydroxypentobarbital concentrations in such patients are generally less than 10% those of the parent drug levels (Cary and Pope, 1983).

Metabolism and Excretion. The biotransformation of pentobarbital proceeds primarily via oxidation of the penultimate carbon of the methylbutyl side-chain with formation of a diastereoisomeric mixture of alcohols, and secondarily by N-hydroxylation (Maynert, 1965; Tang et al., 1977). Unlike hydroxyamobarbital, the alcoholic metabolites of pentobarbital are pharmacologically inactive (Maynert and Dawson, 1952). The existence of a carboxylic acid metabolite resulting from the oxidation of the terminal methylbutyl side-chain carbon atom has also been suggested (Algeri and McBay, 1953; Titus and Weiss, 1955). The oral bioavailability of pentobarbital is 100% (Doluisio et al., 1978).

As much as 86% of a radioactive dose of pentobarbital is excreted in the urine in 6 days; about 1% is present as unchanged drug, up to 73% as the levorotatory and dextrorotatory diastereoisomers of 3'-hydroxypentobarbital (in a 5.4 to 1 ratio), and up to 15% as N-hydroxypentobarbital (Maynert, 1965; Tang et al., 1977). None of the metabolites was found to be eliminated in a conjugated form.

N-hydroxypentobarbital   pentobarbital   3'-hydroxypentobarbital

3'-carboxypentobarbital

Parker et al. (1970) found urine pentobarbital concentrations of only 0.7–1.8 mg/L throughout the 21 hour period after a 600 mg oral dose of the drug, representing less than 0.2% of the total dose.

Toxicity. Although the frequency of pentobarbital involvement in poisoning episodes has declined in recent years, much data has been accumulated on the tissue levels of the drug following overdosage. A plasma concentration of 28 mg/L was achieved by a comatose patient who regained consciousness when the level fell to 13 mg/L after 24 hours (Prescott et al., 1973).

In 61 fatalities attributed to pentobarbital, postmortem blood concentrations ranging from 12–112 mg/L (average, 40) were determined (Rehling, 1967). In another 55 cases, blood concentrations averaged 30 mg/L (range, 5–169) and liver concentrations averaged 130 mg/kg (range, 23–550) (Baselt and Cravey, 1977). The estimated lethal dose as established by investigation of these cases has ranged from 2–10 g (Cravey et al., 1977). In 3 fatal overdoses in which pentobarbital and 3'-hydroxypentobarbital concentrations were measured by gas chromatography, the following tissue distribution was observed (Robinson and McDowall, 1979):

Drug Concentrations in Pentobarbital Fatalities (mg/L or mg/kg)

	Blood	Lung	Liver	Kidney	Urine	Gastric
Pentobarbital						
Average	29	35	77	28	25	325 mg
(Range)	(10–51)	(16–51)	(20–165)	(18–46)	(5–62)	(74–550)
Hydroxypentobarbital						
Average	1.3	8	7	6	74	0
(Range)	(0–4)	(4–10)	(5–9)	(4–7)	(65–82)	(0)

Analysis. Analytical methods for the determination of barbiturate derivatives are discussed in the section on amobarbital.

References

E.J. Algeri and A.J. McBay. The identification of pentobarbital by paper chromatography in a medicolegal death. New Eng. J. Med. 248: 423–424, 1953.

R.C. Baselt and R.H. Cravey. A compendium of therapeutic and toxic concentrations of toxicologically significant drugs in human biofluids. J. Anal. Tox. 1: 81–103, 1977.

D.D. Breimer. Clinical pharmacokinetics of hypnotics. Clin. Pharmacokin. 2: 93–109, 1977.

P.L. Cary and B.E. Pape. Quantitation of 3'-hydroxypentobarbital in serum using high-performance liquid chromatography. J. Chrom. 275: 107–114, 1983.

R.H. Cravey, D. Reed, P.R. Sedgwick and J.E. Turner. Toxicologic data from documented drug-induced or drug-related fatal cases. Clin. Tox. 10: 327–339, 1977.

J.T. Doluisio, R.B. Smith, A.H.C. Chun and L.W. Dittert. Pentobarbital absorption from capsules and suppositories in humans. J. Pharm. Sci. 67: 1586–1588, 1978.

M. Ehrnebo. Pharmacokinetics and distribution properties of pentobarbital in humans following oral and intravenous administration. J. Pharm. Sci. 63: 1114–1118, 1974.

L.F. Marshall, H.M. Shapiro, A. Rauscher and N.M. Kaufman. Pentobarbital therapy for intracranial hypertension in metabolic coma. Crit. Care Med. 6: 1–5, 1978.

L.F. Marshall, R.W. Smith and H.M. Shapiro. The outcome with aggressive treatment in severe head injuries. J. Neurosurg. 50: 26–30, 1979.

E.W. Maynert and J.M. Dawson. Ethyl (3-hydroxy-1-methylbutyl) barbituric acids as metabolites of pentobarbital. J. Biol. Chem. 195: 389–395, 1952.

E.W. Maynert. The alcoholic metabolites of pentobarbital and amobarbital in man. J. Pharm. Exp. Ther. 150: 118–121, 1965.

K.D. Parker, H.W. Elliott, J.A. Wright et al. Blood and urine concentrations of subjects receiving barbiturates, meprobamate, glutethimide, or diphenylhydantoin. Clin. Tox. 3: 131–145, 1970.

L.F. Prescott, P. Roscoe and J.A.H. Forrest. Plasma concentrations and drug toxicity in man. In *Biological Effects of Drugs in Relation to their Plasma Concentrations* (D.S. Davies and B.N.C. Prichard, eds.), University Park Press, Baltimore, 1973, pp. 51–81.

C.J. Rehling. Poison residues in human tissues. In *Progress in Chemical Toxicology*, Vol. 3 (A. Stolman, ed.), Academic Press, New York, 1967, pp. 363–386.

A.E. Robinson and R.D. McDowall. The distribution of amylobarbitone, butobarbitone, pentobarbitone and quinalbarbitone and the hydroxylated metabolites in man. J. Pharm. Pharmac. 31: 357–365, 1979.

R.B. Smith, L.W. Dittert, W.O. Griffen, Jr. and J.T. Doluisio. Pharmacokinetics of pentobarbital after intravenous and oral administration. J. Pharm. Biopharm. 1: 5–16, 1973.

S. Sun and A.H.C. Chun. Determination of pentobarbital in serum by electron-capture GLC. J. Pharm. Sci. 66: 477–480, 1977.

B.K. Tang, T. Inaba and W. Kalow. N-hydroxylation of pentobarbital in man. Drug Met. Disp. 5: 71–74, 1977.

E. Titus and H. Weiss. The use of biologically prepared radioactive indicators in metabolic studies: metabolism of pentobarbital. J. Biol. Chem. 214: 807–820, 1955.

Perphenazine

T½: 8–12 hr
Vd: 10–35 L/kg
Fb: ?
pKa: 7.8

Occurrence and Usage. Perphenazine (Trilafon, ingredient of Etrafon and Triavil) is a chlorpromazine analogue and one of a number of phenothiazine derivatives that contain a piperazine ring. The compound was first synthesized in 1956 and has received considerable clinical usage since that year. It is administered as the free base by intramuscular injection in doses of 5–10 mg, or orally in chronic daily amounts of 12–64 mg; a long-acting enanthate ester is also available for intramuscular administration at a dosage of 100 mg once every 14 days.

Blood Concentrations. Following a single intramuscular injection of 100 mg of perphenazine enanthate, perphenazine concentrations as high as 0.007 mg/L and sulfoxide concentrations averaging 0.001 mg/L are detectable in blood for the 14 day post-drug period (Hansen and Larsen, 1974; Larsen and Naestoft, 1975). A peak plasma concentration of 0.016 mg/L was achieved at 3 hours after a single oral 6 mg dose of the free base by a volunteer (Midha et al., 1981). The average terminal half-life of the drug is 9.4 hours (Hansen et al., 1976).

Patients receiving chronic daily oral doses of 12–48 mg of perphenazine developed plasma concentrations of 0.0004–0.0300 mg/L of the unchanged drug and concentrations of 0.0003–0.0170 mg/L of the sulfoxide; a poor correlation was obtained between drug dosage and steady-state plasma concentrations (Hansen and Larsen, 1977). In 7 patients receiving 24–48 mg daily oral doses for at least 3 weeks, trough plasma levels averaged 0.004 mg/L for perphenazine, 0.004 mg/L for perphenazine sulfoxide, and 0.011 mg/L for N-desalkylperphenazine (Hansen et al., 1979).

Metabolism and Excretion. The known or postulated pathways of perphenazine metabolism in man are oxidation to the sulfoxide, which may have some pharmacologic activity; N-dealkylation; cleavage of the piperazine ring; and phenolic hydroxylation followed by glucuronide conjugation (Huang and Kurland, 1964; Gaertner er al., 1975). Approximately 1% of a daily oral dose is eliminated unchanged in the 24 hour urine; 13% is excreted as the sulfoxide and about 30% is excreted as glucuronide conjugates (Huang and Kurland, 1964; van Kempen, 1971).

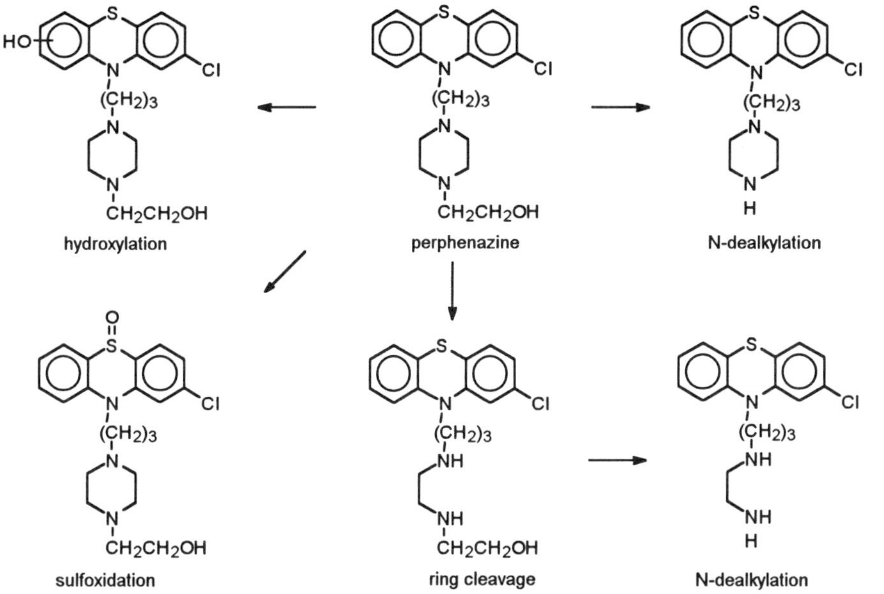

hydroxylation — perphenazine — N-dealkylation

sulfoxidation — ring cleavage — N-dealkylation

Toxicity. Numerous adverse reactions have been reported during perphenazine therapy, including extrapyramidal effects, tardive dyskinesia, anticholinergic effects, drowsiness, postural hypotension, blood dyscrasias, obstructive jaundice, and sudden death.

In an individual who ingested an overdose of a perphenazine-amitriptyline combination, postmortem blood contained 1.9 mg/L perphenazine and 8.5 mg/L amitriptyline (Gottschalk and Cravey, 1980). A 55 year old man ingested approximately 1 g of perphenazine and died unattended; his postmortem blood contained 0.17 g/dL ethanol, while perphenazine concentrations were: blood, 3 mg/L; brain, 11 mg/kg; liver, 149 mg/kg; and gastric contents, 22 mg (Cravey, 1980).

Analysis. Perphenazine and its sulfoxide metabolites have been assayed in urine by fluorometric technique (van Kempen, 1971) and in plasma by electron-capture gas chromatography of the trimethylsilyl derivatives (Larsen and Naestoft, 1975; Cooper et al., 1978, 1979). Liquid chromatographic methods have also been reported (Tjaden et al., 1976; Larsen et al., 1985).

References

S. Cooper, J.M. Albert, R. Dugal and M. Bertrand. Separation of perphenazine, its sulphoxide and its probable phenolic metabolites by electron-capture gas-liquid chromatography. J. Chrom. 150: 263–265, 1978.

S. Cooper, J.M. Albert, R. Dugal et al. Gas chromatographic determination of amitriptyline, nortriptyline and perphenazine in plasma of schizophrenic patients after administration of the combination of amitriptyline with perphenazine. Arz. Forsch. 29: 158–161, 1979.

R.H. Cravey. Personal communication, 1980.

H.J. Gaertner, G. Liomin, D. Villumsen et al. Tissue metabolites of trifluoperazine, fluphenazine, prochlorperazine, and perphenazine. Drug. Met. Disp. 3: 437–444, 1975.

L.A. Gottschalk and R.H. Cravey. *Toxicological and Pathological Studies on Psychoactive Drug-Involved Deaths*, Biomedical Publications, Davis, California, 1980, pp. 74–75.

C.E. Hansen and N. Larsen. Perphenazine concentrations in human whole blood. Psychopharmacologia 37: 31–36, 1974.

C.E. Hansen, T.R. Christensen, J. Elley et al. Clinical pharmacokinetic studies of perphenazine. Brit. J. Clin. Pharm. 3: 915–923, 1976.

L.B. Hansen and N. Larsen. Plasma concentrations of perphenazine and its sulphoxide metabolite during continuous oral treatment. Psychopharmacology 53: 127–130, 1977.

L.B. Hansen, J. Elley, T.R. Christensen et al. Plasma levels of perphenazine and its major metabolites during simultaneous treatment with anticholinergic drugs. Brit. J. Clin. Pharm. 7: 75–80, 1979.

C.L. Huang and A.A. Kurland. Perphenazine (Trilafon) metabolism in psychotic patients. Arch. Gen. Psych. 10: 639–646, 1964.

N. Larsen and J. Naestoft. Determination of perphenazine and its sulphoxide metabolite in human plasma after therapeutic doses by gas chromatography. J. Chrom. 109: 259–264, 1975.

N.F. Larsen, L.B. Hansen and P. Knudsen. Quantitative determination of perphenazine and its dealkylated metabolite using hplc. J. Chrom. 341: 244–250, 1985.

K.K. Midha, C. Mackonka, J.K. Cooper et al. Radioimmunoassay for perphenazine in human plasma. Brit. J. Clin. Pharm. 11: 85–88, 1981.

U.R. Tjaden, J. Lankelma, H. Poppe and R.G. Muusze. Determination of blood levels of perphenazine and fluphenazine. J. Chrom. 125: 275–286, 1976.

G.M.J. van Kempen. Urinary excretion of perphenazine and its sulfoxide during administration in oral and long-acting injectable form. Psychopharmacologia 21: 283–286, 1971.

Phenacetin

T½: 0.6–1.3 hr
Vd: 1–2 L/kg
Fb: 0.33

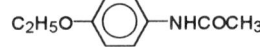

Occurrence and Usage. Phenacetin (acetophenetidin) is always found, in amounts of 100–162 mg, in combination with such other drugs as acetaminophen, aspirin, caffeine, codeine and propoxyphene. This neutral compound has analgesic and antipyretic effects qualitatively and quantitatively similar to acetaminophen, its major active metabolite. The suspected involvement of phenacetin in the development of nephrotoxicity in abusers of non-narcotic analgesics has led to the gradual replacement of the drug in many of these mixtures by acetaminophen.

Blood Concentrations. Two subjects achieved peak plasma phenacetin levels of 0.09–0.22 mg/L within 1–2 hours of a single 250 mg oral dose (Findlay et al., 1979). Ingestion of 650 mg of phenacetin by volunteers resulted in a maximum plasma phenacetin concentration of 2.2 mg/L after 30 minutes and a maximum acetaminophen concentration of 7.1 mg/L after 90 minutes, declining to 2.7 mg/L by 5 hours (Prescott et al., 1970). Following oral administration of 1800 mg of phenacetin, an average peak plasma phenacetin concentration of 8.4 mg/L (range, 0.8–19.2) and a peak acetaminophen concentration of 11.5 mg/L (range, 5.4–18.2) each occurred at 2 hours (Prescott et al., 1968). The particle size of the phenacetin in the dosage form was found to have a dramatic influence on the resulting plasma phenacetin concentrations, although the acetaminophen levels were much less affected by this variable. The elimination half-life of phenacetin has been found to average 48 minutes (Shively and Vesell, 1975).

Metabolism and Excretion. Only about 0.2% of a dose of phenacetin is excreted unchanged in the urine. Acetaminophen is the major metabolite and is formed rapidly following therapeutic doses. Approximately 56% of a dose of phenacetin is excreted in the 24 hour urine as conjugated acetaminophen and 2.5% as free acetaminophen; deacetylation of phenacetin to p-phenetidin followed by 2-hydroxylation and conjugation resulted in the excretion of 1.9% of the dose as 2-hydroxyphenetidin, probably as the sulfate conjugate (Thomas et al., 1972). This latter metabolite is unstable and its degradation products may account for the yellow pigment in the urine of persons receiving phenacetin. Phenacetin itself is oxidized in minor amounts to form 2-hydroxy-, 3-hydroxy- and N-hydroxy-phenacetin, and these metabolites, as well as p-phenetidin, are often implicated in the nephrotoxic, hemolytic and methemoglobinemic effects associated with phenacetin therapy (Prescott et al., 1968).

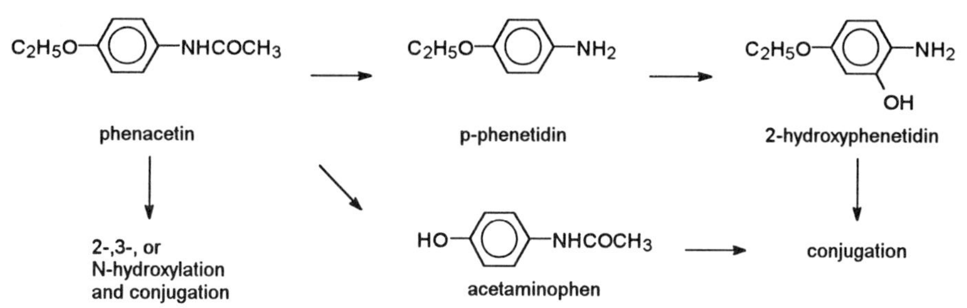

Toxicity. Chronic excessive intake of phenacetin, especially in combination with other analgesics, can lead to nephritis, renal tubular disease, and papillary necrosis (Fifield, 1963; Nanra, 1976). Certain individuals develop methemoglobinemia even after therapeutic amounts of the drug; 2 such patients were found to excrete 16–34% of a dose as conjugated p-hydroxyphenetidin, compared to 3–8% in normal subjects (Shahidi and Hemaidan, 1969). Hemolytic anemia and sulfhemoglobinemia have been produced in persons who abuse the drug (Basset et al., 1981).

Very little information is available on the human distribution of phenacetin or levels to be expected in fatal poisoning. Serum concentrations of total p-aminophenol ranging from 45–250 mg/L have been detected in cases of known or suspected phenacetin overdosage (Clarke, 1969). In addition, a blood phenacetin concentration of 136 mg/L was determined in a case of death due to intentional overdosage of a preparation containing codeine, aspirin, phenacetin and caffeine. The codeine and salicylate blood concentrations were 5.3 and 265 mg/L, respectively (Wright et al., 1975).

Analysis. Phenacetin in biological samples may be estimated colorimetrically following diazotization (Brodie and Axelrod, 1949), or more specifically by gas chromatography after trimethylsilyl derivatization (Prescott, 1971). Recently, both liquid chromatography (Gotelli et al., 1977; Mineshita et al., 1986) and gas chromatography-mass spectrometry (Garland et al., 1977) have been applied to the analysis of phenacetin and its major metabolites.

References

P. Basset, J.P. Bergerat, J.M. Lang et al. Hemolytic anemia and sulfhemoglobinemia due to phenacetin abuse: a case with multivisceral adverse effects. Clin. Tox. 18: 493–499, 1981.

B.B. Brodie and J. Axelrod. Metabolic fate of acetophenetidin in man. J. Pharm. Exp. Ther. 97: 58–67, 1949.

E.G.C. Clarke (ed.). *Isolation and Identification of Drugs*, Pharmaceutical Press, London, 1969, p. 478.

M.M. Fifield. Renal disease associated with prolonged use of acetophenetidin-containing compounds. New Eng. J. Med. 269: 722–726, 1963.

J.W.A. Findlay, R.L. DeAngelis, R.F. Butz et al. Disposition of phenacetin in dog and man determined by a sensitive and specific radioimmunoassay. J. Pharm. Exp. Ther. 210: 127–133, 1979.

W.A. Garland, K.C. Hsiao, E.J. Pantuck and A.H. Conney. Quantitative determination of phenacetin and its metabolite acetaminophen by GLC-chemical ionization mass spectrometry. J. Pharm. Sci. 66: 340–344, 1977.

G.R. Gotelli, P.M. Kabra and L.J. Marton. Determination of acetaminophen and phenacetin in plasma by high-pressure liquid chromatography. Clin. Chem. 23: 957–959, 1977.

S. Mineshita, R. Eggers, N.R. Kitteringham and E.E. Ohnhaus. Determination of phenacetin and its major metabolites in human plasma and urine by high-performance liquid chromatography. J. Chrom. 380: 407–413, 1986.

R.S. Nanra. Analgesic nephropathy. Med. J. Aust. 1: 745–748, 1976.

L.F. Prescott, M. Sansur, W. Levin and A.H. Conney. The comparative metabolism of phenacetin and N-acetyl-p-aminophenol in man, with particular reference to effects on the kidney. Clin. Pharm. Ther. 9: 605–614, 1968.

L.F. Prescott, R.F. Steel and W.R. Ferrier. The effects of particle size on the absorption of phenacetin in man. Clin. Pharm. Ther. 11: 496–504, 1970.

L.F. Prescott. The gas-liquid chromatographic estimation of phenacetin and paracetamol in plasma and urine. J. Pharm. Fharmac. 23: 111–115, 1971.

N.T. Shahidi and A. Hemaidan. Acetophenetidin-induced methemoglobinemia and its relation to the excretion of diazotizable amines. J. Lab. Clin. Med. 74: 581–585, 1969.

C.A. Shively and E.S. Vesell. Temporal variations in acetaminophen and phenacetin half-life in man. Clin. Pharm. Ther. 18: 413–424, 1975.

H.H. Thomas, B.B. Coldwell, W. Zeitz and G. Solomonraj. Effect of aspirin, caffeine, and codeine on the metabolism of phenacetin and acetaminophen. Clin. Pharm. Ther. 13: 906–910, 1972.

J.A. Wright, R.C. Baselt and C.H. Hine. Blood codeine concentrations in fatalities associated with codeine. Clin. Tox. 8: 457–463, 1975.

Phencyclidine

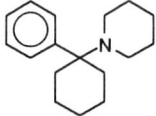

T½: 7–46 hr
Vd: 5.3–7.5 L/kg
Fb: 0.65
pKa: 8.5

Occurrence and Usage. Phencyclidine (1-phenylcyclohexylpiperidine, PCP, Sernyl, Sernylan) is a popular drug of abuse, as well as being a legitimate veterinary tranquilizer. The drug is structurally related to ketamine and was first developed for possible human use as an intravenous anesthetic agent. It is self-administered either by smoking (amounts of 1–3 mg applied to plant material), by nasal insufflation and intravenous injection (1–3 mg) or by oral ingestion (2–6 mg). These doses typically result in lethargy, disorientation, hallucinations and loss of coordination (Lundberg et al., 1976). The compound is prepared from 1-piperidinocyclohexanecarbonitrile in a Grignard reaction, as first performed in 1956. Currently, a number of PCP analogues prepared in the like manner with similar pharmacological effects are in vogue as street drugs, including cyclohexamine (PCE), phenylcyclohexylpyrrolidine (PHP), phenylcyclopentylpiperidine (PCPP), and thienylcyclohexylpiperidine (TCP):

| PCE | PHP | PCPP | TCP |

Blood Concentrations. No controlled pharmacokinetic studies of PCP in humans using psychoactive doses have been performed, although the widespread abuse of this drug has permitted the estimation of several parameters. In 26 subjects arrested for driving under the influence of drugs or of being intoxicated in public, blood phencyclidine concentrations were found to range from 0.007–0.240 mg/L with an average of 0.075 mg/L (Pearce, 1976). The plasma half-life of PCP has been variously estimated at 11–13 hours (Marshman et al., 1976; Wall et al., 1981) and 7–46 hours (average, 21) (Cook et al., 1982), although values of 1–4 days have been observed in cases of severe poisoning (Done et al., 1977). The blood/plasma concentration ratio for the drug averages 1.0 (Cook et al., 1982).

Metabolism and Excretion. Evidence indicates that PCP undergoes oxidative metabolism to at least 2 inactive metabolites, 4-phenyl-4-piperidinocyclohexanol and 1-(1-phenylcyclohexyl)-4-hydroxypiperidine, which are excreted as glucuronide conjugates in the urine (Ober et al., 1963; Lin et al., 1975; Wong and Biemann, 1976). A third metabolite, 5-(1-phenylcyclohexylamino)valeric acid, has been reported present in the urine of asymptomatic PCP users at concentrations of 0.027–

1.388 mg/L, similar to those of the parent drug (Syracuse et al., 1986; Elsohly et al., 1988). From 30–50% of a labeled intravenous dose is eliminated in the 72 hour urine as unchanged drug (4–19%) and conjugated metabolites (25–30%). Only 2% of a dose is excreted in feces. An average of 77% of an intravenous dose is found in urine and feces after 10 days (Wall et al., 1981).

Concentrations of unchanged drug in the urine of ambulatory users of PCP were most frequently between 0.04 and 3.4 mg/L (Green et al., 1976). The renal clearance of PCP is increased markedly with acidification of the urine (Done et al., 1977).

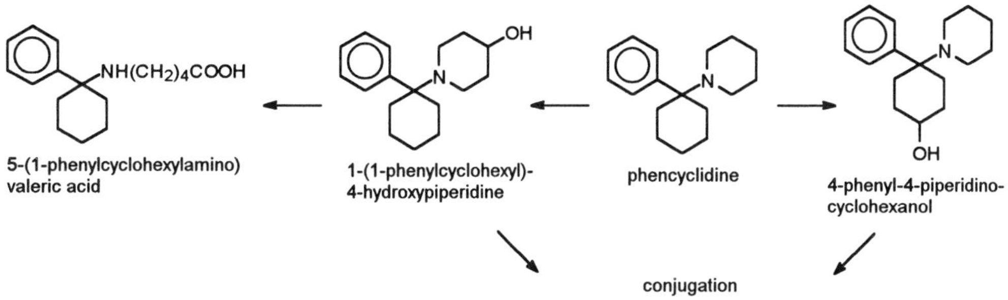

5-(1-phenylcyclohexylamino) valeric acid

1-(1-phenylcyclohexyl)-4-hydroxypiperidine

phencyclidine

4-phenyl-4-piperidino-cyclohexanol

conjugation

Toxicity. Phencyclidine is capable of causing sedation, nystagmus, hypertension, ataxia, agitation, combativeness, seizures, spasticity, coma, and respiratory depression. Four patients exhibiting signs ranging from disorientation to coma had plasma concentrations of 0.09–0.22 mg/L, with an average of 0.18 mg/L (Marshman et al., 1976). Urine concentrations in 19 intoxicated patients ranged from 0.4–340 mg/L (Burns and Lerner, 1976). Neither plasma nor urine phencyclidine concentrations appear to relate to the degree of intoxication in the many patients studied (Bailey, 1979; McCarron et al., 1981). In severe cases, administration of ammonium chloride or ascorbic acid to acidify both blood and urine causes a shift of phencyclidine out of the brain and enhances its renal excretion (Done et al., 1979; Giannini et al., 1987).

The phencyclidine precursor, 1-piperidinocyclohexanecarbonitrile, is found in about 20% of the illicit samples of phencyclidine tested, in amounts of up to 68 mole%. This substance is more toxic than phencyclidine, and is suspected of releasing cyanide *in vivo* (Bailey et al., 1976; Ballinger and Marshman, 1979; Soine et al., 1979; Cone et al., 1980; Soine et al., 1980).

Death has been known to result following the ingestion of only 120 mg of PCP. The following tissue distribution was observed in 17 deaths due to accidental or intentional ingestion of the drug (Reynolds, 1976; Noguchi and Nakamura, 1978; Caplan et al., 1979; Cravey et al., 1979):

Phencyclidine Concentrations in Fatalities (mg/L or mg/kg)

	Blood	Brain	Liver	Urine	Gastric
Average	4.8	7.3	23	35	155 mg
(Range)	(0.3–25)	(0.1–32)	(0.9–170)	(0.4–120)	(0–840)

Analysis. Phencyclidine may be assayed in biological specimens by gas chromatography with detection by flame-ionization (Marshman et al., 1976; Reynolds, 1976; Kammerer et al., 1980), nitrogen-phosphorus (Lewellen et al., 1979; Bailey and Guba, 1980; Miceli et al., 1981; Werner et al., 1986; Kandiko et al., 1990), or mass spectrometry (Lin et al., 1975; Green et al., 1976; Pearce, 1976; Cone et al., 1981; Stevenson et al., 1992). Reagents are commercially available for detection of urinary PCP by immunoassay.

References

D.N. Bailey. Phencyclidine abuse. Am. J. Clin. Path. 72: 795–799, 1979.

D.N. Bailey and J.J. Guba. Gas-chromatographic analysis for phencyclidine in plasma, with use of a nitrogen detector. Clin. Chem. 26: 437–440, 1980.

K. Bailey, A.Y.K. Chow, R.H. Downie and R.K. Pike. 1-Piperidinocyclohexanecarbonitrile, a toxic precursor of phencyclidine. J. Pharm. Pharmac. 28: 713–714, 1976.

J.R. Ballinger and J.A. Marshman. GLC quantitation of 1-piperidinocyclohexanecarbonitrile (PCC) in illicit phencyclidine (PCP). J. Anal. Tox. 3: 158–161, 1979.

R.S. Burns and S.E. Lerner. Perspectives: acute phencyclidine intoxication. Clin. Tox. 9: 477–501, 1976.

Y.H. Caplan, K.G. Orloff, B.C. Thompson and R.S. Fisher. Detection of phencyclidine in medical examiner's cases. J. Anal. Tox. 3: 47–52, 1979.

E.J. Cone, D.B. Vaupel and W.F. Buchwald. Phencyclidine: detection and measurement of toxic precursors and analogs in illicit samples. J. Anal. Tox. 4: 119–123, 1980.

E.J. Cone, W. Buchwald and D. Yousefnejad. Simultaneous determination of phencyclidine and monohydroxylated metabolites in urine of man by gas chromatography-mass fragmentography with methane chemical ionization. J. Chrom. 223: 331–339, 1981.

C.E. Cook, D.R. Brine, A.R. Jeffcoat et al. Phencyclidine disposition after intravenous and oral doses. Clin. Pharm. Ther. 31: 625–634, 1982.

R.H. Cravey, D. Reed and J.L. Ragle. Phencyclidine-related deaths: a report of nine fatal cases. J. Anal. Tox. 3: 199–201, 1979.

A.K. Done, R. Aronow, J.N. Miceli and D.C.K. Lin. Pharmacokinetic observations in the treatment of phencyclidine poisoning. A preliminary report. In *Management of the Poisoned Patient* (B.H. Rumack and A.R. Temple, eds.), Science Press, Princeton, 1977, pp. 79–102.

A. Done, R. Aronow, J. Miceli and S. Cohen. Pharmacokinetic bases for the treatment of phencyclidine (PCP) intoxication. Vet. Hum. Tox. 21: 104–107, 1979.

M.A. ElSohly, T.L. Little, J.M. Mitchell et al. GC/MS analysis of phencyclidine and acid metabolite in human urine. J. Anal. Tox. 12: 180–182, 1988.

A.J. Giannini, R.H. Loiselle, L.R. DiMarzio and M.C. Giannini. Augmentation of haloperidol by ascorbic acid in phencyclidine intoxication. Am. J. Psych. 144: 1207–1209, 1987.

D.E. Green, F.C. Chao, K.O. Loeffler and R. Lemon. Phencyclidine blood levels by probability based matching GC/MS. Proc. West. Pharm. Soc. 19: 355–361, 1976.

R.C. Kammerer, E.D. Stefano and D. Schmitz. A gas-liquid chromatography assay for phencyclidine and its metabolites. J. Anal. Tox. 4: 293–298, 1980.

C.T. Kandiko, S. Browning, T. Cooper and W.A. Cox. Detection of low-nanogram quantities of phencyclidine extracted from human urine. J. Chrom. 528: 208–213, 1990.

L.J. Lewellen, E.T. Solomons and F.L. O'Brien. Nitrogen-sensitive gas chromatographic detection and quantitation of nanogram levels of phencyclidine in whole blood. J. Anal. Tox. 3: 72–75, 1979.

D.C.K. Lin, A.F. Fentiman, Jr. and R.L. Foltz. Quantitation of phencyclidine in body fluids by gas chromatography chemical ionization mass spectrometry and identification of two metabolites. Biomed. Mass Spec. 2: 206–214, 1975.

G.D. Lundberg, R.C. Gupta and S.H. Montgomery. Phencyclidine: patterns seen in street drug analysis. Clin. Tox. 9: 503–511, 1976.

J.A. Marshman, M.P. Ramsay and E.M. Sellers. Quantitation of phencyclidine in biological fluids and application to human overdose. Tox. Appl. Pharm. 35: 129–136, 1976.

M.M. McCarron, B.W. Schulze, G.A. Thompson et al. Acute phencyclidine intoxication: incidence of clinical findings in 1,000 cases. Ann. Emerg. Med. 10: 237–242, 1981.

J.N. Miceli, D.B. Bowman and M.K. Aravind. An improved method for the quantitation of phencyclidine (PCP) in biological samples utilizing nitrogen-detection gas chromatography. J. Anal. Tox. 5: 29–32, 1981.

T.T. Noguchi and G.R. Nakamura. Phencyclidine-related deaths in Los Angeles County, 1976. J. For. Sci. 23: 503–507, 1978.

R.E. Ober, G.W. Gwynn, T. Chang et al. Metabolism of 1-(1-phenylcyclohexyl) piperidine (Sernyl). Fed. Proc. 22: 539, 1963.

D.S. Pearce. Detection and quantitation of phencyclidine in blood by use of (^{2}H$_5$) phencyclidine and select ion monitoring applied to nonfatal cases of phencyclidine intoxication. Clin. Chem. 22: 1623–1626, 1976.

P.C. Reynolds. Clinical and forensic experiences with phencyclidine. Clin. Tox. 9: 547–552, 1976.

W.H. Soine, W.C. Vincek and D.T. Agee. Phencyclidine contaminant generates cyanide. New Eng. J. Med. 301: 438, 1979.

W.H. Soine, W.C. Vincek, D.T. Agee et al. Contamination of illicit phencyclidine with 1-piperidino-cyclohexanecarbonitrile. J. Anal. Tox. 4: 217–221, 1980.

C.C. Stevenson, D.L. Cibull, G.E. Platoff, Jr., et al. Solid phase extraction of phencyclidine from urine followed by capillary gas chromatography/mass spectrometry. J. Anal. Tox. 16: 337–339, 1992.

C.D. Syracuse, B.R. Kuhnert, N.L. Golden and B.S. Bagby. Measurement of the amino acid metabolite of phencyclidine by selected ion monitoring. Biomed. Env. Mass Spec. 13: 113–115, 1986.

M.E. Wall, D.R. Brine, A.R. Jeffcoat et al. Phencyclidine metabolism and disposition in man following a 100 µg intravenous dose. Res. Comm. Sub. Abuse 2: 161–172, 1981.

M. Werner, M. Hertzman and C.J. Pauley. Gas-liquid chromatography of phencyclidine in serum, with nitrogen-phosphorus detection. Clin. Chem. 32: 1921–1924, 1986.

L.K. Wong and K. Biemann. Metabolites of phencyclidine. Clin. Tox. 9: 583–591, 1976.

Phendimetrazine

T½: ?
Vd: ?
Fb: ?
pKa: 7.6

Occurrence and Usage. Phendimetrazine (Bontril, Plegine, Prelu-2, Statobex) is a phenethylamine derivative, synthesized in 1956, in which the ethylamino moiety is contained in a morpholine ring. The compound is used as an anorectic agent and has the sympathomimetic actions common to other drugs in this group. It is available as the tartrate salt of the d-isomer and is administered in single oral doses of 35 mg and total daily doses of up to 210 mg.

Blood Concentrations. After a single oral dose of 35 mg given to 5 adults, serum phendimetrazine concentrations averaged 0.090 mg/L at 1 hour and declined rapidly to 0.045 mg/L by 2 hours and 0.025 mg/L by 4 hours. Following a single oral administration of a sustained-release preparation containing 105 mg of the drug, serum concentrations reached a peak of only 0.052 mg/L at 1 hour, but remained at 0.044 mg/L after 6 hours and 0.036 mg/L after 12 hours (Hundt et al., 1975). With the ingestion of 105 mg of a normal formulation, plasma concentrations rose to 0.240 mg/L after 1 hour (Hadler, 1968).

Metabolism and Excretion. Phendimetrazine is metabolized primarily by N-demethylation to phenmetrazine, which is itself an active anorectic agent. The further biotransformation of this metabolite is discussed under phenmetrazine. Under conditions of acid urine only about 9% of a dose of phendimetrazine is excreted unchanged in the 24 hour urine, and up to 20% is eliminated as phenmetrazine (Beckett, 1969).

phendimetrazine → phenmetrazine

Toxicity. Overdosage with phendimetrazine can produce restlessness, confusion, hallucinations, sweating, dizziness, flushing, tachycardia, hypertension, arrhythmias, convulsions, coma, and circulatory collapse.

Two adult males who died suddenly following recreational use of the drug had postmortem blood phendimetrazine concentrations of 0.3 and 0.7 mg/L (Hood et al., 1988; Kintz et al., 1989).

Analysis. Gas chromatography has been used for the analysis of phendimetrazine, employing either flame-ionization (Beckett et al., 1967; Hundt et al., 1975; Kintz et al., 1989) or nitrogen-specific detection (Rudolph et al., 1983).

References

A.H. Beckett. Kinetics of the absorption and elimination of "amphetamines" in normal humans. In *Abuse of Central Stimulants* (F. Sjoqvist and M. Tottie, eds.), Almqvist and Wiksell, Stockholm, 1969, pp. 375–408.

A.H. Beckett, G.T. Tucker and A.C. Moffat. Routine detection and identification in urine of stimulants and other drugs, some of which may be used to modify performance in sport. J. Pharm. Pharmac. 19: 273–294, 1967.

A.J. Hadler. Sustained-action phendimetrazine in obesity. J. Clin. Pharm. 8: 113–117, 1968.

I. Hood, J. Monforte, R. Gault and H. Mirchandani. Fatality from illicit phendimetrazine use. Clin. Tox. 26: 249–255, 1988.

H.K.L. Hundt, E.C. Clark and F.O. Muller. GLC determination of phendimetrazine in serum. J. Pharm. Sci. 64: 1041–1043, 1975.

P. Kintz, A. Tracqui, P. Mangin et al. A simple gas chromatographic identification and determination of 11 CNS stimulants in biological samples. For. Sci. Int. 40: 153–159, 1989.

G.R. Rudolph, J.R. Miksic and M.J. Levitt. GLC determination of phendimetrazine in human plasma, serum, or urine. J. Pharm. Sci. 72: 519–521, 1983.

Phenelzine

T½: 1.5–4.0 hr
Vd: ?
Fb: ?
pKa: ?

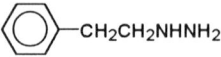

Occurrence and Usage. Phenelzine (beta-phenylethylhydrazine, Nardil) is a monoamine oxidase inhibitor that has been used since the 1960's as an antidepressant agent. It is available as the sulfate in tablets of 15 mg. Daily oral doses of 45–90 mg are recommended, and usually must be continued for at least 4 weeks before a response is apparent.

Blood Concentrations. A single 30 mg oral dose given to a volunteer produced a peak plasma concentration of 2.0 μg/L at 2 hours, which declined to 1.0 μg/L by 3 hours and 0.2 μg/L by 6 hours. Very similar concentrations were observed in a patient who had been receiving 30 mg of the drug daily for 6 weeks, and who had a plasma phenelzine trough level of 0.1 μg/L (Cooper et al., 1978).

Metabolism and Excretion. The instability of phenelzine has made the study of its biotransformation difficult. It is believed to be metabolized by N-acetylation, since patients who are rapid acetylators tend to excrete more phenelzine-related products in the urine. From 0.25–1.1% of a single oral dose is excreted in the 24 hour urine as products that react as phenelzine using nonspecific methods (Gelbicova-Ruzickova et al., 1971; Caddy et al., 1978). From 17–49% of a dose is eliminated as phenylacetic acid and from 16–31% as p-hydroxyphenylacetic acid in the 96 hour urine (Robinson et al., 1985).

Toxicity. Adverse reactions to this drug include postural hypotension, systemic lupus erythematosus, and fatal hepatocellular necrosis. Severe hypertensive reactions have occurred in patients concurrently receiving anticholinergic agents, narcotic analgesics, tricyclic antidepressants, or fermented foods high in tyramine content. Overdosage with phenelzine results in drowsiness, dizziness, irritability, ataxia, hypotension, headache, excessive sweating, tachycardia, rapid and shallow respiration, coma, convulsions, and circulatory collapse.

Two individuals who ingested large amounts of the drug had blood phenelzine concentrations of 1.5 and 2.0 mg/L, while the postmortem urine from a suicide victim contained 58 mg/L (Caddy et al., 1976; Caddy and Stead, 1978). The following concentrations were observed postmortem in an adult male who intentionally ingested up to 2250 mg of phenelzine (Hansson, 1990):

Phenelzine Concentrations in a Fatal Case (mg/L or mg/kg)

Blood	Liver	Urine	Gastric
2.7	89	142	4 mg

Analysis. Phenelzine is extremely unstable at alkaline pH, and so most procedures for its measurement in biological fluids involve derivatization prior to extraction. The drug has been measured in urine by gas chromatography after oxidation (Gelbicova-R·ιzickova et al., 1971; Caddy and Stead, 1977) or acetonide formation (Caddy et al., 1976; Lichtenwainer et al., 1988). Its assay has been accomplished by electron-capture gas chromatography of a halogenated derivative (Cooper et al., 1978; Rao et al., 1987), or by derivatization prior to extraction and gas chromatography-mass spectrometry (Jindal et al., 1980).

References

B. Caddy, W.J. Tilstone and E.C. Johnstone. Phenelzine in urine: assay and relation to acetylator status. Brit. J. Clin. Pharm. 3: 633–637, 1976.

B. Caddy and A.H. Stead. Indirect determination of phenelzine in urine. Analyst 102: 42–49, 1977.

B. Caddy and A.H. Stead. Three cases of poisoning involving the drug phenelzine. J. For. Sci. Soc. 18: 207–208, 1978.

B. Caddy, A.H. Stead and E.C. Johnstone. The urinary excretion of phenelzine. Brit. J. Clin. Pharm. 6: 185–188, 1978.

T.B. Cooper, D.S. Robinson and A. Nies. Phenelzine measurement in human plasma: a sensitive GLC-ECD procedure. Comm. Psychopharm. 2: 505–512, 1978.

J. Gelbicova-Ruzickova, J. Novak and B. Chundela. Determination of β–phenylethylhydrazine in pharmaceuticals and urine by gas chromatography. Biochem. Med. 5: 537–547, 1971.

R.C. Hansson. Personal communication, 1990.

S.P. Jindal, T. Lutz and T.B. Cooper. Determination of phenelzine in human plasma with gas chromatography-mass spectrometry using an isotope labeled internal standard. J. Chrom. 221: 301–308, 1980.

M. Lichtenwainer, M. McMullin, D. Hardy and F. Rieders. Quantitative determination of phenelzine in human fluids by gas chromatography with nitrogen specific detection. J. Anal. Tox. 98–101, 1988.

T.S. Rao, G.B. Baker, R.T. Coutts et al. Analysis of the antidepressant phenelzine in brain tissue and urine using electron-capture gas chromatography. J. Pharm. Meth. 17: 297–304, 1987.

D.S. Robinson, T.B. Cooper, S.P. Jindal et al. Metabolism and pharmacokinetics of phenelzine: lack of evidence for acetylation pathway in humans. J. Clin. Pharm. 5: 333–337, 1985.

Phenformin

T½: 5–15 hr
Vd: 5–10 L/kg
Fb: 0.20
pKa: 11.8

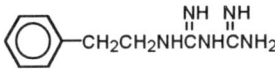

Occurrence and Usage. Phenformin (beta-phenylethylbiguanide, DBI, Dibotin) is a biguanide derivative that has been in clinical use since 1956 as a hypoglycemic agent for the treatment of adult diabetes. It is administered as the hydrochloride in daily oral doses of 25–200 mg as tablets or sustained-release capsules. It was withdrawn from the United States market in 1977 due to its propensity for causing serious, often fatal, lactic acidosis.

Blood Concentrations. A 50 mg capsule of phenformin given orally to one subject produced a maximum plasma concentration of 0.145 mg/L after 3–4 hours, declining to 0.060 mg/L by 10 hours and 0.020 mg/L by 24 hours (Karam et al., 1974). The elimination half-life of the drug averaged 11 hours in 2 volunteers (Alkalay et al., 1975). In 6 volunteers given 50 mg as a sustained-release capsule, plasma concentrations averaged 0.039 mg/L at 3.5 hours and 0.025 mg/L at 9.5 hours (Nattrass et al., 1980). Eight diabetics receiving 50 mg of phenformin every 8 hours had plasma levels averaging 0.178 mg/L (range, 0.102–0.241) at 2 hours after a dose (Karam et al., 1974).

Metabolism and Excretion. Phenformin is inactivated by p-hydroxylation. An average of 45% of a labeled oral dose is eliminated in the 24 hour urine as unchanged drug (about 30%) and as free p-hydroxyphenformin (about 15%). Unabsorbed drug probably represents the remainder of the dose (Beckman, 1968).

phenformin → p-hydroxyphenformin

Toxicity. Severe lactic acidosis has been produced in hundreds of patients who have either become chronically intoxicated or who suffered an acute reaction due to hypersensitivity or an overdose. The survival rate in these individuals has been on the order of 50% (Luft et al., 1978). Seven patients with lactic acidosis had serum phenformin levels of 0.020–0.625 mg/L, and 3 exhibited drug half-lives of 5–30 hours (Conlay et al., 1977).

Postmortem concentrations of 3 mg/L in blood and 60 mg/kg in liver were detected in a fatality that occurred 30 hours after the ingestion of about 1500 mg of phenformin by an adult, who died in a state of hypoglycemia and severe acidosis (Bingle et al., 1970). Another fatality has been recorded in which concentrations of 3.7 mg/L in blood and 24 mg/kg in liver were measured (Registry, 1978).

Analysis. A colorimetric technique for the determination of phenformin in biological specimens has been described (Freedman et al., 1961), but does not have sufficient sensitivity for the measurement of therapeutic plasma concentrations. Electron-capture gas chromatography of an acyl derivative is suitable for this purpose (Matin et al., 1975), as is liquid chromatography (Hill and Chamberlain, 1978). The latter technique has also been applied to the analysis of phenformin and p-hydroxyphenformin in urine (Oates et al., 1980).

References

D. Alkalay, L. Khemani, W.E. Wagner, Jr. and M.F. Bartlett. Pharmacokinetics of phenformin in man. J. Clin. Pharm. 15: 446–448, 1975.

R. Beckmann. The fate of biguanides in man. Ann. N.Y. Acad. Sci. 148: 820–832, 1968.

J.P. Bingle, G.W. Storey and J.M. Winter. Fatal self-poisoning with phenformin. Brit. Med. J. 3: 752, 1970.

L.A. Conlay, J.H. Karam, S.B. Matin and J.E. Loewenstein. Serum phenformin concentrations in patients with phenformin-associated lactic acidosis. Diabetes 26: 628–631, 1977.

L. Freedman, M. Blitz, E. Gunsberg and S. Zak. Determination of phenformin in biologic fluids and tissues. J. Lab. Clin. Med. 58: 662–666, 1961.

H.M. Hill and J. Chamberlain. Determination of oral anti-diabetic agents in human body fluids using high-performance liquid chromatography. J. Chrom. 149: 349–358, 1978.

J. Karam, S. Matin, S. Levin and P.H. Forsham. Circulating phenformin (Pf) levels: implications as to Pf's therapeutic action. Diabetes 23 (Suppl. 1): 375, 1974.

D. Luft, R.M. Schmuelling and M. Eggstein. Lactic acidosis in biguanide-treated diabetics. Diabetologia 14: 75–87, 1978.

S.B. Matin, J.H. Karam and P.H. Forsham. Simple electron capture gas chromatographic method for the determination of oral hypoglycemic biguanides in biological fluids. Anal. Chem. 47: 545–548, 1975.

M. Nattrass, K. Sizer and K.G.M.M. Alberti. Correlation of plasma phenformin concentration with metabolic effects in normal subjects. Clin. Sci. 58: 153–155, 1980.

N.S. Oates, R.R. Shah, J.R. Idle and R.L. Smith. On the urinary disposition of phenformin and 4-hydroxy-phenformin and their rapid simultaneous measurement. J. Pharm. Pharmac. 32: 731–732, 1980.

Registry of Human Toxicology, American Academy of Forensic Sciences, 1978.

Pheniramine

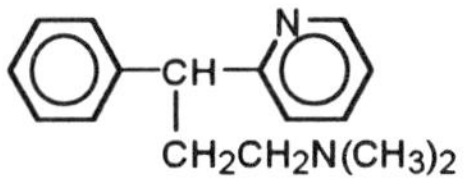

T½: 8–19 hr
Vd: 1.9–3.0 L/kg
Fb: ?
pKa: 4.2, 9.3

Occurrence and Usage. Pheniramine (ingredient of Dristan, Triaminic) is an antihistaminic agent that has been widely used for more than 20 years. The drug is usually found in combination with decongestants, antitussives, expectorants and analgesics. It is available in a variety of forms in single doses of 8–16 mg as the maleate salt.

Blood Concentrations. Blood pheniramine concentrations ranged from 0.01–0.19 mg/L (average, 0.11) 2 hours after oral administration of 75 mg to 6 adults weighing 57–81 kg (Queree et al., 1979). After intravenous administration of 30.5 mg of the free base to 3 subjects, serum pheniramine concentrations were initially as high as 0.23–0.89 mg/L. Following oral administration of the same dose to 3 adults, peak serum pheniramine concentrations of 0.17–0.27 mg/L were reached after 1–2.5 hours. Norpheniramine was present in serum in trace amounts (up to 0.02 mg/L) and was still detectable after 72 hours (Witte et al., 1985).

Metabolism and Excretion. Pheniramine is biotransformed in man to norpheniramine and dinorpheniramine. In a study of one subject following a single dose of pheniramine, 24% of the dose was excreted in the urine unchanged, 26% as norpheniramine and less than 1% as dinorpheniramine (Kabasakalian et al., 1968). The recovery in urine ranged from 68–94% of the dose after intravenous injection and 70–83% after oral administration (Whitte et al., 1985).

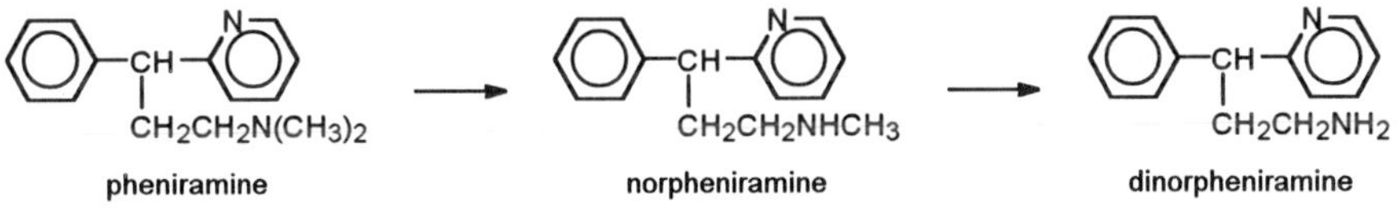

pheniramine   norpheniramine   dinorpheniramine

Toxicity. Adverse reactions to pheniramine in overdosage include agitation, hallucinations, disorientation, delirium, cardiac arrhythmias, coma and death (Bobik and McLean, 1976; Mendelson, 1976; Mendelson, 1977).

The following tissue distribution was noted in 3 fatal cases that involved overdosage of pheniramine (Queree et al., 1979; Chan, 1983):

Pheniramine Concentrations in Fatal Cases (mg/L or mg/kg)

	Blood	Liver	Urine	Gastric
Average	14	52	256	228 mg
(Range)	(1.9–30)	(6.6–115)	(149–362)	(135–320)

Analysis. Pheniramine has been determined in biological samples by gas chromatography with flame-ionization (Bobik and McLean, 1976) and nitrogen-phosphorus detection (Queree et al., 1979).

References

A. Bobik and A.J. McLean. Cardiovascular complications due to pheniramine overdosage. Aust. N.Z. J. Med. 6: 65–67, 1976.

L.F.T. Chan. Personal communication, 1983.

P. Kabasakalian, M. Taggert and E. Townley. Urinary excretion of pheniramine and its N-demethylated metabolites in man—comparison with chlorpheniramine and brompheniramine data. J. Pharm. Sci. 57: 621–623, 1968.

G. Mendelson. Accidental poisoning: pheniramine. Med. J. Aust. 63: 110, 1976.

G. Mendelson. Pheniramine aminosalicylate overdosage. Arch. Neurol. 34: 313, 1977.

E.A. Queree, S.J. Dickson and A.W. Missen. Therapeutic and toxic levels of pheniramine in biological specimens. J. Anal. Tox. 3: 253–255, 1979.

P.U. Witte, R. Irmisch and P. Hajdu. Pharmacokinetics of pheniramine (Avil) and metabolites in healthy subjects after oral and intravenous administration. Int. J. Clin. Pharm. Ther. Tox. 23: 59–62, 1985.

Phenmetrazine

T½: 8 hr
Vd: ?
Fb: ?
pKa: 8.5

Occurrence and Usage. Phenmetrazine (Preludin) is the N-desmethyl analogue of phendimetrazine. It was synthesized in 1958 and is currently used as an anorectic agent. The compound is available for oral use as the hydrochloride salt in single doses of 25 mg and daily doses of up to 75 mg. Like amphetamine, phenmetrazine has a high potential for abuse, and its use in certain countries has been restricted or banned.

Blood Concentrations. Following a single oral 75 mg dose given to 6 volunteers, plasma concentrations reached an average peak of 0.13 mg/L (range, 0.00–0.24) at 2 hours and slowly declined to 0.11 mg/L by 5 hours and 0.06 mg/L after 12 hours. The plasma half-life of the drug was found to average 8 hours. After ingestion of a 75 mg sustained-release tablet, the average peak plasma concentration in 6 volunteers was only about 0.07 mg/L at 5 hours (Quinn et al., 1967).

Metabolism and Excretion. Phenmetrazine is metabolized by p-hydroxylation and conjugation, and also by oxidation at the 3-position in the morpholine ring to a lactam. N-hydroxylation may occur to a certain extent. The morpholine ring appears to be metabolically stable. About 19% of a dose is eliminated unchanged in the 24 hour urine, with another 19% present as the lactam (5-methyl-3-oxo-6-phenylmorpholine), 12% and 10% as free and conjugated p-hydroxyphenmetrazine, respectively, and 5% as an N-hydroxyphenmetrazine nitrone breakdown product (Franklin et al., 1977). During conditions of acid urine, as much as 46% of a dose is eliminated in the urine within 16 hours (Beckett, 1969).

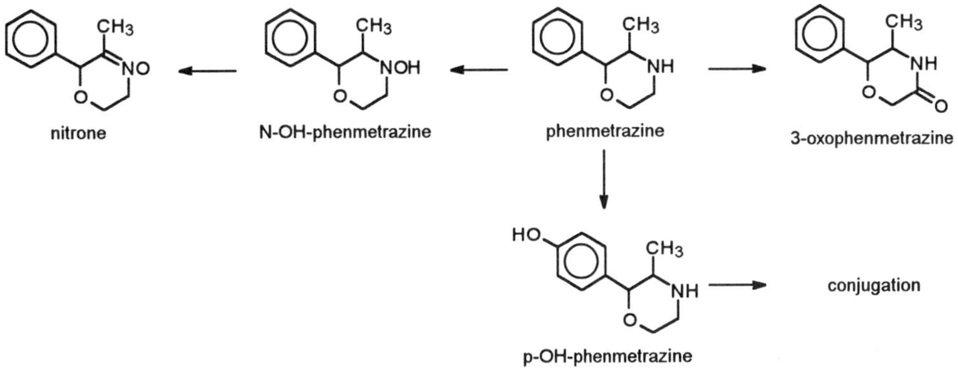

| nitrone | N-OH-phenmetrazine | phenmetrazine | 3-oxophenmetrazine |

p-OH-phenmetrazine

conjugation

Toxicity. Phenmetrazine overdosage produced dizziness, anxiety, tremor, headache, tachycardia, hypertension, confusion, rapid breathing, hallucinations, aggressive behavior, cardiac arrhythmias, convulsions, coma, and circulatory collapse.

Phenmetrazine concentrations of 0.5–4.0 mg/L in blood and 56–290 mg/L in urine have been detected in 7 drug abusers who were arrested while driving motor vehicles (Bonnichsen et al., 1970). Cravey (1978) found the following concentrations in the tissues of an adult who committed suicide by gunfire: blood, 0.7 mg/L; brain, 0.8 mg/kg; liver, 2.5 mg/kg; and urine, 2.5 mg/L. In a fatal case that followed intravenous usage of the drug, a blood concentration of 4 mg/L, liver concentration of 5 mg/kg and urine concentration of 24 mg/L were observed (Norheim, 1973). The following distribution was obtained from a series of 12 fatalities (Gottschalk, 1977):

Phenmetrazine Concentrations in Fatalities (mg/L or mg/kg)

	Blood	Brain	Liver	Bile	Kidney	Urine
Average	1.1	2.9	3.1	5.5	1.5	21
(Range)	(0.1–4.9)	(0.1–15)	(0.1–20)	(0.2–23)	(0.1–8.0)	(0.1–90)

Analysis. Phenmetrazine has been analyzed in biological materials by flame-ionization gas chromatography of the underivatized drug (Beckett et al., 1967) or of the N-acetyl derivative (Franklin et al., 1977), and by radioacetylation (Quinn et al., 1967).

References

A.H. Beckett, G.T. Tucker and A.C. Moffat. Routine detection and identification in urine of stimulants and other drugs, some of which may be used to modify performance in sport. J. Pharm. Pharmac. 19: 273–294, 1967.

A.H. Beckett. Kinetics of the absorption and elimination of "amphetamine" in normal humans. In *Abuse of Central Stimulants* (F. Sjoqvist and M. Tottie, eds.), Almqvist and Wiksell, Stockholm, 1969, pp. 375–408.

R. Bonnichsen, A.C. Maehly, Y. Marde et al. Determination and identification of sympathomimetic amines in blood samples from drivers by a combination of gas chromatography and mass spectrometry. Z. Rechtsmed. 67: 19–26, 1970.

R.H. Cravey. Personal communication, 1978.

R.B. Franklin, L.G. Dring and R.T. Williams. The metabolism of phenmetrazine in man and laboratory animals. Drug Met. Disp. 5: 223–233, 1977.

L. Gottschalk. Personal communication, 1977.

G. Norheim. A fatal case of phenmetrazine poisoning. J. For. Sci. Soc. 13: 287–289, 1973.

G.P. Quinn, M.M. Cohn, M.B. Reid et al. The effect of formulation on phenmetrazine plasma levels in man studied by a sensitive analytical method. Clin. Pharm. Ther. 8: 369–373, 1967.

Phenobarbital

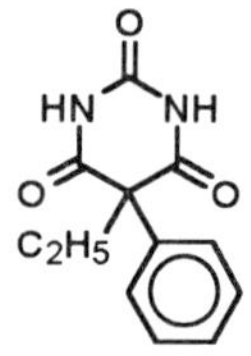

T½: 2–6 days
Vd: 0.5–0.6 L/kg
Fb: 0.50
pKa: 7.2

Occurrence and Usage. Phenobarbital is a barbiturate derivative that has been used as a daytime sedative and very extensively as an anticonvulsant since 1912. Phenobarbital is an excellent inducer of drug-metabolizing microsomal enzymes and its use often results in the lowering of plasma levels of other drugs. Its low oil/water partition coefficient relative to other barbiturates is the basis for its slow accumulation in brain tissue and its limited metabolism. The drug is available as either the free acid or the sodium salt in an elixir or as tablets of 15–65 mg for oral use, or in a 65–130 mg/mL solution for intramuscular or intravenous injection. It is often found in combination with bronchodilators, vasodilators, analgesics, and anticholinergic agents. It is generally administered to epileptic patients in oral doses of 60–200 mg daily, often in combination with other anticonvulsant drugs.

Blood Concentrations. A single 30 mg oral dose given to 3 volunteers produced an average peak serum concentration of about 0.7 mg/L, while the same dose repeated for 21 days resulted in an average peak level of 8.1 mg/L. Rather than inducing its own metabolism, phenobarbital appeared to have a longer half-life after repeated dosing (Viswanathan et al., 1979). Following oral administration of 600 mg of phenobarbital to volunteers, the average peak blood concentration measured 4.5 hours later was 18 mg/L (range, 12–26) (Parker et al., 1970).

With chronic administration of 200 mg daily to epileptic patients, blood concentrations averaged 29 mg/L and ranged from 16–48 mg/L (Plaa and Hine, 1960). Plasma concentrations of 10–30 mg/L are generally considered desirable in patients receiving phenobarbital as an anticonvulsant, and it may require 14–21 days to achieve a steady-state level. The compound has an average plasma half-life of approximately 4 days (Kutt and Penry, 1974).

Metabolism and Excretion. Biotransformation of phenobarbital occurs primarily by N-glucoside formation and by oxidation to p-hydroxyphenobarbital, which is consequently conjugated with glucuronic acid. A dihydrodihydroxyphenyl metabolite has also been identified in minor amounts and is thought to arise from an epoxide intermediate (Harvey et al., 1972). From 78–87% of a single labeled dose is excreted in the urine within 16 days as unchanged drug (25–33%), N-glucosylphenobarbital (24–30%), and free or conjugated p-hydroxyphenobarbital (18–19%) (Tang et al., 1979). In patients on chronic phenobarbital therapy, an average of 25% (range, 12–55%) of the dose is excreted unchanged in the 24 hour urine; 8% is excreted as free p-hydroxyphenobarbital and 9% as the glucuronide conjugate (Whyte and Dekaban, 1977). In volunteers receiving a single dose of 600 mg of phenobarbital, less than 2% was excreted unchanged in urine during the first 21 hours, and peak urine phenobarbital concentrations ranged from 8–22 mg/L (Parker et al., 1970).

The following concentrations are indicative of phenobarbital tissue distribution during therapy in an epileptic patient (Sakata et al., 1985):

Phenobarbital Concentrations During Therapy (mg/L or mg/kg)

Blood	Brain	Lung	Liver	Kidney	Urine
8.9	18	18	33	21	3.9

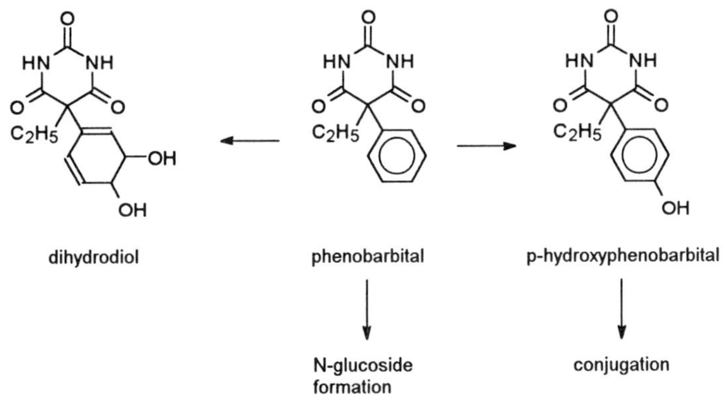

dihydrodiol   phenobarbital   p-hydroxyphenobarbital

N-glucoside   conjugation
formation

Toxicity. Toxic reactions to phenobarbital in chronically dosed subjects generally occur when plasma concentrations exceed 40 mg/L. Patients developing coma with reflexes present exhibited plasma concentrations of 65–117 mg/L, while those lacking deep tendon reflexes had concentrations of 100–134 mg/L (Sunshine, 1957). One patient survived overdosage with the drug after achieving a plasma phenobarbital level of 253 mg/L (Costello and Poklis, 1981).

In acute fatalities that occurred after ingestion of as little as 6 g of phenobarbital, blood concentrations ranged from 78–116 mg/L and liver concentrations from 89–266 mg/kg (Cravey, 1975). The following body distribution of phenobarbital was observed in the death of an epileptic patient (Bruce and Smith, 1977):

Phenobarbital Concentrations in a Fatal Case (mg/L or mg/kg)*

Blood	Brain	Liver	Bile	Kidney	Urine	Fat
64	63	138	75	84	38	46

*By gas chromatography of underivatized drug

Analysis. The classical approach to measurement of phenobarbital in biological specimens involves ultraviolet spectrophotometry (Goldbaum, 1952); this technique has been modified to allow the simultaneous determination of phenytoin, which otherwise would interfere with the assay (Wallace, 1969). Gas chromatography provides a more specific result and is usually performed with flame-ionization or nitrogen-selective detection of the free drug (Ritz and Warren, 1975) or its methylated derivative (Kananen et al., 1972; Vandemark and Adams, 1976). Gas chromatographic procedures have been described for determination of p-hydroxyphenobarbital in plasma and urine (Kallberg et al., 1975; Patel et al., 1980). Phenobarbital has been included in general liquid chromatographic schemes for the common anticonvulsant drugs (Kabra et al., 1978; Rainbow et al., 1990). Reagents are commercially available for determination of the drug by immunoassay.

References

A.M. Bruce and H. Smith. The investigation of phenobarbitone, phenytoin and primidone in the death of epileptics. Med. Sci. Law 17: 195–199, 1977.

J.B. Costello and A. Poklis. Treatment of massive phenobarbital overdose with dopamine diuresis. Arch. Int. Med. 141: 938–940, 1981.

R.H. Cravey. Personal communication, 1975.

L.R. Goldbaum. Determination of barbiturates. Anal. Chem. 24: 1604–1607, 1952.

D.J. Harvey, L. Glazener, C. Stratton et al. Detection of a 5-(3,4-dihydroxy-1,5-cyclohexadien-1-yl)-metabolite of phenobarbital and mephobarbital in rat, guinea pig and human. Res. Comm. Chem. Path. Pharm. 3: 557–565, 1972.

P.M. Kabra, D.M. McDonald and L.J. Marton. A simultaneous high-performance liquid chromatographic analysis of the most common anticonvulsants and their metabolites in the serum. J. Anal. Tox. 2: 127–133, 1978.

N. Kallberg, S. Agurell, O. Ericsson et al. Quantitation of phenobarbital and its main metabolites in human urine. Eur. J. Clin. Pharm. 9: 161–168, 1975.

G. Kananen, R. Osiewicz and I. Sunshine. Barbiturate analysis—a current assessment. J. Chrom. Sci. 10: 283–287, 1972.

H. Kutt and J.K. Penry. Usefulness of blood levels of antiepileptic drugs. Arch. Neurol. 31: 282–288, 1974.

K.D. Parker, H.W. Elliott, J.A. Wright et al. Blood and urine concentrations of subjects receiving barbiturates, meprobamate, glutethimide, or diphenylhydantoin. Clin. Tox. 3: 131–145, 1970.

I.H. Patel, R.H. Levy, J.M. Neal and W.F. Trager. Simultaneous analysis of phenobarbital and p-hydroxyphenobarbital in biological fluids by GLC-chemical-ionization mass spectrometry. J. Pharm. Sci. 69: 1218–1219, 1980.

G.L. Plaa and C.H. Hine. Hydantoin and barbiturate blood levels observed in epileptics. Arch. Int. Pharm. Ther. 128: 375–383, 1960.

S.J. Rainbow, C.M. Dawson and T.R. Tickner. Direct serum injection high-performance liquid chromatographic method for the simultaneous determination of phenobarbital, carbamazepine and phenytoin. J. Chrom. 527: 389–396, 1990.

D.P. Ritz and C.G. Warren. Single extraction of GLC analysis of six commonly prescribed antiepileptic drugs. Clin. Tox. 8: 311–324, 1975.

M. Sakata, K. Sakata, M. Haga et al. Distribution of antiepileptic drugs in human blood and tissue. In *Proceedings of the 21st International Meeting*, International Association of Forensic Toxicologists, Brighton, England, 1985.

I. Sunshine. Chemical evidence of tolerance to phenobarbital. J. Lab. Clin. Med. 50: 127–133, 1957.

B.K. Tang, W. Kalow and A.A. Grey. Metabolic fate of phenobarbital in man. Drug Met. Disp. 7: 315–318, 1979.

F.L. Vandemark and R.F. Adams. Ultramicro gas-chromatographic analysis for anticonvulsants, with use of nitrogen-selective detector. Clin. Chem. 22: 1062–1065, 1976.

C.T. Viswanathan, H.E. Booker and P.G. Welling. Pharmacokinetics of phenobarbital following single and repeated doses. J. Clin. Pharm. 19: 282–289, 1979.

J.E. Wallace. Simultaneous spectrophotometric determination of diphenylhydantoin and phenobarbital in biologic specimens. Clin. Chem. 14: 323–330, 1969.

M.P. Whyte and A.S. Dekaban. Metabolic fate of phenobarbital. Drug Met. Disp. 5: 63–70, 1977.

Phenol

T½: 30 min
Vd: ?
Fb: ?
pKa: 9.9

Occurrence and Usage. Phenol (carbolic acid) is used commercially as a disinfectant and as an intermediate in chemical syntheses. Exposure may occur by inhalation of the vapor, by cutaneous absorption or by oral ingestion. The current threshold limit value for occupational exposure is 5 ppm (19 mg/m³). The chemical is also used to produce sympathetic nerve block in patients with chronic peripheral vascular disease by injection of 5–10 mL of a 7% aqueous solution.

Blood Concentrations. Phenol is present as acid-labile conjugates in the serum of normal persons at an average level of 0.1 mg/L (Wengle and Hellstrom, 1972). The chemical has not been measured in the blood of occupationally exposed individuals. In adult patients receiving 350–720 mg phenol injections for nerve blockade, serum concentrations reached an average maximum level of 3.0 mg/L (range, 1.0–4.9) at 19 minutes for unconjugated phenol and 4.2 mg/L (range, 0.5–8.2) at 55 minutes for conjugated phenol (Nomoto et al., 1987). Pediatric patients receiving 7–70 mg/kg injections for nerve blockade had peak plasma phenol concentrations of 2.0–36 mg/L (average, 12) at 15 minutes post-dose (Morrison et al., 1991).

Metabolism and Excretion. An oral dose of phenol is efficiently eliminated in the 24 hour urine as the sulfate and glucuronide conjugates, representing 77% and 16% of the dose, respectively (Capel et al., 1972). The excretory half-life of phenol has been variously reported to be 1–2 hours and 4.5 hours (Sherwood, 1972; Docter and Zielhuis, 1967).

A subject exposed to phenol vapor at a concentration of 24 mg/m^3 for 6 hours developed a total urine phenol level of 100 mg/L within 2 hours of the end of exposure (Piotrowski, 1971). Urine phenol concentrations of 100–400 mg/L have been observed in workers exposed to phenol at air concentrations of 4.2–12.5 mg/m^3 (Ohtsuji and Ikeda, 1972). By comparison, phenol levels in urine are generally less than 75 mg/L during worker exposure to 10 ppm of benzene, which yields phenol as a metabolite, and endogenous phenol in the urine of normal persons averages 5–10 mg/L (Docter and Zielhuis, 1967; Piotrowski, 1971).

Toxicity. Phenol causes severe irritation and corrosion on contact with skin or other tissue. Absorption of the chemical may produce cyanosis, shock, weakness, cardiac arrhythmia, collapse, convulsions, liver and kidney damage, coma and death. Phenol is rapidly absorbed upon dermal contact; one subject developed a urine phenol concentration of 100 mg/L with 30 minutes of accidental dermal exposure to the substance (Sherwood, 1972).

A workman who fell into a vat of phenol solution up to his thighs was immediately removed and washed, but became drowsy, lost consciousness, and died within half an hour; postmortem blood contained 90 mg/L phenol (Consden, 1967). A 10 year old boy suffered serious burns and was hospitalized; during the next 2.5 days his burns were treated by the application of a total of 7.5 L of an antiseptic solution containing 2% phenol. He developed fever, abdominal pain and distention, and became stuporous and cyanotic. His urine was dark, respiration became labored, and he died in coma. The postmortem urine specimen contained 220 mg/L of conjugated phenol (Cronin and Brauer, 1949). In 2 other fatal cases involving dermal exposure to phenol, postmortem blood concentrations of 4.7 and 56 mg/L were measured (Lewin and Cleary, 1982; Soares and Tift, 1982). A man who drank Lysol in a suicidal gesture and died shortly thereafter exhibited the following levels at autopsy (Briglia, 1981):

Phenol Concentrations in a Fatal Case (mg/L or mg/kg)

Blood	Lung	Liver	Kidney
46	471	269	259

Analysis. Procedures involving both colorimetry and gas chromatography for the analysis of total phenol in urine specimens are cited in the section on benzene. Unconjugated phenol in blood has been measured by gas chromatography with flame-ionization (Handson and Hanrahan, 1983; Nomoto et al., 1987) or mass spectrometric detection (Pierce and Nerland, 1988; Harrison et al., 1991).

References

R. Briglia. Presented at the quarterly meeting of the California Association of Toxicologists, Millbrae, California, February 7, 1981.

I.D. Capel, M.R. French, P. Millburn et al. The fate of (^{14}C) phenol in various species. Xenobiotica 2: 25–34, 1972.

R. Consden. Personal communication, 1967.

T.D. Cronin and R.O. Brauer. Death due to phenol contained in foille. J. Am. Med. Asso. 139: 777–778, 1949.

H.J. Docter and R.L. Zielhuis. Phenol excretion as a measure of benzene exposure. Ann. Occ. Hyg. 10: 317–326, 1967.

P.D. Handson and P.D. Hanrahan. A rapid gas chromatographic method for the determination of free phenol in blood. J. Agr. Food Chem. 31: 447–448, 1983.

L.M. Harrison, J.E. Morrison and P.V. Fennessey. Microtechnique for quantifying phenol in plasma by gas chromatography-mass spectrometry. Clin. Chem. 37: 1739–1742, 1991.

J.F. Lewin and W.T. Cleary. An accidental death caused by the absorption of phenol through skin. A case report. For. Sci. Int. 19: 177–179, 1982.

J.E. Morrison, D. Matthews, R. Washington et al. Phenol motor point blocks in children. Anesthesiology 75: 359–362, 1991.

Y. Nomoto, T. Fujita and Y. Kitani. Serum and urine levels of phenol following phenol blocks. Can. J. Anaesth. 34: 307–310, 1987.

H. Ohtsuji and M. Ikeda. Quantitative relationship between atmospheric phenol vapour and phenol in urine of workers of Bakelite factories. Brit. J. Ind. Med. 29: 70–73, 1972.

W.M. Pierce, Jr. and D.E. Nerland. Qualitative and quantitative analyses of phenol, phenylglucuronide and phenylsulfate in urine and plasma by gas chromatography/mass spectrometry. J. Anal. Tox. 12: 344–347, 1988.

J.K. Piotrowski. Evaluation of exposure to phenol: absorption of phenol vapour in the lungs and through the skin and excretion of phenol in urine. Brit. J. Ind. Med. 28: 172–178, 1971.

R.J. Sherwood. Benzene: the interpretation of monitoring results. Ann. Occ. Hyg. 15: 409–421, 1972.

E.R. Soares and J.P. Jift. Phenol poisoning: three fatal cases. J. For. Sci. 27: 729–731, 1982.

B. Wengle and K. Hellstrom. Volatile phenols in serum of uraemic patients. Clin. Sci. 43: 493–498, 1972.

Phensuximide

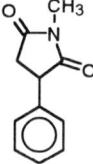

T½: 5–12 hr
Vd: ?
Fb: 0
pKa: ?

Occurrence and Usage. Phensuximide (N-methyl-2-phenyl-succinimide, Milontin) is an anticonvulsant succinimide derivative that has been used clinically since 1952. It is administered as a racemic mixture of the free acid in oral doses of 1–3 g daily. Phensuximide was the first succinimide to be adopted for the treatment of epilepsy, but is used infrequently today due to the availability of more effective agents.

Blood Concentrations. Volunteers who received a single 1 g oral dose of phensuximide exhibited an average peak plasma concentration of 14 mg/L at 1 hour, which declined to 4.5 mg/L by 6 hours (Glazko and Dill, 1972). In subjects who received 1.8 g of phensuximide daily for 8 days, peak serum concentrations of the drug ranged from 6.0–9.4 mg/L on the final day with no apparent drug accumulation during the period (Glazko et al., 1954). Both of these studies utilized a fluorimetric procedure for assaying the compound and it is unknown whether any active metabolites interfere with the determination. Five patients receiving 3 g daily achieved average steady-state plasma concentrations of 5.7 mg/L (range, 3.9–7.9) for phensuximide and 1.7 mg/L (range, 1.4–2.1) for norphensuximide. Both substances exhibited elimination half-lives that averaged 7.8 hours (Porter et al., 1979).

Metabolism and Excretion. The metabolism of phensuximide in man has not been thoroughly investigated. Undoubtedly a substantial portion of a dose is N-demethylated to norphensuximide, a compound that is nearly as active an anticonvulsant as its parent (Chen et al., 1951). A tentative identification of conjugated p-hydroxyphensuximide has been made in human urine (Glazko et al., 1954).

norphensuximide   phensuximide   p-hydroxyphensuximide

Toxicity. Adverse reactions to phensuximide have included nausea, vomiting, drowsiness, ataxia, dizziness, skin eruptions, renal damage, and blood dyscrasias.

Analysis. Analysis of phensuximide has been performed both by the previously mentioned fluorometric method (Glazko et al., 1954) and by gas chromatography of the underivatized drug by flame-ionization (Bonitati, 1976) or mass spectrometric detection (Kupferberg et al., 1977).

References

J. Bonitati. Gas-chromatographic analysis for succinimide anticonvulsants in serum: macro- and micro-scale methods. Clin. Chem. 22: 341–345, 1976.

G. Chen, R. Portman, C.R. Ensor and A.C. Bratton, Jr. The anticonvulsant activity of α–phenyl succinimides. J. Pharm. Exp. Ther. 103: 54–61, 1951.

A.J. Glazko, W.A. Dill, L.M. Wolf and C.A. Miller. The determination and physiological disposition of Milontin (N-methyl-α–phenylsuccinimide). J. Pharm. Exp. Ther. 111: 413–424, 1954.

A.J. Glazko and W.A. Dill. Other succinimides. Methsuximide and phensuximide. In *Antiepileptic Drugs* (D.M. Woodbury, J.K. Penry and R.P. Schmidt, eds.), Raven Press, New York, 1972, pp. 455–464.

H.J. Kupferberg, W.D. Yonekawa, J.R. Lacy et al. Comparison of methsuximide and phensuximide metabolism in epileptic patients. In *Antiepileptic Drug Monitoring* (C. Gardner-Thorpe, D. Janz and H. Meinardi, eds.), Tunbridge Wells, Kent, England, 1977, pp. 173–180.

R.J. Porter, J.K. Penry, J.R. Lacy et al. Plasma concentrations of phensuximide, methsuximide, and their metabolites in relation to clinical efficacy. Neurology 29: 1509–1513, 1979.

Phentermine

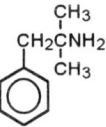

T½: 19–24 hr
Vd: 3–4 L/kg
Fb: ?
pKa: 10.1

Occurrence and Usage. Phentermine (Adipex, Ionamin) was synthesized as early as 1946 and is currently approved for use as an anorectic agent. It is the alpha-methyl derivative of amphetamine and derives its efficacy from the same sympathomimetic properties as other compounds in this class. It is also a metabolite of mephentermine, a related drug. Phentermine is supplied for oral use in 30 mg capsules as the hydrochloride, or as 15 and 30 mg sustained-release preparations. Generally no more than 15–30 mg are consumed daily.

Blood Concentrations. Following a single oral dosage of 0.375 mg/kg (26 mg/70 kg) of the hydrochloride, blood concentrations reached an average peak of about 0.09 mg/L at 4 hours, declining to 0.03 mg/L after 40 hours (Hinsvark et al., 1973). Adult volunteers receiving 30 mg daily oral doses for 2 weeks achieved steady-state plasma concentrations of 0.18–0.51 mg/L (average, 0.36) (Groenewoud et al., 1993).

Metabolism and Excretion. Phentermine is much less susceptible to metabolism than its close relative, amphetamine. The primary pathways for biotransformation are p-hydroxylation and N-oxidation. In acid urine, up to 84% of a dose is eliminated as unchanged phentermine within 24 hours (Beckett and Brookes, 1971). During uncontrolled urine pH conditions, excretion of unchanged drug averages 48% in 24 hours and 89% within 72 hours (Delbeke and Debackere, 1986). Less than 0.7% is excreted as free and conjugated p-hydroxyphentermine in urine within 5 hours (Cho, 1974), while up to 5% is present as N-hydroxyphentermine and other products of N-oxidation (Beckett and Belanger, 1974).

The following distribution was obtained from the tissues of a 70 kg adult on chronic therapy with phentermine (40 mg daily in slow-release form) who died of heart failure (Price, 1974):

Phentermine Concentrations During Therapy (mg/L or mg/kg)*

Blood	Liver	Bile	Urine	Gastric
0.9	4.0	6.5	50	3 mg

* By flame-ionization gas chromatography

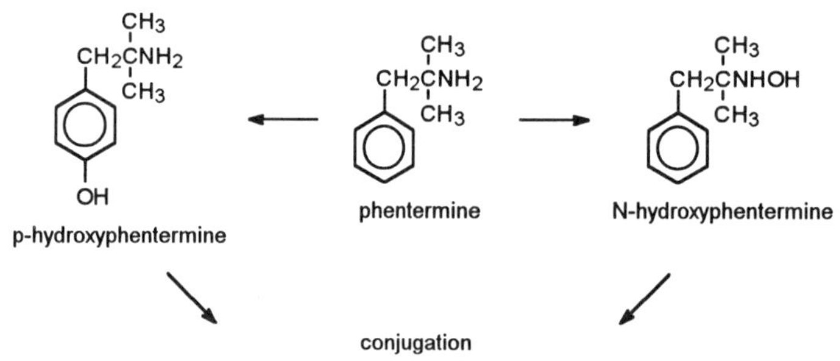

p-hydroxyphentermine   phentermine   N-hydroxyphentermine

conjugation

Toxicity. Adverse reactions to normal or elevated doses of phentermine include nervousness, tremor, confusion, headache, tachycardia, hypertension, hallucinations, psychotic episodes, nausea, vomiting, rapid respiration, cardiac arrhythmias, hyperthermia, convulsions, coma, and circulatory collapse.

The tissues of 3 adults who died following overdosage with phentermine exhibited the following tissue concentrations upon autopsy (Gottschalk and Cravey, 1980; Registry of Human Toxicology, 1980; Levine et al., 1984):

Phentermine Concentrations in Overdosage (mg/L or mg/kg)

	Blood	Liver	Kidney	Urine	Gastric
Average	4.0	10	14	84	13 mg
(Range)	(1.5–7.6)	(1.8–15)	(12–16)	(13–150)	(1.9–22)

Analysis. Phentermine may be determined in biological samples using many of the methods described for amphetamine. Very sensitive techniques involving formation of the N-trifluoroacetamide derivative and gas chromatographic analysis with either flame-ionization (O'Brien et al., 1972) or mass spectrometric detection (Cho et al., 1973) have been reported.

References

A.H. Beckett and L.G. Brookes. The metabolism and urinary excretion in man of phentermine, and the influence of N-methyl and p-chloro-substitution. J. Pharm. Pharmac. 23: 288–294, 1971.

A.H. Beckett and P.M. Belanger. Metabolism of chlorphentermine and phentermine in man to yield hydroxylamino, C-nitroso- and nitro-compounds. J. Pharm. Pharmac. 26: 205–206, 1974.

A.K. Cho, B.J. Hodshon, B. Lindeke and G.T. Miwa. Application of quantitative GC-mass spectrometry to study of pharmacokinetics of amphetamine and phentermine. J. Pharm. Sci. 62: 1491–1494, 1973.

A.K. Cho. The identification of p-hydroxyphentermine as a urinary metabolite of phentermine. Res. Comm. Chem. Path. Pharm. 7: 67–78, 1974.

F.T. Delbeke and M. Debackere. The influence of diuretics on the excretion and metabolism of doping agents. Arz. Forsch. 36: 134–137, 1986.

L.A. Gottschalk and R.H. Cravey. *Toxicological and Pathological Studies on Psychoactive Drug-Involved Deaths*, Biomedical Publications, Davis, California, 1980, p. 389.

G. Groenewoud, R. Schall, H.K.L. Hundt et al. Steady-state pharmacokinetics of phentermine extended-release capsules. Int. J. Clin. Pharm. Ther. Tox. 31: 368–372, 1993.

O.N. Hinsvark, A.P. Truant, D.J. Jenden and J.A. Steinborn. The oral bioavailability and pharmacokinetics of soluble and resin-bound forms of amphetamine and phentermine in man. J. Pharm. Biopharm. 1: 319–328, 1973.

B. Levine, Y.H. Caplan and A.M. Dixon. A fatality involving phentermine. J. For. Sci. 29: 1242–1245, 1984.

J.E. O'Brien, W. Zazulak, V. Abbey and O. Hinsvark. Determination of amphetamine and phentermine in biological fluids. J. Chrom. Sci. 10: 336–341, 1972.

K. Price. Personal communication, 1974.

Registry of Human Toxicology, American Academy of Forensic Sciences, Colorado Springs, CO, 1980.

Phenylbutazone

T½: 29–175 hr (dose-dependent)
Vd: 0.02–0.15 L/kg
Fb: 0.99
pKa: 4.5

Occurrence and Usage. Phenylbutazone (Butazolidin) was introduced in 1949 and is used today for its anti-inflammatory effects. It is structurally related to antipyrine, an analgesic that is rarely used clinically. Phenylbutazone is available as the free acid in 100 mg tablets and is administered orally in daily doses of 100–400 mg. In the early literature on the drug, doses of up to 1600 mg daily were reported.

Blood Concentrations. A single 200 mg oral dose produced in one subject a maximal plasma concentration of nearly 16 mg/L about 3 hours after ingestion, declining to 10 mg/L by 48 hours and 4 mg/L by 144 hours (McGilveray et al., 1974). A single 400 mg oral dose resulted in a peak phenylbutazone plasma concentration of about 60 mg/L shortly after ingestion, with concentrations of 1–3 mg/L still detectable after 16 days; plasma concentrations of oxyphenbutazone, an active metabolite, peaked at 10 mg/L after 72 hours and were also in the range of 1–3 mg/L after 16 days (Midha et al., 1974). Thirty-five subjects who were receiving 400 mg daily doses of the drug on a chronic basis developed steady-state plasma concentrations that averaged 93 mg/L; in an equal number of patients on an 800 mg chronic dosage, these concentrations averaged 107 mg/L (range, 60–150) (Burns et al., 1953). The phenylbutazone/oxyphenbutazone serum concentration ratio for persons on chronic therapy averages 2:1 (Herrmann, 1960). Phenylbutazone exhibits dose-dependent kinetics, probably due to an increase in the free drug fraction in plasma with higher doses, resulting in faster clearance (Higham et al., 1981).

Metabolism and Excretion. Phenylbutazone is metabolized in man by p-hydroxylation of one of the phenyl groups to oxyphenbutazone, which has pharmacologic activity equivalent to that of its parent and probably contributes significantly to the effects of the drug during chronic therapy. Both compounds are highly bound to plasma protein (99%) and have similar plasma half-lives (72 hours). A second metabolite that results from oxidation of the n-butyl side chain, 3'-hydroxyphenylbutazone, is apparently without significant activity, has a half-life of only 12 hours, and reaches plasma concentrations similar to those of oxyphenbutazone during chronic therapy. A dose of phenylbutazone is slowly eliminated in the urine (61%) and feces (27%) over a period of many days. In a 2 day period, urinary excretion products include about 1% of a dose as unchanged drug and 9% as oxyphenbutazone, 3'-hydroxyphenylbutazone and dihydroxyphenylbutazone; the 4-C-glucuronides of phenylbutazone and 3'-hydroxyphenylbutazone comprise about 40% and 12%, respectively. Oxyphenbutazone is primarily eliminated as an O-glucuronide (Burns et al., 1955; Gutman et al., 1960; Midha et al., 1974; Dieterle et al., 1976; Aarbakke et al., 1977).

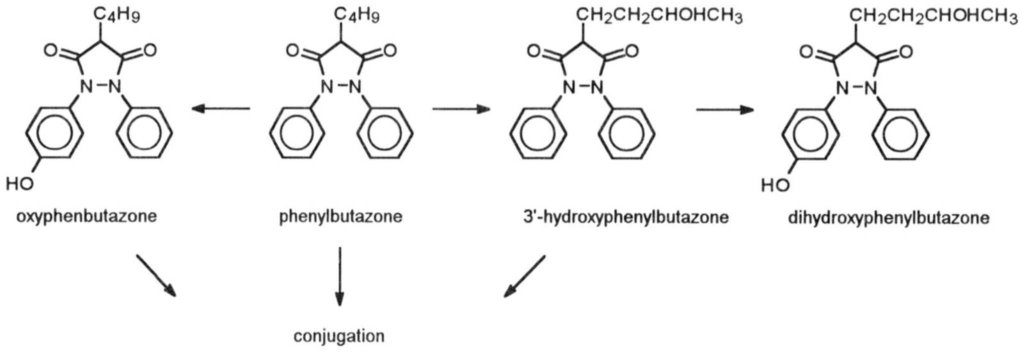

oxyphenbutazone   phenylbutazone   3'-hydroxyphenylbutazone   dihydroxyphenylbutazone

conjugation

Toxicity. This drug is known for its spectrum of serious toxic effects, which include gastrointestinal ulceration, exfoliative dermatitis, hepatitis and agranulocytosis. Toxicity is most frequently associated with serum concentrations of the drug that exceed 100 mg/L (Bruck et al., 1954). A number of deaths have occurred due to blood dyscrasias that occurred following therapeutic administration of phenylbutazone (Mauer, 1955; Inman, 1977).

Acute overdosage with 8 g of the drug in a 17 year old girl produced peak plasma concentrations of 670 mg/L for phenylbutazone, about 400 mg/L for 3'-hydroxyphenylbutazone, and about 60 mg/L for oxyphenbutazone. Symptoms of malaise, drowsiness, vomiting, and jaundice lasted for at least 3 days. The plasma half-life of phenylbutazone was only 23 hours (Prescott et al., 1980). Irritability, rapid respiration, tachycardia and coma were observed in 3 patients who survived the acute ingestion of up to 16 g of the drug after exhibiting peak plasma levels of 120–350 mg/L; hemoperfusion appears to markedly reduce the half-life of phenylbutazone (Juul, 1965; Strong et al., 1979; Berlinger et al., 1982).

The death of a 5 year old, 1 day after accidental ingestion of an unknown quantity of the compound, yielded the following tissue distribution upon toxicological investigation (Lam and Chien, 1976):

Phenylbutazone Concentrations in a Fatal Case (mg/L or mg/kg)

Blood	Liver	Kidney	Bile	Gastric
400	250	250	475	290 mg

Analysis. Phenylbutazone may be determined in body fluids and tissues by ultraviolet spectrophotometry of the drug at 265 nm after heptane extraction from aqueous acid solution (Burns et al., 1953) or of a permanganate oxidation product (Wallace, 1968; Jahnchen and Levy, 1972). Gas chromatographic procedures have been described for the intact drug (McGilveray et al., 1974; Sioufi et al., 1978; Budd, 1982), for phenylbutazone and oxyphenbutazone as methyl derivatives (Midha et al., 1974), and for 3'-hydroxyphenylbutazone as a methyl derivative (Midha et al., 1978). High-pressure liquid chromatographic methods are available for phenylbutazone analysis, several of which are applicable to the major metabolites as well (Pound et al., 1974; Aarons and Higham, 1980; Alvinerie, 1980; Marunaka et al., 1980).

References

J. Aarbakke, O.M. Bakke, E.J. Milde and D.S. Davies. Disposition and oxidative metabolism of phenylbutazone in man. Eur. J. Clin. Pharm. 11: 359–366, 1977.

L. Aarons and C. Higham. An improved HPLC assay for monitoring phenylbutazone and its two major oxidised metabolites in plasma. Clin. Chim. Acta 105: 377–382, 1980.

M. Alvinerie. Reversed-phase high-performance liquid chromatography of phenylbutazone in body fluids. J. Chrom. 181: 132–134, 1980.

W.G. Berlinger, R. Spector, M.J. Flanigan et al. Hemoperfusion for phenylbutazone poisoning. Ann. Int. Med. 96: 334–335, 1982.

E. Bruck, M.E. Fearnley, I. Meanock and H. Patley. Phenylbutazone therapy. Lancet 1: 225–228, 1954.

R.D. Budd. Gas chromatographic determination of Butazolidin (phenylbutazone) in biological fluids. J. Chrom. 243: 368–371, 1982.

J.J. Burns, R.K. Rose, T. Chenkin et al. The physiological disposition of phenylbutazone (Butazolidin) in man and a method for its estimation in biological material. J. Pharm. Exp. Ther. 109: 346–357, 1953.

J.J. Burns, R.K. Rose, S. Goodwin et al. The metabolic fate of phenylbutazone (Butazolidin) in man. J. Pharm. Exp. Ther. 113: 481–489, 1955.

W. Dieterle, J.W. Faigle, F. Fruh et al. Metabolism of phenylbutazone in man. Arz. Forsch. 26: 572–577, 1976.

A.B. Gutman, P.G. Dayton, T.F. Yu et al. A study of the inverse relationship between pKa and rate of renal excretion of phenylbutazone analogs in man and dog. Am. J. Med. 29: 1017–1033, 1960.

B. Herrmann. Ueber den Stoffwechsel des Butazolidin. Med. Exp. 1: 170–178, 1960.

C. Higham, L. Aarons, P.J.L. Holt et al. A chronic dose-ranging study of the pharmacokinetics of phenylbutazone in rheumatoid arthritic patients. Brit. J. Clin. Pharm. 12: 123–129, 1981.

W.H.W. Inman. Study of fatal bone marrow depression with special reference to phenylbutazone and oxyphenbutazone. Brit. Med. J. 1: 1500–1505, 1977.

E. Jahnchen and G. Levy. Determination of phenylbutazone in plasma. Clin. Chem. 18: 984–986, 1972.

J. Juul. Acute poisoning with Butazolidin (phenylbutazone). Acta Paediat. Scand. 54: 503–507, 1965.

K.L. Lam and K. Chien. Personal communication, 1976.

T. Marunaka, T. Shibata, Y. Minami and Y. Umeno. Simultaneous determination of phenylbutazone and its metabolites in plasma and urine by high-performance liquid chromatography. J. Chrom. 183: 331–338, 1980.

E.F. Mauer. The toxic effects of phenylbutazone (Butazolidin). New Eng. J. Med. 253: 404–410, 1955.

I.J. McGilveray, K.K. Midha, R. Brien and L. Wilson. The assay of phenylbutazone in human plasma by a specific and sensitive gas-liquid chromatographic procedure. J. Chrom. 89: 17–22, 1974.

K.K. Midha, I.J. McGilveray and C. Charette. GLC determination of plasma concentration of phenylbutazone and its metabolite oxyphenbutazone. J. Pharm. Sci. 63: 1234–1239, 1974.

K.K. Midha, I.J. McGilveray and J.K. Cooper. GLC determination of plasma concentrations of α−oxo metabolite of phenylbutazone. J. Pharm. Sci. 67: 279–281, 1978.

N.J. Pound, I.J. McGilveray and R.W. Sears. Analysis of phenylbutazone in plasma by high-speed liquid chromatography. J. Chrom. 89: 23–30, 1974.

L.F. Prescott, J.A.J.H. Critchley and M. Balali-Mood. Phenylbutazone overdosage: abnormal metabolism associated with hepatic and renal damage. Brit. Med. J. 2: 1106–1107, 1980.

A. Sioufi, F. Caudal and F. Marfil. GLC determination of phenylbutazone in human plasma. J. Pharm. Sci. 67: 243–245, 1978.

J.E. Strong, J. Wilson, J.F. Douglas and D.L. Coppel. Phenylbutazone self-poisoning treated by charcoal haemoperfusion. Anaesthesia 34: 1038–1040, 1979.

J.E. Wallace. Ultraviolet spectrophotometric determination of phenylbutazone in biologic specimens. J. Pharm. Sci. 57: 2053–2056, 1968.

Phenylephrine

T½: 2–3 hr
Vd: 5 L/kg
Fb: ?
pKa: 8.8

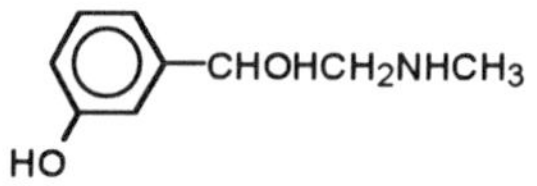

Occurrence and Usage. Phenylephrine (Neo-Synephrine) is a synthetic alpha-receptor stimulant that was first studied in 1910 and is now used frequently as a nasal decongestant and bronchodilator. The compound is the 4-desoxy derivative of epinephrine and, like that drug, causes primarily peripheral effects. It is available as the hydrochloride of the l-isomer, often in combination with other drugs, for oral administration in doses of 2.5–25 mg, for nasal topical administration in 0.125–1.0% solutions, or for parenteral injection in a 1% solution.

Blood Concentrations. Following a single oral dose of 9 mg of the hydrochloride, plasma concentrations in 6 subjects averaged 0.030 mg/L at 1 hour and 0.014 mg/L by 8 hours, expressed as total radioactivity (Cavallito et al., 1963).

Metabolism and Excretion. Phenylephrine is known to be metabolized by conjugation or deamination. Up to 86% of a labeled intravenous dose is excreted in the 48 hour urine as free drug (16%), conjugated phenylephrine (8%), and m-hydroxymandelic acid (over 50%). Oral administration results in excretion of these 3 substances in amounts of 3%, 46%, and less than 33% of the dose, respectively. The oral bioavailability of phenylephrine is 38% (Hengstmann and Goronzy, 1982).

Toxicity. Phenylephrine is capable of causing hypertension and cardiac arrhythmias. Hypertension has been observed in neonates following the administration of ophthalmic solutions to produce pupillary dilation (Lees and Cabal, 1981). Psychosis was reported in a chronic user of phenylephrine nasal drops (Escobar and Karno, 1982).

Analysis. A gas chromatographic method of assaying this compound in biological fluids involves electron-capture detection of a trifluoroacetyl derivative (Dombrowski et al., 1973). Liquid chromatography has also been described (Chien and Schoenwald, 1985; Martinsson et al., 1986).

References

C.J. Cavallito, L. Chafetz and L.D. Miller. Some studies of a sustained release principle. J. Pharm. Sci. 52: 259–263, 1963.

D.S. Chien and R.D. Schoenwald. Fluorometric determination of phenylephrine hydrochloride by liquid chromatography in human plasma. J. Pharm. Sci. 74: 562–564, 1985.

L.J. Dombrowski, P.M. Comi and E.L. Pratt. GLC determination of phenylephrine hydrochloride in human plasma. J. Pharm. Sci. 62: 1761–1763, 1973.

J.I. Escobar and M. Karno. Chronic hallucinosis from nasal drops. J. Am. Med. Asso. 247: 1859–1860, 1982.

J.H. Hengstmann and J. Goronzy. Pharmacokinetics of ³H-phenylephrine in man. Eur. J. Clin. Pharm. 21: 335–341, 1982.

B.J. Lees and L.A. Cabal. Increased blood pressure following pupillary dilation with 2.5% phenylephrine hydrochloride in preterm infants. Pediatrics 68: 231–234, 1981.

A. Martinsson, S. Bevegard and P. Hjemdahl. Analysis of phenylephrine in plasma: initial data about the concentration-effect relationship. Eur. J. Clin. Pharm. 30: 427–431, 1986.

Phenylpropanolamine

T½: 3.0–4.4 hr
Vd: 4.5 L/kg
Fb: ?
pKa: 9.1

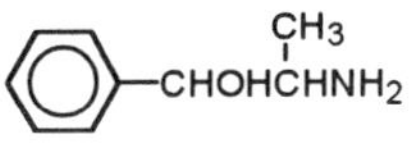

$$\bigcirc\!\!-\!\!CHOH\overset{CH_3}{\underset{|}{C}}HNH_2$$

Occurrence and Usage. Phenylpropanolamine (norephedrine) is a synthetic sympathomimetic drug that is approximately equivalent to ephedrine in its pharmacological properties. It is supplied as the hydrochloride of the racemic mixture; the D-threo form (norpseudoephedrine) occurs naturally in certain plants and is indistinguishable by most analytical procedures. Phenylpropanolamine is available for oral administration in single doses of 6–50 mg for use as a decongestant, and is commonly found in combination with antihistamines and analgesics. It is also an ingredient of numerous nonprescription diet aids, in amounts of 25–75 mg.

Blood Concentrations. Peak plasma concentrations of phenylpropanolamine averaged 0.11, 0.18 and 0.40 mg/L in 5 adult males at 1.0–1.7 hours following a single oral dose of 25, 50 or 100 mg, respectively (Scherzinger et al., 1990). Serum concentrations reached an average peak level of about 0.28 mg/L at 6 hours after oral ingestion of a 150 mg sustained-release preparation by 6 volunteers (Dowse et al., 1983). The serum half-life has been estimated at 3.0–4.4 hours (Dowse et al., 1987).

Metabolism and Excretion. The drug is nearly quantitatively excreted unchanged in the 24 hour urine, a mean of 97% of a dose being recovered. The existence of a p-hydroxy metabolite has been postulated but not confirmed (Heimlich et al., 1961). Acidification of the urine slightly enhanced the rate of phenylpropanolamine excretion, whereas alkalinization significantly reduced the rate (Zimmerman, 1988).

Toxicity. Phenylpropanolamine is capable of causing dizziness, palpitation, tachycardia, nervousness, insomnia, hypertension, and cardiac arrhythmias. Single doses of 50–75 mg have produced anxiety, agitation, hallucinations, and tremor in susceptible persons (Dietz, 1981). Slightly higher doses have caused severe headache and hypertensive crisis in a number of individuals (Ostern and Dodson, 1965; Salmon, 1965; Frewin et al., 1978; Horowitz et al., 1979; Teh, 1979; McEwen, 1983; Mueller, 1983). Hypertension resulted in one patient from the combination of indomethacin and phenylpropanolamine, both in therapeutic amounts (Lee et al., 1979).

Death due to ventricular arrhythmia was ascribed to the simultaneous use of phenylpropanolamine and thioridazine by a schizophrenic patient (Chouinard et al., 1978). The death of a 15 year old girl 32 hours after ingestion of 400–450 mg of phenylpropanolamine was believed due to adult respiratory distress syndrome (Logie and Scott, 1984). A woman taking an over-the-counter diet aid collapsed in seizure and died within a few minutes; postmortem blood contained 2 mg/L phenylpropanolamine and the gastric contents contained 2.2 mg (Cravey, 1981). A 16 year old girl ingested a phenylpropanolamine overdose and displayed agitation, confusion, dyspnea and hypertension; she arrested about 5 hours after ingestion and postmortem blood contained 4.6 mg/L of the drug (Augenstein et al., 1988). The following tissue distribution was observed in the case of a 20 year old man who ingested a large overdose of the drug, apparently for suicidal purposes (Cravey, 1981):

Phenylpropanolamine Concentrations in a Fatal Case (mg/L or mg/kg)

Blood	Brain	Liver	Gastric
48	86	460	20 mg

Analysis. Phenylpropanolamine has been assayed by ultraviolet spectrophotometry after oxidation to benzaldehyde (Heimlich et al., 1961). Gas chromatographic methods have involved flame-ionization (Beckett and Wilkinson, 1965), nitrogen-selective (Neelakantan and Kostenbauder, 1976), electron-capture (Crisologo et al., 1984) and mass spectrometric detection (Thurman et al., 1992). Liquid chromatographic methods have also been described (Mason and Amick, 1981; Dowse et al., 1983; Mason and Mason, 1983; Shi et al., 1985).

References

W.L. Augenstein, P. Bakerman, M. Radetsky et al. Phenylpropanolamine (PPA) overdose resulting in pulmonary edema and death. Vet. Hum. Tox. 30: 365, 1988.

A.H. Beckett and G.R. Wilkinson. Identification and determination of ephedrine and its congeners in urine by gas chromatography. J. Pharm. Pharmac. 17: 104S–106S, 1965.

G. Chouinard, A.M. Ghadirian and B.D. Jones. Death attributed to ventricular arrhythmia induced by thioridazine in combination with a single Contac C capsule. Can. Med. Asso. J. 119: 729–731, 1978.

R.H. Cravey. Personal communication, 1981.

N. Crisologo, D. Dye and W.F. Bayne. Electron-capture capillary gas chromatographic determination of phenylpropanolamine in human plasma following derivatization with trifluoroacetic anhydride. J. Pharm. Sci. 73: 1313–1315, 1984.

A.J. Dietz, Jr. Amphetamine-like reactions to phenylpropanolamine. J. Am. Med. Asso. 245: 601–602, 1981.

R. Dowse, J.M. Haigh and I. Kanfer. Determination of phenylpropanolamine in serum and urine by high-performance liquid chromatography. J. Pharm. Sci. 72: 1018–1020, 1983.

R. Dowse, J.M. Haigh and I. Kanfer. Pharmacokinetics of phenylpropanolamine in humans after a single dose study. Int. J. Pharm. 39: 141–148, 1987.

D.B. Frewin, P.P. Leonello and M.E. Frewin. Hypertension after ingestion of Trimolets. Med. J. Aust. 2: 497–498, 1978.

K.R. Heimlich, D.R. MacDonnell, T.L. Flanagan and P.D. O'Brien. Evaluation of a sustained release form of phenylpropanolamine hydrochloride by urinary excretion studies. J. Pharm. Sci. 50: 232–237, 1961.

J.D. Horowitz, J.J. McNeil, B. Sweet et al. Hypertension and postural hypotension induced by phenylpropanolamine (Trimolets). Med. J. Aust. 1: 175–176, 1979.

K.Y. Lee, L.J. Beilin and R. Vandongen. Severe hypertension after ingestion of an appetite suppressant (phenylpropanolamine) with indomethacin. Lancet 1: 1110–1111, 1979.

A.W. Logie and C.M. Scott. Fatal overdosage of phenylpropanolamine. Brit. Med. J. 289: 591, 1984.

W.D. Mason and E.N. Amick. High-pressure liquid chromatographic analysis of phenylpropanolamine in human plasma following derivatization with o-phthalaldehyde. J. Pharm. Sci. 70: 707–709, 1981.

W.D. Mason and J.S. Mason. Improved high pressure liquid chromatographic method for phenylpropanolamine in human plasma. Anal. Letters 16: 693–699, 1983.

J. McEwen. Phenylpropanolamine-associated hypertension after the use of "over-the-counter" appetite-suppressant products. Med. J. Aust. 2: 71–73, 1983.

S.M. Mueller. Neurologic complications of phenylpropanolamine use. Neurology 33: 650–652, 1983.

L. Neelakantan and H.B. Kostenbauder. Electron-capture GLC determination of phenylpropanolamine as a pentafluorophenyloxazolidine derivative. J. Pharm. Sci. 65: 740–742, 1976.

S. Ostern and W.H. Dodson. Hypertension following Ornade ingestion. J. Am. Med. Asso. 194: 472, 1965.

P.R. Salmon. Hypertensive crisis with Eskornade. Brit. Med. J. 1: 193, 1965.

S.S. Scherzinger, R. Dowse and I. Kanfer. Steady-state pharmacokinetics and dose-proportionality of phenylpropanolamine in healthy subjects. J. Clin. Pharm. 30: 372–377, 1990.

R.J.Y. Shi, W.L. Gee, R.L. Williams et al. Ion-pair liquid chromatographic analysis of phenylpropanolamine in plasma and urine by post-column derivatization with o-phthalaldehyde. J. Liq. Chrom. 8: 1489–1500, 1985.

A.Y.F. Teh. Phenylpropanolamine and hypertension. Med. J. Aust. 2: 425–426, 1979.

E.M. Thurman, M.J. Pedersen, R.L. Stout and T. Martin. Distinguishing sympathomimetic amines from amphetamine and methamphetamine in urine by gas chromatography/mass spectrometry. J. Anal. Tox. 16: 19–27, 1992.

C.L. Zimmerman. The effect of urinary pH modification on the disposition of phenylpropanolamine. Pharm. Res. 5: 120–122, 1988.

Phenytoin

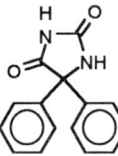

T½: 8–60 hr (dose-dependent)
Vd: 0.5–0.8 L/kg
Fb: 0.87–0.93
pKa: 8.3

Occurrence and Usage. Phenytoin (diphenylhydantoin, Dilantin) was synthesized in 1908 and its efficacy as an anticonvulsant in man was first reported in 1938. It is considered by many to be the drug of choice for most forms of epilepsy. Phenytoin is available as the sodium salt in capsules of 30 and 100 mg, an oral suspension of 30–125 mg/5 mL, and a 50 mg/mL injectable solution. The drug is usually given orally in doses of 300–400 mg daily, but may also be administered by intravenous or intramuscular injection for acute seizure problems.

Blood Concentrations. Following a single 100 mg oral dose of phenytoin, peak serum concentrations of 1.6–2.8 mg/L were observed at 2–4 hours after ingestion (Robinson et al., 1975). After a 600 mg oral dose, peak blood concentrations averaging 9.3 mg/L (range, 7.6–10.8) were achieved at 19.5 hours (Parker et al., 1970). During chronic treatment of patients with 300–400 mg of phenytoin daily, plasma concentrations averaged 13.6 mg/L and ranged from 7.8–17.5 mg/L (Wilder et al., 1973). The desirable range of phenytoin plasma concentrations in patients is generally considered to be 10–20 mg/L, although some patients may require higher levels (Levine and Chang, 1990).

The plasma half-life of phenytoin averages 18–22 hours, but varies widely. Each individual has a threshold dose or plasma concentration, beyond which the drug exhibits zero-order kinetics. The plasma concentration then increases out of proportion to an increase in the dose, due to an increasing elimination half-life (Arnold and Gerber, 1970; Kostenbauder et al., 1975). The blood/plasma concentration ratio for phenytoin has been reported to average 0.50 (Bock and Sherwin, 1971).

Metabolism and Excretion. Phenytoin exhibits capacity-limited metabolism at doses used therapeutically. The major pathway of biotransformation is via p-hydroxylation of the phenyl ring. The resulting metabolite, p-hydroxyphenytoin (known as HPPH), tends to accumulate in the plasma of

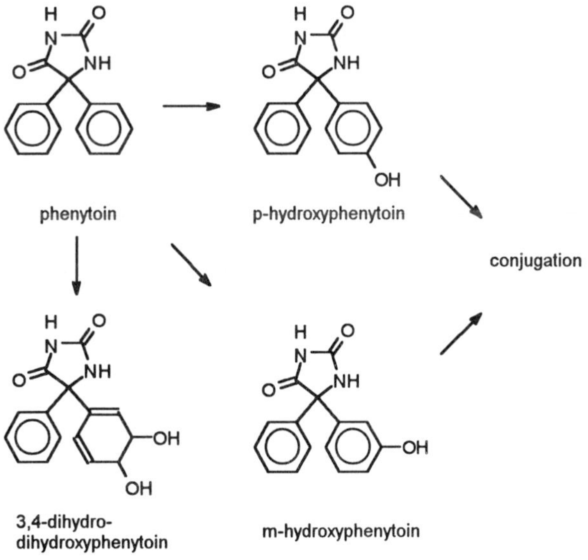

phenytoin

p-hydroxyphenytoin

conjugation

3,4-dihydro-
dihydroxyphenytoin

m-hydroxyphenytoin

uremic patients and may reach concentrations as high as 37 mg/L. This compound is a poor anti-convulsant and is present largely as a glucuronide conjugate (Letteri et al., 1971). Other products of oxidation, including m-hydroxyphenytoin and a 3,4-dihydrodihydroxyphenyl derivative, constitute minor metabolites (Glazko, 1973).

Concentrations of unchanged phenytoin in the urine after a single 600 mg dose did not exceed 5 mg/L, and total excretion of unchanged drug in the 21 hour urine was less than 4% of the dose (Parker et al., 1970). The urinary excretion of p-hydroxyphenytoin as a conjugate accounts for 23–67% of a single dose within 48 hours (Inaba and Brien, 1973). An isomer, m-hydroxyphenytoin, may account for nearly 5% of a dose as a urinary conjugate (Atkinson et al., 1970), although it has been suggested that this compound arises as an artifact from dehydration of the dihydrodiol (Pruitt et al., 1975).

Toxicity. Although relatively few deaths have occurred as a result of phenytoin overdosage, cases of patient intoxication with the drug are not uncommon. The formation of p-hydroxyphenytoin is capacity-limited, and in patients receiving a dosage in excess of their ability to metabolize and excrete it, the parent drug accumulates and causes nystagmus, ataxia, slurred speech and confusion (Garrettson and Jusko, 1975). A viral infection caused a transient increase in the steady-state serum phenytoin level of an adult from 16–51 mg/L, with the development of toxicity (Levine and Jones, 1983). Plasma concentrations as high as 108 mg/L have been detected in patients who developed toxicity after repeated doses (Kutt et al., 1964; Gerber et al., 1972; Pruitt et al., 1975). After acute ingestion of 2.8 g of phenytoin by a 2.5 year old child, a maximal blood concentration of 112 mg/L was observed, at which time the patient was comatose (Tenckhoff et al., 1968). Two cases have been reported of massive acute ingestion in which peak plasma phenytoin concentrations of 95–97 mg/L were not reached until 4–7 days after hospital admission; this is believed due to continued absorption from a concretion of drug within the gastrointestinal tract (Albertson et al., 1981; Matzke et al., 1981).

Death due to ventricular fibrillation or asystole has resulted from too rapid intravenous administration of phenytoin (Gellerman and Martinez, 1967; Goldschlager and Karliner, 1967; Zoneraich et al., 1976). The following tissue concentrations were reported in 2 fatal cases involving oral ingestion of phenytoin (Laubscher, 1966; Bruce and Smith, 1977):

Phenytoin Concentrations in Fatal Cases (mg/L or mg/kg)

Episode	Other Drugs	Blood	Brain	Liver	Kidney
Chronic	Phenobarbital	9.5	34	24	44
Acute*	None	45	78	272	112

*Died 80 hours after ingestion of 2 g of drug; an antemortem blood concentration of 94 mg/L was observed 24 hours after ingestion in this 4.5 year old child.

Analysis. Numerous procedures the plasma-level monitoring of phenytoin have been published. These have included spectrophotometry (Wallace, 1969), flame-ionization gas chromatography of the underivatized drug (Ritz and Warren, 1975) or of its methyl (Kupferberg, 1970) or trimethylsilyl (Chang and Glazko, 1970) derivatives, and nitrogen-selective gas chromatography (Vandemark and Adams, 1976). Liquid chromatography may be used for the simultaneous determination of phenytoin and HPPH in plasma and urine (Slonek et al., 1978; Sawchuk and Cartier, 1980; Lum et al., 1985; Maya et al., 1993). Commercial immunoassays have been found to be rapid and relatively specific, although certain procedures may yield spuriously high values for uremic patients in whom HPPH has accumulated (McDonald and Kabra, 1980; Reeves et al., 1985). Specimens stored in serum separator tubes at room temperature for 24 hours lost 18% of their initial phenytoin concentrations (Parish and Alexander, 1990).

References

T.E. Albertson, C.J. Fisher, Jr., T.A. Shragg and R.C. Baselt. A prolonged severe intoxication after ingestion of phenytoin and phenobarbital. West. J. Med. 135: 418–422, 1981.

K. Arnold and N. Gerber. The rate of decline of diphenylhydantoin. Clin. Pharm. Ther. 11: 121–134, 1970.

A.J. Atkinson, J. MacGee, J. Strong et al. Identification of 5-metahydroxyphenyl-5-phenylhydantoin as a metabolite of diphenylhydantoin. Biochem. Pharm. 19: 2483–2491, 1970.

G.W. Bock and A.L. Sherwin. The rapid quantitative determination of diphenylhydantoin in plasma, serum, and whole blood of patients with epilepsy. Clin. Chim. Acta 34: 97–103, 1971.

A.M. Bruce and H. Smith. The investigation of phenobarbitone, phenytoin and primidone in the death of epileptics. Med. Sci. Law 17: 195–199, 1977.

T. Chang and A.J. Glazko. Quantitative assay of 5,5-diphenylhydantoin (Dilantin) and 5-(p-hydroxyphenyl)-5-phenylhydantoin by gas-liquid chromatography. J. Lab. Clin. Med. 75: 145–155, 1970.

L.K. Garrettson and W.J. Jusko. Diphenylhydantoin elimination kinetics in overdosed children. Clin. Pharm. Ther. 17: 481–491, 1975.

G.L. Gellerman and C. Martinez. Fatal ventricular fibrillation following intravenous sodium diphenylhydantoin therapy. J. Am. Med. Asso. 200: 337–338, 1967.

N. Gerber, R. Lynn and J. Oates. Acute intoxication with 5,5-diphenylhydantoin (Dilantin) associated with impairment of biotransformation. Ann. Int. Med. 77: 765–771, 1972.

A.J. Glazko. Diphenylhydantoin metabolism. Drug Met. Disp. 5: 711–714, 1973.

A.W. Goldschlager and J.S. Karliner. Ventricular standstill after intravenous diphenylhydantoin. Am. Heart J. 74: 410–412, 1967.

T. Inaba and J.F. Brien. Determination of the major urinary metabolite of diphenylhydantoin by high-performance liquid chromatography. J. Chrom. 80: 161–165, 1973.

H.B. Kostenbauder, R.P. Rapp, J.P. McGovren et al. Bioavailability and single-dose pharmacokinetics of intramuscular phenytoin. Clin. Pharm. Ther. 18: 449–456, 1975.

H.J. Kupferberg. Quantitative estimation of diphenylhydantoin, primidone and phenobarbital in plasma by gas-liquid chromatography. Clin. Chim. Acta 29: 283–288, 1970.

H. Kutt, M. Wolk, R. Scherman and F. McDowell. Insufficient parahydroxylation as a cause of diphenylhydantoin toxicity. Neurology 14: 542–548, 1964.

F.A. Laubscher. Fatal diphenylhydantoin poisoning. J. Am. Med. Asso. 198: 1120–1121, 1966.

J.M. Letteri, H. Mellk, S. Louis et al. Diphenylhydantoin metabolism in uremia. New Eng. J. Med. 285: 648–652, 1971.

M. Levine and M.W. Jones. Toxic reaction to phenytoin following a viral infection. Can. Med. Asso. J. 128: 1270–1271, 1983.

M. Levine and T. Chang. Therapeutic drug monitoring of phenytoin: rationale and current status. Clin. Pharmacokin. 19: 341–358, 1990.

J.T. Lum, N.A. Vassanji and P.G. Wells. Analysis of the toxicologically relevant metabolites of phenytoin in biological samples by high-performance liquid chromatography. J. Chrom. 338: 242–248, 1985.

G.R. Matzke, J.C. Cloyd and R.J. Sawchuk. Acute phenytoin and primidone intoxication: a pharmacokinetic analysis. J. Clin. Pharm. 21: 92–99, 1981.

M.T. Maya, A.R. Farinha, A.M. Lucas and J.A. Morais. Sensitive method for the determination of phenytoin in plasma, and phenytoin and 5-(4-hydroxyphenyl)-5-phenylhydantoin in urine by high-performance liquid chromatography. J. Pharm. Biomed. Anal. 10: 1001–1006, 1993.

D.M. McDonald and P.M. Kabra. Renal disease may increase apparent phenytoin in serum as measured by enzyme-multiplied immunoassay. Clin. Chem. 26: 361–362, 1980.

R.C. Parish and T. Alexander. Stability of phenytoin in blood collected in vacuum blood collection tubes. Ther. Drug Mon. 12: 85–89, 1990.

K.D. Parker, H.W. Elliot, J.A. Wright et al. Blood and urine concentrations of subjects receiving barbiturates, meprobamate, glutethimide, or diphenylhydantoin. Clin. Tox. 2: 131–145, 1970.

A.W. Pruitt, G.T. Zwiren, J.H. Patterson et al. A complex pattern of disposition of phenytoin in severe intoxication. Clin. Pharm. Ther. 18: 112–120, 1975.

S.E. Reeves, J.J. Hanyok, S.A. Amon and P.J. Godley. Discrepancy in serum phenytoin concentrations determined by two immunoassay methods in uremic patients. Am. J. Hosp. Pharm. 42: 359–362, 1985.

D.P. Ritz and C.G. Warren. Single extraction GLC analysis of six commonly prescribed antiepileptic drugs. Clin. Tox. 8: 311–324, 1975.

J.D. Robinson, B.A. Morris, G.W. Aherne and V. Marks. Pharmacokinetics of a single dose of phenytoin in man measured by radioimmunoassay. Brit. J. Clin. Pharm. 2: 345–349, 1975.

R.J. Sawchuk and L.L. Cartier. Liquid-chromatographic method for simultaneous determination of phenytoin and 5-(4-hydroxyphenyl)-5-phenylhydantoin in plasma and urine. Clin. Chem. 26: 835–839, 1980.

J.E. Slonek, G.W. Peng and W.L. Chiou. Rapid and micro high-pressure liquid chromatographic determination of plasma phenytoin levels. J. Pharm. Sci. 67: 1462–1464, 1978.

H. Tenckhoff, D.J. Sherrard, R.O. Hickman and R.L. Ladda. Acute diphenylhydantoin intoxication. Am. J. Dis. Child. 116: 422–425, 1968.

F.L. Vandemark and R.F. Adams. Ultramicro gas-chromatographic analysis for anticonvulsants, with use of a nitrogen-selective detector. Clin. Chem. 22: 1062–1065, 1976.

J.E. Wallace. Simultaneous spectrophotometric determination of diphenylhydantoin and phenobarbital in biologic specimens. Clin. Chem. 14: 323–330, 1969.

B.J. Wilder, E.E. Serrano and R.E. Ramsey. Plasma diphenylhydantoin levels after loading and maintenance doses. Clin. Pharm. Ther. 14: 797–801, 1973.

S. Zoneraich, O. Zoneraich and J. Siegel. Sudden death following intravenous sodium diphenylhydantoin. Am. Heart J. 91: 375–377, 1976.

Phosphine

T½: ?
Vd: ?   PH₃
Fb: ?
pKa: ?

Occurrence and Usage. Phosphine (hydrogen phosphide) is a colorless gas with an odor of carbide or decaying fish. It is widely used as an agricultural fumigant and is usually generated by the action of water on metallic phosphides. The current threshold limit value for phosphine is 0.3 ppm (0.42 mg/m³). Commercial rodenticide pellets may contain up to 2% of aluminum or zinc phosphide.

Blood Concentrations. Phosphine has not been measured in the blood of asymptomatic or occupationally exposed individuals.

Metabolism and Excretion. Inhaled phosphine is readily absorbed by the lungs. If a metallic phosphide is ingested, phosphine is released in the acid medium of the stomach and is absorbed through the gut. Little is known of its fate in the body, although a certain portion may be exhaled unchanged (Hayes, 1982).

Toxicity. Phosphine is an extremely poisonous gas. In the workplace, symptoms begin to occur as soon as the odor of phosphine is obvious, usually about 2 ppm. Sixty-seven men so exposed described symptoms of diarrhea, nausea, vomiting, epigastric pain, tightness of the chest, palpitations, breathlessness, headache, dizziness and staggering gait (Jones et al., 1964). After ingestion of aluminum or zinc phosphide tablets, symptoms have included severe abdominal pain, an intolerable burning sensation throughout the body, vomiting and coma. Pulmonary edema appears to be a consequence if exposure is by inhalation or ingestion (Harger and Spolyar, 1958; Hayes, 1982; Rodenberg et al., 1989).

Analysis of tissues from the body of a 27 year old man who ingested an unknown number of aluminum phosphide tablets revealed a blood phosphine concentration of 0.5 µg/L and liver concentration of 3 µg/kg (Chan et al., 1983). Phosphine released during the clandestine synthesis of methamphetamine using the ephedrine/red phosphorus/hydriodic acid process was held responsible for the deaths of 3 individuals (Muto, 1985).

Analysis. Phosphine has been determined in human tissues employing gas chromatography with nitrogen-phosphorus detection (Chan et al., 1983).

References

L.T.F. Chan, R.J. Crowley, D. Delliou et al. Phosphine analysis in post mortem specimens following ingestion of aluminum phosphide. J. Anal. Tox. 7: 165–167, 1983.

R.N. Harger and L.W. Spolyar. Toxicity of phosphine, with a possible fatality from this poison. Arch. Ind. Health 18: 497–504, 1958.

W.J. Hayes, Jr. *Pesticides Studied in Man*, Williams and Wilkins, Baltimore, 1982, pp. 133–135.

A.T. Jones, R.C. Jones and E.O. Longley. Environmental and clinical aspects of bulk wheat fumigation with aluminum phosphide. Am. Ind. Hyg. Asso. J. 25: 376–379, 1964.

J. Muto. Personal communication, 1985.

H.D. Rodenberg, C.C. Chang and W.A. Watson. Zinc phosphide ingestion: a case report and review. Vet. Hum. Tox. 31: 559–562, 1989.

Pindolol

T½: 3–4 hr
Vd: 1–2 L/kg
Fb: 0.40
pKa: 8.8

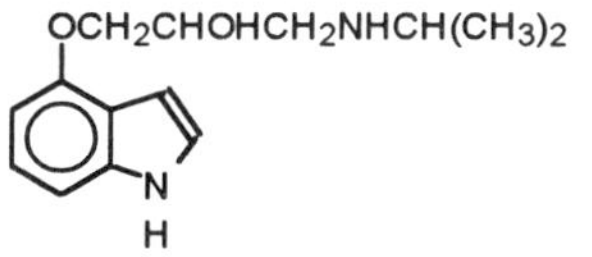

$OCH_2CHOHCH_2NHCH(CH_3)_2$

Occurrence and Usage. Pindolol (Visken) is a potent beta-adrenoceptor blocking agent used in the treatment of hypertension. It is available as the hydrochloride salt in 5 and 10 mg tablets. The recommended initial dose is 5 mg twice daily, alone or in combination with other antihypertensive agents. The dose may be adjusted in increments of 10 mg up to a maximum of 60 mg per day.

Blood Concentrations. Oral administration of a single 5 mg tablet of pindolol to 12 volunteers, 19–30 years of age weighing 50–80 kg, produced an average plasma concentration of 33 µg/L (range, 11–81) 1 hour post-ingestion; by 2 hours post-ingestion, the average plasma concentration was 32 µg/L (range, 18–56) (Gugler et al., 1974). Following the oral administration of a single 10 mg dose of pindolol to 8 healthy subjects aged 20–25 years, maximum plasma concentrations ranged from 23–105 µg/L after 1–2 hours; the mean plasma concentration after 1 hour was 35 µg/L (Gugler et al., 1975). A single oral dose of 20 mg of pindolol given to 15 previously untreated subjects produced a mean plasma pindolol concentration of 12 µg/L after 1 hour, 39 µg/L after 2 hours, and 10 µg/L after 6 hours (Anavekar et al., 1975).

Mean steady-state plasma concentrations ranged from 11–19 µg/L (average, 15) in 6 healthy volunteers aged 23–32 years, weighing 56–71 kg, following 6 days of treatment with 15 mg pindolol per day (Gugler and Bodem, 1978). Ten healthy male subjects, aged 22–30 and weighing 63–82 kg, had average peak plasma concentrations of 49 µg/L on day 1 and 47 µg/L on day 4 following daily treatment with a 20 mg prolonged-release tablet (Aellig et al., 1981).

Metabolism and Excretion. Pindolol is metabolized primarily by hydroxylation; the numerous metabolites are excreted in the urine as glucuronides and ethereal sulfates. Unchanged drug accounts for 30–40% of a dose in the 48 hour urine (Gugler et al., 1974; Ohnhaus et al., 1974, 1982).

Toxicity. In overdose situations, bradycardia, cardiac failure, hypotension and bronchospasm may occur. Fatal bronchospasm has been reported in one case after a single dose of pindolol and a serum concentration of less than 10 µg/L (Schaffer, 1984).

Analysis. Pindolol can be determined in biological specimens by spectrofluorometry (Pacha, 1969; Spahn et al., 1985). Gas chromatography with electron-capture detection has been reported (Guerret, 1980). Liquid chromatography with fluorescence detection has also been employed (Bangah et al., 1980; Schields et al., 1986; Smith, 1987; Chmielowiec et al., 1991).

References

W.H. Aellig, H.H. Narjes, E. Nuesch et al. A pharmacodynamic and pharmacokinetic comparison of pindolol 20 mg retard and a conventional tablet. Eur. J. Clin. Pharm. 20: 179–183, 1981.

W.H. Aellig, E. Nuesch and W. Pacha. Pharmacokinetic comparison of pindolol 30 mg retard and 15 mg normal tablets. Eur. J. Pharm. 21: 451–455, 1982.

S.N. Anavekar, W.J. Louis, T.O. Morgan et al. The relationship of plasma levels of pindolol in hypertensive patients to effects on blood pressure, plasma renin and plasma noradrenaline levels. Clin. Exp. Pharm. Physiol. 2: 203–212, 1975.

M. Bangah, G. Jackman and A. Bobik. Determination of pindolol in human plasma by high-performance liquid chromatography. J. Chrom. 183: 255–259, 1980.

D. Chmielowiec, D. Schuster and F. Gengo. Determination of pindolol in human serum by HPLC. J. Chrom. Sci. 29: 37–39, 1991.

M. Guerret. Determination of pindolol in biological fluids by an electron capture gas-liquid chromatographic method on a wall-coated open tubular column. J. Chrom. 221: 387–392, 1980.

R. Gugler, W. Herold and H.J. Dengler. Pharmacokinetics of pindolol in man. Eur. J. Clin. Pharm. 7: 17–24, 1974.

R. Gugler, W. Hobel, G. Bodem and H.J. Dengler. The effect of pindolol on exercise-induced cardiac acceleration in relation to plasma levels in man. Clin. Pharm. Ther. 17: 127–133, 1975.

R. Gugler and G. Bodem. Single and multiple dose pharmacokinetics of pindolol. Eur. J. Clin. Pharm. 13: 13–16, 1978.

E.E. Ohnhaus, E. Nuesch, J. Meier, and F. Kalberer. Pharmacokinetics of unlabelled and ^{14}C-labelled pindolol in uraemia. Eur. J. Pharm. 7: 25–29, 1974.

E.E. Ohnhaus, H. Heidemann, J. Meier and G. Maurer. Metabolism of pindolol in patients with renal failure. Eur. J. Pharm. 22: 423–428, 1982.

W.L. Pacha. A method for the fluorimetric determination of 4-(2-hydroxy-3-isopropylaminopropoxy)-indole (LB46), a β–blocking agent, in plasma and urine. Experienta 25: 802–803, 1969.

M.I. Schaffer. Personal communication, 1984.

B.J. Schields, J.J. Lima, P.F. Binkley et al. Determination of pindolol in human plasma and urine by high-performance liquid chromatography with ultraviolet detection. J. Chrom. 378: 163–171, 1986.

H.T. Smith. High-performance liquid chromatographic method for the determination of pindolol in human plasma. J. Chrom. 415: 93–103, 1987.

H. Spahn, M. Prinoth and E. Mutschler. Determination of pindolol in plasma and urine by thin-layer chromatography. J. Chrom. 342: 458–464, 1985.

Piroxicam

T½: 45–71 hr
Vd: 0.31 L/kg
Fb: 0.04
pKa: 5.1 (acid), 1.8 (base)

Occurrence and Usage. Piroxicam (Feldene) has anti-inflammatory, analgesic and antipyretic properties. The drug is most commonly prescribed for the relief of signs and symptoms of osteoarthritis and rheumatoid arthritis. It is available for oral use in capsules containing either 10 mg or 20 mg of the free acid. It is recommended that the daily dose not exceed 20 mg.

Blood Concentrations. Twenty-five volunteers given 20 mg of piroxicam orally following an overnight fast demonstrated peak plasma concentrations of 1.5–2.0 mg/L in men and 2.0–3.0 mg/L in women (Richardson et al., 1985). Twenty healthy adult male subjects who received a 40 mg oral dose of piroxicam exhibited plasma concentrations within 1–3 hours that ranged from 3.4–6.4 mg/L (average, 4.5) (Hobbs and Twomey, 1976).

Following administration of 20 mg piroxicam daily to a healthy young adult for a period of 14 days, a plasma concentration of about 8 mg/L was determined by liquid chromatography on the 14th day; the concentration of the major metabolite, 5-hydroxypiroxicam, was less than 3 mg/L (Richardson and Ross, 1986). Steady-state plasma piroxicam concentrations ranging from 3–7 mg/L are found during chronic therapy with 20 mg/day (U.S. Pharmacopeial Convention, 1987).

Metabolism and Excretion. Metabolism of piroxicam occurs by hydroxylation to yield 5'-hydroxypiroxicam, with further biotransformation of this product occurring by conjugation, hydrolysis, decarboxylation, ring contraction, and N-demethylation (Richardson et al., 1986; Twomey and Hobbs, 1978). Up to 66% of a dose of piroxicam is excreted as metabolites in the urine with less than 5% of the dose eliminated unchanged. About 33% of the dose is excreted in the feces (Fourtillan and Dubourg, 1983; Ishizaki et al., 1979; U.S. Pharmacopeial Convention, 1987).

piroxicam → 5-hydroxypiroxicam

Toxicity. Piroxicam may cause leukopenia, eosinophilia, elevation of blood urea nitrogen, gastrointestinal distress, dizziness and rash. With overdosage, central nervous system depression and pulmonary edema can occur. An adult male who intentionally ingested 560 mg of the drug manifested drowsiness and occasional involuntary movements for 2 days; his serum piroxicam levels were 24, 15 and 4.7 mg/L at 14, 38 and 86 hours post-dose, respectively (Lo and Chan, 1983).

Analysis. Piroxicam has been measured in plasma by ultraviolet spectrophotometric (Hobbs and Twomey, 1979) and fluorometric methods (Hobbs and Twomey, 1979; Ishizaki et al., 1979). Due to lack of selectivity and sensitivity, they have been largely replaced by liquid chromatographic techniques (Twomey et al., 1980; Fourtillan and Dubourg, 1983; Richardson and Ross, 1986; Macek and Vacha, 1987; Wanwimolruk et al., 1991).

References

J.B. Fourtillan and D. Dubourg. Etude pharmacocinetique du piroxicam chez l'homme sain, apres administration d'une dose uniquie egale a 20 mg par coie orale. Therapie 38: 163–170, 1983.

D.C. Hobbs and T.M. Twomey. Piroxicam pharmacokinetics in man: aspirin and antacid interaction studies. J. Clin. Pharm. 19: 270–281, 1979.

T. Ishizaki, T. Nomura and T. Abe. Pharmacokinetics of piroxicam, a new nonsteroidal anti-inflammatory agent, under fasting and post-prandial states in man. J. Pharm. Biopharm. 7: 369–381, 1979.

G.C.C. Lo and J.Y.W. Chan. Piroxicam poisoning. Brit. Med. J. 287: 798, 1983.

J. Macek and J. Vacha. Rapid and sensitive method for determination of piroxicam in human plasma by high-performance liquid chromatography. J. Chrom. 420: 445–449, 1987.

C.J. Richardson, K.L.N. Blocka, S.G. Ross and R.K. Verbeeck. Effects of age and sex on piroxicam disposition. Clin. Pharm. Ther. 37: 13–18, 1985.

C.J. Richardson and S.G. Ross. High-performance liquid chromatographic analysis of piroxicam and its major metabolite 5'-hydroxypiroxicam in human plasma and urine. J. Chrom. 382: 382–388, 1986.

T.M. Twomey and D.C. Hobbs. Biotransformation of piroxicam by man. Fed. Proc. 37: 271, 1978.

T.M. Twomey, S.R. Bartolucci and D.C. Hobbs. Analysis of piroxicam in plasma by high pressure liquid chromatography, J. Chrom. 183: 104–108, 1980.

U.S. Pharmacopeial Convention. *Drug Information for the Health Care Provider*, 7th ed., Rockville, Maryland, 1987, p. 303.

S. Wanwimolruk, S.Z. Wanwimolruk and A.R. Zoest. A simple and sensitive hplc assay for piroxicam in plasma and its applicability to bioavailability study. J. Liq. Chrom. 14: 2373–2381, 1991.

Platinum

T½: 59–73 hr Pt^{+2}
Vd: ?
Fb: 0.90–0.95

Occurrence and Usage. Certain coordination complexes of divalent platinum have been found to have anticancer activity. Recently, cisplatin (cis-dichlorodiammine platinum, Platinol) was approved for use in the treatment of metastatic ovarian and testicular tumors. It is administered, usually in combination with other chemotherapeutic agents, by daily intravenous injection of 50–100 mg/m². Dosage schedules vary from once every 4 weeks to 5 times per week. Each mg of cisplatin contains 0.65 mg of platinum. The threshold limit value for occupational exposure is 1 mg/m³ for the metal and 0.002 mg/m³ for its soluble salts in the industrial atmosphere.

Blood Concentrations. Intravenous bolus injection of 50 mg/m² of cisplatin in 6 patients produced average total platinum plasma concentrations of 4.7 mg/L at 5 minutes, 1.8 mg/L at 1 hour, and 1.2 mg/L at 6 hours. The corresponding values for a 100 mg/m² dose were 6.2, 2.5, and 1.6 mg/L. Intact cisplatin represented approximately 50% of the total platinum value at 5 minutes and 25% at 1 hour; the cisplatin half-life averaged 20 minutes (Himmelstein et al., 1981). A 1 hour infusion of 70 mg/m² of cisplatin resulted in an average peak plasma level of platinum, just after the end of infusion, of 5.9 mg/L in 8 patients; the levels declined with an average terminal half-life of 67 hours. By 21 days after infusion, the plasma platinum concentrations averaged 0.3 mg/L (Gormley et al., 1979).

Metabolism and Excretion. An average of 50% of the administered platinum in an intravenous bolus dose of cisplatin was excreted in the 24 hour urine of 3 patients; this excretion of platinum averaged 75% when the drug was given by 6 hour infusion (Patton et al., 1978). From 28–67% of the urinary platinum during the first 6 hours after a dose is unchanged cisplatin (DeConti et al., 1973).

In all animal species examined, kidney contains the highest platinum concentration of any organ after a dose of cisplatin, up to 4 times that of liver. Kidney concentrations declined with a half-life of 8.4 days in rats (Taylor, 1978).

Toxicity. Adverse reactions to cisplatin include nephrotoxicity, ototoxicity, bone marrow depression, nausea, vomiting, peripheral neuropathy, and anaphylactic response. Stark and Howell (1978) demonstrated that nephrotoxicity could be avoided by limiting daily doses to 20 mg/m² and providing adequate hydration.

Analysis. Flameless atomic absorption spectrometry has been used to determine free or total platinum in plasma (LeRoy et al., 1977; Bannister et al., 1978; Hull et al., 1981; Smeyers-Verbeke et al., 1981; Hopfer et al., 1989) and in tissues (Denniston et al., 1981). Liquid chromatographic methods have also been described (Drummer et al., 1984; Reece et al., 1984; Parsons and LeRoy, 1986).

References

S.J. Bannister, Y. Chang, L.A. Sternson and A.J. Repta. Atomic absorption spectrophotometry of free circulating platinum species in plasma derived from cis-dichlorodiammineplatinum. Clin. Chem. 24: 877–880, 1978.

R.C. DeConti, B.R. Toftness, R.C. Lange and W.A. Creasey. Clinical and pharmacological studies with cis-diamminedichloroplatinum (II). Cancer Res. 33: 1310–1315, 1973.

M.L. Denniston, L.A. Sternson and A.J. Repta. Analysis of total platinum derived from cisplatin in tissue. Anal. Letters 14: 451–462, 1981.

O.H. Drummer, A. Proudfoot, L. Howes and W.J. Louis. High-performance liquid chromatographic determination of platinum (II) in plasma ultrafiltrate and urine: comparison with a flameless atomic absorption spectrometric method. Clin. Chim. Acta 136: 65–74, 1984.

P.E. Gormley, J.M. Bull, A.F. LeRoy and R. Cysyk. Kinetics of cis-dichlorodiammineplatinum. Clin. Pharm. Ther. 25: 351–357, 1979.

K.J. Himmelstein, T.F. Patton, R.J. Belt et al. Clinical kinetics of intact cisplatin and some related species. Clin. Pharm. Ther. 29: 658–664, 1981.

S.M. Hopfer, L. Ziebka, F.W. Sunderman, Jr. et al. Direct analysis of platinum in plasma and urine in electrothermal atomic absorption spectrophotometry. Ann. Clin. Lab. Sci. 19: 389–396, 1989.

D.A. Hull, N. Muhammad, J.G. Lanese et al. Determination of platinum in serum and ultrafiltrate by flameless atomic absorption spectrophotometry. J. Pharm. Sci. 70: 500–502, 1981.

A.F. LeRoy, M.L. Wehling, H.L. Sponseller et al. Analysis of platinum in biological materials by flameless atomic absorption spectrophotometry. Biochem. Med. 18: 184-191, 1977.

P.J. Parsons and A.F. LeRoy. Determination of cis-diamminedichloroplatinum (II) in human plasma using ion-pair chromatography with electrochemical detection. J. Chrom. 378: 395–408, 1986.

T.F. Patton, K.J. Himmelstein, R. Belt et al. Plasma levels and urinary excretion of filterable platinum species following bolus injection and IV infusion of cis-dichlorodiammineplatinum(II) in man. Cancer Treat. Rep. 62: 1359–1362, 1978.

P.A. Reece, J.T. McCall, G. Powis and R.L. Richardson. Sensitive high-performance liquid chromatographic assay for platinum in plasma ultrafiltrate. J. Chrom. 306: 417–423, 1984.

J. Smeyers-Verbeke, M.R. Detaevernier, L. Denis and D.L. Massart. The determination of platinum in biological fluid by means of graphite furnace atomic absorption spectrometry. Clin. Chim. Acta 113: 329–333, 1981.

J.J. Stark and S.B. Howell. Nephrotoxicity of cis-platinum (II) dichlorodiammine. Clin. Pharm. Ther. 23: 461–466, 1978.

D.M. Taylor. The pharmacokinetics of cis-diamminodichloro-platinum (II) in animals and man: relation to treatment schedule. Biochimie 60: 949–956, 1978.

Polybrominated Biphenyls

T½: 12 years
Vd: ?
Fb: ?

Occurrence and Usage. Polybrominated biphenyls (PBB), usually with 4–8 bromine atoms per molecule, are used commercially as fire retardants. One such mixture, consisting primarily of 2,2',4,4',5,5'-hexabromobiphenyl, was inadvertently added to cattle feed in Michigan in 1973, leading to widespread contamination. The compounds are believed to be well-absorbed after ingestion or dermal contact. There is no assigned threshold limit value for the polybrominated biphenyls.

Blood Concentrations. In a study conducted in 1976–1977, a group of unexposed farmers had nearly uniformly undetectable serum PBB concentrations, while Michigan farmers and consumers showed concentrations ranging from undetectable to greater than 100 μg/L, with most in the 1–5 μg/L range (Anderson et al., 1979). Serum PBB levels ranged from 1–1530 μg/L in 14 workers at a PBB production plant (Wolff et al., 1979a).

Metabolism and Excretion. PBB metabolites have not been identified in man. The compounds are very lipid soluble and tend to accumulate in fat with continued exposure. In rats, hexabromobiphenyl is apparently not metabolized; it primarily localizes in adipose tissue and is excreted very slowly over a 42 day period in urine (0.1%) and feces (6.6%). It was estimated that less than 10% of a single dose would be excreted by a rat in its lifetime (Matthews et al., 1977).

PBB concentrations in adipose tissue of most members of the general population are below detectable levels, but in 1975 averaged 226 μg/kg in urban residents of Michigan, 516 μg/kg in non-quarantined farmers and 1,965 μg/kg in quarantined farmers. After 1974, fat PBB levels were found to decline by an average of 39% (range, 11–72) in 16 persons over a 6 month period. No consistent relationship was found between PBB concentrations in fat and serum. The ratio of PBB in fat to that in breast milk averaged about 2 (Meester and McCoy, 1977; Meester, 1979). Breast milk concentrations averaged 68 µg/L (range, 0–1200) in 53 women from Michigan's lower peninsula (Brilliant et al., 1978).

Toxicity. Symptoms observed in persons exposed to PBB in their diets have included fatigue, joint pain and stiffness, headache, muscle pain, dizziness, sleepiness and skin rash. Abnormal serum enzyme levels suggestive of liver damage were especially noted in farmers whose serum PBB concentrations exceeded 1 µg/L, and a positive correlation was noted between serum PBB concentrations and urinary porphyrin excretion (Anderson et al., 1979; Meester, 1979). Animals severely poisoned by PBB developed anorexia, alopecia, abnormal growth of the hooves, fatty metamorphosis and cancer of the liver, and kidney damage (Meester and McCoy, 1977; Kimbrough, 1987).

Analysis. PBB in serum and fat is routinely analyzed by gas chromatography with electron-capture (Willett et al., 1978; Wolff et al., 1979b; Burse et al., 1980) or mass spectrometric detection (Bekesi et al., 1979; Lewis and Sovocool, 1982).

References

H.A. Anderson, M.S. Wolff, R. Lilis et al. Symptoms and clinical abnormalities following ingestion of poly-brominated-biphenyl-contaminated food products. Ann. N.Y. Acad. Sci. 320: 684–702, 1979.

J.G. Bekesi, J. Roboz, H.A. Anderson et al. Impaired immune function and identification of polybrominated biphenyls (PBB) in blood compartments of exposed Michigan dairy farmers and chemical workers. Drug Chem. Tox. 2: 179–191, 1979.

L.B. Brilliant, K. Wilcox, G. Van Amburg et al. Breast-milk monitoring to measure Michigan's contamination with polybrominated biphenyls. Lancet 2: 643–646, 1978.

V.W. Burse, L.L. Needham, J.A. Liddle et al. Interlaboratory comparison for results of analyses for polybromi-nated biphenyls in human serum. J. Anal. Tox. 4: 22–26, 1980.

R.D. Kimbrough. Human health effects of polychlorinated biphenyls (PCBs) and polybrominated biphenyls (PBBs). Ann. Rev. Pharm. Tox. 27: 87–111, 1987.

R.G. Lewis and G.W. Sovocool. Identification of polybrominated biphenyls in the adipose tissues of the general population of the United States. J. Anal. Tox. 6: 196–198, 1982.

H.B. Matthews, S. Kato, N.M. Morales and D.B. Tuey. Distribution and excretion of 2,4,5,2',4',5'-hexabromobiphenyl, the major component of firemaster BP-6. J. Tox. Env. Health 3: 599–605, 1977.

W.D. Meester and D.J. McCoy, Sr. Human toxicology of polybrominated biphenyls. In *Management of the Poisoned Patient* (B.H. Rumack and A.R. Temple, eds.), Science Press, Princeton, 1977, pp. 32–61.

W.D. Meester. The effect of polybrominated biphenyls on man: the Michigan PBB disaster. Vet. Hum. Tox. 21: 131–135, 1979.

L.B. Willett, C.J. Brumm and C.L. Williams. Method for extraction, isolation, and detection of free polybro-minated biphenyls (PBBs) from plasma, feces, milk, and bile using disposable glassware. J. Agr. Food Chem. 26: 122–125, 1978.

M.S. Wolff, H.A. Anderson, K.D. Rosenman and I.J. Selikoff. Equilibrium of polybrominated biphenyl (PBB) residues in serum and fat of Michigan residents. Bull. Env. Cont. Tox. 21: 775–781, 1979a.

M.S. Wolff, H.A. Anderson, F. Camper et al. Analysis of adipose tissue and serum from PBB (polybrominated biphenyl)-exposed workers. J. Env. Path. Tox. 2: 1397–1411, 1979b.

Polychlorinated Biphenyls

T½: 7–8 months (Arochlor 1242)
    33–34 months (Arochlor 1260)
Vd: ?
Fb: ?

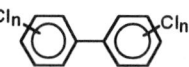

Occurrence and Usage. The polychlorinated biphenyls (PCB) were produced in the United States from 1929 until 1977 for use as coolant and insulator fluids for transformer and capacitors, as heat transfer fluids and as flame retardants for wood products. Their manufacture continues in a number of European countries. The substances are extremely persistent, and heavy industrial usage has led to widespread contamination of the environment. The current FDA limit for PCB in edible freshwater fish is 5 mg/kg, although examples of certain species have been found to contain as much as 900 mg/kg. Exposure can be dietary or by inhalation, dermal contact or ingestion in occupational situations. The current threshold limit value is 1 mg/m^3 for PCB containing 42% chlorine and 0.5 mg/m^3 for mixtures containing 54% chlorine.

Blood Concentrations. PCB residues were found in 43% of 616 plasma specimens from residents of the southeastern United States, in concentrations up to 29 μg/L (Finklea et al., 1972). Other studies have shown an average PCB serum level of 4–7 μg/L in U.S. citizens without any unusual exposure, with a range of 1–37 μg/L (Sahl et al., 1985; Kimbrough, 1987). These levels ranged from 1.8–3.8 μg/L in the blood of 10 members of the Japanese population in 1975 (Fukano and Doguchi, 1977). Blood PCB levels were observed to increase by 50% in 2 volunteers within several hours after the ingestion of a fish meal containing 128–181 μg of PCB (Kuwabara et al., 1979). The serum elimination half-life for Arochlor 1242 has been estimated at 7–8 months, while that for Arochlor 1260 at 33–34 months (Steele et al., 1986).

Metabolism and Excretion. The metabolism of the PCB isomers has not been studied in humans. In animals, the compounds are biotransformed by oxidation and dechlorination, and the hydroxylated metabolites and their conjugates are excreted in urine, feces and milk. The rate of metabolism of each isomer is a function of the number and position of chlorine atoms; the fully chlorinated compound, decachlorobiphenyl, is apparently not metabolized. All of the PCB isomers are highly lipid soluble and tend to accumulate in adipose tissue with repeated exposure (NIOSH, 1977). The extent of elimination of an isomer is a function of its rate of metabolism, such that the more highly chlorinated compounds are extremely long-lived in mammals (Matthews and Anderson, 1975).

Of 637 specimens of adipose tissue obtained from members of the U.S. population, 69% contained less than 1 mg/kg of PCB, 26% contained from 1–2 mg/kg and 5%, more than 2 mg/kg (Yobs, 1972). In 30 Japanese citizens, these levels averaged 1.0 mg/kg and ranged from 0.4–2.5 mg/kg (Fukano and Doguchi, 1977). In 6 Japanese citizens, liver concentrations of PCB averaged 0.09 mg/kg and ranged from 0.03–0.32 mg/kg (Watanabe et al., 1980).

Breast milk PCB concentrations in specimens from 1057 nursing mothers in Michigan averaged 1.5 mg/L, ranging from trace amounts to 5.1 mg/L; 50% of the specimens were in the 1–2 mg/L range (Wickizer and Brilliant, 1981).

Toxicity. Workers exposed to PCB air concentrations of only 0.1 mg/m^3 have developed skin irritation characterized by an acneform eruption (chloracne). In 34 workers, air concentrations of up to 2.2 mg/m^3 produced skin irritation, nausea and an average blood PCB level of 400 μg/L (Ouw et al., 1976). In a study of 326 capacitor manufacturing workers, the most prevalent symptoms of PCB exposure were the dermatologic effects together with such neurologic effects as headache, nervousness, fatigue and dizziness; these workers had total PCB concentrations in plasma that averaged 172 μg/L and ranged up to 2530 μg/L. A positive correlation was found between plasma PCB level and plasma SGOT concentration (Fischbein et al., 1979). One chronically exposed individual developed mental impairment, depression and malaise; a maximal serum PCB level of 414 µg/L was observed (Jackson, 1985).

A mass poisoning in Japan that affected nearly 2000 persons has been attributed to the dietary use of PCB-contaminated rice oil. The symptoms of the disease, known as Yusho, includes those mentioned above as well as brown pigmentation of the skin and nails, increased eye secretions, weakness, swelling of the joints and numbness in the extremities. Five years after the incident, the average blood PCB concentrations in 72 of these patients was 5.9 µg/L (Urabe et al., 1979), and in 6 other patients the PCB fat concentration ranged from 0.7–4.3 mg/kg (Masuda et al., 1974). These concentrations are relatively low, and it has been suggested that polychlorinated dibenzofurans also present in the Japanese oil contributed significantly to the toxic effects observed in these patients (Fischbein et al., 1979). In a very similar mass poisoning in Taiwan, in which analytical measurements were made within 1 year after the outbreak, blood PCB concentrations in 66 patients averaged 49 µg/L and ranged from 11–720 µg/L (Chen et al., 1980).

Analysis. PCB concentrations in serum or adipose tissue are routinely measured by gas chromatography with electron-capture (Price and Welch, 1972; Doguchi and Fukano, 1975; Chen et al., 1980; Needham et al., 1981; Luotamo et al., 1985; Burse et al., 1990) or mass spectrometric detection (Biros et al., 1970). A radioisotope dilution assay has been described (Kohli et al., 1979; Ando et al., 1986). Up to a 100-fold variation in reported serum PCB levels is possible depending on the method used for calculation (Lawton et al., 1985).

References

M. Ando, H. Saito and I. Wakisaka. Gas chromatographic and mass spectrometric analysis of polychlorinated biphenyls in human placenta and cord blood. Env. Res. 41: 14–22, 1986.

F.J. Biros, A.C. Walker and A. Medbery. Polychlorinated biphenyls in human adipose tissue. Bull. Env. Cont. Tox. 5: 317–323, 1970.

P.H. Chen, J.M. Gaw, C.K. Wong and C.J. Chen. Levels of gas chromatographic patterns of polychlorinated biphenyls in the blood of patients after PCB poisoning in Taiwan. Bull. Env. Cont. Tox. 25: 325–329, 1980.

M. Doguchi and S. Fukano. Residue levels of polychlorinated terphenyls, polychlorinated biphenyls and DDT in human blood. Bull. Env. Cont. Tox. 13: 57–63, 1975.

J. Finklea, L.E. Priester, J.P. Creason et al. Polychlorinated biphenyl residues in human plasma expose a major urban pollution problem. Am. J. Pub. Health 62: 645–651, 1972.

A. Fischbein, M.S. Wolff, R. Lilis et al. Clinical findings among PCB-exposed capacitor manufacturing workers. Ann. N.Y. Acad. Sci. 320: 703–714, 1979.

S. Fukano and M. Doguchi. PCT, PCB and pesticide residues in human fat and blood. Bull. Env. Cont. Tox. 17: 613–617, 1977.

J.E. Jackson. Neuropsychiatric manifestations of chronic PCB intoxication. Vet. Hum. Tox. 28: 299, 1985.

R.D. Kimbrough. Human health effects of polychlorinated biphenyls (PCBs) and polybrominated biphenyls (PBBs). Ann. Rev. Pharm. Tox. 27: 87–111, 1987.

K.K. Kohli, P.W. Albro and J.D. McKinney. Radioisotope dilution assay (RIDA) for the estimation of polychlorinated biphenyls (PCBs). J. Anal. Tox. 3: 125–128, 1979.

K. Kuwabara, T. Kakushiji, I. Watanabe et al. Increase in the human blood PCB levels promptly following ingestion of fish containing PCBs. Bull. Env. Cont. Tox. 21: 273–278, 1979.

R.W. Lawton, J.F. Brown, M.R. Ross and J. Feingold. Comparability and precision of serum PCB measurements. Arch. Env. Health 40: 29–37, 1985.

M. Luotama, J. Jarvisalo and A. Aitio. Analysis of polychlorinated biphenyls (PCBs) in human serum. Env. Health Persp. 60: 327–332, 1985.

Y. Masuda, R. Kagawa and M. Kuratsune. Comparison of polychlorinated biphenyls in Yusho patients and ordinary persons. Bull. Env. Cont. Tox. 11: 213–216, 1974.

H.B. Matthews and M.W. Anderson. Effect of chlorination on the distribution and excretion of polychlorinated biphenyls. Drug Met. Disp. 3: 371–380, 1975.

L.L. Needham, V.W. Burse and H.A. Price. Temperature-programmed gas chromatographic determination of polychlorinated and polybrominated biphenyls in serum. J. Asso. Off. Anal. Chem. 64: 1131–1137, 1981.

NIOSH. *Occupational Exposure to Polychlorinated Biphenyls (PCBs)*, National Institute for Occupational Safety and Health, Cincinnati, Ohio, 1977.

H.K. Ouw, G.R. Simpson and D.W. Siyali. Use and health effects of Arochlor 1242, a polychlorinated biphenyl, in an electrical industry. Arch. Env. Health 31: 189–194, 1976.

H.A. Price and R.L. Welch. Occurrence and polychlorinated biphenyls in humans. Env. Health Persp. 1: 73–78, 1972.

J.D. Sahl, T. Crocker, R.J. Gordon et al. Polychlorinated biphenyls in the blood of personnel from an electric utility. J. Occ. Med. 27: 639–643, 1985.

G. Steele, P. Stehr-Green and E. Welty. Estimates of the biologic half-life of polychlorinated biphenyls in human serum. New Eng. J. Med. 314: 926–927, 1986.

H. Urabe, H. Koda and M. Asahi. Present state of Yusho patients. Ann. N.Y. Acad. Sci. 320: 273–276, 1979.

I. Watanabe, T. Yakushiji and N. Kunita. Distribution differences between polychlorinated terphenyls and polychlorinated biphenyls. Bull. Env. Cont. Tox. 25: 810–815, 1980.

T.M. Wickizer and L.B. Brilliant. Testing for polychlorinated biphenyls in human milk. Pediatrics 68: 411–415, 1981.

A.R. Yobs. Levels of polychlorinated biphenyls in adipose tissue of the general population of the nation. Env. Health Persp. 1: 79–81, 1972.

Potassium

T½: ?
Vd: ? K^+
Fb: 0

Occurrence and Usage. Potassium is a highly reactive alkali metal that is found in salt form in nature. Potassium salts are widely used in various industrial processes and are common laboratory chemicals. Potassium is the most abundant intracellular cation and its bioregulation in the mammalian organism is critical to maintenance of proper function. The daily dietary intake for humans has been estimated at 3–5 g, expressed as the metal. Potassium is used therapeutically in the form of the acetate, bicarbonate, bitartrate, chloride, citrate, gluconate, iodide and phosphate salts as gastric antacids, urine acidifiers, dietary supplements and sodium substitutes. A typical 20 mL vial of 15% potassium chloride solution intended for intravenous injection contains 3000 mg of KCl, equivalent to 1572 mg of K^+ (40 mmol or 40 mEq); 1 or 2 such vials could provide the recommended daily adult requirement of 40–80 mmol, at an infusion rate not to exceed 10 mmol/hour. The pediatric maintenance requirement for potassium is 2 mmol/kg/day.

Blood Concentrations. The usual reference range for serum potassium, regardless of age or sex, is 3.5–4.9 mmol/L. Serum potassium may be lowered by malnutrition or certain diuretics and may be elevated by circulatory failure, tissue necosis or renal insufficiency (Hitz, 1985). The normal erythrocyte potassium content is 105 mmol/L, giving a blood/plasma concentration ratio of approximately 13. Hemolysis of a whole blood specimen to the extent of 0.5% produces a rise in serum potassium of approximately 0.5 mmol/L (Tietz, 1983).

Intravenous administration of 100–200 mmol of potassium at the rate of 10 mmol/hour will cause a rise in serum potassium of 1 mmol/L in most adults (Cuddy, 1992).

Metabolism and Excretion. Potassium salts are readily absorbed from the gastrointestinal tract. The ion enters the extracellular pool and becomes available for uptake into cells; intracellular potassium averages 150 mmol/L and represents 98% of total body potassium content. Excess potassium is slowly released to the extracellular fluid and is excreted largely by the kidney; minor routes of elimination include feces, sweat, saliva and tears. The distribution volume and elimination half-life of an administered dose of potassium vary greatly with the dose, rate of administration, potassium and acid-base balance of the individual, and renal and cardiac function. Urine normally contains 25–125 mmol/L of potassium, although this may vary significantly with diet and fluid balance (Tietz, 1983; Hitz, 1985; Cuddy, 1992).

Toxicity. Moderate hyperkalemia, defined as a serum potassium level of 6.5–8.0 mmol/L, may cause electrocardiographic abnormalities and neuromuscular weakness; severe hyperkalemia, associated with serum potassium values exceeding 8.0 mmol/L, may result in skeletal muscle paresthesias and paralysis and cardiac arrhythmias and arrest (Cuddy, 1992). Treatment for hyperkalemia often involves administration of calcium gluconate to antagonize the depressant effect of potassium on muscle function, sodium bicarbonate, glucose and/or insulin to promote the intracellular movement of the ion, and a cation-exchange resin or the use of hemodialysis to remove potassium from the body (Ellenhorn and Barceloux, 1988). Two cases of accidental over-ingestion of potassium chloride salt substitutes have been reported in which the individuals survived, despite developing severe weakness, EKG abnormalities, and serum potassium values of 9.1–10.2 mmol/L (Kallen et al., 1976; Hoyt, 1986). Three individuals survived the intentional ingestion of 12–24 g of potassium chloride in the form of slow-release tablets after developing peak plasma potassium values, about 5–6 hours after ingestion, of 8.9–9.3 mmol/L (Illingworth and Proudfoot, 1980).

Two children who died after accidental oral ingestion of potassium chloride exhibited serum potassium levels of 10.1 and 14 mmol/L (Bacon, 1974; Wetli and Davis, 1978). Since whole blood potassium concentrations are normally on the order of 77–84 mmol/L, it is quite likely that fatal potassium poisoning would not be detected by analysis of a hemolyzed postmortem blood specimen (Bhatkhande and Joglekar, 1977). Vitreous humor, which contains potassium at levels similar to those of serum in living persons, may be indicative of potassium poisoning if allowance is made for the steady increase in potassium concentration that occurs after death. Vitreous humor potassium concentrations of 10.8 mmol/L at 18 hours postmortem and 17.5 mmol/L at 36 hours postmortem were determined to be consistent with fatal potassium poisoning in 2 adults (Wetli and Davis, 1978; Forrest, 1984). Using the regression formula published by Sturner (1963), postmortem interval (hours) = $(7.14 \times K^+) - 39.1$, we can calculate that the expected vitreous humor concentrations in the above cases in the absence of potassium poisoning would have been 8.0 and 10.5 mmol/L, respectively, clearly lower than the measured values.

Analysis. Potassium is normally measured in body fluids by flame photometry or ion-selective potentiometry (Kaplan and Szabo, 1983).

References

C. Bacon. Death from accidental potassium poisoning in childhood. Brit. Med. J. 1: 389–390, 1974.

C.Y. Bhatkhande and V.D. Joglekar. Fatal poisoning by potassium in human and rabbit. For. Sci. 9: 33–36, 1977.

P.G. Cuddy. Fluid and electrolyte disorders. In *Applied Therapeutics* (M.A. Koda-Kimble and L.Y. Young, eds.), Applied Therapeutics, Vancouver, Washington, 1992, pp. 28–7 to 28–11.

A.R.W. Forrest. Personal communication, 1984.

J. Hitz. Potassium and sodium. In *Interpretation of Clinical Laboratory Tests* (G. Siest et al., eds.), Biomedical Publications, Foster City, California, 1985, pp. 366–378.

R.E. Hoyt. Hyperkalemia due to salt substitutes. J. Am. Med. Asso. 256: 1726, 1986.

R.N. Illingworth and A.T. Proudfoot. Rapid poisoning with slow-release potassium. Brit. Med. J. 281: 485–486, 1980.

A. Kaplan and L.L. Szabo. *Clinical Chemistry*, Lea & Febiger, Philadelphia, 1983, pp. 86–88.

R.J. Kallen, C.H.L. Rieger, H.S. Cohen et al. Near-fatal hyperkalemia due to ingestion of salt substitute by an infant. J. Am. Med. Asso. 235: 2125–2126, 1976.

W.Q. Sturner. The vitreous humor: postmortem potassium changes. Lancet 1: 807–808, 1963.

N.W. Tietz. *Clinical Guide to Laboratory Tests*, W.B. Saunders, Philadelphia, 1983, pp. 398–401.

C.V. Wetli and J.H. Davis. Fatal hyperkalemia from accidental overdose of potassium chloride. J. Am. Med. Asso. 240: 1339, 1978.

Prazepam

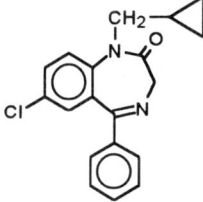

T½: 1.3 hr
Vd: 12–14 L/kg
Fb: ?
pKa: 2.7

Occurrence and Usage. Prazepam (Centrax, Verstran) is the N-cyclopropylmethyl analogue of diazepam. It was synthesized in 1965 and is currently available for use as an antianxiety agent. It is supplied as the free base in tablets or capsules of 5–10 mg. The compound is administered orally in daily doses of 20–60 mg.

Blood Concentrations. After a single 20 mg oral dose given to 12 volunteers, prazepam was not detected in plasma. Nordiazepam concentrations reached peak levels of 0.072–0.174 mg/L (average, 0.138 mg/L) at times of 2.5 to 72 hours (average, 13 hours). The half-life of nordiazepam averaged 69 hours, ranging from 29–193 hours (Allen et al., 1979). In 9 volunteers given a 30 mg tablet, plasma prazepam concentrations reached an average peak of 0.007 mg/L within 30 minutes and declined rapidly, while peak nordiazepam concentrations averaged 0.321 mg/L at a mean time of 4.3 hours. The nordiazepam half-life averaged 96 hours in this study (Smith et al., 1979). Three volunteers given a single 40 mg oral dose achieved an average peak serum level of 0.218 mg/L at an average time of 6.8 hours (Ochs et al., 1984).

Metabolism and Excretion. Prazepam is either dealkylated to nordiazepam, the major plasma species, or oxidized to 3-hydroxyprazepam. This latter compound may be either conjugated directly or first dealkylated to oxazepam, which is then conjugated. Unchanged prazepam has not been detected in urine and only trace amounts of nordiazepam have been found. Over 38% of a dose is excreted as urinary metabolites in 48 hours and nearly 60% after 7 days, primarily as oxazepam glucuronide (30–59% of the total) and 3-hydroxyprazepam glucuronide (3–35%). A number of unidentified metabolites have been observed (DiCarlo et al., 1970; Viau et al., 1973).

prazepam

3-hydroxyprazepam

conjugation

nordiazepam

oxazepam

Toxicity. Adverse reactions to prazepam administration include dizziness, fatigue, drowsiness, ataxia, weakness, confusion, and slurred speech.

Analysis. A method has been briefly described for the flame-ionization gas chromatographic detection of prazepam following its hydrolysis to a benzophenone derivative (Maier and Wehr, 1974). More sensitive and specific procedures involve electron-capture gas chromatography (Nau et al., 1978; Smith et al., 1979). Many of the techniques described in the sections on clorazepate and diazepam are also applicable to determination of prazepam and its active entity, nordiazepam.

References

M.D. Allen, D.J. Greenblatt, J.S. Harmatz and R.I. Shader. Single-dose kinetics of prazepam, a precursor of desmethyldiazepam. J. Clin. Pharm. 19: 445–450, 1979.

F.J. DiCarlo, J.P. Viau, J.E. Epps and L.J. Haynes. Prazepam metabolism by man. Clin. Pharm. Ther. 11: 890–897, 1970.

R.D. Maier and K.H. Wehr. Zum Nachweis von Prazepam, einen neuen Tranquilizer aus der Reihe der Benzodiazepine. Arch. Tox. 32: 341–345, 1974.

H. Nau, C. Liddiard, D. Jesdinsky et al. Quantitative analysis of prazepam and its metabolites by electron capture gas chromatography and selected ion monitoring. J. Chrom. 146: 227–239, 1978.

H.R. Ochs, D.J. Greenblatt, B. Verburg-Ochs and A. Locniskar. Comparative single-dose kinetics of oxazolam, prazepam and clorazepate: three precursors of desmethyldiazepam. J. Clin. Pharm. 24: 446–451, 1984.

M.T. Smith, L.E.J. Evans, M.J. Eadie and J.H. Tyrer. Pharmacokinetics of prazepam in man. Eur. J. Clin. Pharm. 16: 141–147, 1979.

J.P. Viau, J.E. Epps and F.J. DiCarlo. Prazepam metabolism after chronic administration to humans. Xenobiotica 3: 581–587, 1973.

Prazosin

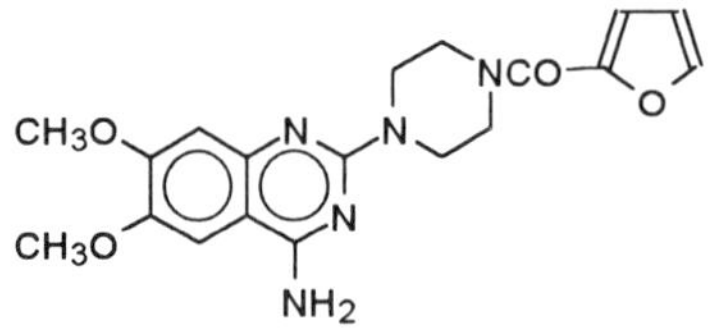

T½: 2–3 hr
Vd: 0.6 L/kg
Fb: 0.97
pKa: 6.5

Occurrence and Usage. Prazosin (Minipress) is a post-synaptic alpha-adrenergic blocking agent used in the treatment of hypertension. It is available as the hydrochloride salt in 1–5 mg capsules. The usual initial dose of prazosin is 1 mg two or three times daily, increased as necessary. Total daily doses as high as 20–40 mg have been given, but the benefit of daily doses exceeding 10 mg is questionable.

Blood Concentrations. After single oral doses of 5 mg given to 24 healthy male subjects, peak plasma concentrations of 6–78 µg/L (average, 36) were attained in 1–4 hours (Hobbs et al., 1978).

Metabolism and Excretion. Animal studies indicate that prazosin is extensively metabolized, primarily by demethylation and conjugation, and excreted mainly via bile and feces. Less extensive human studies indicate similar pathways of metabolism and excretion (Taylor et al., 1977; Hobbs et al., 1978). About 6% of the drug is eliminated unchanged in the urine. The 2 major metabolites are O-methylated and are almost completely excreted in the bile (Lenz et al., 1985).

Toxicity. Faintness and dizziness have been reported in up to one-half the patients receiving prazosin (Stanaszek et al., 1983). Other adverse effects include irregular heartbeat, headache, shortness of breath, water retention, drop in blood pressure, nausea and vomiting. A 75 year old man ingested

80 mg of prazosin and had an admission serum level of 899 µg/L; he manifested only drowsiness and mild hypotension and recovered within 18 hours (Rygnestad and Dale, 1983). A 72 year old man was admitted to hospital in coma with severe hypotension 3 hours after ingestion of 120 mg of the drug in an unsuccessful suicide attempt; a plasma concentration was not obtained until 11 hours after ingestion, at which time it was 48 µg/L (Lenz et al., 1985).

Analysis. The quantitative determination of prazosin in plasma has been accomplished by fluorometry (Wood et al., 1976; Hobbs et al., 1978). High-performance liquid chromatography with fluorescence detection has been used for the determination of prazosin in plasma, blood and urine (Twomey and Hobbs, 1978; Lin et al., 1980; Shen and Pitterman, 1985).

References

D.C. Hobbs, T.M. Twomey and R.F. Palmer. Pharmacokinetics of prazosin in man. J. Clin. Pharm. 18: 402–406, 1978.

K. Lenz, W. Druml, G. Kleinberger et al. Acute intoxication with prazosin: case report. Hum. Tox. 4: 53–56, 1985.

E.T. Lin, R.A. Baughman, Jr. and L.Z. Benet. High-performance liquid chromatographic determination of prazosin in human plasma, whole blood and urine. J. Chrom. 183: 367–371, 1980.

T.K. Rygnestad and O. Dale. Self-poisoning with prazosin. Acta Med. Scand. 213: 157–158, 1983.

D.D. Shen and A.B. Pitterman. High-performance assay for prazosin in serum. In. *Methodology for Analytical Toxicology*, Vol. III (I. Sunshine, ed.), CRC Press, Boca Raton, Florida, 1985, pp. 159–164.

W.F. Stanaszek, D. Kellerman, R.N. Brogden et al. Prazosin update: a review of its pharmacological properties and therapeutic use in hypertension. Drugs 25: 339–384, 1983.

J.A. Taylor, T.M. Twomey and M. Schach von Witteman. The metabolic fate of prazosin. Xenobiotica 7: 357–360, 1977.

T.M. Twomey and D.C. Hobbs. Analysis of prazosin in plasma by a sensitive high-performance liquid chromatographic-fluorescence method. J. Pharm. Sci. 67: 1468–1469, 1978.

A.J. Wood, B. Bolli and F.O. Simpson. Prazosin in normal subjects: plasma levels, blood pressure and heart rate. Brit. J. Clin. Pharm. 1: 199, 1976.

Prilocaine

T½: ?
Vd: 0.7–4.4 L/kg
Fb: 0.30
pKa: 7.9

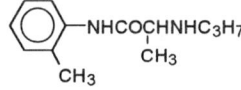

Occurrence and Usage. Prilocaine (Citanest) is a local anesthetic of the amide type, first synthesized in 1960. It is supplied as the hydrochloride in 1–3% solutions for epidural, caudal, peripheral nerve and infiltration anesthesia. Doses of 30–600 mg are commonly used.

Blood Concentrations. Following administration of 200, 400 or 600 mg of prilocaine for epidural anesthesia, plasma concentrations in at least 10 subjects reached average peaks of 1.69, 2.67 and 4.47 mg/L, respectively, at 10–20 minutes; the erythrocyte/plasma concentration ratio for the drug is 1.2 at therapeutic levels (Scott et al., 1972). After intercostal nerve block with 400 mg in 9 subjects, plasma concentrations averaged 4.69 mg/L after 15 minutes and 2.46 mg/L by 1 hour (Braid and Scott, 1965). During obstetric lumbar peridural anesthesia produced by 140 mg of prilocaine, simultaneously determined plasma concentrations in 21 mothers and neonates averaged 0.53 and 0.44 mg/L, respectively (Hook et al., 1971).

Metabolism and Excretion. The metabolism of prilocaine in man has not been investigated. In rats, the drug is rapidly metabolized by hydrolysis of the amide linkage, probably to o-toluidine. One hour after an injection, the highest concentrations of prilocaine are found in lung, kidney, brain, heart, liver, and blood, in decreasing order. Only a small amount is eliminated unchanged in urine (Akerman et al., 1966). Acidification of the urine is known to markedly increase the renal clearance of the drug in man (Eriksson and Granberg, 1965).

Toxicity. Overdosage with prilocaine can produce dizziness, blurred vision, tremors, drowsiness, hypotension, bradycardia, convulsions, coma, and respiratory and cardiac arrest. Methemoglobinemia occurs in all patients who receive the drug, apparently due to the formation of o-toluidine as a metabolite. A patient who received 1650 mg of prilocaine over a 12 hour period developed cyanosis, but this was readily reversed by administration of methylene blue (Poppers, 1967). A 5 year old dental patient developed severe cyanosis, generalized convulsions and coma after administration of only 52 mg of the drug; he was also successfully treated with methylene blue (Ludwig 1981).

In the case of an 83 year old man who died after receiving 864 mg of prilocaine during the course of an hour for dental anesthesia, postmortem concentrations of 13 mg/L in blood, 49 mg/kg in liver and 69 mg/L in urine were determined (Kaliciak and Chan, 1986).

Analysis. Prilocaine has been determined in plasma by a nonspecific dye technique (Braid and Scott, 1965). Flame-ionization gas chromatography is preferred for its greater specificity (Svinhufvud et al., 1965; Keenaghan, 1968; Cameron, 1974). Liquid chromatography has also been described (Whelpton et al., 1990).

References

B. Akerman, A. Astrom, S. Ross and A. Tele. Studies of the absorption, distribution and metabolism of labelled prilocaine and lidocaine in some animal species. Acta Pharm. Tox. 24: 389–403, 1966.

D.P. Braid and D.B. Scott. The systemic absorption of local analgesic drugs. Brit. J. Anaesth. 37: 394–404, 1965.

J.D. Cameron. The gas chromatographic determination of plasma concentrations of some local anaesthetics using a nitrogen detector. Clin. Chim. Acta 56: 307–309, 1974.

E. Eriksson and P. Granberg. Studies on the renal excretion of Citanest and Xylocaine. Acta Anaesth. Scand. (Suppl.) 16: 79–85, 1965.

R. Hook, R.A. Greenberg and F.W. Hehre. Continuous lumbar peridural anesthesia in obstetrics. Anesth. Anal. 50: 693–698, 1971.

H.A. Kaliciak and S.C. Chan. Distribution of prilocaine in body fluids and tissues in lethal overdose. J. Anal. Tox. 10: 75–76, 1986.

J.B. Keenaghan. The determination of lidocaine and prilocaine in whole blood by gas chromatography. Anesthesiology 29: 110–112, 1968.

S.C. Ludwig. Acute toxic methemoglobinemia following dental analgesia. Ann. Emer. Med. 10: 265–266, 1981.

P.J. Poppers. Practical and theoretical considerations on the use of prilocaine in obstetrics. Acta Anaesth. Scand. (Suppl.) 25: 385–388, 1967.

D.B. Scott, P.J.R. Jebson, D.P. Braid et al. Factors affecting plasma levels of lignocaine and prilocaine. Brit. J. Anaesth. 44: 1040–1049, 1972.

G. Svinhufvud, B. Ortengren and S.E. Jacobsson. The estimation of lidocaine and prilocaine in biological material by gas chromatography. Scand. J. Clin. Lab. Invest. 17: 162–164, 1965.

R. Whelpton, P. Dudson, H. Cannell and K. Webster. Determination of prilocaine in human plasma samples using high-performance liquid chromatography with dual-electrode electrochemical detection. J. Chrom. 526: 215–222, 1990.

Primaquine

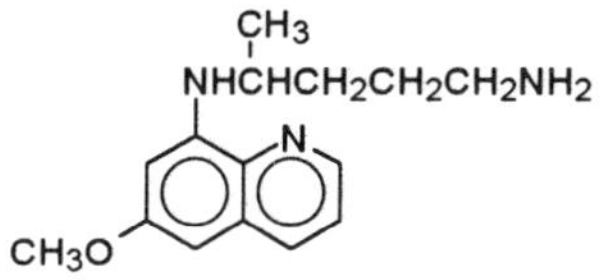

T½: 4–10 hr
Vd: 3–4 L/kg
Fb: ?
pKa: ?

Occurrence and Usage. Primaquine (Aralen) is a 4-aminoquinoline compound that is highly effective against the erythrocytic forms of *Plasmodium vivax* and most strains of *P. falciparum*. It is available as the phosphate in tablets containing 79 mg (equivalent to 45 mg base) in combination with 500 mg (equivalent to 300 mg base) of chloroquine. The usual adult dose is 1 tablet weekly taken on the same day each week.

Blood Concentrations. After oral administration of 45 mg primaquine to 5 healthy male volunteers, a mean peak plasma concentration of 153 µg/L (range, 131–180) was attained in 2–3 hours; a mean peak plasma carboxyprimaquine concentration of 1427 µg/L (range, 1078–1808) was attained in 2–12 hours (Mihaly et al., 1984).

Metabolism and Excretion. Primaquine is extensively metabolized by N-dealkylation to 6-methoxy-8-aminoquinoline and by oxidation to carboxyprimaquine, its major metabolite in plasma. Since negligible amounts of carboxyprimaquine are recovered in the urine, it is probably further metabolized prior to excretion (Baty et al., 1975; Mihaly et al., 1984). Less than 1% of a dose is excreted unchanged over a 24 hour period (Greaves et al., 1980).

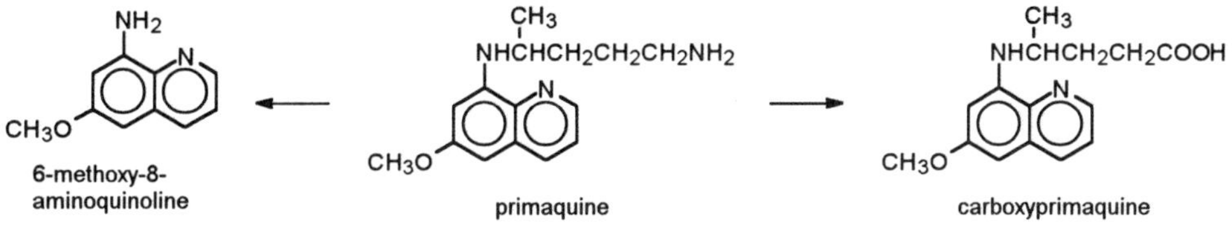

Toxicity. Hemolytic anemia may occur after therapeutic doses of primaquine in persons deficient in glucose-6-phosphate dehydrogenase, while methemoglobinemia may occur in subjects deficient in nicotinamide adenine dinucleotide (NADH). Following overdosage of primaquine, headache, drowsiness, visual disturbances, gastrointestinal distress, cardiovascular collapse, convulsions, and sudden respiratory and cardiac arrest may occur.

Analysis. Primaquine has been determined in biological samples employing electron-capture gas chromatography (Rajagopalan et al., 1981), liquid chromatography (Baker et al., 1982; Parkhurst et al., 1984; Ward et al., 1984; Bhatia et al., 1985), and gas chromatography-mass spectrometry (Baty et al., 1975; Baty et al., 1978; Greaves et al., 1979; Greaves et al., 1980).

References

J.K. Baker, J.D. McChesney, C.D. Hufford and A.M. Clark. High-performance liquid chromatographic analysis of the metabolism of primaquine and the identification of a new mammalian metabolite. J. Chrom. 230: 69–77, 1982.

J.D. Baty, D.A. Price Evans and P.A. Robinson. The identification of 6-methoxy 8-aminoquinoline as a metabolite of primaquine in man. Biomed. Mass Spec. 2: 304–306, 1975.

J.D. Baty, D.A. Price-Evans, H.M. Gilles and J. Greaves. Gas chromatography mass spectrometry studies on biologically important 8-aminoquinoline derivatives. Biomed. Mass Spec. 5: 76–79, 1978.

S.C. Bhatia, S.N. Revankar, E.D. Bharucha et al. Determination of the antimalarial primaquine in whole blood and urine by normal-phase high-performance liquid chromatography. Anal. Letters 18: 1671–1686, 1985.

J. Greaves, D.A. Price-Evans and H.M. Gilles. A selected ion monitoring assay for primaquine in plasma and urine. Biomed. Mass Spec. 6: 109–112, 1979.

J. Greaves, D.A.P. Evans and K.A. Fletcher. Urinary primaquine excretion and red cell methaemoglobin levels in man following a primaquine:chloroquine regimen. Brit. J. Clin. Pharm. 10: 293–295, 1980.

G.W. Mihaly, S.A Ward, E. Edwards et al. Pharmacokinetics of primaquine in man; identification of the carboxylic acid derivative as a major plasma metabolite. J. Clin. Pharm. 17: 441–446, 1984.

G.W. Parkhurst, M.V. Nora, R.W. Thomas and P.E. Carson. High-performance liquid chromatographic-ultra-violet determination of primaquine and its metabolites in human plasma and urine. J. Pharm. Sci. 73: 1329–1331, 1984.

T.G. Rajagopalan, B. Anjaneyulu, V.D. Shanbag and R.S. Grewal. Electron-capture gas chromatographic assay for primaquine in blood. J. Chrom. 224: 265–273, 1981.

S.A. Ward, G. Edwards, M.L.E. Orme and A.M. Breckenridge. Determination of primaquine in biological fluids by reversed-phase high-performance liquid chromatography. J. Chrom. 305: 239–243, 1984.

Primidone

T½: 6–22 hr
Vd: 0.5–1.0 L/kg
Fb: 0
pKa: ?

Occurrence and Usage. Primidone (Mysoline), a desoxy derivative of phenobarbital, was synthesized in 1949 and first evaluated as an anticonvulsant in 1952. It is used frequently for the treatment of grand mal and temporal lobe seizures in daily oral doses of 250–1500 mg. The drug is supplied as the free acid in tablets of 50 and 250 mg and as a 250 mg/5 mL suspension for oral administration.

Blood Concentrations. A single 250 mg oral dose of primidone given to 10 patients who were not receiving other anticonvulsants produced an average peak serum primidone concentration of 4.9 mg/L at 4 hours. Primidone concentrations declined with an average half-life of 15 hours (range, 9–22) in these patients, but patients receiving other anticonvulsant drugs exhibited primidone half-lives averaging 8 hours. The metabolites phenylethylmalonamide and phenobarbital were present at detectable levels within 24 or 48 hours, respectively, of the single primidone dose (Cloyd et al., 1981). After a 500 mg oral dose, one subject achieved a peak serum primidone concentration of about 8 mg/L within 5 hours, while phenylethylmalonamide and phenobarbital concentrations remained below 2 mg/L for at least 24 hours (Gallagher et al., 1972).

Steady-state plasma primidone concentrations were found to correlate well with the chronic daily primidone dose when it was varied over a range of 250–1250 mg; a dose of 500 mg produced an average plasma concentration of 6.7 mg/L (range, 1–14) while 1250 mg gave a concentration of 14.7 mg/L (range, 10–19) (Booker et al., 1970). Patients receiving 1000 mg of the drug daily exhibited serum primidone concentrations of 11–15 mg/L, phenobarbital concentrations of 17–29 mg/L and phenylethylmalonamide concentrations of 7–10 mg/L (Bielman et al., 1974). The plasma half-life of primidone is relatively short compared to its metabolites phenobarbital (3–4 days) and phenylethylmalonamide (29–36 hours) (Gallagher and Baumel, 1972).

Metabolism and Excretion. Primidone is metabolized primarily by oxidative cleavage to phenylethylmalonamide, with a small amount being oxidized to phenobarbital. Although phenobarbital is a minor metabolite, its long half-life results in its accumulation in plasma during chronic primidone therapy. The concurrent administration of phenytoin, an enzyme inducer, produces much higher phenobarbital concentrations than those seen in patients receiving primidone alone (Fincham et al., 1974).

Primidone and metabolically-produced phenobarbital may account for nearly all of the anticonvulsant activity of primidone, since phenylethylmalonamide is a relatively poor anticonvulsant (Baumel et al., 1973). However, a recent study in rats showed that seizure protection correlated best with the summed serum concentrations of phenylethylmalonamide and phenobarbital (Albertson et al., 1980).

During chronic administration of primidone, approximately 92% of the dose is eliminated in the 24 hour urine; 42% is found as primidone, 45% as phenylethylmalonamide and 5% as phenobarbital, its hydroxy metabolites and their conjugates (Kauffman et al., 1977).

Toxicity. Primidone intoxication is manifested by weakness, ataxia, vertigo, nystagmus, drowsiness, nausea, and vomiting. A patient on chronic therapy with primidone developed these symptoms and was found to have serum concentrations of 4 mg/L for primidone, 126 mg/L for phenylethylmalonamide, and 94 mg/L for phenobarbital. Serum half-lives for the latter 2 substances were about 8 days each, substantially longer than in normal subjects (Stern, 1977).

Patients who survived massive acute ingestion of primidone have exhibited maximal serum concentrations of 97–300 mg/L for primidone, 68–155 mg/L for phenylethylmalonamide, and 25–77 mg/L for phenobarbital. The half-lives for the drugs were within the normal ranges for therapeutic doses. A finding common to all such patients was crystalluria, due to precipitation of unchanged drug in urine (Bailey and Jatlow, 1972; Lagenstein et al., 1977; Matzke et al., 1981; van Heijst et al., 1983).

In contrast, a nonfatal suicide attempt involving a 10 year old epileptic patient resulted in serum concentrations of 95 and 175 mg/L for primidone and phenobarbital, respectively, about 12 hours after ingestion; the corresponding urine concentrations were 1570 and 50 mg/L, respectively (Cate and Tenser, 1975). The high phenobarbital concentrations observed in this case are probably a result of both enzyme induction and pre-existing drug due to prior treatment with primidone.

A case of fatal overdosage with primidone in an adult who was not under therapy with the drug was reported in which the blood primidone concentration was 65 mg/L and phenobarbital, 3 mg/L (Wright, 1975).

Analysis. Several gas chromatographic procedures have been reported that are capable of measuring primidone and its 2 metabolites simultaneously in plasma. Baumel and others (1972) described a method in which primidone and phenylethylmalonamide were converted to trimethylsilyl derivatives, and phenobarbital, which does not form a stable silyl derivative, was analyzed underivatized in a second injection. A single-injection analysis described by Couch et al. (1973) involved a treatment of a sample extract with diazomethane, yielding the dimethyl derivative of phenobarbital without affecting primidone or phenylethylmalonamide. Other authors performed the analysis without derivatization on columns with mixed liquid phases (Thoma et al., 1978; Streete and Berry, 1987). Liquid chromatography is well-suited to the simultaneous assay of these 3 drugs (Kabra et al., 1978).

Many analysts consider it sufficient to measure only primidone and phenobarbital concentrations and this is easily accomplished with most comprehensive anticonvulsant assays.

References

T.E. Albertson, S.L. Peterson, L.G. Stark and R.C. Baselt. Barbiturate serum levels and protection against kindled amygdaloid seizures in the rat. Neuropharmacology 19: 1141–1144, 1980.

D.N. Bailey and P.I. Jatlow. Chemical analysis of massive crystalluria following primidone overdose. Am. J. Clin. Pharm. 58: 583–589, 1972.

I.P. Baumel, B.B. Gallagher and R.H. Mattson. Phenylethylmalonamide (PEMA). Arch. Neurol. 27: 34–41, 1972.

I.P. Baumel, B.B. Gallagher, J. DiMicco and H. Goico. Metabolism and anticonvulsant properties of primidone in the rat. J. Pharm. Exp. Ther. 186: 306–314, 1973.

P. Bielmann, T.H. Levac, Y. Langlois and L. Tetreault. Bioavailability of primidone in epileptic patients. Int. J. Clin. Pharm. 9: 132–137, 1974.

H.E. Booker, K. Hosokowa, R.D. Burdette and B. Darcey. A clinical study of serum primidone levels. Epilepsia 11: 395–402, 1970.

J.C. Cate and R. Tenser. Acute primidone overdosage with massive crystalluria. Clin. Tox. 8: 385–389, 1975.

J.C. Cloyd, K.W. Miller and I.E. Leppik. Primidone kinetics: effects of concurrent drugs and duration of therapy. Clin. Pharm. Ther. 29: 402–407, 1981.

M.W. Couch, M. Greer and C.M. Williams. Determination of primidone and its metabolites in biological fluids by gas chromatography. J. Chrom. 87: 559–561, 1973.

R.W. Fincham, D.D. Schottelius and A.L. Sahs. The influence of diphenylhydantoin on primidone metabolism. Arch. Neurol. 30: 259–262, 1974.

B.B. Gallagher and I.P. Baumel. Primidone-biotransformation. In *Antiepileptic Drugs* (D.M. Woodbury, J.K. Penry and R.P. Schmidt, eds.), Raven Press, New York, 1972, pp. 361–366.

B.B. Gallagher, I.P. Baumel and R.H. Mattson. Metabolic disposition of primidone and its metabolites in epileptic subjects after single and repeated administration. Neurology 22: 1186–1192, 1972.

P.M. Kabra, D.M. McDonald and L.J. Marton. A simultaneous high-performance liquid chromatographic analysis of the most common anticonvulsants and their metabolites in the serum. J. Anal. Tox. 2: 127–133, 1978.

R.E. Kauffman, R. Habersang and L. Lansky. Kinetics of primidone metabolism and excretion in children. Clin. Pharm. Ther. 22: 200–205, 1977.

L. Lagenstein, H.J. Sternowsky, E. Iffland and E. Blaschke. Intoxication with primidone: continuous monitoring of serum primidone and its metabolites during forced diuresis. Neuropaediatrie 8: 190–195, 1977.

G.R. Matzke, J.C. Cloyd and R.J. Sawchuk. Acute phenytoin and primidone intoxication: a pharmacokinetic analysis. J. Clin. Pharm. 21: 92–99, 1981.

E.L. Stern. Possible phenylethylmalondiamide (PEMA) intoxication. Ann. Neurol. 2: 356–357, 1977.

J.M. Streete and D.J. Berry. Gas chromatographic analysis of phenylethylmalonamide in human plasma. J. Chrom. 416: 281–291, 1987.

J.J. Thoma, T. Ewald and M. McCoy. Simultaneous analysis of underivatized phenobarbital, carbamazepine, primidone and phenytoin by isothermal gas-liquid chromatography. J. Anal. Tox. 2: 219–225, 1978.

A.N.P. van Heijst, W. de Jong, R. Seldenrijk and A. van Dijk. Coma and crystalluria: a massive primidone intoxication treated with haemoperfusion. Clin. Tox. 20: 307–318, 1983.

J.A. Wright. Personal communication, 1975.

Procainamide

TЅ⁄₂: 2–5 hr
Vd: 3.3–4.8 L/kg
Fb: 0.15
pKa: 9.2

$$H_2N \text{—} \bigcirc \text{—} CONHCH_2CH_2N(C_2H_5)_2$$

Occurrence and Usage. Procainamide (Procan, Pronestyl) has been utilized as an antiarrhythmic drug since 1951. It is the amide analogue of procaine, a local anesthetic with *in vitro* antiarrhythmic efficacy similar to quinidine but which is hydrolyzed too rapidly to be of practical importance. Substitution of an amide linkage for the ester group of procaine produced a longer-acting, clinically

useful drug. Procainamide is normally administered orally as the hydrochloride in daily maintenance doses of 50 mg/kg (3500 mg/70 kg), divided into amounts that are given at 3 hour intervals;
for the initiation of therapy it is sometimes administered by intramuscular and, rarely, intravenous
injection of 200–1000 mg.

Blood Concentrations. With oral administration of 1000 mg to a single subject, the plasma
procainamide concentration peaked at 4.5 mg/L at 1 hour and declined with a half-life of 2.9 hours;
intramuscular injection of 1000 mg to the same subject produced a peak concentration of 5.9 mg/L
at 0.5 hours; intravenous injection of the same dose resulted in an initial concentration of 16 mg/L
at 10 minutes, declining with a distribution half-life of 4.4 minutes to 5.7 mg/L by 0.5 hours (Koch-
Weser and Klein, 1971). Cardiac patients have been shown to exhibit a longer half-life for this drug
(5.5 hours) compared to normal subjects (Giardina et al., 1976). A single oral dose of 6.5 mg/kg
(455 mg/70 kg) to 4 subjects produced peak plasma procainamide concentrations of 2.01–2.51
mg/L at 1–2 hours; peak plasma N-acetylprocainamide concentrations in the 2 subjects who were
slow acetylators ranged from 0.28–0.53 mg/L at 2–4 hours and from 0.86–1.80 mg/L at 2 hours in
the fast acetylators (Gibson et al., 1976). The plasma half-life for N-acetylprocainamide in normal
subjects is 6.2 hours (Dutcher et al., 1977).

Plasma procainamide concentrations of 4–8 mg/L are considered safe and effective in most persons on oral maintenance therapy with the drug, although concentrations of 8–16 mg/L are necessary for occasional patients (Koch-Weser and Klein, 1971). In 20 patients on maintenance therapy,
procainamide concentrations in random plasma specimens averaged 3.7 mg/L (range, 0.8–8.8) and
N-acetylprocainamide concentrations averaged 5.4 mg/L (range, 1.5–10.5), as measured by a specific gas chromatographic method (Frislid et al., 1975).

Metabolism and Excretion. A major metabolite of procainamide in man is N-acetylprocainamide,
a compound nearly as effective in its antiarrhythmic effects as its parent, which may contribute
significantly to the efficacy of procainamide during chronic therapy (Drayer et al., 1974; Elson et
al., 1975). The rate of formation of this metabolite is determined by N-acetyltransferase activity;
slow acetylators exhibit a longer half-life (4.1 hours) for procainamide than fast acetylators (2.5
hours) (Gibson et al., 1976) and tend to excrete less N-acetylprocainamide in urine (Gibson et al.,
1975). Two other metabolites, norprocainamide and N-acetylnorprocainamide, are about one-half
as active as the parent drug; these compounds are found in the plasma of treated patients at concentrations of less than 0.5 mg/L and 0.4–3.9 mg/L, respectively (Ruo et al., 1981).

Up to 91% of a single oral dose of procainamide is eliminated in the 72 hour urine; excretion
products in the 24 hour urine include unchanged drug (31–56%), N-acetylprocainamide (7–24%)
and the 2 dealkylated metabolites (8–14%). Hydrolysis of the amide linkage does not appear to
occur to a significant extent in man (Dreyfuss et al., 1972; Giardina et al., 1976).

H_2N—⟨O⟩—$CONHCH_2CH_2N(C_2H_5)_2$ ⟶ CH_3CONH—⟨O⟩—$CONHCH_2CH_2N(C_2H_5)_2$

procainamide   N-acetylprocainamide

H_2N—⟨O⟩—$CONHCH_2CH_2NHC_2H_5$ ⟶ CH_3CONH—⟨O⟩—$CONHCH_2CH_2NHC_2H_5$

norprocainamide   N-acetylnorprocainamide

Toxicity. Manifestations of procainamide toxicity usually appear at plasma concentrations in excess of 16 mg/L and include hypotension and depression of myocardial contractility. In severe renal
failure, plasma concentrations may be greatly elevated even with normal doses. Procainamide treatment may lead to development of a lupus erythematosus-like syndrome, usually preceded by a
rising serum antinuclear antibody titer. Serious blood dyscrasias may result with chronic adminis-

tration and may have a fatal outcome. A 67 year old woman ingested an overdose and presented with coma, seizures and hypotension; admission serum contained 106 mg/L procainamide and 44 mg/L N-acetylprocainamide, but the patient survived with hemodialysis and supportive treatment (Goldstein et al., 1988).

Four subjects who died as a result of procainamide therapy developed plasma levels of 17.6–25.2 mg/L within 1 hour of death (Koch-Weser, 1971). Four cases of fatal procainamide overdosage were reported in which postmortem blood concentrations of 80–260 mg/L (average, 145) were determined (Registry, 1978). The following concentrations were observed in an adult who apparently died of procainamide overdosage (Kopjak and Jennison, 1976):

Procainamide Concentrations in a Fatal Case (mg/L or mg/kg)

Blood	Liver	Urine	Gastric
114	283	556	99 mg

Analysis. The originally reported colorimetric method for procainamide assay in biological fluids, which involves a diazotization step and appears specific for the unchanged drug (Mark et al., 1951), has been modified to improve sensitivity (Sitar et al., 1976). A very convenient fluorometric technique (Koch-Weser and Klein, 1971) has undergone modifications to allow the sequential measurement of both procainamide and N-acetylprocainamide (Matusik and Gibson, 1975). Gas chromatographic techniques have relied on flame-ionization (Elson et al., 1975; Frislid et al., 1975; Gibson et al., 1975) or nitrogen-selective detection (Yamaji et al., 1987). Liquid chromatographic procedures for procainamide and its metabolite have also been described (Butterfield et al., 1978; Gadalla et al., 1978; Lai et al., 1980; Kessler et al., 1982; Patel, 1983). Commercial immunoassays are now frequently employed in clinical laboratories. Up to a 35% decrease in procainamide concentration and a 24% increase in N-acetylprocainamide concentration were noted during storage of whole blood at room temperature; this effect is prevented by removal of red cells from plasma (Chen et al., 1983).

References

A.G. Butterfield, J.K. Cooper and K.K. Midha. Simultaneous determination of procainamide and N-acetylprocainamide in plasma by high-performance liquid chromatography. J. Pharm. Sci. 67: 839–842, 1978.

M.L. Chen, M.G. Lee and W.L. Chiou. Pharmacokinetics of drugs in blood III: metabolism of procainamide and storage effect of blood samples. J. Pharm. Sci. 72: 572–574, 1983.

D.E. Drayer, M.M. Reidenberg and R.W. Sevy. N-acetylprocainamide: an active metabolite of procainamide. Proc. Soc. Exp. Biol. Med. 146: 358–363, 1974.

J. Dreyfuss, J.T. Bigger, Jr., A.I. Cohen and E.C. Schreiber. Metabolism of procainamide in rhesus monkey and man. Clin. Pharm. Ther. 13: 366–371, 1972.

J.S. Dutcher, J.M. Strong, S.V. Lucas et al. Procainamide and N-acetylprocainamide kinetics investigated simultaneously with stable isotope methodology. Clin. Pharm. Ther. 22: 447–457, 1977.

J. Elson, J.M. Strong, W. Lee and A.J. Atkinson, Jr. Antiarrhythmic potency of N-acetylprocainamide. Clin. Pharm. Ther. 17: 134–140, 1975.

K. Frislid, J.E. Bredesen and P.K.M. Lunde. Fluorometric or gas-liquid chromatographic determination of procainamide? Clin. Chem. 21: 1180–1182, 1975.

M.A.F. Gadalla, G.W. Peng and W.L. Chiou. Rapid and micro high-pressure liquid chromatographic method for simultaneous determination of procainamide and N-acetylprocainamide in plasma. J. Pharm. Sci. 67: 869–871, 1978.

E.V. Giardina, J. Dreyfuss, J.T. Bigger, Jr. et al. Metabolism of procainamide in normal and cardiac subjects. Clin. Pharm. Ther. 19: 339–351, 1976.

T.P. Gibson, J. Matusik, E. Matusik et al. Acetylation of procainamide in man and its relationship to isonicotinic acid hydrazide acetylation phenotype. Clin. Pharm. Ther. 17: 395–399, 1975.

T.P. Gibson, E. Matusik and W.A. Briggs. N-acetylprocainamide levels in patients with end-stage renal failure. Clin. Pharm. Ther. 19: 206–212, 1976.

D.A. Goldstein, D.R. Sawyer, R.E. Garrett and J.W. Rathouz. Successful hemodialysis of procainamide and N-acetylprocainamide in acute overdose. Vet. Hum. Tox. 30: 352, 1988.

K.M. Kessler, P. Ho-Tung, B. Steele et al. Simultaneous quantitation of quinidine, procainamide, and N-acetylprocainamide in serum by gas-liquid chromatography with a nitrogen-phosphorus selective detector. Clin. Chem. 28: 1187–1190, 1982.

J. Koch-Weser and S.W. Klein. Procainamide dosage schedules, plasma concentrations and clinical effects. J. Am. Med. Asso. 215: 1454–1460, 1971.

L. Kopjak and T.A. Jennison. Personal communication, 1976.

C.M. Lai, B.L. Kamath, Z.M. Look and A. Yacobi. Determination of procainamide and N-acetylprocainamide in biological fluids by high-pressure liquid chromatography. J. Pharm. Sci. 69: 982–984, 1980.

L.C. Mark, H.J. Kayden, J.M. Steele et al. The physiological disposition and cardiac effects of procaine amide. J. Pharm. Exp. Ther. 102: 5–15, 1951.

E. Matusik and T.P. Gibson. Fluorometric assay for N-acetylprocainamide. Clin. Chem. 21: 1899–1902, 1975.

C.P. Patel. Improved liquid chromatographic determination of procainamide and N-acetylprocainamide in serum. Ther. Drug Mon. 5: 235–238, 1983.

Registry of Human Toxicology, American Academy of Forensic Sciences, 1978.

T.I. Ruo, Y. Morita, A.J. Atkinson, Jr. et al. Identification of desethyl procainamide in patients: a new metabolite of procainamide. J. Pharm. Exp. Ther. 216: 357–362, 1981.

D.S. Sitar, D.N. Graham, R.E. Rangno et al. Modified colorimetric method for procainamide in plasma. Clin. Chem. 22: 379–380, 1976.

A. Yamaji, K. Kataoka, M. Oishi et al. Simultaneous determination of procainamide and N-acetylprocainamide in serum by gas chromatography with nitrogen-selective detection. J. Chrom. 415: 143–147, 1987.

Procaine

T½: 7–8 min
Vd: 0.3–0.8 L/kg
Fb: ?
pKa: 8.8

$H_2N-\langle\bigcirc\rangle-COOCH_2CH_2N(C_2H_5)_2$

Occurrence and Usage. Procaine (Novocain) is a local anesthetic of the ester type that was synthesized as early as 1905. The drug is frequently used for nerve block, infiltration and spinal anesthesia in doses of 300–600 mg; solutions of 1–10% as the hydrochloride are available in 2 mL ampules and are administered with or without epinephrine as a vasoconstrictor.

Blood Concentrations. The intravenous infusion of 1 mg/kg/min of procaine to 6 patients, also receiving thiamylal and diazepam, produced average maximal plasma procaine concentrations of 12.7 mg/L at the end of the 1 hour infusion; using a dose of 1.5 mg/kg/min for the same period, the maximal concentration was 43 mg/L (range, 22–63). In both cases, procaine disappeared rapidly from plasma when the infusion stopped, with elimination half-lives of 7–8 minutes (Seifen et al., 1979). The intramuscular administration of 2000 mg of procaine penicillin (4.8 million units) resulted in initial plasma procaine concentrations of 3.6–11.0 mg/L (average, 6.6) in 26 patients, with a decline to less than 2 mg/L in each subject after 30 minutes (Green et al., 1974).

Metabolism and Excretion. Procaine is readily hydrolyzed, primarily by plasma esterases, to p-aminobenzoic acid and diethylaminoethanol, both of which are present in plasma at concentrations of up to 15 and 3.7 mg/L, respectively, during constant infusion of the drug. The incubation of procaine at a concentration of 5 mg/L in human plasma results in complete loss of the drug within 2–6 minutes. After intravenous infusion, about 2% of a dose is excreted unchanged in the 24 hour urine; approximately 80% is found as free or conjugated p-aminobenzoic acid. Diethylaminoethanol is apparently further metabolized, since only 30% of a dose of procaine may be accounted for as this metabolite in the urine (Brodie et al., 1948).

$$H_2N-\langle\bigcirc\rangle-COOCH_2CH_2N(C_2H_5)_2 \longrightarrow HOCH_2CH_2N(C_2H_5)_2 + H_2N-\langle\bigcirc\rangle-COOH \longrightarrow \text{conjugation}$$

procaine   diethylaminoethanol   p-aminobenzoic acid

Toxicity. Adverse reactions to procaine include nervousness, dizziness, blurred vision, tremor, drowsiness, bradycardia, hypotension or hypertension, coma, and respiratory and cardiac arrest. The co-administration of central nervous system depressants may inhibit many of these reactions in patients receiving anesthesia (Seifen et al., 1979).

Ten subjects who were taken to the point of toxicity (generalized convulsions) with intravenous procaine received from 18–55 mg/kg (1260–3850 mg/70 kg) of the drug within 2–15 minutes and developed peak plasma procaine concentrations of 21–86 mg/L (average, 49); the subjects recovered within 17–44 minutes, at which time plasma levels had declined to 1–13 mg/L (Usubiaga et al., 1966). An adult who inadvertently received 400 mg of procaine by intravenous injection following the administration of succinylcholine and a plasma cholinesterase inhibitor developed a maximal blood procaine concentration of 96 mg/L; convulsions did not develop due to the protective effect of succinylcholine, but hypertension, tachycardia and mydriasis were apparent. Muscle tone returned after about 45 minutes and the patient recovered uneventfully (Wikinski et al., 1970).

Analysis. Procaine has been determined in blood or plasma by a colorimetric procedure (Brodie et al., 1948) and by flame-ionization gas chromatography (Green et al., 1974; Smith et al., 1978). Liquid chromatography has also been described (Stevenson et al., 1992). The *in vitro* hydrolysis of the drug has been prevented by the addition of sodium arsenite (2 drops of 50% solution/mL of blood) (Brodie et al., 1948). However, echothiophate iodide is much more efficient, causing 100% inhibition of esterase activity at a concentration of 1 mg/mL, which is equivalent to 250 mg/mL of sodium arsenite (Smith et al., 1978).

References

B.B. Brodie, P.A. Lief and R. Poet. The fate of procaine in man following its intravenous administration and methods for the estimation of procaine and diethylaminoethanol. J. Pharm. Exp. Ther. 94: 359–366, 1948.

R.L. Green, J.E. Lewis, S.J. Kraus and E.L. Frederickson. Elevated plasma procaine concentrations after administration of procaine penicillin G. New Eng. J. Med. 291: 223–226, 1974.

A.B. Seifen, A.A. Ferrari, E.E. Seifen et al. Pharmacokinetics of intravenous procaine infusion in humans. Anesth. Anal. 58: 382–386, 1979.

R.H. Smith, M.A. Brewster, J.A. MacDonald and D.S. Thompson. Measurement of chloroprocaine and procaine in plasma by flame ionization gas-liquid chromatography. Clin. Chem. 24: 1599–1602, 1978.

A.J. Stevenson, M.P. Weber, F. Todi et al. Determination of procaine in equine plasma and urine by hplc. J. Anal. Tox. 16: 93–96, 1992.

J.E. Usubiaga, J. Wikinski, R. Ferrero et al. Local anesthetic-induced convulsions in man. Anesth. Anal. 45: 611–620, 1966.

A. Wikinski, J.E. Usubiaga and R.W. Wikinski. Cardiovascular and neurological effects of 4000 mg of procaine. J. Am. Med. Asso. 213: 621–623, 1970.

Procyclidine

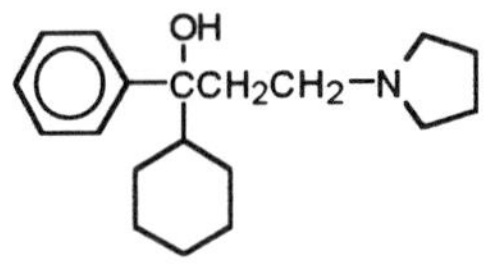

T½: 8–18 hr
Vd: 0.7–1.3 L/kg
Fb: ?
pKa: ?

Occurrence and Usage. Procyclidine (Kemadrin) is an anticholinergic agent used since 1965 in the treatment of idiopathic and drug-induced Parkinsonism. It is available as the hydrochloride in tablets of 2 and 5 mg. Daily oral doses range from 6–20 mg.

Blood Concentrations. After a 10 mg oral dose, a volunteer achieved a peak plasma procyclidine concentration of about 0.078 mg/L within 2 hours; the level declined to 0.048 mg/L by 6 hours and 0.015 mg/L by 24 hours (Dean et al., 1980). Six volunteers receiving the same oral dose developed an average peak plasma level of 0.116 mg/L at an average time of 1.1 hours (Whiteman et al., 1985). Steady-state plasma concentrations ranged from 0.15–0.63 mg/L in 6 patients receiving the drug in daily doses of 10–30 mg (Missen et al., 1978).

Metabolism and Excretion. The disposition of procyclidine in man has not been reported. A metabolite, believed to be p-hydroxylated on the benzene ring, was isolated from blood, liver and urine in a case of fatal overdosage (Ashton, 1980). A second metabolite, believed to be m-hydroxylated on the cyclohexane ring, was isolated from urine (Paeme et al., 1980).

Toxicity. Adverse reactions to procyclidine include nausea, dryness of the mouth, weakness, pupillary dilation, blurred vision, confusion, agitation, hallucinations and psychotic episodes.

In 5 fatal cases of overdosage, most of which involved other drugs, the following concentrations were observed (Bailey, 1976; Liddy, 1977; Missen et al., 1978; Ashton, 1980; Rousseau, 1983):

Procyclidine Concentrations in Fatal Cases (mg/L or mg/kg)

	Blood	Liver	Urine	Gastric
Average	3.7	10	4.6	3.8 mg
(Range)	(0.4–7.8)	(6–15)	(1.8–7)	(0.4–13)

Analysis. Procyclidine has been assayed in biological specimens by gas chromatography with nitrogen-phosphorus detection (Missen et al., 1978; Dean et al., 1980).

References

P.G. Ashton. Personal communication, 1980.

M. Bailey. Personal communication, 1976.

K. Dean, G. Land and A. Bye. Analysis of procyclidine in human plasma and urine by gas-liquid chromatography. J. Chrom. 221: 408–413, 1980.

M. Liddy. Personal communication, 1977.

A.W. Missen, S.J. Dickson and W.T. Cleary. Analysis of procyclidine in blood by gas-liquid chromatography with nitrogen-phosphorus detector. J. Anal. Tox. 2: 238–240, 1978.

G. Paeme, W. Sonck, D. Tourwe et al. 1-(3-Hydroxycyclohexyl)-1-phenyl-3-(1-pyrrolidinyl)-1-propanol, a procyclidine metabolite. Drug Met. Disp. 8: 115-116, 1980.

M. Rousseau. Personal communication, 1983.

P.D. Whiteman, A.S.E. Fowle, M.J. Hamilton et al. Pharmacokinetics and pharmacodynamics of procyclidine in man. Eur. J. Clin. Pharm. 28: 73–78, 1985.

Promethazine

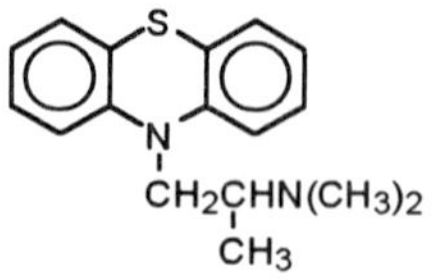

T½: 9–16 hr
Vd: 9–19 L/kg
Fb: 0.93
pKa: 9.1

Occurrence and Usage. Promethazine (Phenergan, Remsed, Zipan) is a phenothiazine derivative that is widely used for its antihistaminic, antiemetic, and sedative effects. It is available as the hydrochloride in 12.5–50 mg tablets and a 6.25 mg/5 mL syrup for oral use, solutions of 25 and 50 mg/mL for parenteral injection, and 12.5–50 mg rectal suppositories. It is also found in combination with a number of narcotic and non-narcotic analgesics. Daily oral doses range from 25–150 mg.

Blood Concentrations. A 30 mg oral dose given to a volunteer produced a peak plasma concentration of 0.011 mg/L at 2 hours, with a decline to 0.005 mg/L by 12 hours (Taylor et al., 1979). In 2 subjects given a 50 mg oral dose, serum concentrations reached peak levels of 0.008 and 0.023 mg/L at 3 hours and declined to 0.003 and 0.004 mg/L by 12 hours (Wallace et al., 1981a, 1981b). Peak serum promethazine concentrations of 0.006–0.099 mg/L (average, 0.029) occurred at an average of 3.3 hours after a 50 mg oral dose in 20 volunteers (Stavchansky et al., 1987). The elimination half-life averages 12 hours. Promethazine sulfoxide concentrations in plasma are several times those of the parent after oral dosing (Taylor et al., 1983). The whole blood/plasma concentration ratio for promethazine has been reported as 0.66 (Osselton et al., 1980).

Metabolism and Excretion. The metabolism of promethazine has not been thoroughly investigated in man. The drug is believed to be extensively biotransformed, with only 0.2% of a dose excreted unchanged in the 72 hour urine (Taylor et al., 1979). Norpromethazine and promethazine sulfoxide have been identified in human plasma (Patel and Welling, 1981; Taylor et al., 1983). Both N-demethylation and sulfoxidation are known to occur in rats (Reddrop et al., 1980).

Toxicity. Adverse reactions to promethazine include drowsiness, extrapyramidal reactions, dizziness, tinnitus, ataxia, blurred vision, tremor, anxiety, hysteria, hypotension, and tachycardia or bradycardia. Overdosage can cause coma, convulsions, respiratory depression, and circulatory failure. Physostigmine has been found to reverse many of these effects (Cleghorn and Bourke, 1980).

Promethazine was found postmortem in the case of a 14 month old infant who died unexpectedly at concentrations of 0.16 mg/L in blood and 1.0 mg/kg in liver (Degouffe and Rice, 1982). The following concentrations were determined in 3 fatalities believed due to promethazine overdosage (Allender and Archer, 1984; Farr, 1986):

Promethazine Concentrations in Fatalities (mg/L or mg/kg)

	Blood	Liver	Urine	Gastric
Average	6.5	66	10	137 mg
(Range)	(2.4–12)	(23–143)	(6–14)	(23–360)

Promethazine may exhibit postmortem redistribution; in a series of 5 fatal cases, heart blood/femoral blood concentration ratios averaged 1.6 (range, 1.0–2.0) (Prouty and Anderson, 1990).

Analysis. Promethazine has been determined in biological fluids by nitrogen-specific gas chromatography (Taylor et al., 1979; Reddrop et al., 1980; Patel and Welling, 1981) and liquid chromatography (Wallace et al., 1981a, 1981b; Patel and Welling, 1982; Taylor and Houston, 1982; Melethil et al., 1983; Allender and Archer, 1984; Fox and McLoughlin, 1993). The second, delayed rise in plasma promethazine concentrations reported by some authors may be due to thermal degradation of promethazine sulfoxide to promethazine when gas chromatographic procedures are employed (Patel and Welling, 1981).

References

W.J. Allender and A.W. Archer. Liquid chromatographic analysis of promethazine and its major metabolites in human postmortem material. J. For. Sci. 29: 515–526, 1984.

G. Cleghorn and G. Bourke. Physostigmine for promethazine poisoning. Lancet 2: 368–369, 1980.

M. Degouffe and J. Rice. Possible involvement of promethazine in a sudden unexpected infant death. Can. Soc. For. Sci. J. 15: 166–168, 1982.

L.M. Farr. Personal communication, 1986.

A.R. Fox and D.A. McLoughlin. Rapid, sensitive high-performance liquid chromatographic method for the quantitation of promethazine in human serum with electrochemical detection. J. Chrom. 631: 255–260, 1993.

S. Melethil, A. Dutta, V. Chungi and L. Dittert. Liquid chromatographic assay for promethazine in plasma using electrochemical detection. Anal. Letters 16: 701–709, 1983.

M.D. Osselton, M.D. Hammond and A.C. Moffat. Distribution of drug and toxic chemicals in blood. J. For. Sci. Soc. 20: 187–193, 1980.

R.B. Patel and P.G. Welling. On-column reduction of promethazine metabolite during gas chromatography. Clin. Chem. 27: 1780–1781, 1981.

R.B. Patel and P.G. Welling. High-pressure liquid chromatographic determination of promethazine plasma levels in the dog after oral, intramuscular, and intravenous dosage. J. Pharm. Sci. 71: 529–532, 1982.

R.W. Prouty and W.H. Anderson. The forensic science implications of site and temporal influences on postmortem blood-drug concentrations. J. For. Sci. 35: 243–270, 1990.

C.J. Reddrop, W. Riess and T.F. Slater. Rapid, sensitive determination of unchanged promethazine in biological material using a nitrogen-selective flame ionization detector. J. Chrom. 192: 375–386, 1980.

S. Stavchansky, J.E. Wallace, R. Geary et al. Bioequivalence and pharmacokinetic profile of promethazine hydrochloride suppositories in humans. J. Pharm. Sci. 76: 441–445, 1987.

G. Taylor, R.T. Calvert and J.B. Houston. Determination of promethazine in biological fluids. Anal. Letters 12: 1435–1442, 1979.

G. Taylor and J.B. Houston. Simultaneous determination of promethazine and two of its circulating metabolites by high-performance liquid chromatography. J. Chrom. 230: 194–198, 1982.

G. Taylor, J.B. Houston, J. Schaffer and G. Mawer. Pharmacokinetics of promethazine and its sulphoxide metabolite after intravenous and oral administration to man. Brit. J. Clin. Pharm. 15: 287–293, 1983.

J.E. Wallace, E.L. Shimek, Jr., S.C. Harris and S. Stavchansky. Determination of promethazine in serum by liquid chromatography. Clin. Chem. 27: 253–255, 1981a.

J.E. Wallace, E.L. Shimek, Jr., S. Stavchansky and S.C. Harris. Determination of promethazine and other phenothiazine compounds by liquid chromatography with electrochemical detection. Anal. Chem. 53: 960–962, 1981b.

Propafenone

T½: 2–10 hr (normal metabolizers)
    10–32 hr (slow metabolizers)
Vd: 2.5–4.0 L/kg
Fb: 0.77–0.97
pKa: ?

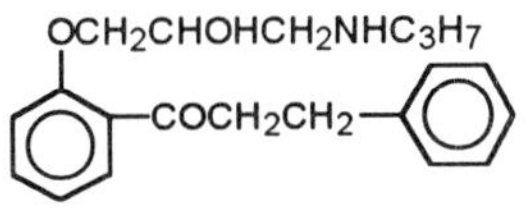

OCH$_2$CHOHCH$_2$NHC$_3$H$_7$

—COCH$_2$CH$_2$—

Occurrence and Usage. Propafenone (Rythmol) is a class 1C antiarrhythmic drug synthesized in 1970 and marketed in West Germany since 1977. It has now been approved in the United States for therapy of ventricular arrhythmias. The drug is administered orally in doses of 150 mg every 8 hours, with some patients receiving as much as 300 mg every 8 hours. It is available in tablets of 150 and 300 mg as the hydrochloride salt.

Blood Concentrations. Following oral doses of either 300 or 450 mg of propafenonone to 8 healthy volunteers, peak serum concentrations of the parent drug ranged from 37–256 µg/L (average, 278); values for 5-hydroxypropafenone ranged from 101–288 µg/L (average, 178), and for norpropafenone, from 7.8–40 µg/L (average, 23) (Vozeh et al., 1990). It has been determined that, with food, the maximum plasma propafenone concentration will be reached earlier and will be significantly increased; following oral doses of 300 mg to 24 healthy fasting males aged 19–38 years and weighing 62–82 kg, peak plasma propafenone concentrations ranged from 25–1204 µg/L (average, 324), while those after the postprandial state ranged from 38–1680 µg/L (average, 472) (Axelson et al., 1987).

In 7 subjects with normal P-450 enzyme activity who were receiving 150 mg of propafenone 3 times daily, steady-state plasma concentrations averaged 408, 242 and 91 µg/L for the parent drug, 5-hydroxypropafenone and norpropafenone, respectively; on the other hand, 2 subjects deficient in the metabolizing enzyme receiving the same dosage reached steady-state plasma concentrations averaging 2885, 15 and 197 µg/L for the drug and its 2 metabolites, respectively (Funck-Brentano et al., 1989). The mean plasma propafenone concentration associated with adequate therapeutic effect has been reported to be approximately 750 µg/L, with a range of 176–1648 µg/L (Hammill et al., 1986).

Metabolism and Excretion. Propafenone undergoes extensive metabolism via N-dealkylation, aryl-hydroxylation and conjugation. The major metabolites, 5-hydroxypropafenone and norpropafenone, are pharmacologically active (Von Philipsborn et al., 1984; Valenzuela et al., 1987; Malfatto et al., 1988; Thompson et al., 1988). Other metabolites have not been found to be quantitatively important. In 90% of patients, the drug is rapidly and extensively metabolized, but about 10% of the Caucasian population has a reduced metabolic capacity, leading to significant differences in plasma drug levels and elimination half-lives (Hii et al., 1991).

Less than 1% of a dose is excreted unchanged in the urine. Virtually all of the drug and its metabolites recovered from the feces (53% of a dose) and urine are in their conjugated form. At 8 hours post-dose, urinary excretion of conjugated parent drug and 5-hydroxypropafenone accounted for 1.6% and 3.3% of the dose, respectively (Seipel and Breithardt, 1980; Hollman et al., 1983; Leloux and Maes, 1991).

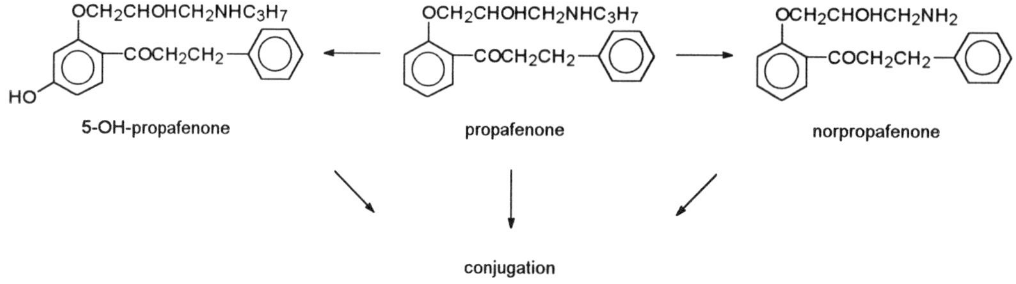

OCH2CHOHCH2NHC3H7 — COCH2CH2 — 5-OH-propafenone ← OCH2CHOHCH2NHC3H7 — COCH2CH2 — propafenone → OCH2CHOHCH2NH2 — COCH2CH2 — norpropafenone

conjugation

Toxicity. Adverse reactions to propafenone include dizziness, nausea, vomiting, headache, blurred vision, confusion and cardiac arrhythmias. Overdosage may cause hypotension, somnolence, convulsions and sustained ventricular tachycardia. Central nervous system side-effects appear to be more common at plasma propafenone concentrations exceeding 900 µg/L, regardless of the rate of metabolism (Funck-Brentano et al., 1990).

In a case involving a 14 year old who died in hospital following intentional overdose, a postmortem blood concentration of 800 µg/L was reported (Dimopoulos, 1987). In another case in which a

37 year old woman may have taken as much as 4800 mg in a single dose, the following concentrations were found at autopsy (Brzezinka, 1988):

Propafenone Concentrations in a Fatal Case (mg/L or mg/kg)

Blood	Brain	Kidney	Liver	Gastric
7.7	3.4	40	258	6.9

Analysis. Propafenone has been determined in biological samples by liquid chromatography (Harapat and Kates, 1982; Kannan et al., 1983). Propafenone and its major metabolites have also been analyzed by gas chromatography-mass spectrometry (Leloux and Maes, 1991).

References

J.E. Axelson, G.L.Y. Chan, E.B. Kirsten et al. Food increases the bioavailability of propafenone. Brit. J. Clin. Pharm. 23: 735–741, 1987.

H. Brzezinka. Personal communication, 1988.

G. Dimopoulos. Personal communication, 1987.

C. Funck-Brentano, H.K. Kroemer, H. Pavlou et al. Genetically-determined interaction between propafenone and low dose quinidine: role of active metabolites in modulating net drug effect. Brit. J. Clin. Pharm. 27: 435–444, 1989.

C. Funck-Brentano, H.K. Kroemer, J.T. Lee and D.M. Roden. Propafenone. New Eng. J. Med. 322: 518–525, 1990.

S.C. Hammill, P.B. Sorenson, D.L. Wood et al. Propafenone for the treatment of refractory complex ventricular ectopic activity. Mayo Clinic Proc. 61: 98–103, 1986.

S.R. Harapat and R.E. Kates. High performance liquid chromatographic analysis of propafenone in human plasma samples. J. Chrom. 230: 448–453, 1982.

J.T.Y. Hii, H.J. Duff and E.D. Burgess. Clinical pharmacokinetics of propafenone. Clin. Pharmacokin. 21: 1–10, 1991.

M. Hollmann, E. Brode, D. Hotz et al. Investigations on the pharmacokinetics of propafenone in man. Arz. Forsch. 33: 763–770, 1983.

R. Kannan, D. Tidwell and B.N. Singh. High performance liquid chromatographic procedure for the quantitation of propafenone in serum and tissues. J. Chrom. 272: 428–431, 1983.

M.S. Leloux and R.A.A. Maes. Identification and determination of propafenone and its principal metabolites in human urine using capillary gas chromatography/mass spectrometry. Bio. Mass Spec. 20: 382–388, 1991.

G. Malfatto, A. Zaza, M. Forster et al. Electrophysiologic, inotropic and antiarrhythmic effects of propafenone, 5-hydroxypropafenone and N-depropylpropafenone. J. Pharm. Exp. Ther. 246: 419–426, 1988.

L. Seipel and G. Breithardt. Propafenone—a new anti-arrhythmic drug. Eur. Heart J. 1: 309–313, 1980.

K.A. Thompson, D.H.S. Iansmith, L.A. Dissoway et al. Potent electrophysiologic effects of the major metabolites of propafenone in canine Purkinje fibers. J. Pharm. Exp. Ther. 244: 950–955, 1988.

C. Valenzuela, C. Delgado and J. Tamargo. Electrophysiological effects of 5-hydroxypropafenone on guinea pig ventricular muscle fibers. J. Cardiovasc. Pharm. 25: 831–833, 1987.

G. Von Philipsborn, J. Bries, H.P. Hofmann et al. Pharmacological studies on propafenone and its main metabolite 5-hydroxypropafenone. Arz. Forsch. 34: 1489–1497, 1984.

S. Vozeh, W. Haefeli, H.R. Ha et al. Nonlinear kinetics of propafenonone metabolites in healthy man. Eur. J. Clin. Pharm. 38: 509–513, 1990.

Propofol

T½: 1–3 days
Vd: 60 L/kg
Fb: 0.99
pKa: 11.0

$(CH_3)_2CH$ ⬡ $CH(CH_3)_2$ (OH)

Occurrence and Usage. Propofol (2,6-diisopropylphenol, Diprivan) is a sedative-hypnotic used as an intravenous anesthetic agent. Most patients require 2.0–2.5 mg/kg for induction followed by an infusion of 0.2 mg/kg/hour for maintenance of anesthesia. Propofol is available as an oil/water emulsion in 20–100 mL vials containing 10 mg/mL as the free acid.

Blood Concentrations. For induction of anesthesia, blood concentrations of about 6–10 mg/L are necessary, but during maintenance of anesthesia levels of approximately 2–4 mg/L are sufficient (Kanto and Gepts, 1989).

In 50 surgical patients administered a 2 mg/kg (140 mg/70 kg) intravenous bolus dose followed by a variable-rate infusion of 0–20 mg/min, it was determined that patients required an average blood propofol concentration of 4.0 mg/L for major surgery and 3.0 mg/L for minor surgery; blood concentrations at which 50% of the patients were awake and oriented after surgery were 1.07 and 0.95 mg/L, respectively (Shafer et al., 1988).

Adult patients requiring prolonged mechanical ventilation were given an initial intravenous bolus dose of 1–3 mg/kg, followed by continuous infusion of 3 mg/kg/hour for 72 hours; after an initial peak blood level ranging from 0.8–16 mg/L from the loading dose, there was a decrease in blood propofol concentration to an average of 1.3 mg/L at the sixth hour, which in turn was followed by a further gradual decrease (Albanese et al., 1990).

Metabolism and Excretion. Propofol rapidly undergoes oxidation and conjugation to inactive metabolites. Approximately 60% of a single dose was excreted in the urine as the 1- and 4-glucuronide and 4-sulfate conjugates of 2,6-diisopropyl-1,4-quinol, and the remainder consisted of propofol glucuronide (Simons et al., 1985, 1988). The extensive tissue partitioning of the drug causes rapid distribution out of the vascular space once administration has ceased, accounting for the short duration of action; the early distribution half-life of 5–7 minutes is in stark contrast to the terminal elimination half-life of 1–3 days (PDR, 1994).

Toxicity. Adverse reactions to propofol include bradycardia, hypotension, fever, cardiac arrhythmia, somnolence and seizures. Overdosage causes cardiorespiratory depression. A 29 year old female radiographer who committed suicide by intravenous injection of 400 mg of propofol had postmortem levels of 0.22 mg/L in femoral blood and 1.4 mg/kg in liver (Drummer, 1992).

Analysis. Propofol has been determined in biological fluids by gas chromatography (Yu and Liau, 1993) and liquid chromatography (Adam et al., 1981; Plummer, 1987; Vree et al., 1987; Mazzi and Schivella, 1990; Pavan et al., 1992; Altmayer et al., 1993).

References

H.K. Adam, E.J. Douglas, G.F. Plummer and M.B. Cosgrove. Estimation of ICI 35868 (Diprivan) in blood by high performance liquid chromatography, following coupling with Gibb's reagent. J. Chrom. 223: 232–236, 1981.

J. Albanese, C. Martin, B. Lacarelle et al. Pharmacokinetics of long-term propofol infusion used for sedation in ICU patients. Anesthesiology 73: 214–217, 1990.

P. Altmayer, U. Buch, H.P. Buch and R. Larsen. Rapid and sensitive pre-column extraction high-performance liquid chromatographic assay for propofol in biological fluids. J. Chrom. 612: 326–330, 1993.

O.H. Drummer. A fatality due to propofol poisoning. J. For. Sci. 37: 1168–1189, 1992.

J. Kanto and E. Gepts. Pharmacokinetic implications for the clinical use of propofol. Clin. Pharmacokin. 17: 308–326, 1989.

G. Mazzi and M. Schivella. Simple and practical high-performance liquid chromatographic assay of propofol in human blood by phenyl column chromatography with electrochemical detection. J. Chrom. 528: 537–541, 1990.

I. Pavan, E. Buglione, M. Massiccio et al. Monitoring propofol serum levels by rapid and sensitive reversed-phase high-performance liquid chromatography during prolonged sedation in ICU patients. J. Chrom. Sci. 30: 164–166, 1992.

Physicians' Desk Reference, Medical Economics, Montvale, New Jersey, 1994, pp. 2328–2332.

G.F. Plummer. Improved method for the determination of propofol in blood by high-performance liquid chromatography with fluorescence detection. J. Chrom. 421: 171–176, 1987.

A. Shafer, V.A. Doze, S.L. Shafer and P.F. White. Pharmacokinetics and pharmacodynamics of propofol infusions during general anesthesia. Anesth. Anal. 69: 348–356, 1988.

P.J. Simons, I.D. Cockshott, E.J. Douglas et al. Blood concentrations, metabolism and elimination after a subanaesthetic intravenous dose of ^{14}C-propofol ('Diprivan') to male volunteers. Postgrad. Med. J. 61: 64, 1985.

P.J. Simons, I.D. Cockshott, E.J. Douglas et al. Disposition in male volunteers of a subanaesthetic intravenous dose of an oil in water emulsion of ^{14}C-propofol. Xenobiotica 18: 429–440, 1988.

T.B. Vree, A.M. Baars and P.M.R.M. Grood. High-performance liquid chromatographic determination and preliminary pharmacokinetics of propofol and its metabolites in human plasma and urine. J. Chrom. 417: 458–464, 1987.

H.Y. Yu and J.K. Liau. Quantitation of propofol in plasma by capillary gas chromatography. J. Chrom. 615: 77–82, 1993.

Propoxyphene

T½: 8–24 hr
Vd: 12–26 L/kg
Fb: 0.78
pKa: 6.3

$C_2H_5COOCCHCH_2N(CH_3)_2$
CH_3

Occurrence and Usage. d-Propoxyphene (Darvon, Wygesic) is a mildly effective narcotic analgesic, somewhat less potent than codeine, that bears a close structural relationship to methadone. It is available in oral formulations either as the hydrochloride (32 or 65 mg) or as the napsylate salt (50 or 100 mg), and is often found in combination with aspirin or acetaminophen. Like methadone, it causes local tissue irritation following parenteral administration. The l-isomer, which is ostensibly devoid of narcotic effects, is commercially available as an antitussive (Novrad). Daily oral doses of propoxyphene range from 128–390 mg for the hydrochloride and 200–600 mg for the napsylate. The use of large daily doses (800–1400 mg) of propoxyphene napsylate for the maintenance or withdrawal of heroin addicts has been investigated with apparent success.

Blood Concentrations. Following a single 130 mg oral dose of propoxyphene hydrochloride, an average peak plasma concentration of 0.23 mg/L occurred at 2 hours, while the peak norpropoxyphene concentration, 0.27 mg/L, occurred at 4 hours (Verebely and Inturrisi, 1974). Chronic daily doses of 195 mg of hydrochloride were shown to produce average plasma concentrations of 0.42 mg/L propoxyphene and 1.45 mg/L norpropoxyphene 2 hours after the last administration (Verebely and Inturrisi, 1973). Elimination half-lives were found to average 15 hours (range, 8–24) for propoxyphene and 27 hours (range, 24–34) for norpropoxyphene (Gram et al., 1979). Other authors have reported average half-lives of 31 hours for propoxyphene and 34 hours for norpropoxyphene; acidification or alkalinization of the urine had little effect on the elimination half-life (Karkainnen and Neuvonen, 1985). The blood/plasma concentration ratio for propoxyphene averages 1.0 (Baselt, 1975).

Opiate addicts maintained on 800–1600 mg of propoxyphene napsylate daily developed serum levels of 0.13–1.07 mg/L for propoxyphene and 0.81–2.64 mg/L for norpropoxyphene; the subjects were asymptomatic at these levels (Hartmann et al., 1988).

Metabolism and Excretion. Propoxyphene is metabolized primarily via N-demethylation to norpropoxyphene, which is one-fourth to one-half as active an analgesic as propoxyphene, but which tends to accumulate in plasma due to a longer half-life. The contribution of norpropoxyphene to the efficacy or toxicity of the parent drug has not been thoroughly established (Nickander et al., 1977). Norpropoxyphene may undergo further N-demethylation to dinorpropoxyphene, which is in turn dehydrated to yield cyclic dinorpropoxyphene. Ring hydroxylation and ester hydrolysis are 2 additional pathways of propoxyphene metabolism and may be followed by conjugation to produce highly water soluble metabolites (McMahon et al., 1973).

The amounts of metabolites excreted in the 20 hour urine following a 130 mg single oral dose of propoxyphene hydrochloride were (expressed as a percentage of the dose): 1.1% propoxyphene, 13.2% norpropoxyphene, and 0.7% dinorpropoxyphene (McMahon et al., 1973). Since ingestion of an identical dose of labeled propoxyphene resulted in the excretion of 34% of the administered radioactivity in a similar time period, it is apparent that other metabolites account for a substantial portion of the dose (McMahon et al., 1971). Up to 75% of a labeled dose is excreted in the urine over a 7 day period (Gram et al., 1979).

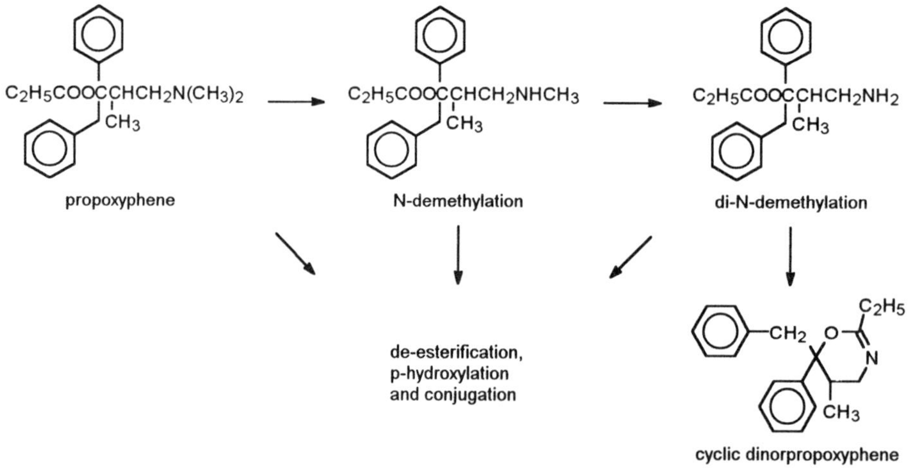

Toxicity. Overdosage with propoxyphene can result in stupor, coma, convulsions, respiratory depression, cardiac arrhythmias, hypotension, pulmonary edema, and circulatory collapse. While the acute toxic effects of propoxyphene may be prevented in animals by administration of the narcotic antagonist, naloxone (Nickander et al., 1977), and although naloxone has been recommended for use in the treatment of propoxyphene overdosage in man (Kersh, 1973), its use in clinical situations has been reported as ineffective (Karliner, 1967; Bogartz and Miller, 1971; Warren et al., 1974; Mauer et al., 1975). Based on norpropoxyphene's toxicity in animals and its resistance to naloxone (Nickander et al., 1977), it is conceivable that norpropoxyphene is at least partially responsible for the toxic effects of propoxyphene in man, especially the cardiotoxicity (Holland and Steinberg, 1979; Amsterdam et al., 1981). Instances of abuse of and psychic dependence on the drug have been reported but significant physical dependence is rare. Seven acutely intoxicated patients who survived due to hospital treatment were found to have average plasma propoxyphene and norpropoxyphene concentrations of 1.6 and 2.0 mg/L, respectively (Schou et al., 1978).

The minimum lethal dose of propoxyphene in adults has been estimated at 500–800 mg. Numerous reports of fatalities involving hundreds of cases exist in the literature. Generally, blood propoxyphene concentrations exceeding 1 mg/L are considered indicative of serious toxicity, and concentrations of 2 mg/L or more are consistent with death, although fatalities have been reported in which no other drugs were involved and in which the blood propoxyphene concentrations were less than 1 mg/L (Sturner and Garriott, 1973; Cravey et al., 1974; Baselt et al., 1975; Finkle et al., 1976; McBay, 1976; Caplan et al., 1977; Finkle et al., 1981). The following distribution of propoxyphene and its major metabolite was noted in 7 cases of fatal overdosage of the drug:

Propoxyphene Concentrations in Fatalities (mg/L or mg/kg)

	Blood	Brain	Liver	Urine
Propoxyphene				
Average	4.7	21	59	20
(Range)	(1.0–17)	(8.8–40)	(7.3–119)	(2.5–35)
Norpropoxyphene				
Average	8.4	20	125	82
(Range)	(1.7–30)	(10–30)	(53–280)	(34–192)

In most specimens norpropoxyphene concentrations exceed those of propoxyphene, except in brain where the reverse is usually true. After acute overdosage, the liver concentrations of both compounds exceed the respective blood concentrations by a factor of 10 or more, making it possible to distinguish this situation from chronic therapeutic administration, in which liver concentrations are on the same order of magnitude as those in the blood (Baselt et al., 1975). Propoxyphene and norpropoxyphene may exhibit postmortem redistribution; in a series of 14 fatal cases, heart blood/femoral blood concentration ratios averaged 3.5 (range, 0.9–11) and 2.6 (range, 0.8–12), respectively (Anderson and Prouty, 1989).

Analysis. Propoxyphene has been determined in biological specimens by ultraviolet spectrophotometry of a hydrolysis product (Wallace et al., 1965; McBay et al., 1974). There are a number of specific gas chromatographic procedures for the assay of propoxyphene and norpropoxyphene in the literature (Norheim, 1976; Serfontein and de Villiers, 1976; Angelo and Christensen, 1977; Christensen, 1977; Cleemann, 1977; Kintz et al., 1990), most of which are modifications of the original methods of Wolen and Gruber (1968) or Verebely and Inturrisi (1973). In the latter procedure, norpropoxyphene is treated with strong base before the final extraction, converting it into an internal amide in order to improve its chromatographic properties. Under certain analytical conditions, the minor metabolites dinorpropoxyphene and its cyclic dehydration product may be included in a gas chromatographic analysis (Nash et al., 1975). Mass fragmentography has been successfully used in the kinetic analysis of propoxyphene disposition in man (Wolen et al., 1975). Several reports have dealt with the problem of thermal decomposition of propoxyphene during gas chromatographic analysis. Sparacino et al. (1973) found that the use of Chromosorb W-HP or Gas Chrom Q as solid supports plus occasional column silanization gave the best results; Millard et al. (1980) claimed that only the routine use of bis(trimethylsilyl)acetamide as an injection solvent will prevent decomposition from occurring; and Margot et al. (1983) suggested the use of separate extraction schemes and different internal standards for propoxyphene and norpropoxyphene. Liquid chromatography has been reported (Angelo et al., 1985; Kunka et al., 1985; Rio et al., 1987; Rop et al., 1993). The d- and l-isomers of propoxyphene may be differentiated by a commercial immunoassay (Slightom, 1982).

References

E.A. Amsterdam, S.V. Rendig, G.L. Henderson and D.T. Mason. Depression of myocardial contractile function by propoxyphene and norpropoxyphene. J. Cardiovasc. Pharm. 3: 129–138, 1981.

W.H. Anderson and R.W. Prouty. Postmortem redistribution of drugs. In *Advances in Analytical Toxicology* (R.C. Baselt, ed.), Vol. 2, YearBook Medical, Chicago, 1989, pp. 70–102.

H.R. Angelo and J.M. Christensen. Gas chromatographic method for the determination of dextropropoxyphene and nordextropropoxyphene in human plasma, serum and urine. J. Chrom. 140: 280–283, 1977.

H.R. Angelo, T. Kranz, J. Strom et al. High-performance liquid chromatographic method for the determination of dextropropoxyphene and nordextropropoxyphene in serum. J. Chrom. 345: 413–418, 1985.

R.C. Baselt. Unpublished results, 1975.

R.C. Baselt, J.A. Wright, J.E. Turner and R.H. Cravey. Propoxyphene and norpropoxyphene tissue concentrations in fatalities associated with propoxyphene hydrochloride and propoxyphene napsylate. Arch. Tox. 34: 145–152, 1975.

L.J. Bogartz and W.C. Miller. Pulmonary edema associated with propoxyphene intoxication. J. Am. Med. Asso. 215: 259–262, 1971.

Y.H. Caplan, B.C. Thompson and R.S. Fisher. Propoxyphene fatalities: blood and tissue concentrations of propoxyphene and norpropoxyphene and a study of 115 medical examiner cases. J. Anal. Tox. 1: 27–35, 1977.

H. Christensen. Determination of dextropropoxyphene and norpropoxyphene in autopsy material. Acta Pharm. Tox. 40: 289–297, 1977.

M. Cleemann. Gas chromatographic determination of propoxyphene and norpropoxyphene in plasma. J. Chrom. 132: 287–294, 1977.

R.H. Cravey, R.F. Shaw and G.R. Nakamura. Incidence of propoxyphene poisoning: a report of fatal cases. J. For. Sci. 19: 72–80, 1974.

B.S. Finkle, K.L. McCloskey, G.F. Kiplinger and I.F. Bennett. A national assessment of propoxyphene in postmortem medicolegal investigation, 1972–1975. J. For. Sci. 21: 706–742, 1976.

B.S. Finkle, Y.H. Caplan, J.C. Garriott et al. Propoxyphene in postmortem toxicology. J. For. Sci. 26: 739–757, 1981.

L.F. Gram, J. Schou, W.L. Way et al. d-Propoxyphene kinetics after single oral and intravenous doses in man. Clin. Pharm. Ther. 26: 473–482, 1979.

B. Hartmann, D.S. Miyada, H. Pirkle et al. Serum propoxyphene concentrations in a cohort of opiate addicts on long-term propoxyphene maintenance therapy. J. Anal. Tox. 12: 25–29, 1988.

D.R. Holland and M.I. Steinberg. Electrophysiologic properties of propoxyphene and norpropoxyphene in canine cardiac conducting tissues *in vitro* and *in vivo*. Tox. Appl. Pharm. 47: 123–133, 1979.

S. Karkkainen and P.J. Neuvonen. Effect of oral charcoal and urine pH on dextropropoxyphene pharmacokinetics. Int. J. Clin. Pharm. Ther. Tox. 23: 219–225, 1985.

J.S. Karliner. Propoxyphene hydrochloride poisoning. J. Am. Med. Asso. 199: 1006–1009, 1967.

E.S. Kersh. Treatment of propoxyphene overdosage with naloxone. Chest 63: 112–114, 1973.

P. Kintz, A. Tracqui, P. Mangin et al. Simultaneous determination of dextropropoxyphene, norpropoxyphene and methaqualone in plasma by gas chromatography with selective nitrogen detection. J. Tox. Clin. Exp. 10: 89–94, 1990.

R.L. Kunka, C.L. Yong, C.F. Ladik and T.R. Bates. Liquid chromatographic determination of propoxyphene and norpropoxyphene in plasma and breast milk. J. Pharm. Sci. 74: 103–104, 1985.

S.M. Mauer, C.L. Paxson, B. von Hartizsch et al. Hemodialysis in an infant with propoxyphene intoxication. Clin. Pharm. Ther. 17: 88–92, 1975.

P.A. Margot, D.J. Crouch, B.S. Finkle et al. Capillary and packed column GC determination of propoxyphene and norpropoxyphene in biological samples: analytical problems and improvements. J. Chrom. Sci. 21: 201–204, 1983.

A.J. McBay, R.F. Turk, B.W. Corbett and P. Hudson. Determination of propoxyphene in biological materials. J. For. Sci. 19: 81–89, 1974.

A.J. McBay. Propoxyphene and norpropoxyphene concentrations in blood and tissues in cases of fatal overdosage. Clin. Chem. 22: 1319–1321, 1976.

R.E. McMahon, A.S. Ridolfo, H.W. Culp et al. The fate of radiocarbon-labelled propoxyphene in rat, dog, and human. Tox. Appl. Pharm. 19: 427–444, 1971.

R.E. McMahon, H.R. Sullivan, S.L. Due and F.J. Marshall. The metabolite pattern of d-propoxyphene in man. The use of heavy isotopes in drug disposition studies. Life Sci. 12: 463–473, 1973.

B.J. Millard, E.B. Sheinin and W.R. Benson. Thermal decomposition of propoxyphene during GLC analysis. J. Pharm. Sci. 69: 1177–1179, 1980.

J.F. Nash, I.F. Bennett, R.J. Bopp et al. Quantitation of propoxyphene and its major metabolites in heroin addict plasma after large dose administration of propoxyphene napsylate. J. Pharm. Sci. 64: 429–433, 1975.

R. Nickander, S.E. Smits and M.I. Steinberg. Propoxyphene: pharmacologic and toxic effects in animals. J. Pharm. Exp. Ther. 200: 245–253, 1977.

G. Norheim. Determination of dextropropoxyphene and norpropoxyphene in autopsy material by gas chromatography. Arch. Tox. 36: 89–95, 1976.

J. Rio, N. Hodnett and J.H. Bidanset. The determination of propoxyphene, norpropoxyphene, and methadone in postmortem blood and tissues by high-performance liquid chromatography. J. Anal. Tox. 11: 222–224, 1987.

P.P. Rop, F. Grimaldi, M. Bresson et al. Simultaneous determination of dextromoramide, propoxyphene and norpropoxyphene in necropsic whole blood by liquid chromatography. J. Chrom. 615: 357–364, 1993.

J. Schou, H. Angelo, W. Dam et al. Pharmacokinetics of dextropropoxyphene in acute poisoning. Arch. Tox. (Suppl. 1): 343–346, 1978.

W.J. Serfontein and L.S. de Villiers. A new g.c. procedure, based on nitrosation, for the simultaneous determination of propoxyphene and norpropoxyphene in biological material. J. Pharm. Pharmac. 28: 718–719, 1976.

E.L. Slightom. Differentiation of levo and dextropropoxyphene using a homogenous enzyme immunoassay. Presented at the annual meeting of the American Academy of Forensic Sciences, Orlando, Florida, February 10, 1982.

C.M. Sparacino, E.D. Pellizzari, C.E. Cook and M.W. Wall. A re-examination of the gas chromatographic determination of α-d-propoxyphene. J. Chrom. 77: 413–418, 1973.

W.Q. Sturner and J.C. Garriott. Deaths involving propoxyphene. A study of 41 cases over a two-year period. J. Am. Med. Asso. 22: 1125–1130, 1973.

K. Verebely and C.E. Inturrisi. The simultaneous determination of propoxyphene and norpropoxyphene in human biofluids using gas-liquid chromatography. J. Chrom. 75: 195–205, 1973.

K. Verebely and C.E. Inturrisi. Disposition of propoxyphene and norpropoxyphene in man after a single oral dose. Clin. Pharm. Ther. 15: 302–309, 1974.

J.E. Wallace, J.D. Biggs and E.V. Dahl. A rapid and specific spectrophotometric method for determining propoxyphene. J. For. Sci. 10: 179–191, 1965.

R.D. Warren, D.S. Meyers, B.A. Pape and J.F. Maher. Fatal overdose of propoxyphene napsylate and aspirin. J. Am. Med. Asso. 230: 259–260, 1974.

R.L. Wolen and C.M. Gruber, Jr. Determination of propoxyphene in human plasma by gas chromatography. Anal. Chem. 40: 1243–1246, 1968.

R.L. Wolen, E.A. Ziege and C.M. Gruber, Jr. Determination of propoxyphene and norpropoxyphene by chemical ionization mass fragmentography. Clin. Pharm. Ther. 17: 15–20, 1975.

Propranolol

T½: 2–4 hr
Vd: 3–5 L/kg
Fb: 0.93
pKa: 9.5

$OCH_2CHOHCH_2NHCH(CH_3)_2$

Occurrence and Usage. Propranolol (Inderal) is a beta-adrenergic blocking agent that was synthesized in 1964. It is currently used as an antihypertensive and antiarrhythmic agent in man, being administered as the hydrochloride salt in daily oral doses of 30–320 mg or by intravenous injection of 1–3 mg. The compound is supplied as the racemic mixture, although most of the activity resides in the l-isomer. It is available as 10–80 mg tablets, 60–160 mg sustained-release capsules and ampules of 1 mg/mL; some oral dosage forms also contain hydrochlorothiazide.

Blood Concentrations. Following a single oral administration of 80 mg to 5 subjects, plasma propranolol concentrations peaked at 0.097 mg/L (range, 0.036–0.212) at 1.5–2 hours and declined with a half-life of 3.1 hours (range, 2.2–4.0). During an intravenous infusion of 10 mg (1 mg/min), plasma concentrations were initially as high as 0.100–0.200 mg/L (Shand et al., 1970). Plasma half-lives of 2.0 and 3.2 hours were determined for the d- and l-isomers, respectively (George et al.,

1972). The drug is 93% bound to plasma protein at therapeutic concentrations (Evans et al., 1973) and exhibits an average blood/plasma ratio of 1.33 in hypertensive patients (Sawchuk et al., 1974).

Plasma levels of 0.100 mg/L were found effective against exercise-induced tachycardia with intravenously administered propranolol, whereas levels of only 0.040 mg/L were effective after oral dosing (Coltart and Shand, 1970). Steady-state peak plasma concentrations in patients receiving 40, 80, 160, or 320 mg of the drug daily by mouth averaged 0.010, 0.023, 0.046, and 0.335 mg/L, respectively (Walle et al., 1978). Four patients on chronic oral therapy with 160 mg daily had plasma concentrations 2 hours after the last dose that averaged 0.115 mg/L (range, 0.031–0.262) for propranolol and 0.027 mg/L (range, 0.008–0.063) for 4-hydroxypropranolol (Walle et al., 1975). Propranolol glucuronide is present in plasma during oral therapy at about 6 times the propranolol concentration (Walle et al., 1976), while naphthoxylactic acid levels are about 10 times as high (Walle et al., 1979).

Metabolism and Excretion. Propranolol undergoes a complex pattern of biotransformation in man, with production of several active metabolites. 4-Hydroxypropranolol has beta-blocking activity comparable to that of propranolol and is present in plasma after oral administration of the drug, but has a shorter half-life than its parent. Norpropranolol and alpha-naphthoxy-2,3-propyleneglycol (NPG) also have biological activity, but the extent of their contribution to the effects of the drug is uncertain. Most of the propranolol metabolites, including propranolol itself, are excreted in the urine in both conjugated and free form; about 84–92% of an oral dose is eliminated in the 48 hour urine, with 20% as naphthoxylactic acid, up to 25% as propranolol glucuronide and only trace amounts of unchanged drug (Bond, 1967; Paterson et al., 1970; Walle and Gaffney, 1972; Walle, 1974; Walle et al., 1976).

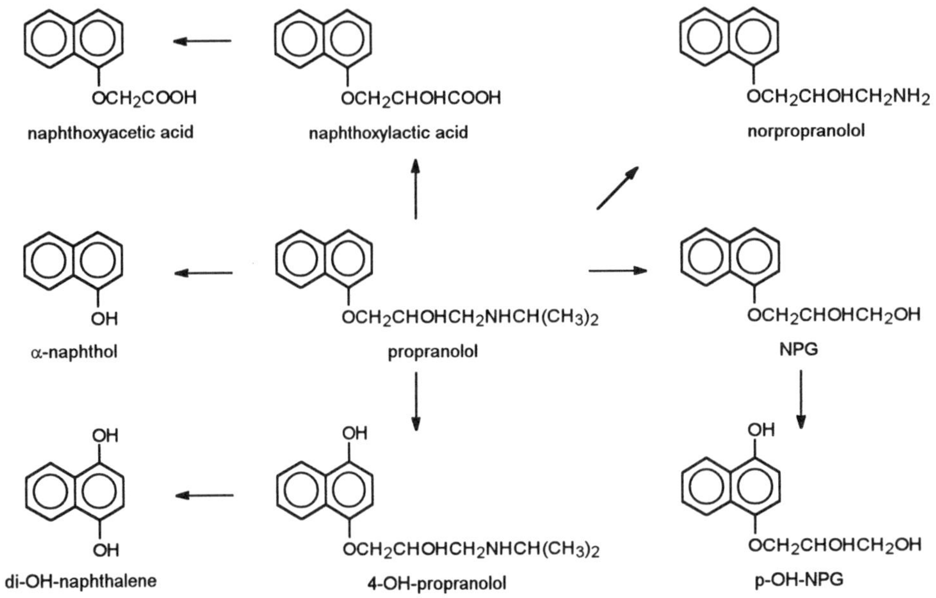

OCH$_2$COOH   OCH$_2$CHOHCOOH   OCH$_2$CHOHCH$_2$NH$_2$
naphthoxyacetic acid   naphthoxylactic acid   norpropranolol

OH   OCH$_2$CHOHCH$_2$NHCH(CH$_3$)$_2$ OCH$_2$CHOHCH$_2$OH
α-naphthol   propranolol   NPG

OH / OH   OH / OCH$_2$CHOHCH$_2$NHCH(CH$_3$)$_2$ OH / OCH$_2$CHOHCH$_2$OH
di-OH-naphthalene   4-OH-propranolol   p-OH-NPG

Toxicity. Adverse reactions to propranolol include nausea, vomiting, lightheadedness, weakness, visual disturbances, hallucinations, disorientation, memory loss, catatonia, bradycardia, hypotension, paresthesias, congestive heart failure, and bronchospasm. Up to 2 g of propranolol have been ingested acutely without obvious signs of toxicity (Wermut and Wojcicki, 1973). Fatal bronchospasm may result in asthmatic patients after even a single therapeutic dose (Schaffer et al., 1984). A 20 year old woman who ingested 2 g of propranolol became unresponsive, without pulse or blood pressure; her admission serum level exceeded 4.5 mg/L, but she survived with extracorporeal circulatory support (McVey and Corke, 1991).

A woman who ingested 3.1 g of drug collapsed, had a seizure and became hypotensive; a plasma propranolol level of 1.5 mg/L was measured 13 hours after ingestion and she eventually expired after 20 days (Chen et al., 1985). The deaths of 12 persons have been reported following ingestion of up to 6 g of the drug, with postmortem propranolol concentrations averaging 14 mg/L (range, 4–29) in blood and 198 mg/kg (range, 60–451) in liver (Robinson, 1973; Turner and Cravey, 1975; Piper and Smith, 1976; Gault et al., 1977; Kristinsson and Johannesson, 1977; Registry, 1978; Rousseau, 1981; Jones et al., 1982; Suarez et al., 1988). One additional case was reported with a blood level of 167 mg/L and liver of 958 mg/kg (Stevenson, 1979). Two of the above cases exhibited the following tissue distribution of the drug (Turner and Cravey, 1975; Kristinsson and Johannesson, 1977):

Propranolol Concentrations in Fatal Cases (mg/L or mg/kg)*

Blood	Brain	Liver	Kidney	Urine	Gastric
14	67	171		0.9	85 mg
16	41	254	71	2	320 mg

*By flame-ionization gas chromatography

Analysis. Propranolol has been frequently determined in plasma by a fluorometric method (Shand et al., 1970) that has undergone several modifications (Kraml and Robinson, 1978; Vasiliades et al., 1978); one variation allows measurement of both the parent drug and 4-hydroxypropranolol (Rao et al., 1978). Gas chromatographic procedures have utilized electron-capture detection of various halogenated derivatives (Di Salle et al., 1973; Walle, 1974; Kates and Jones, 1977). Propranolol and 4-hydroxypropranolol have been simultaneously analyzed in plasma by mass fragmentography of their trifluoroacetyl derivatives; the addition of sodium bisulphite to plasma prior to extraction was necessary to prevent the decomposition of the metabolite (Walle et al., 1975). Numerous liquid chromatographic techniques have been developed for the drug and its metabolites (Hackett and Dusci, 1979; Lo and Riegelman, 1980; Drummer et al., 1981; Rosseel and Bogaert, 1981; Albani et al., 1982; Harrison et al., 1985; Koshakji and Wood, 1987; Fu and Mason, 1989). Gas chromatography-mass spectrometry has also been employed (Quaglio et al., 1993). Certain brands of blood collection tubes may cause lowering of plasma propranolol due to interference with plasma protein binding by a contaminant (Cotham and Shand, 1975).

References

F. Albani, R. Riva and A⸱ Baruzzi. Simple and rapid determination of propranolol and its active metabolite, 4-hydroxypropranolol, in human plasma by liquid chromatography with fluorescence detection. J. Chrom. 228: 362–365, 1982.

P.A. Bond. Metabolism of propranolol ('Inderal'), a potent, specific β-adrenergic receptor blocking agent. Nature 213: 721, 1967.

T.W. Chen, T.P. Huang, W.C. Yang and C.Y. Hong. Propranolol intoxication: three cases' experiences. Vet. Hum. Tox. 27: 528–530, 1985.

D.J. Coltart and D.G. Shand. Plasma propranolol levels in the quantitative assessment of β-adrenergic blockade in man. Brit. Med. J. 3: 731–734, 1970.

R.H. Cotham and D. Shand. Spuriously low plasma propranolol concentrations resulting from blood collection methods. Clin. Pharm. Ther. 18: 535–538, 1975.

E. Di Salle, K.M. Baker, S.R. Bareggi et al. A sensitive gas chromatographic method for the determination of propranolol in human plasma. J. Chrom. 84: 347–353, 1973.

O.H. Drummer, J. McNeil, E. Pritchard and W.J. Louis. Combined high-performance liquid chromatographic procedure for measuring 4-hydroxypropranolol and propranolol in plasma: pharmacokinetic measurements following conventional and slow-release propranolol administration. J. Pharm. Sci. 70: 1030–1032, 1981.

G.H. Evans, A.S. Nies and D.G. Shand. The disposition of propranolol. III. Decreased half-life and volume of distribution as a result of plasma binding in man, monkey, dog and rat. J. Pharm. Exp. Ther. 186: 114–122, 1973.

C.J. Fu and W.D. Mason. Determination of propranolol and 4-hydroxypropranolol in human plasma by high-performance liquid chromatography. Analyst 114: 1219–1223, 1989.

R. Gault, J.R. Monforte and S. Khasnabis. A death involving propranolol (Inderal). Clin. Tox. 11: 295–299, 1977.

C.F. George, T. Fenyvesi, M.E. Conolly and C.T. Dollery. Pharmacokinetics of dextro-, laevo- and racemic propranolol in man. Eur. J. Clin. Pharm. 4: 74–76, 1972.

L.P. Hackett and L.J. Dusci. The analysis of propranolol in human serum using high-performance liquid chromatography. Clin. Tox. 15: 63–66, 1979.

P.M. Harrison, A.M. Tonkin, C.M. Cahill and A.J. McLean. Rapid and simultaneous extraction of propranolol, its neutral and basic metabolites from plasma and assay by high-performance liquid chromatography. J. Chrom. 343: 349–358, 1985.

J.W. Jones, M.A. Clark and B.L. Mullen. Suicide by ingestion of propranolol. J. For. Sci. 27: 213–216, 1982.

R.E. Kates and C.L. Jones. Rapid GLC determination of propranolol in human plasma samples. J. Pharm. Sci. 66: 1490–1492, 1977.

R.P. Koshakji and A.J.J. Wood. Improved high-performance liquid chromatographic method for the simultaneous determination of propranolol and 4-hydroxypropranolol in plasma with fluorescence detection. J. Chrom. 422: 294–300, 1987.

M. Kraml and W.T. Robinson. Fluorimetry of propranolol and its glucuronide: applicability, specificity, and limitations. Clin. Chem. 24: 169–171, 1978.

J. Kristinsson and J. Johannesson. A case of fatal propranolol intoxication. Acta Pharm. Tox. 41: 190–192, 1977.

M. Lo and S. Riegelman. Determination of propranolol and its major metabolites in plasma and urine by high-performance liquid chromatography without solvent extraction. J. Chrom. 183: 213–220, 1980.

F.K. McVey and C.F. Corke. Extracorporeal circulation in the management of massive propranolol overdose. Anaesthesia 46: 744–746, 1991.

J.W. Paterson, M.E. Connolly, C.T. Dollery et al. The pharmacodynamics and metabolism of propranolol in man. Pharm. Clin. 2: 127–133, 1970.

N. Piper and D. Smith. Personal communication, 1976.

M.P. Quaglio, A.M. Bellini, L. Minozzi et al. Simultaneous determination of propranolol or metoprolol in the presence of butyrophenones in human plasma by gas chromatography with mass spectrometry. J. Pharm. Sci. 82: 87–90, 1993.

P.S. Rao, L.C. Quesada and H.S. Mueller. A simple micromethod for simultaneous determination of plasma propranolol and 4-hydroxypropranolol. Clin. Chim. Acta 88: 355–361, 1978.

Registry of Human Toxicology, American Academy of Forensic Sciences, 1978.

R. Robinson. Personal communication, 1973.

M.T. Rosseel and M.G. Bogaert. High-performance liquid chromatographic determination of propranolol and 4-hydroxypropranolol in plasma. J. Pharm. Sci. 70: 688–689, 1981.

M. Rousseau. Personal communication, 1981.

R.J. Sawchuk, J. Robayo and K.W. Miller. The distribution of propranolol between blood and plasma in hypertensive patients. Brit. J. Clin. Pharm. 1: 440–442, 1974.

M.I. Shaffer, L.F. Beamer and R.H. Kirschner. Acute, fatal bronchospasm caused by single dose of β-adrenergic blocking agents: report of 3 cases. Presented at the annual meeting of the American Academy of Forensic Sciences, Anaheim, California, February 23, 1984.

D.G. Shand, E.M. Nuckolls and J.A. Oates. Plasma propranolol levels in adults with observations in four children. Clin. Pharm. Ther. 11: 112–120, 1970.

A.J. Stevenson. Personal communication, 1979.

R.V. Suarez, M.S. Greenwald and E. Geraghty. Intentional overdosage with propranolol. Am. J. For. Med. Path. 9: 45–47, 1988.

J.E. Turner and R.H. Cravey. A fatal case involving propranolol and codeine. Clin. Tox. 8: 271–275, 1975.

J. Vasiliades, T. Turner and C. Owens. A modified sensitive spectrofluorometric method for the determination of propranolol in serum. Am. J. Clin. Path. 70: 793–799, 1978.

T. Walle and T.E. Gaffney. Propranolol metabolism in man and dog: mass spectrometric identification of six new metabolites. J. Pharm. Exp. Ther. 182: 83–92, 1972.

T. Walle. GLC determination of propranolol, other beta-blocking drugs, and metabolites in biological fluids and tissues. J. Pharm. Sci. 63: 1885–1891, 1974.

T. Walle, J. Morrison, K. Walle and E. Conradi. Simultaneous determination of propranolol and 4-hydroxypropranolol in plasma by mass fragmentography. J. Chrom. 114: 351–359, 1975.

T. Walle, E.C. Conradi, U.K. Walle and T.E. Gaffney. Steady-state plasma concentrations and urinary excretion of propranolol-O-glucuronide and propranolol in patients during chronic oral propranolol therapy. Fed. Proc. 35: 665, 1976.

T. Walle, E.C. Conradi, U.K. Walle et al. The predictable relationship between plasma levels and dose during chronic propranolol therapy. Clin. Pharm. Ther. 24: 668–677, 1978.

T. Walle, E.C Conradi, U.K. Walle et al. Naphthoxylactic acid after single and long-term doses of propranolol. Clin. Pharm. Ther. 26: 548–554, 1979.

W. Wermut and M. Wojcicki. Suicidal attempt with propranolol. Brit. Med. J. 3: 591, 1973.

Propylene Glycol

T½: 2–5 hr
Vd: 0.55 L/kg
Fb: ?

$HOCH_2CHOHCH_3$

Occurrence and usage. Propylene glycol (1,2-propanediol) is used extensively as a preservative, emollient and vehicle for both oral and intravenous medications. These medications in their intravenous form may contain as much as 80% propylene glycol.

Blood Concentrations. Propylene glycol serum concentrations in 5 patients receiving intravenous medications containing propylene glycol ranged from 6–711 mg/L (Kelner and Bailey, 1985). In a study involving adults who received 41.4 g propylene glycol every 12 hours as a solvent in an oral phenytoin solution, peak plasma concentrations of over 1000 mg/L were observed (Yu et al., 1985).

Metabolism and Excretion. About 45% of absorbed propylene glycol is excreted unchanged by the kidneys and the remainder is oxidized by alcohol dehydrogenase to lactate, pyruvate and acetate (Ruddick, 1972).

Toxicity. Although propylene glycol has been considered relatively nontoxic, there have been reports that its use in pharmaceuticals has produced a decreased level of consciousness (Martin and Finberg, 1970; Cate and Hedrick, 1980), seizures (Arulanantham and Genel, 1978), and lactic acidosis (Cate and Hedrick, 1980; Kelner and Bailey, 1985). Two infants who ingested propylene glycol developed drowsiness, transient acidosis and osmolal gap and exhibited peak serum propylene glycol levels of 3670 and 3740 mg/L (McKinney et al., 1992). A woman who received intravenous diazepam and lorazepam for sedation developed lactic acidosis and a peak serum propylene glycol levels of 1240 mg/L; the 2 medications were noted to contain 40% and 80%, respectively, by weight of the chemical (Apple et al., 1993).

Analysis. Propylene glycol has been determined in biological specimens by gas chromatography with flame-ionization detection (Yu and Sawchuk, 1983; Fligner et al., 1985; Kelner and Bailey, 1985). It has been reported that propylene glycol cannot be separated from ethylene glycol by gas chromatography using an OV-17 column, but that separation is possible using an OV-1 column (Robinson et al., 1982).

References

F.S. Apple, M.K. Googins and D. Resen. Propylene glycol interference in gas-chromatography assay of ethylene glycol. Clin. Chem. 39: 167: 1993.

K. Arulanantham and M. Genel. Central nervous system toxicity associated with ingestion of propylene glycol. J. Pediat. 93: 515–516, 1978.

J.C. Cate and R. Hedrick. Propylene glycol intoxication and lactic acidosis. New Eng. J. Med. 303: 1237, 1980.

C.L. Fligner, R. Jack, G.A. Twiggs and V.A. Raisys. Hyperosmolality induced by propylene glycol. J. Am. Med. Asso. 253: 1606–1609, 1985.

M.J. Kelner and D.N. Bailey. Propylene glycol as the cause of lactic acidosis. J. Anal. Tox. 9: 40–42, 1985.

G. Martin and I. Finberg. Propylene glycol: a potentially toxic vehicle in liquid dosage form. J. Pediat. 77: 877–878, 1970.

P. McKinney, S. Phillips, H.F. Gomez et al. Acute propylene glycol ingestion: 2 cases. Vet. Hum. Tox. 34: 338, 1992.

C.A. Robinson, J.W. Scott and C. Ketchum. Propylene glycol interference with ethylene glycol procedures. Clin. Chem. 28: 727, 1982.

J.A. Ruddick. Toxicology, metabolism, and biochemistry of 1,2-propanediol. Tox. Appl. Pharm. 21: 102–111, 1972.

D.K. Yu and R.J. Sawchuk. Gas-liquid determination of propylene glycol in plasma and urine. Clin. Chem. 29: 2088–2090, 1983.

D.K. Yu, W.F. Elmquist and R.J. Sawchuk. Pharmacokinetics of propylene glycol in humans during multiple dosing regimens. J. Pharm. Sci. 74: 876–879, 1985.

Propylhexedrine

T½: ?
Vd: ?
Fb: ?
pKa: 10.4

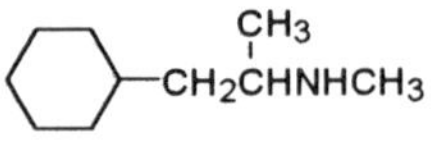

Occurrence and Usage. Propylhexedrine (Benzedrex, Obesin) is the cyclohexyl analogue of meth-amphetamine. It is available without prescription for use as a nasal decongestant; plastic inhalers contain 250 mg of the free base and deliver approximately 0.25 mg/inhalation. The compound has been widely abused for its central nervous system stimulant properties.

Blood Concentrations. Blood concentrations of propylhexedrine after normal therapeutic usage are believed to be on the order of 0.01 mg/L (Di Maio and Garriott, 1977).

Metabolism and Excretion. Propylhexedrine is known to be metabolized in man by N-demethylation, N-oxidation, and p-hydroxylation. Urinary excretion products (not quantified) included parent drug, norpropylhexedrine, cyclohexylacetoxime, and 4-hydroxypropylhexedrine (Midha et al., 1974). Urine concentrations of the parent drug, following a brief period of inhaler use by a volunteer, ranged from 0.04 mg/L after 10 minutes to 0.60 mg/L after 2.3 hours (Di Maio and Garriott, 1977).

4-OH-propylhexedrine   ←   propylhexedrine   →   norpropylhexedrine

cyclohexylacetoxime

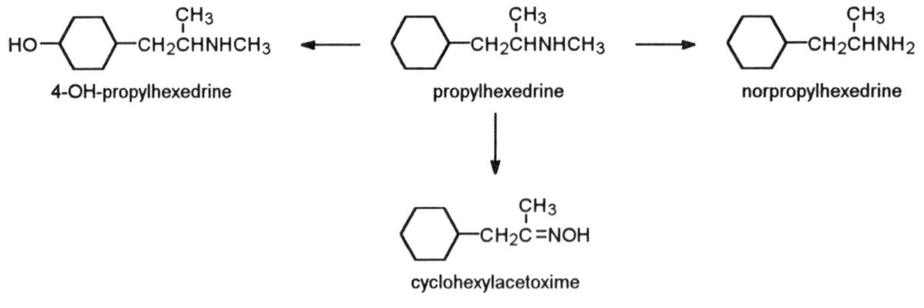

Toxicity. Several individuals have exhibited psychotic behavior during chronic oral ingestion of propylhexedrine; usually, amounts of 250–500 mg (the content of 1–2 inhalers) were taken daily by chewing or dissolving in a beverage (Anderson, 1970; Johnson et al., 1972; Pallis et al., 1972). The acute ingestion of 250 mg by an adult and 375 mg by a 3 year old child caused headache, tremor, chest pain, palpitation, rapid respiration, cold and clammy skin, dilated pupils and tachycardia. The adult experienced myocardial infarction and progressed to severe hypotension and pulmonary edema, while the child exhibited hyperactivity for several days; both patients recovered with supportive treatment (Polster, 1965; Marsden and Sheldon, 1972). Intravenous administration of the drug may cause vasospasm, local tissue necrosis and neurological impairment (Mancusi-Ungaro et al., 1984; Fornazzari et al., 1986). Three adult intravenous abusers of propylhexedrine who exhibited hyperactivity, rapid speech, dilated pupils and rapid pulse had urine concentrations of the drug ranging from 37–224 mg/L (Meeker, 1991).

A 30 year old man who died following acute oral overdosage with propylhexedrine had postmortem drug concentrations of 30 mg/L in blood, 36 mg/kg in liver and 60 mg/L in urine (Riddick and Reisch, 1981). The following tissue concentrations were determined in 12 victims of intravenous abuse of propylhexedrine (Sturner et al., 1974; DiMaio and Garriott, 1977; Anderson et al., 1979):

Propylhexedrine Concentrations in Fatalities (mg/L or mg/kg)

	Blood	Liver	Kidney	Urine
Average	1.7	5.6	3.2	41
(Range)	(0.3–2.7)	(1.3–11.8)	(0.5–9.5)	(13–70)

Analysis. Propylhexedrine may be analyzed in biological specimens by many of the techniques described for amphetamine. Flame-ionization gas chromatography has been used in cases of overdosage (Sturner et al., 1974).

References

E.D. Anderson. Propylhexedrine (Benzedrex) psychosis. New Zeal. Med. J. 71: 302, 1970.

R.J. Anderson, H.R. Garza, J.C. Garriott and V. DiMaio. Intravenous propylhexedrine (Benzedrex) abuse and sudden death. Am. J. Med. 67: 15–20, 1979.

V.J.M. DiMaio and J.C. Garriott. Intravenous abuse of propylhexedrine. J. For. Sci. 22: 152–158, 1977.

L. Fornazzari, P.L. Carlen and B.M. Kapur. Intravenous abuse of propylhexedrine (Benzedrex) and the risk of brainstem dysfunction in young adults. Can. J. Neurol. Sci. 13: 337–339, 1986.

J. Johnson, D.A.W. Johnson and A.J. Robins. Propylhexedrine chewing and psychosis. Brit. Med. J. 2: 529–530, 1972.

H.R. Mancusi-Ungaro, W.J. Decker, V.R. Forshan et al. Tissue injuries associated with parenteral propylhexedrine abuse. Clin. Tox. 21: 359–372, 1984.

P. Marsden and J. Sheldon. Acute poisoning by propylhexedrine. Brit. Med. J. 1: 730, 1972.

J. Meeker. Personal communication, 1991.

K.K. Midha, A.H. Beckett and A. Saunders. Identification of the major metabolites of propylhexedrine *in vivo* (in man) and *in vitro* (in guinea pig and rabbit). Xenobiotica 4: 627–635, 1974.

D.J. Pallis, B.M. Barraclough and J. Tsiantis. Psychosis and nasal decongestants. Practitioner 209: 676–678, 1972.

H. Polster. Ueber eine Vergiftung mit dem Appetitzuegler Propylhexedrin, "Obesin", bei einem 3 jaehrigen Kinde. Arch. Tox. 20: 271–273, 1965.

L.R. Riddick and R. Reisch. Oral overdose of propylhexedrine. J. For. Sci. 26: 834–839, 1981.

W.Q. Sturner, F.G. Spruill and J.C. Garriott. Two propylhexedrine-associated fatalities: benzedrine revisited. J. For. Sci. 19: 572–574, 1974.

Protriptyline

T½: 54–92 hr
Vd: 15–31 L/kg
Fb: 0.92
pKa: ?

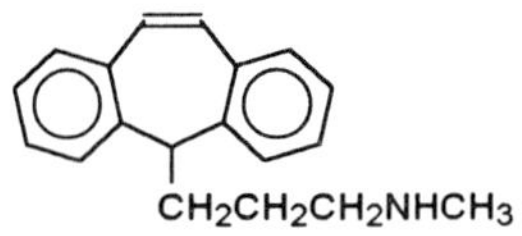

Occurrence and Usage. Protriptyline (Vivactil) is a tricyclic antidepressant similar in structure to nortriptyline. It is available as the hydrochloride in tablets of 5 and 10 mg; daily oral doses range from 15–60 mg.

Blood Concentrations. Eight volunteers given a single 30 mg oral dose of protriptyline achieved peak plasma concentrations of 0.010–0.022 mg/L (average, 0.014) at times of 6–12 hours after ingestion; the elimination half-life averaged 74 hours (Ziegler et al., 1978).

Steady-state protriptyline plasma concentrations in 21 patients receiving 20 mg/day ranged from 0.022–0.167 mg/L, averaging 0.069 mg/L; patients with concentrations greater than 0.070 mg/L demonstrated the best clinical response (Biggs and Ziegler, 1977). Thirty patients receiving 40 mg/day had steady-state levels after 27 days of 0.113–0.376 mg/L, averaging 0.217 mg/L; the investigators suggested a therapeutic range for this drug of 0.083–0.110 mg/L, measured after 7 days of therapy (Moody et al., 1977). After 27 days of therapy, the plasma concentrations should optimally be in the range of 0.131–0.247 mg/L (Whyte et al., 1976).

Metabolism and Excretion. An average of 50% of a labeled oral dose of protriptyline is excreted in urine over a 16 day period, with about 2% in feces (Charalampous and Johnson, 1967). Analysis of urinary metabolites revealed unchanged drug, 10-hydroxyprotriptyline, 10,11-dihydro-dihydroxyprotriptyline, and a rearrangement product (5,10-dihydro-10-formylanthracene-5-propylamine). The two hydroxylated metabolites existed in both free and conjugated form (Sisenwine et al., 1970).

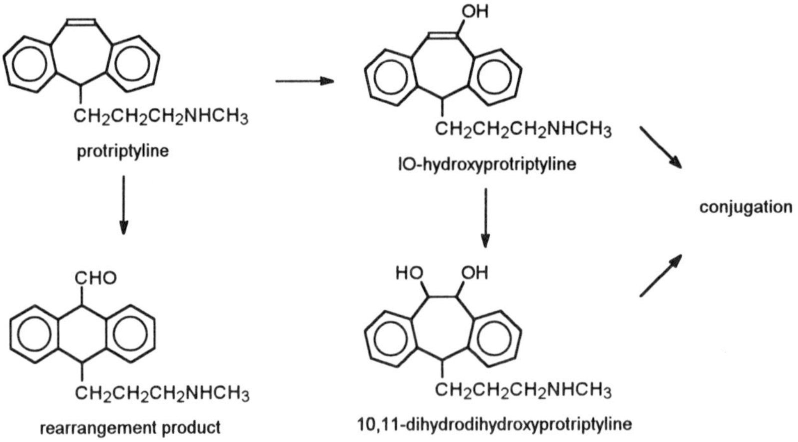

Toxicity. Overdosage with protriptyline may cause vomiting, drowsiness, confusion, hypothermia, tachycardia, arrhythmias, congestive heart failure, convulsions, coma and severe hypotension. Physostigmine is considered to be a specific antidote for many of these symptoms.

Analysis. Plasma protriptyline has been measured by fluorometry (Moody et al., 1973). Many of the chromatographic procedures cited in the section on amitriptyline are also applicable.

References

J.T. Biggs and V.E. Ziegler. Protriptyline plasma levels and antidepressant response. Clin. Pharm. Ther. 22: 269–273, 1977.

K.D. Charalampous and P.C. Johnson. Studies of C^{14}-protriptyline in man: plasma levels and excretion. J. Clin. Pharm. 7: 93–96, 1967.

J.P. Moody, S.F. Whyte and G.J. Naylor. A simple method for the determination of protriptyline in plasma. Clin. Chim. Acta 43: 355–359, 1973.

J.P. Moody, S.F. Whyte, A.J. MacDonald and G.J. Naylor. Pharmacokinetic aspects of protriptyline plasma levels. Eur. J. Clin. Pharm. 11: 51–56, 1977.

S.F. Sisenwine, C.O. Tio, S.R. Shrader and H.W. Ruelius. The biotransformation of protriptyline in man, pig and dog. J. Pharm. Exp. Ther. 175: 51–59, 1970.

S.F. Whyte, A.J. MacDonald, G.J. Naylor and J.P. Moody. Plasma concentrations of protriptyline and clinical effects in depressed women. Brit. J. Psych. 128: 384–390, 1976.

V.E. Ziegler, J.T. Biggs, L.T. Wylie et al. Protriptyline kinetics. Clin. Pharm. Ther. 23: 580–584, 1978.

Pseudoephedrine

T½: 3–16 hr (urine pH-dependent)
Vd: ?
Fb: ?
pKa: 9.7

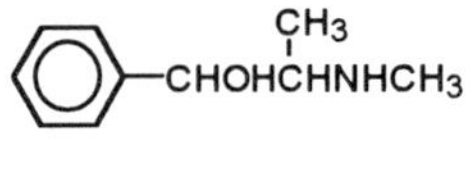

Occurrence and Usage. Pseudoephedrine (Sudafed) occurs naturally in various *Ephedra* species as the d-isomer, in combination with l-ephedrine. Pseudoephedrine is administered orally for use as a nasal decongestant and bronchodilator in single doses of 15–60 mg as the hydrochloride. Up to 240 mg may be taken daily. It is commonly found in nonprescription cold and allergy formulations in conjunction with antihistamines and analgesics.

Blood Concentrations. A 60 mg oral dose of the drug administered to 10 subjects produced an average peak plasma concentration of 0.21 mg/L at 3 hours (Bye et al., 1975). Following an oral dose of 180 mg to 3 subjects, peak plasma levels occurred at 2–3 hours and averaged 0.77 mg/L; plasma half-lives of 5.2–8.0 hours were observed in normal subjects, but ranged from 3.0–16.0 hours when the urine was maintained acidic or alkaline, respectively (Kuntzman et al., 1971). A single dose of 5 mg/kg (350 mg/70 kg) given to a volunteer resulted in a maximal serum concentration of about 1.1 mg/L at 2.5 hours after ingestion (Lin et al., 1977). The chronic administration of 360 mg daily resulted in steady-state plasma concentrations that averaged 0.50–0.64 mg/L in 10 subjects over a 14 day period (Bye et al., 1975).

Metabolism and Excretion. Pseudoephedrine is metabolized to only a minor extent, by N-demethylation to norpseudoephedrine (D-threo-phenylpropanolamine). Up to 88% of a dose is excreted unchanged in the 36 hour urine, with less than 1% present as norpseudoephedrine (Bye et al., 1975). A single 120 mg oral dose produced urine concentrations during the first 24 hours of 4–50 mg/L for pseudoephedrine and 0.07–0.52 mg/L for norpseudoephedrine (Baaske et al., 1979; Lo et al., 1981).

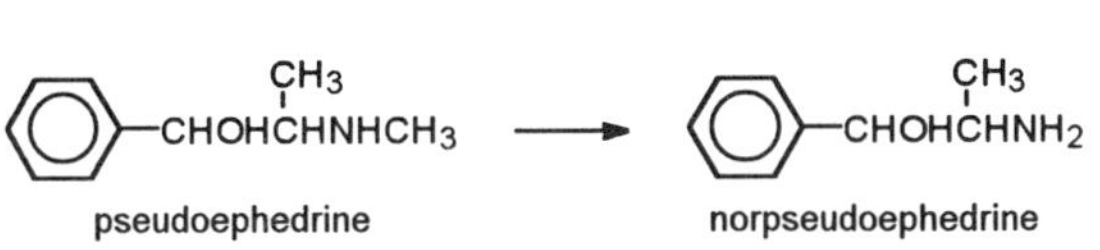

pseudoephedrine → norpseudoephedrine

Toxicity. Adverse reactions to pseudoephedrine may include headache, dizziness, palpitations, tachycardia, restlessness, tremor, anxiety, insomnia, dyspnea, hallucinations, pallor, weakness, convulsions, arrhythmias, hypotension, and cardiovascular collapse. A woman who habitually ingested 3000–4500 mg of the drug daily as a psychic stimulant exhibited tachycardia, lethargy, mild delerium, irritability, and bizarre behavior without frank psychosis (Diaz et al., 1979). A patient with renal tubular acidosis and persistently alkaline urine exhibited increasingly bizarre behavior with hallucinations and personality changes while on chronic pseudoephedrine therapy; her serum half-life was found to be 50 hours, apparently as a result of her high urinary pH (Brater et al., 1980).

A 2 year old child believed to have ingested at least seven 60 mg pseudoephedrine tablets was found dead; a postmortem blood level of 66 mg/L was measured (Reynolds, 1983). The following distribution of pseudoephedrine was noted in a case of fatal overdosage (Registry, 1978):

Pseudoephedrine Concentrations in a Fatal Case (mg/L or mg/kg)

Blood	Brain	Liver	Urine	Gastric
19	22	33	105	102 mg

Analysis. Gas chromatographic techniques for the determination of pseudoephedrine and norpseudoephedrine in plasma and urine have relied on flame-ionization detection (Beckett and Wilkinson, 1965) or nitrogen-selective detection (Bye et al., 1975) of the native drugs, or electron-capture detection of halogenated derivatives (Cummins and Fourier, 1969; Lin et al., 1977; Sun and Leveque, 1979; Lo et al., 1981). Liquid chromatographic methods have also been reported (Lai et al., 1979; Brendel et al., 1988; Veals et al., 1988).

References

D.M. Baaske, C.M. Lai, L. Klein et al. Comparison of GLC and high-pressure liquid chromatographic methods for analysis of urinary pseudoephedrine. J. Pharm. Sci. 68: 1472, 1979.

A.H. Beckett and G.R. Wilkinson. Identification and determination of ephedrine and its congeners in urine by gas chromatography. J. Pharm. Pharmac. 17: 104S–106S, 1965.

D.C. Brater, S. Kaojarern, L.Z. Benet et al. Renal excretion of pseudoephedrine. Clin. Pharm. Ther. 28: 690–694, 1980.

E. Brendel, L. Meineke, E.M. Henne et al. Sensitive high-performance liquid chromatographic determination of pseudoephedrine in plasma and urine. J. Chrom. 426: 406–411, 1988.

C. Bye, H.M. Hill, D.T.D. Hughes and S.W. Peck. A comparison of plasma levels of L(+) pseudoephedrine following different formulations, and their relation to cardiovascular and subjective effects in man. Eur. J. Clin. Pharm. 8: 47–53, 1975.

L.M. Cummins and M.J. Fourier. GLC determination of pseudoephedrine and related ephedrines in serum as the heptafluorobutyryl derivatives. Anal. Letters 2: 403–409, 1969.

M.A. Diaz, T.N. Wise and G.O. Semchyshyn. Self-medication with pseudoephedrine in a chronically depressed patient. Am. J. Psych. 136: 1217–1218, 1979.

R.G. Kuntzman, I. Tsai, L. Brand and L.C. Mark. The influence of urinary pH on the plasma half-life of pseudoephedrine in man and dog and a sensitive assay for its determination in human plasma. Clin. Pharm. Ther. 12: 62–67, 1971.

C.M. Lai, R.G. Stoll, Z.M. Look and A. Yacobi. Urinary excretion of chlorpheniramine and pseudoephedrine in humans. J. Pharm. Sci. 68: 1243–1246, 1979.

E.T. Lin, D.C. Brater and L.Z. Benet. Gas-liquid chromatographic determination of pseudoephedrine and norpseudoephedrine in human plasma and urine. J. Chrom. 140: 275–279, 1977.

L.Y. Lo, G. Land and A. Bye. Sensitive assay for pseudoephedrine and its metabolite, norpseudoephedrine in plasma and urine using gas-liquid chromatography with electron-capture detection. J. Chrom. 222: 297–302, 1981.

Registry of Human Toxicology, American Academy of Forensic Sciences, 1978.

P. Reynolds. Personal communication, 1983.

S.R. Sun and M.J. Leveque. Electron-capture GLC determination of pseudoephedrine in serum. J. Pharm. Sci. 68: 1567–1568, 1979.

J. Veals, H. Kim, C. Korduba et al. Determination of plasma pseudoephedrine by fluorescence detection and high performance liquid chromatography. J. Liq. Chrom. 11: 417–433, 1988.

Pyrilamine

T½: ?
Vd: ?
Fb: ?
pKa: ?

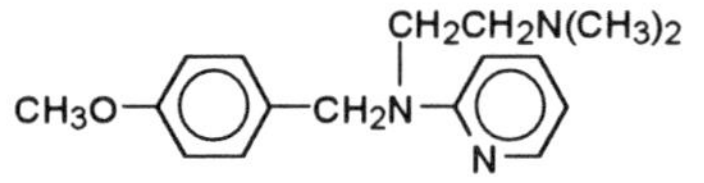

CH_3O—〈○〉—CH_2N—〈○〉 with $CH_2CH_2N(CH_3)_2$ and N

Occurrence and Usage. Pyrilamine (ingredient of Midol-PMS, Robitussin Night Relief) is an antihistamine used frequently in prescription and non-pre cription cold, allergy, and sleep aids. It is available as the maleate or tannate salt in tablets, capsules or elixirs. The usual oral dose is 25 mg taken up to 4 times daily.

Blood Concentrations. Blood concentrations of pyrilamine following therapeutic administration have not been reported.

Metabolism and Excretion. The disposition of pyrilamine has not been studied in man. Preliminary studies have suggested the drug may be N-demethylated (Haley, 1983). Two metabolites, pyrilamine N-oxide and N-desmethylpyrilamine, have been identified in the urine of rats (Korfmacher et al., 1986). High concentrations of unchanged drug have been found in the bile and urine of man following overdose (Wu Chen et al., 1983b).

Toxicity. A 46 year old woman who survived the ingestion of 10 g of pyrilamine suffered grand mal seizures, tachycardia, pulmonary congestion, anuria and cardiogenic shock (Freedberg et al., 1987). The following values were obtained in 4 fatalities due to acute pyrilamine ingestion (Cravey, 1981; Johnson, 1981; Wu Chen et al., 1983b; Cravey, 1984):

Pyrilamine Concentrations in Fatal Cases (mg/L or mg/kg)

	Blood	Brain	Liver	Bile	Urine
Average	13	71	69	83	80
(Range)	(5–27)	(71)	(18–239)	(83)	(80)

Analysis. Pyrilamine has been determined in biological specimens by gas chromatography with flame-ionization (Johnson, 1981; Wu Chen et al., 1983a) and mass spectrometric detection (Wu Chen et al., 1983b; Korfmacher et al., 1986). Liquid chromatography has also been described (Billedeau et al., 1990).

References

S.M. Billedeau, C.L. Holder and T.A. Getek. High-performance liquid chromatography of the antihistamine pyrilamine and its N-oxide using electrochemical detection. J. Chrom. 534: 151–160, 1990.

R.H. Cravey. Unpublished results, 1981.

R.H. Cravey. Unpublished results, 1984.

R.S. Freedberg, G.R. Friedman, R.N. Paul and F. Feit. Cardiogenic shock due to antihistamine overdose. J. Am. Med. Asso. 257: 660–661, 1987.

T.J. Haley. Physical and biological properties of pyrilamine. J. Pharm. Sci. 72: 3–12, 1983.

G.R. Johnson. A fatal case involving pyrilamine. Clin. Tox. 18: 907–909, 1981.

W.A. Korfmacher, C.L. Holder, A.B. Gosnell et al. Identification of pyrilamine metabolites by ammonia chemical ionization mass spectrometry. J. Anal. Tox. 10: 142–146, 1986.

N.B. Wu Chen, M.I. Schaffer, R.L. Lin et al. The general toxicology unknown. I. The systematic approach. J. For. Sci. 28: 391–397, 1983a.

N.B. Wu Chen, M.I. Schaffer, R.L. Lin et al. The general toxicology unknown II. A case report: doxylamine and pyrilamine intoxication. J. For. Sci. 28: 398–403, 1983b.

Quazepam

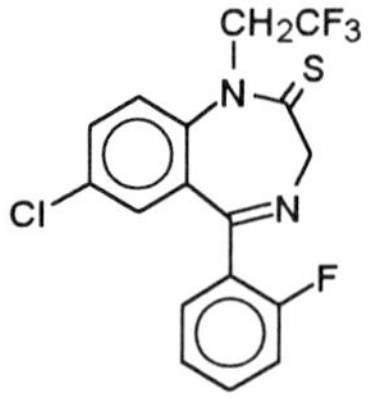

T½: 39–53 hr
Vd: ?
Fb: ?
pKa: ?

Occurrence and Usage. Quazepam (Doral) is a benzodiazepine derivative with hypnotic effects in animals and man. The drug is is available in tablet form containing 7.5–15 mg of the free base for oral use. A single tablet is to be taken prior to bedtime for sleep induction.

Blood Concentrations. Ten healthy geriatric subjects, aged 65–77 and weighing 50–93 kg (average, 58), received a single 15 mg dose following an overnight fast; the average maximum plasma concentrations were 29 µg/L for quazepam achieved at 2.7 hours, 14 µg/L for 2-oxoquazepam at 3.0 hours, and 15 µg/L for N-desalkyl-2-oxoquazepam at 43 hours (Hilbert et al., 1984a). Six healthy male volunteers, 20–32 years of age and weighing 68–87 kg (average, 78), were given 25 mg of quazepam orally following an overnight fast; the average maximum plasma concentrations were 148 µg/L for quazepam in 1.5 hours, 46 µg/L for 2-oxoquazepam in 1.6 hours, and 41 µg/L for N-desalkyl-2-oxoquazepam in 14 hours (Zampaglione et al., 1985).

Eleven healthy adult men (average age, 27 years) weighing 63–89 kg (average, 75) received a 15 mg quazepam tablet once daily for 14 days; steady-state plasma concentrations of 11 µg/L for quazepam and 8 µg/L for 2-oxoquazepam were reached by the seventh day, while a level of 92 µg/L for N-desalkyl-2-oxoquazepam was achieved by the thirteenth day (Chung et al., 1984).

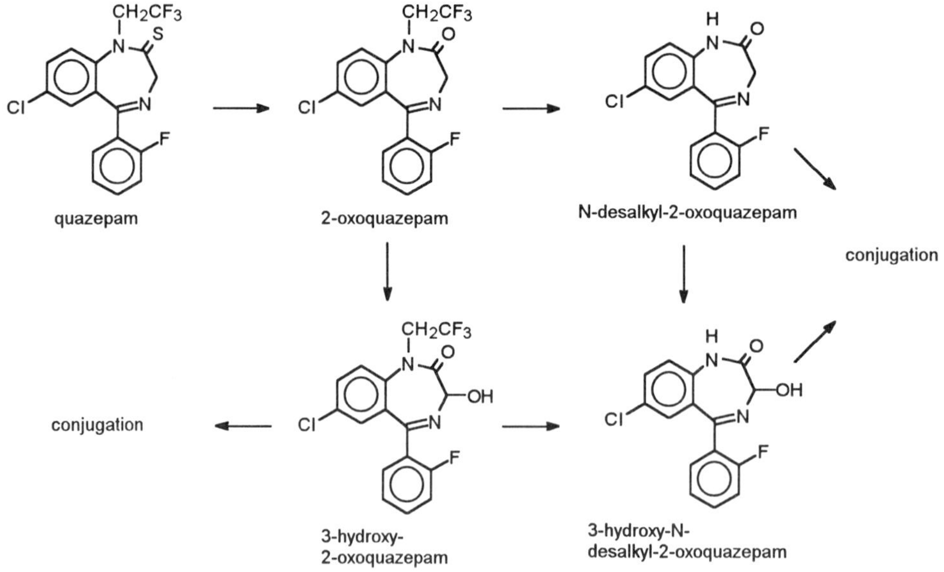

Metabolism and Excretion. Quazepam undergoes rapid and extensive biotransformation in man to 2-oxoquazepam, obtained by replacement of the sulfur group with oxygen; this metabolite, in turn, is metabolized by N-dealkylation to N-desalkyl-2-oxoquazepam or by hydroxylation to 3-hydroxy-2-oxoquazepam, which is excreted as a glucuronide. 2-Oxoquazepam and N-desalkyl-2-oxoquazepam are pharmacologically active (Zampaglione et al., 1985; Hilbert et al., 1984b). Only trace amounts of quazepam are excreted as unchanged drug. Over a 5 day period, 31% of a single dose is excreted as metabolites in the urine and 23% in feces (Zampaglione et al., 1984).

Toxicity. Adverse effects associated with quazepam administration include daytime sleepiness, drowsiness, slurred speech and poor coordination (Kales et al., 1982).

Analysis. Quazepam and its major metabolites have been determined in plasma by gas chromatography with packed (Hilbert et al., 1984c) or capillary columns (Bun et al., 1986) employing electron-capture detection. Liquid chromatography and gas chromatography-mass spectrometry have been used to identify the major metabolites in urine (Zampaglione et al., 1985).

References

H. Bun, P. Coassolo, B. Ba et al. Plasma quantification of quazepam and its 2-oxo and N-desmethyl metabolites by capillary gas chromatography. J. Chrom. 378: 137–145, 1986.

M. Chung, J.M. Hilbert, R.P. Gural et al. Multiple-dose quazepam kinetics. Clin. Pharm. Ther. 35: 520–524, 1984.

J.M. Hilbert, M. Chung, E. Radwanski et al. Quazepam kinetics in the elderly. Clin. Pharm. Ther. 36: 566–569, 1984a.

J. Hilbert, B. Pramanik, S. Symchowicz and N. Zampaglione. The disposition and metabolism of a hypnotic benzodiazepine, quazepam, in the hamster and mouse. Drug Met. Disp. 12: 453–459, 1984b.

J.M. Hilbert, J.M. Ning, G. Murphy et al. Gas chromatographic determination of quazepam and two major metabolites in human plasma. J. Pharm. Sci. 73: 516–519, 1984c.

A. Kales, E.O. Bixler, C.R. Soldatos et al. Quazepam and flurazepam: long-term use and extended withdrawal. Clin. Pharm. Ther. 32: 781–788, 1982.

N. Zampaglione, J.M. Hilbert, J. Ning et al. Disposition and metabolic fate of ^{14}C-quazepam in man. Drug Met. Disp. 13: 25–29, 1985.

Quinidine

T½: 5–12 hr
Vd: 1.8–3.0 L/kg
Fb: 0.74–0.88
pKa: 4.2, 8.3

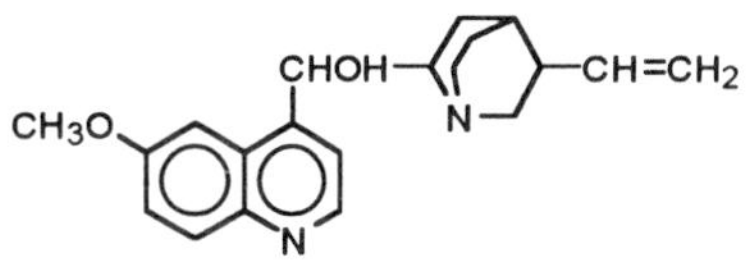

Occurrence and Usage. Quinidine (Duraquin, Quinaglute, Quinora) is a dextrorotatory stereoisomer of quinine that occurs together with that drug in cinchona bark in a concentration of 0.25–3.0%. It is commonly prepared today by the isomerization of quinine and has been used as an antiarrhythmic agent since 1918. It may be administered on an acute basis by intramuscular or intravenous injection of 200–750 mg of the gluconate salt, or for maintenance therapy in oral doses of 600–4000 mg daily, usually as the sulfate salt.

Blood Concentrations. A single oral 600 mg dose of quinidine sulfate given to 6 patients produced an average peak plasma concentration of 3.2 mg/L at 2.25 hours; intramuscular injection of 650 mg of quinidine lactate resulted in a maximal plasma level of 2.7 mg/L after 2.3 hours (Kalmansohn and Sampson, 1950a). In a number of studies the mean elimination half-life has ranged from 5–12 hours (Ochs et al., 1980).

The chronic ingestion of 500 mg of quinidine bisulfate every 12 hours (1000 mg daily) by 6 volunteers produced a mean steady-state serum concentration of 2.6 mg/L (range, 1.8–3.1) (Henning and Nyberg, 1973). Plasma concentrations associated with therapeutic effectiveness are considered to lie between 2 and 5 mg/L for most patients (Kessler et al., 1974). Quinidine exhibits 74–88% plasma protein binding at normally encountered concentrations (Wosilait, 1975) and distributes between erythrocytes and plasma in a 45/55 ratio (Hughes et al., 1975). In cardiac patients on quinidine therapy, serum concentrations of 3-hydroxyquinidine and 2'-quinidinone average 20–34% and 4–14%, respectively, of the quinidine concentrations (Drayer et al., 1978, 1980). Plasma concentrations of quinidine-N-oxide and quinidine-10,11-dihydrodiol average about 14% of the steady-state quinidine level (Rakhit et al., 1984).

Metabolism and Excretion. The metabolism of quinidine in man has not been thoroughly investigated. Its oral bioavailability is 70% or greater (Ochs et al., 1980). It is known that the compound is oxidized to 2'-quinidinone, 3-hydroxyquinidine, quinidine-N-oxide and quinidine-10,11-dihydrodiol and that these metabolites are present in urine in concentrations less than that of the parent drug (Brodie et al., 1951; Carroll et al., 1974; Rakhit et al., 1984). Quinidinone and 3-hydroxyquinidine have antiarrhythmic potency equivalent to that of quinidine (Drayer et al., 1978). Some commercial preparations of quinidine contain up to 15% dihydroquinidine as an impurity, and this compound, which has equivalent activity, will also give rise to urinary metabolites (Hartel and Korhonen, 1968). The urinary elimination of unchanged quinidine is highly pH dependent; urine quinidine concentrations in subjects receiving 800 mg on a chronic daily basis averaged 115 mg/L with a urine pH less than 6, and 13 mg/L when the urine pH exceeded 7.5 (Gerhardt et al., 1969). Persons receiving chronic therapy excrete an average of 16% (range, 9–24) of the daily dose as unchanged drug in the 24 hour urine (Sokolow and Edgar, 1950). Quinidine-N-oxide has been reported as a minor urinary metabolite (Bonora et al., 1979). The following tissue distribution was observed in a patient who died while on therapy with quinidine (Geyer, 1983):

Quinidine Concentrations During Therapy (mg/L or mg/kg)

Blood	Brain	Liver	Urine	Gastric
2.5	0.3	8.8	64	0.9 mg

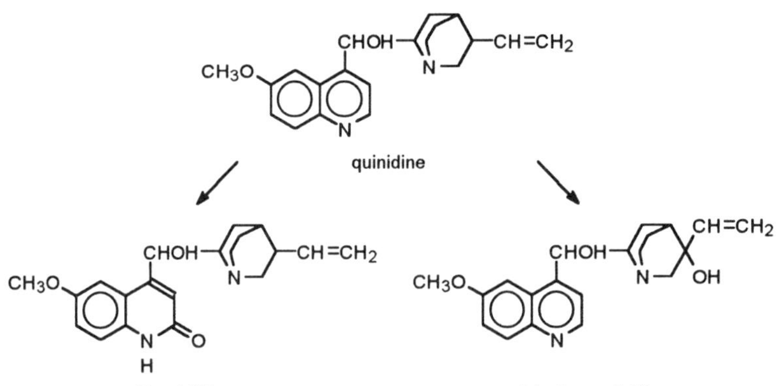

quinidine

2'-quinidinone   3-hydroxyquinidine

Toxicity. Quinidine toxicity is manifested by gastrointestinal disturbances, giddiness, tinnitus, diplopia and hypotension; such symptoms occur primarily at plasma concentrations exceeding 8 mg/L. Concentrations as high as 24 mg/L have been found necessary for successful antiarrhythmic therapy in some patients (Kalmansohn and Sampson, 1950b; Conn and Luchi, 1964). Quinidine-induced syncope occurs in about 5% of the patients receiving the drug, due to hypotension, ventricular tachycardia or an idiosyncratic reaction; it is associated with an 11% mortality rate, but has been successfully treated with bretylium (Luchi, 1978; VanderArk et al., 1976).

A 16 year old girl who ingested 8 g of quinidine sulfate became comatose and exhibited convulsions, arrhythmias, shallow respiration, severe hypotension, and a maximal serum quinidine level of 21 mg/L measured about 10 hours after ingestion. She recovered within several days with supportive therapy (Shub et al., 1978). In 3 similar cases, peak serum quinidine levels ranged from 9.7–28 mg/L; hemodialysis has been shown to double the elimination rate of the drug, markedly improving clinical status (Kerr et al., 1971; Reimold et al., 1973; Woie and Oyri, 1974).

A 2 year old child who ingested about 5 g of a sustained-release preparation of the drug and died after 28.5 hours was found to have developed the following tissue concentrations (McBay and Turk, 1972):

Quinidine Concentrations in a Fatal Case (mg/L or mg/kg)

Blood	Myocardium	Liver*	Kidney
45	80	220	180

*Fixed tissue

Analysis. Quinidine has commonly been determined in body fluids by fluorometry, which is either performed directly on a protein-free filtrate or after solvent extraction (Edgar and Sokolow, 1950). A fluorometric technique utilizing benzene extraction (Cramer and Isaksson, 1963) has been found to yield 40% lower values than the former method, as a result of greater specificity (Hartel and Harjanne, 1969). Gas chromatographic techniques have also been described for the flame-ionization detection of a methyl derivative of quinidine (Midha and Charette, 1974) and nitrogen-specific detection of the intact drug (Moulin and Kinsun, 1977). Recently, liquid chromatography has been shown to be specific for the drug in the presence of its metabolites (Kates et al., 1978; Powers and Sadee, 1978; Guentert et al., 1979; Kline et al., 1979; Weidner et al., 1979; Reece and Peikert, 1980; Patel, 1982; Mackichan and Shields, 1987; Hoyer et al., 1991). An enzyme immunoassay is commercially available; it yields values for serum quinidine that are approximately 10% lower than fluorometry with benzene extraction, and 10% higher than liquid chromatography (Batra et al., 1981; Ha et al., 1981). Serum quinidine values were found to be reduced by 9–24% after contact of the specimen with the stoppers of Vacutainer tubes (Vinet, 1981).

References

K.K. Batra, J. Omand and R.C. Baselt. Serum quinidine concentrations as measured by direct fluorometry, double-extraction fluorometry, and enzyme immunoassay. Clin. Chem. 27: 780–781, 1981.

M.R. Bonora, T.W. Guentert, R.A Upton and S. Riegelman. Determination of quinidine and metabolites in urine by reverse-phase high-pressure liquid chromatography. Clin. Chim. Acta 91: 277–284, 1979.

B.B. Brodie, J.E. Baer and L.C. Craig. Metabolic products of the cinchona alkaloids in human urine. J. Biol. Chem. 188: 567–581, 1951.

F.I. Carroll, D. Smith, M.E. Wall and C.G. Moreland. Carbon-13 magnetic resonance study. Structure of the metabolites of orally administered quinidine in humans. J. Med. Chem. 17: 985–987, 1974.

H.L. Conn, Jr. and R.J. Luchi. Some cellular and metabolic considerations relating to the action of quinidine as a prototype antiarrhythmic agent. Am. J. Med. 37: 685–699, 1964.

G. Cramer and B. Isaksson. Quantitative determination of quinidine in plasma. Scand. J. Clin. Lab. Invest. 15: 553–556, 1963.

D.E. Drayer, D.T. Lowenthal, K.M. Restivo et al. Steady-state serum levels of quinidine and active metabolites in cardiac patients with varying degress of renal function. Clin. Pharm. Ther. 24: 31–39, 1978.

D.E. Drayer, M. Hughes, B. Lorenzo and M.M. Reidenberg. Prevalence of high (3S)-3-hydroxyquinidine/ quinidine ratios in serum, and clearance of quinidine in cardiac patients with age. Clin. Pharm. Ther. 27: 72–75, 1980.

A.L. Edgar and M. Sokolow. Experiences with the photofluorometric determination of quinidine in blood. J. Lab. Clin. Med. 36: 478–484, 1950.

R.E. Gerhardt, R.F. Knouss, P.T. Thyrum et al. Quinidine excretion in aciduria and alkaluria. Ann. Int. Med. 71: 927–933, 1969.

R. Geyer. Personal communication, 1983.

T.W. Guentert, P.E. Coates, R.A. Upton et al. Determination of quinidine and its major metabolites by high-performance liquid chromatography. J. Chrom. 162: 59–70, 1979.

H.R. Ha, G. Kewitz, M. Wenk and F. Follath. Quinidine determination in serum: enzyme immunoasay (EIA) v HPLC. Brit. J. Clin. Pharm. 11: 312–314, 1981.

G. Hartel and A. Korhonen. Thin-layer chromatography for the quantitative separation of quinidine and quinidine metabolites from biological fluids and tissues. J. Chrom. 37: 70–75, 1968.

G. Hartel and A. Harjanne. Comparison of two methods for quinidine determination and chromatographic analysis of the difference. Clin. Chim. Acta 23: 289–294, 1969.

R. Henning and G. Nyberg. Serum quinidine levels after administration of three different quinidine preparations. Eur. J. Clin. Pharm. 6: 239–244, 1973.

G.L. Hoyer, D.C. Clawson, L.A. Brookshier et al. High-performance liquid chromatographic method for the quantitation of quinidine and selected quinidine metabolites. J. Chrom. 572: 159–169, 1991.

I.E. Hughes, K.F. Ilett and L.B. Jellett. The distribution of quinidine in human blood. Brit. J. Clin. Pharm. 2: 521–525, 1975.

R.W. Kalmansohn and J.J. Sampson. Studies of plasma quinidine control. I. Relation to single dose administration by three routes. Circulation 1: 564–568, 1950a.

R.W. Kalmansohn and J.J. Sampson. Studies of plasma quinidine content. II. Relation to toxic manifestations and therapeutic effect. Circulation 1: 569–575, 1950b.

R.E. Kates, D.W. McKennon and T.J. Comstock. Rapid high-pressure liquid chromatographic determination of quinidine and dihydroquinidine in plasma samples. J. Pharm. Sci. 67: 269–270, 1978.

F. Kerr, G. Kenoyer and M. Bilitch. Quinidine overdosage. Brit. Heart J. 33: 629–631, 1971.

K.M. Kessler, D.T. Lowenthal, H. Warner et al. Quinidine elimination in patients with congestive heart failure or poor renal function. New Eng. J. Med. 290: 706–709, 1974.

B.J. Kline, V.A. Turner and W.H. Barr. Determination of quinidine and dihydroquinidine in plasma by high performance liquid chromatography. Anal. Chem. 51: 449–451, 1979.

R.J. Luchi. Intoxication with quinidine. Chest 73: 129–131, 1978.

J.J. MacKichan and B.J. Shields. Specific high performance liquid chromatographic determination of quinidine in serum, blood, and urine. Ther. Drug Mon. 9: 104–112, 1987.

A.J. McBay and R.F. Turk. Personal communication, 1972.

K.K. Midha and C. Charette. GLC determination of quinidine from plasma and whole blood. J. Pharm. Sci. 63: 1244–1247, 1974.

M.A. Moulin and H. Kinsun. A gas-liquid chromatographic method for the quantitative determination of quinidine in blood. Clin. Chim. Acta 75: 491–495, 1977.

H.R. Ochs, D.J. Greenblatt and E. Woo. Clinical pharmacokinetics of quinidine. Clin. Pharmacokin. 5: 150–168, 1980.

C.P. Patel. Liquid chromatographic determination of quinidine in serum and urine. Ther. Drug Mon. 4: 213–217, 1982.

J.L. Powers and W. Sadee. Determination of quinidine by high-performance liquid chromatography. Clin. Chem. 24: 299–302, 1978.

A. Rakhit, N.H.G. Holford, T.W. Guentert et al. Pharmacokinetics of quinidine and three of its metabolites in man. J. Pharmacokin. Biopharm. 12: 1–21, 1984.

P.A. Reece and M. Peikert. Simple and selective high-performance liquid chromatographic method for estimating plasma quinidine levels. J. Chrom. 181: 207–217, 1980.

E.W. Reimold, W.J. Reynolds, D.E. Fixler and L. McElroy. Use of hemodialysis in the treatment of quinidine poisoning. Pediatrics 52: 111–115, 1973.

C. Shub, G.T. Gau, P.M. Sidell and L.A. Brennan, Jr. The management of acute quinidine intoxication. Chest 73: 173–178, 1978.

M. Sokolow and A.L. Edgar. Blood quinidine concentrations as a guide in the treatment of cardiac arrhythmias. Circulation 1: 576–592, 1950.

C.R. VanderArk, E.W. Reynolds, D.R. Kahn and G. Tullett. Quinidine syncope. J. Thor. Cardiovasc. Surg. 72: 464–467, 1976.

B. Vinet. Evaluation des tubes Vacutainer a bouchon bleu royal pour la determination de la quinidine plasmatique. Clin. Biochem. 14: 105, 1981.

N. Weidner, J.H. Ladenson, L. Larson et al. A high-pressure liquid chromatography method for serum quinidine and (3S)-3-hydroxyquinidine. Clin. Chim. Acta 91: 7–13, 1979.

L. Woie and A. Oyri. Quinidine intoxication treated with hemodialysis. Acta Med. Scand. 195: 237–239, 1974.

W.D. Wosilait. A theoretical analysis of the distribution of quinidine in the plasma: the relationship between protein binding and therapeutic drug levels. Res. Comm. Chem. Path. Pharm. 12: 147–154, 1975.

Quinine

T½: 3–15 hr
Vd: 1.8–3.0 L/kg
Fb: 0.90
pKa: 4.3, 8.4

Occurrence and Usage. Quinine (Quinamm), a stereoisomer of quinidine, is the primary alkaloid of cinchona bark, which has been used for centuries in the treatment of malaria. It has been replaced to a large extent in modern therapy by the synthetic agents, but is still used for the relief of skeletal muscle cramps. It is often found as an adulterant in illicit heroin sold in the eastern United States, and is also present in small amounts (30–80 mg/L) in quinine water. When administered as an antimalarial, daily doses of 600–2000 mg as the hydrochloride or sulfate salts are taken orally.

Blood Concentrations. Persons drinking tonic water containing quinine develop blood quinine concentrations that generally do not exceed 0.3 mg/L (McCloskey et al., 1978). A single oral 650 mg dose of quinine sulfate in capsule form given to 11 subjects produced plasma concentrations that averaged 2.8 mg/L at 2 hours and 1.9 mg/L at 8 hours (Hall et al., 1973). The plasma half-life of quinine averages 7.3 hours in normal volunteers; the drug is evenly distributed between erythrocytes and plasma in healthy subjects, but apparently accumulates in plasma during malarial illness (Trenholme et al., 1976). Plasma concentrations measured 8 hours after the last dose during chronic therapy with 1950 mg of quinine sulfate daily averaged 4.9–5.2 mg/L in 100 healthy subjects; in malarial patients, plasma levels averaged initially as high as 9.7 mg/L and declined to 6.4 mg/L after 9 or 10 days of therapy (Powell and McNamara, 1972). The recommended range for plasma quinine levels in the treatment of falciparum malaria is 5–15 mg/L, usually obtained by a dose of 15–30 mg/kg/day (Franke et al., 1987).

Metabolism and Excretion. Quinine is metabolized by oxidation to several more polar hydroxy metabolites. An average of 17% of a dose is eliminated unchanged in the 24 hour urine during chronic therapy; about the same amount is present as 3-hydroxyquinine and about one-third that amount as 2'-hydroxyquinine. A nonphenolic dihydroxy derivative has also been isolated but not quantitated (Brodie et al., 1951; Brooks et al., 1969; Liddle et al., 1981). Urine quinine concentrations in 5 subjects who ingested 41–55 mg in the form of tonic water ranged from 4.8–7.2 mg/L after 12 hours and from 0–3.2 mg/L after 24 hours (McCloskey et al., 1978).

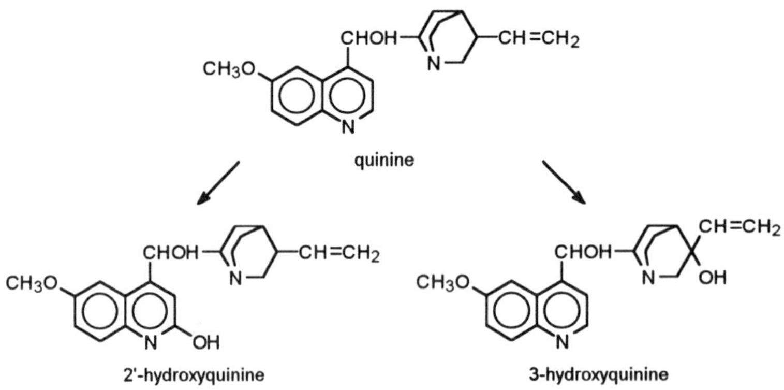

quinine

2'-hydroxyquinine   3-hydroxyquinine

Toxicity. Adverse reactions to quinine include tinnitus, deafness, dizziness, visual difficulties, and gastrointestinal disturbances; this spectrum of effects is known as cinchonism. Plasma quinine levels of 10 mg/L or greater generally result in toxicity in persons on chronic therapy with the drug (Powell and McNamara, 1972). Plasma concentrations of 6.8–26 mg/L have been noted in 8 cases of nonfatal acute poisoning. Convulsions, cyanosis, hypotension, cardiac arrhythmias, coma, blindness, and renal damage were noted in the patients; hemodialysis or peritoneal dialysis was usually effective in attenuating the intoxication, but relatively small amounts of drug were actually removed by these procedures (Hillman and Harpur, 1961; Markham et al., 1967; Clarke, 1969; Frisius and Beyer, 1969; Held, 1972; Floyd et al., 1974; Boscoe et al., 1983). Repeated administration of oral charcoal has been effective in hastening the elimination of quinine in poisoned patients (Prescott et al., 1989).

Blood quinine concentrations of 0.4–11 mg/L were noted in 186 cases of death due to overdosage of heroin that was adulterated with quinine, but it was not felt that quinine contributed significantly to the deaths (Monforte, 1977). The following tissue distribution was observed in 4 fatalities that occurred after the acute ingestion of as little as 6 g of quinine (Rauschke and Burger, 1957; Clarke, 1969; Winek, 1974; Coutselinis and Boukis, 1977):

Quinine Concentrations in Fatal Cases (mg/L or mg/kg)

	Blood	Brain	Liver	Kidney	Urine
Average	13	63	107	116	140
(Range)	(6–24)	(63)	(39–185)	(70–224)	(140)

Analysis. Quinine is generally assayed in biological fluids by fluorometry after protein precipitation (Brodie and Udenfriend, 1943) or after solvent extraction (Hall et al., 1973). Ultraviolet spectrophotometry with measurement of the 250 nm absorbance maximum is also used, and thin-layer chromatography allows the differentiation of quinine and quinidine (Clarke, 1969). Liquid chromatography has also been reported (Edstein et al., 1983; Mihaly et al., 1987; Rauch et al., 1988).

References

M.J. Boscoe, D.M. Calver, C. Keyte and J.G. Ayres. Quinine overdose. Anaesthesia 38: 669–671, 1983.

B.B. Brodie and S. Udenfriend. The estimation of quinine in human plasma with a note on the estimation of quinidine. J. Pharm. Exp. Ther. 78: 154–158, 1943.

B.B. Brodie, J.E. Baer and L.C. Craig. Metabolic products of the cinchona alkaloids in human urine. J. Biol. Chem. 188: 567–581, 1951.

M.H. Brooks, J.P. Malloy, P.J. Bartelloni et al. Quinine, pyrimethamine, and sulphorthodimethoxine: clinical response, plasma levels, and urinary excretion during the initial attack of naturally acquired falciparum malaria. Clin. Pharm. Ther. 10: 85–91, 1969.

E.G.C. Clarke (ed.). In *Isolation and Identification of Drugs*, Pharmaceutical Press, London, 1969, pp. 532–533.

A. Coutselinis and D. Boukis. Quinine concentrations in blood and viscera in a case of acute fatal intoxication. Clin. Chem. 23: 914, 1977.

M. Edstein, J. Stace and F. Shann. Quantification of quinine in human serum by high-performance liquid chromatography. J. Chrom. 278: 445–451, 1983.

M. Floyd, A.V.L. Hill, B.J. Ormston et al. Quinine amblyopia treated by hemodialysis. Clin. Nephrol. 2: 44–46, 1974.

V. Franke, B. Proksch, M. Muller et al. Drug monitoring of quinine by hplc in cerebral malaria with acute renal failure treated by haemofiltration. Eur. J. Clin. Pharm. 33: 293–296, 1987.

H. Frisius and K.H. Beyer. Klinik, Toxikologie und Therapie einer schweren Chininvergiftung. Arch. Tox. 24: 201–213, 1969.

A.P. Hall, A.W. Czerwinski, E.C. Madonia and K.L. Evensen. Human plasma and urine quinine levels following tablets, capsules, and intravenous infusion. Clin. Pharm. Ther. 14: 580–585, 1973.

H. Held. Ueber die Wirksamkeit der Peritonealdialyse bei der Behandlung der Chininvergiftung. Deut. Med. Wochenshr. 97: 1793–1795, 1972.

E. Hillman and E.R. Harpur. Quinine poisoning. New Eng. J. Med. 264: 138–139, 1961.

C. Liddle, G.G. Graham, R.K. Christopher et al. Identification of new urinary metabolites in man of quinine using methane chemical ionization gas chromatography-mass spectrometry. Xenobiotica 11: 81–87, 1981.

T.N. Markham, V.N. Dodson and D.L. Eckberg. Peritoneal dialysis in quinine sulfate intoxication. J. Am. Med. Asso. 202: 1102–1103, 1967.

K.L. McCloskey, J.C. Garriott and S.M. Roberts. Quinine concentrations in blood following the consumption of gin and tonic preparations in a social setting. J. Anal. Tox. 2: 110–112, 1978.

G.W. Mihaly, K.M. Hyman, R.A. Smallwood and K.J. Hardy. High-performance liquid chromatographic analysis of quinine and its diastereoisomer quinidine. J. Chrom. 415: 177–182, 1987.

J.R. Monforte. Some observations concerning blood morphine concentrations in narcotic addicts. J. For. Sci. 22: 718–724, 1977.

R.D. Powell and J.V. McNamara. Quinine: side-effects and plasma levels. Proc. Helminth. Soc. Wash. 39: 331–338, 1972.

L.F. Prescott, A.R. Hamilton and R. Heyworth. Treatment of quinine overdosage with repeated oral charcoal. Brit. J. Clin. Pharm. 27: 95–97, 1989.

K. Rauch, J. Ray and G. Graham. Improved hplc method for the determination of quinine in plasma. J. Chrom. 430: 170–174, 1988.

J. Rauschke and E. Burger. Toedliche Vergiftung mit Chinin bei gleichzeitiger Atebrineinwirkung. Arch. Tox. 16: 320–322, 1957.

G.M. Trenholme, R.L. Williams, K.H. Rieckmann et al. Quinine disposition during malaria and during induced fever. Clin. Pharm. Ther. 19: 459–567, 1976.

C.L. Winek, E.R. Davis, W.D. Collom and S.P. Shanor. Quinine fatality—case report. Clin. Tox. 7: 129–132, 1974.

Ranitidine

T½: 2–3 hr
Vd: 1.6–2.4 L/kg
Fb: 0.15
pKa: 2.3, 8.2

$$(CH_3)_2NCH_2 -\!\!\!\!\!\!\langle\rangle\!\!\!\!\!\!- CH_2SCH_2CH_2NH\overset{\overset{\text{CHNO}_2}{\|}}{C}NHCH_3$$

Occurrence and Usage. Ranitidine (Zantac) is a histamine H-2 receptor antagonist that is used to inhibit gastric acid secretion in ulcer patients. It is available as the hydrochloride in 25 mg/mL solutions for intravenous or intramuscular injection and in 150 and 300 mg tablets. Parenterally, the drug may be given in single doses of 50 mg up to a maximum of 400 mg/day; oral doses generally range from 150–300 mg/day, but patients with severe disease have received up to 6000 mg/day.

Blood Concentrations. Intravenous administration of 1 mg/kg (70 mg/70 kg) of ranitidine to 7 adults produced plasma concentrations that averaged 3.5 mg/L at 0.5 hours, 0.2 mg/L at 2 hours and 0.1 mg/L at 4 hours. A 150 mg oral dose in the same subjects resulted in average plasma levels of 0.2 mg/L at 2 hours, 0.3 mg/L at 4 hours and 0.1 mg/L at 8 hours (Chau et al., 1982). Single 250 and 400 mg oral doses given to 6 adult males produced average peak serum concentrations of 0.84 and 1.43 mg/L, respectively, at an average time of 2.3 hours. Twice daily dosing for up to 28 days did not change the drug's kinetics or increase the serum ranitidine concentrations at 1 hour post-dose (Garg et al., 1985).

Metabolism and Excretion. Ranitidine undergoes biotransformation via N- and S-oxidation and N-demethylation. The oral bioavailability of ranitidine has been found to average 60%. A single oral dose is excreted in the 24 hour urine as unchanged drug (40%), ranitidine-N-oxide (6.0%), ranitidine-S-oxide (1.8%) and N-desmethylranitidine (2.6%). Plasma levels of the metabolites are generally less than 20% those of the parent drug (Van Hecken et al., 1982; Lant et al., 1985; Prueksaritanont et al., 1989).

Toxicity. Side effects of ranitidine administration include nausea, dizziness, confusion, agitation and hallucinations. Overdosage may cause muscular tremor and rapid breathing. Blood or tissue concentrations in such instances have not been reported.

Analysis. Ranitidine is routinely analyzed in biological specimens by liquid chromatography (Carey and Martin, 1979; Carey et al., 1981; Mullersman and Derendorf, 1986; Guiso et al., 1987; Rustum et al., 1987; Prueksaritanont et al., 1989; Rahman et al., 1989).

References

P.F. Carey and L.E. Martin. A high-performance liquid chromatography method for the determination of ranitidine in plasma. J. Liq. Chrom. 2: 1291–1303, 1979.

P.F. Carey, L.E. Martin and P.E. Owen. Determination of ranitidine and its metabolites in human urine by reversed-phase ion pair high-performance liquid chromatography. J. Chrom. 225: 161–168, 1981.

N.P. Chau, P.Y. Zech, N. Pozet et al. Ranitidine kinetics in normal subjects. Clin. Pharm. Ther. 31: 770–774, 1982.

D.C. Garg, F.N. Eshelman and D.J. Weidler. Pharmacokinetics of ranitidine following oral administration with ascending doses and with multiple-fixed doses. J. Clin. Pharm. 25: 437–443, 1985.

G. Guiso, C. Fracasso, S. Caccia and A. Abbiati. Determination of ranitidine in rat plasma and brain by high-performance liquid chromatography. J. Chrom. 413: 363–369, 1987.

M.S. Lant, L.E. Martin and J. Oxford. Qualitative and quantitative analysis of ranitidine and its metabolites by high-performance liquid chromatography-mass spectrometry. J. Chrom. 323: 143–152, 1985.

G. Mullersman and H. Derendorf. Rapid analysis of ranitidine in biological fluids and determination of its erythrocyte partitioning. J. Chrom. 381: 385–391, 1986.

T. Prueksaritanont, N. Sittichai, S. Prueksaritanont and R. Vongsaroj. Simultaneous determination of ranitidine and its metabolites in human plasma and urine by high-performance liquid chromatography. J. Chrom. 490: 175–185, 1989.

A. Rahman, N.E. Hoffman and A.M. Rustum. Determination of ranitidine in plasma by high-performance liquid chromatography. J. Pharm. Biomed. Anal. 7: 747–753, 1989.

A.M. Rustum, A. Rahman and N.E. Hoffman. High-performance liquid chromatographic determination of ranitidine in whole blood and plasma by using a short-polymeric column. J. Chrom. 421: 418–424, 1987.

A.M. Van Hecken, T.B. Tjandramaga, A. Mullie et al. Single dose pharmacokinetics and absolute bioavailability in man. Brit. J. Clin. Pharm. 14: 195–200, 1982.

Salicylamide

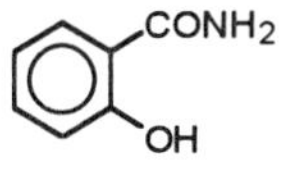

T½: 26–35 min
Vd: ?
Fb: ?
pKa: 8.2

Occurrence and Usage. Salicylamide is the amide derivative of salicylic acid. It is used as an analgesic and antipyretic agent, always in combination with other drugs such as acetaminophen, chlorpheniramine, codeine, phenylpropanolamine, and aspirin. Because it causes drowsiness, it was at one time included in nonprescription sleeping preparations. The oral medications currently available contain from 200–400 mg of salicylamide as the free acid; by following the label recommendations, it is possible to ingest up to 3200 mg daily.

Blood Concentrations. A 1000 mg oral dose of salicylamide given to 6 subjects produced serum concentrations of total drug that averaged 19 mg/L (range, 3–32) at 1 hour, 11 mg/L (range, 0–22) at 3 hours, and 7 mg/L (range, 0–15) at 5 hours. These values were obtained after acid hydrolysis using a colorimetric method with a detectability limit of 2–5 mg/L; no free salicylamide was found in serum (Weikel, 1958). The oral administration of 1500 mg of drug to 5 volunteers resulted in peak plasma levels of 22–45 mg/L (average, 31) occurring at an average time of 12 minutes; a specific gas chromatographic analysis was used (de Boer et al., 1983).

Metabolism and Excretion. Salicylamide is rapidly metabolized in man, primarily by sulfate or glucuronide conjugation and to a lesser extent by hydroxylation to gentisamide. Only traces of parent drug are eliminated in urine. About 40% of a dose is present in the 24 hour urine as salicylamide sulfate, 50% as salicylamide glucuronide, and 10% as gentisamide glucuronide. With larger doses, saturation of the sulfate pathway occurs, and a greater proportion is excreted as glucuronide (Levy and Matsuzawa, 1967).

salicylamide → gentisamide → conjugation

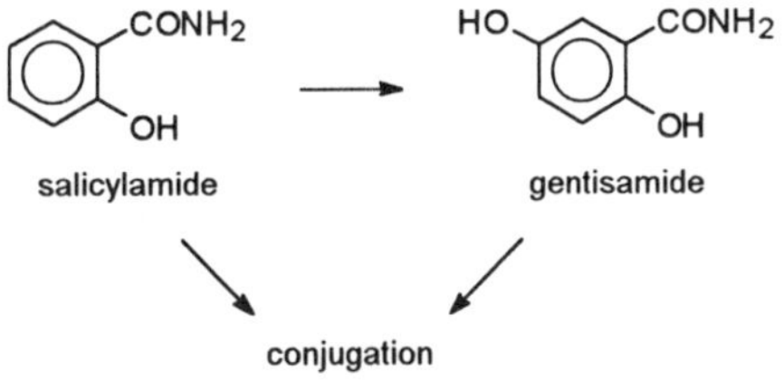

Toxicity. The analgesic efficacy of salicylamide is questionable due to its rapid elimination. Gastrointestinal irritation, drowsiness, and dizziness are exhibited by 10–20% of the patients taking the drug in normal amounts, although doses of up to 20 g daily have been tolerated by some individuals.

In a suicide due to ingestion of a nonprescription sleeping preparation containing salicylamide and methapyrilene, the postmortem blood contained 27 mg/L salicylamide and 9 mg/L methapyrilene. Salicylamide was isolated by chloroform extraction of the blood at pH 2 and quantitated by ultraviolet spectrophotometry (Gottschalk and Cravey, 1980).

Analysis. Unconjugated salicylamide may be determined in plasma or urine by colorimetry (Levy and Matsuzawa, 1967), fluorometry (Veresh et al., 1971), or nitrogen-selective gas chromatography (de Boer et al., 1979). Total salicylamide is measurable with these methods following acid or enzyme hydrolysis of conjugates. Liquid chromatographic methods capable of simultaneously analyzing for salicylamide and its metabolites have been described (Morris and Levy, 1983; Fielding et al., 1984; Xu and Pang, 1987).

References

A.G. de Boer, J.M. Gubbens-Stibbe, F.H. de Koning et al. Assay of underivatized salicylamide in plasma, saliva and urine. J. Chrom. 162: 457–460, 1979.

A.G. de Boer, D.D. Breimer, J.M. Gubbens-Stibbe and A. Bosma. First-pass elimination of salicylamide in man following oral and rectal administration. Biopharm. Drug Disp. 4: 321–330, 1983.

R.M. Fielding, J.A. Waschek, G.M. Rubin et al. Analysis of salicylamide and its metabolites in blood and urine by hplc. J. Liq. Chrom. 7: 1221–1234, 1984.

L.A. Gottschalk and R.H. Cravey. *Toxicological and Pathological Studies on Psychoactive Drug-Involved Deaths*, Biomedical Publications, Davis, California, 1980, pp. 429–430.

G. Levy and T. Matsuzawa. Pharmacokinetics of salicylamide elimination in man. J. Pharm. Exp. Ther. 156: 285–293, 1967.

M.E. Morris and G. Levy. Determination of salicylamide and five metabolites in biological fluids by high-performance liquid chromatography. J. Pharm. Sci. 72: 612–617, 1983.

S.A. Veresh, F.S. Hom and J.J. Miskel. Spectrophotofluorometric determination of salicylamide in blood serum and urine. J. Pharm. Sci. 60: 1092–1095, 1971.

J.H. Weikel, Jr. A comparison of human serum levels of acetylsalicylic acid, salicylamide, and N-acetyl-p-aminophenol following oral administration. J. Am. Pharm. Asso. 47: 477–479, 1958.

X. Xu and K.S. Pang. High-performance liquid chromatographic method for the quantitation of salicylamide and its metabolites in biological fluids. J. Chrom. 420: 313–327, 1987.

Scopolamine

T½: 1–3 hr
Vd: 1.4–2.0 L/kg
Fb: ?
pKa: 7.5

Occurrence and Usage. Scopolamine (hyoscine, Transderm Scop) is an alkaloid that occurs in the shrub *Hyoscyamus niger* (henbane) and in *Datura stramonium* (jimsonweed). It differs from atropine only in the oxygen bridge on the scopine moiety. Because of its antimuscarinic properties and central nervous system depressant actions, scopolamine has diverse therapeutic applications, including use as a preanesthetic medication, treatment of Parkinsonism and gastrointestinal disorders, and prevention of motion sickness. It is available in a variety of forms in single doses of 0.01–0.5 mg, usually as the hydrobromide salt. Dermal patches contain 1.5 mg scopolamine and are intended to deliver 0.5 mg of the drug over a 3 day period.

Blood Concentrations. In one subject given a 0.9 mg oral dose of scopolamine as the free base, a peak plasma concentration of 1.1 μg/L was observed at about 1 hour, declining to 0.3 μg/L by 4 hours (Bayne et al., 1975). A 0.005 mg/kg (0.35 mg/70 kg) intramuscular dose in 6 surgical patients produced an average peak serum concentration of 1.7 μg/L at 10 minutes (Kanto et al., 1989). A 0.5 mg transdermal patch applied to 8 subjects produced plasma scopolamine concentrations that increased gradually to an average of 0.13 μg/L (range, 0.08–0.24) by 24 hours (Cintron and Chen, 1987).

Metabolism and Excretion. About 4–5% of a single oral dose of scopolamine is excreted unchanged in the urine within 2 days (Bayne et al., 1975). In animals, the major metabolite is a glucuronide conjugate.

Toxicity. Scopolamine overdosage may cause double vision, dryness of the throat, dilated pupils, skin flushing, hallucinations, coma and death. The estimated fatal dose of scopolamine for a child is as low as 10 mg, but survival following the ingestion of as much as 1,000 mg has been reported in an adult male (Thakkar and Lasser, 1972). An adult male who accidentally ingested as much as

435 mg of the drug developed dyspnea and partial paralysis, but recovered within several hours (Smith et al., 1991). Scopolamine readily crosses the placenta within 15 minutes of maternal administration and one case of severe scopolamine toxicity has been reported in the newborn (Evens and Leopold, 1980).

In a fatal case attributed to scopolamine intoxication in a 30 year old male, drug concentrations in blood, bile and liver were 1890 µg/L, 110 µg/L and 360 µg/kg, respectively (Lin, 1984).

Analysis. Scopolamine has been analyzed in plasma and urine at therapeutic concentrations by radioreceptor assay (Cintron and Chen, 1987) and by gas chromatography-mass spectrometry of a halogenated derivative (Bayne et al., 1975; Deutsch et al., 1990). Liquid chromatography has also been described (Whelpton et al., 1992).

References

W.F. Bayne, F.T. Tao and N. Crisologo. Submicrogram assay for scopolamine in plasma and urine. J. Pharm. Sci. 64: 288–291, 1975.

N.M. Cintron and Y. Chen. A sensitive radioreceptor assay for determining scopolamine concentrations in plasma and urine. J. Pharm. Sci. 76: 328–332, 1987.

J. Deutsch, T.T. Soncrant, N.H. Greig and S.I. Rapoport. Electron-impact ionization detection of scopolamine by GC-MS in rat plasma and brain. J. Chrom. 528: 325–331, 1990.

R.P. Evens and J.C. Leopold. Scopolamine toxicity in a newborn. Pediatrics 66: 329–330, 1980.

J. Kanto, C. Kentala, T. Kaila and K. Pihlajamaki. Pharmacokinetics of scopolamine during caesarean section. Acta Anaesth. Scand. 33: 482–486, 1989.

R. Lin. A fatal scopolamine intoxication. Presented at the annual meeting of the American Academy of Forensic Sciences, Anaheim, California, February 23, 1984.

E.A. Smith, C.E. Meloan, J.A. Pickell and F.W. Oehme. Scopolamine poisoning from homemade 'moon flower' wine. J. Anal. Tox. 15: 216–219, 1991.

M.K. Thakkar and R.P. Lasser. Scopolamine intoxication from nonprescription sleeping pill. N.Y. State J. Med. 72: 725–726, 1972.

R. Whelpton, P.R. Hurst, R.F. Metcalfe and S.A. Saunders. Liquid chromatographic determination of hyoscine (scopolamine) in urine using solid phase extraction. Biomed. Chrom. 6: 198–204, 1992.

Secobarbital

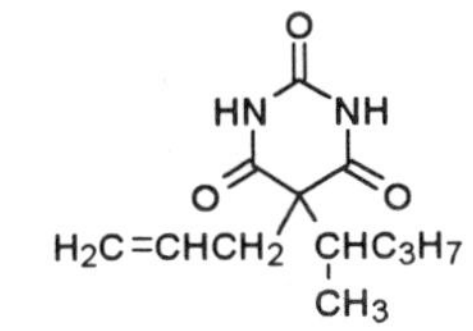

T½: 22–29 hr
Vd: 1.6–1.9 L/kg
Fb: 0.46–0.70
pKa: 7.9

Occurrence and Usage. Secobarbital (quinalbarbitone, Seconal) is a barbiturate derivative of short duration of action first prepared in 1934. It is available in amounts of 8–250 mg alone or in combination with other drugs for use as either a sedative or hypnotic. Both the free acid and sodium salt are utilized and may be administered rectally, orally or by intravenous and intramuscular injection.

Blood Concentrations. Employees passively exposed to secobarbital in a manufacturing process had end-of-shift blood concentrations averaging 0.4 mg/L (range, 0.1–0.9) (Baxter et al., 1986). A 3.3 mg/kg (231 mg/70 kg) oral dose of secobarbital given to 6 subjects produced an average maximal blood concentration of 2.0 mg/L (range, 1.8–2.2) at 3 hours, diminishing to 1.3 mg/L by 20 hours and 0.8 mg/L by 40 hours. The average half-life of the drug in these subjects was determined to be 29 hours (Clifford et al., 1974). Other workers have reported a value of 23 hours for the plasma half-life of secobarbital (Dalton et al., 1976). The oral administration of 600 mg of the drug over a 3 hour period to 5 volunteers resulted in an average peak blood concentration of 4.3 mg/L (range, 3.4–5.3) at 0.5 hours after the last dose, with a decline to 2.7 mg/L (range, 2.1–3.3) by 18 hours (Parker et al., 1970).

Metabolism and Excretion. Secobarbital undergoes extensive biotransformation by oxidation of both side-chains to a series of more polar and pharmacologically inactive compounds. Three metabolites, 5-(2,3-dihydroxypropyl)-5-(1-methylbutyl)barbituric acid (referred to as secodiol) and the 2 diastereoisomeric pairs of 3'-hydroxysecobarbital, accounted for about 50% of a single dose of the drug in the 48 hour urine. The presence of 5-(1-methylbutyl)barbituric acid in the urine was also established, and it was suggested that a carboxylic acid metabolite resulting from the oxidation of the terminal carbon atom in the methylbutyl side-chain might be formed. Only about 5% of the drug is excreted unchanged in the urine within 2 days (Waddell, 1965). Secobarbital concentrations in urine ranged from 0.7–1.8 mg/L in the 21 hour period following a single 600 mg dose and represented less than 0.2% of the total dose (Parker et al., 1970).

3'-hydroxysecobarbital   secobarbital   secodiol

5-(1-methylbutyl) barbituric acid

Toxicity. A group of 11 barbiturate abusers who were titrated to the point of mild toxicity (ataxia, slurred speech, drowsiness) with 100–200 mg of secobarbital orally each hour achieved blood concentrations of 5–12 mg/L with total doses of 400–1100 mg (Faulkner et al., 1978). Blood concentrations of 2–11 mg/L (average, 6) were observed in 498 conscious secobarbital abusers, while in 25 comatose patients a blood level range of 3–12 mg/L (average, 7) was reported (Finkle, 1971). A plasma concentration of 67 mg/L was attained by a comatose individual following overdosage; the patient awoke when the level fell to 8 mg/L after 42 hours, during which time the half-life of the drug diminished by 50% (Prescott et al., 1973). One patient survived the ingestion of 4–5 g of secobarbital with hospital treatment; she achieved a plasma level of 102 mg/L, which declined to 14 mg/L 2 days later (O'Donnell et al., 1978).

In 103 fatal cases that followed the ingestion of as little as 2 g of secobarbital, blood concentrations averaged 21 mg/L (range, 5–52) and liver, 115 mg/kg (range, 15–330) (Baselt and Cravey, 1977). The following values for secobarbital (S) and 3'-hydroxysecobarbital (HS) were determined in the tissues of 2 victims of fatal overdosage (Robinson and McDowall, 1979):

Drug Concentrations in Secobarbital Fatalities (mg/L or mg/kg)

Drug	Blood	Lung	Liver	Kidney	Urine	Gastric
S	12–13	28–33	44–77	25–37	6–32	11–824
HS	0–2	2–18	4–25	3–17	0–33	0

Secobarbital may exhibit postmortem redistribution, as shown with an animal model (Quatrehomme et al., 1990). In 2 fatal cases, heart blood/femoral blood concentration ratios averaged 1.5 (range, 1.2–1.8) (Prouty and Anderson, 1990).

Analysis. Techniques for the determination of barbiturate derivatives in fluids and tissues are cited in the section on amobarbital.

References

R.C. Baselt and R.H. Cravey. A compendium of therapeutic and toxic concentrations of toxicologically significant drugs in human biofluids. J. Anal. Tox. 1: 81–103, 1977.

P.J. Baxter, A.M. Samuel, T.C. Aw and J. Cocker. Exposure to quinalbarbitone sodium in pharmaceutical workers. Brit. Med. J. 292: 660–661, 1986.

J.M. Clifford, J.H. Cookson and P.E. Wickham. Absorption and clearance of secobarbital, heptabarbital, methaqualone, and ethinamate. Clin. Pharm. Ther. 16: 376–389, 1974.

W.S. Dalton, R. Martz, B. Rodda et al. Influence of cannabinol on secobarbital effects and plasma kinetics. Clin. Pharm. Ther. 20: 695–700, 1976.

T.P. Faulkner, J.W. McGinty, J.H. Hayden et al. Pharmacokinetic studies on tolerance to sedative-hypnotics in a poly-drug abuse population I. Secobarbital. Clin. Pharm. Ther. 23: 36–46, 1978.

B.S. Finkle. Ubiquitous reds: a local perspective on secobarbital abuse. Clin. Tox. 4: 253–264, 1971.

C.M. O'Donnell, R. Smith and D.O. Rodgerson. Letter to the editors. J. Anal. Tox. 2: 75, 1978.

K.D. Parker, H.W. Elliott, J.A. Wright et al. Blood and urine concentrations of subjects receiving barbiturates, meprobamate, glutethimide, or diphenylhydantoin. Clin. Tox. 3: 131–145, 1970.

L.F. Prescott, P. Roscoe and J.A.H. Forrest. Plasma concentrations and drug toxicity in man. In *Biological Effects of Drugs in Relation to their Plasma Concentrations* (D.S. Davies and B.N.C. Prichard, eds.), University Park Press, Baltimore, 1973, pp. 51–81.

R.W. Prouty and W.H. Anderson. The forensic science implications of site and temporal influences on postmortem blood-drug concentrations. J. For. Sci. 35: 243–270, 1990.

G. Quatrehomme, F. Bourret, M. Zhioua et al. Post mortem kinetics of secobarbital. For. Sci. Int. 44: 117–123, 1990.

A.E. Robinson and R.D. McDowall. The distribution of amylobarbitone, butobarbitone, pentobarbitone and quinalbarbitone and the hydroxylated metabolites in man. J. Pharm. Pharmac. 31: 357–365, 1979.

W.J. Waddell. The metabolic fate of 5-allyl-5-(1-methylbutyl) barbituric acid (secobarbital). J. Pharm. Exp. Ther. 149: 23–28, 1965.

Selegiline

T½: 9 min
Vd: 4.3 L/kg
Fb: 0.94
pKa: ?

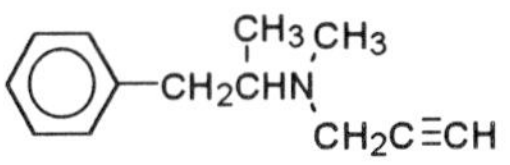

Occurrence and Usage. Selegiline (Deprenyl, Eldepryl) is a levorotatory derivative of methamphetamine that acts as a selective monoamine oxidase inhibitor. It has proven effective in the treatment of Parkinson's disease and has shown promise in alleviating the symptoms of dementia and schizophrenia. The drug is available as the hydrochloride salt in 5 mg tablets; the recommended total daily dose is 10 mg.

Blood Concentrations. Average peak serum levels for 4 patients receiving 10 mg of selegiline daily for 22 months were 19 µg/L for l-methamphetamine, 7.5 µg/L for l-amphetamine and 7.4 µg/L for N-desmethylselegiline; selegiline itself did not reach detectable concentrations in the serum (Heinonen et al., 1989). The elimination half-lives of the 3 metabolites have been reported to average 21, 18 and 2.0 hours, respectively (PDR, 1994).

Metabolism and Excretion. Selegiline is metabolized by N-dealkylation to l-methamphetamine, l-amphetamine and N-desmethylselegiline. On the usual regimen of a 5–10 mg/day oral dose, urinary elimination of l-methamphetamine and l-amphetamine accounts for most of the dose (Schacter et al., 1980; Reynolds et al., 1978). These metabolites are probably responsible for most of the activity of the parent drug. They may be inactivated by oxidation to the corresponding p-hydroxy derivatives, which are available for conjugation with glucuronic acid. No unchanged selegiline has been detected in urine following chronic therapeutic administration (Heinonen et al., 1989).

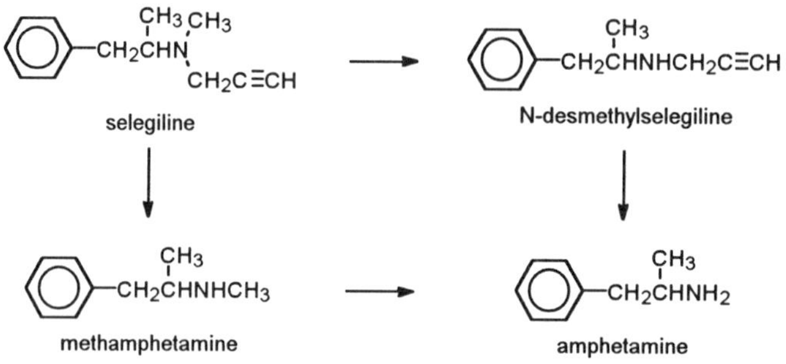

$$\text{(phenyl)}-CH_2CHN(CH_3)(CH_2C{\equiv}CH)\;\;[\text{CH}_3] \longrightarrow \text{(phenyl)}-CH_2CHNHCH_2C{\equiv}CH\;\;[\text{CH}_3]$$

selegiline → N-desmethylselegiline

$$\downarrow \qquad\qquad \downarrow$$

$$\text{(phenyl)}-CH_2CHNHCH_3\;\;[\text{CH}_3] \longrightarrow \text{(phenyl)}-CH_2CHNH_2\;\;[\text{CH}_3]$$

methamphetamine → amphetamine

Toxicity. Adverse reactions to selegiline include confusion, agitation, insomnia, delusions, hallucinations and cardiac arrhythmia. Severe hypotension and psychomotor agitation have been associated with overdosage.

In the death of a 72 year old female who left a note suggesting suicidal intentions and who ingested as many as 12 selegiline tablets, selegiline itself was not detected in postmortem blood; concentrations of the metabolites are as follows (Meeker and Reynolds, 1990):

Selegiline Metabolites in a Fatality (mg/L or mg/kg)*

Drug	Femoral Blood	Heart Blood	Urine	Liver
l-Methamphetamine	0.17	0.28	2.38	0.71
l-Amphetamine	0.07	0.08	0.72	0.36

*Other drugs include ethanol, methyprylon, nortriptyline and trazodone.

Analysis. Selegiline and its major metabolites have been determined in biological samples by gas chromatography (Juvancz et al., 1984; Salonen, 1990) and gas chromatography-mass spectrometry (Maurer and Kraemer, 1992; Patrick et al., 1992; Reimer et al., 1993). The levorotatory metabolites of selegiline may be differentiated from their illicit dextrorotatory enantiomers, d-methamphetamine and d-amphetamine, by immunoassay or stereoselective chromatographic methods (Maurer and Kraemer, 1992).

References

E.H. Heinonen, V. Myllyla, K. Sotaniemi et al. Pharmacokinetics and metabolism of selegiline. Acta Neurol. Scand. 126: 93–99, 1989.

Z. Juvancz, I. Ratonyi, A. Toth and M. Vajda. Chromatographic determination of nanogram levels of 2-(methylpropargylamino)-1-phenylpropane (Jumex, Deprenyl) in plasma. J. Chrom. 286: 363–369, 1984.

H.H. Maurer and T. Kraemer. Toxicological detection of selegiline and its metabolites in urine using fluorescence polarization immunoassay (FPIA) and gas-chromatography mass-spectrometry (GC-MS) and differentiation by enantioselective GC-MS of the intake of selegiline from abuse of methamphetamine or amphetamine. Arch. Tox. 66: 675–678, 1992.

J.E. Meeker and P.C. Reynolds. Postmortem tissue methamphetamine concentrations following selegiline administration. J. Anal. Tox. 14: 330–331, 1990.

K.S. Patrick, B.L. Nguyen and J.D. McCallister. Gas chromatographic-mass spectrometric determination of plasma selegiline using a deuterated internal standard. J. Chrom. 583: 254–258, 1992.

M.L.J. Reimer, O.A. Mamer, A.P. Zavitsanos et al. Determination of amphetamine, methamphetamine and desmethyldeprenyl in human plasma by gas chromatography/negative ion chemical ionization mass spectrometry. Biol. Mass Spec. 22: 235–242, 1993.

G.P. Reynolds, J.D. Elsworth, K. Blau et al. Deprenyl is metabolized to methamphetamine and amphetamine in man. Brit. J. Clin. Pharm. 12: 542–544, 1978.

J.S. Salonen. Determination of the amine metabolites of selegiline in biological fluids by capillary gas chromatography. J. Chrom. 527: 163–168, 1990.

M. Schacter, C.D. Marsden, J.D. Parkes et al. Deprenyl in the management of response fluctuations in patients with Parkinson's disease on levodopa. J. Neurol. Neurosurg. Psych. 43: 1016–1021, 1980.

Selenium

T½: 69–77 days
Vd: ?
Fb: ?

Se

Occurrence and Usage. Selenium is produced largely as a by-product of copper refining. It has numerous applications in industry, including its use in electronic semiconductors, as a decolorizer for ceramics and glass, a vulcanizing agent for rubber and an antidandruff agent in shampoos. It is considered an essential trace element and is supplied in the diet at an average rate of 60–150 µg/day. The current threshold limit value for occupational exposure to selenium, as the metal or its compounds, is 0.2 mg/m^3.

Blood Concentrations. Selenium concentrations in the blood and plasma of 250 normal subjects have been found to average 0.182 mg/L and 0.144 mg/L, respectively, by neutron activation analysis (Dickson and Tomlinson, 1967). In a study of 210 residents of various areas of the United States, blood selenium concentrations averaged 0.206 mg/L and ranged from 0.100–0.340 mg/L (Allaway et al., 1968). Blood selenium concentrations did not correlate with domestic water selenium content in a community where selenium levels in water (range, 26–1800 µg/L) were substantially elevated over the U.S. standard of 10 µg/L (Valentine et al., 1978). More recent data from European citizens has shown that normal serum or plasma selenium concentrations average 0.066–0.104 mg/L (Ducros and Favier, 1992).

Metabolism and Excretion. An average of 59% of a labeled oral dose of selenite was absorbed by 3 volunteers; over a 2 week period, 7–14% was excreted in urine and 33–58% in feces. The long plasma half-life observed, 69–77 days, may represent selenium incorporated into serum proteins (Thomson and Stewart, 1974). The body burden of selenium in normal humans has been estimated to range from 13–20 mg, with the highest concentrations found in kidney, liver and spleen. Nearly all of the daily dietary intake of selenium can be accounted for in the daily urine (20–50 µg), feces (8–30 µg) and miscellaneous excreta (32–80 µg). The selenium body burden does not appear to increase with age (Schroeder et al., 1970).

In animals given relatively large doses of selenium, urinary and pulmonary excretion became increasingly important; from 50–80% of a dose may be excreted in urine, largely as trimethylselenonium ion, and up to 30% in the exhaled air, largely as dimethylselenium. These organic metabolites of selenium are formed regardless of the original nature of the selenium administered and are much less toxic than either selenite or selenate (Subcommittee on Selenium, 1976).

Urine selenium concentrations have been found to range from undetectable to 150 µg/L (average, 34) in normal persons, from 22–203 µg/L (average, 79) in persons living in an area with high water selenium content, and from 120–350 µg/L in asymptomatic selenium workers. Urine concentrations of the metal correlate well with dietary intake and with air concentrations of selenium; the urine concentrations decline rapidly when exposure to selenium is curtailed (Glover, 1967; Glover, 1970; Valentine et al., 1978).

Hair selenium has been found to average 0.33–1.47 mg/kg in studies conducted in various geographical locations, but is not considered a reliable guide to exposure due to the use of selenium sulfide in antidandruff shampoos (Howe, 1979). The following selenium concentrations were determined in the tissues of normal Japanese subjects by neutron activation analysis (Yukawa et al., 1980):

Selenium Concentrations in Normal Tissues (mg/kg)

	Brain	Heart	Lung	Liver	Kidney
Average	1.7	1.9	7.8	2.3	1.5
(Range)	(0.2–5.0)	(0.4–5.0)	(0.5–15)	(0.9–6.2)	(0.5–4.8)

Toxicity. Selenium and its compounds cause irritation of the skin and mucous membranes on contact. Workers in a selenium plant exposed to air concentrations of 0.2–3.6 mg/m^3 and excreting urine containing up to 430 µg/L selenium had symptoms limited to garlic odor of the breath (probably due to *in vivo* formation of dimethylselenium), metallic taste, dermatitis and indigestion (Glover, 1967; Glover, 1970; Alderman and Bergin, 1986). Acute exposure to selenium fumes in a group of workers at a smelting plant produced irritation of the mucous membranes, headache, sore throat and, in one worker, severe dyspnea (Clinton, 1947).

Selenium that accumulates in certain plants growing in alkaline soil has been held responsible for a chronic disease in cattle known as "blind staggers," causing impaired vision, stumbling and respiratory distress. Alkaline disease in domestic animals is believed due to excessive amounts of selenium in feed, and is manifested by lameness, loss of hair and hoof malformation (Subcommittee on Selenium, 1976).

Five persons who unintentionally ingested large amounts of a poultry food supplement containing sodium selenite developed nausea, vomiting, diarrhea, chills, abdominal pain, and tremor within a short time of ingestion but improved within 24 hours. Serum levels of 0.41–0.89 mg/L and urine levels of 1.18–4.37 mg/day were measured initially, but these returned to normal within a week (Sioris et al., 1980). A teenage girl survived the ingestion of 2 g of sodium selenate after exhibiting EKG changes and abnormal liver function tests; a serum selenium level of 3.1 mg/L was observed (Civil and McDonald, 1978). Selenium as a dietary supplement has caused toxicity and death in cystic fibrosis patients (Snodgrass et al., 1981).

Three children became comatose, cyanotic, and died within 2 hours to 17 days of ingesting a selenious acid solution intended as gun-blueing compound (Carter, 1966; Normann et al., 1984; Nantel et al., 1985). A young man ingested selenium dioxide as a suicidal gesture and died within 3 hours; the unusually high blood and liver concentrations of 38 mg/L and 741 mg/kg were found (Koppel et al., 1986). The following concentrations were determined in 4 fatalities after ingestion of sodium selenite or selenious acid (Pentel et al., 1985; Matoba et al., 1986; Schellmann et al., 1986; Farago, 1988):

Selenium Concentrations in Fatal Cases (mg/L or mg/kg)

	Blood	Brain	Lung	Liver	Kidney	Urine
Average	5.9	0.9	6.7	2.3	7.7	2.1
(Range)	(0.5–18)	(0.5–1.2)	(1.4–13)	(0.8–5.4)	(1.5–14)	(2.1)

Analysis. Selenium has been frequently determined in biological fluids by fluorometry (Watkinson, 1966; Olson et al., 1973; Geahchan and Chambon, 1980; Lalonde et al., 1982; Tamari et al., 1986; Sheehan and Gao, 1990). Atomic absorption spectrometry after digestion and extraction (Tully and Lehmann, 1982), with hydride generation (Schmidt and Royer, 1973; Ihnat, 1976; Cox and Bibb, 1981; Welz et al., 1984) or direct electrothermal analysis (Saeed and Thomassen, 1982; Morisi et al., 1988) is also useful. Gas chromatography has received attention as a sensitive and specific means of determination (Bycroft and Clegg, 1978; Cappon and Smith, 1978; Kurahashi et al., 1980; McCarthy et al., 1981; Uchida et al., 1981; Ducros and Favier, 1992) as has liquid chromatography (Handelman et al., 1989).

References

L.C. Alderman and J.J. Bergin. Hydrogen selenide poisoning: an illustrative case with review of the literature. Arch. Env. Health 41: 354–358, 1986.

W.H. Allaway, J. Kubota, F. Losee and M. Roth. Selenium, molybdenum, and vanadium in human blood. Arch. Env. Health 16: 342–348, 1968.

B.M. Bycroft and D.E. Clegg. Gas-liquid chromatographic determination of selenium in biological materials, using 4-bromo- and 4-chloro-1,2-diaminobenzene as derivatizing reagents. J. Asso. Off. Anal. Chem. 61: 923–926, 1978.

C.J. Cappon and J.C. Smith. Determination of selenium in biological materials by gas chromatography. J. Anal. Tox. 2: 114–120, 1978.

R.F. Carter. Acute selenium poisoning. Med. J. Aust. 1: 525–528, 1966.

I.D.S. Civil and M.J.A. McDonald. Acute selenium poisoning: case report. New Zeal. Med. J. 87: 354–356, 1978.

M. Clinton, Jr. Selenium fume exposure. J. Ind. Hyg. Tox. 29: 225–226, 1947.

D.H. Cox and A.E. Bibb. Hydrogen selenide evolution-electrothermal atomic absorption method for determining nanogram levels of total selenium. J. Asso. Off. Anal. Chem. 64: 265–269, 1981.

R.C. Dickson and R.H. Tomlinson. Selenium in blood and human tissues. Clin. Chim. Acta 16: 311–321, 1967.

V. Ducros and A. Favier. Gas chromatographic-mass spectrometric method for the determination of selenium in biological samples. J. Chrom. 583: 35–44, 1992.

E. Farago. Personal communication, 1988.

A. Geahchan and P. Chambon. Fluorometry of selenium in urine. Clin. Chem. 26: 1272–1274, 1980.

J.R. Glover. Selenium in human urine: a tentative maximum allowable concentration for industrial and rural populations. Ann. Occ. Hyg. 10: 3–14, 1967.

J.R. Glover. Selenium and its industrial toxicology. Ind. Med. 39: 50–54, 1970.

G.J. Handelman, P. Kosted, S. Short and E.A. Dratz. Determination of selenium in human blood by high-performance liquid chromatography with fluorescence detection. Anal. Chem. 61: 2244–2249, 1989.

M. Howe. Selenium in the blood of South Dakotans. Arch. Env. Health 34: 444–448, 1979.

M. Ihnat. Atomic absorption spectrometric determination of selenium with carbon furnace atomization. Anal. Chim. Acta 82: 293–309, 1976.

C. Koppel, H. Baudisch, K.H. Beyer et al. Fatal poisoning with selenium dioxide. Clin. Tox. 24: 21–35, 1986.

K. Kurahashi, S. Inoue, S. Yonekura et al. Determination of selenium in human blood by gas chromatography with electron-capture detection. Analyst 105: 690–695, 1980.

L. Lalonde, Y. Jean, K.D. Roberts et al. Fluorometry of selenium in serum or urine. Clin. Chem. 28: 172–174, 1982.

R. Matoba, H. Kimura, E. Uchima et al. An autopsy case of acute selenium (selenious acid) poisoning and selenium levels in human tissues. For. Sci. Int. 31: 87–92, 1986.

T.P. McCarthy, B. Brodie, J.A. Milner and R.F. Bevill. Improved method for selenium determination in biological samples by gas chromatography. J. Chrom. 225: 9–16, 1981.

G. Morisi, M. Patriarca and A. Menotti. Improved determination of selenium in serum by Zeeman atomic
absorption spectrometry. Clin. Chem. 34: 127–130, 1988.

A.J. Nantel, M. Brown, P. Dery and M. Lefebvre. Acute poisoning by selenious acid. Vet. Hum. Tox. 27: 531–
533, 1985.

S.A. Normann, K. Nisbet and M.S. Manoguerra. Acute selenious acid poisoning—case report. Vet. Hum. Tox.
26: 406, 1984.

P. Pentel, D. Fletcher and J. Jentzen. Fatal acute selenium poisoning. J. For. Sci. 30: 556–562, 1985.

O.E. Olson, I.S. Palmer and E.I. Whitehead. Determination of selenium in biological materials. Meth. Biochem.
Anal. 21: 39–78, 1973.

K. Saeed and Y. Thomassen. Electrothermal atomic absorption spectrometric determination of selenium in
blood serum and seminal fluid after protein precipitation with trichloroacetic acid. Anal. Chim. Acta 143:
223–228, 1982.

B. Schellmann, H.J. Raithel and K.H. Schaller. Acute fatal selenium poisoning. Arch. Tox. 59: 61–63, 1986.

F.J. Schmidt and J.L. Royer. Sub microgram determination of arsenic, selenium, antimony and bismuth by
atomic absorption utilizing sodium borohydride reduction. Anal. Letters 6: 17–23, 1973.

H.A. Schroeder, D.V. Frost and J.J. Balassa. Essential trace metals in man: selenium. J. Chron. Dis. 23: 227–
243, 1970.

T.M.T. Sheehan and M. Gao. Simplified fluorometric assay of total selenium in plasma and urine. Clin. Chem.
36: 2124–2126, 1990.

L.J. Sioris, K. Guthrie and P.R. Pentel. Acute selenium poisoning. Vet. Hum. Tox. 22: 364, 1980.

W. Snodgrass, B.H. Rumack, J.B. Sullivan, Jr. et al. Selenium: childhood poisoning and cystic fibrosis. Clin.
Tox. 18: 211–220, 1981.

Subcommittee on Selenium. *Selenium*, National Academy of Sciences, Washington, DC, 1976, pp. 60–61.

Y. Tamari, S. Ohmori and K. Hiraki. Fluorometry of nanogram amounts of selenium in biological samples.
Clin. Chem. 32: 1464–1467, 1986.

C.D. Thomson and R.D.H. Stewart. The metabolism of (^{75}Se)selenite in young women. Brit. J. Nutri. 32: 47–
57, 1974.

R.T. Tulley and H.P. Lehmann. Flameless atomic absorption spectrophotometry of selenium in whole blood.
Clin. Chem. 28: 1448–1450, 1982.

H. Uchida, Y. Shimoishi and K. Toei. Rapid determination of trace amounts of selenium in biological samples
by gas chromatography with electron-capture detection. Analyst 106: 757–762, 1981.

J.L. Valentine, H.K. Kang and G.H. Spivey. Selenium levels in human blood, urine, and hair in response to
exposure via drinking water. Env. Res. 17: 347–353, 1978.

J.H. Watkinson. Fluorometric determination of selenium in biological material with 2,3-diaminonaphthalene.
Anal. Chem. 38: 92–97, 1966.

B. Welz, M. Melcher and J. Neve. Determination of selenium in human body fluids by hydride-generation
atomic absorption spectrometry. Anal. Chim. Acta 165: 131–140, 1984.

M. Yukawa, M. Suzuki-Yasumoto, K. Amano and M. Terai. Distribution of trace elements in the human body
determined by neutron activation analysis. Arch. Env. Health 35: 36–44, 1980.

Sertraline

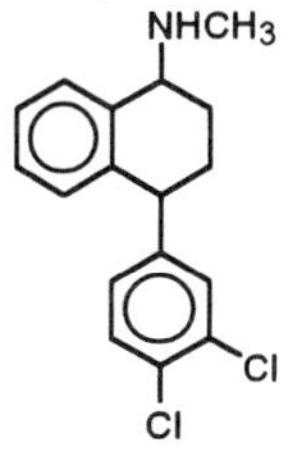

T½: 24–26 hr
Vd: ?
Fb: 0.99
pKa: ?

Occurrence and Usage. Sertraline (Zoloft) is a selective inhibitor of serotonin uptake that has been available since 1992 for the treatment of mental depression. Other drugs in this pharmacological category include fluoxetine and paroxetine. It is marketed in 50–100 mg tablets as the hydrochloride for oral administration; daily doses range from 50–200 mg.

Blood Concentrations. Single and oral doses of 50, 100 and 200 mg given to 3 adult males resulted in average peak plasma sertraline concentrations of 9.5, 16 and 56 µg/L, respectively, at times of 6–8 hours (Fouda et al., 1987). Patients maintained on chronic oral daily doses of 100, 200 or 300 mg achieved steady-state plasma sertraline concentrations averaging 32 µg/L (range, 20–48), 91 µg/L (range, 40–187) and 206 µg/L (range, 99–309), respectively. Plasma concentrations of norsertraline in these patients averaged 167% of the parent drug concentration (Gupta and Dziurdzy, 1994).

Metabolism and Excretion. Sertraline is known to undergo N-demethylation to norsertraline, a metabolite that has only 10–20% of the pharmacological activity of the parent drug but which accumulates in plasma due to slow elimination (half-life estimated at 62–104 hours). Both sertraline and norsertraline undergo deamination, hydroxylation and conjugation; about 40–45% of a radiolabeled dose is excreted in the urine over a 9 day period, with unchanged drug representing less than 0.2% of the dose (Tremaine et al., 1989). Both sertraline and norsertraline were undetectable in the urine of a patient receiving the drug chronically (Logan et al., 1994).

Toxicity. Adverse reactions to sertraline include dry mouth, headache, dizziness, tremor, nausea, diarrhea, fatigue, insomnia and somnolence. Sertraline in overdosage is considered to be less sedating and to result in fewer cardiovascular effects than the tricyclic antidepressants; up to 4500 mg has been acutely ingested by an adult without profound toxicity (Myers et al., 1993). In a study of 31 overdosed patients averaging 31 years of age with an average acute dose of 1109 mg, plasma sertraline concentrations averaged 245 µg/L at a mean time of 4.8 hours post-ingestion; all patients survived the event, after manifesting symptoms that included vomiting, lethargy and ataxia (Kassner and Woolf, 1993).

Postmortem blood sertraline and norsertraline concentrations of 0.61 and 1.6 mg/L were measured in an adult male who apparently committed suicide by drug overdose; diphenhydramine was also present at a blood level of 0.58 mg/L (Logan et al., 1994).

Analysis. Sertraline has been analyzed in biological fluids by gas chromatography with electron-capture (Tremaine and Joerg, 1989) or mass spectrometric detection (Fouda et al., 1987; Logan et al., 1994). Liquid chromatography has also been described (Gupta and Dziurdzy, 1994; Logan et al., 1994).

References

H.G. Fouda, R.A. Ronfeld and D.J. Weidler. Gas chromatographic-mass spectrometric analysis and preliminary human pharmacokinetics of sertraline, a new antidepressant drug. J. Chrom. 417: 197–202, 1987.

R.N. Gupta and S.A. Dziurdzy. Therapeutic monitoring of sertraline. Clin. Chem. 40: 498–499, 1994.

J. Kassner and A. Woolf. Sertraline hydrochloride: correlation of clinical presentation with plasma concentration. Vet. Hum. Tox. 35: 341, 1993.

B.K. Logan, P.N. Friel and G.A. Case. Analysis of sertraline (Zoloft) and its major metabolite in postmortem specimens by gas and liquid chromatography. J. Anal. Tox. 18: 139–142, 1994.

L.B. Myers, B.S. Dean and E.P. Krenzelok. Sertraline (Zoloft): overdose assessment of a new antidepressent. Vet. Hum. Tox. 35: 341, 1993.

L.M. Tremaine and E.A. Joerg. Automated gas chromatographic-electron capture assay for the selective serotonin uptake blocker sertraline. J. Chrom. 496: 423–429, 1989.

L.M. Tremaine, W.M. Welch and R.A. Ronfeld. Metabolism and disposition of the 5-hydroxytryptamine uptake blocker sertraline in the rat and dog. Drug Met. Disp. 17: 542–550, 1989.

Sotalol

T½: 7–18 hr
Vd: 1.6–2.4 L/kg
Fb: 0
pKa: 8.3, 9.8

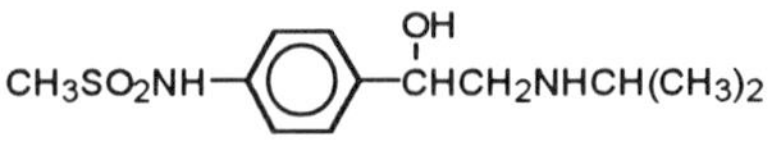

$$CH_3SO_2NH-\!\!\bigcirc\!\!-\overset{\overset{OH}{|}}{C}HCH_2NHCH(CH_3)_2$$

Occurrence and Usage. Sotalol (Betapace) is a beta-adrenergic blocking agent without intrinsic sympathomimetic activity that exerts both class II and III antiarrhythmic effects. Sotalol is available as the hydrochloride salt in 80–240 mg tablets for oral administration. The initial dose is generally 160 mg daily, but may be increased to a recommended maximum of 320 mg daily.

Blood Concentrations. A single oral 160 mg dose of sotalol administered to 12 healthy volunteers resulted in peak sotalol serum concentrations of 1.4–1.7 within 2–3 hours (Sundquist et al., 1979). Following daily oral doses of 400 mg of sotalol for 5 days in 5 subjects, an average plasma concentration of 6 mg/L was found 3 hours after the last dose (McDevitt and Shanks, 1977).

Metabolism and Excretion. No metabolites of sotalol have been detected in plasma or urine from animals or humans (Tjandramaga et al., 1976; Blair et al., 1981). Labeled metabolites of sotalol were detected in the bile of dogs, but accounted for less than 1% of the dose (Schnelle and Garrett, 1973). After oral administration of single doses ranging from 5–160 mg, the mean urinary recovery of sotalol was 80% of the dose, with 12.5% in feces. After intravenous administration, 77% of the dose was recovered in the urine and only 1% in the feces (Antonaccio and Gomoll, 1990).

Toxicity. Adverse reactions to sotalol include dyspnea, bradycardia, chest pain, fatigue, dizziness, lightheadedness and muscle weakness. Toxic effects such as hypotension and cardiac arrhythmias are said to appear above the threshold concentration of 5 mg/L (Montagna and Groppi, 1980).

Two fatalities due to acute overdosage have been reported, with tissue concentrations as shown below. A 58 year old woman who ingested 14.4 g of the drug and presented in coma with a serum sotalol level of 65 mg/L died of irreversible cardiovascular failure 3.5 hours after admission (Perrot et al., 1988). The second case was that of a male adult who ingested approximately 3 g of sotalol and was found dead (Montagna and Groppi, 1980).

Sotalol Concentrations in Fatal Cases (mg/L or mg/kg)

	Blood	Brain	Liver	Kidney	Urine
Case 1	40	12	103	103	
Case 2	40	0.6	88	116	416

Analysis. Sotalol has been determined in body fluids by a spectrofluorometric assay (Garrett and Schnelle, 1971), but the method lacks specificity. The drug is most often analyzed by liquid chromatography (Bartek et al., 1987; Gluth et al., 1988; Hoyer, 1988; Poirier et al., 1989; Urech et al., 1990; Boutagy and Shenfield, 1991).

References

A.J. Antonaccio and A. Gomoll. Pharmacology, pharmacodynamics and pharmacokinetics of sotalol. Am. J. Cardiol. 65: 12A–21A, 1990.

M.J. Bartek, M. Vekshteyn, M.P. Boarman and D.G. Gallo. Liquid chromatographic determination of sotalol in plasma and urine employing solid-phase extraction of fluorescence detection. J. Chrom. 421: 309–318, 1987.

A.D. Blair, E.D. Burgess, B.M. Maxwell and R.E. Cutler. Sotalol kinetics in renal insufficiency. Clin. Pharm. Ther. 29: 457–463, 1981.

J. Boutagy and G.M. Shenfield. Simplified method for the determination of sotalol in plasma by high-performance liquid chromatography. J. Chrom. 565: 523–528, 1991.

E.R. Garrett and K. Schnelle. Separation and spectrofluorometric assay of beta-adrenergic blocker sotalol from blood and urine. J. Pharm. Sci. 60: 833–839, 1971.

W.P. Gluth, F. Sorgel, B. Gluth et al. Determination of sotalol in human body fluids for pharmacokinetic and toxicokinetic studies using high-performance liquid chromatography. Arz. Forsch. 38: 408–411, 1988.

G.L. Hoyer. Improved high-performance liquid chromatographic method for the analysis of serum sotalol. J. Chrom. 427: 181–187, 1988.

D.G. McDevitt and R.G. Shanks. Evaluation of once daily sotalol administration in man. Brit. J. Clin. Pharm. 4: 153–156, 1977.

M. Montagna and A. Groppi. Fatal sotalol poisoning. Arch. Tox. 43: 221–226, 1980.

D. Perrot, B. Bui-Xuan, J. Lang et al. A case of sotalol poisoning with fatal outcome. Clin. Tox. 26: 389–396, 1988.

J.M. Poirier, M. Lebot and G. Chrymol. Rapid and sensitive column liquid chromatographic determination of sotalol in plasma. J. Chrom. 493: 409–413, 1989.

K. Schnelle and E.R. Garrett. Pharmacokinetics of the beta-blocker sotalol in dogs. J. Pharm. Sci. 62: 362–375, 1973.

H. Sundquist, M. Anttila, A. Simon and J.W. Reich. Comparative bioavailability and pharmacokinetics of sotalol administered alone and in combination with hydrochlorothiazide. J. Clin. Pharm. 19: 557–564, 1979.

T.B. Tjandramaga, T.J. Verbeeck, R. Verbesselt et al. The effect of end-stage renal failure and haemodialysis on the elimination kinetics of sotalol. Brit. J. Clin. Pharm. 3: 259–265, 1976.

R. Urech, L. Chan and P. Duffy. High-performance liquid chromatographic assay of sotalol—improved procedure and investigation of peak broadening. J. Chrom. 534: 271–278, 1990.

Strychnine

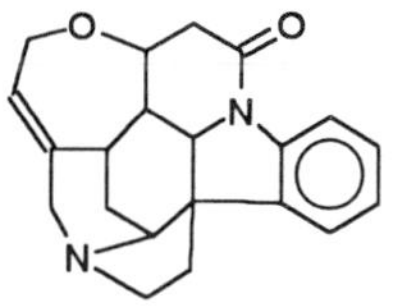

T½: 10–11 hr
Vd: 13 L/kg
Fb: ?
pKa: 2.3, 8.0

Occurrence and Usage. Strychnine is an alkaloid found together with the less active brucine in the seeds of *Strychnos nux-vomica*, a tree indigenous to India. It is a potent central nervous stimulant and convulsant, acting by the selective blockade of post-synaptic neuronal inhibition. Strychnine was used therapeutically for hundreds of years as a tonic to improve circulation and muscle tone; in certain countries it continues to be administered for this purpose, in oral or intramuscular doses of 0.05–8 mg as the nitrate or sulfate salt. It is also available commercially as bait in concentrations of 0.3–3.0% for the extermination of rodents and predatory animals.

Blood Concentrations. There are no published data regarding concentrations of strychnine in body fluids following therapeutic administration.

Metabolism and Excretion. Very little information is available on the disposition of this drug in man. From 10–20% is excreted in the 24 hour urine unchanged, and the remainder undergoes oxidative biotransformation in the liver to unknown metabolites (Adamson and Fouts, 1959).

In rats, approximately 30% of a labeled dose is eliminated in the urine by 7 days, with unchanged drug representing 6% of the dose. The metabolites are of relatively low toxicity, and include products of N-oxidation, hydroxylation, epoxidation and conjugation (Oguri et al., 1989).

Toxicity. Strychnine continues to cause episodes of accidental or intentional poisoning. Death may occur after the ingestion of 60–100 mg by an adult and is due to paralysis of the muscles of respiration. In persons who survive poisoning, convulsions generally subside within 12–24 hours after ingestion. Intravenous diazepam is usually effective in preventing convulsions without depressing respiration (Jackson et al., 1971; Maron et al., 1971; Herishanu and Landau, 1972). A urine strychnine concentration of 37 mg/L was observed in a teenage boy who inhaled the drug, believing it to be cocaine; his convulsions were controlled with intravenous phenobarbital and diazepam. A companion, who had also sampled the substance but remained asymptomatic, had a urine concentration of 4 mg/L (Baselt, 1980).

Postmortem blood concentrations of 5–90 mg/L (average, 26) were observed in 6 adults who died within an hour of ingesting unknown quantities of the poison (Baselt and Cravey, 1977). The following data are taken from the analytical results seen in 14 fatal cases that resulted from the ingestion of as much as 14 g of strychnine (Bogan et al., 1966; Rehling, 1967; Sedgwick, 1973; Alha et al., 1974; Mohseni and Ahbab, 1975; Bailey, 1976; Schepens, 1984; Winek, 1986):

Strychnine Concentrations in Fatalities (mg/L or mg/kg)

	Blood	Brain	Liver	Kidney	Urine	Gastric
Average	21	14	122	46	9.1	61 mg
(Range)	(0.5–61)	(0.5–26)	(2–257)	(0.07–106)	(1–33)	(7.5–107)

In 2 cases in which death occurred rapidly after ingestion, liver concentrations of strychnine were very low (0.8 and 1.6 mg/kg), even though the blood concentrations (2.4 and 12 mg/L) were in the lethal range (Drost, 1979).

Analysis. Strychnine may be assayed in biological fluids and tissues by colorimetry (El Darawy and Tompsett, 1956) or ultraviolet spectrophotometry at 254 nm after solvent extraction (Bogan et al., 1966). Gas chromatography on OV-1 at 250° C. has been reported (Oliver et al., 1979). Liquid chromatography has also been described (Alliot et al., 1982; Hoogenboom and Rammell, 1985).

References

R.H. Adamson and J.R. Fouts. Enzymatic metabolism of strychnine. J. Pharm. Exp. Ther. 127: 87–91, 1959.

A. Alha, T. Korte and I. Lukkari. Personal communication, 1974.

L. Alliot, G. Bryant and P.S. Guth. Measurement of strychnine by high-performance liquid chromatography. J. Chrom. 232: 440–442, 1982.

M. Bailey. Personal communication, 1976.

R.C. Baselt. Unpublished results, 1980.

R.C. Baselt and R.H. Cravey. A compendium of therapeutic and toxic concentrations of toxicologically significant drugs in human biofluids. J. Anal. Tox. 1: 81–103, 1977.

J. Bogan, E. Rentoul, H. Smith and W.P. Weir. Homicidal poisoning by strychnine. J. For. Sci. Soc. 6: 166–169, 1966.

M.L. Drost. Strychnine overdose in man. Can. Soc. For. Sci. J. 12: 125–131, 1979.

Z.I. El Darawy and S.L. Tompsett. The determination of alkaloids in biological material by compound forma-tion with indicators. Analyst 81: 601–606, 1956.

Y. Herishanu and H. Landau. Diazepam in the treatment of strychnine poisoning. Brit. J. Anaesth. 44: 747–748, 1972.

J.J.L. Hoogenboom and C.G. Rammell. Liquid chromatographic determination of strychnine in stomach con-tents. J. Asso. Off. Anal. Chem. 68: 1131–1133, 1985.

G. Jackson, S.H. Ng, G.E. Diggle and I.G. Bourke. Strychnine poisoning treated successfully with diazepam. Brit. Med. J. 2: 519–520, 1971.

B.J. Maron, J.R. Krupp and B. Tune. Strychnine poisoning successfully treated with diazepam. J. Pediat. 78: 697–699, 1971.

H. Mohseni and M. Ahbab. Personal communication, 1975.

J.S. Oliver, H. Smith and A.A. Watson. Poisoning by strychnine. Med. Sci. Law 19: 134–137, 1979.

K. Oguri, Y. Tanimoto, M. Mishima and H. Yoshimura. Metabolic fate of strychnine in rats. Xenobiotica 19: 171–178, 1989.

C.J. Rehling. Poison residues in human tissues. In *Progress in Chemical Toxicology*, Vol. 3 (A. Stolman, ed.), Academic Press, New York, 1967, pp. 363–386.

P.J.C. Schepens. Personal communication, 1984.

P. Sedgwick. Personal communication, 1973.

C.L. Winek, W.W. Wahba, F.M. Esposito and W.D. Collom. Fatal strychnine ingestion. J. Anal. Tox. 10: 120–121, 1986.

Styrene

T½: 13 hr
Vd: 1.4 L/kg
Fb: ?

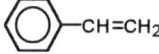

Occurrence and Usage. Styrene (phenylethylene, vinylbenzene) is used as an intermediate for chemical synthesis, a solvent for synthetic resins and in the manufacture of polymeric plastics. The compound is volatile (b.p., 146° C.) and is readily absorbed following inhalation or dermal contact. The current threshold limit value for styrene in the industrial atmosphere is 50 ppm (213 mg/m³).

Blood Concentrations. Blood styrene concentrations in non-occupationally exposed persons aver-aged 0.2 µg/L (range, 0–0.9) (Brugnone et al., 1989). Three volunteers exposed to styrene at an air concentration of approximately 50 ppm for 1 hour developed blood styrene concentrations of 0.2–0.7 mg/L; exposure to approximately 100 ppm for 8 hours produced maximal blood concentrations of 0.9–1.4 mg/L (Stewart et al., 1968). Blood styrene concentrations in 22 workers exposed at air concentrations of 120–684 ppm ranged from 0.5–3.7 mg/L in specimens collected at the end of the work shift (Apostoli et al., 1983). The elimination half-life of styrene averages 13 hours (Ramsey and Young, 1978).

Metabolism and Excretion. Styrene is extensively metabolized in man by oxidation of the vinyl side-chain. Mandelic acid and phenylglyoxylic acid are produced as major metabolites and repre-sent 85% and 10%, respectively, of an inhaled dose of styrene as urinary excretion products. About 1–2% of a dose is exhaled unchanged. The half-life of styrene as determined by mandelic acid excretion is 4–7 hours, whereas by excretion in breath it varies from 1–7 hours (Stewart et al., 1968; Bardodej and Bardodejova, 1970). Other authors have found that mandelic acid elimination fol-lows biphasic kinetics, with an initial half-life of 4 hours and a terminal half-life of 25 hours (Guillemin and Bauer, 1979); this model is consistent with the known prolonged storage of styrene in body fat (Engstrom et al., 1978). Hippuric acid may be a minor metabolite of styrene in man (Ikeda et al., 1974), as may 4-vinylphenol (Pfaffli et al., 1981).

Mandelic acid concentrations in the urine of exposed workers have ranged from physiological levels (less than 5 mg/L) to as high as 3000 mg/L. The concentrations tend to increase during the exposure period and usually reach a peak within an hour after the end of exposure. Phenylglyoxylic acid concentrations are often 15–50% of the mandelic acid concentrations (Piotrowski, 1977; Apostoli et al., 1983). Breath styrene concentrations average about 25% of the corresponding air styrene concentration during constant exposure, but decline very rapidly after cessation of exposure (Stewart et al., 1968).

Toxicity. At lower atmospheric concentrations, styrene produces irritation of the mucous membranes. The substance is absorbed upon dermal contact and may cause dermatitis (Dutkiewicz and Tyras, 1968). Higher concentrations cause central nervous system depression, nausea, headache, and fatigue. Organ toxicity due to chronic exposure is rare, although the compound is potentially hepatotoxic on the basis of its metabolism to an epoxide intermediate (Leibman, 1975).

A group of 27 exposed workers, whose blood styrene concentrations averaged 0.55 mg/L (range, 0.16–1.67) at the end of a day, reported a significant impairment in physical, mental and general health status compared to unexposed control workers (Cherry et al., 1980).

Analysis. Styrene in blood has been analyzed by headspace gas chromatography (Astrand et al., 1974). Methods for mandelic acid and phenylglyoxylic acid in urine include colorimetry (Ohtsuji and Ikeda, 1970), gas chromatography after derivatization (Guillemin and Bauer, 1976; Van Roosmalen and Drummond, 1978; Flek and Sedivec, 1980; Dills et al., 1991) and liquid chromatography (Ogata and Sugihara, 1978; Will et al., 1980; Poggi et al., 1982; Kivisto et al., 1993). Urine specimens should be analyzed or frozen immediately after collection to avoid a steady loss of phenylglyoxylic acid by spontaneous decarboxylation.

References

P. Apostoli, F. Brugnone, L. Perbellini et al. Occupational styrene exposure: environmental and biological monitoring. Am. J. Ind. Med. 4: 741–754, 1983.

I. Astrand, A. Kilbom, P. Ovrum et al. Exposure to styrene. Work Env. Health 11: 69–85, 1974.

Z. Bardodej and E. Bardodejova. Biotransformation of ethyl benzene, styrene, and alpha-methylstyrene in man. Am. Ind. Hyg. Asso. J. 31: 206–209, 1970.

F. Brugnone, L. Perbellini, G.B. Faccini et al. Breath and blood levels of benzene, toluene, cumene and styrene in non-occupational exposure. Int. Arch. Occ. Env. Health 61: 303–311, 1989.

N. Cherry, H.A. Waldron, G.G. Wells et al. An investigation of the acute behavioural effects of styrene on factory workers. Brit. J. Ind. Med. 37: 234–240, 1980.

R.L. Dills, R.L. Wu, H. Checkoway and D.A. Kalman. Capillary gas chromatographic method for mandelic and phenylglyoxylic acids in urine. Int. Arch. Occ. Env. Health 62: 603–606, 1991.

T. Dutkiewicz and H. Tyras. Skin absorption of toluene, styrene, and xylene by man. Brit. J. Ind. Med. 25: 243, 1968.

J. Engstrom, R. Bjurstrom, J. Astrand and P. Ovrum. Uptake, distribution and elimination of styrene in man. Scand. J. Work Env. Health 4: 315–323, 1978.

J. Flek and V. Sedivec. Simultaneous gas chromatographic determination of urinary mandelic and phenylglyoxylic acids using diazomethane derivatization. Int. Arch. Occ. Env. Health 45: 181–188, 1980.

M. Guillemin and D. Bauer. Human exposure to styrene. II. Quantitative and specific gas chromatographic analysis of urinary mandelic and phenylglyoxylic acids as an index of styrene exposure. Int. Arch. Occ. Env. Health 37: 57–64, 1976.

M.P. Guillemin and D. Bauer. Human exposure to styrene. III. Elimination kinetics of urinary mandelic and phenylglyoxylic acids after single experimental exposure. Int. Arch. Occ. Env. Health 44: 249–263, 1979.

M. Ikeda, T. Imamura, M. Hayashi et al. Evaluation of hippuric, phenylglyoxylic and mandelic acids in urine as indices of styrene exposure. Int. Arch. Arbeitsmed. 32: 93–101, 1974.

H. Kivisto, K. Pekari and A. Aitio. Analysis and stability of phenylglyoxylic and mandelic acids in the urine of styrene-exposed persons. Int. Arch. Occ. Env. Health 64: 399–403, 1993.

K.C. Leibman. Metabolism and toxicity of styrene. Env. Health Persp. 11: 115–119, 1975.

H. Ohtsuji and M. Ikeda. A rapid colorimetric method for the determination of phenylglyoxylic and mandelic acids. Brit. J. Ind. Med. 27: 150–154, 1970.

M. Ogata and R. Sugihara. High performance liquid chromatographic procedure for quantitative determination of urinary phenylglyoxylic, mandelic, and hippuric acids as indices of styrene exposure. Int. Arch. Occ. Env. Health 42: 11–19, 1978.

P. Pfaffli, A. Hesso, H. Vainio and M. Hyvonen. 4-Vinylphenol excretion suggestive of arene oxide formation in workers occupationally exposed to styrene. Tox. Appl. Pharm. 60: 85–90, 1981.

J.K. Piotrowski. *Exposure Tests for Organic Compounds in Industrial Toxicology,* U.S. Government Printing Office, Washington, D.C., 1977, pp. 60–65.

G. Poggi, M. Giusiani, U. Palagi et al. High-performance liquid chromatography for the quantitative determination of the urinary metabolites of toluene, xylene, and styrene. Int. Arch. Occ. Env. Health 50: 25–31, 1982.

J.C. Ramsey and J.D. Young. Pharmacokinetics of inhaled styrene in rats and humans. Scand. J. Work Env. Health 4: 84–91, 1978.

R.D. Stewart, H.C. Dodd, E.D. Baretta and A.W. Schaffer. Human exposure to styrene vapor. Arch. Env. Health 16: 656–662, 1968.

P.B. Van Roosmalen and I. Drummond. Simultaneous determination by gas chromatography of the major metabolites in urine of toluene, xylenes and styrene. Brit. J. Ind. Med. 35: 56–60, 1978.

W. Will, W. Zschiesche, K. Gossler et al. Quantitative Bestimmung der Styrol-Metaboliten Mandelsaeure und Phenylglyoxylsaeure in Urin mit Hochdruck-Fluessigkeits-Chromatographie und Gas-Chromatographie. Fresenius Z. Anal. Chem. 303: 401–405, 1980.

Succinylcholine

T½: 2–6 min (dogs)
Vd: 0.7–3.1 L/kg (dogs)
Fb: ?

$$(CH_3)_3N^+CH_2CH_2OCOCH_2CH_2COOCH_2CH_2N^+(CH_3)_3$$

Occurrence and Usage. Succinylcholine (suxamethonium, succinyldicholine, Anectine) was first synthesized in 1906, although its ability to produce neuromuscular blockade was not recognized until 1949. It is a depolarizing agent with a brief duration of action, attributed to its rapid hydrolysis in plasma. This quaternary ammonium compound is supplied as the dichloride for intravenous or intramuscular administration in single doses of 20–80 mg; for lengthy procedures the drug is given by intravenous infusion at a rate of 0.5–10 mg/minute.

Blood Concentrations. Due to its rapid disappearance, succinylcholine has not been determined in plasma after administration to man. Experiments with labeled drug in dogs indicated that within 5 minutes of administration 80% of the radioactivity was cleared from the plasma, primarily by extravascular redistribution (Dal Santo, 1968). A 5 mg/kg intravenous dose in dogs produced an average peak plasma succinylcholine concentration of 132 mg/L, declining to 1.1 mg/L by 35 minutes when recovery from paralysis began, with a further decline to 0.43 mg/L by 1 hour (Baldwin and Forney, 1988). A 2 mg/kg (140 mg/70 kg) intravenous dose in a human patient produced plasma levels of approximately 40 mg/L at 0.5 minute, 2.4 mg/L at 4.5 minutes and 0.5 mg/L at 15 minutes (Lagerwerf et al., 1991).

Metabolism and Excretion. Biotransformation of the drug proceeds largely via hydrolysis by plasma cholinesterase and liver esterases initially to succinylmonocholine, which is 20–50 times less potent than its parent, and then more slowly to succinic acid and choline. The compound will also undergo rapid hydrolysis in aqueous alkaline solution, or even in acid solution at elevated temperature (Gibb, 1972). Acetylcholinesterase, present at the neuromuscular junction, does not hydrolyze succinylcholine (Foldes, 1975). Unchanged drug appears in the urine immediately after intravenous injection, and accounts for 2.2% of a dose within 30 minutes; no further excretion was found to occur after that time. After the administration of succinylmonocholine, an average of 12% of the dose was found unchanged in the 30 minute urine (Foldes et al., 1955). Urine samples collected 10–15 minutes after therapeutic drug injection contained up to 16 mg/L of succinylcholine, whereas a sample that had been retained in the bladder for 22 hours measured only 0.2 mg/L. An occasional urine specimen had esterase activity that resulted in total loss of drug (Stevens and Moffat, 1974).

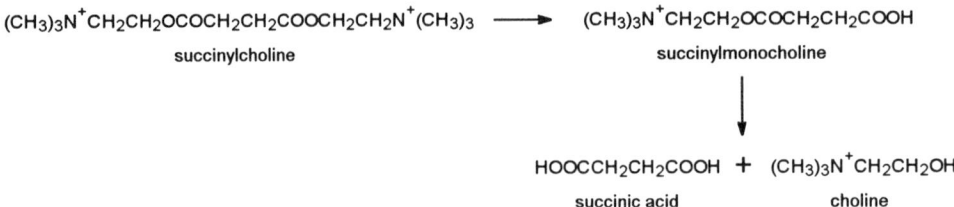

Toxicity. Succinylcholine toxicity is occasionally encountered in patients with genetically-determined atypical plasma cholinesterase or in those who have received cholinesterase inhibitors; prolonged periods of apnea may result, requiring assisted respiration (Foldes et al., 1955; Foldes, 1975; Benzer et al., 1991). Succinylcholine has been isolated from the area of injection in a fatal poisoning, although no unchanged drug was detected in the blood, liver or kidney (Gajdzinska and Szczepanski, 1967). A succinic acid level of 12 mg/kg in postmortem brain tissue was used to prove antemortem administration of succinylcholine in a case of suspected homicidal poisoning (Holmes, 1968). However, Fiorese (1969) has shown that endogenous succinic acid concentrations in fresh or embalmed brain (range, 19–200 mg/kg) and liver (range, 182–2000 mg/kg) are so variable as to preclude any meaningful distinction between normal subjects and persons who have received the drug prior to death.

Analysis. The analysis of succinylcholine in urine has been accomplished by extraction of an ion-pair complex with bromothymol blue, followed by thin-layer chromatography, hydrolysis of the isolated drug to succinic acid, esterification of the liberated acid to one or more derivatives and quantitation by gas chromatography (Stevens and Moffat, 1974). A procedure involving ion-exchange purification with quantitation by visible spectrophotometry of a reineckate salt has also been described, although the practical application of the technique was not demonstrated (Fiori and Marigo, 1967). Thin-layer chromatographic separation of succinylcholine, succinylmonocholine, and choline was reported as part of a procedure to assay serum cholinesterase activity (Agarwal and Goedde, 1976). More recently, succinylcholine in tissue has been measured by gas chromatography/mass spectrometry of a demethylated derivative (Forney et al., 1982; Balkon et al., 1983). Liquid chromatography with fluorescence detection has also been employed (Lagerwerf et al., 1991). The drug may disappear entirely from tissue specimens within 20 days unless preserved with embalming fluid or physostigmine (Baldwin and Forney, 1988). Attempts to assay blood or plasma for succinylcholine immediately after *in vitro* addition of the drug at a concentration of 5 mg/L without a cholinesterase inhibitor have not been successful (Stevens and Moffat, 1974).

References

D.P. Agarwal and H.W. Goedde. Thin-layer chromatographic separation of ^{14}C-labelled succinyldicholine, succinylmonocholine and choline. J. Chrom. 121: 170–172, 1976.

K.A. Baldwin and R. Forney, Jr. The influence of storage temperature and chemical preservation on the stability of succinylcholine in canine tissue. J. For. Sci. 33: 462–469, 1988.

K.A. Baldwin and R. Forney, Jr. Correlation of plasma concentration and effects of succinylcholine in dogs. J. For. Sci. 33: 470–479, 1988.

J. Balkon, B. Donnelly and T.A. Rejent. Determination of succinylcholine in tissues by TLC, GC/NPD, and GC/MS. J. Anal. Tox. 7: 237–240, 1983.

A. Benzer, G. Luz, E. Oswald et al. Succinylcholine-induced prolonged apnea in a 3-week-old newborn: treatment with human plasma cholinesterase. Anesth. Anal. 74: 137–138, 1992.

G. Dal Santo. Kinetics of distribution of radioactive labeled muscle relaxants. Anesthesiology 29: 435–443, 1968.

F. Fiorese. Method for the evaluation of succinic acid in liver and brain and its importance in medico-legal cases. Presented at the 3rd Triennial Meeting of the International Association of Forensic Toxicologists, Toronto, June, 1969.

A. Fiori and M. Marigo. A method for the detection of d-tubocurarine, gallamine, decamethonium and succinylcholine in biological materials. J. Chrom. 31: 171–176, 1967.

F.F. Foldes, R.S. Vandervort and S.P. Shanor. The fate of succinylcholine in man. Anesthesiology 16: 11–21, 1955.

F.F. Foldes. Distribution and biotransformation of succinylcholine. Int. Anesth. Clin. 13 (4): 101–115, 1975.

R.B. Forney, Jr, F.T. Carroll, I.K. Nordgren et al. Extraction, identification and quantitation of succinylcholine in embalmed tissue. J. Anal. Tox. 6: 115–119, 1982.

H. Gajdzinska and J. Szczepanski. Detection of scoline in autopsy material. Acta Polon. Pharm. 24: 639–642, 1967.

D.B. Gibb. Suxamethonium—a review. Anaesth. Int. Care 1: 109–118, 1972.

P. Holmes. *The Trials of Doctor Coppolino*, New American Library, New York, 1968.

A.J. Lagerwerf, L.E.H. Vanlinthout and T.B. Vree. Rapid determination of succinylcholine in human plasma by hplc with fluorescence detection. J. Chrom. 570: 390–395, 1991.

H.M. Stevens and A.C. Moffat. A rapid screening procedure for quaternary ammonium compounds in fluids and tissues with special reference to suxamethonium (succinylcholine). J. For. Sci. Soc. 14: 141–148, 1974.

Sufentanil

T½: 1.6–5.7 hr
Vd: 1.5–3.9 L/kg
Vb: 0.93
pKa: 8.0

Occurrence and Usage. Sufentanil (Sufenta) is a potent synthetic narcotic analgesic used in surgical procedures. It is about 5–7 times as potent as fentanyl and 500–800 times as potent as morphine. As an adjunct to general anesthesia, 1–2 μg/kg is the usual adult dose, with supplemental doses of 10–25 μg given as needed. Doses of 2–8 μg/kg produce profound analgesia, while doses of 8–30 μg/kg cause deep general anesthesia. Sufentanil citrate is supplied for intravenous use in solutions containing 50 μg/mL of the free base.

Blood Concentrations. Following intravenous sufentanil administration of 1.5 μg/kg to an adult male, a serum sufentanil concentration of 11 μg/L was found at 10 minutes, 5 μg/L at 30 minutes and 2 μg/L at 60 minutes (Weldon et al., 1985). After a bolus intravenous injection of 5 μg/kg to 10 surgical patients, plasma sufentanil concentrations declined to an average of about 1 μg/L at 60 minutes; an elimination half-life averaging 2.7 hours (range, 1.6–5.7) was observed over an 8 hour period (Bovill et al., 1984). In 10 surgical patients aged 53–81 years who received a total sufentanil dose of 12.5 μg/kg by intravenous infusion at the rate of 2.5 μg/kg/min, serum concentrations initially exceeded 20 μg/L; hemodynamic responses to surgical stimulation first occurred at an average of 61 minutes after induction of anesthesia, when the serum levels had declined to an average of 3.1 μg/L (Hudson et al., 1989).

Metabolism and Excretion. Sufentanil readily crosses the blood-brain barrier and is rapidly and extensively distributed to body tissues. About 80% of a dose is excreted in the urine in 24 hours, with only about 2% present as unchanged drug. The 2 primary metabolites of sufentanil are N-desalkylsufentanil and O-desmethylsufentanil (Meuldermans et al., 1980; Weldon et al., 1985). Up to 30% of a dose appears as conjugates in both urine and feces; presumably these are conjugates of O-desmethylsufentanil (Wiggum et al., 1985).

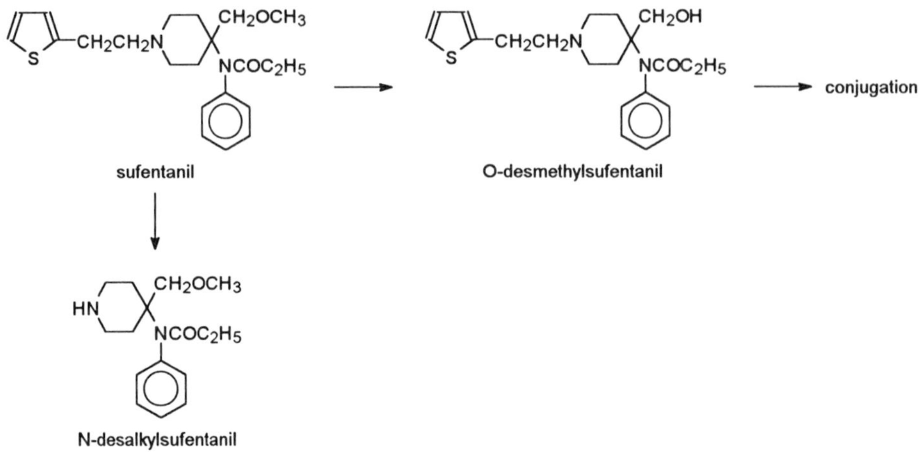

Toxicity. Sufentanil is capable of causing respiratory depression, hypotension, muscle rigidity, euphoria, dizziness, drowsiness, nausea, vomiting and slow or irregular heartbeat. Sudden hypotension after therapeutic administration has been reported (Spiess et al., 1986), as have seizures (Molbegott et al., 1987) and acute respiratory arrest (Chang and Fish, 1985). A 68 year old 80 kg man with renal failure was given a single bolus injection of 120 µg of sufentanil (1.5 µg/kg) for induction of anesthesia and later exhibited postoperative respiratory depression; sufentanil plasma concentrations of 2.6, 1.2 and 0.6 µg/L were observed at 5, 9 and 13 hours, respectively, after drug administration (Wiggum et al., 1985).

The self-administration of sufentanil by intravenous injection was responsible for the deaths of 2 male adults, whose postmortem specimens contained 1.1 and 7.0 µg/L in blood and 1.8 and 3.4 µg/kg in liver (Cravey, 1987; Ferslew et al., 1989).

Analysis. A radioimmunoassay has been developed in which sufentanil metabolites are said not to interfere (Michiels et al., 1983). Sufentanil has been analyzed by gas chromatography with nitrogen-specific detection (Gillespie et al., 1981); this method has been modified using a capillary column to enhance sensitivity (Weldon et al., 1985). A method employing gas chromatography-mass spectrometry has also been reported (Woestenborghs et al., 1994).

References

J.G. Bovill, P.S. Sebel, C.L. Blackburn et al. The pharmacokinetics of sufentanil in surgical patients. Anesthesiology 61: 502–506, 1984.

J. Chang and K.J. Fish. Acute respiratory arrest and rigidity after anesthesia with sufentanil: a case report. Anesthesiology 63: 710–711, 1985.

R.H. Cravey. Personal communication, 1987.

K.E. Ferslew, A.N. Hagardorn and W.F. McCormick. Postmortem determination of the biological distribution of sufentanil and midazolam after an acute intoxication. J. For. Sci. 34: 249–257, 1989.

T.J. Gillespie, A.J. Gandolfi, R.J. Maiorino and R.V. Vaughn. Gas chromatographic determination of fentanyl and its analogues in human plasma. J. Anal. Tox. 5: 133–137, 1981.

R.J. Hudson, R.G. Bergstrom, I.R. Thomson et al. Pharmacokinetics of sufentanil in patients undergoing abdominal aortic surgery. Anesthesiology 70: 426–431, 1989.

W. Meuldermans, R. Hurmans, J. Hendricks et al. Plasma levels, excretion, and metabolism of tritium-labeled sufentanil after intravenous administration in dogs. Janssen Preclinical Research Report R33, Janssen Pharmaceutica, Brussels, Belgium, November, 1980, pp. 800–808.

M. Michiels, R. Hendriks and J. Heykants. Radioimmunoassay of the new opiate analgesics alfentanil and sufentanil. Preliminary pharmacokinetic profile in man. J. Pharm. Pharmac. 35: 86–93, 1983.

L.P. Molbegott, M.H. Flashburg, H.L. Farasic and B.L. Karlin. Probable seizures after sufentanil. Anesth. Anal. 66: 91–93, 1987.

B.D. Spiess, R.H. Stahoff, A.R.S. El-Ganzouri and A.D. Ivankovich. High-dose sufentanil; four cases of sudden hypotension on induction. Anesth. Anal. 65: 703–705, 1986.

S.T. Weldon, D.F. Perry, R.C. Cork and A.J. Gandolfi. Detection of picogram levels of sufentanil by capillary gas chromatography. Anesthesiology 63: 684–687, 1985.

D.C. Wiggum, R.C. Cork, S.T. Weldon et al. Postoperative respiratiory depression and elevated sufentanil levels in a patient with chronic renal failure. Anesthesiology 63: 708–710, 1985.

R.J.H. Woestenborghs, P.M.M.B.L. Timmerman, M.L.J.E. Cornelissen et al. Assay methods for sufentanil in plasma. Anesthesiology 80: 666–670, 1994.

Sulindac

T½: 7 hr
Vd: ?
Fb: 0.93
pKa: ?

Occurrence and Usage. Sulindac (Clinoril) is a non-steroidal, anti-inflammatory indene derivative that also possesses analgesic and antipyretic activity. It is used for acute or long-term relief of signs and symptoms of osteoarthritis, rheumatoid arthritis, ankylosing spondylitis and other rheumatic disorders. The drug is supplied in tablets containing 150 or 200 mg of the free acid and is taken in daily oral doses of 300-400 mg.

Blood Concentrations. A single oral dose of 200 mg of sulindac given to 14 healthy adults produced an average peak plasma concentration of 4 mg/L after 1 hour; the average peak plasma concentration for the sulfide metabolite was 3 mg/L and, for the sulfone metabolite, 2 mg/L, both attained after 2 hours (Duggan et al. 1977). Steady-state plasma concentrations determined in 12 adult volunteers following daily oral doses of 400 mg were 5 mg/L for sulindac, 7 mg/L for the sulfide metabolite and 2.6 mg/L for the sulfone metabolite (Swanson et al., 1982).

Metabolism and Excretion. Sulindac is an inactive prodrug that is metabolized by reversible reduction to a pharmacologically active sulfide metabolite and by irreversible oxidation to an inactive sulfone. Both metabolites undergo conjugation, principally with glucuronic acid, as does the parent drug. The sulfone and its conjugates account for 28% of a dose as urinary excretion products, sulindac and its glucuronide account for about 20%, and polar metabolites account for about 25% of the dose. No significant concentrations of the sulfide metabolite, either free or conjugated, can be detected in the urine (Hucker et al., 1973; Duggan et al., 1977; Kwan and Duggan, 1977; Verbeeck et al., 1983; Gallanose and Spyker, 1985; Vale and Meredith, 1986). Although the primary route of excretion in man is via the urine, approximately 25% of a dose is found in the feces, primarily as the sulfone and sulfide metabolites (Hucker et al., 1973; Kwan and Duggan, 1977; Dujovne et al., 1983).

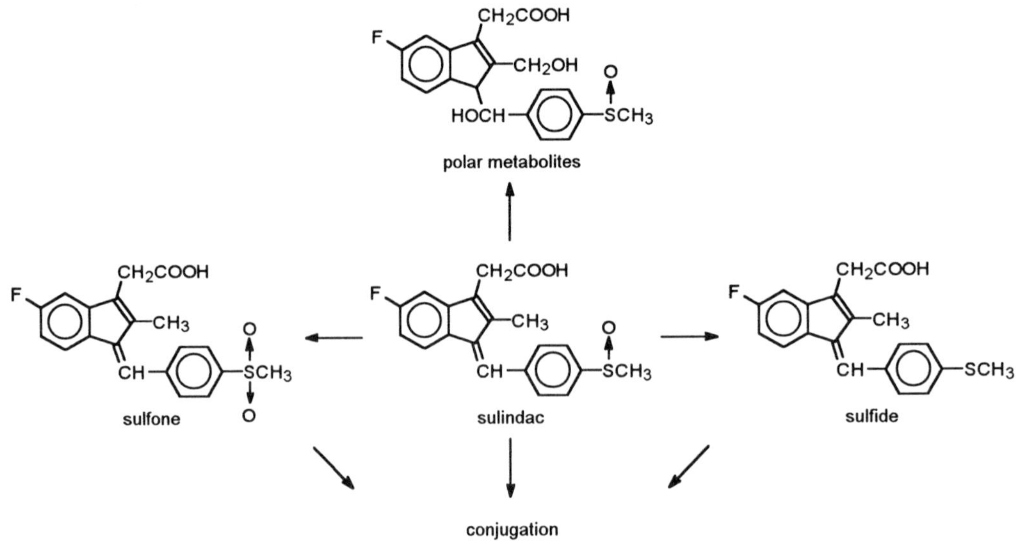

Toxicity. Acute but reversible granulocytosis (Gross, 1982) and hepatotoxicity (Gallanosa and Spyker, 1985) have been reported following sulindac use. Stupor, hypotension, coma and death may occur in overdose situations.

In the sudden death of a 58 year old woman after ingestion of an unknown quantity of sulindac tablets, the following concentrations were found (Archibald, 1984):

Sulindac Concentrations in a Fatal Case (mg/L or mg/kg)

Blood	Liver	Bile	Kidney
130	136	2810	125

Analysis. Ultraviolet spectrophotometry may be used for the determination of sulindac in blood (Archibald, 1984). Gas chromatographic (Archibald, 1984) as well as liquid chromatographic methods (Shinek et al., 1981; Musson et al., 1984; Stubbs et al., 1987) have been reported. Gas chromatography/mass spectrometry offers a sensitive and specific means of determining sulindac and its metabolites in biological specimens (Archibald, 1984).

References

J.T. Archibald. A case report of suspected sulindac poisoning. Can. Soc. For. Sci. J. 17: 71–76, 1984.

D.E. Duggan, L.E. Hare, C. Ditzler et al. The disposition of sulindac. Clin. Pharm. Ther. 21: 326–355, 1977.

C.A. Dujovne, A. Pitterman, W.C. Vincek et al. Enterophepatic circulation of sulindac and metabolites. Clin. Pharm. Ther. 33: 172–177, 1983.

A.G. Gallanosa and D.A. Spyker. Sulindac hepatotoxicity: a case report and review. Clin. Tox. 23: 205–238, 1985.

G.E. Gross. Granulocytosis and sulindac overdose. Ann. Int. Med. 96: 793–794, 1982.

H.B. Hucker, S.C. Stauffer, S.D. White et al. Physiologic disposition and metabolic fate of a new anti-inflammatory agent, cis-5-fluoro-2-methyl-1(p-methylsulfinylbenzylidenyl)-indene-3-acetic acid in the rat, dog, rhesus monkey, and man. Drug Met. Disp. 1: 721–736, 1973.

K.C. Kwan and D.E. Duggan. Pharmacokinetics of sulindac. Acta Rheum. Belg. 1: 168–178, 1977.

D.G. Musson, W.C. Vincek, M.L. Constanzer and T.E. Detty. Analytical methods for the determination of sulindac and metabolites in plasma, urine, bile and gastric fluid by liquid chromatography using ultraviolet detection. J. Pharm. Sci. 73: 1270–1273, 1984.

J.L. Shimek, N.G.S. Rao and S.K.W. Khalil. High performance liquid chromatographic analysis of tolmetin, indomethacin and sulindac in plasma. J. Liq. Chrom. 4: 1987–2013, 1981.

R.J. Stubbs, L.L. Ng, L.A. Entwistle and W.F. Bayne. Analysis of sulindac and metabolites in plasma and urine by high-performance liquid chromatography. J. Chrom. 413: 171–180, 1987.

B.N. Swanson, V.K. Boppana, P.H. Vlasses et al. Sulindac disposition when given once or twice daily. Clin. Pharm. Ther. 32: 397–403, 1982.

J.A. Vale and T.J. Meredith. Acute poisoning due to non-steroidal anti-inflammatory drugs, clinical features and management. Med. Tox. 1: 12–31, 1986.

R.K. Verbeeck, J.L. Blackburn and G.R. Loewen. Clinical pharmacokinetics of non-steroidal anti-inflammatory drugs. Clin. Pharmacokin. 8: 297–331, 1983.

Temazepam

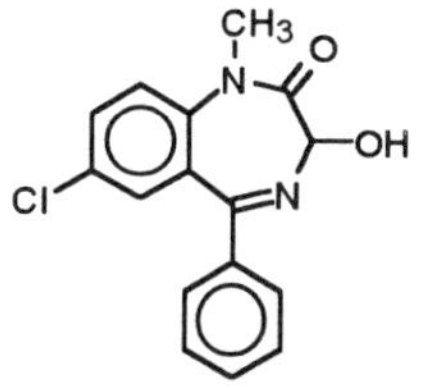

T½: 3–13 hr
Vd: 0.8–1.0 L/kg
Fb: 0.97
pKa: 1.3

Occurrence and Usage. Temazepam (methyloxazepam, Normison, Restoril), the 3-hydroxylated metabolite of diazepam, has been available as a hypnotic drug since 1979. It is supplied as the free base in 15 and 30 mg capsules intended for oral administration on a once-nightly basis.

Blood Concentrations. Ten elderly subjects given a single 10 mg oral dose of temazepam developed peak plasma levels of 0.205–0.430 mg/L (average, 0.305) within 15–90 minutes (Klem et al., 1986). Plasma temazepam concentrations in 6 volunteers reached peak levels of 0.363–0.856 mg/L (average, 0.668) within 15–75 minutes of ingestion of 20 mg (Bittencourt et al., 1979). Following a single 30 mg oral dose of temazepam to 24 healthy volunteers, an average peak plasma concentration of 0.87 mg/L (range, 0.5–1.1) occurred at an average time of 1.4 hours (Locniskar and Greenblatt, 1990). The average elimination half-life of 7–8 hours does not change significantly after 1 week of nightly dosing (Fuccella et al., 1977).

Metabolism and Excretion. An average of 82% of a labeled dose of temazepam is excreted in urine, with about 12% in feces. The urinary excretion products include unchanged drug (1.5% of a dose), conjugated temazepam (73%), and free (1.0%) and conjugated (5.8%) oxazepam (Schwarz, 1979).

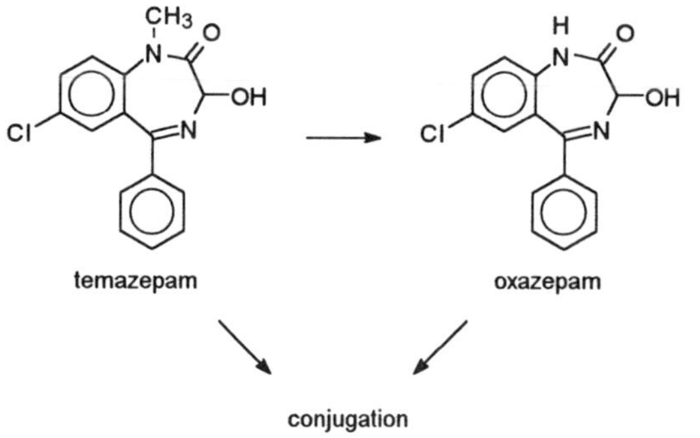

temazepam → oxazepam

conjugation

Toxicity. Temazepam causes sedation and drowsiness in normal doses. A single oral 20 mg dose at night has been shown to impair driving performance the next morning (Betts and Birtle, 1982). Overdoses may produce loss of consciousness, coma and mild to moderate respiratory depression.

Twelve fatalities involving temazepam and at least one other drug were reported in which temazepam blood levels ranged from 0.9–14 mg/L (Forrest et al., 1986). Two individuals who died after ingesting only temazepam had blood levels of 3.8–9.0 mg/L and liver levels of 39–107 mg/kg (Martin and Chan, 1986).

Analysis. Temazepam may be assayed in biological specimens by electron-capture gas chromatography of the native drug (Divoll and Greenblatt, 1981) or a silyl derivative (Belvedere et al., 1972) or by liquid chromatography (Huggett et al., 1979; Ho et al., 1983; Patterson, 1986; Kunsman et al., 1991). Many of the methods cited in the section on diazepam are also applicable.

References

G. Belvedere, G. Tognoni, A. Frigerio and P.L. Morselli. A specific, rapid and sensitive method for gas-chromatographic determination of methyloxazepam in small samples of blood. Anal. Letters 5: 531–541, 1972.

T.A. Betts and J. Birtle. Effect of two hypnotic drugs on actual driving performance next morning. Brit. Med. J. 285: 852, 1982.

P. Bittencourt, A. Richens, P.A. Toseland et al. Pharmacokinetics of the hypnotic benzodiazepine, temazepam. Brit. J. Clin. Pharm. 8: 37S–38S, 1979.

M. Divoll and D.J. Greenblatt. Plasma concentrations of temazepam, a 3-hydroxy benzodiazepine, determined by electron-capture gas-liquid chromatography. J. Chrom. 222: 125–128, 1981.

A.R.W. Forrest, I. Marsh, C. Bradshaw and S.K. Brnach. Fatal temazepam overdoses. Lancet 2: 226, 1986.

L.M. Fuccella, G. Bolcioni, V. Tamassia et al. Human pharmacokinetics and bioavailability of temazepam administered in soft gelatin capsules. Eur. J. Clin. Pharm. 12: 383–386, 1977.

P.C. Ho, E.J. Triggs, V. Heazlewood and D.W.A. Bourne. Determination of nitrazepam and temazepam in plasma by high-performance liquid chromatography. Ther. Drug Mon. 5: 303–307, 1983.

A. Huggett, G.C.A. Storey and R.J. Flanagan. Rapid high-performance liquid chromatographic method for the measurement of temazepam in blood-plasma or serum. In *Forensic Toxicology* (J.S. Oliver, ed.), Croom Helm, London, 1979, pp. 259–267.

K. Klem, G.R. Murray and K. Laake. Pharmacokinetics of temazepam in geriatric patients. Eur. J. Clin. Pharm. 30: 745–747, 1986.

G.W. Kunsman, J.E. Manno, M.A. Przekop et al. Determination of temazepam and temazepam glucuronide by reversed-phase high-performance liquid chromatography. J. Chrom. 568: 427–436, 1991.

A. Locniskar and D.J. Greenblatt. Oxidative versus conjugative biotransformation of temazepam. Biopharm. Drug Disp. 11: 499–506, 1990.

H.J. Schwarz. Pharmacokinetics and metabolism of temazepam in man and several animal species. Brit. J. Clin. Pharm. 8: 23S–29S, 1979.

C.D. Martin and S.C. Chan. Distribution of temazepam in body fluids and tissues in lethal overdose. J. Anal. Tox. 10: 77–78, 1986.

S.E. Patterson. Determination of temazepam in plasma and urine by high-performance liquid chromatography using disposable solid-phase extraction columns. J. Pharm. Biomed. Anal. 4: 271–274, 1986.

Terbutaline

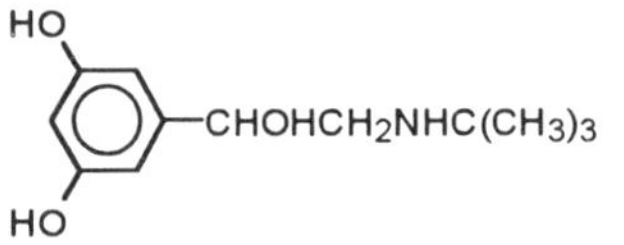

T½: 3–4 hr
Vd: 1–2 L/kg
Fb: 0.15–0.25
pKa: 8.7 (phenol), 10.0 (amine), 11.0 (phenol)

Occurrence and Usage. Terbutaline (Brethine, Bricanyl) is a beta-adrenergic receptor agonist used for the relief of reversible bronchospasm in patients with obstructive airway diseases such as asthma, bronchitis and emphysema. The sulfate salt is available as an aerosol, an injectable solution (1 mg/mL), or in tablet form (2.5–5 mg). The usual dose by inhalation is 0.4 mg (2 inhalations) every 4–6 hours, by subcutaneous injection, 0.25 mg repeated after 15–30 minutes if necessary, and by oral administration, 2.5–5 mg 3 times daily.

Blood Concentrations. Following a single oral dose of 5 mg of terbutaline to 8 subjects, an average peak plasma concentration of 3 µg/L (range, 2–5) occurred in 2–4 hours. After a single subcutaneous injection of 0.5 mg to the same subjects, an average peak plasma concentration of 7 µg/L (range, 5–11) was attained in 12–36 minutes (Leferink et al., 1982). After a subcutaneous injection of 0.75 mg of terbutaline to an adult patient, a peak plasma concentration of approximately 10 µg/L was attained in about 30 minutes, falling to 4 µg/L in 1 hour (Oosterhuis et al., 1986). A 5 minute intravenous infusion of 5–6 µg/kg in 7 children produced plasma terbutaline levels that were initially as high as 20–30 µg/L, but declined to an average of 2.7 µg/L by 1 hour (Hultquist et al., 1989).

Metabolism and Excretion. Terbutaline is extensively biotransformed, principally by sulfate and glucuronide conjugation. After oral administration, approximately 10% of a dose is eliminated in urine and up to 60% in feces as parent drug; most of the remainder appears in urine as conjugates (Hornblad et al., 1976). With intravenous administration, an average of 62% of a dose is excreted in the 36 hour urine as unchanged drug, with an additional 14% present in conjugated form (Hultquist et al., 1989).

The following concentrations of terbutaline were measured in the tissues of a subject who received 2.5–5 mg daily and who died in an accident: liver, 8.5 µg/kg; lung, 7.0 µg/kg; heart, 3.6 µg/kg (Leferink et al., 1978).

Toxicity. Side-effects from terbutaline include headache, increased heart rate, palpitations, sweating, muscle cramps and drowsiness. In overdosage, myocardial ischemia, ventricular tachycardia, pulmonary edema, cerebral hemorrhage and seizures may occur (Friedman et al., 1982).

Leferink et al. (1978) reported the case of an asthmatic who suffered a severe night attack of asthma, took an unknown quantity of terbutaline and died the following morning:

Terbutaline Concentrations in a Fatal Case (µg/L or µg/kg)

Serum	Lung	Heart	Liver	Kidney	Muscle
14	26	36	55	54	63

Analysis. Terbutaline has been determined in serum and plasma employing thin-layer fluorimetry (Tripp et al., 1978), liquid chromatography with electrochemical detection (Oosterhuis et al., 1986), and gas chromatography-mass spectrometry (Martin et al., 1979; Jacobsson et al., 1980; Lindberg and Jonsson, 1982; Maes, 1985; Leis et al., 1990).

References

R. Friedman, B. Zitelli, D. Jardine and P. Fireman. Seizures in a patient receiving terbutaline. Am. J. Dis. Child. 136: 1091–1092, 1982.

Y. Hornblad, E. Ripe, P.O. Magnusson and K. Tegner. The metabolism and clinical activity of terbutaline and its prodrug ibuterol. Eur. J. Clin. Pharm. 10: 9–18, 1976.

C. Hultquist, C. Lindberg, L. Nyberg et al. Pharmacokinetics of intravenous terbutaline in asthmatic children. Dev. Pharm. Ther. 13: 11–20, 1989.

S.E. Jacobsson, S. Jonsson, C. Lindberg and L.A. Svensson. Determination of terbutaline in plasma by gas chromatography chemical ionization mass spectrometry. Biomed. Mass Spec. 7: 265–268, 1980.

J.G. Leferink, I. Wagemaker-Engels and R.A. Maes. Determination of terbutaline in postmortem human tissues by gas chromatography-mass spectrometry. J. Anal. Tox. 2: 86–88, 1978.

J.G. Leferink, W. van den Berg, J. Wagemaker-Engels et al. Pharmacokinetics of terbutaline, a β_2-sympatho-mimetic, in healthy volunteers and asthmatic patients. Arz. Forsch. 32: 159–164, 1982.

H.J. Leis, H. Bleispach, V. Nitsche and E. Malle. Quantitative determination of terbutaline and orciprenaline in human plasma by gas chromatography/negative ion chemical ionization mass spectrometry. Biomed. Env. Mass Spec. 19: 382–386, 1990.

C. Lindberg and S. Jonsson. Simultaneous determination of terbutaline and salbutamol in plasma by selected ion monitoring. Biomed. Mass Spec. 6: 493–494, 1982.

R.A.A. Maes. Terbutaline, salbutamol and fenoterol using C-18 extraction and mass fragmentography. In *Methodology for Analytical Toxicology* (I. Sunshine, ed.), CRC Press, Boca Raton, Florida, 1985, pp. 175–179.

L.E. Martin, J. Oxford, R.J.N. Tanner and M.J. Hetheridge. The determination of terbutaline in human plasma by selected ion monitoring of the t-butyldimethylsilyl ether. Biomed. Mass Spec. 6: 460–461, 1979.

B. Oosterhuis, M.C.P. Braat, C.M. Roos et al. Pharmacokinetic-pharmacodynamic modeling of terbutaline bronchodilation in asthma. Clin. Pharm. Ther. 40: 469–475, 1986.

S.L. Tripp, E. Williams, W.J. Roth et al. Analysis of terbutaline in human serum by thin-layer fluorimetry. Anal. Letters B11: 727–740, 1978.

Terfenadine

T½: 3–6 hr (acid metabolite)
Vd: ?
Fb: 0.98
pKa: ?

Occurrence and Usage. Terfenadine (Seldane) is a peripherally-acting histamine H_1-receptor antagonist that is purported to be free of the sedative and anticholinergic side-effects generally associated with antihistamines. It is intended for the relief of symptoms of allergic rhinitis such as sneezing, watery eyes and nasal sinus inflammation. It is available as the free base in tablets of 60 mg; the usual dosage is 1 tablet every 12 hours.

Blood Concentrations. A single 60 mg oral dose of terfenadine suspension given to 14 healthy adult volunteers resulted in an average peak plasma terfenadine concentration of 1.5 µg/L at 0.8 hours; following the unusually large single dose of 180 mg, the peak plasma level averaged 4.5 µg/L at 1.1 hours (Garteiz et al., 1982). In a study of 8 healthy elderly women (average age, 68 years) given a 1 mg/kg (70 mg/70 kg) oral terfenadine dose, the average peak serum acid metabolite concentration was 190 µg/L at 2.0 hours (Simons et al., 1990).

Following 60 mg of terfenadine given orally twice daily for 6 days to 6 healthy adults, the average maximum plasma concentration of the acid metabolite was 277 µg/L (range, 184–385) at 2–4 hours (Honig et al., 1993).

Metabolism and Excretion. Terfenadine has been shown to undergo oxidation of the tert-butyl sidechain to a carboxylic acid derivative known as the acid metabolite; it also undergoes oxidative fission at the piperdinyl nitrogen, forming azacyclonol. Other metabolites include alcohol and aldehyde oxidative precursors to the acid metabolite. The acid metabolite, which greatly exceeds the concentration of the parent drug in plasma, has been found to have about one third the antihistaminic activity of terfenadine and an elimination half-life of 3–6 hours. Azacyclonol (Ataractan, Frenquel) is prescribed as a sedative in some European countries.

An average of 32 percent of a dose of terfenadine is eliminated in the 24 hour urine, largely as the acid metabolite (11.8%) and azacyclonol (10.7%). Approximately 60 percent of a dose can be accounted for in the 5 day feces, with about half of that being represented by the acid metabolite. Only trace amounts of unchanged drug are present in urine or feces. Altogether, urinary and fecal excretion account for 99.5 percent of a dose as products of biotransformation (Garteiz et al., 1982; Chen et al., 1991).

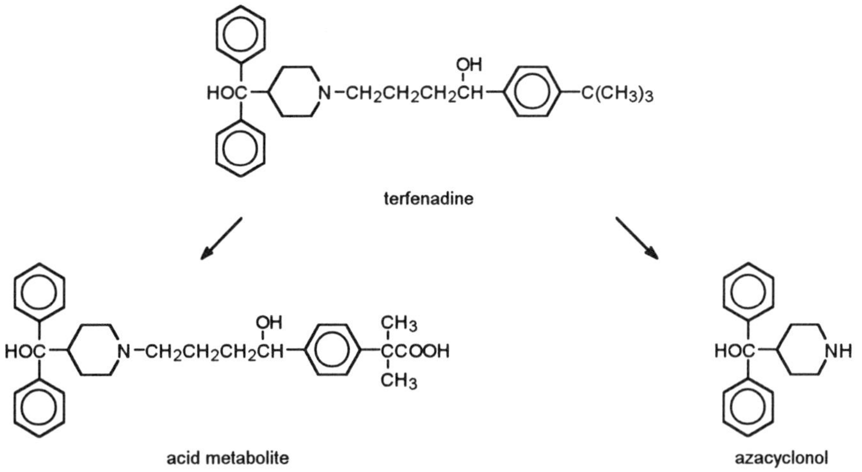

terfenadine

acid metabolite

azacyclonol

Toxicity. Most instances of overdosage with terfenadine result in only mild symptomatology. A study of 28 children aged 1–5 years who accidentally ingested 60–900 mg of the drug showed that no significant morbidity was produced in any of the victims. Several adults who have ingested up to 1500 mg of terfenadine have experienced only mild symptoms of headache, nausea, confusion and hypotension (Spiller et al., 1989). However, one person who ingested 3360 mg of the drug in combination with 7000 mg of cephalexin (an antibiotic) developed severe ventricular arrhythmia 15 hours later; the patient survived with treatment (PDR, 1991). A 21 year old woman apparently ingested an overdose and exhibited seizures and electrocardiographic abnormalities; serum concentrations on admission were 43 μg/L for terfenadine and 1504 μg/L for the acid metabolite (Davies et al., 1989).

Recently, there have been several reports of serious interaction between terfenadine and ketoconazole, an oral antifungal agent. A 39 year old woman who had been taking 120 mg/day of terfenadine for 10 days and 400 mg/day of ketoconazole for 2 days developed palpitations, dyspnea, diaphoresis, lightheadedness and syncope; while in hospital for observation, she exhibited ventricular arrhythmia (Torsade de pointes) and near syncope. Admission serum contained 57 μg/L terfenadine and 385 μg/L of the acid metabolite (Monahan et al., 1990). Explanations that have been offered regarding this effect of ketoconazole on the drugs with which it interacts include a reduction in the rate of metabolism and/or alteration in the body distribution of the other agent (Brown et al., 1985). The concomitant administration of erythromycin may cause similar toxic effects, since it has been shown to result in a doubling of the serum concentration of the acid metabolite in persons taking terfenadine chronically (Honig et al., 1992).

Analysis. Terfenadine has been measured in biological fluids using a specific radioimmunoassay (Cook et al., 1980). Liquid chromatography has been applied to the detection of the parent drug and its major metabolite (Alkaysi et al., 1987; Coutant et al., 1991). Gas chromatography (Neill et al., 1991, 1992) as well as liquid chromatography (Chen et al., 1992) combined with mass spectrometry have also been employed.

References

H. Alkaysi, M. Sheikhsalem and A. Badwan. Reverse-phase high-performance liquid chromatographic analysis of terfenadine. J. Pharm. Biomed. Anal. 5: 729–733, 1987.

M.W. Brown, A.L. Maldonado, C.G. Meredith and K.V. Speeg, Jr. Effect of ketoconazole on hepatic oxidative drug metabolism. Clin. Pharm. Ther. 37: 290–297, 1985.

T.M. Chen, K.Y. Chan, J.E. Coutant and R.A. Okerholm. Determination of the metabolites of terfenadine in human urine by thermospray liquid chromatography-mass spectrometry. J. Pharm. Biomed. Anal. 9: 929–934, 1992.

C.E. Cook, D.L. Williams, M. Myers et al. Radioimmunoassay for terfenadine in human plasma. J. Pharm. Sci. 69: 1419–1423, 1980.

J.E. Coutant, P.A. Westmark, P.A. Nardella et al. Determination of terfenadine and terfenadine acid metabolite in plasma using solid-phase extraction and high-performance liquid chromatography with fluorescence detection. J. Chrom. 570: 139–148, 1991.

A.J. Davies, V. Harindra, A. McEwan and R.R. Ghose. Cardiotoxic effect with convulsions in terfenadine overdose. Brit. Med. J. 298: 325, 1989.

D.A. Garteiz, R.H. Hook, B.J. Walker and R.A. Okerholm. Pharmacokinetics and biotransformation studies of terfenadine in man. Arz. Forsch. 32: 1185–1190, 1982.

P.K. Honig, R.L. Woosley, K. Zamani et al. Changes in the pharmacokinetics and electrocardiographic pharmacodynamics of terfenadine with concomitant administration of erythromycin. Clin. Pharm. Ther. 52: 231–238, 1992.

P.K. Honig, D.C. Wortham, K. Zamani et al. Effect of concomitant administration of cimetidine and ranitidine on the pharmacokinetics and electrocardiographic effects of terfenadine. Eur. J. Clin. Pharm. 45: 41–46, 1993.

J.J. Kuhlman, B. Levine, K.L. Klette et al. Measurement of azacyclonol in urine and serum of humans following terfenadine (Seldane) administration using gas chromatography-mass spectrometry. J. Chrom. 578: 207–214, 1992.

B.P. Monahan, C.L. Ferguson, E.S. Killeavy et al. Torsades de pointes occurring in association with terfenadine use. J. Am. Med. Asso. 264: 2788–2790, 1990.

G.P. Neill, N.W. Davies and S. McLean. Automated screening procedure using gas chromatography-mass spectrometry for identification of drugs after their extraction from biological samples. J. Chrom. 565: 207–224, 1991.

Physician's Desk Reference, Medical Economics, Oradell, N.J., 1991.

K.J. Simons, T.J. Martin, W.T.A. Watson and F.S.R. Simons. Pharmacokinetics and pharmacodynamics of terfenadine and chlorpheniramine in the elderly. J. Aller. Clin. Immun. 85: 540–547, 1990.

H.A. Spiller, M. Picciotti and E. Perez. Accidental terfenadine ingestion in children. Vet. Hum. Tox. 31: 154–156, 1989.

Tetrachloroethylene

T½: 33–72 hr
Vd: 8.2 L/kg $Cl_2C=CCl_2$
Fb: ?

Occurrence and Usage. Tetrachloroethylene (perchloroethylene, tetrachloroethene) is widely used as a solvent, dry-cleaning agent and degreasing fluid. Pulmonary absorption constitutes the primary route of entry into the body under industrial conditions, although the liquid is also known to penetrate the intact skin. The current threshold limit value for tetrachloroethylene in the industrial atmosphere is 50 ppm (339 mg/m³).

Blood Concentrations. Blood tetrachloroethylene concentrations in 21 neighbors living on the floor above a dry-cleaning shop averaged 0.15 mg/L (range, 0–1.77) (Popp et al., 1992). Blood concentrations averaged 1.2 mg/L (range, 0.4–3.1) in 26 workers exposed to an average air concentration of 21 ppm (range, 9–38) for 30 minutes (Lauwerys et al., 1983). Blood concentrations in 6 subjects reached an average peak level of 2.6 mg/L at the end of a 3 hour exposure to 194 ppm of the vapor; the compound was rapidly cleared from the blood when the exposure ended and was not detectable (at a sensitivity limit of 1 mg/L) after 30 minutes (Stewart et al., 1961a). Blood concentrations were found to correlate with the atmospheric tetrachloroethylene concentration as well as the degree of physical activity of an individual (Monster et al., 1979).

Metabolism and Excretion. The disposition of tetrachloroethylene in man is poorly understood. Of an inhaled dose, about 25% is eliminated unchanged in the breath during the 40 hours after exposure and only a very minor amount through the skin (Bolanowska and Golacka, 1972). The biological half-life of the compound has been estimated from pulmonary excretion data as 72 hours (Guberan and Fernandez, 1974), and it is therefore likely that the major portion of a dose (at least 80%) is eventually exhaled unchanged. Urinary metabolites, consisting of trichloroacetic acid and an unknown compound, have been found to account for less than 3% of a dose over a 67 hour period (Ogata et al., 1971). Trichloroethanol as determined by colorimetry was thought to be a minor urinary metabolite (Ikeda and Ohtsuji, 1972), but other investigators using a gas chromatographic technique have not found this compound in human urine (Fernandez et al., 1976).

Alveolar breath concentrations of tetrachloroethylene approach 50% of the atmospheric concentration of the chemical during constant exposure (Guberan and Fernandez, 1974). In subjects exposed to 100 ppm of the vapor, breath concentrations averaged 15 ppm during the first hour after exposure, 8 ppm after 15 hours and 4.5 ppm after 71 hours (Stewart et al., 1961a; Stewart et al., 1970).

Urinary tetrachloroethylene concentrations average 0.12 mg/L in workers exposed to 50 ppm of the chemical for 4 hours (Imbriani et al., 1988). Urinary concentrations of trichloroacetic acid are not considered a reliable index of worker exposure to tetrachloroethylene (Popp et al., 1992).

Toxicity. Acute exposure to tetrachloroethylene may cause blistering of the skin on contact and symptoms of central nervous system depression, including confusion, irritability, nausea, numbness and coma, upon absorption of the compound into the body. Chronic exposure has been associated with peripheral neuropathy, chemical hepatitis and damage to liver, kidneys and spleen. Tetrachloroethylene is known to cause hepatocellular carcinoma in mice and is suspected of being a human carcinogen (NIOSH, 1978).

Breath tetrachloroethylene concentrations of 85–110 ppm were measured shortly after accidental inhalation exposure to the chemical in 2 subjects who developed unconsciousness as a result; in one of these situations it was estimated that exposure to 1100 ppm of the vapor for 30 minutes had been sufficient to produce coma (Stewart et al., 1961b; Stewart, 1969). In experimental human exposures, it has been found that vapor concentrations of 1000 ppm may be tolerated for up to 1.5 hours, but that levels of 1500 ppm and above quickly produce faintness and dizziness (Carpenter, 1937). A 6 year old child became comatose after orally ingesting 8–10 mL of tetrachloroethylene; he developed a peak blood level of 22 mg/L, but survived with treatment (Koppel et al., 1985).

Hepatitis has been reported in several chronically exposed individuals (Hughes, 1954; Meckler and Phelps, 1966), while one man exhibited confusion, disorientation, muscle cramps, fatigue, and agitation after 3 years of industrial exposure (Gold, 1969).

A woman found dead after intentionally inhaling tetrachloroethylene fumes had a postmortem blood level of 115 mg/L (Sims, 1993). Two adults who died shortly after massive exposure to tetrachloroethylene fumes in dry cleaning establishments were found to have the following tissue concentrations of the chemical (Lukaszewski, 1979; Levine et al., 1981):

Tetrachloroethylene Concentrations in Fatal Cases (mg/L or mg/kg)

Blood	Brain	Lung	Liver	Kidney
44	360	3		
4.5	69	30	240	71

Analysis. Tetrachloroethylene may be determined in biological specimens by gas chromatography with flame-ionization (Baselt, 1980) or mass spectrometric detection (Lukaszewski, 1979; Levine et al., 1981). Methods for determination of trichloroacetic acid in urine are cited in the section on trichloroethylene.

References

R.C. Baselt. *Biological Monitoring Methods for Industrial Chemicals*, Biomedical Publications, Davis, California, 1980, pp. 39–40.

W. Bolanowska and J. Golacka. Absorption and excretion of tetrachloroethylene in humans under experimental conditions. Med. Prac. 23: 109–119, 1972.

C.P. Carpenter. The chronic toxicity of tetrachloroethylene. J. Ind. Hyg. Tox. 19: 323–336, 1937.

F. Fernandez, E. Guberan and J. Caperos. Experimental human exposures to tetrachloroethylene vapor and elimination in breath after inhalation. Am. Ind. Hyg. Asso. J. 37: 143–150, 1976.

J.H. Gold. Chronic perchlorethylene poisoning. Can. Psych. Asso. J. 14: 627–630, 1969.

E. Guberan and J. Fernandez. Control of industrial exposure to tetrachloroethylene by measuring alveolar concentrations: theoretical approach using a mathematical model. Brit. J. Ind. Med. 31: 159–167, 1974.

J.P. Hughes. Hazardous exposure to some so-called safe solvents. J. Am. Med. Asso. 156: 234–237, 1954.

M. Ikeda and H. Ohtsuji. Comparative study of the excretion of Fujiwara reaction-positive substances in urine of humans and rodents given trichloro- or tetrachloro-derivatives of ethane and ethylene. Brit. J. Ind. Med. 29: 99–104, 1972.

M. Imbriani, S. Ghittori, G. Pezzagno and E. Capodaglio. Urinary excretion of tetrachloroethylene (perchloroethylene) in experimental and occupational exposure. Arch. Env. Health 43: 292–298, 1988.

C. Koppel, I. Arendt, U. Arendt and P. Koeppe. Acute tetrachloroethylene poisoning—blood elimination kinetics during hyperventilation therapy. Clin. Tox. 23: 103–115, 1985.

A. Lauwerys, J. Herbrand, J.P. Buchet et al. Health surveillance of workers exposed to tetrachloroethylene in dry-cleaning shops. Int. Arch. Occ. Env. Health 52: 69–77, 1983.

B. Levine, M.F. Fierro, S.W. Goza and J.C. Valentour. A tetrachloroethylene fatality. J. For. Sci. 26: 206–209, 1981.

T. Lukaszewski. Acute tetrachloroethylene fatality. Clin. Tox. 15: 411–415, 1979.

L.C. Meckler and D.K. Phelps. Liver disease secondary to tetrachloroethylene exposure. J. Am. Med. Asso. 197: 144–145, 1966.

A.C. Monster, G. Boersma and H. Steenweg. Kinetics of tetrachloroethylene in volunteers; influence of exposure concentration and work load. Int. Arch. Occ. Env. Health 42: 303–309, 1979.

NIOSH. Current Intelligence Bulletin 20, *Tetrachloroethylene*, National Institute for Occupational Safety and Health, Cincinnati, Ohio, January 20, 1978.

M. Ogata, Y. Takatsuka and K. Tomokuni. Excretion of organic chlorine compounds in the urine of persons exposed to vapours of trichloroethylene and tetrachloroethylene. Brit. J. Ind. Med. 28: 386–391, 1971.

J.K. Piotrowski. *Exposure Tests for Organic Compounds in Industrial Toxicology*, U.S. Government Printing Office, Washington, D.C., 1977, pp. 98–101.

W. Popp, G. Muller, B. Baltes-Schmitz et al. Concentrations of tetrachloroethene in blood and trichloroacetic acid in urine in workers and neighbours of dry-cleaning shops. Int. Arch. Occ. Env. Health 63: 393–395, 1992.

D.N. Sims. Personal communication, 1993.

R.D. Stewart, H.H. Gay, D.S. Erley et al. Human exposure to tetrachloroethylene vapor. Arch. Env. Health 2: 40–46, 1961a.

R.D. Stewart, D.S. Erley, A.W. Schaffer and H.H. Gay. Accidental vapor exposure to anesthetic concentrations of a solvent containing tetrachloroethylene. Ind. Med. Surg. 30: 327–330, 1961b.

R.D. Stewart. Acute tetrachloroethylene intoxication. J. Am. Med. Asso. 208: 1490–1492, 1969.

R.D. Stewart, E.D. Baretta, H.C. Dodd and T.R. Torkelson. Experimental human exposure to tetrachloroethylene. Arch. Env. Health 20: 224–229, 1970.

Tetraethyllead

T½: ?
Vd: ?
Fb: ?

$(C_2H_5)_4Pb$

Occurrence and Usage. Tetraethyllead is a volatile (b.p., 199° C.) and flammable liquid that has been used to improve the octane rating of automotive and aviation gasoline. Prior to the establishment of environmental controls, it was found in most premium grade fuels at a concentration not exceeding 0.1%. The compound slowly decomposes in the atmosphere to inorganic lead, although most atmospheric lead is derived from tetraethyllead that is oxidized in automotive engines and is discharged as inorganic lead salts. The average urban adult inhales 20–40 μg of lead daily, retaining 30–45%, and ingests about 300 μg in the diet, absorbing only 5–10%. The current threshold limit value for tetraethyllead is 0.1 mg/m³. It is well-absorbed after inhalation, ingestion or dermal contact.

Blood Concentrations. Intact tetraethyllead has not been measured in blood. In healthy suburban adults, a range of 0.07–0.22 mg/L was observed for total blood lead, 7–14% of which was derived from atmospheric sources (Manton, 1977). Blood lead concentrations in 104 healthy tetraethyllead workers averaged 0.43 mg/L (range, 0.10–1.19) over an 8–10 year period (Robinson, 1976). Generally, 0.40 mg/L is considered the upper limit for blood lead levels in normal subjects.

Metabolism and Excretion. The disposition of tetraethyllead in man has been only briefly studied. The compound is quite lipid-soluble and is well distributed throughout the body, tending to localize in liver, kidney, brain and adipose tissue. Tetraethyllead is known to be slowly metabolized to triethyllead, to which is attributed the toxic effects of the parent compound. Triethyllead undergoes further dealkylation to diethyllead, which is the primary urinary species. It is believed that eventually the alkyl compounds are converted to inorganic lead and largely excreted in urine (Kehoe, 1976; Zhang et al., 1994).

Urinary lead concentrations averaged 0.04 mg/L (range, 0.01–0.19) in 60 urban adult males (Barry, 1975) and 0.09 mg/L (range, 0.03–0.17) in 153 healthy tetraethyllead workers (Robinson, 1976). Urine lead concentrations did not exceed 0.15 mg/L in workers exposed to an average atmospheric tetraethyllead level of 0.121 mg/m³ (ACGIH, 1971). Urinary diethyllead concentrations averaged 0.07 mg/L in 16 gasoline depot workers exposed to an average air tetraethyllead concentration of 0.107 mg/m³ (Zhang et al., 1994). Normal tissue lead concentrations are shown in the section on lead.

Toxicity. Acute exposure to tetraethyllead causes symptoms of central nervous system toxicity that include insomnia, anxiety, lassitude, tremor, hallucinations, psychotic behavior and convulsions. Absorption of only 1 g of the chemical may be sufficient to cause death within 3–30 days due to the slow degradation of the compound to triethyllead. In intoxicated workers, blood lead concentrations are rarely elevated to significant levels yet urine lead concentrations generally exceed 0.2 mg/L (Fleming, 1964).

Numerous cases of acute and chronic poisoning due to the inhalation of tetraethyllead have occurred, usually as a result of accidental or intentional exposure to gasoline. Subjects with chronic exposure may demonstrate symptoms of inorganic lead poisoning as well as the central nervous system effects of organic lead intoxication. No residual symptoms have been observed in those who survive tetraethyllead intoxication (Machle, 1935; Sanders, 1964). Dimercaprol, penicillamine, and calcium EDTA have each been used in the treatment of this illness, with apparent success.

Urine lead concentrations in 27 workers intoxicated during gasoline storage tank cleaning operations ranged from 0.11–0.48 mg/L (Cassells and Dodds, 1946), while blood lead concentrations in 8 similar workers ranged from 0.51–0.93 mg/L (Boyd et al., 1957; Beattie et al., 1972). Blood lead concentrations in 6 intoxicated gasoline sniffers have ranged from 1.00–1.69 mg/L (Law and Nelson, 1968; Boeckx et al., 1977; Hansen and Sharp, 1978; Robinson, 1978).

Two persons who died following accidental inhalation of tetraethyllead vapor had total blood lead concentrations of 3.33 and 4.00 mg/L, and triethyllead blood concentrations of 0.15 and 2.43 mg/L (Stasik et al., 1969). Triethyllead constituted 50–100% of the total lead content in the visceral organs of these victims (Bolanowska et al., 1967). Tissue lead concentrations have been determined in 3 workers fatally poisoned by tetraethyllead (Cassells and Dodds, 1946; Kehoe, 1976):

Lead Concentrations in Tetraethyllead Fatalities (mg/kg)

	Brain	Lung	Liver	Spleen	Kidney
Average	7.8	2.2	30	4.0	11
(Range)	(6–10)	(2.2)	(24–41)	(2.7–6.5)	(7.9–12)

Analysis. Intact tetraethyllead has not been reported to have been measured in human biological specimens. The alkyl metabolites may be determined by colorimetry (Bolanowska et al., 1967), atomic absorption spectrometry (Yamauchi et al., 1981) or liquid chromatography (Blaszkewicz et al., 1984). Procedures for total blood and urine lead are cited in the section on lead.

References

ACGIH. *Documentation of the Threshold Limit Values*, American Conference of Governmental Industrial Hygienists, Cincinnati, Ohio, 1971, pp. 251–252.

P.S.I. Barry. A comparison of concentrations of lead in human tissues. Brit. J. Ind. Med. 32: 119–139, 1975.

A.D. Beattie, M.R. Moore and A. Goldberg. Tetraethyl-lead poisoning. Lancet 2: 12–15, 1972.

M. Blaszkewicz, G. Baumhoer and B. Neidhart. Kopplung von HPLC und chemischem Reaktionsdetektor zur Trennung und Bestimmung von bleiorganischen Verbindungen. Fresenius Z. Anal. Chem. 317: 221–225, 1984.

R.L. Boeckx, B. Posti and F.J. Coodin. Gasoline sniffing and tetraethyl lead poisoning in children. Pediatrics 60: 140–145, 1977.

W. Bolanowska, J. Piotrowski and H. Garczynski. Triethyllead in the biological material in cases of acute tetraethyllead poisoning. Arch. Tox. 22: 278–282, 1967.

P.R. Boyd, G. Walker and I.N. Henderson. The treatment of tetraethyl lead poisoning. Lancet 1: 181–185, 1957.

D.A.K. Cassells and E.C. Dodds. Tetra-ethyl lead poisoning. Brit. Med. J. 2: 681–685, 1946.

A.J. Fleming. Industrial hygiene and medical control procedures. Arch. Env. Health 8: 266–270, 1964.

K.S. Hansen and F.R. Sharp. Gasoline sniffing, lead poisoning, and myoclonus. J. Am. Med. Asso. 240: 1375–1376, 1978.

R.A. Kehoe. Pharmacology and toxicology of heavy metals: lead. Pharm. Ther. A 1: 161–188, 1976.

W.R. Law and E.R. Nelson. Gasoline-sniffing by an adult. J. Am. Med. Asso. 204: 1002–1004, 1968.

W.F. Machle. Tetra-ethyl lead intoxication and poisoning by related compounds of lead. J. Am. Med. Asso. 105: 578–585, 1935.

W.I. Manton. Sources of lead in blood. Arch. Env. Health 32: 149–159, 1977.

T.R. Robinson. The health of long service tetraethyl lead workers. J. Occ. Med. 18: 31–40, 1976.

R.O. Robinson. Tetraethyl lead poisoning from gasoline sniffing. J. Am. Med. Asso. 240: 1373–1374, 1978.

L.W. Sanders, Sr. Tetraethyllead intoxication. Arch. Env. Health 8: 270–277, 1964.

M. Stasik, Z. Byczkowska, S. Szendzikowski and Z. Fiedorczuk. Acute tetraethyllead poisoning. Arch. Tox. 24: 283–291, 1969.

H. Yamauchi, F. Arai and Y. Yamamura. Determination of triethyllead, diethyllead and inorganic ions by hydride generation flameless atomic absorption spectrometry. Ind. Health 19: 113–124, 1981.

W. Zhang, G.G. Zhang, H.Z. He and H.M. Bolt. Early health effects and biological monitoring in persons occupationally exposed to tetraethyl lead. Int. Arch. Occ. Env. Health 65: 395–399, 1994.

Tetrahydrocannabinol

T½: 20–57 hr (infrequent users)
    3–13 days (frequent users)
Vd: 4–14 L/kg
Fb: 0.97
pKa: 10.6

Occurrence and Usage. Tetrahydrocannabinol (Δ^9-THC, Δ^1-THC, THC) is the most active of the principle constituents of marijuana (*Cannabis sativa*) and is contained in various parts of the plant in amounts that vary from only traces to as high as 12% by weight. It is administered either orally or by smoking in approximate doses of 5–20 mg, which result in sedation, euphoria, hallucinations and temporal distortion. Only about 22% of the THC contained in a cigarette may be recovered from the smoke; during the smoking process, portions of the inactive constituents such as tetrahydrocannabinol carboxylic acid and cannabidiol are converted to THC (Mikes and Waser, 1971).

Blood Concentrations. Peak plasma THC concentrations ranged from 46–188 µg/L in 6 subjects during a 10 minute smoking period with a cigarette containing 8.8 mg of THC (Perez-Reyes et al., 1981). In 6 male adults who smoked cigarettes containing 15.8 mg of THC in 11 minutes, peak plasma concentrations averaged 84 µg/L (range, 50–129) for THC at an average time of 0.14 hours, 6.7 µg/L (range, 3.3–10) for 11-hydroxy-THC at 0.25 hours, and 25 µg/L (range, 15–54) for 11-carboxy-THC at 2.4 hours. The plasma concentrations of THC and 11-hydroxy-THC declined rapidly, reaching average levels of 1.2 and 0.7 µg/L, respectively, by 3.0 hours; those of 11-carboxy-THC declined more slowly, averaging 8.8 µg/L at 12 hours (Huestis et al., 1992).

Following oral administration of THC, peak plasma levels are not reached until 1–3 hours after ingestion and are considerably lower than after smoking or intravenous injection, averaging 6 µg/L after ingestion of 20 mg; absorption from the gut is believed to be 90–95% complete (Lemberger et al., 1972; Hollister et al., 1981). The maximum psychological effect persists for 4–8 hours but lags behind the time of peak THC plasma level by 10–30 minutes for smoking and by 1–3 hours for oral administration (Hollister et al., 1981; Chiang and Barnett, 1984).

After intravenous infusion of 4–5 mg of THC in 7 subjects, the following average peak plasma concentrations were observed: 62 µg/L of THC at 20 minutes, 3 µg/L of 11-hydroxy-THC at 25 minutes, 4 µg/L of 8-beta-hydroxy-THC at 25 minutes, and 14 µg/L of unconjugated 11-carboxy-THC at 40 minutes (Wall and Perez-Reyes, 1981).

The whole blood/plasma concentration ratio for THC is 0.55 (Widman et al., 1974); estimates of its elimination half-life have ranged from 20–57 hours in infrequent users (Hunt and Jones, 1980; Wall and Perez-Reyes, 1981; Agurell et al., 1986) and from 3–13 days in frequent users (Johansson et al., 1989). The elimination half-life of 11-carboxy-THC averaged 33 hours in infrequent users of marijuana and 40 hours in frequent users (Peat et al., 1985).

Metabolism and Excretion. THC is metabolized to 2 monohydroxy compounds, 11-hydroxy-THC and 8-beta-hydroxy-THC, which, although active, do not achieve appreciable plasma concentrations and probably do not contribute significantly to the acute effects of the drug after smoking. Two other compounds, 8-alpha-OH-THC and 8,11-dihydroxy-THC, are apparently without activity (Perez-Reyes et al., 1973). A fifth metabolite, 11-carboxy-THC, has been identified and is believed to be a product of further oxidation of 11-hydroxy-THC (Kanter and Hollister, 1977). About 70% of a dose of THC is excreted within 72 hours in the feces (40%) and urine (30%). Unchanged THC is present in only trace amounts in urine and 11-hydroxy-THC (as a conjugate) accounts for only 2% of a dose. The remainder of the urinary metabolites consist largely of conjugates of 11-carboxy-THC and other unidentified acidic compounds, which persist in the urine for several weeks after a single dose (Lemberger and Rubin, 1975; Kanter and Hollister, 1977; Wall et al., 1983). After a single 10 mg dose of THC by smoking, urinary 11-carboxy-THC concentrations measured by a specific technique reached peak levels of 6–129 µg/L in 10 volunteers and occurred at various times within 16 hours of smoking (McBurney et al., 1986). Concentrations of 11-carboxy-THC as high as 2705 µg/L have been observed in frequent users (Baselt, 1984). The urinary elimination half-life of 11-carboxy-THC averaged 3.0 days (range, 0.8–9.8) in heavy smokers of marijuana (Johansson and Halldin, 1989).

Passive inhalation of marijuana smoke has resulted in plasma THC levels of 1–7 µg/L and urine 11-carboxy-THC levels as high as 39 µg/L, as measured by a specific assay (Mason et al., 1983; Morland et al., 1985; Cone and Johnson, 1986; Cone et al., 1987).

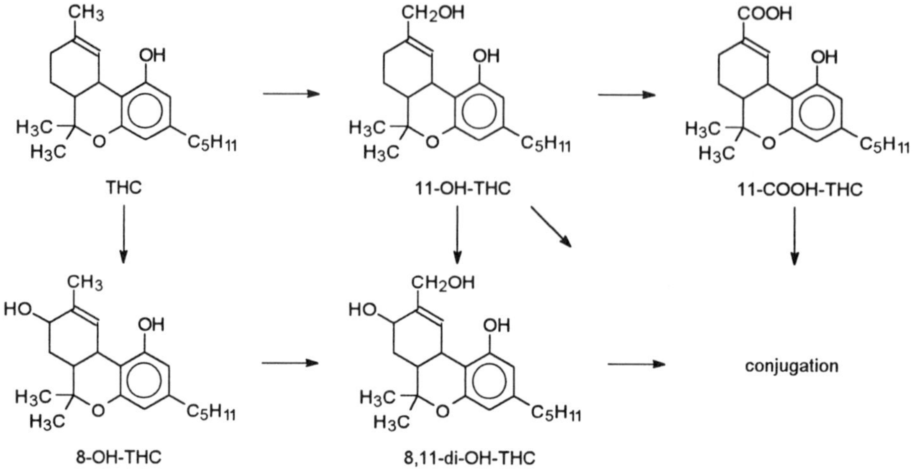

Toxicity. THC was found present in the blood of 10 of 159 victims of fatal auto accidents during a 1 year period, at concentrations of 4–14 µg/L (McBay, 1981). Six of 66 similar blood specimens were positive for cannabinoids by radioimmunoassay, and 3 were found to contain THC at levels of 2–4 µg/L (Teale et al., 1977; Law, 1981).

A 19 year old student was found comatose, sweating and with muscular rigidity after smoking a substance alleged to be THC; he was responsive to pain within 12 hours, but suffered hallucinations and became quite violent over the next 2 days, finally improving 4 days after onset of symptoms. An admission blood specimen contained 180 µg/L of cross-reacting cannabinoid by radioimmunoassay (Garrett et al., 1977). THC concentrations of 38 and 42 mg/kg were found in liver and kidney, respectively, of a man believed to have died of acute oral overdosage with THC (Tewari and Sharma, 1980).

Analysis. A number of techniques are now available for measuring THC and other cannabinols in body fluids; it is obvious that with the number of related cannabinoids present in marijuana, as well as the various metabolites of all of these produced *in vivo*, that a high degree of specificity is mandatory for meaningful results. Published techniques have involved the flame photometric-gas chromatographic detection of phosphate ester derivatives of THC and cannabinol (McCallum et al., 1978; McCallum and Shaw, 1981), electron-capture gas chromatography of fluorinated derivatives of THC (Garrett and Hunt, 1973; Fenimore et al., 1973; Bachmann et al., 1979) and gas chromatography-mass spectrometry of underivatized THC (Agurell et al., 1973; Pirl et al., 1979; Wall et al., 1979) or its methyl (Rosenfeld et al., 1974) or silyl derivative (Foltz et al., 1979; Foltz, 1984). Gas chromatography-mass spectrometry is also widely used for the analysis of 11-carboxy-THC in urine (Karlsson et al., 1983; Foltz, 1984; Paul et al., 1987; Nakamura et al., 1990; Dixit and Dixit, 1991; Clouette et al., 1993). Liquid chromatography has been employed as a method of analysis of THC or 11-carboxy-THC in biological fluids, with detection by radioimmunoassay (Williams et al., 1979), electron-capture gas chromatography (Garrett and Hunt, 1977), mass spectrometry (Valentine et al., 1977; Foltz et al., 1979), electrochemistry (Isenschmid and Caplan, 1986; Bourquin and Brenneisen, 1987) or ultraviolet spectrophotometry (Posey and Kimble, 1984; Thompson and Cone, 1987). Thin-layer chromatography has been reported for analysis of urine (Forrest et al., 1971; Kogan et al., 1984). Numerous immunoassay methods are now commercially available for the analysis of cannabinoids in body fluids.

THC in blood or plasma is relatively stable at refrigerator or freezer temperature in glass containers for up to 4–6 months; if stored longer, however, or if stored at room temperature or in plastic containers, losses may be extensive (Wong et al., 1982; Johnson et al., 1984; Christophersen, 1986). Loss of 11-carboxy-THC occurs in urine specimens over time (Cody, 1988) and through the use of plastic pipettes or containers during specimen processing (Blanc et al., 1993).

References

S. Agurell, B. Gustafson, B. Holmstedt et al. Quantitation of delta-1-tetrahydrocannabinol in plasma from cannabis smokers. J. Pharm. Pharmac. 25: 554–558, 1973.

S. Agurell, M. Halldin, J.E. Lindgren et al. Pharmacokinetics and metabolism of Δ1-tetrahydrocannabinol and other cannabinoids with emphasis on man. Pharm. Rev. 38: 21–43, 1986.

E.W. Bachmann, A.A. Hofmann and P.G. Waser. Identification of delta-9-tetrahydrocannabinol in human plasma by gas chromatography. J. Chrom. 178: 320–323, 1979.

R.C. Baselt. Unusually high cannabinoid concentrations in urine. J. Anal. Tox. 8: 16A, 1984.

J.A. Blanc, V.A. Manneh, R. Ernst et al. Adsorption losses from urine-based cannabinoid calibrators during routine use. Clin. Chem. 39: 1705–1712, 1993.

D. Bourquin and R. Brenneisen. Confirmation of cannabis abuse by the determination of 11-nor-Δ9-tetrahydrocannabinol-9-carboxylic acid in urine with high-performance liquid chromatography and electrochemical detection. J. Chrom. 414: 187–191, 1987.

C.N. Chiang and G. Barnett. Marijuana effect and delta-9-tetrahydrocannabinol plasma level. Clin. Pharm. Ther. 36: 234–238, 1984.

A.S. Christophersen. Tetrahydrocannabinol stability in whole blood; plastic versus glass containers. J. Anal. Tox. 10: 129–131, 1986.

J. Clouette, M. Jacob, P. Koteel and M. Spain. Confirmation of 11-nor-Δ9-tetrahydrocannabinol in urine as its t-butyldimethylsilyl derivative using GC/MS. J. Anal. Tox. 17: 1–4, 1993.

J.T. Cody. Evaluation of THC-COOH stability in urine. Presented at the annual meeting of the American Academy of Forensic Sciences, Philadelphia, February 19, 1988.

E.J. Cone and R.E. Johnson. Contact highs and urinary cannabinoid excretion after passive exposure to marijuana smoke. Clin. Pharm. Ther. 40: 247–256, 1986.

E.J. Cone, R.E. Johnson, W.D. Darwin et al. Passive inhalation of marijuana smoke: urinalysis and room air levels of delta-9-tetrahydrocannabinol. J. Anal. Tox. 11: 89–96, 1987.

V. Dixit and V.M. Dixit. Solid-phase extraction of 11-nor-Δ9-tetrahydrocannabinol-9-carboxylic acid from human urine with gas chromatography-mass spectrometric confirmation. J. Chrom. 567: 81–91, 1991.

D.C. Fenimore, R.R. Freeman and P.R. Loy. Determination of delta-9-tetrahydrocannabinol in blood by electron capture gas chromatography. Anal. Chem. 45: 2331–2335, 1973.

R.L. Foltz, P.A. Clarke, B.J. Hidy et al. Quantitation of delta-9-tetrahydrocannabinol and 11-nor-delta-9-tetrahydrocannabinol-9-carboxylic acid in body fluids by GC/CI-MS. In *Cannabinoid Analysis in Physiological Fluids* (J. Vinson, ed.), American Chemical Society, Washington, D.C., 1979, pp. 59–71.

R.L. Foltz. Analysis of cannabinoids in physiological specimens by gas chromatography/mass spectrometry. In *Advances in Analytical Toxicology*, Volume 1 (R.C. Baselt, ed.), Biomedical Publications, Foster City, California, 1984, pp. 125–157.

I.S. Forrest, D.E. Green, S.D. Rose et al. Fluorescent-labeled cannabinoids. Res. Comm. Chem. Path. Pharm. 2: 787–792, 1971.

C.P.O. Garrett, R.A. Braithwaite and J.D. Teale. Unusual case of tetrahydrocannabinol intoxication confirmed by radioimmunoassay. Brit. Med. J. 2: 166, 1977.

E.R. Garrett and C.A. Hunt. Picogram analysis of tetrahydrocannabinol and application to biological fluids. J. Pharm. Sci. 62: 1211–1214, 1973.

E.R. Garrett and C.A. Hunt. Separation and analysis of delta-9-tetrahydrocannabinol in biological fluids by high-pressure liquid chromatography and GLC. J. Pharm. Sci. 66: 20–26, 1977.

V.W. Hanson, M.H. Buonarati, R.C. Baselt et al. Comparison of [3]H- and ^{125}I-radioimmunoassay and gas chromatography/mass spectrometry for the determination of Δ^9-tetrahydrocannabinol and cannabinoids in blood and serum. J. Anal. Tox. 7: 96–102, 1983.

L.E. Hollister, H.K. Gillespie, A. Ohlsson et al. Do plasma concentrations of delta-9-tetrahydrocannabinol reflect the degree of intoxication? J. Clin. Pharm. 21: 171S–177S, 1981.

M.A. Huestis, J.E. Henningfield and E.J. Cone. Blood cannabinoids. I. Absorption of THC and formation of 11-OH-THC and THCCOOH during and after smoking marijuana. J. Anal. Tox. 16: 276–282, 1992.

C.A. Hunt and R.T. Jones. Tolerance and disposition of tetrahydrocannabinol in man. J. Pharm. Exp. Ther. 215: 35–44 1980.

D.S. Isenschmid and Y.H. Caplan. A method for the determination of 11-nor-delta-9-tetrahydrocannabinol-9-carboxylic acid in urine using high performance liquid chromatography with electrochemical detection. J. Anal. Tox. 10: 170–174, 1986.

E. Johansson and M.M. Halldin. Urinary excretion half-life of Δ^1-tetrahydrocannabinol-7-oic acid in heavy marijuana users after smoking. J. Anal. Tox. 13: 218–223, 1989.

E. Johansson, M.M. Halldin, S. Agurell et al. Terminal elimination plasma half-life of Δ^1-tetrahydrocannabinol (Δ^1-THC) in heavy users of marijuana. Eur. J. Clin. Pharm. 37: 273–277, 1989.

J.R. Johnson, T.A. Jennison, M.A. Peat and R.L. Foltz. Stability of Δ^9-tetrahydrocannabinol (THC), 11-hydroxy-THC and 11-nor-9-carboxy-THC in blood and plasma. J. Anal Tox. 8: 202–204, 1984.

S.L. Kanter and L.E. Hollister. Marihuana metabolites in urine of man. Res. Comm. Chem. Path. Pharm. 17: 421–431, 1977.

L. Karlsson, J. Jonsson, K. Aberg and C. Roos. Determination of Δ^9-tetrahydrocannabinol-11-oic acid in urine as its pentafluoropropyl-pentafluoropropionyl derivative by GC-MS utilizing negative chemical ionization. J. Anal. Tox. 7: 198–202, 1983.

M.J. Kogan, E. Newman and N.J. Willson. Detection of marijuana metabolite 11-nor-Δ^9-tetrahydrocannabinol-9-carboxylic acid in human urine by bonded-phase adsorption and thin-layer chromatography. J. Chrom. 306: 441–443, 1984.

B. Law. Cases of cannabis abuse detected by analysis of body fluids. J. For. Sci. Soc. 21: 31–39, 1981.

L. Lemberger, J.L. Weiss and A.M. Watanabe. Delta-9-tetrahydrocannabinol. New Eng. J. Med. 286: 685–688, 1972.

L. Lemberger and A. Rubin. The physiologic disposition of marihuana in man. Life Sci. 17: 1637–1642, 1975.

A.P. Mason, M. Perez-Reyes, A.J. McBay and R.L. Foltz. Cannabinoid concentrations in plasma after passive inhalation of marijuana smoke. J. Anal. Tox. 7: 172–174, 1983.

A.J. McBay. Personal communication, 1981.

L.J. McBurney, B.A. Bobbie and L.A. Sepp. GC/MS and EMIT analyses for Δ^9-tetrahydrocannabinol metabolites in plasma and urine of human subjects. J. Anal. Tox. 10: 56–64, 1986.

N.K. McCallum, E.R. Cairns, D.G. Ferry and R.J. Wong. A simple gas chromatographic method for routine delta-1-tetrahydrocannabinol analyses of blood and brain. J. Anal. Tox. 2: 89–93, 1978.

N.K. McCallum and S.M. Shaw. Chromatographic analysis for delta-1-tetrahydrocannabinol in blood and brain. J. Anal. Tox. 5: 148–149, 1981.

F. Mikes and P.G. Waser. Marihuana components: effects of smoking on delta-9-tetrahydrocannabinol and cannabidiol. Science 172: 1158–1159, 1971.

J. Morland, A. Bugge, B. Skuterand et al. Cannabinoids in blood and urine after passive inhalation of *Cannabis* smoke. J. For. Sci. 30: 997–1002, 1985.

G.R. Nakamura, R.D. Meeks and W.J. Stall. Solid-phase extraction, identification, and quantitation of 11-nor-Δ^9-tetrahydrocannabinol-9-carboxylic acid. J. For. Sci. 34: 792–796, 1990.

B.D. Paul, L.D. Mell, J.M. Mitchell et al. Detection and quantitation of urinary 11-nor-delta-9-tetrahydrocannabinol-9-carboxylic acid, a metabolite of tetrahydrocannabinol, by capillary gas chromatography and electron impact mass fragmentography. J. Anal. Tox. 11: 1–5, 1987.

M.A. Peat, K.M. McGinnis, J.R. Johnson et al. Concentrations of Δ^9-tetrahydrocannabinol and its metabolites in plasma and urine in "light" and "heavy" marijuana users. In *Proceedings of the 21st International Meeting*, September 13–17, Brighton, UK, International Association of Forensic Toxicologists, 1985, pp. 219–227.

M. Perez-Reyes, M.C. Timmons, M.A. Lipton et al. A comparison of the pharmacological activity of delta-9-tetrahydrocannabinol and its monohydroxylated metabolites in man. Experientia 29: 1009–1010, 1973.

M. Perez-Reyes, S.M. Owens and S.Di Guiseppi. The clinical pharmacology and dynamics of marihuana cigarette smoking. J. Clin. Pharm. 21: 201S–207S, 1981.

J.N. Pirl, V.M. Papa and J.J. Spikes. The detection of delta-9-tetrahydrocannabinol in postmortem blood samples. J. Anal. Tox. 3: 129–132, 1979.

B.L. Posey and S.N. Kimble. Quantitative determination of 11-nor-Δ^9-tetrahydrocannabinol-9-carboxylic acid in urine by HPLC. J. Anal. Tox. 8: 234–238, 1984.

J.J. Rosenfeld, B. Bowins and J. Roberts. Mass fragmentographic assay for delta-9-tetrahydrocannabinol in plasma. Anal. Chem. 46: 2232–2233, 1974.

J.D. Teale, J.M. Clough, L.J. King et al. The incidence of cannabinoids in fatally injured drivers: an investigation by radioimmunoassay and high pressure liquid chromatography. J. For. Sci. Soc. 17: 177–183, 1977.

S.N. Tewari and J.D. Sharma. Detection of delta-9-tetrahydrocannabinol in the organs of a suspected case of cannabis poisoning. Tox. Letters 5: 279–281, 1980.

L.K. Thompson and E.J. Cone. Determination of Δ^9-tetrahydrocannabinol in human blood and saliva by high-performance liquid chromatography with amperometric detection. J. Chrom. 421: 91–97, 1987.

J.L. Valentine, P.J. Bryant, P.L. Gutshall et al. High-pressure liquid chromatographic-mass spectrometric determination of delta-9-tetrahydrocannabinol in human plasma following marijuana smoking. J. Pharm. Sci. 66: 1263–1266, 1977.

M.E. Wall, D.R. Brine, J.T. Bursey and D. Rosenthal. Detection and quantitation of tetrahydrocannabinol in physiological fluids. In *Cannabinoid Analysis in Physiological Fluids* (J. Vinson, ed.), American Chemical Society, Washington, D.C. 1979, pp. 39–57.

M.E. Wall and M. Perez-Reyes. The metabolism of delta-9-tetrahydrocannabinol and related cannabinoids in man. J. Clin. Pharm. 21: 178S–189S, 1981.

M.E. Wall, B.M. Sadler, D. Brine et al. Metabolism, disposition, and kinetics of delta-9-tetrahydrocannabinol in men and women. Clin. Pharm. Ther. 34: 352–363, 1983.

M. Widman, S. Agurell, M. Ehrnebo and G. Jones. Binding of (+)- and (-)-delta-1-tetrahydrocannabinols and (-)-7-hydroxy-delta-1-tetrahydrocannabinol to blood cells and plasma proteins in man. J. Pharm. Pharmac. 26: 914–916, 1974.

P.L. Williams, A.C. Moffat and L.J. King. Combined high-performance liquid chromatography and radioimmunoassay method for the analysis of delta-9-tetrahydrocannabinol metabolites in human urine. J. Chrom. 186: 595–603, 1979.

A.S. Wong, M.W. Orbanowsky, V.C. Reeve and J.D. Beede. Stability of delta-9-tetrahydrocannabinol in stored blood and serum. In *Analysis of Cannabinoids* (R. Hawks, ed.), NIDA Research Monograph No. 42, National Institute on Drug Abuse, Rockville, Maryland, 1982, pp. 119–124.

Thallium

T½: 2–4 days
Vd: ?
Fb: ?

Tl

Occurrence and Usage. Thallium salts are currently used as insecticides and rodenticides; the amount of the monovalent metal, usually as the sulfate, in these commercially available products is limited to 1% in the United States. Thallium also has a number of minor industrial uses, and has been employed externally as a depilatory. It was once administered orally to children in doses of 8 mg/kg as the acetate salt to produce alopecia during treatment of ringworm of the scalp. The current threshold limit value for soluble thallium salts in the industrial atmosphere is 0.1 mg/m³.

Blood Concentrations. In 320 young urban children, normal thallium concentrations averaged 0.003 mg/L, with a range of 0–0.080 mg/L; over 79% of the blood specimens contained less than 0.005 mg/L of thallium (Singh et al., 1975). The half-life of thallium in blood ranges from 2–4 days (Hologgitas et al., 1980; Chandler et al., 1990).

Metabolism and Excretion. Thallium salts are well-absorbed after inhalation, ingestion or dermal contact. When thallium was administered orally in small doses to an adult, it was found to localize primarily in the soft tissues, with the highest concentrations in scalp hair, kidney and heart. Excretion was primarily via the kidney and proceeded at the rate of about 3% daily of the amount remaining in the body (Barclay et al., 1953). The slow elimination of thallium from the body has been attributed to a persistent cycle of intestinal secretion and reabsorption (Rauws, 1974). Following thallium overdosage, elimination is largely via the feces (Stevens et al., 1974). Thallium, if present in normal urine, is in concentrations of less than 0.002 mg/L (Kubasik and Volosin, 1973). Urine thallium concentrations in residents living near a cement plant that emitted thallium-containing dust averaged 0.005 mg/L (range, 0.0001–0.077) (Dolgner et al., 1983). Normal liver concentrations range from 0.4–0.9 mg/kg (Johnson, 1976).

Toxicity. Many fatal and non-fatal poisonings have resulted from the medicinal, cosmetic and pesticidal application of thallium salts. Symptoms of intoxication include colic, nausea, vomiting, tremors and paralysis, with alopecia occurring only after a period of approximately 1–3 weeks. The average lethal dose in an adult is about 1 g of a soluble thallium salt. No single chelating agent has been shown to be especially effective in treating thallium poisoning, although dithiocarb and Prussian blue hasten excretion of the metal; dithiocarb is contraindicated, however, since the chelate that is formed redistributes to the brain, causing deterioration of cerebral function (Kamerbeek et al., 1971). Trihexyphenidyl is frequently used to control tremors in victims. Since thallium competes with potassium in many biological processes, forced diuresis with potassium loading has been employed to encourage urinary elimination of thallium (Mulkey and Oehme, 1993).

Industrial exposure to excessive amounts of thallium has caused albuminuria, sensory changes, polyneuritis, speech impairment, weakness and visual disturbances to the point of permanent blindness. Workers who manifested symptoms of chronic thallium intoxication had urine thallium concentrations of 0.2–1.0 mg/L (Richeson, 1958).

Blood thallium concentrations of 1.0–8.0 mg/L and urine concentrations of 1.8–20 mg/L have been measured 1–21 days after hospital admission in several young children who survived the poisoning episode (Grossman, 1955; Chamberlain et al., 1958; Stein and Perlstein, 1959; Taber, 1964; Arena et al., 1965). In 9 adults who survived the accidental or intentional ingestion of thallium sulfate, blood concentrations of 0.08–1.9 mg/L and urine concentrations of 1.4–10 mg/L were observed within 1–30 days after admission (Gettler and Weiss, 1943b; Grunfeld and Hinostroza, 1964; Koshy and Lovejoy, 1981; de Backer et al., 1982; Nogue et al., 1982; Heath et al., 1983; Chandler et al., 1990).

The following tissue concentrations of thallium were determined in 5 adults who died within 4–15 days of ingestion of up to 17 g of the metal (Grunfeld and Hinostroza, 1964; Smith and Doherty, 1964; van Peteghem, 1974; de Wolff, 1979; Hologgitas et al., 1980):

Thallium Concentrations in Fatal Cases (mg/L or mg/kg)

	Blood	Brain	Liver	Kidney	Urine
Average	4.0	7.8	15	11	5.2
(Range)	(0.5–11)	(3–15)	(5–29)	(6–20)	(1.7–11)

Analysis. Several convenient but somewhat nonspecific colorimetric methods have been applied to the determination of thallium in biological materials (Gettler and Weiss, 1943a; Campbell et al., 1959; de Wolf and Lenstra, 1964). Flame atomic absorption procedures involve acid digestion and solvent extraction (Savory et al., 1968) or chelation and extraction (Berman, 1967; Curry et al., 1969; Amore, 1974). Flameless atomic absorption techniques for thallium in urine have involved chelation and extraction (Kubasik and Volosin, 1973) or direct sample introduction (Paschal and Bailey, 1986).

References

F. Amore. Determination of cadmium, lead, thallium, and nickel in blood by atomic absorption spectrometry. Anal. Chem. 46: 1597–1599, 1974.

J.M. Arena, G.A. Watson and S.S. Sakhadeo. Fatal thallium poisoning. Clin. Pediat. 4: 267–270, 1965.

R.K. Barclay, W.C. Peacock and D.A. Karnofsky. Distribution and excretion of radioactive thallium in the chick embryo, rat, and man. J. Pharm. Exp. Ther. 107: 178–187, 1953.

E. Berman. Determination of cadmium, thallium and mercury in biological materials by atomic absorption. At. Abs. Newsl. 6: 57–60, 1967.

E.E. Campbell, M.F. Milligan and J.A. Lindsey. The determination of thallium in urine and air. Am. Ind. Hyg. Asso. J. 20: 23–25, 1959.

P.H. Chamberlain, W.B. Stavinoha, H. Davis et al. Thallium poisoning. Pediatrics 22: 1170–1182, 1958.

H.A. Chandler, G.P.R. Archbold, J.M. Gibson et al. Excretion of a toxic dose of thallium. Clin. Chem. 36: 1506–1509, 1990.

A.S. Curry, J.F. Read and A.R. Knott. Determination of thallium in biological material by flame spectropho-tometry and atomic absorption. Analyst 94: 744–753, 1969.

W. de Backer, P. Zachee, G.A. Verpooten et al. Thallium intoxication treated with combined hemoperfusion-hemodialysis. Clin. Tox. 19: 259–264, 1982.

J.N.M. de Wolf and J.B. Lenstra. The determination of thallium in urine. Pharm. Weekblad. 99: 377–382, 1964.

F.A. de Wolff. Personal communication, 1979.

R. Dolgner, A. Brockhaus, U. Evers et al. Repeated surveillance of exposure to thallium in a population living in the vicinity of a cement plant emitting dust containing thallium. Int. Arch. Occ. Env. Health 52: 79–94, 1983.

A.O. Gettler and L. Weiss. Thallium poisoning. II. The quantitative determination of thallium in biologic material. Am. J. Clin. Path. 13: 368–377, 1943a.

A.O. Gettler and L. Weiss. Thallium poisoning. III. Clinical toxicology of thallium. Am. J. Clin. Path. 13: 422–429, 1943b.

H. Grossman. Thallotoxicosis. Report of a case and a review. Pediatrics 16: 868–872, 1955.

O. Grunfeld and G. Hinostroza. Thallium poisoning. Arch. Int. Med. 114: 132–138, 1964.

A. Heath, J. Ahlmen, B. Branegard et al. Thallium poisoning-toxin elimination and therapy in three cases. Clin. Tox. 20: 451–463, 1983.

J. Hologgitas, P. Ullucci, J. Driscoll et al. Thallium elimination kinetics in acute thallotoxicosis. J. Anal. Tox. 4: 68–73, 1980.

C.A. Johnson. The determination of some toxic metals in human liver as a guide to normal levels in New Zealand. Part I. Determination of Bi, Cd, Cr, Co, Cu, Pb, Mn, Ni, Ag, Tl and Zn. Anal. Chim. Acta 81: 69–74, 1976.

H.H. Kamerbeek, A.G. Rauws, M.T. Ham and A.N.P. van Heijst. Dangerous redistribution of thallium by treatment with sodium diethyldithiocarbamate. Acta Med. Scand. 189: 149–154, 1971.

K.M. Koshy and F.H. Lovejoy. Thallium ingestion with survival: ineffectiveness of peritoneal dialysis and potassium chloride diuresis. Clin. Tox. 18: 521–525, 1981.

N.P. Kubasik and M.T. Volosin. A simplified determination of urinary cadmium, lead, and thallium, with use of carbon rod atomization and atomic absorption spectrophotometry. Clin. Chem. 19: 954–958, 1973.

J.P. Mulkey and F.W. Oehme. A review of thallium toxicity. Vet. Hum. Tox. 35: 445–453, 1993.

S. Nogue, A. Mas, A. Pares et al. Acute thallium poisoning: an evaluation of different forms of treatment. Clin. Tox. 19: 1015–1021, 1982.

D.C. Paschal and G.G. Bailey. Determination of thallium in urine with Zeeman effect graphite furnace atomic absorption. J. Anal. Tox. 10: 252–254, 1986.

A.G. Rauws. Thallium pharmacokinetics and its modification by Prussian blue. Naunyn-Schmiedeberg's Arch. Pharm. 284: 295–306, 1974.

E.M. Richeson. Industrial thallium intoxication. Ind. Med. Surg. 27: 607–619, 1958.

J. Savory, N.O. Roszel, P. Mushak and F.W. Sunderman, Jr. Measurements of thallium in biologic materials by atomic absorption spectrometry. Am. J. Clin. Path. 50: 505–509, 1968.

N.P. Singh, J.D. Bodgen and M.M. Joselow. Distribution of thallium and lead in children's blood. Arch. Env. Health 30: 557–558, 1975.

D.H. Smith and R.A. Doherty. Thallitoxicosis: report of three cases in Massachusetts. Pediatrics 34: 480–490, 1964.

M.D. Stein and M.A. Perlstein. Thallium poisoning. Am. J. Dis. Child. 98: 80–85, 1959.

W. Stevens, C. van Peteghem, A. Heyndrickx and F. Barbier. Eleven cases of thallium intoxication treated with Prussian blue. Int. J. Clin. Pharm. 10: 1–22, 1974.

P. Taber. Chronic thallium poisoning: rapid diagnosis and treatment. J. Pediat. 65: 461–463, 1964.

C. van Peteghem. Personal communication, 1974.

Theophylline

T½: 3–11 hr
Vd: 0.3–0.7 L/kg
Fb: 0.53–0.65
pKa: 8.6

Occurrence and Usage. Theophylline (1,3-dimethylxanthine, Bronkodyl, Quibron, Somophyllin, Theodur) has been used as a bronchodilator in the control of asthma since 1936. It occurs naturally in tea leaves, together with caffeine. Theophylline is administered by intravenous injection, orally or rectally as the free acid or as one of a number of salts. The ethylenediamine salt, aminophylline, contains about 85% anhydrous theophylline and is one of the most widely used preparations. Intravenous doses of 500 mg and daily oral doses of 300–1000 mg are frequently employed.

Blood Concentrations. A single intravenous injection of 170 mg of aminophylline to 3 adults produced an average peak plasma concentration of 4.5 mg/L (range, 4.3–4.8) at 1 hour (Mitenko and Ogilvie, 1972). A single oral 500 mg dose of aminophylline administered to 3 non-fasting adults produced average blood levels of 1.4, 4.5 and 7.7 mg/L at 1, 2 and 4 hours, respectively (Lillehei, 1968). The ingestion of 470 mg of aminophylline as a syrup by 10 subjects resulted in an average peak serum theophylline concentration of 9.0 mg/L at 1.5 hours, which decreased to 6.0 mg/L by 6 hours (Sherter and Denefrio, 1974).

An intravenous loading dose of 5.6 mg/kg (392 mg/70 kg) of aminophylline, followed by constant infusion of 0.9 mg/kg/hour, has been shown to produce an effective plasma theophylline level of 5–15 mg/L in 95% of patients (Mitenko and Ogilvie, 1973). To achieve therapeutic serum theophylline concentrations of 10–20 mg/L (measured just before the morning dose) during chronic oral therapy in 83 patients, daily doses of 400–3200 mg (average, 1200) of aminophylline were required; plasma half-lives of the drug in 10 patients averaged 5.2 hours (range, 3.0–9.5) (Jenne et al., 1972). The kinetics of theophylline are best described by a 2 compartment open model (Chrzanowski et al., 1977). The whole blood/plasma concentration ratio averages 0.76 in children and 0.81 in adults (Koup and Hart, 1979).

Children of less than 6 months of age tend to exhibit longer plasma half-lives for theophylline (average, 6.9 hours) than older children (average, 4.1 hours) (Rosen et al., 1979). Certain medical disorders may prolong the half-life of this drug by directly or indirectly inhibiting its metabolism. Children with viral infections had half-lives of 10–20 hours (Woo et al., 1980), while half-lives averaged 23 hours in 9 adults with acute cardiogenic pulmonary edema (Piafsky et al., 1977) and 65 hours in 7 patients with decompensated liver cirrhosis (Staib et al., 1980).

Metabolism and Excretion. Theophylline is metabolized by oxidation to 1,3-dimethyluric acid, and by N-demethylation of both this metabolite and the parent drug. About 77% of an oral dose is excreted in the 48 hour urine as unchanged drug (10%), 3-methylxanthine (13%), 1,3-dimethyluric acid (35%) and 1-methyluric acid (19%) (Cornish and Christman, 1957). With chronic dosing, 3-methylxanthine accounts for 36% of a dose while other urinary excretion products remain at about the same levels (Jenne et al., 1976). The urine of premature infants given theophylline contains only unchanged drug (Grygiel and Birkett, 1980). Caffeine has been reported as a minor urinary metabolite in adults (Tang-Liu and Riegelman, 1981), but may represent a significant portion of a dose (average, 8.5%) in neonates (Kraus et al., 1993).

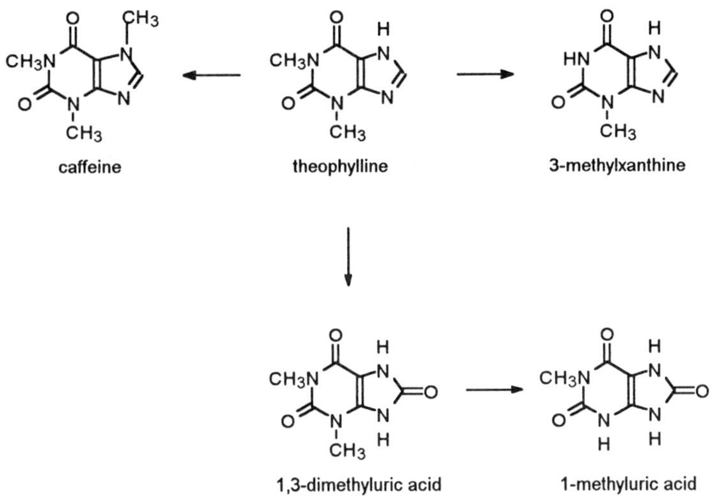

caffeine   theophylline   3-methylxanthine

1,3-dimethyluric acid   1-methyluric acid

Toxicity. Toxic signs such as nausea and vomiting are commonly associated with serum theophylline concentrations in excess of 20 mg/L (Jenne et al., 1972). Four patients undergoing intravenous aminophylline therapy who suffered from nausea, epigastric pain or headache were found to have serum theophylline levels of 31–38 mg/L (average, 35); another 8 patients developed grand mal seizures at concentrations of 25–70 mg/L (average, 53) (Zwillich et al., 1975). An impaired ability to metabolize theophylline has been implicated in patients with either liver cirrhosis or chronic obstructive pulmonary disease who developed toxicity during chronic oral therapy with the drug; serum levels of 42–86 mg/L were determined and, after discontinuation of the drug, elimination half-lives of 28–134 hours were noted (Jacobs and Senior, 1974; Baselt and Albertson, 1982). Five other patients exhibited toxicity due to accumulation of theophylline while on chronic therapy and had plasma levels of 33–56 mg/L (Loughnan and McNamara, 1978; Gotz et al., 1979; Woo et al., 1980).

Six patients survived the accidental or intentional acute ingestion of theophylline after developing plasma concentrations of 86–300 mg/L (average, 170); "coffee-ground" emesis, tachycardia, seizures, and respiratory arrest were common manifestations. In one adult, nonlinear elimination kinetics were evident at plasma theophylline concentrations exceeding 35 mg/L (Ehlers et al., 1978; Kadlec et al., 1978; Baltassat et al., 1979; Rose, 1979; Wells and Ferlauto, 1979; Miceli et al., 1980). Reduction of serum theophylline levels may be accomplished by oral charcoal administration or hemoperfusion (Radomski et al., 1984; Woo et al., 1984).

Five patients who died of seizures while on theophylline therapy had serum drug concentrations prior to death of 25–62 mg/L, averaging 46 mg/L (Zwillich et al., 1975; Vincent, 1978). Three patients who died after acute ingestion of 10–12 g of theophylline had antemortem plasma levels of 66, 85, and 120 mg/L (Helliwell and Berry, 1979). The following postmortem tissue concentrations were determined in 7 adults who died within 1 day of ingesting overdoses (Loveland, 1974; Winek et al., 1980; Burgan et al., 1982; Donnelly, 1983; Ryall, 1985; Robins, 1988):

Theophylline Concentrations in Fatal Cases (mg/L or mg/kg)

	Blood	Brain	Liver	Kidney	Urine
Average	154	156	180	160	246
(Range)	(63–250)	(118–231)	(108–275)	(108–212)	(150–342)

Analysis. The original ultraviolet spectrophotometric method for the determination of theophylline in biologic specimens (Schack and Waxler, 1949) has been modified to improve specificity (Jatlow,

1975; Hohnadel et al., 1978; Schwertner et al., 1978). Gas chromatographic techniques have involved flame-ionization detection of the native drug (Schwertner, 1979) or of a derivative (Dusci et al., 1975; Bailey et al., 1976; Pranskevich et al., 1978). Liquid chromatographic methods are now in routine use in many laboratories (Peng et al., 1978; Manno et al., 1979; Tin et al., 1979; Broussard et al., 1981; Kabra and Marton, 1982; Kester et al., 1987; Lauff, 1987; Blanchard et al., 1990). Reagents for immunoassay are commercially available; falsely high results in uremic patients may be obtained with these assays (Opheim et al., 1983).

References

D.G. Bailey, H.L. Davis and G.E. Johnson. Improved theophylline serum analysis by an appropriate internal standard for gas chromatography. J. Chrom. 121: 263–268, 1976.

P. Baltassat, E. Hartmann, C. Bory and A. Frederich. Theophylline acute poisoning in a child: evidence for biotransformation of theophylline into caffeine. Vet. Hum. Tox. 21: 211–213, 1979.

R.C. Baselt and T.E. Albertson. Markedly prolonged theophylline half-life in liver failure. J. Anal. Tox. 6: 62–63, 1982.

J. Blanchard, S. Harvey and W.J. Morgan. A rapid and specific high-performance liquid chromatographic assay for theophylline in biological fluids. J. Chrom. Sci. 28: 303–306, 1990.

L.A. Broussard, F.M. Stearns, R. Tulley and C.S. Frings. Theophylline determination by "high-pressure" liquid chromatography. Clin. Chem. 27: 1931–1933, 1981.

T.H.S. Burgan, I. Gupta and C.M. Bate. Fatal overdose of theophylline simulating acute pancreatitis. Brit. Med. J. 284: 939–940, 1982.

F.A. Chrzanowski, P.J. Niebergall, R.L. Mayock et al. Kinetics of intravenous theophylline. Clin. Pharm. Ther. 22: 188–195, 1977.

H.H. Cornish and A.A. Christman. A study of the metabolism of theobromine, theophylline, and caffeine in man. J. Biol. Chem. 228: 315–323, 1957.

B. Donnelly. Personal communication, 1983.

L.J. Dusci, L.P. Hackett and I.A. McDonald. Gas-liquid chromatographic determination of theophylline in human plasma. J. Chrom. 104: 147–150, 1975.

S.M. Ehlers, D.E. Zaske and R.J. Sawchuk. Massive theophylline overdose. J. Am. Med. Asso. 240: 474–475, 1978.

V.P. Gotz, D.E. Drayer, E.S. Schned and M.M. Reidenberg. Unusual cause of theophylline toxicity. N.Y. State J. Med. 79: 1232–1234, 1979.

J. Grygiel and D.J. Birkett. Effect of age on patterns of theophylline metabolism. Clin. Pharm. Ther. 28: 456–462, 1980.

M. Helliwell and D. Berry. Theophylline poisoning in adults. Brit. Med. J. 2: 1114, 1979.

D.C. Hohnadel, T.H. Grove and P. Alonzo. A micro method for the ultraviolet spectrophotometric determination of theophylline. J. Anal. Tox. 2: 141–145, 1978.

M.H. Jacobs and R.M. Senior. Theophylline toxicity due to impaired theophylline degradation. Am. Rev. Resp. Dis. 110: 342–345, 1974.

P. Jatlow. Ultraviolet spectrophotometry of theophylline in plasma in the presence of barbiturates. Clin. Chem. 21: 1518–1520, 1975.

J.W. Jenne, E. Wyze, F.S. Rood and F.M. MacDonald. Pharmacokinetics of theophylline. Clin. Pharm. Ther. 13: 349–360, 1972.

J.W. Jenne, H.T. Nagasawa and R.D. Thompson. Relationship of urinary metabolites of theophylline to serum theophylline levels. Clin. Pharm. Ther. 19: 375–381, 1976.

P.M. Kabra and L.J. Marton. Liquid-chromatographic analysis for serum theophylline in less than 70 seconds. Clin. Chem. 28: 687–689, 1982.

G.J. Kadlec, C.H. Jarboe, S.J. Pollard and J.L. Sublett. Acute theophylline intoxication. Biphasic first order elimination kinetics in a child. Ann. Allergy 41: 337–339, 1978.

M.B. Kester, C.L. Saccar, and H.C. Mansmann, Jr. A new simplified micro-assay for the quantitation of theophylline in serum by high-performance liquid chromatography. J. Liq. Chrom. 10: 957–975, 1987.

J.R. Koup and B.A. Hart. Relationship between plasma and whole blood theophylline concentration in neonates. J. Pediat. 94: 320–321, 1979.

D.M. Kraus, J.H. Fischer, S.J. Reitz et al. Alterations in theophylline metabolism during the first year of life. Clin. Pharm. Ther. 54: 351–359, 1993.

J.J. Lauff. Ion-pair high-performance liquid chromatographic procedure for the quantitation analysis of theophylline in serum samples. J. Chrom. 417: 99–110, 1987.

J.P. Lillehei. Aminophylline. Oral vs rectal administration. J. Am. Med. Asso. 205: 530–533, 1968.

P.M. Loughnan and J.M. Mc Namara. Paroxysmal supraventricular tachycardia during theophylline therapy in a premature infant. J. Pediat. 92: 1016–1018, 1978.

M.R. Loveland. Personal communication, 1974.

B.R. Manno, J.E. Manno and B.C. Hilman. A direct injection HPLC procedure for the quantitation of theophylline in blood and saliva. J. Anal. Tox. 3: 81–86, 1979.

J.N. Miceli, B. Clay, L.E. Fleischmann et al. Pharmacokinetics of severe theophylline intoxication managed by peritoneal dialysis. Dev. Pharm. Ther. 1: 16–25, 1980.

P.A. Mitenko and R.I. Ogilvie. Rapidly achieved plasma concentration plateaus, with observations on theophylline kinetics. Clin. Pharm. Ther. 13: 329–335, 1972.

P.A. Mitenko and R.I. Ogilvie. Rational intravenous doses of theophylline. New Eng. J. Med. 289: 600–603, 1973.

K.E. Opheim, V. Ainardi and V.A. Raisys. Increase in apparent theophylline concentration in the serum of two uremic patients as measured by some immunoassay methods (caused by 1,3-dimethyluric acid?). Clin. Chem. 29: 1698–1699, 1983.

G.W. Peng, M.A.F. Gadalla and W.L. Chiou. High-performance liquid-chromatographic determination of theophylline in plasma. Clin. Chem. 24: 357–360, 1978.

K.M. Piafsky, D.S. Sitar, R.E. Rangno and R.I. Ogilvie. Theophylline kinetics in acute pulmonary edema. Clin. Pharm. Ther. 21: 310–316, 1977.

C.A. Pranskevich, J.I. Swihart and J.J. Thoma. Serum theophylline determination by isothermal gas-liquid chromatography on 3% SP2250-DB. J. Anal. Tox. 2: 3–6, 1978.

L. Radomski, G.D. Park, M.J. Goldberg et al. Model for theophylline overdose treatment with oral activated charcoal. Clin. Pharm. Ther. 35: 402–408, 1984.

A.J. Robins. Personal communication, 1988.

C. Rose. Theophylline toxicity. West. J. Med. 130: 466–467, 1979.

J.P. Rosen, M. Danish, M.C. Ragni et al. Theophylline pharmacokinetics in the young infant. Pediatrics 64: 248–251, 1979.

J.E. Ryall. Personal communication, 1985.

J.A. Schack and S.H. Waxler. An ultraviolet spectrophotometric method for the determination of theophylline and theobromine in blood and tissues. J. Pharm. Exp. Ther. 97: 283–291, 1949.

C. Sherter and J. Denefrio. Comparative serum theophylline levels following the oral administration of Elixophyllin and Somophyllino-O, a new preparation of aminophylline. Curr. Ther. Res. 16: 239–242, 1974.

H.A. Schwertner, J.E. Wallace and K. Blum. Improved ultraviolet spectrophotometry of serum theophylline. Clin. Chem. 24: 360–361, 1978.

H.A. Schwertner. Analysis for underivatized theophylline by gas-chromatography on a silicone stationary phase, SP-2510-DA. Clin. Chem. 25: 212–214, 1979.

A.H. Staib, D. Schuppan, R. Lissner et al. Pharmacokinetics and metabolism of theophylline in patients with liver disease. Int. J. Clin. Pharm. Ther. Tox. 18: 500–502, 1980.

D.D.S. Tang-Liu and S. Riegelman. Metabolism of theophylline to caffeine in adults. Res. Comm. Chem. Path. Pharm. 34: 371–380, 1981.

A.A. Tin, S.M. Somani, H.S. Bada and N.N. Khanna. Caffeine, theophylline and theobromine determinations in serum, saliva and spinal fluid. J. Anal. Tox. 3: 26–29, 1979.

F.M. Vincent. Fatal theophylline induced seizures. Postgrad. Med. 63: 76–77, 1978.

D.H. Wells and J.J. Ferlauto. Survival after massive aminophylline overdose in a premature infant. Pediatrics 64: 252–253, 1979.

C.L. Winek, J.D. Bricker, W.D. Collom and F.W. Fochtman. Theophylline fatalities. For. Sci. Int. 15: 233–236, 1980.

O.F. Woo, J.R. Koup, M. Kraemer and W.O. Robertson. Acute intoxication with theophylline while on chronic therapy. Vet. Hum. Tox. 22 (Suppl. 2): 48–51, 1980.

O.F. Woo, S.M. Pond, N.L. Benowitz and K.R. Olson. Benefit of hemoperfusion in acute theophylline intoxication. Clin. Tox. 22: 411–424, 1984.

C.W. Zwillich, F.D. Sutton, Jr., T.A. Neff et al. Theophylline-induced seizures in adults. Ann. Int. Med. 82: 784–787, 1975.

Thiopental

T½: 6–46 hr
Vd: 1.4–6.7 L/kg
Fb: 0.72–0.86
pKa: 7.6

Occurrence and Usage. Thiopental (thiopentone, Pentothal) was introduced for use as an intravenous anesthetic in 1935, and has since achieved popularity as an induction agent. It is an ultrashort-acting thiobarbiturate with a rapid onset of action. It is supplied as the sodium salt and is usually administered in 100–250 mg initial doses, with rarely more than 1 g being given during a single procedure.

Blood Concentrations. In a subject receiving 400 mg of thiopental by intravenous injection over a 2 minute period, a maximal plasma concentration of 28 mg/L was observed immediately after administration, with a decline to 7 mg/L after 15 minutes (at which time the patient awoke) and to 3 mg/L by 90 minutes (Brodie et al., 1950). In a random study of 22 surgical patients, plasma thiopental concentrations ranged from 4.2–134 mg/L with a mean of 28 mg/L (Becker, 1976). By monitoring the corneal reflex and trapezius muscle response, Becker (1978) found that plasma thiopental levels of 39–42 mg/L were suitable for surgical anesthesia; the thiopental requirement is reduced by 70% with the co-administration of 67% nitrous oxide. The blood/plasma concentration ratio of thiopental is 1.0; the terminal elimination half-life of the drug has been found to average 11.5 hours in surgical patients (Morgan et al., 1981a) and 26 hours in women undergoing caesarian section (Morgan et al., 1981b).

Thiopental is used in the treatment of cranial injury to lower intracranial pressure and to reduce cerebral oxygen demand. Doses of 2–10 mg/kg by intravenous bolus injection are often given, followed by constant infusion of 3–5 mg/kg/hour, to maintain plasma thiopental concentrations between 40 and 100 mg/L for several days; concentrations of pentobarbital, a metabolite, usually average 10% of the thiopental value. The elimination kinetics of the drug become non-linear with these high doses, such that half-lives of up to 60 hours are observed. After termination of the infusion, assessment of neurologic function is usually possible when plasma thiopental levels fall to 20–30 mg/L (Stanski et al., 1980; Turcant et al., 1985).

Metabolism and Excretion. The rapid initial decline of thiopental plasma concentrations has been shown to be due to redistribution to other tissues, primarily the lean body mass, rather than metabolism of the drug, which is extensive but slow. At 30 minutes after an intravenous injection, the highly perfused viscera contain about 5% of the drug, the fat, 18%, and the lean body mass, 75% (Price et al., 1960). Only 0.3% of an administered dose of thiopental is excreted unchanged in urine over a 48 hour period. The biotransformation of the compound has not been well investigated in man, but it is known that 10–25% of a dose is excreted in the urine as a carboxylic acid product of side-chain oxidation, and that a lesser amount undergoes desulfuration to pentobarbital (Brodie et al., 1950).

Toxicity. Thiopental causes fewer side-effects than many other anesthetic agents, but occasionally anaphylaxis occurs in sensitive individuals (Barjenbruch and Jones, 1972; Baldwin, 1979; Dolovich et al., 1980).

Numerous fatalities have resulted due to accidental or intentional overdosage of thiopental; the following tissue distribution was noted in 4 anesthetic deaths in which adequate ventilation was not maintained (Campbell, 1960):

Thiopental Concentrations in Anesthetic Fatalities (mg/L or mg/kg)

	Blood	Brain	Liver	Kidney	Urine	Fat
Average	19	20	53	23	13	30
(Range)	(11–26)	(8–70)	(32–79)	(16–41)	(13)	(2–124)

In self-administered overdosage, blood thiopental concentrations as high as 279 and 392 mg/L and as low as 6–14 mg/L have been reported (Winek et al., 1969; Yip, 1974; Backer et al., 1975; Bruce et al., 1977; Noirfalise, 1979).

Analysis. Thiopental may be conveniently analyzed in biological fluids and tissues by ultraviolet spectrophotometry (Brodie et al., 1950; Bruce et al., 1977). Gas chromatography has employed flame-ionization (Becker, 1976; Bruce et al., 1977; Van Hamme and Ghoneim, 1978; Kulpmann et al., 1983) or nitrogen-selective detection (Sennello and Kohn, 1974; Jung et al., 1981). Liquid chromatography offers a convenient and sensitive means of measuring this drug (Freeman, 1981; Salvadori et al., 1981; Kelner and Bailey, 1983; Levine et al., 1983; Houdret et al., 1985; Schmid and Wolf, 1989; Celardo and Bonati, 1990).

References

R.C. Backer, Y.H. Caplan and C.E. Duncan. Thiopental suicide—case report. Clin. Tox. 8: 282–287, 1975.

A.C. Baldwin. Thiopentone anaphylaxis. Anaesthesia 34: 333–335, 1979.

K.P. Barjenbruch and J.R. Jones. Thiopental anaphylaxis: a case report. Anesth. Anal. 51: 113–116, 1972.

K.E. Becker, Jr. Gas chromatographic assay for free and total plasma levels of thiopental. Anesthesiology 45: 656–660, 1976.

K.E. Becker, Jr. Plasma levels of thiopental necessary for anesthesia. Anesthesiology 49: 192–196, 1978.

G.L. Blackman, G.J. Jordan and J.D. Paull. Analysis of thiopentone in human plasma by high-performance liquid chromatography. J. Chrom. 145: 492–495, 1978.

B.B. Brodie, L.C. Mark, E.M. Papper et al. The fate of thiopental in man and a method for its estimation in biological materials. J. Pharm. Exp. Ther. 98: 85–96, 1950.

A.M. Bruce, J.S. Oliver and H. Smith. A suicide by thiopentone injection. For. Sci. 9: 205–207, 1977.

J.E. Campbell. Deaths associated with anesthesia. J. For. Sci. 5: 501–549, 1960.

A. Celardo and M. Bonati. Determination of thiopental measured in human blood by reversed-phase high-performance liquid chromatography. J. Chrom. 527: 220–225, 1990.

J.H. Christensen and F. Andreasen. Determination of thiopental by high pressure liquid chromatography. Acta Pharm. Tox. 44: 260–263, 1979.

J. Dolovich, S. Evans, D. Rosenbloom et al. Anaphylaxis due to thiopental sodium anesthesia. Can. Med. Asso. J. 123: 292–294, 1980.

D.J. Freeman. Monitoring serum thiopental concentrations by liquid chromatography. Clin Chem. 27: 1942–1943, 1981.

N. Houdret, M. Lhermitte, G. Lalau et al. Determination of thiopental and pentobarbital in plasma using high-performance liquid chromatography. J. Chrom. 343: 437–442, 1985.

D. Jung, M. Mayersohn and D. Perrier. Gas-chromatographic assay for thiopental in plasma, with use of a nitrogen-specific detector. Clin. Chem. 27: 113–115, 1981.

M. Kelner and D.N. Bailey. Reversed-phase liquid-chromatographic simultaneous analysis for thiopental and pentobarbital in serum. Clin. Chem. 29: 1097–1100, 1983.

W.R. Kulpmann, R. Fitzlaff, A. Spring and H. Dietz. Thiopental monitoring by gas-chromatography. J. Clin. Chem. Clin. Biochem. 21: 181–184, 1983.

B. Levine, R. Blanke and J. Valentour. Liquid chromatographic analysis of thiopental in blood and tissues. J. Anal. Tox. 7: 207–208, 1983.

D.J. Morgan, G.L. Blackman, J.D. Paull and L.J. Wolf. Pharmacokinetics and plasma binding of thiopental. I: studies in surgical patients. Anesthesiology 54: 468–473, 1981a.

D.J. Morgan, G.L. Blackman, J.D. Paull and L.J. Wolf. Pharmacokinetics and plasma binding of thiopental. II: studies at cesarean section. Anesthesiology 54: 474–480, 1981b.

A. Noirfalise. Fatal intoxication by thiopental. For. Sci. 11: 167, 1978.

H.L. Price, P.J. Kovnat, J.N. Safer et al. The uptake of thiopental by body tissues and its relation to the duration of narcosis. Clin. Pharm. Ther. 1: 16–22, 1960.

C. Salvadori, R. Farinotti, P. Duvaldestin and A. Dauphin. Liquid chromatography determination of thiopentone in human plasma. Ther. Drug Mon. 3: 171–176, 1981.

R.W. Schmid and C. Wolf. Simultaneous determination of thiopental and its metabolite, pentobarbital, in blood by high-performance liquid chromatography and post-column photochemical reaction. J. Pharm. Biomed. Anal. 7: 1749–1756, 1989.

L.T. Sennello and F.E. Kohn. Gas chromatographic determination of thiopental in plasma using an alkali flame ionization detector. Anal. Chem. 46: 752–754, 1974.

D.R. Stanski, F.G. Mihm, M.H. Rosenthal and S.M. Kalman. Pharmacokinetics of high-dose thiopental used in cerebral resuscitation. Anesthesiology 53: 169–171, 1980.

A. Turcant, A. Delhumeau, A. Premel-Cabic et al. Thiopental pharmacokinetics under conditions of long-term infusion. Anesthesiology 63: 50–54, 1985.

M.J. Van Hamme and M.M. Ghoneim. A sensitive gas chromatograph assay for thiopentone in plasma. Brit. J. Anaesth. 50: 143–145, 1978.

C.L. Winek, W.D. Collom and E.R. Davis. Death from rectal thiopental. Clin. Tox. 2: 75–79, 1969.

M.W. Yip. Personal communication, 1974.

Thioridazine

T½: 26–36 hr
Vd: 18 L/kg
Fb: 0.96
pKa: 9.5

Occurrence and Usage. Thioridazine (Mellaril, Melleril) is an effective antipsychotic phenothiazine derivative that was first synthesized in 1958 and made clinically available in 1959. The drug is administered as the hydrochloride in daily oral doses of 100–800 mg in tablet form or as a liquid concentrate.

Blood Concentrations. Young adults given a single 25 mg oral dose developed average serum concentrations of thioridazine, mesoridazine and sulforidazine of 0.05, 0.17 and 0.05 mg/L, respectively, at 4 hours post-dose (Cohen and Sommer, 1988). Following a single oral 100 mg dose of thioridazine administered to 5 volunteers, maximal serum concentrations of the unchanged drug averaged 0.24 mg/L at 1.7 hours; of mesoridazine, 0.32 mg/L at 4 hours; of sulforidazine, 0.08 mg/L at 6.9 hours; and of thioridazine ring sulfoxide, 0.18 mg/L at 5 hours. During chronic oral administration of 400 mg daily of the drug to patients, the following steady-state serum concentrations were observed: thioridazine, 0.64 mg/L (range, 0.14–2.60); mesoridazine, 0.49 mg/L (range, 0.10–1.37); sulforidazine, 0.18 mg/L (range, 0.03–0.52); and ring sulfoxide, 1.20 mg/L (range, 0.04–3.76). Proportionate changes were seen in these levels with changes in daily dosages (Axelsson and Martensson, 1977). Using a nonspecific fluorometric method, it was found that steady-state plasma concentrations averaged 3.9 mg/L in patients who were maintained on a daily oral thioridazine dosage of 437 mg (deJonghe et al., 1973). The whole blood/plasma concentration ratio of the parent drug ranged from 0.64–0.86 in 12 patients (Shvartsburd et al., 1984).

Metabolism and Excretion. Metabolism of thioridazine is known to proceed primarily via oxidation of the side-chain sulfur atom to a sulfoxide (mesoridazine) and a sulfone (sulforidazine), both of which are active antipsychotics; and via corresponding oxidation of the ring sulfur atom, which may result in loss of activity. N-demethylation and ring hydroxylation are relatively minor pathways (Vanderheeren and Muusze, 1977; Papadopoulos et al., 1985). Only 2.5–17% of a daily dose is excreted as thioridazine or its known metabolites in the 24 hour urine; 0.5% is excreted as thioridazine, an equal amount as mesoridazine, and about 1% as the ring sulfoxide. A number of other minor metabolites are also present (Martensson et al., 1975).

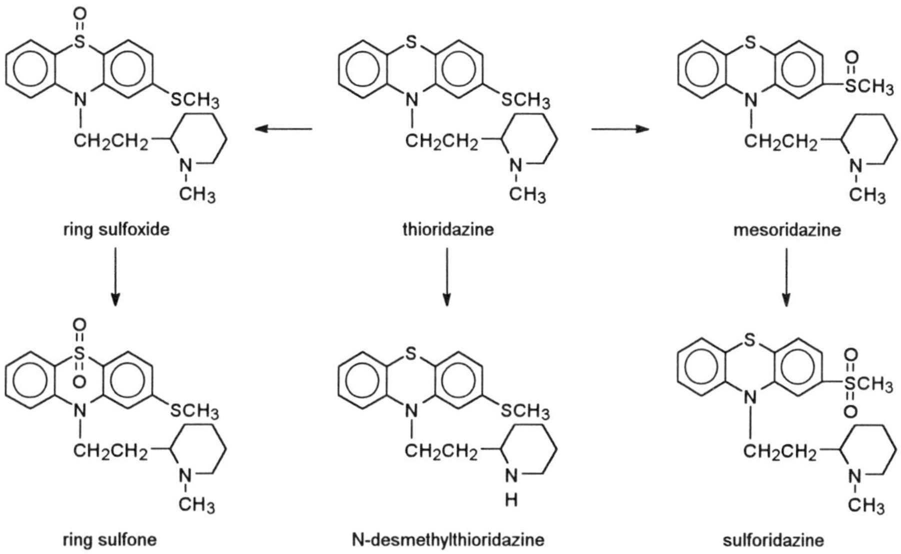

ring sulfoxide   thioridazine   mesoridazine

ring sulfone   N-desmethylthioridazine   sulforidazine

Toxicity. Adverse reactions to thioridazine include drowsiness, confusion, blurred vision, dry mouth, blood dyscrasias, convulsive seizures, hypotension, and electrocardiographic changes. No relationship has been observed between EKG changes and plasma levels of thioridazine or its metabolites (Gottschalk et al., 1978a). Ventricular arrhythmias, occasionally fatal, have been noted in patients receiving therapeutic doses (Rosenquist et al., 1971; Sydney, 1973).

Overdosage with thioridazine is not an infrequent event and a fair number of nonfatal and fatal cases have been reported. Thioridazine blood or plasma concentrations obtained with nonspecific spectrophotometric or fluorometric methods even after massive overdosage are not greatly elevated over concentrations observed during therapeutic administration, and diagnosis of thioridazine intoxication is best made on the basis of gas chromatography results, clinical history or liver concentrations in fatal cases. Serum concentrations ranging from 2.4–11.8 mg/L have been recorded during nonfatal intoxications, using a spectrophotometric method (Tompsett, 1968; Hassoun, 1976).

Blood concentrations of 0.8–13 mg/L (average, 4.8) and liver concentrations of 25–513 mg/kg (average, 109) were observed using fluorometry in 8 cases of fatal overdosage, whereas in 6 psychiatric patients receiving thioridazine who died of causes other than drug overdosage, blood concentrations of 0.6–3.6 mg/L (average, 1.7) and liver concentrations of 1.0–12 mg/kg (average, 5.7) were found (Baselt et al., 1978). In 8 other acute fatalities, concentrations have ranged from 1–18 mg/L (average, 5.4) in blood, 35–110 mg/kg (average, 69) in liver, and 18–70 mg/kg (average, 47) in kidney (Curry, 1962; Bonnichsen et al., 1970; Joubert and Olivier, 1974; McCutcheon, 1976; Donlon and Tupin, 1977; Yamarellos, 1981). The following data from 8 fatal cases illustrate the distribution of thioridazine and its metabolites as determined by a specific liquid chromatographic technique (Allender, 1985):

Thioridazine Concentrations in Fatal Cases (mg/L or mg/kg)

Drug	Blood	Liver	Urine	Gastric
Thioridazine	2.5	39	1.4	390 mg
	(0.3–8.5)	(3.6–154)	(0.7–2.0)	(0.3–2500)
Thioridazine ring sulfoxide	2.8	9.2	2.1	8.6 mg
	(0.2–11)	(1.0–29)	(0–5.1)	(0.03–37)
Thioridazine disulfoxide	2.3	4.1	3.1	3.6 mg
	(0.7–7.0)	(0.3–15)	(0.9–5.2)	(2.4–4.8)
Mesoridazine	2.2	7.7	12	3.8 mg
	(0.07–7.2)	(0.2–28)	(7.3–16)	(1.9–6.8)
Sulforidazine	0.1	1.0	1.3	1.8
	(0–0.5)	(0–2.0)	(0–7.8)	(0–2.1)
Northioridazine	0.2	0.7	0	0
	(0–1)	(0–1.5)	(0)	(0)

Thioridazine may occasionally exhibit postmortem redistribution; in 9 decedents, heart blood/femoral blood concentration ratios averaged 1.4 (range, 0.4–2.8), but in only 3 of the cases did the ratio exceed 1.0 (Prouty and Anderson, 1990).

Analysis. Fluorimetry has been a popular method for the analysis of thioridazine (Pacha, 1969), but has the disadvantage of measuring the sum of the drug and its non-phenolic metabolites. Several gas chromatographic procedures have been developed for the quantitation of thioridazine and its major metabolites in biological fluids, all of which utilize flame-ionization detection (Martensson et al., 1975; Vanderheeren et al., 1976; Dinovo et al., 1976; Ng and Crammer, 1977). Liquid chromatographic methods have also been described (McCutcheon, 1979; Skinner et al., 1981; Kilts et al., 1982; Wells et al., 1983; Allender, 1985; Svensson et al., 1990). Thioridazine and its metabolites are stable in plasma stored frozen for up to 1 year (Gottschalk et al., 1978b). However, upon exposure of spiked plasma specimens to indirect sunlight during the analytical extraction process, thioridazine concentrations decreased by 17–22% (Eap et al., 1993).

References

W.J. Allender. High-pressure liquid chromatographic determination of thioridazine and its major metabolites in biological tissues and fluids. J. Chrom. Sci. 24: 541–545, 1985.

R. Axelsson and E. Martensson. The concentration pattern of nonconjugated thioridazine metabolites in serum by thioridazine treatment and its relationship to physiological and clinical variables. Curr. Ther. Res. 20: 561–586, 1977.

R.C. Baselt, J.A. Wright and E.M. Gross. Human tissue distribution of thioridazine during therapy and after poisoning. J. Anal. Tox. 2: 41–43, 1978.

R. Bonnichsen, P. Geertinger and A.C. Maehly. Toxicological data on phenothiazine drugs in autopsy cases. Z. Rechtsmed. 67: 158–169, 1970.

B.M. Cohen and B.R. Sommer. Metabolism of thioridazine in the elderly. J. Clin. Psychopharm. 8: 336–339, 1988.

A.S. Curry. Twenty-one uncommon cases of poisoning. Brit. Med. J. 1: 687, 1962.

F.E.R.E.R. deJonghe, H.J. van der Helm, H.F.A. Schalken and J.H. Thiel. Therapeutic effect and plasma level of thioridazine. Acta Psych. Scand. 19: 535–545, 1973.

E.C. Dinovo, L.A. Gottschalk, B.R. Nandi and P.G. Geddes. GLC analysis of thioridazine, mesoridazine, and their metabolites. J. Pharm. Sci. 65: 667–669, 1976.

P.T. Donlon and J.P. Tupin. Successful suicides with thioridazine and mesoridazine. Arch. Gen. Psych. 34: 955–957, 1977.

C.B. Eap, L. Koeb and P. Baumann. Artifacts in the analysis of thioridazine and other neuroloptics. J. Pharm. Biomed. Anal. 11: 451–457, 1993.

L.A. Gottschalk, E. Dinovo, R. Biener and B.R. Nandi. Plasma concentrations of thioridazine metabolites and ECG abnormalities. J. Pharm. Sci. 67: 155–157, 1978a.

L.A. Gottschalk, E.C. Dinovo and B.R. Nandi. The assay of plasma concentration of thioridazine and its metabolites as a function of time. Comm. Psychopharm. 2: 475–479, 1978b.

A. Hassoun. Personal communication, 1976.

P.H. Joubert and J.A. Olivier. Fatal suicidal ingestion of thioridazine. Clin. Tox. 133–138, 1974.

C.D. Kilts, K.S. Patrick, G.R. Breese and R.B. Mailman. Simultaneous determination of thioridazine and its S-oxidized and N-demethylated metabolites using high-performance liquid chromatography on radially compressed silica. J. Chrom. 231: 377–391, 1982.

E. Martensson, G. Nyberg, R. Axelsson and K. Serck-Hansen. Quantitative determination of thioridazine and nonconjugated thioridazine metabolites in serum and urine of psychiatric patients. Curr. Ther. Res. 18: 687–700, 1975.

J.R. McCutcheon. Personal communication, 1976.

J.R. McCutcheon. Reverse-phase HPLC determination of thioridazine and mesoridazine in whole blood. J. Anal. Tox. 3: 105–107, 1979.

C.H. Ng and J.L. Crammer. Measurement of thioridazine in blood and urine. Brit. J. Clin. Pharm. 4: 173–183, 1977.

W.L. Pacha. A method for the fluorimetric determination of thioridazine (Mellaril) or mesoridazine (Lidanil) in plasma. Experientia 25: 103–104, 1969.

A.S. Papadopoulos, J.L. Crammer and D.A. Cowan. Phenolic metabolites of thioridazine in man. Xenobiotica 15: 309–316, 1985.

R.W. Prouty and W.H. Anderson. The forensic science implications of site and temporal influences on post-mortem blood-drug concentrations. J. For. Sci. 35: 243–270, 1990.

R.J. Rosenquist, W.W. Brauer and J.N. Mork. Recurrent major ventricular arrhythmias. Minn. Med. 54: 877–879, 1971.

A. Shvartsburd, V. Nwokeafo and R.C. Smith. Red blood cell and plasma levels of thioridazine and mesoridazine in schizophrenic patients. Psychopharmacology 82: 55-61, 1984.

T. Skinner, R. Gochnauer and M. Linnoila. Liquid chromatographic method to measure thioridazine and its active metabolites in plasma. Acta Pharm. Tox. 48: 223–226, 1981.

C. Svensson, G. Nyberg, M. Soomagi and E. Martensson. Determination of the serum concentrations of thioridazine and its main metabolites using a solid-phase extraction technique and high-performance liquid chromatography. J. Chrom. 529: 229–236, 1990.

M.A. Sydney. Ventricular arrhythmias associated with use of thioridazine hydrochloride in alcohol withdrawal. Brit. Med. J. 4: 467, 1973.

S.L. Tompsett. The spectrophotometric determination of phenothiazine drugs in blood serum. Acta Pharm. Tox. 26: 298–302, 1968.

F.A.J. Vanderheeren, D.J.C.J. Theunis and M.T. Rosseel. Gas-liquid chromatographic determination of perazine, thioridazine and thioridazine metabolites in human plasma. J. Chrom. 120: 123–128, 1976.

F.A.J. Vanderheeren and R.G. Muusze. Plasma levels and half lives of thioridazine and some of its metabolites. Eur. J. Clin. Pharm. 11: 135–140, 1977.

C.E. Wells. E.C. Juenge and W.B. Furman. Simultaneous assay of thioridazine and its major metabolites in plasma at single dosage levels with a novel report of two ring sulfoxides of thioridazine. J. Pharm. Sci. 72: 622–625, 1983.

P. Yamarellos. Personal communication, 1981.

Thiothixene

T½: 12–36 hr
Vd: ?
Fb: ?
pKa: ?

Occurrence and Usage. Thiothixene (Navane) is a sulfonated thioxanthene derivative that was synthesized in 1964 and made available as an antipsychotic drug in 1965. It is administered as the hydrochloride orally or by intramuscular injection in doses of 20–60 mg daily.

Blood Concentrations. Following administration of a single oral 20 mg dose to 5 volunteers, plasma concentrations of thiothixene determined by a fluorometric method averaged about 0.050 mg/L at 1.5 hours and declined to about 0.015 mg/L by 12 hours. Less than 10% of the plasma fluorescence was due to the N-demethyl metabolite (Mjorndal and Oreland, 1971). With the same method, plasma concentrations ranging from 0.010–0.100 mg/L were observed in patients receiving chronic daily therapy with 0.1–0.9 mg/kg (7–63 mg/70 kg) of the drug (Bergling et al., 1975). In patients receiving 15–60 mg on a chronic daily oral basis, plasma concentrations measured with a highly specific method were found to range from 0.010–0.023 mg/L at 2 hours after the last dose (Hobbs et al., 1974). Mavroidis et al. (1984) suggest that the optimal range for plasma levels in schizophrenic patients is 0.002–0.015 mg/L, as measured by gas chromatography. Erythrocyte thiothixene concentrations are only 15–33% of serum levels (Yesavage et al., 1983).

Metabolism and Excretion. The only known metabolite of thiothixene in man is the N-demethylated compound resulting from loss of the piperazine methyl group; comparison with other related compounds suggests that sulfoxidation, piperazine ring fission and phenolic hydroxylation are possible pathways for metabolism of this drug. In rats given a single oral labeled dose, 3% was excreted in urine over a 4 day period and the balance in feces, largely as unidentified metabolites (Hobbs, 1968).

Toxicity. Adverse reactions to thiothixene include drowsiness, dry mouth, blurred vision, tachycardia, EKG changes, hypotension, syncope, extrapyramidal symptoms, tardive dyskinesia and blood dyscrasias. Patients with higher steady-state plasma thiothixene levels tend to be at risk for developing tardive dyskinesia (Yesavage et al., 1987). An adult survived the ingestion of 800 mg of the drug after developing a blood level of 0.52 mg/L (Kemal and Imami, 1985).

In a case of fatal intoxication following ingestion of 250 mg of thiothixene and an unknown amount of doxepin, the thiothixene concentration in blood (the only specimen available) was 0.13 mg/L as determined by a fluorometric method (Baselt, 1977).

Analysis. The fluorometric procedure for the determination of thiothixene in biological fluids (Mjorndal and Oreland, 1971) is highly sensitive and convenient, although it yields concentrations approximately twice those obtained with a more specific mass fragmentographic technique (Hobbs et al., 1974). Liquid chromatographic methods have also been described (Narasimhachari et al., 1982; Dilger et al., 1988).

References

R.C. Baselt. Unpublished results, 1977.

R. Bergling, T. Mjorndal, L. Oreland et al. Plasma levels and clinical effects of thioridazine and thiothixene. J. Clin. Pharm. 15: 178–186, 1975.

C. Dilger, Z. Salama and H. Jaeger. Improved high performance liquid chromatographic method for the determination of thiothixene in human serum. Arz. Forsch. 38: 1522–1525, 1988.

D.C. Hobbs. Metabolism of thiothixene. J. Pharm. Sci. 57: 105–111, 1968.

D.C. Hobbs, W.M. Welch, M.J. Short et al. Pharmacokinetics of thiothixene in man. Clin. Pharm. Ther. 16: 473–478, 1974.

M. Kemal and R.H. Imami. Acute thiothixene overdose. J. Anal. Tox. 9: 94–95, 1985.

M.L. Mavroidis, D.R. Kanter, J. Hirschowitz and D.L. Garver. Clinical relevance of thiothixene plasma levels. J. Clin. Psychopharm. 4: 155–157, 1984.

T. Mjorndal and L. Oreland. Determination of thioxanthenes in plasma at therapeutic concentrations. Acta Pharm. Tox. 29: 295–302, 1971.

N. Narasimhachari, M. Mumtaz, S. Golden and R.O. Friedel. Separation and quantitation of cis- and trans-thiothixene in human plasma by high-performance liquid chromatography. J. Chrom. 233: 257–267, 1982.

J.A. Yesavage, C.A. Holman, R. Cohn and L. Lombrozo. Correlation of initial thiothixene serum levels and clinical response. Arch. Gen. Psych. 40: 301–304, 1983.

J.A. Yesavage, E.D. Tanke and J.I. Sheikh. Tardive dyskinesia and steady-state serum levels of thiothixene. Arch. Gen. Psych. 44: 913–915, 1987.

Timolol

T½: 2–6 hr
Vd: 1–3 L/kg
Fb: 0.10
pKa: 8.8

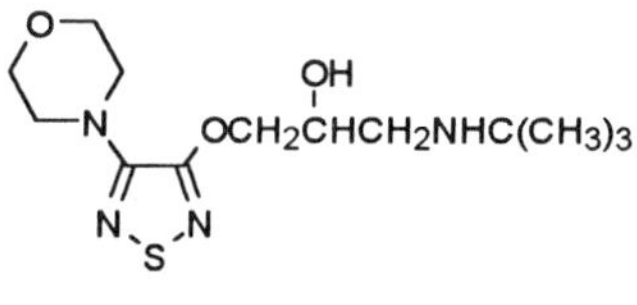

Occurrence and usage. Timolol (Blocadren) is a potent non-selective beta-adrenoceptor antagonist used for the treatment of systemic hypertension, angina pectoris and glaucoma. Timolol is available as the maleate salt in ophthalmic solutions in concentrations of 0.25–0.5% and in tablets of 5–20 mg for oral administration. Daily doses of up to 60 mg are given.

Blood Concentrations. Following a single oral dose of 20 mg of timolol to 5 healthy volunteers, peak plasma concentrations ranging from 0.05–0.11 mg/L (average, 0.08) occurred within 0.5–3 hours (Fourtillan et al., 1981). Steady-state plasma concentrations ranging from 0.04–0.23 mg/L (average, 0.11) were attained following daily oral doses of 15 mg 3 times daily to 8 adults aged 21–40 and weighing 56–79 kg (Singh et al., 1980).

Metabolism and Excretion. Timolol is almost completely absorbed after oral administration. It is metabolized in the liver primarily by oxidation and hydrolytic cleavage of the morpholine ring. After oral administration, approximately 72% of a dose is excreted in urine and 6% in feces over a 3 day period; urinary excretion products include unchanged drug (20%) and 2 products of ring cleavage, metabolite I (10%) and metabolite II (30%) (Tocco et al., 1975a, 1980).

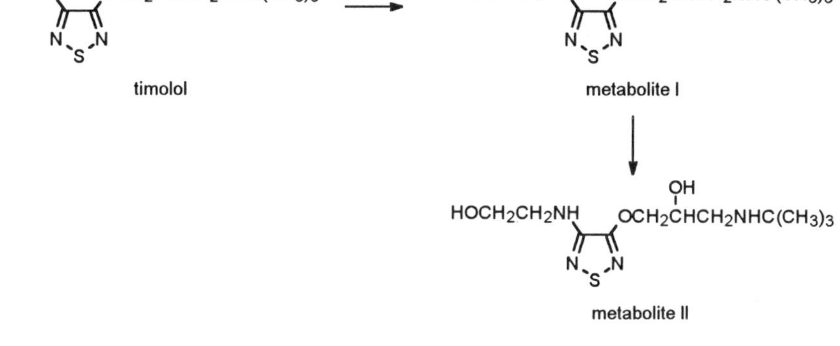

timolol

metabolite I

metabolite II

Toxicity. Timolol is capable of producing dizziness, headache, itching, bradycardia, hallucinations, bronchospasm, hypotension, cardiac arrest and death in overdosage.

Analysis. Timolol and its metabolites may be measured in biological fluids by gas chromatography with electron-capture (Tocco et al., 1975b; Sutton and Richardson, 1992) or mass spectrometric detection (Tocco et al., 1980; Fourtillan et al., 1981). Liquid chromatographic techniques have also been reported (Gregg and Jack, 1983; Lennard and Parkin, 1985; Kubota et al., 1990).

References

J.B. Fourtillan, M.A. Lefebvre, J. Girault et al. Mass fragmentographic determination of timolol in human plasma and urine. J. Pharm. Sci. 70: 573–575, 1981.

M.R. Gregg and D.B. Jack. Determination of timolol in plasma and breast milk using high-performance liquid chromatography with electrochemical detection. J. Chrom. 305: 244–249, 1984.

K. Kubota, H. Nakamura, E. Koyama et al. Simple and sensitive determination of timolol in human plasma and urine by high-performance liquid chromatography with ultraviolet detection. J. Chrom. 533: 255–263, 1990.

M.S. Lennard and S. Parkin. Timolol determination in plasma and urine by high-performance liquid chromatography with ultraviolet detection. J. Chrom. 338: 249–252, 1985.

B.N. Singh, F.M. Williams, R.M.L. Whitlock et al. Plasma timolol levels and systolic time intervals. Clin. Pharm. Ther. 28: 159–166, 1980.

B.M. Sutton and R.A. Richardson. Assay of timolol in human plasma using gas chromatography with electron-capture detection. J. Chrom. 581: 277–280, 1992.

D.J. Tocco, A.E.W. Duncan, F.A. Deluna et al. Physiological disposition and metabolism of timolol in man and laboratory animals. Drug Met. Disp. 3: 361–370, 1975a.

D.J. Tocco, F.A. Deluna and A.E.W. Duncan. Electron-capture GLC determination of timolol in human plasma and urine. J. Pharm. Sci. 64: 1879–1881, 1975b.

D.J. Tocco, A.E.W. Duncan, F.A. Deluna et al. Timolol metabolism in man and laboratory animals. Drug Met. Disp. 8: 236–240, 1980.

Tin

T½: ?
Vd: ?   Sn
Fb: ?

Occurrence and Usage. In man, tin is a trace element for which there is no apparent biological requirement. The metal and its inorganic salts have numerous applications in metallurgy and other industries, including their use as tanning agents, polishing compounds and metal coatings ("tin" cans). The organic compounds of tin, usually ethyl, butyl or phenyl derivatives, are widely used as fungicides, pesticides, antihelmintics and stabilizers for plastics. The current threshold limit values (expressed as Sn) for industrial usage are 10 mg/m^3 for tin oxide, 2 mg/m^3 for other inorganic compounds and 0.1 mg/m^3 for organic compounds of tin. The soluble compounds are well-absorbed after ingestion or inhalation, and the organic forms are known to be absorbed through the skin as well.

Blood Concentrations. The average concentration of tin in the blood of normal subjects is 0.14 mg/L, although not all specimens contain detectable amounts of the metal. Most or all of this amount, which resides primarily in the erythrocytes, is believed to originate in the daily diet. A typical daily diet contains 3.6 mg of tin, the major portion of which is derived from canned foods (Schroeder et al., 1964). Serum tin concentrations average 0.0005 mg/L in normal subjects (Versieck and Vanballenberghe, 1991).

Metabolism and Excretion. Of an approximate 4 mg of tin that is ingested daily in the diet by urban adults, over 99% is excreted unabsorbed in the feces and less than 1% is eliminated in the urine. Tin accumulates to only a small extent in the body with age and, when present in tissues, is rather randomly distributed. Lung, liver and kidney specimens from Americans usually contain from 0.2–1.2 mg/kg of the metal. Specimens from primitive peoples may contain little or none. Tin concentrations in the urine of Americans have been estimated to average 0.023 mg/L, with a range of 0–0.040 mg/L (Schroeder et al., 1964).

The organic forms of tin behave as liposoluble compounds and, unlike inorganic tin, are rapidly distributed to the central nervous system. The compounds are believed to undergo slow degradation via oxidative dealkylation (Barnes and Stoner, 1959).

Toxicity. Tin and its inorganic compounds are relatively nontoxic and are not considered important industrial hazards. Some of the compounds cause skin and mucous membrane irritation due to their acidity or alkalinity in aqueous solution. Exposure to tin oxide dusts has caused benign pneumoconiosis in workers (Oyanguren et al., 1958; Schuler et al., 1958). Nausea, vomiting, and diarrhea were produced in volunteers who ingested canned juice containing 1370 mg/L of tin, whereas no effects were observed at concentrations of 498–730 mg/L (Benoy et al., 1971).

The organotin compounds, especially the tri- and tetraalkyl derivatives, present a more serious hazard. Exposure to these substances can cause local irritation, cerebral edema, hepatic necrosis and death. Severe skin lesions have been observed in workers exposed to butyl tin derivatives (Lyle, 1958). A clinical trial of a diethyltin preparation for the treatment of furunculosis ended in disaster when 217 subjects developed tin poisoning and 100 of these persons died. The medication, found to contain the more toxic triethyltin as an impurity, was administered orally in doses of 90 mg/day for 8 days. The symptoms of poisoning appeared after a period of 4 days and included persistent head-ache, vertigo, visual disturbances, abdominal pain, vomiting and psychic disturbances. The more severely poisoned subjects developed partial paralysis and convulsions and died of respiratory or cardiac failure. Interstitial edema of the white matter of the brain was a characteristic finding at autopsy (Barnes and Stoner, 1959). Similar effects were produced by trimethyltin in 2 subjects who survived the poisoning episode (Fortemps et al., 1978) and by a dimethyltin-trimethyltin combination in 6 workers who developed urine tin concentrations of 555–1600 µg/L (Rey et al., 1984).

Analysis. Colorimetric methods are used routinely to determine total tin (Corbin, 1973) or organotin (Sherman and Carlson, 1980) in urine. Gas chromatography has been used to assay alkyltin compounds in biological specimens (Arakawa et al., 1981; Ohhira and Matsui, 1990). Tin has been determined in blood and other tissues employing atomic absorption spectrometry after wet ashing (Chiba, 1987; Itami et al., 1991). Neutron activation analysis has also been described (Versieck and Vanballenberghe, 1991).

References

Y. Arakawa, O. Wada, T.H. Yu and H. Iwai. Rapid method for the determination of tetraakyltin compounds in various kinds of biological material by gas chromatography. J. Chrom. 207: 237–244, 1981.

J.M. Barnes and H.B. Stoner. The toxicology of tin compounds. Pharm. Rev. 11: 211–231, 1959.

C.J. Benoy, P.A. Hooper and R. Schneider. The toxicity of tin in canned fruit juices and solid foods. Food Cosmet. Tox. 9: 645–656, 1971.

M. Chiba. Determination of tin in biological materials by atomic-absorption spectrometry with a graphite furnace. J. Anal. Tox. 11: 125–130, 1987.

H.B. Corbin. Rapid and selective pyrocatechol violet method for tin. Anal. Chem. 45: 534–537, 1973.

E. Fortemps, G. Amand, A. Bomboir et al. Trimethyltin poisoning: report of two cases. Int. Arch. Occ. Env. Health 41: 1–6, 1978.

T. Itami, M. Ema, H. Amano and H. Kawasaki. Simple determination of tin in biological materials by atomic absorption spectrometry with a graphite furnace. J. Anal. Tox. 15: 119–122, 1991.

W.H. Lyle. Lesions of the skin in process workers caused by contact with butyl tin compounds. Brit. J. Ind. Med. 15: 193–196, 1958.

S. Ohhira and H. Matsui. Simultaneous determination of triphenyltin and its metabolites, mono- and diphenyltin, in biological materials by capillary gas chromatography. Bull. Env. Cont. Tox. 44: 294–301, 1990.

H. Oyanguren, R. Haddad and H. Maass. Stannosis. I. Environmental and experimental studies. Ind. Med. Surg. 27: 427–431, 1958.

C. Rey, H.J. Reinecke and R. Besser. Methyltin intoxication in six men: toxicologic and clinical aspects. Vet. Hum. Tox. 26: 121–122, 1984.

H.A. Schroeder, J.J. Balassa and I.H. Tipton. Abnormal trace metals in man: tin. J. Chron. Dis. 17: 483–502, 1964.

P. Schuler, E. Cruz, C. Guijon et al. Stannosis. II. Clinical study. Ind. Med. Surg. 27: 432–435, 1958.

L.R. Sherman and T.L. Carlson. A modified phenylfluorone method for determining organotin compounds in the ppb and sub-ppb range. J. Anal. Tox. 4: 31–33, 1980.

J. Versieck and L. Vanballenberghe. Determination of tin in human blood serum by radiochemical neutron activation analysis. Anal. Chem. 63: 1143–1146, 1991.

Tobramycin

T½: 2–4 hr
Vd: 0.22–0.31 L/kg
Fb: 0–0.10
pKa: 6.7, 8.3, 9.9

Occurrence and Usage. Tobramycin (Nebcin) is an aminoglycoside antibiotic used clinically since 1972 in the treatment of serious gram-negative bacillary infections. It is supplied as the sulfate in 20–40 mg/mL solutions for intramuscular or intravenous injection in doses of 3–5 mg/kg per day, which are usually divided into 3 equal portions and administered at 8 hour intervals.

Blood Concentrations. Serum tobramycin concentrations in 10 patients with normal renal function averaged 6.8 mg/L at 0.5 hour, 3.9 mg/L at 2 hours, and 1.6 mg/L at 6 hours after the intravenous injection of 1 mg/kg (70 mg/70 kg) of the drug; the elimination half-life averaged 3.0 hours (Naber et al., 1973). After intramuscular administration of the same dose, peak serum concentrations in 4 volunteers ranged from 3.8–7.8 mg/L and occurred after 30–70 minutes (Pechere et al., 1976).

The half-life of tobramycin correlates directly with renal function impairment, and may be estimated (in hours) by multiplying the serum creatinine concentration (in mg/dL) by 2 (Naber et al., 1973). In 64 patients for whom the dosage schedule was individually adjusted to produce a peak tobramycin level of 6–10 mg/L (30 minutes after a 1 hour infusion) and a trough level of 0.5–2.0 mg/L, dosing intervals ranged from 4–48 hours and doses ranged from 0.3–15 mg/kg/day. Half-lives ranged from 0.5–8.6 hours in patients with normal serum creatinine, and up to 43 hours in those with elevated creatinine (Cipolle et al., 1980). Although the kinetic behavior of tobramycin is usually described by a one-compartment model, Schentag et al. (1978) found that a second, tissue compartment accumulates drug during multiple dosing; drug is eliminated from this compartment with an average half-life of 146 hours, causing a steady increase in peak and trough serum concentrations with repeated administration.

Metabolism and Excretion. Tobramycin is not known to be metabolized, but is eliminated in the urine as the parent drug by glomerular filtration. About 60% of an intravenous dose is eliminated within 6 hours in patients with normal renal function, and the complete dose is recoverable if the urine is collected for at least 10 days. Urine concentrations of 30–260 mg/L are produced during the first 3 hours after a 1 mg/kg intravenous dose. In 4 patients who died during tobramycin therapy, concentrations of the drug in renal cortex were found to exceed 20 mg/kg (Naber et al., 1973; Schentag et al., 1978).

Toxicity. Tobramycin produced ototoxicity, characterized by tinnitus, dizziness, or hearing loss, in only 21 of 3,506 patients receiving the drug. In most cases the effects were reversible. Ototoxicity is associated with doses of greater than 3 mg/kg/day given for 10 days or more (Neu and Bendush, 1976). Impairment of renal function, manifested by oliguria and azotemia, occurred in 5 of 33 tobramycin-treated patients but was usually reversible. The drug is considered to be much less nephrotoxic than gentamicin (Kumin, 1980).

Analysis. Microbiological assays for tobramycin and other aminoglycoside antibiotics have largely been supplanted by more sensitive and specific tests involving enzyme immunoassay, radioimmunoassay, and enzymatic radiochemical assay (Maitra et al., 1979a). Fluorometry (Csiba, 1979), gas chromatography (Mayhew and Gorback, 1978), and liquid chromatography (Anhalt and Brown, 1978; Maitra et al., 1979b; Barends et al., 1981; Kabra et al., 1983) have also been investigated. Serum specimens for tobramycin analysis from patients receiving concurrent therapy with carbenicillin or ticarcillin should be refrigerated or frozen, if not analyzed immediately, due to *in vitro* inactivation of the drug by these beta-lactam antibiotics (Pickering and Gearhart, 1979).

References

.P. Anhalt and S.D. Brown. High-performance liquid-chromatographic assay of aminoglycoside antibiotics in serum. Clin. Chem. 24: 1940–1947, 1978.

D.M. Barends, C.L. Zwaan and A. Hulshoff. Micro-determination of tobramycin in serum by high-performance liquid chromatography with ultraviolet detection. J. Chrom. 225: 417–426, 1981.

R.J. Cipolle, R.D. Seifert, D.E. Zaske and R.G. Strate. Systematically individualizing tobramycin dosage regimens. J. Clin. Pharm. 20: 570–580, 1980.

A. Csiba. Spectrofluorimetric method for aminoglycoside antibiotics. J. Pharm. Pharmac. 31: 115–116, 1979.

P.M. Kabra, P.K. Bhatnagar, M.A. Nelson et al. Liquid-chromatographic determination of tobramycin in serum with spectrophotometric detection. Clin. Chem. 29: 672–674, 1983.

G.D. Kumin. Clinical nephrotoxicity of tobramycin and gentamicin. J. Am. Med. Asso. 244: 1808–1810, 1980.

S.K. Maitra, T.T. Yoshikawa, L.B. Guze and M.C. Schotz. Determination of aminoglycoside antibiotics in biological fluids: a review. Clin. Chem. 25: 1361–1367, 1979a.

S.K. Maitra, T.T. Yoshikawa, J.L. Hansen et al. Quantitation of serum tobramycin concentration using high-pressure liquid chromatography. Am. J. Clin. Path. 71: 428–432, 1979b.

J.W. Mayhew and S.L. Gorbach. Gas-liquid chromatographic method for the assay of aminoglycoside antibiotics in serum. J. Chrom. 151: 133–146, 1978.

K.G. Naber, S.R. Westenfelder and P.O. Madsen. Pharmacokinetics of the aminoglycoside antibiotic tobramycin in humans. Antimicrob. Agents Chemother. 3: 469–473, 1973.

H.C. Neu and C.L. Bendush. Ototoxicity of tobramycin: a clinical overview. J. Infect. Dis. 134 (Suppl.): 206–218, 1976.

J.C. Pechere, B. Roy and R. Dugal. Distribution and elimination kinetics of intravenously and intramusculary administered tobramycin in man. Int. J. Clin. Pharm. 14: 313–318, 1976.

L.K. Pickering and P. Gearhart. Effect of time and concentration upon interaction between gentamicin, tobramycin, netilmicin, or amikacin and carbenicillin or ticarcillin. Antimicrob. Agents Chemother. 15: 592–596, 1979.

J.J. Schentag, G. Lasezkay, T.J. Cumbo et al. Accumulation pharmacokinetics of tobramycin. Antimicrob. Agents Chemother. 13: 649–656, 1978.

Tocainide

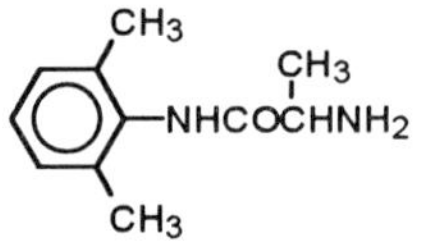

T½: 12–15 hr
Vd: 1.4 L/kg
Fb: 0.10–0.15
pKa: 7.7

Occurrence and Usage. Tocainide (Tonocard) is a primary amine analog of lidocaine with antiarrhythmic properties useful in the treatment of ventricular arrhythmias. It is available for oral administration as the hydrochloride in tablets containing 400 mg. The usual adult dose is between 1200 and 1800 mg/day in divided doses.

Blood Concentrations. Three normal subjects given a single oral dose of 400 mg of tocainide attained peak plasma concentrations of 1.6–1.8 mg/L in 0.5–2 hours. Following oral administration of 1200 mg/day in divided doses to 4 subjects, an average steady-state plasma concentration of 5.9 mg/L (range, 4.9–7.1) was reported (Graffner et al., 1980).

Metabolism and Excretion. The oral bioavailability of tocainide is virtually 100%. Its primary biotransformation pathway involves N-carboxy formation and conjugation with glucuronic acid (Elvin et al., 1980a). Approximately 30% of a dose is excreted in this form together with 39–52% of a dose as unchanged tocainide in the 72 hour urine (Elvin et al., 1980b).

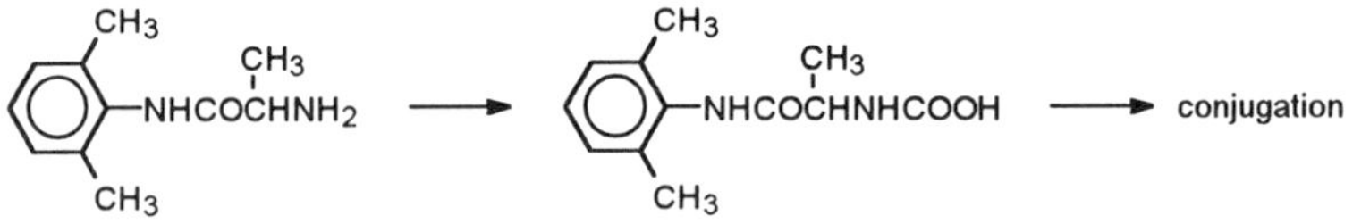

tocainide   tocainide carbaminic acid

Toxicity. Following overdose with tocainide, coma, seizures, ventricular fibrillation, pulmonary edema and respiratory arrest may occur.

A blood tocainide concentration of 78 mg/L was reported in a 26 year old comatose woman who ingested an unknown quantity of drug in a suicide attempt; death occurred within an hour after admission to hospital and a vitreous humor tocainide concentration of 9.3 mg/L and bile of 11 mg/L were found in postmortem specimens (Sperry et al., 1987). A 70 year old severely depressed man died following an overdose of tocainide tablets; the following distribution was noted (Barnfield and Kemmenoe, 1986):

Tocainide Concentrations in a Fatality (mg/L or mg/kg)

Blood	Liver	Urine	Gastric
74	80	550	3 mg

Analysis. Tocainamide has been determined in body fluids by gas chromatography with flame-ionization (Gettings et al., 1981; Smith, 1986), electron-capture (Venkataramanan and Axelson, 1978; Pillai et al. 1982), nitrogen-phosphorus (Beijnen et al., 1990) and mass spectrometric detection (Jones, 1986; Sperry et al., 1987). Liquid chromatography (Meffin et al., 1977; Wolshin et al., 1978; Reece and Stanley, 1980; Proelss and Townsend, 1986; Boutagy and O'Shea, 1987; Sperry et al., 1987) has also been employed.

References

C. Barnfield and A.V. Kemmenoe. A sudden death due to tocainide overdose. Hum. Tox. 5: 337–340, 1986.

J.H. Beijnen, R. Van Gijn and W.J.M. Underberg. Gas chromatographic analysis, with nitrogen detection, of tocainide in plasma. J. Pharm. Biomed. Anal. 8: 1101–1103, 1990.

J. Boutagy and K. O'Shea. Liquid-chromatographic determination of tocainide in plasma with N-acyl derivatives of tocainide as internal standards. Clin. Chem. 33: 1069, 1987.

A.T. Elvin, J.B. Keenaghan, E.W. Byrnes et al. Tocainide conjugation in humans. Novel biotransformation pathway for a primary amine. J. Pharm. Sci. 69: 47–49, 1980a.

S.D. Gettings, R.J. Flanagan and D.W. Holt. Simple method for the measurement of tocainide and lignocaine in blood plasma or serum using gas-liquid chromatography with flame ionization detection. J. Chrom. 225: 469–475, 1981.

C. Graffner, T. Conradson, S. Hofvendahl and L. Ryden. Tocainide kinetics after intravenous and oral administration in healthy subjects and in patients with acute myocardial infarction. Clin. Pharm. Ther. 27: 64–71, 1980.

C.W. Jones. Mass-spectrometric assay of tocainide in serum. Clin. Chem. 32: 503–505, 1986.

P.R. Meffin, S.R. Harapat and D.C. Harrison. High-pressure liquid chromatographic analysis of drugs in biological fluids II: Determination of an antiarrhythmic drug, tocainide, as its dansyl derivative using a fluorescence detector. J. Pharm. Sci. 66; 583–586, 1977.

G.K. Pillai, J.E. Aselson and K.M. McErlane. Electron-capture gas-liquid chromatographic determination of tocainide in biological fluids using fused silica capillary columns. J. Chrom. 229: 103–109, 1982.

H.F. Proelss and T.B. Townsend. Simultaneous liquid-chromatographic determination of five antiarrhythmic drugs and their major active metaboites in serum. Clin. Chem. 32: 1311–1317, 1986.

P.A. Reece and P.E. Stanley. High-performance liquid chromatographic assay for tocainide in human plasma: comparison with gas-liquid chromatographic assay. J. Chrom. 183: 109–114, 1980.

P.J. Smith. Measurement of tocainide in serum by capillary gas chromatography. Ther. Drug Mon. 8: 361–364, 1986.

K. Sperry, N. Wohlenberg and J.C. Standefer. Fatal intoxication by tocainide. J. For. Sci. 32: 1440–1446, 1987.

R. Venkataramanan and J.E. Axelson. Electron-capture detector GLC technique for estimating tocainide in biological fluids. J. Pharm. Sci. 67: 201–205, 1978.

E.M. Wolshin, M.H. Cavanaugh, C.V. Manion et al. Assay of tocainide in blood by high-pressure liquid chromatography. J. Pharm. Sci. 67: 1692–1695, 1978.

Tolbutamide

T½: 5–11 hr
Vd: 0.10–0.15 L/kg
Fb: 0.95–0.97
pKa: 5.3

CH_3

$SO_2NHCONHC_4H_9$

Occurrence and Usage. Tolbutamide (Orinase) is a sulfonylurea derivative that was synthesized in 1956 and is now used frequently as an oral hypoglycemic agent in the treatment of maturity-onset diabetes. Tablets for oral administration contain 250 or 500 mg of the free acid. It is administered in single or divided doses of 250–2000 mg daily.

Blood Concentrations. A single 500 mg oral dose given to 5 subjects resulted in an average peak serum concentration of about 43 mg/L after 8 hours (West and Johnson, 1960). A single 4000 mg oral dose in 2 subjects produced an average peak serum level of 183 mg/L by 5.5 hours, declining to 18 mg/L by 24 hours (Bladh and Norden, 1958). The serum half-life of the drug has been estimated at 7.2 hours (range, 5.1–11.1) in 10 healthy persons (Held et al., 1973). Serum concentrations of tolbutamide in 8 controlled diabetic patients receiving 1000–2000 mg on a chronic daily basis averaged 78 mg/L (range, 53–96) at 3–5 hours after the morning dose (Sheldon et al., 1965).

Metabolism and Excretion. Tolbutamide is extensively metabolized in man by oxidation of the p-methyl group. One of the metabolites, carboxytolbutamide, accumulates in plasma to the extent of 10–28% of the parent drug level (Stowers et al., 1958) but is pharmacologically inert (Louis et al., 1956). Up to 85% of a dose is excreted in the urine over a 48 hour period as carboxytolbutamide (57%) and hydroxymethyltolbutamide (28%), with little or no intact tolbutamide found present. An additional 9% of the dose is eliminated in the feces during this period (Nelson et al., 1960; Thomas and Ikeda, 1966).

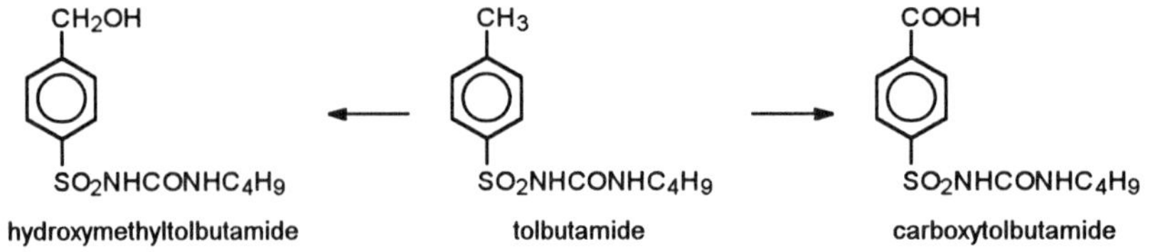

hydroxymethyltolbutamide   tolbutamide   carboxytolbutamide

Toxicity. Adverse reactions observed during tolbutamide therapy include nausea, headache, allergic skin manifestations, blood dyscrasias, and severe hypoglycemia. Irreversible cerebral damage occurred in one woman who ingested an overdose and became comatose; she survived for 6 months, never regaining consciousness (Cosnett, 1961).

At least 8 persons have died as a result of hypoglycemia induced by this drug (Seltzer, 1972). A nondiabetic young woman, who ingested 50 g of the drug for suicidal purposes and died in a hypoglycemic state after 18 hours, showed the following tissue concentrations at autopsy (Pribilla, 1968):

Tolbutamide Concentrations in a Fatal Case (mg/L or mg/kg)

Blood	Liver	Kidney	Urine	Gastric
640	930	1073	3510	80 mg

Analysis. Tolbutamide may be analyzed in biologic fluids by a colorimetric procedure (Spingler, 1957), which has been modified to allow its use in the determination of the metabolite (Nelson et al., 1960). A more convenient assay for tolbutamide involves the ultraviolet spectrophotometric measurement of the intact compound at 228 nm (Spingler and Kaiser, 1956; Forist et al., 1957; Bladh and Norden, 1958). Gas chromatographic procedures for the determination of tolbutamide have required the formation of a methyl derivative (Prescott and Redman, 1972; Simmons et al., 1972; Aggarwal and Sunshine, 1974; Schlicht et al., 1978; Hartvig et al., 1980). High-pressure liquid chromatography has also received attention as a means of assaying this compound and its metabolite in serum (Hill and Crechiolo, 1978; Hill and Chamberlain, 1978; Nation et al., 1978; Raghow and Meyer, 1981; Csillag et al., 1989).

References

V. Aggarwal and I. Sunshine. Determination of sulfonylureas and metabolites by pyrolysis gas chromatography. Clin. Chem. 20: 200–204, 1974.

E. Bladh and A. Norden. A method for determining 1-butyl-3-tolylsulphonylurea (Tolbutamide) in human blood serum. Acta Pharm. Tox. 14: 188–194, 1958.

J.E. Cosnett. Tolbutamide overdosage and irreversible cerebral damage. S. African Med. J. 35: 43–44, 1961.

K. Csillag, L. Vereczkey and B. Gachalyi. Simple high-performance liquid chromatographic method for the determination of tolbutamide and its metabolites in human plasma and urine using photodiodide-array detection. J. Chrom. 490: 355–363, 1989.

A.A. Forist, W.L. Miller, Jr., J. Krake and W.A. Struck. Determination of plasma levels of tolbutamide (1-butyl-3-tolylsulfonylurea, Orinase). Proc. Soc. Exp. Biol. Med. 96: 180–183, 1957.

P. Hartvig, C. Fagerlund and O. Gyllenhaal. Electron-capture gas chromatography of plasma sulphonylureas after extractive methylation. J. Chrom. 181: 17–24, 1980.

H. Held, R. Eisert and H.F. von Oldershausen. Pharmakokinetik von Glymidine (Glycodiazin) und Tolbutamid bei akuten und chronischen Leberschaeden. Arz. Forsch. 23: 1801–1807, 1973.

H.M. Hill and J. Chamberlain. Determination of oral anti-diabetic agents in human body fluids using high-performance liquid chromatography. J. Chrom. 149: 349–358, 1978.

R.E. Hill and J. Crechiolo. Determination of serum tolbutamide and chlorpropamide by high-performance liquid chromatography. J. Chrom. 145: 165–168, 1978.

L.H. Louis, S.S. Fajans, J.W. Conn et al. The structure of a urinary excretion product of 1-butyl-3-p-tolylsulfonylurea (Orinase). J. Am. Chem. Soc. 78: 5701–5702, 1956.

R.L. Nation, G.W. Peng and W.L. Chiou. Simple, rapid and micro high-pressure liquid chromatographic method for the simultaneous determination of tolbutamide and carboxytolbutamide in plasma. J. Chrom. 146: 121–131, 1978.

E. Nelson, I. O'Reilly and T. Chulski. Determination of carboxytolbutamide in urine. Clin. Chim. Acta 5: 774–776, 1960.

L.F. Prescott and D.R. Redman. Gas-liquid chromatographic estimation of tolbutamide and chlorpropamide in plasma. J. Pharm. Pharmac. 24: 713–716, 1972.

O. Pribilla. Ueber eine letale Vergiftung mit Tolbutamid (Rastinon) bei einer Nichtdiabetikerin. Arch. Tox. 23: 153–159, 1968.

G. Raghow and M.C. Meyer. High-performance liquid chromatographic assay of tolbutamide and carboxytolbutamide in human plasma. J. Pharm. Sci. 70: 1166–1168, 1981.

H.J. Schlicht, H.P. Gelbke and G. Schmidt. Gas chromatographic procedure for the simultaneous determination of five common antidiabetic drugs in blood. J. Chrom. 155: 178–181, 1978.

H.S. Seltzer. Drug-induced hypoglycemia. Diabetes 21: 955–966, 1972.

J. Sheldon, J. Anderson and L. Stoner. Serum concentration and urinary excretion of oral sulfonylurea compounds. Diabetes 14: 362–367, 1965.

D.L. Simmons, R.J. Ranz and P. Picotte. Determination of serum tolbutamide by gas chromatography. J. Chrom. 71: 421–426, 1972.

H. Spingler and F. Kaiser. Die Bestimmung von N-(4-Methyl-benzolsulfonyl)-N'-butyl-harnstoff in Serum. Arz. Forsch. 6: 760–762, 1956.

H. Spingler. Ueber einen Moeglichkeit zur Colorimetrischen Bestimmung von N-(4-Methyl-benzolsulfonyl)-N'-butyl-harnstoff in Serum. Klin. Wochenschr. 35: 533–535, 1957.

J.M. Stowers, R.F. Mahler and R.B. Hunter. Pharmacology and mode of action of the sulphonylureas in man. Lancet 1: 278–283, 1958.

R.C. Thomas and G.J. Ikeda. The metabolic fate of tolbutamide in man and in the rat. J. Med. Chem. 9: 507–510, 1966.

K.M. West and P.C. Johnson. Metabolism and relative hypoglycemic potencies of four sulfonylureas in man. Diabetes 9: 454–458, 1960.

Tolmetin

T½: 4–6 hr
Vd: 0.1–0.2 L/kg
Fb: 0.99
pKa: 3.5

Occurrence and Usage. Tolmetin (Tolectin) is a nonsteroidal anti-inflammatory agent effective in the treatment of rheumatoid arthritis and osteoarthritis. In addition to anti-inflammatory effects, analgesic and antipyretic activity have been documented. Tolmetin is available for oral administration in tablets or capsules containing from 200–600 mg of the sodium salt. Doses of 600–1800 mg may be taken daily in divided doses.

Blood Concentrations. Five volunteers weighing 70–98 kg given a single oral 300 mg dose developed peak plasma tolmetin concentrations of 32–49 mg/L (average, 39) in 20–60 minutes; peak l-methyl-5-(4-carboxybenzoyl)-lH-pyrrole-2-acetic acid (MCPA) plasma concentrations ranged from 3.9–5.8 mg/L (average, 5.3) after 40–90 minutes (Grindel et al., 1979).

Following the oral administration of 400 mg of tolmetin 4 times daily (1600 mg/day) to 5 volunteers for 7 days, steady-state plasma concentrations ranged from 8.3–79 mg/L (average, 45) for tolmetin and from 4.1–14 mg/L (average, 10) for MCPA (Dromgoole et al., 1982).

Metabolism and Excretion. Tolmetin undergoes extensive oxidation to MCPA, a pharmacologically inactive metabolite; the parent drug may also be conjugated prior to excretion. Nearly an entire dose is eliminated in the 24 hour urine as MCPA (72%), free tolmetin (11%) and conjugated tolmetin (14%) (Sumner et al., 1975; Ayres et al., 1977a; Grindel et al., 1979).

Toxicity. Adverse reactions from tolmetin often include nausea, vomiting, abdominal pain and dizziness. However, more serious conditions such as high fever, reversible renal failure and anaphylaxis have been reported (Brown and Weir, 1978; Restivo and Paulus, 1978; McCall and Cooper, 1980; Katz et al., 1981; Bretza, 1985).

Analysis. Tolmetin has been determined in biological specimens by both gas chromatography (Selley et al., 1974; Cressman et al., 1975) and liquid chromatography (Ayres et al., 1977b; Shimek et al., 1981; Desiraju et al., 1982; Giachetti et al., 1983).

References

J.W. Ayres, D.J. Weidler, E. Sakmar and J.G. Wagner. Linear and nonlinear assessment of tolmetin pharmacokinetics. Res. Comm. Chem. Path. Pharm. 17: 583–593, 1977a.

J.W. Ayres, E. Sakmar, M.R. Hallmark and J.G. Wagner. High-pressure liquid chromatographic (HPLC) determination of tolmetin and its major metabolite in plasma. Res. Comm. Chem. Path. Pharm. 16: 475–483, 1977b.

M. Bretza. Anaphylactoid reactions to tolmetin. West. J. Med. 143: 55–59, 1985.

J.R. Brown and A.B. Weir. Drug fever from tolmetin administration. J. Am. Med. Asso. 239: 24, 1978.

W.A. Cressman, B. Lopez and D. Sumner. Determination of tolmetin in human plasma by GLC and spectrophotometric procedures. J. Pharm. Sci. 64: 1965–1967, 1975.

R.K. Desiraju, D.C. Sedberry, Jr. and K.T. Ng. Simultaneous determination of tolmetin and its metabolite in biological fluids by high-performance liquid chromatography. J. Chrom. 232: 119–128, 1982.

S.H. Dromgoole, D.E. Furst, R.K. Desiraju et al. Tolmetin kinetics and synovial fluid prostaglandin E levels in rheumatoid arthritis. Clin. Pharm. Ther. 32: 371–377, 1982.

C. Giachetti, S. Canali and G. Zanolo. Separation of nonsteroidal antiinflammatory agents by high-resolution gas chromatography: preliminary trials to perform pharmacokinetic studies. J. Chrom. 279: 587–592, 1983.

J.M. Grindel, B.H. Migdalof and J. Plostinieks. Absorption and excretion of tolmetin in arthritic patients. Clin. Pharm. Ther. 2: 122–128, 1979.

S.M. Katz, R. Capaido, E.A. Everts and J.G. Gregorio. Tolmetin: association with reversible renal failure and acute interstitial nephritis. J. Am. Med. Asso. 246: 243–245, 1981.

C.Y. McCall and J.W. Cooper. Tolmetin anaphylactoid reaction. J. Am. Med. Asso. 243: 1263, 1980.

C. Restivo and H.E. Paulus. Anaphylaxis from tolmetin. J. Am. Med. Asso. 240: 246, 1978.

M.L. Selley, J. Thomas and E.J. Triggs. A gas-liquid chromatographic method for the quantitative determination of tolmetin in plasma and tolmetin and its major metabolite in urine. J. Chrom. 94: 143–149, 1974.

J.L. Shimek, N.G.S. Rao and S.K.W. Khalil. High-performance liquid chromatographic analysis of tolmetin, indomethacin and sulindac in plasma. J. Liq. Chrom. 4: 1987–2013, 1981.

D.D. Sumner, P.G. Dayton, S.A. Cucinell and J. Plostnieks. Metabolism of tolmetin in rat, monkey and man. Drug Met. Disp. 3: 283-286, 1975.

Toluene

T½: 72 hr (whole blood)
Vd: ?
Fb: ?

Occurrence and Usage. Toluene (toluol) is an aromatic petroleum hydrocarbon that has many important commercial and industrial applications as a solvent and starting material for organic syntheses. It is present in numerous paints, paint thinners, glues, and other products likely to be found in the household. The acute narcotic effects of toluene are similar to those of benzene, although chronic toxicity is much less a problem. The current threshold limit value for atmospheric toluene is 50 ppm (188 mg/m^3). Industrial exposure generally occurs by inhalation of the vapor or dermal contact with the liquid.

Blood Concentrations. Blood toluene concentrations in 37 nonexposed hospital workers averaged 0.47 µg/L in nonsmokers and 1.14 µg/L in smokers (Brugnone et al., 1989). Blood toluene concentrations in workers exposed to air concentrations of 38 ppm for 8 hours averaged 0.59 mg/L (Foo et al., 1991). Subjects exposed for 30 minutes to a level of 100 ppm toluene had blood concentrations that averaged 0.4 mg/L when resting and 1.2 mg/L during light exercise (Astrand et al., 1972). Workers exposed to toluene concentrations of 191–309 ppm for 8 hours daily had pre-shift blood toluene concentrations that rose, on average, 5 fold within a working week; average post-shift concentrations rose from 3.6–6.7 mg/L during the first week, but declined from 11.6–5.9 mg/L during the second week. Individual post-shift concentrations ranged as high as 20.3 mg/L (Konietzko et al., 1980). The whole blood elimination half-life for toluene initially averages 4.5 hours, with a range of 3–6 hours (Brugnone et al., 1986), but a terminal phase approximating 72 hours has been observed and is thought to represent elimination from adipose tissue (Nise and Orbaek, 1988).

Metabolism and Excretion. Approximately 80% of an absorbed dose of toluene is oxidized to benzoic acid, which is then conjugated with glucuronic acid or glycine and excreted in the urine. The glycine conjugate (hippuric acid) accounts for about 68% of a dose in the 24 hour urine, and has an excretion half-life of 2–3 hours. Glucuronic acid conjugation of the metabolically produced benzoic acid is relatively unimportant until large amounts of toluene are absorbed. Up to 20% of a dose is eliminated unchanged in the expired air and less than 0.1% in the urine (Piotrowski, 1977).

Urinary hippuric acid concentrations were found to average 0.8 g/L (range, 0.4–1.4) in nonexposed persons (Pagnotto and Lieberman, 1967) and were found to parallel the intensity of the toluene exposure in industrial workers. For instance, workers exposed to an average daily level of 50 ppm developed urinary concentrations of 1.26–2.93 g/L (average, 1.92) by late afternoon, and those exposed to 200 ppm had hippuric acid concentrations of 4.12–8.65 g/L (average, 5.97). These urine values are uncorrected for specific gravity (Ikeda and Ohtsuji, 1969).

Toluene is also believed to be oxidized to a very minor degree to o-, m-, and p-cresol, which are probably excreted in the urine as conjugates. p-Cresol is a normal constituent of human urine, often present at concentrations of 20–200 mg/L; exposure to 200 ppm of toluene raises these levels by only 10 mg/L. o-Cresol and m-cresol are not normally found in urine, however, and their presence (at concentrations on the order of 1–3 mg/L) seems to correlate with the intensity of the toluene exposure (Angerer, 1979; Pfaffli et al., 1979; Woiwode et al., 1979; Woiwode and Drysch, 1981; Nise, 1992). A minor metabolite, S-benzyl-N-acetyl-L-cysteine, has been identified in human urine and may represent a more specific marker of toluene exposure (Takahashi et al., 1994).

Alveolar air concentrations of toluene reach a plateau within 15–30 minutes after the start of an exposure and decline rapidly after cessation of exposure; in persons exposed to 100 ppm of toluene, these levels were found to average 18 ppm at rest, 31 ppm during light exercise and 38 ppm during moderate exercise (Astrand et al., 1972). The blood:breath ratio for toluene has been found to range from 7–15 (Brugnone et al., 1976).

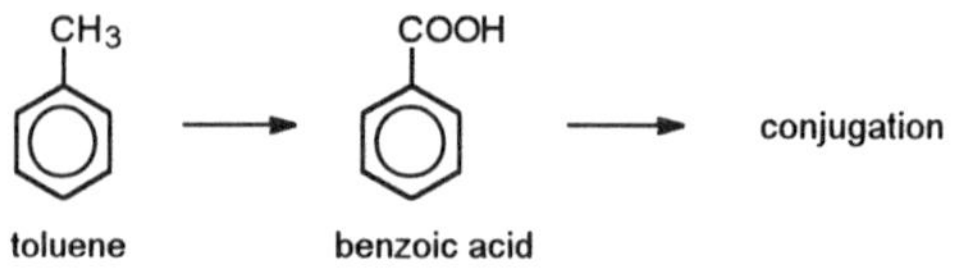

Toxicity. Concern over excessive exposure to toluene has been based primarily on the acute depressant effects of the chemical rather than on any chronic or residual effects on organ systems (von Oettingen et al., 1942). Employee exposure to toluene vapor at concentrations of 200–500 ppm for several weeks produced symptoms of headache, nausea, lassitude, impairment of coordination and loss of memory; concentrations of 500–1500 ppm caused similar but more severe effects (Wilson, 1943). Exposure to air concentrations of 10,000–30,000 ppm of toluene may cause mental confusion, drunkenness and unconsciousness within a few minutes (Longley et al., 1967).

Toluene has been frequently abused for its intoxicating effects by teenagers or adults who inhale the vapors of paint and glue solvents. Reports of 136 such persons who were either hospitalized or arrested while intoxicated showed blood toluene concentrations of 0.3–30 mg/L and urine concentrations of 0–5.0 mg/L (Bonnichsen et al., 1966; Kapur et al., 1986; Gjerde et al., 1990). In a study of 53 young toluene abusers, it was found that those with blood toluene concentrations of less than 1.0 mg/L gave evidence of abuse by the odor of the chemical on their breath; those with concentrations of 1.0–2.5 mg/L showed some signs of intoxication; half of those with levels of 2.5–10 mg/L were hospitalized for marked intoxication, including hallucinations; and those exhibiting levels greater than 10 mg/L were unconscious or had died (Lush et al., 1979). Six toluene abusers, allowed free access to the chemical in controlled circumstances, developed blood toluene concentrations of 9.8–31 mg/L measured within a few minutes of cessation of inhalation. Intoxication was manifested by slurred speech, slow movements, and inability to concentrate (Garriott et al., 1981).

Three cases of long-term habituation to toluene were shown to result in electroencephalographic abnormalities, encephalopathy and, in 2 cases, permanent cerebral atrophy (Satran and Dodson, 1963; Knox and Nelson, 1966; Boor and Hurtig, 1977). Such abuse has also led to hepatic and renal damage (O'Brien et al., 1971) and severe metabolic acidosis with hypokalemia and hyperchloremia (Taher et al., 1974; Fischman and Oster, 1979; Bennett and Forman, 1980; Streicher et al., 1981).

Three persons who died of acute toluene inhalation were found to have postmortem blood concentrations of 50, 60, and 79 mg/L (Nomiyama and Nomiyama, 1978). Another 8 persons who died as a result of accidental or intentional acute exposure to toluene fumes exhibited the following concentrations in postmortem specimens (Bonnichsen et al., 1966; Collom and Winek, 1970; Bidanset, 1973; Luskus et al., 1977; Takeichi et al., 1986; DeLuca et al., 1990):

Toluene Concentrations in Fatal Cases (mg/L or mg/kg)

	Blood	Brain	Lung	Liver	Kidney	Urine
Average	22	47	12	43	21	3
(Range)	(10–48)	(10–182)	(3–35)	(13–73)	(11–39)	(1–5)

Analysis. Techniques for toluene determination in biologic specimens include gas chromatography with adsorption sampling (Peterson and Bruckner, 1978; Garriott et al., 1981), headspace sampling (Collom and Winek, 1970; Sato et al., 1975; Engstrom et al., 1976; Lush et al., 1979; Pekari et al.,

1989) or solvent extraction (Jones et al., 1994). Toluene losses of up to 25% have been noted in glass blood tubes stored unopened for 7 days at room temperature, while refrigeration reduced this loss to 15% (Saker et al., 1991). With storage for 49 days in rubber-stoppered glass tubes, losses of 94% at room temperature and 80% at refrigerator temperature were noted (Gill et al., 1988).

Hippuric acid in urine has been measured by direct colorimetry (Tomokuni and Ogata, 1972), ultraviolet spectrophotometry (Pagnotto and Lieberman, 1967), colorimetry after thin-layer chromatographic separation (Ogata et al., 1969) and gas chromatography of the methyl (Buchet and Lauwerys, 1973; Caperos and Fernandez, 1977) or trimethylsilyl derivatives (Engstrom et al., 1976; Van Roosmalen and Drummond, 1978). Liquid chromatography has also been described (Tardif et al., 1989; Astier, 1992). The cresol metabolites of toluene are determined in urine by hydrolysis of the conjugates and flame-ionization gas chromatography (Pfaffli et al., 1979; Woiwode et al., 1979).

References

J. Angerer. Occupational chronic exposure to organic solvents. VII. Metabolism of toluene in man. Int. Arch. Occ. Env. Health 43: 63–67, 1979.

A. Astier. Simultaneous hplc determination of urinary metabolites of benzene, nitrobenzene, toluene, xylene and sytrene. J. Chrom. 573: 318–322, 1992.

I. Astrand, H. Ehrner-Samuel, A. Kilbom and P. Ovrum. Toluene exposure I. Concentration in alveolar air and blood at rest and during exercise. Work Env. Health 9: 119–130, 1972.

R.H. Bennett and H.R. Forman. Hypokalemic periodic paralysis in chronic toluene exposure. Arch. Neurol. 37: 673, 1980.

J. Bidanset. Presented at the 25th annual meeting of the American Academy of Forensic Sciences, Las Vegas, February 22, 1973.

R. Bonnichsen, A.C. Maehly and M. Moeller. Poisoning by volatile compounds. I. Aromatic hydrocarbons. J. For. Sci. 11: 186–204, 1966.

J.W. Boor and H.I. Hurtig. Persistent cerebellar ataxia after exposure to toluene. Ann. Neurol. 2: 440–442, 1977.

F. Brugnone, L. Perbellini, L. Grigolini et al. Alveolar air and blood toluene concentration in rotogravure workers. Int. Arch. Occ. Env. Health 38: 45–54, 1976.

F. Brugnone, E. deRosa, L. Perbellini and G.B. Bartolucci. Toluene concentrations in the blood and alveolar air of workers during the workshift and the morning after. Brit. J. Ind. Med. 43: 56–61, 1986.

F. Brugnone, L. Perbellini, G.B. Faccini et al. Breath and blood levels of benzene, toluene, cumene and styrene in non-occupational expsorue. Int. Arch. Occ. Env. Health 61: 303–311, 1989.

J.P. Buchet and R.R. Lauwerys. Measurement of urinary hippuric and m-methylhippuric acids by gas chromatography. Brit. J. Ind. Med. 30: 125–128, 1973.

J.R. Caperos and J.G. Fernandez. Simultaneous determination of toluene and xylene metabolites in urine by gas chromatography. Brit. J. Ind. Med. 34: 229–233, 1977.

W.D. Collom and C.L. Winek. Detection of glue constituents in fatalities due to "glue sniffing." Clin. Tox. 3: 125–130, 1970.

R. DeLuca, J. Vogel and C.N. Hodnett. Presented at the annual meeting of the Society of Forensic Toxicologists, Melville, New York, September 12, 1990.

K. Engstrom, K. Husman and J. Rantanen. Measurement of toluene and xylene metabolites by gas chromatography. Int. Arch. Occ. Env. Health 36: 153–160, 1976.

C.M. Fischman and J.R. Oster. Toxic effects of toluene. J. Am. Med. Asso. 241: 1713–1715, 1979.

S.C. Foo, J. Jeyaratnam, C.N. Ong et al. Biological monitoring for occupational exposure to toluene. Am. Ind. Hyg. Asso. J. 52: 212–217, 1991.

J.C. Garriott, E. Foerster, L. Juarez et al. Measurement of toluene in blood and breath in cases of solvent abuse. Clin. Tox. 18: 471–479, 1981.

R. Gill, S.E. Hatchett, M.D. Osselton et al. Sample handling and storage for the quantitative analysis of volatile compounds in blood. J. Anal. Tox. 12: 141–146, 1988.

H. Gjerde, A. Smith-Kielland, P.T. Normann and J. Morland. Driving under the influence of toluene. For. Sci. Int. 44: 77–83, 1990.

M. Ikeda and H. Ohtsuji. Significance of urinary hippuric acid determination as an index of toluene exposure. Brit. J. Ind. Med. 26: 244–246, 1969.

A.D. Jones, M.R. Dunlap and S.M. Gospe, Jr. Stable-isotope dilution GC-MS for determination of toluene in submilliliter volumes of whole blood. J. Anal. Tox. 18: 251–254, 1994.

B. Kapur, E. Wong, P.L. Carlen and L. Fornazzari. Biochemical changes and pharmacokinetics of toluene in inhalant abusers. Clin. Chem. 32: 1055, 1986.

J.W. Knox and J.R. Nelson. Permanent encephalopathy from toluene inhalation. New Eng. J. Med. 275: 1494–1496, 1966.

H. Konietzko, J. Keilbach and K. Drysch. Cumulative effects of daily toluene exposure. Int. Arch. Occ. Env. Health 46: 53–58, 1980.

E.O. Longley, A.T. Jones, R. Welch and O. Lomaev. Two acute toluene episodes in merchant ships. Arch. Env. Health 14: 481–487, 1967.

M. Lush, J.S. Oliver and J.M. Watson. The analysis of blood in cases of suspected solvent abuse, with a review of results during the period October 1977 to July 1979. In *Forensic Toxicology* (J.S. Oliver, ed.), Croom Helm, London, 1979, pp. 304–313.

L.J. Luskus, H.J. Kilian, W.W. Lackey and J.D. Biggs. Gases released from tissue and analyzed by infrared and gas chromatography/mass spectroscopy techniques. J. For. Sci. 22: 500–507, 1977.

G. Nise and P. Orbaek. Toluene in venous blood during and after work in rotogravure printing. Int. Arch. Occ. Env. Health 60: 31–35, 1988.

G. Nise. Urinary excretion of o-cresol and hippuric acid after toluene exposure in rotogravure printing. Int. Arch. Occ. Env. Health 63: 377–381, 1992.

K. Nomiyama and H. Nomiyama. Three fatal cases of thinner-sniffing, and experimental exposure to toluene in human and animals. Int. Arch. Occ. Env. Health 41: 55–64, 1978.

E.T. O'Brien, W.B. Yeoman and J.A.E. Hobby. Hepatorenal damage from toluene in a "glue sniffer." Brit. Med. J. 2: 29–30, 1971.

M. Ogata, K. Tomokuni and Y. Takatsuka. Quantitative determination in urine of hippuric acid and m- or p-methylhippuric acid, metabolites of toluene and m- or p-xylene. Brit. J. Ind. Med. 26: 330–334, 1969.

L.D. Pagnotto and L.M. Lieberman. Urinary hippuric acid excretion as an index of toluene exposure. Am. Ind. Hyg. Asso. J. 28: 129–134, 1967.

K. Pekari, M.L. Riekkola and A. Aitio. Simultaneous determination of benzene and toluene in the blood using head-space gas chromatography. J. Chrom. 491: 309–320, 1989.

R.G. Peterson and J.V. Bruckner. A rapid analytical method for measuring toluene in biological specimens. J. Chrom. 152: 69–78, 1978.

P. Pfaffli, H. Savolainen, P.L. Kalliomaki and P. Kalliokoski. Urinary o-cresol in toluene exposure. Scand. J. Work Env. Health 5: 286–289, 1979.

J.K. Piotrowski. *Exposure Tests for Organic Compounds in Industrial Toxicology*, U.S. Government Printing Office, Washington, D.C., 1977, pp. 48–54.

E.G. Saker, A.E. Eskew and J.W. Panter. Stability of toluene in blood: its forensic relevance. J. Anal. Tox. 15: 246–249, 1991.

A. Sato, T. Nakajima and F. Fujiwara. Determination of benzene and toluene in blood by means of syringe-equilibration method using a small amount of blood. Brit. J. Ind. Med. 32: 210–214, 1975.

R. Satran and V.N. Dodson. Toluene habituation—report of a case. New Eng. J. Med. 268: 719–721, 1963.

H.Z. Streicher, P.A. Gabow, A.H. Moss et al. Syndromes of toluene sniffing in adults. Ann. Int. Med. 94: 758–762, 1981.

S.M. Taher, R.J. Anderson, R. McCartney et al. Renal tubular acidosis associated with toluene "sniffing." New Eng. J. Med. 290: 765–768, 1974.

S. Takahashi, M. Kagawa, K. Shiwaku and K. Matsubara. Determination of S-benzyl-N-acetyl-L-cysteine by GC/MS as a new marker of toluene exposure. J. Anal. Tox. 18: 78–80, 1994.

S. Takeichi, T. Yamada and I. Skikata. Acute toluene poisoning during painting. For. Sci. Int. 32: 109–115, 1986.

R. Tardif. J. Brodeur and G.L. Plaa. Simultaneous hplc analysis of hippuric acid and ortho- meta-, and para-methylhippuric acids in urine. J. Anal. Tox. 13: 313–316, 1989.

K. Tomokuni and M. Ogata. Direct colorimetric determination of hippuric acid in urine. Clin. Chem. 18: 349–351, 1972.

P.B. Van Roosmalen and I. Drummond. Simultaneous determination by gas chromatography of the major metabolites in urine of toluene, xylenes and styrene. Brit. J. Ind. Med. 35: 56–60, 1978.

W.F. von Oettingen, P.A. Neal and D.D. Donahue. The toxicity and potential dangers of toluene. J. Am. Med. Asso. 118: 579–584, 1942.

R.H. Wilson. Toluene poisoning. J. Am. Med. Asso. 123: 1106–1108, 1943.

W. Woiwode, R. Wodarz, K. Drysch and H. Weichardt. Metabolism of toluene in man: gas-chromatographic determination of o-, m- and p-cresol in urine. Arch. Tox. 43: 93–98, 1979.
W. Woiwode and K. Drysch. Experimental exposure to toluene: further consideration of cresol formation in man. Brit. J. Ind. Med. 38: 194–197, 1981.

Tranylcypromine

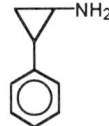

T½: 1.5–3.5 hr
Vd: 1.1–5.7 L/kg
Fb: ?
pKa: 8.2

Occurrence and Usage. Tranylcypromine (Parnate, ingredient of Parstelin) is a close structural analogue of amphetamine currently marketed as an antidepressant agent. Its effects are apparently due to its ability to inhibit cerebral monoamine oxidase, thus increasing biogenic amine levels. The drug is supplied for oral use as the sulfate salt of the racemate in 10 mg tablets. A chronic dosage of 20–40 mg daily is usual.

Blood Concentrations. An average peak serum concentration of 0.039 mg/L was found 1 hour after the oral ingestion of 30 mg of the drug by 2 subjects; the level declined with a half-life of 1.9 hours to less than 0.008 mg/L by 24 hours (Baselt et al., 1977b). Following a single oral 50 mg dose given to 3 volunteers, peak plasma concentrations of 0.076–0.089 mg/L were achieved between 1.5 and 2.3 hours after ingestion (Bailey and Barron, 1980).

Twelve adult patients receiving 0.43 mg/kg (30 mg/70 kg) daily oral doses had an average plasma tranylcypromine concentration at 5 hours after the last dose of 0.029 mg/L (Mallinger et al., 1990). In subjects receiving 10–30 mg on a chronic daily basis, serum concentrations averaged 0.005–0.010 mg/L 12 hours after the last dose (Baselt et al., 1977b).

Metabolism and Excretion. The biotransformation of this drug has not been investigated in man. On the basis of animal studies, the major route of metabolism probably involves cleavage of the cyclopropyl ring with some deamination, and excretion as benzoic acid conjugates (Alleva, 1963). Only 1–2% of a dose is excreted unchanged in the urine over a 24 hour period (Baselt et al., 1977b; Bailey and Barron, 1980). This value may be increased to as much as 11% by acidification of the urine (Turner et al., 1967).

Toxicity. Adverse reactions to tranylcypromine include nausea, headache, restlessness, anxiety, confusion, dizziness, blurred vision, chills, tachycardia and hypotension or hypertension. Overdosage usually results in hyperpyrexia, convulsions, shock, skeletal muscle rigidity and coma. Tranylcypromine was temporarily withdrawn from the U.S. market in 1964 following a series of reports on its clinical toxicity. Hypertensive crises, occasionally fatal, have occurred in patients receiving therapeutic dosages, especially when in conjunction with other monoamine oxidase inhibitors or pressor agents. In one such case involving the co-administration of wine and cheese (containing tyramine), the blood tranylcypromine concentration prior to death was 0.102 mg/L (Mirchandani and Reich, 1985).

Several persons have survived the ingestion of 200–900 mg of the drug following treatment with muscle relaxants, beta-blocking agents, chlorpromazine, or hemodialysis (Matter et al., 1965; Coulter et al., 1971; Robertson, 1972; Shepherd and Whiting, 1974). In a patient who ingested 250 mg of the drug and became comatose, plasma tranylcypromine concentrations reached a level of 1.0 mg/L at about 30 hours after ingestion and declined with a half-life of 3.5 hours (Youdim et al., 1979).

A number of instances of fatal overdosage involving the ingestion of 130–850 mg of the drug have been recorded (Babiak, 1961; Bateman, 1961; Bacon, 1962; Cuthill et al., 1964; Mawdsley, 1968; Griffiths, 1973; Mackell et al., 1979). Postmortem blood concentrations of 1.7 and 5.0 mg/L were measured in 2 such cases (Boniface, 1991). The following distribution was observed in a death that resulted from the ingestion of 300 mg of tranylcypromine together with several other drugs (Baselt et al., 1977a):

Tranylcypromine Concentrations in a Fatal Case (mg/L or mg/kg)

Blood	Brain	Liver	Urine
3.7	1.0	7.3	25

Analysis. Tranylcypromine may be included in many of the analytical schemes designed for the determination of amphetamine. A fluorometric method was developed for the assay of the drug in urine, but suffers from a lack of sensitivity (Turner et al., 1966). Gas chromatography has been applied successfully, using flame-ionization detection of the N-acetyl derivative for toxic levels (Baselt et al., 1977a) and electron-capture or mass spectrometric detection of a halogenated derivative for therapeutic concentrations (Baselt et al., 1977b; Bailey and Barron, 1980; Edwards et al., 1985). A radioenzymatic assay was described for the assay of the drug in brain tissue (Fuentes et al., 1975). Boniface (1991) commented on the volatility of the free base at 50° C. during analytical manipulations.

References

J.J. Alleva. Metabolism of tranylcypromine-C^{14} and dl-amphetamine-C^{14} in the rat. J. Med. Chem. 6: 621–624, 1963.

W. Babiak. Case fatality due to overdosage of a combination of tranylcypromine (Parnate) and imipramine (Tofranil). Can. Med. Asso. J. 85: 377, 1961.

G.A. Bacon. Successful suicide with tranylcypromine sulfate. Am. J. Psych. 119: 585, 1962.

E. Bailey and E.J. Barron. Determination of tranylcypromine in human plasma and urine using high-resolution gas-liquid chromatography with nitrogen-sensitive detection. J. Chrom. 183: 25–31, 1980.

R.C. Baselt, E. Shaskan and E.M. Gross. Tranylcypromine concentrations and monoamine oxidase activity in tissues from a fatal poisoning. J. Anal. Tox. 1: 168–170, 1977a.

R.C. Baselt, C.B. Stewart and E. Shaskan. Determination of serum and urine concentrations of tranylcypromine by electron-capture gas-chromatography. J. Anal. Tox. 1: 215–217, 1977b.

C.R. Bateman. Fatalities from overdosage of antidepressant drugs. Can. Med. Asso. J. 85: 759, 1961.

P.J. Boniface. Two cases of fatal intoxication due to tranylcypromine overdose. J. Anal. Tox. 15: 38–40, 1991.

C. Coulter, J. Edmunds and P.O. Pyle. An overdose of Parstelin. Anaesthesia 26: 500–501, 1971.

J.M. Cuthill, A.B. Griffiths and D.E.B. Powell. Death associated with tranylcypromine and cheese. Lancet 1: 1076–1077, 1964.

D.J. Edwards, A.G. Mallinger, S. Knopf and J.F. Himmelhoch. Determination of tranylcypromine in plasma using gas chromatography-chemical ionization mass spectrometry. J. Chrom. 344: 356–361, 1985.

J.A. Fuentes, M.A. Oleshansky and N.H. Neff. A sensitive enzymatic assay for dextro- or levo-tranylcypromine in brain. Biochem. Pharm. 24: 1971–1973, 1975.

G.J. Griffiths. Overdose of Parstelin (tranylcypromine). Med. Sci. Law 13: 93–94, 1973.

M.A. Mackell, M.E. Case and A. Poklis. Fatal intoxication due to tranylcypromine. Med. Sci. Law 19: 66–68, 1979.

A.G. Mallinger, J.M. Himmelhoch, M.E. Thase et al. Plasma tranylcypromine: relationship to pharmacokinetic variables and clinical antidepressant actions. J. Clin. Pharm. 10: 176–183, 1990.

B.J. Matter, P.E. Donat, M.L. Brill and H.E. Ginn, Jr. Tranylcypromine sulfate poisoning. Arch. Int. Med. 116: 18–20, 1965.

J.A. Mawdsley. "Parstelin": a case of fatal overdose. Med. J. Aust. 2: 292, 1968.

H. Mirchandani and L.E. Reich. Fatal malignant hyperthermia as a result of ingestion of tranylcypromine (Parnate) combined with white wine and cheese. J. For. Sci. 30: 217–220, 1985.

J.C. Robertson. Recovery after massive MAOI overdose complicated by malignant hyperpyrexia, treated with chlorpromazine. Postgrad. Med. J. 48: 64–65, 1972.

J.T. Shepherd and B. Whiting. Beta-adrenergic blockade in the treatment of M.A.O.I. self-poisoning. Lancet 2: 1021, 1974.

P. Turner, J.H. Young and E.F. Scowen. Fluorimetric detection of tranylcypromine in urine. J. Pharm. Pharmac. 18: 550–551, 1966.

P. Turner, J.H. Young and J. Paterson. Influence of urinary pH on the excretion of tranylcypromine sulphate. Nature 215: 881–882, 1967.

M.B.H. Youdim, J.K. Aronson, K. Blau et al. Tranylcypromine ("Parnate") overdose: measurement of tranylcypromine concentrations and MAO inhibitory activity and identification of amphetamines in plasma. Psych. Med. 9: 377–382, 1979.

Trazodone

T½: 4–7 hr
Vd: 0.9–1.5 L/kg
Fb: 0.90
pKa: ?

Occurrence and Usage. Trazodone (Desyrel) is a triazolopyridine derivative used as an antidepressant agent. It is chemically unrelated to other tricyclic or tetracyclic antidepressants. The drug is available for oral administration in 50, 100 and 150 mg tablets as the hydrochloride salt.

Blood Concentrations. After a single 100 mg oral dose of trazodone to fasting volunteers (median age, 24 years; median weight, 63 kg), an average peak plasma concentration of 1.1 mg/L was observed after 2 hours, declining to 0.7 mg/L after 4 hours and 0.3 mg/L after 8 hours (Bayer et al., 1983). Following a single 150 mg oral dose given to 4 adult subjects aged 21–30 years and weighing 49–80 kg, an average peak plasma concentration of 2.1 mg/L of trazodone and 0.01 mg/L of its major metabolite, 1-(3-chlorophenyl)piperazine, were attained in 2–4 hours (Caccia et al., 1982).

Three female patients, aged 20–40, treated with 400 mg of trazodone daily, developed average trough serum concentrations of 0.9–1.1 mg/L, ranging from 0.7–1.6 mg/L (Baxter et al., 1986). Steady-state plasma trazodone concentrations ranged from 0.49–1.21 mg/L (average, 0.80) in 5 patients treated for depression, while concentrations of the major metabolite, 1-(3-chlorophenyl)piperazine, ranged from 0.01–0.03 mg/L (average, 0.02) (Suckow, 1983). Plasma steady-state trazodone concentrations averaged 1.47 mg/L (range, 0.24–4.89) in 23 depressed patients aged 70–88 treated with an average dose of 354 mg/day (range, 150–500) (Spar, 1987).

Metabolism and Excretion. Trazodone is extensively biotransformed, with the major metabolites being beta-(3-oxo-s-triazolic(4-3α)pyridin-2-yl)propionic acid (OTPA), 1-(3-chlorophenyl)piperazine (pharmacologically active), and their glucuronides. Only about 1% of the dose is excreted unchanged in the urine within 24 hours; about 75% of a dose is excreted as urinary metabolites and 15% in the feces within 72 hours (Bajocchi et al., 1974; Caccia et al., 1981a; Caccia et al., 1981b; Suckow, 1983; di Tella et al., 1986).

1-(3-chlorophenyl)piperazine   trazodone   OPTA

conjugation

Toxicity. Adverse effects related to trazodone overdosage include hallucinations, delusions, slurred speech, seizures, respiratory arrest and death. Plasma trazodone concentrations as high as 19 mg/L were observed in poisoned patients who exhibited only drowsiness and ataxia (Henry et al., 1984). A 49 year old woman who collapsed 2 hours after ingestion of 2–8 g of the drug was lethargic and mildly hypotensive upon arrival at hospital; she survived despite attaining a blood concentration of 26 mg/L (Root and Ohlson, 1984).

A 48 year old woman was found dead in her bathtub following an estimated dose of 2–4 g of trazodone; postmortem concentrations are shown below as case 1 (Demorest, 1983). A 44 year old woman who ingested as much as 3.4 g of the drug was found dead in bed with a suicide note nearby; toxicological findings are shown below as case 2 (Kemmenoe et al., 1984).

Trazodone Concentrations in Fatal Cases (mg/L or mg/kg)

	Blood	Brain	Liver	Urine	Bile
Case 1	15	—	57	2.5	45
Case 2	23	25	67	23	—

Trazodone may exhibit postmortem redistribution; the heart blood/femoral blood concentration ratio for the drug was 1.7 in a single decedent (Anderson and Prouty, 1989).

Analysis. Trazodone has been determined by gas chromatography in therapeutic (Caccia et al., 1981b; Abernathy et al., 1984; Gammans et al., 1985; Rifal et al., 1988) and in toxic concentrations (Anderson and Archuleta, 1984). The drug has also been analyzed by liquid chromatography using ultraviolet (Ankier et al., 1981; Root and Ohlson, 1984; Wong et al., 1984; Wong and Marzouk, 1985; di Tella et al., 1986; Miller and Devane, 1986), electrochemical (Suckow, 1983) and fluorescence detection (Gupta and Lew, 1985).

References

D.R. Abernathy, D.J. Greenblatt and R.I. Shader. Plasma levels of trazodone: methodology and applications. Pharmacology 28: 42–45, 1984.

W.H. Anderson and M.M. Archuleta. The capillary gas chromatographic determination of trazodone in biological specimens. J. Anal. Tox. 8: 217–219, 1984.

W.H. Anderson and R.W. Prouty. Postmortem redistribution of drugs. In *Advances in Analytical Toxicology* (R.C. Baselt, ed.), Vol. 2, YearBook Medical, Chicago, 1989, pp. 70–102.

S.I. Ankier, B.K. Morton, M.S. Rogers et al. Trazodone—a new assay procedure and some pharmacokinetic parameters. Brit. J. Clin. Pharm. 11: 505, 1981.

L.R. Baxter, J.N. Wilkins and G.B. Smith. A possible diurnal variation in trazodone clearance. J. Clin. Psychopharm. 6: 223–226, 1986.

A.J. Bayer, M.S.J. Pathy and S.I. Ankier. Pharmacokinetic and pharmacodynamic characteristics of trazodone in the elderly. Brit. J. Clin. Pharm. 16: 371–376, 1983.

L. Baiocchi, A. Frigerio, M. Giannangeli and G. Palazzo. Basic metabolites of trazodone in humans. Arz. Forsch. 24: 1699–1706, 1974.

S. Caccia, M. Ballabio, R. Samanin et al. m-Chlorophenyl-piperazine, a central 5-hydroxytryptamine agonist, is a metabolite of trazodone. J. Pharm. Pharmac. 33: 477–478, 1981a.

S. Caccia, M. Ballabio, R. Fanelli et al. Determination of plasma and brain concentrations of trazodone and its metabolite, 1-m-chlorophenylpiperazine, by gas liquid chromatography. J. Chrom. 210: 311–318, 1981b.

S. Caccia, M.H. Fong, S. Garattini and M.G. Zanini. Plasma concentrations of trazodone and 1-(3-chlorophenyl)piperazine in man after a single oral dose of trazodone. J. Pharm. Pharmac. 34: 605–606, 1982.

D. Demorest. Death involving trazodone. J. Anal. Tox. 7: 63, 1983.

A.S. di Tella, C. diNunzio, P. Ricci and G. Parisi. Determination of trazodone and its metabolite, m-CPP, in serum and urine by HPLC. J. Anal. Tox. 10: 233–235, 1986.

R.E. Gammans, E.H. Kerns, W.W. Bullen et al. Gas chromatographic-mass spectrometric method for trazodone and a deuterated analogue in plasma. J. Chrom. 339: 303–312, 1985.

R.N. Gupta and M. Lew. Determination of trazodone in human plasma by liquid chromatography with fluorescence detection. J. Chrom. 342: 442–446, 1985.

J.A. Henry, C.J. Ali, R. Caldwell and R.J. Flanagan. Acute trazodone poisoning: clinical signs and plasma concentrations. Psychopathology 17 (Suppl. 2): 77–81, 1984.

A.V. Kemmenoe. Personal communication, 1984.

R.L. Miller and C.L. Devane. Analysis of trazodone and m-chlorophenyl-piperazine in plasma and brain tissue by high-performance liquid chromatography. J. Chrom. 374: 388–393, 1986.

N. Rifal, C.B. Levtzow, C.M. Howlett et al. Measurement of trazodone using solid-phase extraction and wide-bore capillary gas chromatography with nitrogen-selective detection. J. Anal. Tox. 12: 150–152, 1988.

I. Root and G.B. Ohlson. Trazodone overdose: report of two cases. J. Anal. Tox. 8: 91–94, 1984.

J.E. Spar. Plasma trazodone concentrations in elderly depressed inpatients: cardiac effects and short-term efficacy. J. Clin. Psychopharm. 7: 406–409, 1987.

R.F. Suckow. A simultaneous determination of trazodone and its metabolite 1-m-chlorophenylpiperazine in plasma by liquid chromatography with electrochemical detection. J. Liq. Chrom. 6: 2195–2208, 1983.

S.H.Y. Wong and N. Marzouk. Determination of a trazodone metabolite, 1-m-chlorophenylpiperazine in plasma by liquid chromatography. J. Liq. Chrom. 8: 1379–1395, 1985.

S.H.Y. Wong, S.W. Waugh, M. Draz and N. Jain. Liquid-chromatographic determination of two antidepressants, trazodone and mianserin, in plasma. Clin. Chem. 302: 230–233, 1984.

Triazolam

T½: 1.8–3.9 hr
Vd: 1.1–2.7 L/kg
Fb: 0.78
pKa: ?

Occurrence and Usage. Triazolam (Halcion), a triazolobenzodiazepine hypnotic agent, is used for short-term management of insomnia. The drug differs from most benzodiazepines in regard to its short plasma half-life. The hypnotic activity of triazolam in doses as low as 0.125 mg has been well-established in controlled studies. It is available in tablets containing 0.125 or 0.25 mg as the free base.

Blood Concentrations. Following an oral dose of 0.25 mg in 6 healthy subjects weighing 48–74 kg (average, 62), a mean peak plasma concentration of 3.0 µg/L (range, 2.3–3.7) was achieved within 0.75–1.5 hours (Baktir et al., 1983). After administration of a single 0.5 mg oral dose of triazolam to 54 healthy men aged 20–44 with a mean body weight of 77 kg, a mean peak plasma concentration of 4.4 µg/L (range, 1.7–9.4) was measured at 0.5–4.0 hours (Friedman et al., 1986). Following a single oral dose of 0.88 mg of ^{14}C-labelled triazolam to 6 men aged 21–46 and within 20% of desirable weight, peak plasma concentrations of 5.6–17 µg/L (average, 8.7) were attained in 0.5–2.9 hours. Peak plasma concentrations of 1-hydroxymethyltriazolam ranged from 2.7–10 µg/L (average, 6.1) after 0.75–2.5 hours, while peak plasma concentrations of 4-hydroxytriazolam ranged from 2.0–9.1 µg/L (average, 6.1) after 1.5–5.0 hours (Eberts et al., 1981). Six normal healthy male subjects, 20–30 years of age and weighing 64–86 kg, given an oral dose of 1 mg of triazolam developed an average peak serum concentration of 8.6 µg/L after 1.0–1.5 hours (Adams et al., 1980).

In a study of 8 geriatric patients (average age, 80 years), a single tablet of 0.25 mg was administered to each patient as a daytime sedative for 7 days; peak serum concentrations averaged 2.0 µg/L and were achieved at 1.5 and 1.4 hours after administration on days 1 and 7, respectively (Dehlin et al., 1983).

Metabolism and Excretion. Triazolam is rapidly absorbed after oral administration and is extensively metabolized in man by hydroxylation and conjugation. Its major metabolite, 1-hydroxymethyltriazolam, has from 50–100% of the pharmacological activity of the parent compound. Other metabolites include 4-hydroxytriazolam and 1-hydroxymethyl-4-hydroxytriazolam. Only trace amounts of unmetabolized triazolam appear in the urine and the hydroxylated metabolites are present largely as glucuronide conjugates. About 80% of the dose is excreted in the urine within 48 hours and approximately 7% is eliminated in the feces in 72 hours (Eberts et al., 1981; Coassolo et al., 1983; Inoue and Suzuki, 1987).

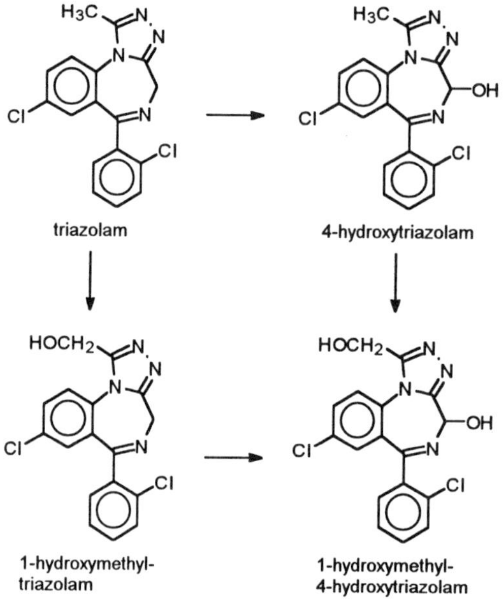

triazolam → 4-hydroxytriazolam

1-hydroxymethyl-triazolam → 1-hydroxymethyl-4-hydroxytriazolam

Toxicity. Triazolam side-effects involving agitation, disorientation, sleepwalking, anger and panic have been observed in a number of patients (van der Kroef, 1979; Einarson and Yoder, 1982; Regestein and Reich, 1985). Overdosage may occur at 4 times the maximum recommended dose; manifestations include somnolence, confusion, impaired coordination, slurred speech and, ultimately, coma, cardiopulmonary collapse and death. A woman who ingested 5 mg of the drug developed coma and an admission serum triazolam level of 31 μg/L, but regained consciousness within 8 hours (Olson et al., 1985). Blood triazolam concentrations averaging 23 μg/L (range, 4–40) were measured in 8 persons arrested for driving under the influence of drugs (Joynt, 1993).

One individual drowned himself in the bathtub after taking 11 triazolam tablets; postmortem concentrations of 6.7 μg/L in blood and 38 μg/kg in liver were detected (Wong, 1984). Six victims of fatal overdosage with triazolam as the sole agent had postmortem blood concentrations averaging 39 μg/L (range, 10–57); postmortem blood concentrations in another 12 victims who also had ethanol present averaged 62 μg/L (range, 10–220) (Reynolds, 1988; Joynt, 1993; Steentoft and Worm, 1993).

Analysis. Triazolam may be determined by gas chromatography with electron-capture (Greenblatt et al., 1981; Jochemsen and Breimer, 1981; Coassolo et al., 1983; Baktir et al., 1985; Edeki et al., 1992) or nitrogen-phosphorus detection (Kudo et al., 1991). Liquid chromatography has also been utilized for the analysis of triazolam and its metabolites (Adams, 1979; Adams et al. 1980; Eberts et al., 1981; Wong, 1984; Inoue and Suzuki, 1987). Gas chromatography-mass spectrometry offers a sensitive and specific means of determining triazolam and its metabolites in biological specimens (Eberts et al., 1981; Caossolo et al., 1983; Koves and Wells, 1986; Fraser et al., 1992; Cairns et al., 1994).

References

W.J. Adams. Specific and sensitive high performance liquid chromatographic determination of alprazolam or triazolam. Anal. Letters 12: 657–671, 1979.

W.J. Adams, U.M. Rykert and P.A. Bombardt. High performance liquid chromatographic determination of triazolam in human serum. Anal. Letters 13: 149–161, 1980.

G. Baktir, H.U. Fisch, P. Huguenin and J. Bircher. Triazolam concentration-effect relationships in healthy subjects. Clin. Pharm. Ther. 34: 195–201, 1983.

G. Baktir, J. Bircher, H.U. Fisch and G. Karlaganis. Capillary gas-liquid chromatographic determination of the benzodiazepine triazolam in plasma using a retention gap. J. Chrom. 339: 192–197, 1985.

E.R. Cairns, B.R. Dent, J.C. Duwerkerk and L.J. Porter. Quantitative analysis of alprazolam and triazolam in hemolysed whole blood and liver digest by GC/MS/NICI with deuterated internal standards. J. Anal. Tox. 18: 1–6, 1994.

P. Coassolo, C. Aubert and J.P. Cano. Simultaneous assay of triazolam and its main hydroxy metabolite in plasma and urine by capillary gas chromatography. J. Chrom. 274: 161–170, 1983.

O. Dehlin, G. Bjornson, L. Borjesson et al. Pharmacokinetics of triazolam in geriatric patients. Eur. J. Clin. Pharm. 25: 91–94, 1983.

F.S. Eberts, Jr., Y. Philopoulos, L.M. Reineke and R.W. Vliek. Triazolam disposition. Clin. Pharm. Ther. 29: 81–93, 1981.

T. Edeki, D.W. Robin, C. Prakash et al. Sensitive assay for triazolam in plasma following low oral doses. J. Chrom. 577: 190–194, 1992.

T.R. Einarson and E.S. Yoder. Triazolam psychosis—a syndrome? Drug Int. Clin. Pharm. 16: 330, 1982.

A.D. Fraser, W. Bryan and A.F. Isner. Urinary screening for α-OH triazolam by FPIA and EIA with confirmation by GC/MS. J. Anal. Tox. 16: 347–350, 1992.

H. Friedman, D.J. Greenblatt, E.S. Burstein et al. Population study of triazolam pharmacokinetics. Brit. J. Clin. Pharm. 22: 639–642, 1986.

D.J. Greenblatt, M. Divoll, L.J. Moschitto and R.I. Shader. Electron-capture gas chromatographic analysis of the triazolobenzodiazepines alprazolam and triazolam. J. Chrom. 225: 202–207, 1981.

T. Inoue and S.I. Suzuki. High-performance liquid chromatographic determination of triazolam and its metabolites in human urine. J. Chrom. 422: 197–204, 1987.

R. Jochemsen and D.D. Breimer. Assay of triazolam in plasma by capillary gas chromatography. J. Chrom. 223: 438–444, 1981.

B.P. Joynt. Triazolam blood concentrations in forensic cases in Canada. J. Anal. Tox. 17: 171–177, 1993.

G. Koves and J. Wells. The quantitation of triazolam in postmortem blood by gas chromatography/negative ion chemical ionization mass spectrometry. J. Anal. Tox. 10: 241–244, 1986.

K. Kudo, T. Nagata, T. Imamura et al. Forensic analysis of triazolam in human tissues using capillary gas chromatography. Int. J. Leg. Med. 104: 67–69, 1991.

K.R. Olson, L. Yin, J. Osterloh et al. Coma caused by trivial triazolam overdose. Ann. Emer. Med. 14: 210–211, 1985.

Q.R. Regestein and P. Reich. Agitation observed during treatment with newer hypnotic drugs. J. Clin. Psych. 46: 280–283, 1985.

P. Reynolds. Personal communication, 1988.

R.B. Smith, P.D. Kroboth and J.P. Phillips. Temporal variation in triazolam pharmacokinetics and pharmacodynamics after oral administration. J. Clin. Pharm. 26: 120–124, 1986.

A. Steentoft and K. Worm. Cases of triazolam poisoning. J. For. Sci. Soc. 33: 45–48, 1993.

C. van der Kroef. Reactions to triazolam. Lancet 2: 526, 1979.

R.J. Wong. The determination of the triazolobenzodiazepine triazolam in post mortem samples. J. Anal. Tox. 8: 10–13, 1984.

Trichloroethane

T½: 53 hr (whole blood)
Vd: ?   CCl3CH3
Fb: ?

Occurrence and Usage. 1,1,1-Trichloroethane (methyl chloroform) was introduced commercially in 1954 as a substitute for the more toxic carbon tetrachloride. It is encountered frequently in both industrial and domestic use as a degreaser, dry cleaning agent, and solvent in paints, glues and aerosol products. The compound has received clinical trials as an inhalation anesthetic, but is not currently used for this purpose. Air concentrations of trichloroethane in the workplace are not to exceed an average 8 hour level of 350 ppm (1910 mg/m³), which is approximately 3 times the odor threshold for this chemical.

Blood Concentrations. Trichloroethane blood concentrations in 12 resting subjects averaged 1.4 mg/L during a 30 minute exposure to 250 ppm of the vapor (Astrand et al., 1973). Blood concentrations of trichloroethane ranged from 1.5–6.5 mg/L (average, 3–4) during a 78 minute exposure to 500 ppm, but fell to 1 mg/L or less within 25 minutes after cessation of exposure. Maximum blood concentrations of 7–10 mg/L were achieved 65 minutes after the start of a 73 minute exposure to 955 ppm by asymptomatic subjects (Stewart et al., 1961).

Metabolism and Excretion. Trichloroethane is slowly metabolized in man by oxidation to trichloroethanol, which is excreted as a glucuronide conjugate (urochloralic acid) in urine over a period of 5–12 days and which accounts for only about 2% of an absorbed dose. Trichloroacetic acid is formed from trichloroethanol as a further oxidation product and is also found in urine to the extent of about 0.5% of a dose. Both of these metabolites are also biotransformation products of chloral hydrate, tetrachloroethylene and trichloroethylene. Trichloroethane is largely exhaled unchanged, 60–80% of a dose appearing within 1 week, and traces may be found in the post-exposure expired breath for as long as 1 month. The terminal elimination half-life averages 53 hours (Stewart et al., 1969; Monster et al., 1979; Nolan et al., 1984). In the rat, 98.7% of a single dose is exhaled unchanged in 25 hours, with 0.5% as carbon dioxide, and much of the balance is found as urinary trichloroethanol glucuronide (Hake et al., 1960).

Alveolar air concentrations in subjects exposed to 350 ppm of trichloroethane were found to average 179 ppm at rest and 239 ppm during light exercise; these concentrations were measured within 20–30 minutes after the start of exposure and declined rapidly upon cessation of exposure (Astrand et al., 1973).

Urinary concentrations of trichloroethanol in workers exposed daily to 53 ppm of trichloroethane were found to average 9.9 mg/L (range, 6.8–14.5) in specimens collected toward the end of the week; the corresponding values for trichloroacetic acid were 3.6 mg/L and a range of 2.4–5.5 mg/L. The half-life of trichloroethane as calculated from urinary metabolite excretion data was 8.7 hours (Seki et al., 1975).

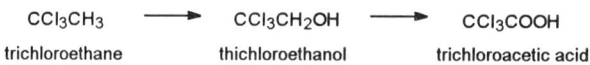

CCl3CH3 ⟶ CCl3CH2OH ⟶ CCl3COOH
trichloroethane   thichloroethanol   trichloroacetic acid

Toxicity. The anesthetic effects of trichloroethane, such as lightheadedness and loss of coordination, are displayed by persons exposed to vapor concentrations exceeding 1000 ppm. The compound has only slight capacity to cause liver or kidney damage with repeated exposure to high concentrations (Torkelson et al., 1958). However, there is some indication that liver abnormalities may be experienced by abusers of trichloroethane (Litt and Cohen, 1969), and one worker developed transient hepatic and renal damage after a single acute overexposure to the chemical (Halevy et al., 1980). Chronic exposure has been associated with peripheral neuropathy in several individuals (House et al., 1994).

Only a small number of non-fatal and fatal acute episodes of poisoning have been reported (Stewart and Andrews, 1966; Stewart, 1971). A postmortem trichloroethane blood concentration of 60 mg/L was determined in a man who succumbed while exposed to a vapor concentration of 500 ppm (Hatfield and Maykoski, 1970). The tissue concentrations found in 10 fatal cases show a wide variation; it is conceivable that, in certain instances, cardiac arrest following ventricular fibrillation may occur prior to the absorption of significant quantities of the vapor (Hall and Hine, 1966; Stahl et al., 1969; Bidanset, 1973; Caplan et al., 1976; Jones and Winter, 1983):

Trichloroethane Concentrations in Fatal Cases (mg/L or mg/kg)

	Blood	Brain	Lung	Liver	Kidney	Urine
Average	126	277	14	102	56	1.6
(Range)	(1.5–720)	(3.2–590)	(1.8–31)	(4.9–220)	(2.6–120)	(0.9–3)

Analysis. The determination of trichloroethane in body fluids and tissues has been performed by flame-ionization gas chromatography using a headspace sampling method (Hall and Hine, 1966; Caplan et al., 1976). Methods for determination of trichloroethanol and trichloroacetic acid in urine are cited in the section on trichloroethylene.

References

I. Astrand, A. Kilbom, I. Wahlberg and P. Ovrum. Methylchloroform exposure. Work Env. Health 10: 69–81, 1973.

J. Bidanset. Presented at the 25th annual meeting of the American Academy of Forensic Sciences, Las Vegas, February 22, 1973.

Y.H. Caplan, R.C. Backer and J.Q. Whitaker. 1,1,1-Trichloroethane: report of a fatal intoxication. Clin. Tox. 9: 69–74, 1976.

C.L. Hake, T.B. Waggoner, D.N. Robertson and V.K Rowe. The metabolism of 1,1,1-trichloroethane by the rat. Arch. Env. Health 1: 101–105, 1960.

J. Halevy, S. Pitlik, J. Rosenfeld and B.D. Eitan. 1,1,1-Trichloroethane intoxication: a case report with transient liver and renal damage. Review of the literature. Clin. Tox. 16: 467–472, 1980.

F.B. Hall and C.H. Hine. Trichloroethane intoxication: a report of two cases. J. For. Sci. 11: 404–413, 1966.

T.R. Hatfield and R.T. Maykoski. A fatal methyl chloroform (trichloroethane) poisoning. Arch. Env. Health 20: 279–281, 1970.

R.A. House, G.M. Liss and M.C. Wills. Peripheral sensory neuropathy associated with 1,1,1-trichloroethane. Arch. Env. Health 49: 196–199, 1994.

R.D. Jones and D.P. Winter. Two case reports of deaths on industrial premises attributed to 1,1,1-trichloroethane. Arch. Env. Health 38: 59–61, 1983.

I.F. Litt and M.I. Cohen. "Danger...vapor harmful": spot-remover sniffing. New Eng. J. Med. 281: 543–544, 1969.

A.C. Monster, G. Boersma and H. Steenweg. Kinetics of 1,1,1-trichloroethane in volunteers; influence of exposure concentration and work load. Int. Arch. Occ. Env. Health 42: 293–301, 1979.

R.J. Nolan, N.L. Freshour, D.L. Rick et al. Kinetics and metabolism of inhaled methyl chloroform (1,1,1-trichloroethane) in male volunteers. Fund. Appl. Tox. 4: 654–662, 1984.

Y. Seki, Y. Urashima, H. Aikawa et al. Trichloro-compounds in the urine of humans exposed to methyl chloroform at sub-threshold levels. Int. Arch. Arbeitsmed. 34: 39–49, 1975.

C.J. Stahl, A.V. Fatteh and A.M. Dominguez. Trichloroethane poisoning: observations on the pathology and toxicology in six fatal cases. J. For. Sci. 14: 393–397, 1969.

R.D. Stewart, H.H. Gay, D.S. Erley et al. Human exposure to 1,1,1-trichloroethane vapor: relationship of expired air and blood concentrations to exposure and toxicity. Am. Ind. Hyg. Asso. J. 22: 252–262, 1961.

R.D. Stewart and J.T. Andrews. Acute intoxication with methylchloroform. J. Am. Med. Asso. 195: 904–906, 1966.

R.D. Stewart, H.H. Gay, A.W. Schaffer et al. Experimental human exposure to methyl chloroform vapor. Arch. Env. Health 19: 467–472, 1969.

R.D. Stewart. Methyl chloroform intoxication. J. Am. Med. Asso. 215: 1789–1792, 1971.

T.R. Torkelson, F. Oyen, D.D. McCollister and V.K. Rowe. Toxicity of 1,1,1-trichloroethane as determined on laboratory animals and human subjects. Am. Ind. Hyg. Asso. J. 19: 353–362, 1958.

Trichloroethylene

T½: 30–38 hr
Vd: ? $Cl_2C=CHCl$
Fb: ?

Occurrence and Usage. Trichloroethylene (Tri, Trilene), first described in 1864, has been used industrially as a solvent, degreaser and dry cleaning agent for over 60 years; since 1934 it has also been employed as an induction agent and sole anesthetic in surgical procedures, but has largely been replaced by the less toxic fluorinated ethers. The current threshold limit value for trichloroethylene is 50 ppm (269 mg/m^3), which is approximately the odor threshold for the compound.

Blood Concentrations. Blood concentrations of trichloroethylene and trichloroethanol, a metabolite, reached average peak levels of 1 and 6 mg/L, respectively, in 5 subjects exposed to 100 ppm trichloroethylene for 6 hours; this was approximately the same trichloroethanol level seen 2 hours after the ingestion of a hypnotic dose (15 mg/kg) of chloral hydrate by 2 subjects (Mueller et al., 1974). During a 3 hour exposure to a vapor concentration of 211 ppm, blood trichloroethylene concentrations in 7 subjects rose to an average maximum of 6 mg/L (range, 4.5–7) within 2 hours (Stewart et al., 1962). Trichloroethylene blood concentrations in 22 surgical patients anesthetized with an induction level of 1% trichloroethylene for 30 minutes averaged 64 mg/L (range, 33–90); blood concentrations upon waking ranged from 16–57 mg/L (Prior, 1972).

Metabolism and Excretion. Trichloroethylene is extensively metabolized in man, probably via an epoxide intermediate that rearranges with migration of a chlorine atom; chloral hydrate has been identified as a transient metabolite, achieving a blood concentration of 0.17 mg/L during trichloroethylene anesthesia (Cole et al., 1975). The major urinary metabolites are trichloroacetic acid and trichloroethanol, the latter appearing largely as a glucuronide conjugate (urochloralic acid). Both chloral hydrate and free trichloroethanol have hypnotic activity in man. Trichloroacetic acid is a hypnotically inactive metabolite, but its presence in plasma should be recognized due to its possible interference in colorimetric assays for trichloroethylene or trichloroethanol; plasma trichloroacetic acid concentrations of 9–40 mg/L (average, 24) were observed on the third day after exposure of subjects to a trichloroethylene concentration of 194 ppm for 5 hours (Bartonicek, 1962).

From 51–64% of an inhaled dose of trichloroethylene is retained; of this, an average of 45% is slowly excreted as trichloroethanol glucuronide and 32% as trichloroacetic acid in the urine over a 3 week period. The excretion half-lives of these metabolites in persons exposed to trichloroethylene are 12 and 100 hours, respectively (Mueller et al., 1974). An additional 8% as both metabolites is eliminated in feces (Bartonicek, 1962), and a small amount (4%) is reportedly found as monochloroacetic acid in urine (Soucek and Vlachova, 1960). Approximately 16% of a dose is excreted unchanged in the expired breath (Nomiyama and Nomiyama, 1971).

Urine concentrations of trichloroethanol and trichloroacetic acid in subjects chronically exposed to trichloroethylene air concentrations of 120–250 ppm averaged 133 and 72 mg/L, respectively, in specimens obtained on a Friday afternoon (Tanaka and Ikeda, 1968). Other investigators using similar conditions have found average values of 682 and 230 mg/L for trichloroethanol and trichloroacetic acid, respectively, in urine of workers exposed to an average air concentration of 120 ppm (Ikeda et al., 1972).

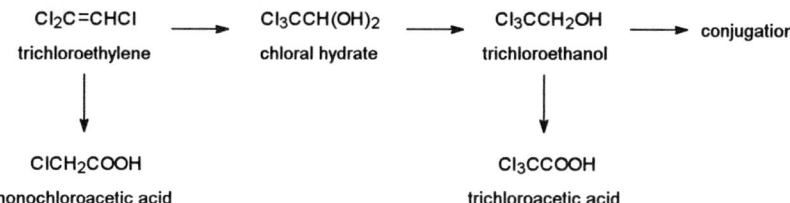

Toxicity. Trichloroethylene has been implicated in numerous chronic and acute poisonings. The compound is addicting in chronic usage (Ikeda et al., 1971), and is known to produce hepatic and renal abnormalities in abusers, probably as a result of its metabolites (Baerg and Kimberg, 1970). Acute toxic episodes may be due to the anesthetic effects of trichloroethylene, the hypnotic effects of trichloroethanol or to cardiac arrhythmia produced by high concentrations of the vapor (Kleinfeld and Tabershaw, 1954; Ertle et al., 1972; McCarthy and Jones, 1983). A man who had intentionally inhaled trichloroethylene developed double vision, ataxia and cranial nerve palsies; on admission, his serum trichloroethanol level was 119 mg/L, while his urinary trichloroethanol and trichloroacetic acid concentrations were 51 and 26 mg/L, respectively (Szlatenyi and Wang, 1994).

Workers chronically exposed to trichloroethylene vapor concentrations of 40–270 ppm often exhibit symptoms of fatigue, headache, irritability, vomiting, flushing of the skin, intolerance to alcohol and electrocardiographic changes. These symptoms are first noted when urinary trichloroacetic acid concentrations are on the order of 100 mg/L, and become pronounced at concentrations of 200 mg/L (ACGIH, 1971). Peripheral neurotoxicity has also been noted (Feldman et al., 1970; McCunney, 1988).

The following tissue concentrations of trichloroethylene were compiled from 20 fatal cases due to the ingestion or inhalation of this agent (James, 1963; Le Breton et al., 1963; Bonnichsen and Maehly, 1966; Cravey and Baselt, 1968; McAuley, 1970; Alha, 1974; Tadjer, 1977; Franc, 1983):

Trichloroethylene Concentrations in Fatal Cases (mg/L or mg/kg)

	Blood	Brain	Lung	Liver	Kidney	Urine
Average	27	62	16	64	31	23
(Range)	(3–110)	(2–270)	(1–45)	(5–250)	(11–112)	(0–73)

Analysis. Trichloroethylene concentrations in body fluids and tissues are usually estimated by gas chromatography with solvent extraction (Stewart et al., 1964) or headspace sampling procedures (Prior, 1972). Colorimetric and gas chromatographic techniques for the determination of trichloroethanol and trichloroacetic acid are cited in the section on chloral hydrate. Additionally, electron-capture gas chromatographic methods have been described for conjugated trichloroethanol in urine (Ertle et al., 1972; Ikeda et al., 1984), for trichloroacetic acid as its methyl derivative (Ehrner-Samuel et al., 1973), and for comprehensive analysis of trichloroethylene and its major metabolites in various specimens (Kimmerle and Eben, 1973; Ogata and Saeki, 1974; Monster and Boersma, 1975). A loss of 50% of the trichloroethylene content was observed in serum specimens stored frozen for 24 hours prior to analysis (Gorski et al., 1990).

References

ACGIH. *Documentation of the Threshold Limit Values*, American Conference of Governmental Industrial Hygienists, Cincinnati, Ohio, 1971, pp. 263–265.

A. Alha. Personal communication, 1974.

R.D. Baerg and D.V. Kimberg. Centrilobular hepatic necrosis and acute renal failure in "solvent sniffers." Ann. Int. Med. 73: 713–720, 1970.

V. Bartonicek. Metabolism and excretion of trichloroethylene after inhalation by human subjects. Brit. J. Ind. Med. 19: 134–141, 1962.

R. Bonnichsen and A.H. Maehly. Poisoning by volatile compounds. II. Chlorinated aliphatic hydrocarbons. J. For. Sci. 11: 414–427, 1966.

W.J. Cole, R.G. Mitchell and R.F. Salamonsen. Isolation, characterization and quantitation of chloral hydrate as a transient metabolite of trichloroethylene in man using electron capture gas chromatography and mass fragmentography. J. Pharm. Pharmac. 27: 167–171, 1975.

R.H. Cravey and R.C. Baselt. Unpublished results, 1968.

H. Ehrner-Samuel, K. Balmer and W. Thorsell. Determination of trichloroacetic acid in urine by a gas chromatographic method. Am. Ind. Hyg. Asso. J. 34: 93–96, 1973.

T. Ertle, D. Henschler, G. Mueller and M. Spassowski. Metabolism of trichloroethylene in man. Arch. Tox. 29: 171–188, 1972.

R.G. Feldman, R.M. Mayer and A. Taub. Evidence for peripheral neurotoxic effect of trichloroethylene. Neurology 20: 599–606, 1970.

A. Franc. Personal communication, 1983.

T. Gorski, T.J. Goehl, C.W. Jameson and B.J. Collins. Sources of error in the determination of trichloroethylene in blood. Bull. Env. Cont. Tox. 45: 1–5, 1990.

M. Ikeda, H. Ohtsuji, H. Kawai and M. Kuniyoshi. Excretion kinetics of urinary metabolites in a patient addicted to trichloroethylene. Brit. J. Ind. Med. 28: 203–206, 1971.

M. Ikeda, H. Ohtsuji, T. Imamura and Y. Komoike. Urinary excretion of total trichloro-compounds, trichloroethanol, and trichloroacetic acid as a measure of exposure to trichloroethylene and tetrachloroethylene. Brit. J. Ind. Med. 29: 328–333, 1972.

M. Ikeda, H. Hattori, Y. Koyama and S. Ohmori. Determination of urochloralic acid, the glucuronic acid conjugate of trichloroethanol, by gas chromatography with electron-capture detection and its application to urine, plasma and liver. J. Chrom. 307: 111–119, 1984.

W.R.L. James. Fatal addiction to trichloroethylene. Brit. J. Ind. Med. 20: 47–49, 1963.

G. Kimmerle and A. Eben. Metabolism, excretion and toxicology of trichloroethylene after inhalation. Arch. Tox. 30: 115–126, 1973.

M. Kleinfeld and I.R. Tabershaw. Trichloroethylene toxicity. Arch. Ind. Hyg. Occ. Med. 10: 134–141, 1954.

R. Le Breton, J. Le Bourhis and J. Garat. Un cas d'empoisonnement criminel par le trichlorethylene. Ann. Med. Leg. 43: 281–283, 1963.

F. McAuley. Personal communication, 1970.

T.B. McCarthy and R.D. Jones. Industrial gassing poisonings due to trichloroethylene, perchlorethylene, and 1-1-1 trichloroethane, 1961–80. Brit. J. Ind. Med. 40: 450–455, 1983.

R.J. McCunney. Diverse manifestations of trichloroethylene. Brit. J. Ind. Med. 45: 122–126, 1988.

A.C. Monster and G. Boersma. Simultaneous determination of trichloroethylene and metabolites in blood and exhaled air by gas chromatography. Int. Arch. Occ. Env. Health 35: 155–163, 1975.

G. Mueller, M. Spassovski and D. Henschler. Metabolism of trichloroethylene in man. Arch. Tox. 32: 283–295, 1974.

K. Nomiyama and H. Nomiyama. Metabolism of trichloroethylene in human. Int. Arch. Arbeitsmed. 28: 37–48, 1971.

M. Ogata and T. Saeki. Measurement of chloral hydrate, trichloroethanol, trichloroacetic acid and monochloroacetic acid in the serum and the urine by gas chromatography. Int. Arch. Arbeitsmed. 33: 49–58, 1974.

F.N. Prior. Blood levels of trichloroethylene during major surgery. Anaesthesia 27: 379–389, 1972.

B. Soucek and D. Vlachova. Excretion of trichloroethylene metabolites in human urine. Brit. J. Ind. Med. 17: 60–64, 1960.

R.D. Stewart, H.H. Gay, D.S. Erley et al. Observations on the concentrations of trichloroethylene in blood and expired air following exposure of humans. Am. Ind. Hyg. Asso. J. 23: 167–170, 1962.

R.D. Stewart, S.E. Sadek, J.D. Swank and H.C. Dodd. Diagnosis of trichloroethylene exposure after death. Arch. Path. 77: 101–104, 1964.

C.S. Szlatenyi and R.Y. Wang. Encephalopathy and cranial nerve palsies due to intentional trichloroethylene inhalation. Vet. Hum. Tox. 36: 348, 1994.

G. Tadjer. Personal communication, 1977.

S. Tanaka and M. Ikeda. A method for determination of trichloroethanol and trichloroacetic acid in urine. Brit. J. Ind. Med. 25: 214–219, 1968.

2,4,5-Trichlorophenoxyacetic Acid

T½: 11–23 hr
Vd: 6.1 L/kg
Fb: 0.99
pKa: 3.1

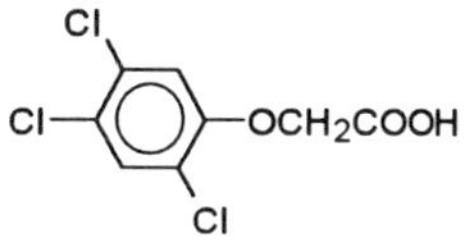

Occurrence and Usage. 2,4,5-Trichlorophenoxyacetic acid (2,4,5-T) and its salts have been extensively used as herbicides for the control of broadleaf plants, often in combination with 2,4-dichlorophenoxyacetic acid. 2,4,5-T in pure form is of relatively low toxicity, but some commercial preparations have been found to contain traces of the highly toxic dioxin. For this reason, the U.S. Environmental Protection Agency banned most major uses of 2,4,5-T in early 1979. The current threshold limit value for occupational exposure to 2,4,5-T is 10 mg/m³.

Blood Concentrations. A single oral 150 mg dose given to a volunteer produced a peak plasma 2,4,5-T concentration of 21 mg/L at 4 hours after administration; the levels declined with a half-life of 11 hours (Matsumura, 1970). A single oral dose of 5 mg/kg (350 mg/70 kg) given to volunteers who remained asymptomatic produced maximal plasma concentrations of 40–88 mg/L, averaging about 60 mg/L, within 4 hours. The levels declined with an average half-life of 23 hours. Approximately 65% of whole blood 2,4,5-T resides in plasma, and of this amount 98.7% is protein bound (Gehring et al., 1973).

Metabolism and Excretion. An average of 89% of a single 5 mg/kg dose of 2,4,5-T was excreted in the urine of asymptomatic volunteers over a 4 day period as unchanged compound. The urine collected during the first 12 hours after administration contained 27% of the dose, producing estimated urine concentrations of 100–300 mg/L. No metabolites are known, although it is possible that a small amount is eliminated as a glucuronide conjugate. Less than 1% of a dose is excreted in feces (Gehring et al., 1973).

Urine concentrations of 2,4,5-T in 8 asymptomatic herbicide spray operators were found to range from 0.05–3.6 mg/L (Shafik et al., 1971). Workers in a chemical factory exposed to 2,4,5-T at levels of 0.2–0.7 mg/m³ had urine concentrations of 1.0–3.5 mg/L (Matsumura, 1970).

Toxicity. 2,4,5-T in pure form is considered to be of relatively low toxicity. In overdosage, the compound causes muscular weakness and stiffness, nausea, vomiting and diarrhea. Workers in a 2,4,5-T factory had an 18% incidence of chloracne, but other organ systems were not significantly affected (Poland et al., 1971).

2,4,5-T itself is not believed to be carcinogenic or teratogenic in animals or man; these effects, produced by technical grades of the chemical, are believed due to the dioxin that is present as an impurity. Early technical grades of 2,4,5-T contained up to 30 ppm of dioxin, although recent samples have contained as little as 0.04 ppm (Courtney and Moore, 1971; American Farm Bureau Federation, 1980). An epidemiological study of an area where 2,4,5-T was sprayed found no evidence of any association with birth defects of the central nervous system (Hanify et al., 1981).

The following tissue concentrations were observed in a young woman who died 16 hours after ingesting a 3:2 mixture of 2,4-D and 2,4,5-T (Coutselinis et al., 1977):

2,4-D and 2,4,5-T Concentrations in a Fatal Case (mg/L or mg/kg)

Chemical	Blood	Liver	Kidney
2,4-D	826	21	82
2,4,5-T	182	5	22

Analysis. 2,4,5-T may be determined in biological specimens by colorimetry (Matsumura, 1970), ultraviolet spectrophotometry (Coutselinis et al., 1977), or electron-capture gas chromatography (Shafik et al., 1971). The procedures cited in the section on 2,4,-dichlorophenoxyacetic acid are also applicable.

References

American Farm Bureau Federation. Dispute resolution conference on 2,4,5-T. Vet. Hum. Tox. 22: 40–42, 1980.

K.D. Courtney and J.A. Moore. Teratology studies with 2,4,5-trichlorophenoxyacetic acid and 2,3,7,8-tetrachlorodibenzo-p-dioxin. Tox. Appl. Pharm. 20: 396–403, 1971.

A. Coutselinis, R. Kentarchou and D. Boukis. Concentration levels of 2,4-D and 2,4,5-T in forensic material. For. Sci. 10: 203–204, 1977.

P.J. Gehring, C.G. Kramer, B.A. Schwetz et al. The fate of 2,4,5-trichlorophenoxyacetic acid (2,4,5-T) following oral administration to man. Tox. Appl. Pharm. 26: 352–361, 1973.

J.A. Hanify, P. Metcalf, C.L. Nobbs and K.J. Worsley. Aerial spraying of 2,4,5-T and human birth malformations: an epidemiological investigation. Science 212: 349–351, 1981.

A. Matsumura. The fate of 2,4,5-trichlorophenoxyacetic acid in man. Jap. J. Ind. Health 12: 20–25, 1970.

A.P. Poland, D. Smith, G. Metter and P. Possick. A health survey of workers in a 2,4-D and 2,4,5-T plant. Arch. Env. Health 22: 316–327, 1971.

M.T. Shafik, H.C. Sullivan and H.F. Enos. A method for determination of low levels of exposure to 2,4-D and 2,4,5-T. Int. J. Env. Anal. Chem. 1: 23–33, 1971.

Trifluoperazine

T½: 7–18 hr
Vd: ?
Fb: ?
pKa: 8.1

Occurrence and Usage. Trifluoperazine (Stelazine) is a phenothiazine derivative used frequently to control the manifestations of psychotic disorders. It is a close chemical relative of fluphenazine and prochlorperazine. The drug is supplied as the hydrochloride in 1–10 mg tablets and a 10 mg/mL concentrate for oral use, and a 2 mg/mL injectable solution. Oral maintenance doses range from 2–40 mg daily, whereas intramuscular doses usually do not exceed 6 mg per day.

Blood Concentrations. Five volunteers who ingested a 5 mg tablet of trifluoperazine developed an average maximal plasma concentration of 1.4 µg/L (range, 0.5–3.1) within 1.5–4.5 hours (Midha et al., 1983). A single 20 mg oral dose given to 4 subjects resulted in peak plasma levels of 0.9–4.0 µg/L by 3–6 hours; the levels declined with an average half-life of 11 hours (Gillespie and Sipes, 1981). An 80 mg oral dose given to a patient, whose pre-dose plasma trifluoperazine level was 2.1 µg/L, produced a peak plasma level of 28 µg/L at 8 hours, declining to 3.8 µg/L by 24 hours (Curry et al., 1981).

Metabolism and Excretion. In patients on chronic therapy, from 0.3–1.0% of the daily dose is excreted unchanged in the 24 hour urine, with 1.3–6.2% present as trifluoperazine sulfoxide (West et al., 1974). Plasma concentrations of 7-hydroxytrifluoperazine, believed to be an active metabolite, are about 50% of those of the parent after a single oral dose, and the elimination half-life is similar (Aravagiri et al., 1985).

In rats, an average of 6% of an oral dose is excreted in the 24 hour urine, with 91% in feces, largely as metabolites. The drug is known to be extensively metabolized in animals by N-demethylation, sulfoxidation, piperazine-ring fission, and N-oxidation. Aromatic ring hydroxylation and conjugation are believed to occur (Huang and Bhansali, 1968; Spirtes, 1974; Gaertner et al., 1975; West and Vogel, 1975).

Toxicity. Overdosage with trifluoperazine produces somnolence, agitation, convulsions, fever, coma, hypotension, and cardiac arrest. A woman who died of suspected overdose while on daily therapy with 40 mg of the drug had postmortem blood and liver concentrations of 60 µg/L and 310 µg/kg, respectively (Street, 1981). A woman who committed suicide by oral ingestion of trifluoperazine had postmortem concentrations of 400 µg/L in blood, 198,000 µg/kg in liver and 83,000 µg/kg in kidney; similar levels of 7-hydroxytrifluoperazine and N-desmethyltrifluoperazine were found in the liver and kidney (Quai et al., 1985).

Analysis. A fluorometric procedure was used to assay trifluoperazine and its sulfoxide in urine (West et al., 1974). Plasma levels of the parent drug have been measured by gas chromatography with nitrogen-phosphorus (Gillespie and Sipes, 1981; Javaid et al., 1982; Roscoe et al., 1982), or mass spectrometric detection (Midha et al., 1982; Whelpton et al., 1982). Liquid chromatography has also been employed (Curry et al., 1981).

References

M. Aravagiri, E.M. Hawes and K.K. Midha. Radioimmunoassay for the 7-hydroxy metabolite of trifluoperazine and its application to a kinetic study in human volunteers. J. Pharm. Sci. 74: 1196–1202, 1985.

S.H. Curry, R.B. Stewart, P.K. Springer and J.E. Pope. Plasma-trifluoperazine concentrations during high dose therapy. Lancet 1: 395–396, 1981.

H.J. Gaertner, G. Liomin, D. Villumsen et al. Tissue metabolites of trifluoperazine, fluphenazine, prochlorperazine, and perphenazine. Drug Met. Disp. 3: 437–444, 1975.

T.J. Gillespie and I.G. Sipes. Sensitive gas chromatographic determination of trifluoperazine in human plasma. J. Chrom. 223: 95–102, 1981.

J.I. Javaid, H. Dekirmenjian and J.M. Davis. GLC analysis of trifluoperazine in human plasma. J. Pharm. Sci. 71: 63–66, 1982.

C.L. Huang and K.G. Bhansali. Nonpolar metabolites of trifluoperazine in rats. J. Pharm. Sci. 57: 1511–1513, 1968.

K.K. Midha, R.H.M. Roscoe, K. Hall et al. A gas chromatographic mass spectrometric assay for plasma trifluoperazine concentrations following single doses. Biomed. Mass Spec. 9: 186–190, 1982.

K.K. Midha, E.D. Korchinski, R.K. Verbeeck et al. Kinetics of oral trifluoperazine disposition in man. Brit. J. Clin. Pharm. 15: 380–382, 1983.

I. Quai, M. Fagarasan and E. Fagarasan. A fatal case of trifluoperazine poisoning. J. Anal. Tox. 9: 43–44, 1985.

R.H.M. Roscoe, J.K. Cooper, E.M. Hawes and K.K. Midha. A glc-nitrogen phosphorus detector assay for trifluoperazine in plasma. J. Pharm. Sci. 71: 625–627, 1982.

M.A. Spirtes. Two types of metabolically produced trifluoperazine N-oxides. In *Phenothiazines and Structurally Related Drugs* (I.S. Forrest, C.J. Carr and E. Usdin, eds.), Raven Press, New York, 1974, pp. 399–404.

E. Street. Personal communication, 1981.

N.R. West, M.P. Rosenblum, H. Sprince et al. Assay procedures for thioridazine, trifluoperazine, and their sulfoxides and determination of urinary excretion of these compounds in mental patients. J. Pharm. Sci. 63: 417–419, 1974.

N.R. West and W.H. Vogel. Absorption, distribution and excretion of trifluoperazine in rats. Arch. Int. Pharm. 215: 318–335, 1975.

R. Whelpton, S.H. Curry and G.M. Watkins. Analysis of plasma trifluoperazine by gas chromatography and selected ion monitoring. J. Chrom. 228: 321–326, 1982.

Trihexyphenidyl

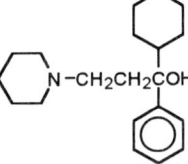

T½: 5–11 hours
Vd: ?
Fb: ?
pKa: ?

Occurrence and Usage. Trihexyphenidyl (benzhexol, Artane) is a synthetic antispasmodic drug that exerts a direct inhibitory effect on the parasympathetic nervous system. It is used in the treatment of Parkinsonism and in the control of extrapyramidal symptoms associated with phenothiazine therapy. Its therapeutic properties are similar to those of atropine, although its adverse effects are ordinarily less frequent and less severe. The drug is available as the hydrochloride salt in 2 and 5 mg tablets, sustained-release capsules of 5 mg, and an elixir containing 2 mg/5 mL.

Blood Concentrations. Twenty-four healthy, young males were given single oral doses of trihexyphenidyl in either a 5 mg immediate-release or a 10 mg sustained-release form; peak plasma concentrations averaged 31 µg/L at 2.0 hours and 15 µg/L at 3.7 hours, respectively (Cheung et al., 1988).

Metabolism and Excretion. Very little information is available regarding the fate of trihexyphenidyl in man. Significant quantities of both the parent drug and a hydroxylated metabolite have been reported in urine (Dawling, 1989; Kintz et al., 1989).

Toxicity. Adverse effects include blurred vision, drowsiness, tachycardia, nausea, weakness and restlessness. The drug has been frequently abused for its euphorigenic, delusional and hallucinogenic effects (Pakes and Brotman, 1978; Goggin and Soloman, 1979).

In a drowning case following ingestion of a 20 mg dose by a teenager, a postmortem blood concentration of 33 µg/L was found (Kopjak, 1976). A male adult who ingested as much as 125 mg of trihexyphenidyl for suicidal purposes had a postmortem blood level of 800 µg/L; the specimen also contained 0.10 g/dL ethanol and 270 µg/L amitriptyline (Dawling, 1989).

Analysis. Trihexyphenidyl has been determined in biological fluids using gas chromatography (Kintz et al., 1989; Owen et al., 1989) and by gas chromatography-mass spectrometry (Maurer, 1992).

References

W.K. Cheung, S.S. Stravinski, S.I. Engel et al. Pharmacokinetic evaluation of a sustained-release formulation of trihexyphenidyl in healthy volunteers. J. Pharm. Sci. 77: 748–750, 1988.

S. Dawling. Personal communication, 1989.

D.A. Goggin and G.F. Solomon. Trihexyphenidyl abuse for euphorigenic effect. Am. J. Psych. 136: 459–460, 1979.

P. Kintz, B. Godelar, P. Mangin et al. Identification and quantification of trihexyphenidyl and its hydroxylated metabolite by gas chromatography with nitrogen-phosphorus detection. J. Anal. Tox. 13: 47–49, 1989.

L. Kopjak. Personal communication, 1976.

H.H. Maurer. Systematic toxicological analysis of drugs and their metabolites by gas chromatography-mass spectrometry. J. Chrom. 580: 3–41, 1992.

J.A. Owen, M. Sribney, J.S. Lawson et al. Capillary gas chromatography of trihexylphenidyl, procyclidine and cycrimine in biological fluids. J. Chrom. 494: 135–142, 1989.

G.E. Pakes and D.M. Brotman. Abuse of trihexyphenidyl. J. Am. Med. Asso. 240: 2434, 1978.

Trimipramine

T½: 16–39 hr
Vd: 17–48 L/kg
Fb: 0.95
pKa: ?

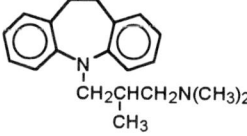

Occurrence and Usage. Trimipramine (Surmontil, Stangyl) is a tricyclic antidepressant, closely related to imipramine, that has been used since 1960 for the treatment of depression. It is marketed in the United States as the maleate salt in 25 and 50 mg capsules for oral administration. Daily doses range from 50–300 mg.

Blood Concentrations. Nine subjects given a single 50 mg oral dose of trimipramine developed an average peak plasma level of 0.028 mg/L (range, 0.015–0.051) at times ranging from 1–6 hours (Abernethy et al., 1984). A single 75 mg oral dose given to 12 subjects produced an average peak plasma concentration of 0.019 mg/L (range, 0.008–0.034) at 2.5 hours (Caille et al., 1980).

A group of 29 patients receiving chronic daily doses of 75–150 mg exhibited average plasma concentrations of 0.086 mg/L (range, 0.011–0.241) for trimipramine, 0.065 mg/L (range, 0.003–0.382) for N-desmethyltrimipramine, and 0.016 mg/L (range, 0.003–0.040) for unconjugated 2-hydroxytrimipramine (Suckow and Cooper, 1984).

Metabolism and Excretion. Trimipramine is known to be metabolized in man by N-demethylation, N-dealkylation, 2-hydroxylation, phenyl hydroxylation, N-oxidation and conjugation. The conjugates of the hydroxylated metabolites tend to accumulate in plasma during chronic therapy. At least 9 metabolites have been identified in urine in addition to the parent drug (Suckow and Cooper, 1984; Koppel and Tenczer, 1988).

Toxicity. Overdosage with trimipramine may cause drowsiness, ataxia, agitation, muscle rigidity, convulsions, coma, tachycardia, hypotension, cardiac arrhythmias, hyperpyrexia, and shock. Physostigmine by intravenous infusion is capable of reversing many of these toxic effects.

Five adults who died after trimipramine overdosage had average blood concentrations of 7.6 mg/L (range, 0.4–12) and liver concentrations of 173 mg/kg (range, 42–544) (Ryall, 1974; Ulrich, 1974; Hucker, 1983; Meatherall et al., 1983; Fraser et al., 1987). Trimipramine may exhibit postmortem redistribution; heart blood/femoral blood concentration ratios of 3.2 and 4.6 were observed in 2 decedents (Anderson and Prouty, 1989).

Analysis. Trimipramine has been assayed in plasma at therapeutic concentrations by gas chromatography with nitrogen-phosphorus (Caille et al., 1980; Abernethy et al., 1984) or mass spectrometric detection (Bougerolle et al., 1988; Eap et al., 1994). Liquid chromatography has also been described (Wong and Stolarum, 1981; Suckow and Cooper, 1984; Gulaid et al., 1991).

References

D.R. Abernethy, D.J. Greenblatt and R.I. Shader. Trimipramine kinetics and absolute bioavailability: use of gas-liquid chromatography with nitrogen-phosphorus detection. Clin. Pharm. Ther. 35: 348–353, 1984.

W.H. Anderson and R.W. Prouty. Postmortem redistribution of drugs. In *Advances in Analytical Toxicology* (R.C. Baselt, ed.), Vol. 2, YearBook Medical, Chicago, 1989, pp. 70–102.

A.M. Bougerolle, J.L. Chabard, M. Jbilou et al. Simultaneous determination of trimipramine and its demethylated metabolites in plasma by gc-ms. J. Chrom. 434: 232–238, 1988.

G. Caille, J.G. Besner, Y. Lacasse and M. Vezina. Pharmacokinetic characteristics of two different formulations of trimipramine determined with a new GLC method. Biopharm. Drug Disp. 1: 187–194, 1980.

C.B. Eap, L. Koeb and P. Baumann. Determination of trimipramine and its demethylated and hydroxylated metabolites in plasma by gas chromatography-mass spectrometry. J. Chrom. 652: 97–103, 1994.

A.D. Fraser, A.F. Isner and R.A. Perry. Distribution of trimipramine and its major metabolites in a fatal overdose case. J. Anal. Tox. 11: 168–170, 1987.

A.A. Gulaid, G.A. Jahn, C. Maslen and M.J. Dennis. Simultaneous determination of trimipramine and its major metabolites by hplc. J. Chrom. 566: 228–233, 1991.

R.S. Hucker. Personal communication, 1983.

C. Koppel and J. Tenczer. Gas chromatographic-mass spectrometric study of the urinary metabolism of trimipramine. J. Chrom. 431: 197–202, 1988.

R.C. Meatherall, D.R.P. Guay, J.M. Nokes and J.R. Keenan. Toxicological findings in a death resulting from the ingestion of trimipramine. J. For. Sci. 28: 1023–1029, 1983.

J. Ryall. Personal communication, 1974.

R.F. Suckow and T.B. Cooper. Determination of trimipramine and metabolites in plasma by liquid chromatography with electrochemical detection. J. Pharm. Sci. 73: 1745–1748, 1984.

R.J. Ulrich. Personal communication, 1974.

S.H. Wong and S.L. Stolarum. Liquid chromatographic assay of trimipramine in plasma. Clin. Chem. 27: 1101–1103, 1981.

Tripelennamine

T½: 2.9–5.3
Vd: 9–12 L/kg
Fb: ?
pKa: 4.2, 8.7

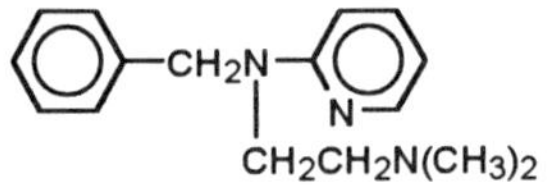

Occurrence and Usage. Tripelennamine (PBZ, Pyribenzamine) is an ethylenediamine derivative that was synthesized in 1946 and is currently used as a topical and oral antihistamine. It is available as the hydrochloride and citrate salts, either alone or in combination with ephedrine and/or codeine. The drug is administered orally in doses of 25–50 mg every 4–6 hours, or as a sustained-release preparation in doses of 50–100 mg every 8–12 hours.

Blood Concentrations. Plasma concentrations of the drug after a 100 mg oral dose reached a maximum of 0.06 mg/L at 2 and 3 hours (Bayley et al., 1975). In 6 volunteers given a single intramuscular dose, plasma levels reached an average peak of 0.105 mg/L at 0.5 hours after 50 mg and 0.199 mg/L at 0.25 hours after 100 mg (Yeh et al., 1986).

Metabolism and Excretion. Tripelennamine has been shown to be metabolized by N-demethylation, hydroxylation, conjugation, and N-oxide formation. Major urinary metabolites include tripelennamine-N-glucuronide (4.4% of a dose), conjugated α-hydroxytripelennamine (23%), con-

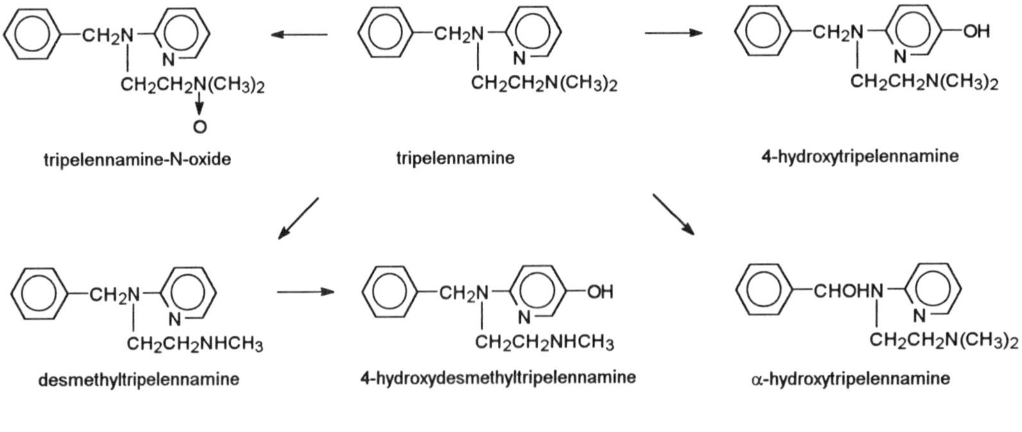

tripelennamine-N-oxide   tripelennamine   4-hydroxytripelennamine

desmethyltripelennamine   4-hydroxydesmethyltripelennamine   α-hydroxytripelennamine jugated 4-hydroxytripelennamine and conjugated 4-hydroxydesmethyltripelennamine. Tripelennamine-N-oxide is a minor urinary metabolite, while very little unchanged drug (1.2%) and no detectable desmethyltripelennamine are present (Perlman, 1949; Chaudhuri et al., 1976; Yeh, 1991).

Toxicity. Adverse reactions to this drug include chills, confusion, nervousness, irritability, hysteria, nausea, blurred vision, hypotension, dizziness, tachycardia, convulsions, and blood dyscrasias. Moderate overdosage in children has caused central nervous system stimulation and hallucinations (Hays et al., 1980).

Postmortem blood tripelennamine concentrations ranged from 0.1–3.0 mg/L in 13 fatalities attributed to combined abuse of tripelennamine and pentazocine (Monforte et al., 1983). One fatality has been reported following the ingestion of 1000 mg of the drug by a 19 year old male; death occurred 7 hours after ingestion, and the following levels were noted in the postmortem specimens (Bayley et al., 1975):

Tripelennamine Concentrations in a Fatal Case (mg/L or mg/kg)

Blood	Brain	Liver	Kidney	Urine
10	43	83	35	287

Analysis. Both ultraviolet spectrophotometry (Bayley et al., 1975) and gas chromatography (Yeh, 1991) have been applied to the analysis of tripelennamine in human tissues.

References

M. Bayley, F.M. Walsh and M.J. Valaske. Report of a fatal, acute tripelennamine intoxication. J. For. Sci. 20: 539–543, 1975.

N.K. Chaudhuri, O.A. Servando, M.J. Manniello et al. Metabolism of tripelennamine in man. Drug Met. Disp. 4: 372–378, 1976.

D.P. Hays, B.F. Johnson and R. Perry. Prolonged hallucinations following a modest overdose of tripelennamine. Clin. Tox. 16: 331–333, 1980.

J.R. Monforte, R. Gault, J. Smialek and T. Goodin. Toxicological and pathological findings in fatalities involving pentazocine and tripelennamine. J. For. Sci. 28: 90–101, 1983.

E. Perlman. A quantitative method for the determination of antihistaminic compounds containing the pyridine radical. J. Pharm. Exp. Ther. 95: 465–481, 1949.

S.Y. Yeh, G.D. Todd, R.E. Johnson et al. The pharmacokinetics of pentazocine and tripelennamine. Clin. Pharm. Ther. 39: 669–676, 1986.

S.Y. Yeh. Metabolic profile of tripelennamine in humans. J. Pharm. Sci. 80: 815–819, 1991.

Tubocurarine

T½: 2.5–3.9 hr
Vd: 0.28–0.56 L/kg
Fb: 0.44
pKa: 8.1, 9.1

Occurrence and Usage. Tubocurarine is one of the curare alkaloids, derived primarily from the South American plant *Chondrodendron tomentosum*. It is a mono-quaternary ammonium compound that, as the d-isomer, is utilized as a neuromuscular blocking agent. The semisynthetic dimethyl ether is also employed clinically and has about 3 times the potency. When tubocurarine is administered in intravenous doses of 5–15 mg it produces a non-depolarizing blockade that lasts for 0.5–1.5 hours. The drug is supplied as the chloride salt in 10 mL ampules of 3 mg/mL.

Blood Concentrations. Five subjects given doses of 0.3 mg/kg (21 mg/70 kg) by intravenous injection developed serum concentrations as high as 6 mg/L initially, with a decline to about 1 mg/L by 20 minutes and 0.5 mg/L by 2 hours; after 24 hours tubocurarine could still be detected in serum at a range of 0.025–0.083 mg/L (Horowitz and Spector, 1973). In a study of 48 patients, it was found that recovery from the effects of tubocurarine did not begin until the mean serum level reached 0.70 mg/L; 50% recovery of muscle tension occurred at a level of 0.45 mg/L, and complete recovery at a mean serum concentration of 0.20 mg/L (Matteo et al., 1974). The plasma protein binding of tubocurarine is approximately 44% at therapeutic concentrations (Ghoneim et al., 1973) and in whole blood the drug is restricted to the plasma (Mahfouz, 1949). Only small amounts of the compound appear in cerebrospinal fluid, with gradual accumulation after a single dose to an average of 0.025 mg/L at 6 hours in 9 surgical patients (Matteo et al., 1977).

Metabolism and Excretion. Tubocurarine is believed to be largely excreted unchanged in the urine and, although no human studies have been performed to elucidate possible products of biotransformation, experiments in dogs suggest that only 1% of a dose is metabolized (Cohen et al., 1967). From 33–41% is eliminated in the urine within 3 hours of an intravenous dose (Mahfouz, 1949; Marsh, 1952), and 43% in 24 hours (Miller et al., 1977). Concentrations of the drug in liver after therapeutic administration decline in conjunction with the plasma levels, but are always lower than plasma; kidney concentrations, however, increase as plasma levels fall and may exceed the plasma concentration by a factor of 5 at 2 hours after injection (Cohen et al., 1965). The plasma half-life is increased about 43% in patients with renal failure (Miller et al., 1977).

Toxicity. Accidental overdosage with this drug, causing hypotension and respiratory failure, is usually controlled by the antidotal administration of neostigmine. The use of tubocurarine as a homicidal poison has been suspected in a series of deaths in which the drug was detected in decomposed tissue (Altman, 1976). A fresh liver specimen in a fatality due to injection of the drug was found to contain 0.8 mg/kg of tubocurarine (Stevens and Fox, 1971).

Analysis. Tubocurarine may be efficiently extracted from biological fluids and tissues with ethylene dichloride in the presence of large amounts of potassium iodide, and quantitated by a methyl orange dye technique (Quinn and Woislawski, 1950), ultraviolet spectrophotometry (Kalow, 1953; Elert, 1956; Elert and Cohen, 1962; Stevens and Fox, 1971) or fluorometry (Cohen, 1963). Fluorometry has also been applied to the quantitation of tubocurarine and other quaternary ammonium compounds after ion-pair extraction and thin-layer chromatographic purification (Wittmer et al., 1975). A highly sensitive radioimmunoassay employing a tritium label was developed and has been used for the direct determination of the drug in serum (Horowitz and Spector, 1973). Liquid chromatography with ultraviolet detection has been described (Meulemans et al., 1981).

References

L.K. Altman. Collaboration and complex techniques led to discovery of curare in tissues. New York Times, March 8, 1976.

E.N. Cohen. Quantitative determination of d-tubocurarine in body tissues and fluids. J. Lab. Clin. Med. 62: 979–984, 1963.

E.N. Cohen, A. Corbascio and G. Fleischli. The distribution and fate of d-tubocurarine. J. Pharm. Exp. Ther. 147: 120–129, 1965.

E.N. Cohen, H.W. Brewer and D. Smith. The metabolism and elimination of d-tubocurarine-H$_3$. Anesthesiology 28: 309–317, 1967.

B.T. Elert. A new ultraviolet spectrophotometric method for the determination of d-tubocurarine chloride in plasma. Am. J. Med. Tech. 22: 331–338, 1956.

B.T. Elert and E.N. Cohen. A micro spectrophotometric method for the analysis of minute concentrations of d-tubocurarine chloride in plasma. Am. J. Med. Tech. 28: 125–134, 1962.

M.M. Ghoneim, E. Kramer, R. Bannow et al. Binding of d-tubocurarine to plasma proteins in normal man and in patients with hepatic or renal disease. Anesthesiology 39: 410–415, 1973.

P.E. Horowitz and S. Spector. Determination of serum d-tubocurarine concentration by radioimmunoassay. J. Pharm. Exp. Ther. 185: 94–100, 1973.

W. Kalow. Urinary excretion of d-tubocurarine in man. J. Pharm. Exp. Ther. 109: 74–82, 1953.

M. Mahfouz. The fate of tubocurarine in the body. Brit. J. Pharm. 4: 295–303, 1949.

D.F. Marsh. The distribution, metabolism, and excretion of d-tubocurarine chloride and related compounds in man and other animals. J. Pharm. Exp. Ther. 105: 299–316, 1952.

R.S. Matteo, S. Spector and P.E. Horowitz. Relation of serum d-tubocurarine concentration to neuromuscular blockade in man. Anesthesiology 41: 440–443, 1974.

R.S. Matteo, E.K. Pua, H.J. Khambatta and S. Spector. Cerebrospinal fluid levels of d-tubocurarine in man. Anesthesiology 46: 396–399, 1977.

A. Meulemans, J. Mohler, D. Henzel and P. Duvaldestin. Quantitation of d-tubocuraine in human plasma using high-performance liquid chromatography. J. Chrom. 226: 255–258, 1981.

R.D. Miller, R.S. Matteo, L.Z. Benet and Y.J. Sohn. The pharmacokinetics of d-tubocurarine in man with and without renal failure. J. Pharm. Exp. Ther. 202: 1–7, 1977.

G.P. Quinn and S. Woislawski. A method for the quantitative estimation of small amounts of d-tubocurarine chloride in plasma. Proc. Soc. Exp. Biol. Med. 74: 365–367, 1950.

H.M. Stevens and R.H. Fox. A method for detecting tubocurarine in tissues. J. For. Sci. Soc. 11: 177–182, 1971.

D. Wittmer, S. Atwell and W.G. Haney, Jr. Quantitative extraction of tubocurarine, gallamine, and decamethonium from biological materials. J. For. Sci. 20: 86–90, 1975.

Valproic Acid

T½: 8–12 hr
Vd: 0.1–0.4 L/kg
Fb: 0.90–0.95
pKa: 4.8

$$C_3H_7$$
$$CH_3CH_2CH_2CHCOOH$$

Occurrence and Usage. Valproic acid (dipropylacetic acid, sodium valproate, Depakene), a carboxylic acid derivative synthesized in 1881, has been used since 1967 as an anticonvulsant drug. At room temperature, it is a colorless liquid with a characteristic odor. The drug is supplied as the free acid in 250 mg capsules or as the sodium salt in a 250 mg/5 mL syrup. Daily oral doses range from 250–2500 mg.

Blood Concentrations. A single oral 400 mg dose of valproic acid given to 4 patients produced peak plasma levels of approximately 32–42 mg/L at times of 1.5–3 hours (Mihaly et al., 1979). Following the oral administration of 800 mg to 6 patients, peak serum concentrations of 66–90 mg/L (average, 72) were observed at times ranging from 0.5–2 hours; the levels declined with an average half-life of 9 hours (Perucca et al., 1978). The blood/plasma concentration ratio for the drug is 0.55 (Loescher, 1978).

Predose steady-state plasma concentrations in patients receiving daily doses of 20–36 mg/kg (1400–2520 mg/70 kg) ranged from 81–106 mg/L. The suggested therapeutic range for plasma valproic acid is 50–100 mg/L (Mihaly et al., 1979).

Metabolism and Excretion. Up to 86% of a labeled dose of valproic acid is eliminated in urine within 24 hours, but only 1–4% of the dose is excreted unchanged. The major urinary metabolite is the glucuronide conjugate of the parent drug, accounting for up to 59% of a dose. Other metabolites include 3-ketovalproic acid (23%), 3-, 4-, and 5-hydroxyvalproic acid (3% each), and 2-propylglutaric acid (PGA) (5%); each of these, as well as the parent drug, may be excreted in conjugated form. Valproic acid also undergoes desaturation, with production of minor amounts of 2-en- and 4-en-valproic acid (Merits, 1977; Schaefer et al., 1980; Dickinson et al., 1989). Most of these substances are found in plasma of patients receiving the drug, but due to their lower potencies and lower concentrations, it is believed that valproic acid itself accounts for at least 90% of the anticonvulsant activity (Loescher, 1981).

Brain concentrations of valproic acid in 9 patients on therapy ranged from 7–28% of the respective plasma drug concentration (Vajda et al., 1981). The following concentrations were measured in the tissues of a patient who died while on therapy with the drug (Sakata et al., 1985):

Valproic Acid Concentrations During Therapy (mg/L or mg/kg)

Blood	Brain	Liver	Kidney	Urine
60	15	100	36	180

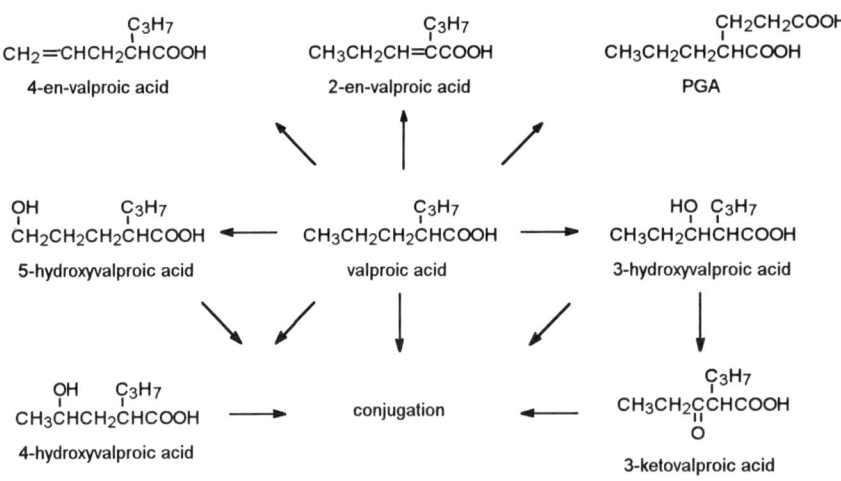

Toxicity. Adverse reactions to valproic acid therapy include nausea, vomiting, sedation, weakness, blood dyscrasias, pancreatitis and hepatic damage. Stupor has resulted in several patients following addition of this drug to a regimen including other anticonvulsants (Sackellares et al., 1979). Tremor and other toxic signs were noted in several patients when aspirin was added to a valproic acid regimen (Goulden et al., 1987). Hepatotoxicity has been noted in 11 patients with plasma valproic acid concentrations of 52–148 mg/L (Willmore et al., 1978; Sussman and McLain, 1979), while fatal hepatitis was reported in 3 pediatric patients, one of whom developed a serum valproic acid level of 166 mg/L (Donat et al., 1979; Suchy et al., 1979). Two young women developed coma and serum valproic acid concentrations of 709–2120 mg/L after ingesting doses of 30–75 g of the drug, but survived without injury (Karlsen et al., 1983; Mortensen et al., 1983).

A teenage girl died in coma after intentional ingestion of an overdose of valproic acid; a peak plasma level of 1969 mg/L was reported (Garnier et al., 1982). An adult male who died after ingesting an overdose was found to have postmortem levels of 720 mg/L in blood and 800 mg/kg in liver (Lokan and Dinan, 1988).

Analysis. Gas chromatographic procedures for the determination of valproic acid in plasma usually involve flame-ionization detection of the native drug (Loescher, 1977; Balkon, 1978; Berry and Clarke, 1978; Jakobs et al., 1978; Levy et al., 1978; Hershey et al., 1979; Peyton et al., 1979; Sioufi et al., 1980; Odusote and Sherwin, 1981; Tosoni et al., 1983) or of an ester derivative (Gyllenhaal and Albinsson, 1978; Tupper et al., 1978; Willox and Foot·, 1978; Gupta et al., 1979a; Calendrillo and Reynoso, 1980; Morita et al., 1981; Nishioka et al., 1983). Liquid chromatography has also been reported (Gupta et al., 1979b; Alric et al., 1981; Lucarelli et al., 1992) and an enzyme immunoassay is commercially available.

References

R. Alric, M. Cociglio, J.H. Blayac and R. Puech. Performance evaluation of a reversed-phase, high-performance liquid chromatographic assay of valproic acid involving a "solvent demixing" extraction procedure and precolumn derivatisation. J. Chrom. 224: 289–299, 1981.

J. Balkon. Rapid determination of valproic acid in biological specimens. J. Anal. Tox. 2: 207–209, 1978.

D.J. Berry and L.A. Clarke. Determination of valproic acid (dipropylacetic acid) in plasma by gas-liquid chromatography. J. Chrom. 156: 301–307, 1978.

B.A. Calendrillo and G. Reynoso. A micromethod for the on-column methylation of valproic acid by gas-liquid chromatography. J. Anal. Tox. 4: 272–274, 1980.

R.G. Dickinson, W.D. Hooper, P.R. Dunstan and M.J. Eadie. Urinary excretion of valproate and some metabolites in chronically treated patients. Ther. Drug Mon. 11: 127–133, 1989.

J.F. Donat, J.A. Bocchini, Jr., E. Gonzalez and R.N. Schwendimann. Valproic acid and fatal hepatitis. Neurology 29: 273–274, 1979.

R. Garnier, O. Boudignat and P.E. Fournier. Valproate poisoning. Lancet 2: 97, 1982.

K.J. Goulden, J.M. Dooley, P.R. Camfield and A.D. Fraser. Clinical valproate toxicity induced by acetylsalicylic acid. Neurology 37: 1392–1394, 1987.

R.N. Gupta, F. Eng and M.L. Gupta. Gas-chromatographic analysis for valproic acid as phenacyl esters. Clin. Chem. 25: 1303–1305, 1979a.

R.N. Gupta, P.M. Keane and M.L. Gupta. Valproic acid in plasma, as determined by liquid chromatography. Clin. Chem. 25: 1984–1985, 1979b.

O. Gyllenhaal and A. Albinsson. Gas chromatographic determination of valproate in minute serum samples after extractive methylation. J. Chrom. 161: 343–346, 1978.

A.E. Hershey, J.R. Patton and K.H. Dudley. Gas chromatographic method for the determination of valproic acid in human plasma. Ther. Drug Mon. 1: 217–241, 1979.

C. Jakobs, M. Bojasch and F. Hanefeld. New direct micro-method for determination of valproic acid in serum by gas chromatography. J. Chrom. 146: 494–497, 1978.

R.L. Karlsen, K. Kett and O. Henriksen. Intoxication with sodium valproate. Acta Med. Scand. 213: 405–406, 1983.

R.H. Levy, L. Martis and A.A. Lai. GLC determination of valproic acid in plasma. Anal. Letters 11: 257–267, 1978.

W. Loescher. Rapid determination of valproate sodium in serum by gas-liquid chromatography. Epilepsia 18: 225–227, 1977.

W. Loescher. Serum protein binding and pharmacokinetics of valproate in man, dog, rat and mouse. J. Pharm. Exp. Ther. 204: 255–261, 1978.

W. Loescher. Concentration of metabolites of valproic acid in plasma of epileptic patients. Epilepsia 22: 169–178, 1981.

R.J. Lokan and A.C. Dinan. An apparent fatal valproic acid poisoning. J. Anal. Tox. 12: 35–37, 1988.

C. Lucarelli, P. Villa, E. Lombaradi et al. HPLC method for the simultaneous analysis of valproic acid and other common anticonvulsant drugs in plasma of serum. Chromatographia 33: 37–40, 1992.

I. Merits. Metabolic fate of valproate sodium in dog, rat, rabbit, monkey and human. Epilepsia 18: 289–290, 1977.

G.W. Mihaly, F.J. Vajda, J.L. Miles and W.J. Louis. Single and chronic dose pharmacokinetic studies of sodium valproate in epileptic patients. Eur. J. Clin. Pharm. 16: 23–29, 1979.

Y. Morita, T.I. Ruo, M.L. Lee and A.J. Atkinson, Jr. On-column propylation method for measuring plasma valproate concentrations by gas chromatography. Ther. Drug Mon. 3: 193–199, 1981.

P.B. Mortensen, H.E. Hansen, B. Pedersen et al. Acute valproate intoxication: biochemical investigations and hemodialysis treatment. Int. J. Clin. Pharm. Ther. Tox. 21: 64–68, 1983.

R. Nishioka, S. Kawai and S. Toyoda. New method for the gas chromatographic determination of valproic acid in serum. J. Chrom. 277: 356–360, 1983.

K.A. Odusote and A.L. Sherwin. A simple, direct extraction method for gas-liquid chromatographic determination of valproic acid in plasma. Ther. Drug Mon. 3: 103–106, 1981.

E. Perucca, G. Gatti, G.M. Frigo et al. Disposition of sodium valproate in epileptic patients. Brit. J. Clin. Pharm. 5: 495–499, 1978.

G.A. Peyton, S.C. Harris and J.E. Wallace. Determination of valproic acid by flame-ionization gas-liquid chromatography. J. Anal. Tox. 3: 108–110, 1979.

J.C. Sackellares, S.I. Lee and F.E. Dreifuss. Stupor following administration of valproic acid to patients receiving other antiepileptic drugs. Epilepsia 20: 697–703, 1979.

M. Sakata, K. Sakata, M. Haga et al. Distribution of antiepileptic drugs in human blood and tissue. In *Proceedings of the 21st International Meeting*, September 13–17, Brighton, UK (N. Dunnett and K.J. Kimber, eds.), International Association of Forensic Toxicologists, 1985, pp. 211–214.

H. Schaefer, R. Luhrs and H. Reith. Chemistry, pharmacokinetics, and biological activity of some metabolites of valproic acid. In *Antiepileptic Therapy: Advances in Drug Monitoring* (S.I. Johannessen, ed.), Raven Press, New York, 1980, pp. 103–110.

A. Sioufi, D. Colussi and F. Marfil. Gas chromatographic determination of valproic acid in human plasma. J. Chrom. 182: 241–245, 1980.

F.J. Suchy, W.F. Balistreri, J.J. Buchino et al. Acute hepatic failure associated with the use of sodium valproate. New Eng. J. Med. 300: 962–966, 1979.

N.M. Sussman and L.W. McLain, Jr. A direct hepatotoxic effect of valproic acid. J. Am. Med. Asso. 242: 1173–1174, 1979.

S. Tosoni, C. Signorini and A. Albertini. Gas-chromatographic determination of valproic acid in serum without derivatization. Clin. Chem. 29: 990, 1983.

N.L. Tupper, E.B. Solow and C.P. Kenfield. A method for esterification of valproic acid for gas-liquid chromatography: clinical data from epileptic patients. J. Anal. Tox. 2: 203–206, 1978.

F.J.E. Vajda, G.A. Donnan, J. Phillips and P.F. Bladin. Human brain, plasma, and cerebrospinal fluid concentration of sodium valproate after 72 hours of therapy. Neurology 31: 486–487, 1981.

L.J. Willmore, B.J. Wilder, J. Bruni and H.J. Villarreal. Effect of valproic acid on hepatic function. Neurology 28: 961–964, 1978.

S. Willox and S.E. Foote. Simple method for measuring valproate (Epilim) in biological fluids. J. Chrom. 151: 67–70, 1978.

Vanadium

T½: ?   v
Vd: ?
Fb: ?

Occurrence and Usage. Vanadium has many minor industrial uses, including its incorporation into dyes, paints and insecticides, but its primary use is as an alloying agent in the production of hard steel. In this process it is encountered as vanadium pentoxide, which may be inhaled by workers as a dust or fume. The current threshold limit value for vanadium as a dust or fume is 0.05

mg/m³. Vanadium is a trace element in biological systems, but is not considered essential for higher animals. The estimated average daily dietary intake of the metal is 20 µg.

Blood Concentrations. Blood vanadium (90% of which resides in plasma) concentrations in normal persons range from 0.4–2.8 µg/L (Gylseth et al., 1979), while serum concentrations range from 2–4 µg/L (Stroop et al., 1982). More recent data indicate that the serum vanadium concentration in healthy subjects is less than 0.24 µg/L (Ishida et al., 1989). In workers exposed to vanadium, blood concentrations were found to average 1.8 µg/L (range, 0.6–3.8) in one group (Gylseth et al., 1979) and serum concentrations averaged 11 µg/L in another (Kiviluoto et al., 1979). Eight healthy vanadium pentoxide workers, exposed for periods of 2–3 years, had serum vanadium levels averaging 20 µg/L during a working period and 13 µg/L at the end of their summer holidays (Kiviluoto et al., 1981).

Metabolism and Excretion. Of the 20 µg of vanadium that is ingested in the daily diet, most is believed to be excreted in feces, apparently unabsorbed. Normal urine averages less than 8 µg/24 hours of the metal, with an upper concentration limit of 22 µg/L. Vanadium is found in only trace amounts in most tissues in the body and data regarding body accumulation with age are inconclusive. Fat contains up to 90% of the total body burden of vanadium (Schroeder et al., 1963; Myron et al., 1978).

In subjects given 4.5 mg daily of a soluble form of vanadium, urinary excretion over 24 hours accounted for 5% of a dose; urine vanadium concentrations ranged from 53–296 µg/L in the asymptomatic subjects (Schroeder et al., 1963). Urinary vanadium concentrations in healthy workers cleaning oil-fired boilers ranged from <0.4–2.3 µg/L prior to beginning work and from 2–11 µg/L after 2 or 3 days of such work (White et al., 1987).

Toxicity. Vanadium compounds are irritants of the skin and mucous membranes, and when encountered in toxic amounts cause primarily symptoms of pulmonary dysfunction. Workers exposed to vanadium pentoxide for only a few days may develop irritation of the conjunctivae, rhinitis, dryness of the throat, hoarseness, bronchitis with coughing and wheezing, dyspnea and pneumonitis (Sjoberg, 1956). Green coloration of the tongue is also associated with vanadium toxicity and is believed to be due to the deposition of vanadium salts (Lewis, 1959). Few systemic effects are seen in this disease and, once the worker has been removed from exposure, the prognosis is very favorable (Sjoberg, 1951).

Eighteen workers who were exposed to vanadium pentoxide dust at concentrations in excess of 0.5 mg/m³ for a period of up to 2 weeks developed acute respiratory symptoms that persisted for nearly 2 weeks after removal from exposure; vanadium was demonstrated in urine at elevated levels, and it continued to be excreted for up to 14 days after exposure had ended (Zenz et al., 1962). Controlled human exposure to vanadium pentoxide at a concentration of 0.1 mg/m³ for 8 hours produced mucous formation in the lungs and cough that subsided within 3 days, while a concentration of 0.25 mg/m³ caused a loose cough that persisted for 7–10 days. The peak urinary vanadium concentration observed was 130 µg/L at 3 days after exposure; vanadium was undetectable in all urine specimens by 7 days following exposure (Zenz and Berg, 1967). Vanadium is a natural component of fuel oil, and workers have developed vanadium poisoning during cleaning operations on oil-fired furnaces. Several of the most severely affected men were found to have urine vanadium concentrations of 43–380 µg/L (Williams, 1952; Thomas and Stiebris, 1956).

Volunteers given daily oral doses of 50–125 mg of ammonium vanadyl tartrate for periods of up to 6 weeks developed green tongue, intestinal cramps, diarrhea and black stools; urinary vanadium concentrations ranged from 38–1300 µg/L and correlated roughly with the dosage administered (Dimond et al., 1963).

Analysis. Vanadium may be determined in urine by colorimetry (Rockhold and Talvitie, 1956; Welch and Allaway, 1972). Atomic absorption spectrometry, of greater sensitivity and specificity, is preferred for the analysis of both serum and urine (Kiviluoto et al., 1981; Buchet et al., 1982;

Stroop et al., 1982; White et al., 1987; Ishida et al., 1989). Liquid chromatography has also been investigated (Godin, 1990).

References

J.P. Buchet, E. Knepper and R. Lauwerys. Determination of vanadium in urine by electrothermal atomic absorption spectrometry. Anal. Chim. Acta 136: 243–248, 1982.

E.G. Dimond, J. Caravaca and A. Benchimol. Vanadium. Excretion, toxicity, lipid effect in man. Am. J. Clin. Nutri. 12: 49–53, 1963.

J. Godin. Hplc method for the determination of vanadium in serum. J. Chrom. 532: 445–448, 1990.

B. Gylseth, H.L. Leira, E. Steinnes and Y. Thomassen. Vanadium in the blood and urine of workers in a ferroalloy plant. Scand. J. Work Env. Health 5: 188–194, 1979.

O. Ishida, K. Kihara, Y. Tsukamoto and F. Marumo. Improved determination of vanadium in biological fluids by electrothermal atomic absorption spectrometry. Clin. Chem. 35: 127–130, 1989.

M. Kiviluoto, L. Pyy and A. Pakarinen. Serum and urinary vanadium of vanadium-exposed workers. Scand. J. Work Env. Health 5: 362–367, 1979.

M. Kiviluoto, L. Pyy and A. Pakarinen. Serum and urinary vanadium of workers processing vanadium pentoxide. Int. Arch. Occ. Env. Health 48: 251–256, 1981.

C.E. Lewis. The biological effects of vanadium. II. The signs and symptoms of occupational vanadium exposure. Arch. Ind. Health 19: 497–503, 1959.

D.R. Myron, T.J. Zimmerman, T.R. Shuler et al. Intake of nickel and vanadium by humans. A survey of selected diets. Am. J. Clin. Nutri. 31: 527–531, 1978.

W.T. Rockhold and N.A. Talvitie. Vanadium concentration of urine. Clin. Chem. 2: 188–194, 1956.

H.A. Schroeder, J.J. Balassa and I.H. Tipton. Abnormal trace metals in man—vanadium. J. Chron. Dis. 16: 1047–1071, 1963.

S.G. Sjoberg. Health hazards in the production and handling of vanadium pentoxide. Arch. Ind. Health 3: 631–646, 1951.

S.G. Sjoberg. Vanadium dust, chronic bronchitis and possible risk of emphysema. Acta Med. Scand. 154: 381–386, 1956.

S.D. Stroop, G. Helinek and H.L. Greene. More sensitive flameless atomic absorption analysis of vanadium in tissue and serum. Clin. Chem. 28: 79–82, 1982.

D.L.G. Thomas and K. Stiebris. Vanadium poisoning in industry. Med. J. Aust. 43: 607–609, 1956.

R.M. Welch and W.H. Allaway. Vanadium determination in biological materials at nanogram levels by a catalytic method. Anal. Chem. 44: 1644–1647, 1972.

M.A. White, G.D. Reeves, S. Moore et al. Sensitive determination of urinary vanadium as a measure of occupational exposure during cleaning of oil-fired boilers. Ann. Occ. Hyg. 31: 339–343, 1987.

N. Williams. Vanadium poisoning from cleaning oil-fired boilers. Brit. J. Ind. Med. 9: 50–55, 1952.

C. Zenz, J.P. Bartlett and W.H. Thiede. Acute vanadium pentoxide intoxication. Arch. Env. Health 5: 542–546, 1962.

C. Zenz and B.A. Berg. Human response to controlled vanadium pentoxide exposure. Arch. Env. Health 14: 709–712, 1967.

Vancomycin

T½: 2.6–7.8 hr
Vd: 0.3–0.7 L/kg
Fb: 0.30
pKa: ?

Occurrence and Usage. Vancomycin (Vancocin) is a glycopeptide antibiotic first isolated from *Streptomyces orientalis* in 1956. It is used frequently in hospitals to treat staphylococcus and other gram-positive bacterial infections. The drug is supplied as the hydrochloride salt in the form of 125 or 250 mg capsules or a 1 or 10 g vial (the contents to be dissolved in 20 or 115 mL water, respectively) for oral administration or in a 500 or 1000 mg vial (for reconstitution with 10 or 20 mL water, respectively) for intravenous injection. The usual daily dose is 500–2000 mg orally given in 3–4 divided doses or 2000 mg intravenously given in 2 or 4 divided doses by slow (1 hour) infusion; lower doses are often necessary in patients with impaired renal function.

Blood Concentrations. Eight adult surgical patients receiving an average daily dose of 26 mg/kg (1820 mg/70 kg) of vancomycin by 1 hour intravenous infusion every 12 hours developed average peak and trough serum concentrations of 31 and 7.9 mg/L, respectively; 9 adult burn patients with similar renal function required a daily dose of 47 mg/kg (3290 mg/70 kg) to produce equivalent peak and trough serum levels (Garrelts and Peterie, 1988). For efficacy, the drug should be given at a dose that will yield peak serum values of 30–40 mg/L at the end of infusion and trough values of 5–10 mg/L just prior to the next dose (Rotschafer et al., 1982). Rodvald et al. (1988) have shown a direct correlation between creatinine clearance (as a measure of renal function) and the dose of vancomycin necessary to attain effective serum concentrations.

Metabolism and Excretion. Vancomycin is believed to be poorly absorbed after oral administration. From 80–90% of an intravenous dose is eliminated unchanged in the 24 hour urine (Knoben et al., 1979).

Toxicity. The adverse effects of vancomycin administration include skin rash, fever, thrombophlebitis, neutropenia, nephrotoxicity and ototoxicity. Nephrotoxicity is associated with serum drug concentrations in excess of 30 mg/L (Farber and Moellering, 1983), while ototoxicity is associated with levels in excess of 80 mg/L (Kirby et al., 1960). The accidental intravenous administration of 1476 mg of the drug to a neonate over a 5 day period produced a peak serum vancomycin level of 427 mg/L, but caused only reversible nephrotoxicity (Burkhart et al., 1992).

Analysis. Reagents are commercially available for determination of vancomycin serum levels by immunoassay. Other techniques include bioassay (Walker and Kopp, 1978) and liquid chromatography (McCain et al., 1982; Hoagland et al., 1984; Rosenthal et al., 1986).

References

K.K. Burkhart, S. Metcalf, E. Shurnas et al. Exchange transfusion and multidose activated charcoal following vancomycin overdose. Clin. Tox. 30: 285–294, 1992.

B.F. Farber and R.C. Moellering. Retrospective study of the toxicity of preparations of vancomycin from 1974 to 1981. Antimicrob. Agents Chemother. 23: 138–141, 1983.

J.C. Garrelts and J.D. Peterie. Altered vancomycin dose vs. serum concentration relationship in burn patients. Clin. Pharm. Ther. 44: 9–13, 1988.

R.J. Hoagland, J.E. Sherwin and J.M. Phillips, Jr. Vancomycin: a rapid HPLC assay for a potent antibiotic. J. Anal. Tox. 8: 75–77, 1984.

W.M.M. Kirby, D.M. Perry and A.W. Bauer. Treatment of staphyloccal septicemia with vancomycin. New Eng. J. Med. 262: 49–55, 1960.

J.E. Knoben, P.O. Anderson and A.S. Watanabe. *Handbook of Clinical Drug Data*, 4th ed., Drug Intelligence Publications, Hamilton, Illinois, 1979, pp. 254–255.

J.B.L. McClain, R. Bongiovanni and S. Brown. Vancomycin quantitation by high-performance liquid chromatography in human serum. J. Chrom. 231: 463–466, 1982.

K.A. Rodvald, R.A. Blum, J.H. Fischer et al. Vancomycin pharmacokinetics in patients with various degrees of renal function. Antimicrob. Agents Chemother. 32: 848–852, 1988.

A.F. Rosenthal, I. Sarfati and E. A'Zary. Simplified liquid-chromatographic determination of vancomycin. Clin. Chem. 32: 1016–1019, 1986.

J.C. Roschafer, K. Crossley, D.E. Zaske et al. Pharmacokinetics of vancomycin: observation in 28 patients and dosage recommendations. Antimicrob. Agents Chemother. 22: 391–394, 1982.

C.A. Walker and B. Kopp. Sensitive bioassay for vancomycin. Antimicrob. Agents Chemother. 13: 30–33, 1978.

Venlafaxine

T½: 3–7 hr
Vd: 4–12 L/kg
Fb: 0.27
pKa: ?

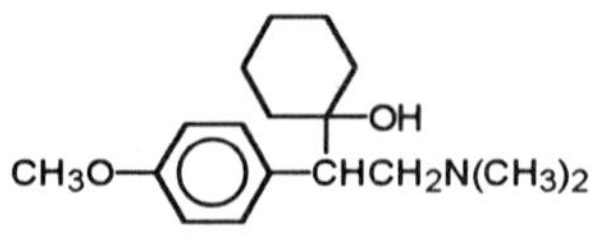

CH₃O—⬡—CHCH₂N(CH₃)₂
with OH and cyclohexyl ring substituents

Occurrence and Usage. Venlafaxine (WY-45030, Effexor) is a phenethylamine derivative that inhibits the reptake of certain neurotransmitters, including serotonin and norepinephrine. It is available for use as an antidepressant and is administered orally as the hydrochloride salt in daily doses of 75–150 mg.

Blood Concentrations. Normal adult subjects receiving a single 50 mg oral dose developed average peak plasma concentrations of 71 µg/L for venlafaxine at 2.2 hours and 106 µg/L for O-desmethylvenlafaxine at 3.9 hours. Predicted steady-state plasma concentrations of the drug and its metabolite in normal subjects receiving 150 mg daily are 70 and 254 µg/L, respectively (Troy et al., 1994).

Metabolism and Excretion. Venlafaxine is known to undergo O- and N-demethylation. An average of 87% of a labeled oral dose is excreted in the 48 hour urine; approximately 5% of a dose is eliminated as parent drug, 29–48% as O-desmethylvenlafaxine, 0.2–7.4% as mono-N-desmethylvenlafaxine and 6–19% as di-N-desmethylvenlafaxine. The O-desmethyl metabolite is believed to exhibit antidepressant activity similar to that of the parent drug, but has a longer elimination half-life (12 vs. 3.9 hours) (Sisenwine et al., 1989; Muth et al., 1991; Troy et al., 1994).

Toxicity. Adverse effects resulting from venlafaxine administration include nausea, vomiting, dizziness, nervousness, anxiety, tremor and blurred vision. Overdosage may cause hypertension or hypotension, cardiac arrhythmia, seizures and coma.

Analysis. Venlafaxine and its O-desmethyl metabolite have been assayed in biological specimens by liquid chromatography (Hicks et al, 1994).

References

D.R. Hicks, D. Wokaniuk, A. Russell et al. A hplc method for the simultaneous detection of venlafaxine and O-desmethylvenlafaxine in biological fluids. Ther. Drug Mon. 16: 100–107, 1994.

E.A. Muth, J.A. Moyer, J.T. Haskins et al. Biochemical, neurophysiological, and behaviorial effects of WY-45,233, its enantiomers, and other identified metabolites of the antidepressant venlafaxine. Drug Dev. Res. 23: 191–199, 1991.

S.F. Sisenwine, J. Politowski, K. Birk et al. A prefatory investigation of the metabolic disposition of WY-45,030 in man. Acta Pharm. Tox. 59 (Suppl. 5, part 2): 312, 1989.

S.M. Troy, R.W. Schulz, V.D. Parker et al. The effect of renal disease on the disposition of venlafaxine. Clin. Pharm. Ther. 56: 14–21, 1994.

Verapamil

T½: 3–7 hr
Vd: 2.5–6.5 L/kg
Fb: 0.90
pKa: ?

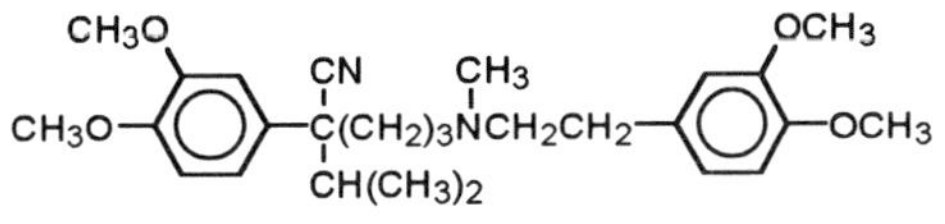

$$CH_3O-\bigcirc\overset{\underset{CH(CH_3)_2}{|}}{\underset{|}{C}}\overset{CN}{\underset{}{}}(CH_2)_3\overset{CH_3}{\underset{}{N}}CH_2CH_2-\bigcirc\overset{OCH_3}{\underset{}{}}-OCH_3$$

Occurrence and Usage. Verapamil (Calan, Isoptin, Verelan) is a synthetic papaverine derivative, first introduced in 1962 as an antianginal agent. It has since been found to have antiarrhythmic and antihypertensive properties, attributable to its ability to inhibit transmembrane calcium flux in excitable tissues. The drug is supplied as the hydrochloride for oral or intravenous administration. Single intravenous doses of 5–10 mg are used for hypertensive crises, while daily oral maintenance doses range from 240–480 mg.

Blood Concentrations. A single 80 mg oral dose of verapamil given to 6 subjects produced peak plasma concentrations averaging 0.055 mg/L (range, 0.029–0.125) at times of 0.5–3 hours; the levels declined with an average half-life of 3.5 hours (Eichelbaum et al., 1981). The oral administration of 120 mg to 6 volunteers resulted in peak plasma levels averaging 0.219 mg/L (range, 0.142–0.262) and occurring between 1.4 and 2.5 hours. The oral bioavailability of the drug ranged from 19–27% (Koike et al., 1979). An intravenous infusion of 13–16 mg, lasting 3.3–5.3 minutes, yielded plasma verapamil concentrations in 8 subjects that averaged 0.274 mg/L at 2 minutes after the infusion and 0.115 mg/L at 10 minutes (Dominic et al., 1981).

Twenty patients receiving long-term oral maintenance therapy with 480 mg of the drug daily exhibited average peak (1 hour after a 160 mg dose) plasma verapamil and norverapamil levels of 0.355 and 0.207 mg/L, respectively, while average trough levels were 0.091 and 0.160 mg/L, respectively (Woodcock et al., 1980). The half-life of verapamil averaged 14 hours in 7 patients with liver cirrhosis (Somogyi et al., 1981).

Metabolism and Excretion. After intravenous or oral administration of a labeled dose of verapamil, from 66–71% is excreted in urine and about 9–16% in feces over a 5 day period. The urine contains only 3–4% of the dose as unchanged drug and about 6% as norverapamil; other metabolites include products of O-demethylation and conjugation, and oxidative cleavage of the C-N-C linkage (Schomerus et al., 1976; Eichelbaum et al., 1979). Norverapamil has been shown to have only 20% of the pharmacological activity of its parent (Neugebauer, 1978).

Toxicity. Adverse effects associated with verapamil administration include nausea, weakness, dizziness, bradycardia, hypotension, and atrioventricular block. These effects were observed in 3 patients who acutely ingested 2.0–5.6 g of the drug and survived; intravenous calcium gluconate reversed the cardiac toxicity in one patient, who was noted to achieve a 4 mg/L blood verapamil concentration at 5 hours after ingestion of 3.2 g (de Faire and Lundman, 1977; Perkins, 1978; Candell et al., 1979).

The following tissue concentrations were obtained in 19 deaths due to acute overdosage with verapamil (Ryall, 1978; Thomson and Pannell, 1981; Picotte, 1985; Crouch et al., 1986; Chan et al., 1987; Hansson, 1987; Koepke and McBay, 1987):

Verapamil Concentrations in Fatal Cases (mg/L or mg/kg)

	Blood	Liver	Kidney	Gastric
Average	11	102	19	436 mg
(Range)	(0.9–85)	(3.2–280)	(10–28)	(0–2470)

Analysis. Verapamil has been assayed in plasma by fluorometry (McAllister and Howell, 1976) and by gas chromatography with flame-ionization (McAllister et al., 1979), nitrogen-phosphorus (Hege, 1979; Todd et al., 1980; Vasiliades et al., 1982), or mass spectrometric detection (Spiegelhalder and Eichelbaum, 1977). Liquid chromatographic methods, usually allowing the simultaneous determination of verapamil and norverapamil, are widely used (Harapat and Kates, 1980; Todd et al., 1980; Kuwada et al., 1981; Lim et al., 1983; Johnson and Khalil, 1987; Bremseth et al., 1988; Rustum, 1990; Koppel and Wagemann, 1991).

References

D.L. Bremseth, J.J. Lima and J.J. MacKichan. Specific HPLC method for the separation of verapamil and four major metabolites after oral dosing. J. Liq. Chrom. 11: 2731–2750, 1988.

J. Candell, V. Valle, M. Soler and J. Rius. Acute intoxication with verapamil. Chest 75: 200–201, 1979.

L.F.T. Chan, L.H. Chhuy and R.J. Crowley. Verapamil tissue concentrations in fatal cases. J. Anal. Tox. 11: 171–174, 1987.

D.J. Crouch, C. Crompton, D.E. Rollins et al. Toxicological findings in a fatal overdose of verapamil. J. For. Sci. 31: 1505–1508, 1986.

U. de Faire and T. Lundman. Attempted suicide with verapamil. Eur. J. Card. 6: 195–198, 1977.

J.A. Dominic, D.W.A. Bourne, T.G. Tan et al. The pharmacology of verapamil. III. Pharmacokinetics in normal subjects after intravenous drug administration. J. Cardiovasc. Pharm. 3: 25–38, 1981.

M. Eichelbaum, M. Ende, G. Remberg et al. The metabolism of dl-(^{14}C)verapamil in man. Drug Met. Disp. 7: 145–148, 1979.

M. Eichelbaum, A. Somogyi, G.E. von Unruh and H.J. Dengler. Simultaneous determination of the intravenous and oral pharmacokinetic parameters of d,l-verapamil using stable isotope-labelled verapamil. Eur. J. Clin. Pharm. 19: 133–137, 1981.

R.C. Hansson. Personal communication, 1987.

S.R. Harapat and R.E. Kates. High-performance liquid chromatographic analysis of verapamil. II. Simultaneous quantitation of verapamil and its active metabolite, norverapamil. J. Chrom. 181: 484–489, 1980.

H.G. Hege. Gas chromatographic determination of verapamil in plasma and urine. Arz. Forsch. 29: 1681–1684, 1979.

S.M. Johnson and S.K.W. Khalil. An HPLC method for the determination of verapamil and norverapamil in human plasma. J. Liq. Chrom. 10: 1187–1201, 1987.

J.F. Koepke and A.J. McBay. Fatal verapamil poisoning. J. For. Sci. 32: 1431–1434, 1987.

Y. Koike, K. Shimamura, I. Shudo and H. Saito. Pharmacokinetics of verapamil in man. Res. Comm. Chem. Path. Pharm. 24: 37–47, 1979.

D. Koppel and A. Wagemann. Plasma level monitoring of d,l-verapamil and three of its metabolites by reversed-phase hplc. J. Chrom. 570: 229–234, 1991.

M. Kuwada, T. Tateyama and J. Tsutsumi. Simultaneous determination of verapamil and its seven metabolites by high-performance liquid chromatography. J. Chrom. 222: 507–511, 1981.

C.K. Lim, J.M. Rideout and J.W.S. Sheldon. Determination of verapamil and norverapamil in serum by high-performance liquid chromatography. J. Liq. Chrom. 6: 887–893, 1983.

R.G. McAllister and S.M. Howell. Fluorometric assay of verapamil in biological fluids and tissues. J. Pharm. Sci. 65: 431–432, 1976.

R.G. McAllister, Jr., T.G. Tan and D.W.A. Bourne. GLC assay of verapamil in plasma: identification of fluorescent metabolites after oral drug administration. J. Pharm. Sci. 68: 574–577, 1979.

G. Neugebauer. Comparative cardiovascular actions of verapamil and its major metabolites in the anaesthetised dog. Cardiovasc. Res. 12: 247–254, 1978.

C.M. Perkins. Serious verapamil poisoning: treatment with intravenous calcium gluconate. Brit. Med. J. 2: 1127, 1978.

P. Picotte. Personal communication, 1985.

A.M. Rustum. Measurement of verapamil in human plasma by reversed-phase high-performance liquid chromatography using a short octyl column. J. Chrom. 528: 480–486, 1990.

J.E. Ryall. Personal communication, 1978.

M. Schomerus, B. Spiegelhalder, B. Stieren and M. Eichelbaum. Physiological disposition of verapamil in man. Cardiovasc. Res. 10: 605–612, 1976.

A. Somogyi, M. Albrecht, G. Kliems et al. Pharmacokinetics, bioavailability and ECG response of verapamil in patients with liver cirrhosis. Brit. J. Clin. Pharm. 12: 51–60, 1981.

B. Spiegelhalder and M. Eichelbaum. Determination of verapamil in human plasma by mass fragmentography using stable isotope-labelled verapamil as internal standard. Arz. Forsch. 27: 94–97, 1977.

B.M. Thomson and L.K. Pannell. The analysis of verapamil in postmortem specimens by HPLC and GC. J. Anal. Tox. 5: 105–109, 1981.

G.D. Todd, D.W.A. Bourne and R.C. McAllister, Jr. Measurement of verapamil concentrations in plasma by gas chromatography and high pressure liquid chromatography. Ther. Drug Mon. 2: 411–416, 1980.

J. Vasiliades, K. Wilkerson, D. Ellul et al. Gas-chromatographic determination of verapamil and norverapamil, with a nitrogen-selective detector. Clin. Chem. 28: 638–641, 1982.

B.G. Woodcock, R. Hopf and M. Kaltenbach. Verapamil and norverapamil plasma concentrations during long-term therapy in patients with hypertrophic obstructive cardiomyopathy. J. Cardiovasc. Pharm. 2: 17–23, 1980.

Vinyl Chloride

T½: ?
Vd: ?
Fb: ?

$$CH_2=CHCl$$

Occurrence and Usage. Vinyl chloride (chloroethylene) is an intermediate in the synthesis of several major commercial chemicals, including polyvinyl chloride, and has been used as an aerosol propellant. The compound is a gas at room temperature and therefore industrial exposure is by inhalation. Prior to recognition of the carcinogenic effect of vinyl chloride, the threshold limit value was set as high as 500 ppm. Currently, this value is 5 ppm (13 mg/m³).

Blood Concentrations. Vinyl chloride has not been measured in the blood of exposed workers.

Metabolism and Excretion. The disposition kinetics of vinyl chloride have not been studied in humans. In rats, 69% of an absorbed dose of the compound is excreted in the 24 hour urine as products of metabolism, and an additional 1.7% is found in the 24–48 hour urine (Bolt et al., 1976). The half-life for urinary excretion in rats is about 4 hours. As much as 12% of a dose is excreted unchanged in the breath after exposure to 1000 ppm of the chemical in air, while only 2% is exhaled after exposure to 10 ppm. The urinary excretion products were found to consist of N-acetyl-S-(2-hydroxyethyl)cysteine, thiodiglycolic acid and an unidentified compound (Watanabe et al., 1976).

Urinary thiodiglycolic acid concentrations average 0.5–0.7 mg/L in unexposed persons and range up to 4 mg/L in workers exposed to 1–7 ppm of vinyl chloride (Mueller et al., 1978). An ethanol dose of 0.8 g/kg has been reported to result in a urinary thiodiglycolic acid concentration of 10 mg/L within 3–5 hours of consumption (Draminski and Trojanowska, 1981).

Vinyl chloride concentrations in the breath of exposed workers, when measured from 1–20 hours post-exposure, tend to decline relatively slowly; the initial 1 hour post-exposure concentrations in workers exposed to 25, 50 or 100 ppm of the chemical for 8 hours were less than 0.6, 1.5 and 3.0 ppm, respectively (Baretta et al., 1969).

Toxicity. Acute exposure to high concentrations (over 10,000 ppm) of vinyl chloride causes central nervous system depression in man, with symptoms of dizziness, lightheadedness, nausea, dulling of the senses and headache (Lester et al., 1963). At least 2 fatalities have occurred in workers exposed for only a few minutes to vinyl chloride vapor while cleaning polymerization tanks; the chemical was not found in postmortem specimens of tissue during toxicological testing (Danziger, 1960).

Chronic exposure to lower levels of vinyl chloride has been found to cause degenerative bone changes in workers (Cook et al., 1971). Other significant chronic effects include circulatory disturbances, thrombocytopenia, splenomegaly, hepatomegaly and hepatic fibrosis; this condition is quite persistent following removal from exposure to vinyl chloride (Veltman et al., 1975; Berk et al., 1975). Angiosarcoma of the liver was first reported in vinyl chloride workers in 1974; the very high incidence of this rare disease prompted the reduction of the TLV for vinyl chloride to the current level of 5 ppm (Falk et al., 1974; Lloyd, 1975).

Analysis. Flame-ionization gas chromatography has been found suitable for measuring blood and breath vinyl chloride concentrations as low as 0.01 ppm (Baretta et al., 1969; Zuccato et al., 1979). It may be necessary to use more sensitive detection methods, such as electron-capture or mass spectrometric detectors, in order to apply this technique to exposures at the level of 5 ppm of vinyl chloride in the atmosphere. Gas chromatography has been used in the determination of thiodiglycolic acid in urine (Mueller et al., 1978, 1979; Draminski and Trojanowska, 1981; Chen et al., 1983). However, this metabolite is found as a normal urinary component and is also a metabolite of other industrial chemicals and some drugs.

References

E.D. Baretta, R.D. Stewart and J.E. Mutchler. Monitoring exposures to vinyl chloride vapor: breath analysis and continuous air sampling. Am. Ind. Hyg. Asso. J. 30: 537–544, 1969.

P.D. Berk, J.F. Martin and J.G. Waggoner. Persistence of vinyl chloride-induced liver injury after cessation of exposure. Ann. N.Y. Acad. Sci. 246: 70–77, 1975.

H.M. Bolt, H. Kappus, A. Buchter and W. Bolt. Disposition of (1,2-^{14}C) vinyl chloride in the rat. Arch. Tox. 35: 153–162, 1976.

Z.Y. Chen, X.R. Gu, M.Z. Cui and X.X. Zhu. Sensitive flame-photometric-detector analysis of thiodiglycolic acid in urine as a biological monitor of vinyl chloride. Int. Arch. Occ. Env. Health 52: 281–284, 1983.

W.A. Cook, P.M. Giever, B.D. Dinman and H.J. Magnuson. Occupational acroosteolysis. II. An industrial hygiene study. Arch. Env. Health 22: 74–82, 1971.

H. Danziger. Accidental poisoning by vinyl chloride: report of two cases. Can. Med. Asso. J. 82: 828–830, 1960.

W. Draminski and B. Trojanowska. Chromatographic determination of thiodiglycolic acid—a metabolite of vinyl chloride. Arch. Tox. 48: 289–292, 1981.

H. Falk, J.L. Creech, Jr., C.W. Heath, Jr. et al. Hepatic disease among workers at a vinyl chloride polymerization plant. J. Am. Med. Asso. 230: 59–63, 1974.

D. Lester, L.A. Greenberg and W.R. Adams. Effects of single and repeated exposures of humans and rats to vinyl chloride. Am. Ind. Hyg. Asso. J. 24: 265–275, 1963.

J.W. Lloyd. Angiosarcoma of the liver in vinyl chloride/polyvinyl chloride workers. J. Occ. Med. 17: 333–334, 1975.

G. Mueller, K. Norpoth, E. Kusters et al. Determination of thiodiglycolic acid in urine specimens of vinyl chloride exposed workers. Int. Arch. Occ. Env. Health 41: 199–205, 1978.

G. Mueller, K. Norpoth and R.H. Wickramasinghe. An analytical method, using GC-MS, for the quantitative determination of urinary thiodiglycolic acid. Int. Arch. Occ. Env. Health 44: 185–191, 1979.

P.G. Watanabe, G.R. McGowan, E.O. Madrid and P.J. Gehring. Fate of (^{14}C) vinyl chloride following inhalation exposure in rats. Tox. Appl. Pharm. 37: 49–59, 1976.

G. Veltman, C.E. Lange, S. Juehe et al. Clinical manifestations and course of vinyl chloride disease. Ann. N.Y. Acad. Sci. 246: 6–17, 1975.

E. Zuccato, F. Marcucci, R. Fanelli and E. Mussini. Head-sp~ce gas-chromatographic analysis of vinyl chloride monomer in rat blood and tissues. Xenobiotica 9: 27–31, 1979.

Warfarin

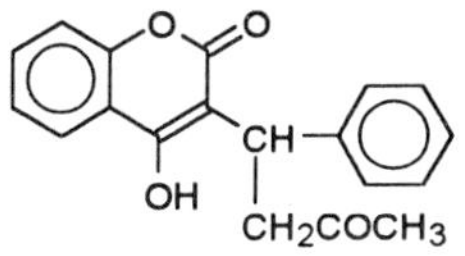

T½: 15–70 hr
Vd: 0.1–0.2 L/kg
Fb: 0.99
pKa: 5.1

Occurrence and Usage. Warfarin (Coumadin, Panwarfin) is a synthetic vitamin K antagonist that was first developed at the Wisconsin Alumni Research Foundation in 1947. It is available as the sodium salt of the racemic mixture for use as an anticoagulant, in oral doses of 2–25 mg daily; loading doses of 40–75 mg are sometimes administered when initiating therapy. The compound is also found in commercial animal baits in a concentration of 0.025%. Industrial exposure is generally by inhalation or absorption through the skin. The current threshold limit value is 0.1 mg/m^3.

Blood Concentrations. A single oral dose of 20 mg of warfarin produced a plasma concentration of 2.7 mg/L at 1 hour, declining to 2.1 mg/L by 5 hours and 1.2 mg/L by 24 hours (Midha et al., 1974). Following a single oral loading dose of 1.5 mg/kg (105 mg/70 kg) administered to 30 subjects, plasma warfarin concentrations averaged 8.8 mg/L (range, 6.4–11.8) after 24 hours and 4.3 mg/L (range, 2.4–6.0) after 72 hours, with a mean half-life of 47 hours.

Fifteen subjects who received chronic oral doses of 10 or 15 mg of the drug daily developed steady-state plasma concentrations of 2.0 mg/L (range, 1.4–3.5) and 3.1 mg/L (range, 1.7–6.8), respectively, by the fourth day (O'Reilly and Aggeler, 1968). Steady-state plasma concentrations in 23 controlled patients on long-term therapy with warfarin (0.04–0.22 mg/kg/day) ranged from 0.6–3.1 mg/L (Breckenridge and Orme, 1973). In a subject with inherited resistance to anticoagulant drugs, a chronic daily dose of 75–80 mg of warfarin was necessary to achieve hypoprothrombinemia and resulted in an average plasma concentration of 25 mg/L (O'Reilly, 1970).

Metabolism and Excretion. Warfarin is metabolized in man by oxidation to 6- and 7-hydroxy derivatives, which are without anticoagulant activity, and by reduction to a pair of diastereoisomeric alcohols, which are apparently active (Trager et al., 1970). The R-isomer of warfarin, which is known to be less potent than its enantiomer and to have a longer half-life in man, gives rise to significant amounts of the alcoholic metabolite. Concentrations of this metabolite in plasma have reached 2.6 mg/L by 36 hours after a 100 mg oral dose of the R-isomer, compared to a metabolite concentration of only 0.5 mg/L after the same dose of the S-isomer. No evidence was found for the presence of conjugated metabolites in plasma (Hewick and McEwen, 1973). Less than 1% of a dose is excreted unchanged in urine, and essentially no unchanged warfarin is found in the feces (O'Reilly et al., 1962). Urinary excretion accounted for 16–43% of a single dose of the drug over a 6 day period, apparently as the 7-hydroxy metabolite (O'Reilly et al., 1963).

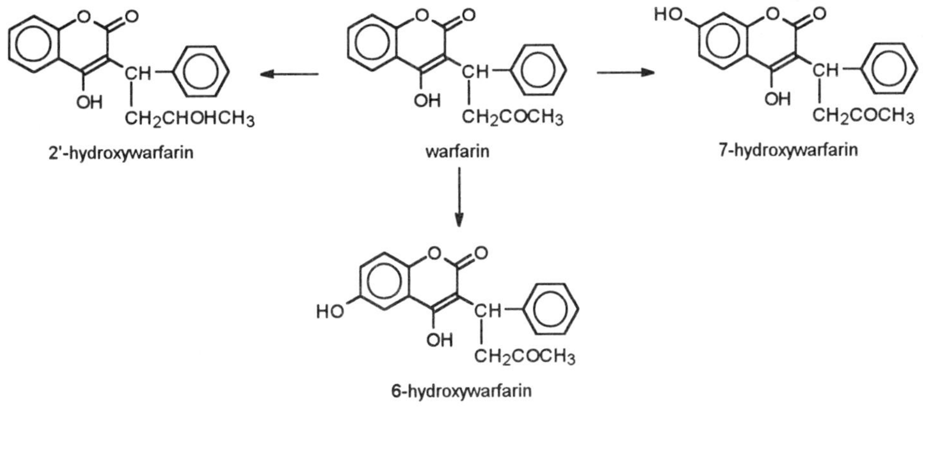

2'-hydroxywarfarin

warfarin

7-hydroxywarfarin

6-hydroxywarfarin

Toxicity. Warfarin inhibits the synthesis of prothrombin and several other clotting factors by the liver, resulting in reduced blood clotting activity and leading to internal hemorrhage in overdosage. Poisoning with warfarin is an infrequent event, since a single dose is usually insufficient to cause significant depression of prothrombin time, and continuous intentional administration of the drug over a long period of time requires a great deal of perseverance.

An amount of 567 mg taken as a suicidal gesture over a 6 day period resulted in a state of intoxication that was successfully treated by vitamin K administration (Holmes and Love, 1952). Dermal contact with warfarin solution on multiple occasions caused hematuria, hematomas, epistaxis and bleeding of the lip in a farmer who subsequently recovered (Fristedt and Sterner, 1965). Inhalation or dermal absorption of warfarin was believed responsible for multiple acute hemorrhagic episodes in a woman who frequently prepared rat poison for domestic use (Green, 1955). Warfarin was also involved in 2 unsuccessful attempts at criminal poisoning by relatives of the victims (Nilsson, 1957; Ikkala et al., 1964).

Fourteen cases of accidental poisoning were described that involved the eating of corn meal containing 0.25% warfarin for a period of 15 days, with only 2 deaths (Lange and Terveer, 1954). A death due to warfarin was reported that resulted from the ingestion of 1 g of the substance over a 13 day period, with death occurring on the 15th day (Pribilla, 1966).

Analysis. Warfarin has been assayed in biological specimens by a variety of methods. Ultraviolet spectrophotometry with measurement of the absorption maximum at 308 nm has found wide application (O'Reilly et al., 1962) and has been shown to be specific for unchanged warfarin (Welling et al., 1970). A rapid fluorometric technique has also been described (Corn and Berberich, 1967) that is apparently subject to interference by metabolites; in order to improve specificity, a thin-layer chromatographic separation was employed prior to fluorometric quantitation (Lewis et al., 1970). Gas chromatographic procedures have involved flame-ionization detection of the intact drug (Hanna et al., 1978) or its methyl derivative (Midha et al., 1974; Loomis and Racz, 1979) and electron-capture detection of either a methyl (Odam and Townsend, 1976) or pentafluorobenzyl derivative (Kaiser and Martin, 1974). Liquid chromatography techniques that can distinguish warfarin from its metabolites have been developed (Vesell and Shively, 1974; Bjornsson et al., 1977; Wong et al., 1977; Fasco et al., 1979; Tasker and Nakatsu, 1982; Riley and Koves, 1992).

References

T.D. Bjornsson, T.F. Blaschke and P.J. Meffin. High-pressure liquid chromatographic analysis of drugs in biological fluids I: warfarin. J. Pharm. Sci. 66: 142–144, 1977.

A. Breckenridge and M.L. Orme. Measurement of plasma warfarin concentrations in clinical practice. In *Biological Effects of Drugs in Relation to Their Plasma Concentrations* (D.S. Davies and B.N.C. Prichard, eds.), University Park Press, Baltimore, 1973, pp. 145–154.

M. Corn and R. Berberich. Rapid fluorometric assay for plasma warfarin. Clin. Chem. 13: 126–131, 1967.

M.J. Fasco, M.J. Cashin and L.S. Kaminsky. A novel method for the quantitation of warfarin and its metabolites in plasma. J. Liq. Chrom. 2: 565–575, 1979.

B. Fristedt and N. Sterner. Warfarin intoxication from percutaneous absorption. Arch. Env. Health 11: 205–208, 1965.

P. Green. Haemorrhagic diathesis attributed to "warfarin" poisoning. Can. Med. Asso. J. 72: 769–770, 1955.

S. Hanna, M. Rosen, P. Eisenberger et al. GLC determination of warfarin in human plasma. J. Pharm. Sci. 67: 84–86, 1978.

D.S. Hewick and J. McEwen. Plasma half-lives, plasma metabolites and anticoagulant efficacies of the enantiomers of warfarin in man. J. Pharm. Pharmac. 25: 458–465, 1973.

R.W. Holmes and J. Love. Suicide attempt with warfarin, a bishydroxycoumarin-like rodenticide. J. Am. Med. Asso. 148: 935–937, 1952.

E. Ikkala, G. Myllyla, H.R. Nevanlinna et al. Haemorrhagic diathesis due to criminal poisoning with warfarin. Acta Med. Scand. 176: 201–203, 1964.

D.G. Kaiser and R.S. Martin. GLC determination of warfarin in human plasma. J. Pharm. Sci. 63: 1579–1581, 1974.

P.F. Lange and J. Terveer. Warfarin poisoning. U.S. Armed Forces Med. J. 5: 872–877, 1954.

R.J. Lewis, L.P. Ilnicki and M. Carlstrom. The assay of warfarin in plasma or stool. Biochem. Med. 4: 376–382, 1970.

C.W. Loomis and W.J. Racz. Determination of warfarin in plasma by gas-liquid chromatography. Anal. Chim. Acta 106: 155–159, 1979.

K.K. Midha, I.J. McGilveray and J.K. Cooper. GLC determination of plasma levels of warfarin. J. Pharm. Sci. 63: 1725–1729, 1974.

I.M. Nilsson. Recurrent hypoprothrombinaemia due to poisoning with a dicumarol-containing rat-killer. Acta Haemat. 17: 176–182, 1957.

E.M. Odam and M.G. Townsend. The determination of warfarin in animal tissues by electron-capture gas-liquid chromatography. Analyst 101: 478–484, 1976.

R.A. O'Reilly, P.M. Aggeler, M.S. Hoag and L. Leong. Studies on the coumarin anticoagulant drugs: the assay of warfarin and its biologic application. Thromb. Diath. Haemat. 8: 82–95, 1962.

R.A. O'Reilly, P.M. Aggeler and L.S. Leong. Studies on the coumarin anticoagulant drugs: the pharmacodynamics of warfarin in man. J. Clin. Invest. 42: 1542–1551, 1963.

R.A. O'Reilly and P.M. Aggeler. Studies on coumarin anticoagulant drugs. Circulation 38: 169–177, 1968.

R.A. O'Reilly. The second reported kindred with hereditary resistance to oral anticoagulant drugs. New Eng. J. Med. 282: 1448–1451, 1970.

O. Pribilla. Mord durch Warfarin. Arch. Tox. 21: 235–249, 1966.

D.A. Riley and E.M. Koves. HPLC identification and quantitation of warfarin in postmortem blood. Can. Soc. For. Sci. J. 25: 191–199, 1992.

R.A.R. Tasker and K. Nakatsu. Rapid, reliable and sensitive assay for warfarin using normal-phase high-performance liquid chromatography. J. Chrom. 228: 346–349, 1982.

W.F. Trager, R.J. Lewis and W.A. Garland. Mass spectral analysis in the identification of human metabolites of warfarin. J. Med. Chem. 13: 1196–1204, 1970.

E.S. Vesell and C.A. Shively. Liquid chromatographic assay of warfarin: similarity of warfarin half-lives in human subjects. Science 184: 466–468, 1974.

P.G. Welling, K.P. Lee, U. Khanna and J.G. Wagner. Comparison of plasma concentrations of warfarin measured by both simple extraction and TLC methods. J. Pharm. Sci. 59: 1621–1625, 1970.

L.T. Wong, G. Solomonraj and B.H. Thomas. Analysis of warfarin in plasma by high-pressure liquid chromatography. J. Chrom. 135: 149–154, 1977.

Xylene

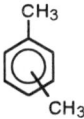

T½: 20–30 hr
Vd: ?
Fb: ?

Occurrence and Usage. The 3 isomers of xylene (xylol) are often found as components of the petroleum hydrocarbon solvents used in paints, lacquers, cleaning agents, pesticides and gasoline. A frequent source of laboratory exposure is in the preparation of tissue specimens for histological purposes. Commercial xylene consists of 75–85% of the m-isomer and only about 5% of the p-isomer. Xylene is quite similar to toluene in its spectrum of toxicity and is well-absorbed after both inhalation and dermal contact. The current threshold limit value for atmospheric vapor concentrations of xylene is 100 ppm (434 mg/m³).

Blood Concentrations. Blood xylene concentrations in non-exposed German citizens averaged 1.6 µg/L in nonsmokers and 1.7 µg/L in smokers (Hajimiragha et al., 1989). Blood xylene concentrations of 16 workers occupationally exposed to xylene-containing paint ranged up to 1.1 mg/L at the end of an 8 hour working day (Engstrom et al., 1976). Volunteers exposed daily to 100 ppm of xylene developed blood concentrations of 1.0 mg/L; during exposure to 200 ppm blood concentrations reached 2.1 mg/L (Savolainen et al., 1979). Blood xylene concentrations decline with an early half-life of 0.5–1 hour and with a terminal half-life of 20–30 hours (Riihimaki and Savolainen, 1980).

Metabolism and Excretion. The 3 xylenes are rapidly metabolized in man primarily by oxidation of a methyl group to the corresponding o-, m- or p-toluic acid; an average of 72% of an absorbed dose is excreted as these metabolites in the 18 hour urine in the form of glycine conjugates, o-, m- and p-methylhippuric acid. Ring hydroxylation of the xylenes also occurs, with about 2% of a dose excreted in urine as the corresponding xylenols, probably in conjugated form. Only about 5% of a dose is excreted unchanged in the breath and less than 0.01% unchanged in urine.

The extent and rate of excretion of the major urinary metabolites have been used as indices of exposure to xylene. Unlike hippuric acid, methylhippuric acid is not a normal urinary constituent. Urine concentrations of m-methylhippuric acid in persons exposed to m-xylene at concentrations of 100 and 200 ppm for 8 hours averaged 1.9 and 4.6 mg/L, respectively, in specimens representative of the whole period of exposure (Ogata et al., 1970; Sedivec and Flek, 1976). The excretion of m-methylhippuric acid in urine continues to increase during an 8 hour exposure, but declines rapidly at the termination of exposure; the half-life of xylene as estimated by urinary metabolite excretion is about 1.5 hours (Senczuk and Orlowski, 1978).

| xylene | toluic acid | methylhippuric acid |

Toxicity. Xylene concentrations of 200 ppm and above produce mucous membrane irritation, nausea, vomiting, dizziness and incoordination. Blood xylene concentrations that exceed 3 mg/L, produced by exposure of sedentary subjects to 300–400 ppm of xylene, cause significant impairment of equilibrium (Savolainen et al., 1979). Air concentrations of about 10,000 ppm of xylene have caused unconsciousness in workers due to central nervous system depression and at least one acute death (Morley et al., 1970). Chronic organ toxicity has not been noted in man, but xylene does cause mild hematopoietic system toxicity in experimental animals exposed to high vapor concentrations for 1–2 months.

A lethal dose by ingestion may be as little as 15 mL of the fluid. In 3 fatalities due to the ingestion of gasoline or other xylene-containing products, blood xylene concentrations ranged from 3–40 mg/L (average, 21) and liver concentrations were all 1 mg/kg (Bonnichsen et al., 1966). An adult who intentionally drank a large quantity of xylene had a postmortem blood level of 110 mg/L (Al Ragheb et al., 1986).

Analysis. Xylene may be specifically determined in biological specimens by headspace gas chromatography (Dubowski, 1975; Engstrom et al., 1976). Gas chromatographic procedures have been described for the methylhippuric acids in urine as their methyl (Caperos and Fernandez, 1977; Morin et al., 1981) or trimethylsilyl derivatives (Engstrom et al., 1976; Van Roosmalen and Drummond, 1978). Liquid chromatography has also been used for this purpose (Ogata et al., 1980; Tardif et al., 1989). Certain commercial serum separator tubes may contain xylene as a component of the separator gel (Streete and Flanagan, 1993).

References

S.A. Al Ragheb, A.S. Salhab and S.S. Amr. Suicide by xylene ingestion. Am. J. For. Med. Path. 7: 327–329, 1986.

R. Bonnichsen, A.C. Maehly and M. Moeller. Poisoning by volatile compounds. I. Aromatic hydrocarbons. J. For. Sci. 11: 186–204, 1966.

J.R. Caperos and J.G. Fernandez. Simultaneous determination of toluene and xylene metabolites in urine by gas chromatography. Brit. J. Ind. Med. 34: 229–233, 1977.

K.M. Dubowski. Organic volatile substances. In *Methodology for Analytical Toxicology* (I. Sunshine, ed.), CRC Press, Cleveland, 1975, pp. 407–411.

K. Engstrom, K. Husman and J. Rantanen. Measurment of toluene and xylene metabolites by gas chromatography. Int. Arch. Occ. Env. Health 36: 153–160, 1976.

H. Hajimiragha, U. Ewers, A. Brockhaus and A. Boetlger. Levels of benzene and other volatile aromatic compounds in the blood of non-smokers and smokers. Int. Arch. Occ. Env. Health 61: 513–518, 1989.

M. Morin, P. Chambon, R. Chambon and N. Bichet. Measurement of exposure to xylenes by separate determination of m- and p-methylhippuric acids in urine. J. Chrom. 210: 346–349, 1981.

R. Morley, D.W. Eccleston, C.P. Douglas et al. Xylene poisoning: a report on one fatal case and two cases of recovery after prolonged unconsciousness. Brit. Med. J. 3: 442–443, 1970.

M. Ogata, K. Tomokuni and Y. Takatsuka. Urinary excretion of hippuric acid and m- or p-methylhippuric acid in urine of persons exposed to vapours of toluene and m- or p-xylene as a test of exposure. Brit. J. Ind. Med. 27: 43–50, 1970.

M. Ogata, Y. Yamazaki, R. Sugihara et al. Quantitation of urinary o-xylene metabolites of rats and human beings by high performance liquid chromatography. Int. Arch. Occ. Env. Health 46: 127–139, 1980.

V. Riihimaki and K. Savolainen. Human exposure to m-xylene. Kinetics and acute effects on the central nervous system. Ann. Occ. Hyg. 23: 411–422, 1980.

K. Savolainen, V. Riihimaki and M. Linnoila. Effects of short-term xylene exposure on psychophysiological functions in man. Int. Arch. Occ. Env. Health 44: 201–211, 1979.

V. Sedivec and J. Flek. The absorption, metabolism, and excretion of xylenes in man. Int. Arch. Occ. Env. Health 37: 205–217, 1976.

W. Senczuk and J. Orlowski. Absorption of m-xylene vapours through the respiratory tract and excretion of m-methylhippuric acid in urine. Brit. J. Ind. Med. 35: 50–55, 1978.

P.J. Streete and R.J. Flanagan. Ethylbenzene and xylene from Sarstedt Monovette serum gel blood-collection tubes. Clin. Chem. 39: 1344–1345, 1993.

R. Tardif, J. Brodeur and G.L. Plaa. Simultaneous hplc analysis of hippuric acid and ortho-, meta-, and para-methylhippuric acids in urine. J. Anal. Tox. 13: 313–316, 1989.

P.V. Van Roosmalen and I. Drummond. Simultaneous determination by gas chromatography of the major metabolites in urine of toluene, xylene and styrene. Brit. J. Ind. Med. 35: 56–60, 1978.

Yohimbine

T½: 0.2–1.1 hr
Vd: 0.3–3.9 L/kg
Fb: ?
pKa: ?

Occurrence and Usage. Yohimbine (Yohimex) is an indole alkaloid obtained from a number of biological sources including *Corynanthe* yohimbe, *Rubiaceae* trees and *Rauwolfia* root. The drug is widely used for its α_2-adrenergic antagonist and mydriatic properties. Urologists are now using yohimbine experimentally for the treatment of certain types of male erectile impotence. It is commercially available as the hydrochloride in tablets of 5 mg for oral administration. For the treatment of impotence, 5 mg is given 3 times daily.

Blood Concentrations. Four healthy volunteers given a 125 µg/kg (8.75 mg/70 kg) intravenous bolus of yohimbine followed by a 1 µg/kg/minute infusion reached an approximate steady-state plasma level averaging 66 µg/L within 30 minutes; after 2 hours of infusion, plasma yohimbine concentrations had dropped to an average of 46 µg/L (Goldberg et al., 1984). Following a 10 mg oral dose of yohimbine in a 27 year old male weighing 64 kg, a peak plasma concentration of about 75 µg/L was attained in 45 minutes (Owen et al., 1987). Nine patients who received a 10 mg oral dose had plasma yohimbine concentrations averaging 289 µg/L at 1 hour, declining to 115 µg/L by 4 hours (Bagheri et al., 1994).

Metabolism and Excretion. Yohimbine is rapidly absorbed after oral administration (absorption half-life, 11 min) and rapidly eliminated. Less than 1% of a dose is recovered unchanged in the urine within 24 hours and the remainder is largely unaccounted for (Owen et al., 1987). Two phenolic metabolites, 10- and 11-hydroxyyohimbine, have been identified in urine (Le Verge et al., 1992).

Toxicity. Adverse effects from yohimbine administration include antidiuresis, increased heart rate, elevated blood pressure, tremor, irritabliity, dizziness, headache, flushing of the skin and nausea. A 16 year old girl who ingested 500 mg of the drug orally developed weakness, loss of coordination, anxiety, pallor, elevated vital signs, and a dissociative state that persisted for more than 18 hours (Linden et al., 1984).

Analysis. Yohimbine has been determined in plasma and other biological fluids using liquid chromatography with amperometric (Diquet et al., 1984), electrochemical (Goldberg et al., 1984), fluorescence (Owen et al., 1985; Reimer et al., 1993) and mass spectrometric detection (Le Verge et al., 1992).

References

H. Bagheri, P. Picault, L. Schmitt et al. Pharmacokinetic study of yohimbine and its pharmacodynamic effects on salivary secretion in patients treated with tricyclic antidepressants. Brit. J. Clin. Pharm. 37: 93–96, 1994.

B. Diquet, L. Doare and G. Gaudel. New method for the determination of yohimbine in biological fluids by high-performance liquid chromatography with amperometric detection. J. Chrom. 311: 449–455, 1984.

M.R. Goldberg, L. Speier and D. Robertson. Assay of yohimbine in human plasma using high performance liquid chromatography with electro-chemical detection. J. Liq. Chrom. 7: 1003–1012, 1984.

R. Le Verge, P. Le Corre, F. Chevanne et al. Determination of yohimbine and its two hydroxylated metabolites in humans by high-performance liquid chromatography and mass spectral analysis. J. Chrom. 574: 283–292, 1992.

C.H. Linden, W.P. Vellman and B.H. Rumack. Yohimbine: a new street drug. Vet. Hum Tox. 26: 407, 1984.

J.A. Owen, S.L. Nakatsu, M. Condra et al. Sub-nanogram analysis of yohimbine and related compounds by high-performance liquid chromatography. J. Chrom. 342: 333–340, 1985.

J.A. Owen, S.L. Nakatsu, J. Fenemore et al. The pharmacokinetics of yohimbine in man. Eur. J. Clin. Pharm. 32: 577–582, 1987.

G. Reimer, A. Suarez and Y.C. Chui. A liquid chromatographic procedure for the analysis of yohimbine in equine serum and urine. J. Anal. Tox. 17: 178–181, 1993.

Zidovudine

T½: 0.7–1.5 hr
Vd: 0.8–1.4 L/kg
Fb: 0.34–0.38
pKa: ?

Occurrence and Usage. Zidovudine (azidothymidine, AZT, Retrovir) is a thymidine analog that has been in clinical use since 1985 for the treatment of immunodeficiency virus infection. The drug is believed to inhibit viral reverse transcriptase, resulting in DNA-chain termination. It is available as 100 mg capsules for oral administration and as a 20 mg/mL solution for intravenous injection. Recommended adult doses are 200 mg every 4 hours orally or 0.5 mg/kg/hour by continuous intravenous infusion.

Blood Concentrations. Chronic oral administration of 250 mg of zidovudine every 4 hours to 21 adults resulted in average peak serum concentrations at 1.5 hours post-dose of 0.62 mg/L (range, 0.05–1.46) and average trough concentrations of 0.16 mg/L (range, 0–0.84) (Barnhart, 1989). In a group of children aged 5 months to 14 years, average steady-state plasma concentrations of 0.75–0.83 mg/L were produced by the continuous intravenous infusion of 0.9–1.4 mg/kg/hour of the drug (Pizzo et al., 1988). Balis et al. (1989) are of the opinion that plasma zidovudine levels should be maintained between 0.27–0.80 mg/L for optimal therapeutic efficacy.

Metabolism and Excretion. The oral bioavailability of zidovudine averages 68% (Balis et al., 1989). The drug is extensively metabolized by glucuronide conjugation. Urinary excretion of the unchanged drug and the glucuronide account for 14% and 74%, respectively, of an oral dose (Barnhart, 1989).

Toxicity. Adverse reactions to zidovudine administration include anxiety, confusion, dizziness, muscle pain and spasm, chills, anemia and granulocytopenia. Neutropenia is a frequent finding when plasma drug levels are allowed to exceed 0.80 mg/L on a continuous basis (Balis et al., 1989). Two adult patients taking chronic oral doses of the drug developed manic disorders characterized by agitation, flight of ideas, pressure of speech and grandiose beliefs; these symptoms resolved after treatment with either lithium or chlorpromazine (Wright et al., 1989). An adult patient who ingested 3.6 g of zidovudine was treated with ipecac; he attained a serum drug level of 1.4 mg/L at 1.5 hours post-dose but remained asymptomatic (Heard and Slovis, 1988).

Analysis. Zidovudine may be measured in biological fluids by commercially available immunoassays. Liquid chromatography has also been reported (Good et al., 1988; Unadkat et al., 1988; Kamali and Rawlins, 1990; Nebinger and Koel, 1994).

References

F. Balis, P. Pizzo, R. Murphy et al. The pharmacokinetics of zidovudine administered by continuous intravenous infusion in children. Ann. Int. Med. 110: 279–285, 1989.

E.R. Barnhart (ed). *Physician's Desk Reference*, Medical Economics Company, Oradell, New Jersey, 1989, pp. 793–795.

S.S. Good, D.J. Reynolds and P. de Miranda. Simultaneous quantification of zidovudine (AZT) and its glucuronide in serum by high performance liquid chromatography. J. Chrom. 431: 123–133, 1988.

J.M. Heard and C.M. Slovis. Zidovudine (AZT) (Retrovir) overdose. Vet. Hum. Tox. 30: 365–366, 1988.

F. Kamili and M.D. Rawlins. Simple and rapid assay for zidovudine and zidovudine glucuronide in plasma using high-performance lqiuid chromatography. J. Chrom. 530: 474–479, 1990.

P. Nebinger and M. Koel. Determination of serum zidovudine by ultrafiltration and high–performance liquid chromatography. J. Pharm. Biomed. Anal. 12: 141–145, 1994.

P.A. Pizzo, J. Eddy, J. Fallon et al. Administration of azidothymidine by continuous intravenous infusion in children with symptomatic HIV infection. New Eng. J. Med. 319: 889–896, 1988.

J.D. Unadkart, S.S. Crosby, J.P. Wong and C.C. Hertel. Simple and rapid high-performance liquid chromatographic assay for zidovudine (azidothymidine) in plasma and urine. J. Chrom. 430: 420–423, 1988.

J.M. Wright, P.S. Sachder, R.J. Perkins and P. Rodriguez. Zidovudine-related mania. Med. J. Aust. 150: 339–341, 1989.

Zimelidine

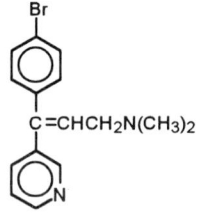

T½: 4–9 hr
Vd: 4 L/kg
Fb: 0.90
pKa: 3.8, 8.6

Occurrence and Usage. Zimelidine (zimeldine, Zelmid) is a bicyclic derivative of the antihistamine pheniramine that has been used as an antidepressant in European countries. It has recently been withdrawn from commercial distribution due to reported hypersensitivity reactions in a few individuals. The drug is usually administered as the dihydrochloride in daily doses of 150–300 mg.

Blood Concentrations. An average peak zimelidine plasma concentration of 0.10 mg/L (range, 0.01–0.14) was attained in 10 healthy male volunteers 2–3 hours after a single oral 100 mg dose; an average peak norzimelidine concentration of 0.04 mg/L (range, 0.01–0.09) was found in the same subjects after 3–8 hours (Caille et al., 1983). The average peak plasma concentration in 5 subjects, 22–30 years of age weighing 64–80 kg, after oral administration of 150 mg of zimelidine was 0.220 mg/L (range, 0.125–0.332) within 1–1.5 hours; norzimelidine concentrations reached a maximum within 3–5 hours and ranged from 0.075–0.116 mg/L (Love et al., 1981).

Two patients were given 300 mg of zimelidine daily for a period of 14 days; plasma taken 10 hours after the last dose contained 0.08–0.14 mg/L zimelidine and 0.21–0.25 mg/L norzimelidine (Caille et al., 1983). The plasma half-life for norzimelidine has been estimated at 15–25 hours.

Metabolism and Excretion. Zimelidine is completely absorbed after oral administration and rapidly demethylated to norzimelidine, which is more active than its parent. N-oxide formation may occur in the gut. The bioavailability of zimelidine averages 26% and norzimelidine, 66%. The excretion of unchanged drug in urine is about 1.3% of an intravenous dose and 0.6% of an oral dose (Brown et al., 1980; Love et al., 1981).

The body distribution of zimelidine during drug therapy was studied in a 30 year old woman who died as a result of a self-inflicted gunshot wound (Semple, 1984):

Drug Concentrations During Zimelidine Therapy (mg/L or mg/kg)

Drug	Blood	Brain	Liver	Bile	Urine
Zimelidine	0.7	0.8	24	1.4	1.5
Norzimelidine	2.2	3.7	8.2	5.2	11

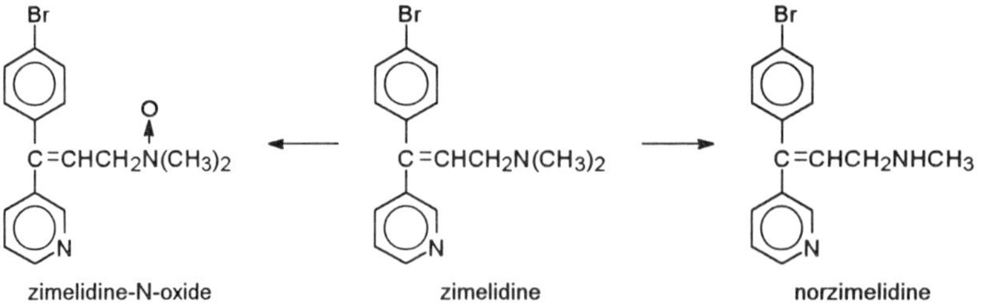

zimelidine-N-oxide   zimelidine   norzimelidine

Toxicity. Zimelidine was withdrawn from the market due to reports of hypersensitivity reactions in some patients, who developed characteristic signs of the Guillain-Barre syndrome (Linnoila et al., 1985). A 28 year old woman was admitted 3 hours after ingestion of 5.2 g of zimelidine; she was alert and oriented but complained of nausea and dizziness. Eight hours after ingestion, a serum zimelidine concentration of 3.7 mg/L and norzimelidine level of 1.3 mg/L was found; she was discharged on the sixth day, at which time her serum zimelidine concentration was undetectable and norzimelidine, 0.2 mg/L (Judd et al., 1983). A 35 year old woman was admitted to hospital in an alert state 2 hours after ingestion of 5 g zimelidine; peak plasma levels of 2.0 mg/L for both zimelidine and norzimelidine occurred 4 hours later. Twelve hours after ingestion, the plasma levels dropped to 0.4 mg/L zimelidine and 1.2 mg/L norzimelidine; no treatment was administered during hospitalization and the patient remained conscious (Ansseau et al., 1985).

Analysis. Zimelidine has been determined in biological specimens by gas chromatography with electron-capture (Caille et al., 1983) and nitrogen-phosphorus detection (Semple, 1984). Liquid chromatography has also been employed (Westerlund and Erixson, 1979).

References

M. Ansseau, C.F. Reynolds, D.J. Kupfer et al. Extrapyramidal signs following zimelidine overdose. J. Clin. Psychopharm. 5: 347–349, 1985.

D. Brown, D.H.T. Scott, D.B. Scott et al. Pharmacokinetics of zimelidine. Eur. J. Clin. Pharm. 17: 111–116, 1980.

G. Caille, E. Kouassi and C. de Montigny. Pharmacokinetic study of zimelidine using a new GLC method. Clin. Pharmacokin. 8: 530–540, 1983.

F.J. Judd, T.R. Norman and G.D. Burrows. Safety of zimeldine in overdose. Brit. Med. J. 287: 1592–1593, 1983.

M. Linnoila, K.V. Dubyoski, R.R. Rawlings et al. Effects of chronic zimelidine and ethanol on psychomotor performance. J. Clin. Pharm. 5: 148–153, 1985.

B.L. Love, R.G. Moore, J. Thomas and S. Chaturvedi. Pharmacokinetics of zimelidine in humans—plasma levels and urinary excretion of zimelidine and norzimelidine after intravenous and oral administration of zimelidine. Eur. J. Clin. Pharm. 20: 135–139, 1981.

D.J. Semple. Zimelidine distribution in a sudden death. J. Anal. Tox. 8: 285–287, 1984.

D. Westerlund and E. Erixson. Reversed-phase chromatography of zimelidine and similar dibasic amines. J. Chrom. 185: 593–603, 1979.

Zinc

T½: 5–16 months (whole body)
Vd: ?   Zn
Fb: 0.99

Occurrence and Usage. Zinc is extensively used as an alloying agent in brass and other alloys, in metal plating (galvanizing) and for numerous minor industrial applications. Zinc chloride in finely divided form is produced by chemical smoke generators that are used for military and other purposes. It is also a component of many soldering fluxes. Exposure to zinc or its compounds is generally by inhalation of dusts or fumes. Zinc is an essential trace metal and is supplied in the daily human diet in amounts of 10–15 mg. The current threshold limit values for exposure to fumes of zinc chloride and zinc oxide are 1 and 5 mg/m^3, respectively.

Blood Concentrations. Serum zinc concentrations in 17 healthy volunteers ranged from 0.66–1.02 mg/L, averaging 0.83 mg/L; plasma concentrations did not differ significantly from those of serum, although erythrocyte zinc concentrations averaged 12.25 mg/L in normal volunteers (Kosman and Henkin, 1979). Low plasma zinc levels have been observed in dietary zinc deficiency as well as in various other disease states (Prasad, 1979). Whole blood and plasma zinc concentrations in healthy brass foundry workers were noted to be 46% and 22% higher, respectively, than those concentrations in healthy control subjects; the investigator concluded that excess zinc that is not immediately excreted is stored in erythrocytes (Hamdi, 1969). The daily ingestion of 300 mg of zinc as a dietary supplement by 11 men raised their average plasma zinc from a baseline level of 0.83–2.00 mg/L after 6 weeks; the levels returned to baseline within 10 weeks after cessation (Chandra, 1984).

Metabolism and Excretion. About 20–30% of the zinc ingested in the diet is absorbed from the gastrointestinal tract. Of the amount absorbed, about 20% is excreted in the daily urine and up to 60% is excreted in feces (Prasad, 1979). Zinc distributes to all tissues, notably the liver, muscles and bone. Normal urine zinc concentrations are from 0.3–0.4 mg/24 hours, but may increase to as much as 2.1 mg/24 hours in patients with albuminuria (Vallee, 1957). Urinary zinc concentrations of 0.6–0.7 mg/L were observed in workers exposed to zinc oxide at levels of 3–5 mg/m³ (ACGIH, 1971). Healthy brass foundry workers exposed to zinc fumes excreted zinc in the urine at an average rate of 0.4 mg/24 hours (range, 0.3–0.6), an increase of only 14% over normal control subjects (Hamdi, 1969).

Toxicity. Poisoning from zinc compounds is primarily a result of acute exposure. Symptoms of inhalation exposure to zinc oxide dust or fume include respiratory tract irritation, chest pain and cough; after several hours, typical symptoms of metal fume fever occur, such as chills, fatigue, headache, nausea, fever, respiratory difficulty and muscle pain. The effects rarely last more than 24 hours, and no fatalities are known to have occurred (Drinker et al., 1927; Sturgis et al., 1927; Rohrs, 1957; McCord, 1960). Urinary zinc concentrations of 0.4–0.6 mg/24 hours were noted in workers who suffered mild gastrointestinal distress due to zinc oxide poisoning (ACGIH, 1971).

Acute exposure to zinc chloride fume, while causing similar symptoms, has produced fatal poisoning in a number of persons exposed to high concentrations of the chemical during the generation of chemical smoke. Severe respiratory inflammation was observed in these patients, who developed fever and a pale cyanotic color. Death was a result of acute pulmonary edema, bronchopneumonia or interstitial pulmonary fibrosis (Evans, 1945; Milliken et al., 1963).

Chronic excessive ingestion of a zinc supplement led to development of sideroblastic anemia and a serum zinc concentration of 2.38 mg/L in an adult male (Broun et al., 1990). A case of chronic poisoning due to dermal exposure to zinc chloride was reported in which the patient suffered leg pains, fatigue, loss of appetite and loss of weight. The patient's condition improved following removal from the job (du Bray, 1937). Three persons survived the acute ingestion of zinc chloride after developing serum zinc levels of 1.46, 12 and 19 mg/L; the patients exhibited lethargy, nausea, vomiting, and erosion of the gastrointestinal mucosa. Calcium EDTA was successful in lowering the serum zinc to normal levels (Chobanian, 1981; Potter, 1981; McKinney et al., 1991). A fourth person, a 6 year old child, died of corrosive gastritis and hepatic necrosis 9 days after ingesting a zinc chloride soldering solution (Jacobziner and Raybin, 1962).

The accidental intravenous administration of 7.4 g of zinc sulfate to a 72 year old woman produced a serum zinc level of 41.8 mg/L; hypotension, pulmonary edema, vomiting, diarrhea, jaundice, and renal failure were manifested prior to her death after 47 days (Brocks et al., 1977).

Analysis. The determination of zinc in serum or urine is commonly performed by atomic absorption spectrometry using flame (Allan et al., 1968; Kelson and Shamberger, 1978; Smith et al., 1979; Kiilerich et al., 1980; Perry, 1990) or graphite furnace (Vieira and Hansen, 1981; Whitehouse et al., 1982; D'Haese et al., 1992). Hemolysis of blood specimens must be avoided to prevent false elevation of serum zinc, and contact with the rubber parts of syringes and collection tubes must be minimized to avoid contamination by zinc (Guillard et al., 1979; Handy, 1979; Saleh et al., 1981).

References

ACGIH. *Documentation of the Threshold Limit Values*, American Conference of Governmental Industrial Hygienists, Cincinnati, Ohio, 1971, pp. 284–285.

R.E. Allan, J.O. Pierce and D. Yeager. Determination of zinc in food, urine, air, and dust by atomic absorption. Am. Ind. Hyg. Asso. J. 29: 469–473, 1968.

A. Brocks, E. Reid and G. Glazer. Acute intravenous zinc poisoning. Brit. Med. J. 1: 1390–1391, 1977.

E.R. Broun, A. Greist, G. Tricot and R. Hoffman. Excessive zinc ingestion. J. Am. Med. Asso. 264: 1441–1443, 1990.

R.K. Chandra. Excessive intake of zinc impairs immune responses. J. Am. Med. Asso. 252: 1443–1446, 1984.

S.J. Chobanian. Accidental ingestion of liquid zinc chloride: local and systemic effects. Ann. Emer. Med. 10: 91–93, 1981.

P.C. D'Haese, L.V. Lamberts, A.O. Vanheule and M.E. DeBroe. Direct determination of zinc in serum by Zeeman atomic absorption spectrometry with a graphite furnace. Clin. Chem. 38: 2439–2492, 1992.

P. Drinker, R.M. Thomson and J.L. Finn. Metal fume fever: IV. Threshold doses of zinc oxide, preventive measures, and the chronic effects of repeated exposure. J. Ind. Hyg. Tox. 9: 331–345, 1927.

E.S. du Bray. Chronic zinc intoxication. An instance of chronic zinc poisoning from zinc chloride used in the pillow manufacturing industry. J. Am. Med. Asso. 108: 383–385, 1937.

E.H. Evans. Casualties following exposure to zinc chloride smoke. Lancet 2: 368–370, 1945.

O. Guillard, A. Piriou, P. Mura and D. Reiss. Zinc contamination of control serum. Clin. Chem. 25: 1867, 1979.

E.A. Hamdi. Chronic exposure to zinc of furnace operators in a brass foundry. Brit. J. Ind. Med. 26: 126–134, 1969.

R.W. Handy. Zn contamination in Vacutainer tubes. Clin. Chem. 25: 197–198, 1979.

H. Jacobziner and H.W. Raybin. Zinc chloride poisoning (solder). N.Y. State J. Med. 62: 1848–1852, 1962.

J.R. Kelson and R.J. Shamberger. Methods compared for determining zinc in serum by flame atomic absorption spectroscopy. Clin. Chem. 24: 240–244, 1978.

S. Kiilerich, M.S. Christensen, J. Naestoft and C. Christiansen. Determination of zinc in serum and urine by atomic absorption spectrophotometry; relationship between serum levels of zinc and proteins in 104 normal subjects. Clin. Chim. Acta 105: 231–239, 1980.

D.J. Kosman and R.I. Henkin. Plasma and serum zinc concentrations. Lancet 1: 1410, 1979.

C.P. McCord. Metal fume fever as an immunological disease. Ind. Med. Surg. 29: 101–107, 1960.

P. McKinney, J. Brent, K. Kulig and B. Rumack. Zinc chloride soldering flux ingestion in a child. Vet. Hum. Tox. 33: 366, 1991.

J.A. Milliken, D. Waugh and M.E. Kadish. Acute interstitial pulmonary fibrosis caused by smoke bomb. Can. Med. Asso. J. 88: 36–39, 1963.

D.F. Perry. Flame atomic absorption spectrometric determination of serum zinc: collaborative study. J. Asso. Off. Anal. Chem. 73: 619–621, 1990.

J.L. Potter. Acute zinc chloride ingestion in a young child. Ann. Emer. Med. 10: 267–269, 1981.

A.S. Prasad. Clinical, biochemical, and pharmacological role of zinc. Ann. Rev. Pharm. Tox. 20: 393–426, 1979.

L.C. Rohrs. Metal-fume fever from inhaling zinc oxide. Arch. Ind. Health 16: 42–47, 1957.

A. Saleh, J.N. Udall and N.W. Solomons. Minimizing contamination of specimens for zinc determination. Clin. Chem. 27: 338–339, 1981.

J.C. Smith, Jr., G.P. Butrimovitz, W.C. Purdy et al. Direct measurement of zinc in plasma by atomic absorption spectroscopy. Clin. Chem. 25: 1487–1491, 1979.

C.C. Sturgis, P. Drinker and R.M. Thomson. Metal fume fever: I. Clinical observations on the effect of the experimental inhalation of zinc oxide by two apparently normal persons. J. Ind. Hyg. Tox. 9: 88–97, 1927.

B.L. Vallee. Zinc and its biological significance. Arch. Ind. Health 16: 147–154, 1957.

N.E. Vieira and J.W. Hansen. Zinc determined in 10-μL serum or urine samples by flameless atomic absorption spectrometry. Clin. Chem. 27: 73–77, 1981.

R.C. Whitehouse, A.S. Prasad, P.I. Rabbani and R.T. Cossack. Zinc in plasma, neutrophils, lymphocytes, and erythrocytes as determined by flameless atomic absorption spectrophotometry. Clin. Chem. 28: 475–480, 1982.

Zolpidem

T½: 1.4–4.5
Vd: ?
Fb: 0.93
pKa: 6.2

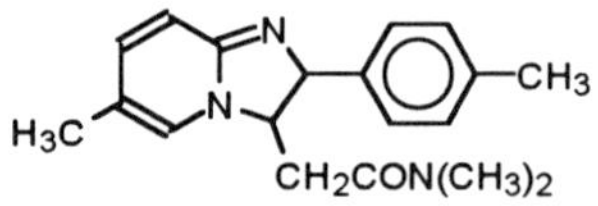

Occurrence and Usage. Zolpidem (Ambien) is an imidazopyridine derivative used since 1986 in European countries and since 1993 in the United States as a hypnotic agent. The drug is available in 5–10 mg tablets as the tartrate salt for oral administration. It is intended for once-nightly consumption for the short-term treatment of insomnia.

Blood Concentrations. Peak plasma zolpidem concentrations in 45 healthy adults following a 5 or 10 mg oral dose averaged 59 µg/L (range, 29–113) and 121 µg/L (range, 58–272), respectively, at 1.6 hours; the average elimination half-life was 2.6 hours. The elimination half-life for the drug may be significantly prolonged in the elderly (average, 2.9 hours) and in patients with hepatic cirrhosis (average, 9.9 hours), but not in those with renal failure (average, 2.4 hours) (PDR, 1994).

Metabolism and Excretion. Zolpidem is converted to pharmacologically inactive metabolites that are eliminated via renal excretion (PDR, 1994).

Toxicity. Adverse effects resulting from zolpidem usage include daytime drowiness, dizziness, amnesia, headache and nausea. A woman who mistakenly ingested a 10 mg tablet in the morning prior to driving to work was arrested by police; she exhibited ataxia, confusion, somnolence and a blood zolpidem concentration of 119 µg/L (Baselt, 1994). In a series of 35 acute intoxications with zolpidem, most patients were asymptomatic while only 2 were classified as mild to moderate toxicity that presented as deep sedation persisting for 8–16 hours (Mercurio et al., 1994).

An adult woman who died after ingesting 600 mg of zolpidem together with other depressants had a postmortem blood zolpidem concentration of 1120 µg/L (Garnier et al., 1994).

Analysis. Zolpidem has been assayed in biological specimens by liquid chromatography with fluorescence detection (Guinebault et al., 1986).

References

R.C. Baselt. Unpublished data, 1994.

R. Garnier, E. Guerault, D. Muzard et al. Acute zolpidem poisoining—analysis of 344 cases. Clin. Tox. 32: 391–404, 1994.

P. Guinebault, C. Dubruc, P. Hermann and J.P. Thenot. High-performance liquid chromatographic determination of zolpidem, a new sleep inducer, in biological fluids with fluorimetric detection. J. Chrom. 383: 206–211, 1986.

M. Mercurio, F. DeRoos and R.S. Hoffman. Zolpidem (Ambien): exposure assessment of a new nonbenzodiazepine GABA agonist. Vet. Hum. Tox. 36: 371, 1994.

Physicians' Desk Reference, Medical Economics Company, Montvale, New Jersey, 1994, pp. 2189–2192.

Zomepirac

T½: 4–10 hr
Vd: 0.6 L/kg
Fb: 0.99
pKa: 4.5

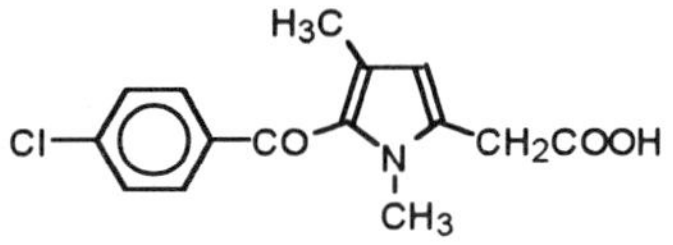

Occurrence and Usage. Zomepirac (Zomax) is a nonsteroidal anti-inflammatory agent with both analgesic and antipyretic properties. It is intended for oral use as the sodium salt. The recommended dose is 100 mg every 4–6 hours, not to exceed 600 mg per day. Zomepirac was withdrawn from the U.S. market in 1983 due to its potential for causing life-threatening allergic reactions.

Blood Concentrations. After a single oral dose of 100 mg of zomepirac to 21 healthy adults, peak plasma concentrations averaging 4.7 mg/L were attained in about 1 hour.

Following the administration of 400 mg daily to 10 healthy adults, steady-state plasma concentrations ranging from 3–4 mg/L were observed (Nayak et al., 1980). Three volunteers who received 400 mg daily doses for 5 days developed peak and trough plasma concentrations of 1.1–2.4 mg/L and 0.14–0.31 mg/L, respectively; the drug did not accumulate in the plasma of any of the volunteers when given in divided doses of 100 mg every 6 hours (Welch et al., 1982).

Metabolism and Excretion. Urinary excretion accounts for 94% of a dose of zomepirac in the first 24 hours, with 57% present as zomepirac glucuronide, 22% as unchanged drug, 6% as hydroxyzomepirac, and less than 1% as 4-chlorobenzoic acid (Muschek and Grindel, 1980).

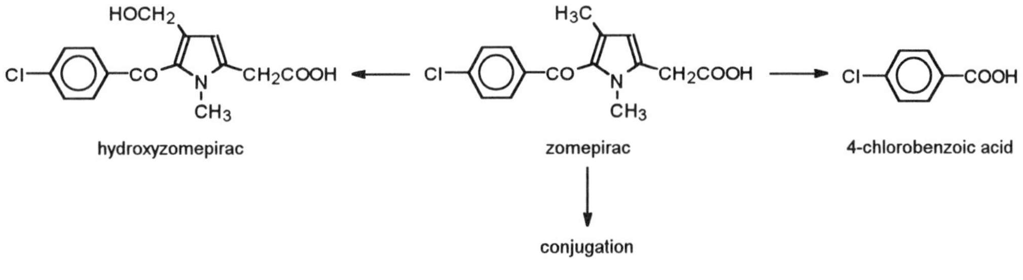

Toxicity. Adverse reactions to zomepirac may be manifested as nausea, gastrointestinal distress, diarrhea, edema, dizziness, rash, elevated blood pressure, tinnitus and cardiac irregularity (Andelman et al., 1980; Honig, 1980; Lewis, 1981). Acute allergic reactions involving severe bronchospasm, toxic eruptions, fever, lymphoadenopathy and eosinophilia have been reported (Ross et al., 1982; Kiani and Kushner, 1983). The death of a 36 year old woman resulting from suicidal ingestion of 9 g of zomepirac occurred after 17 hours of coma; blood taken 9 hours before death contained 286 mg/L of the drug, while postmortem blood contained 152 mg/L (Backer et al., 1983).

Analysis. Zomepirac has been analyzed by gas chromatography with detection by flame-ionization (Backer et al., 1983) or electron-capture (Ng and Kalbron, 1983). Liquid chromatography employing ultraviolet detection is also used (Ng and Silverman, 1979; Welch et al., 1982; Grindel et al., 1983; Langendijk et al., 1984; Welch, 1985).

References

S. Andelman, J. Levin, J. Simpson et al. A double-blind crossover comparison of zomepirac and placebo in pain secondary to osteoarthritis of the knee. J. Clin. Pharm. 20: 364–370, 1980.

R.C. Backer, V.H. Kshirsagar and I.M. Sopher. Case report—zomepirac suicide. J. Anal. Tox. 7: 223–224, 1983.

J.M. Grindel, J.F. Hills and N.L. Renzi. Reversed-phase high-performance liquid chromatographic assay for zomepirac. J. Chrom. 272: 210–215, 1983.

S. Honig. Preliminary report: long-term safety of zomepirac. J. Clin. Pharm. 20: 392–396, 1980.

R. Kiani and M. Kushner. Zomepirac-induced serum sickness. A report of two cases. J. Am. Med. Asso. 249: 2812–2813, 1983.

P.N.J. Langendijk, P.C. Smith, J. Hasegawa and L.Z. Benet. Simultaneous determination of zomepirac and its major metabolite zomepirac glucuronide in human plasma and urine. J. Chrom. 307: 371–379, 1984.

J.R. Lewis. Zomepirac sodium. A new nonaddicting analgesic. J. Am. Med. Asso. 246: 377–379, 1981.

L.D. Muschek and J.M. Grindel. Review of the pharmacokinetics and metabolism of zomepirac in man and animals. J. Clin. Pharm. 20: 223–229, 1980.

R.K. Nayak, K.T. Ng, S. Gottlieb and J. Plostnieks. Zomepirac kinetics in healthy males. Clin. Pharm. Ther. 27: 395–401, 1980.

K.T. Ng and T. Silverman. Determination of zomepirac in plasma by high pressure liquid chromatography. J. Chrom. 178: 241–247, 1979.

K.T. Ng and J.J. Kalbron. Sensitive gas chromatographic quantitation of zomepirac in plasma using an electron-capture detector. J. Chrom. 276: 311–318, 1983.

S.R. Ross, C.J. Friedman and E.J. Lesnefsky. Near fatal bronchospasm induced by zomepirac sodium. Ann. Allergy 48: 233–234, 1982.

C.L. Welch, T.M. Annesley, H.S. Luthra and T.P. Moyer. Liquid-chromatographic determination of zomepirac in serum and plasma. Clin. Chem. 28: 481–484, 1982.

C.L. Welch. Reversed-phase liquid chromatographic analysis of zomepirac in serum and plasma. In *Methodology for Analytical Toxicology*, Vol. III (I. Sunshine, ed.), CRC Press, Boca Raton, Florida, 1985, pp. 225–232.

Index